Exotic Animal Laboratory Diagnosis

Exotic Animal Laboratory Diagnosis

Edited by

J. Jill Heatley DVM, MS, DABVP (Avian, Reptilian, Amphibian), DACZM

Department of Small Animal Clinical Sciences
College of Veterinary Medicine & Biomedical Sciences
Texas A&M University
College Station
Texas, USA

Karen E. Russell DVM, PhD, DACVP (Clinical Pathology)

Department of Veterinary Pathobiology
College of Veterinary Medicine & Biomedical Sciences
Texas A&M University
College Station
Texas, USA

WILEY Blackwell

This edition first published 2020

Registered Office
John Wiley & Sons, Inc., 111 River Street, Hoboken, NJ 07030, USA

Editorial Office
111 River Street, Hoboken, NJ 07030, USA

For details of our global editorial offices, customer services, and more information about Wiley products visit us at www.wiley.com.

Wiley also publishes its books in a variety of electronic formats and by print-on-demand. Some content that appears in standard print versions of this book may not be available in other formats.

Library of Congress Cataloging-in-Publication Data

Names: Heatley, J. Jill, editor. | Russell, Karen (Karen E.), editor.
Title: Exotic animal laboratory diagnosis / edited by J. Jill Heatley, Karen Russell.
Description: Hoboken, NJ : Wiley Blackwell, 2020. | Includes bibliographical references and index. |
Identifiers: LCCN 2018024345 (print) | LCCN 2018025477 (ebook) | ISBN 9781118814246 (Adobe PDF) | ISBN 9781118814277 (ePub) | ISBN 9780470960356 (hardcover)
Subjects: LCSH: Exotic animals–Diseases–Diagnosis. | MESH: Animals, Exotic | Animal Diseases–diagnosis | Clinical Laboratory Techniques–veterinary | Laboratory Manuals
Classification: LCC SF997.5.E95 (ebook) | LCC SF997.5.E95 E94 2018 (print) | NLM SF 997.5.E95 | DDC 636.089/6–dc23 LC record available at https://lccn.loc.gov/2018024345

Cover Design: Wiley
Cover Images: © J. Jill Heatley

Set in 10/12pt Warnock by SPi Global, Pondicherry, India

Contents

Contributors

Megan A. Albertelli DVM, PhD, DACLAM
Department of Comparative Medicine
Stanford University
Stanford, California
USA

Matthew Allender DVM, MS, PhD, DACZM
Wildlife Epidemiology Laboratory
College of Veterinary Medicine University of Illinois
Urbana, Illinois
USA

Jill Arnold MS, MT (ASCP)
National Aquarium Baltimore
Baltimore, Maryland
USA

Christopher J. Bonar VMD, DACZM
Dallas Zoo
Dallas, Texas
USA

Rosemary J. Booth BVSc, MS
David Fleay Wildlife Park
SE Regions Terrestrial Parks
Queensland Parks & Wildlife Service Department
of Environment & Resource Management (DERM)
Queensland, Australia

Jen Brown DVM, DACVP (Clinical Pathology)
Rochester, New York
USA

Melinda S. Camus DVM, DACVP
Department of Veterinary Pathology
College of Veterinary Medicine
University of Georgia
Athens, Georgia
USA

Rosely Gioia-Di Chiacchio PhD
Department of Animal Pathology
Universidade Paulista
São Paulo
Brazil

John Chitty MRCVS
Anton Vets
Andover
Hants
UK

Sabrina D. Clark DVM, DACVP (Clinical Pathology)
Department of Pathobiology
College of Veterinary Medicine & Biomedical Sciences
Texas A&M University
College Station, Texas
USA

Jennifer R. Cook DVM, MS, DACVP (Clinical Pathology)
Idexx Laboratories, Inc.
Bloomfield Hills, Michigan
USA

Stephen J. Divers DECZM (Zoo Health Management, Herpetology) DACZM, FRCVS
Department of Small Animal Medicine
and Surgery
College of Veterinary Medicine
University of Georgia
Athens, Georgia
USA

Stephen A. Felt DVM, MPH, DACVPM, DACLAM
Department of Comparative Medicine
Stanford University School of Medicine
Stanford, California
USA

Christine Fiorello DVM, PhD, DACZM
Wildlife Health Center
School of Veterinary Medicine
University of California Davis
Davis, California
USA

María J. Forzán PhD, DACVP
College of Veterinary Medicine
University of Long Island
Brookvale, New York
USA

Jordan Gentry DVM
Downtown Aquarium, Houston
Montgomery County Animal Shelter
Conroe, Texas
USA

Cheryl B. Greenacre DVM, DABVP (Avian and Exotic Companion Mammal)
Department of Small Animal Clinical Sciences
College of Veterinary Medicine
University of Tennessee
Knoxville, Tennessee
USA

J. Jill Heatley DVM, MS, DABVP (Avian, Reptilian, Amphibian), DACZM
Department of Small Animal Clinical Sciences
College of Veterinary Medicine & Biomedical Sciences
Texas A&M University
College Station, Texas
USA

Sylvia Hester MFA
Freelance Illustrator
Glen Carbon, Illinois
USA

Jessica Hokamp DVM, PhD, DACVP (Clinical Pathology)
College of Veterinary Medicine & Biomedical Sciences
Texas A&M University
College Station, Texas
Clinical Department of Veterinary Biosciences
International Veterinary Renal Pathology Service
The Ohio State University
Columbus, Ohio
USA

Barbara S. Horney DVM, PhD, DACVP (Clinical Pathology)
Department of Pathology and Microbiology
University of Prince Edward Island
Charlottetown
Canada

Charles Innis VMD, DABVP (Reptilian and Amphibian)
Department of Animal Health
New England Aquarium
Boston, Massachusetts
USA

Michael P. Jones DVM, DABVP
Avian and Zoological Medicine
College of Veterinary Medicine
The University of Tennessee
Knoxville, Tennessee
USA

Ann B. Kier DVM, PhD, DACLAM
Department of Veterinary Pathobiology
College of Veterinary Medicine & Biomedical Sciences
Texas A&M University
College Station, Texas
USA

Melissa Kling DVM
Mercer University School of Medicine
Macon, Georgia
USA

Zdenek Knotek DVM, PhD, DECZM
Avian & Exotic Animal Clinic
Faculty of Veterinary Medicine
University of Veterinary & Pharmaceutical Sciences
Brno
Czech Republic

Frank J. Krupka DVM
Avon Lake Animal Clinic
Avon Lake, Ohio
USA

James Kusmeirczyk VMD
Cameron Park Zoo
Waco, Texas
USA

R. Scott Larsen DVM, DACZM
Denver Zoo
Denver, Colorado
USA

Kemba Marshall DVM, DABVP (Avian)
Purina Animal Nutrition Center
Gray Summit, Missouri
USA

Eliana Reiko Matushima FMVZ, USP
Pathology Department
Sáo Paulo University
São Paulo
Brazil

Gabriel P. McKeon DVM, DACLAM
North Carolina State College of Veterinary Medicine
Raleigh, North Carolina
USA

Sherrelle M. Milligan DVM
Department of Veterinary Pathobiology
College of Veterinary Medicine & Biomedical Sciences
Texas A&M University
College Station, Texas
USA

Claude M. Nagamine DVM, PhD
Department of Comparative Medicine
Stanford University School of Medicine
Stanford, California
USA

Barbara L. Oglesbee DVM, DABVP (Avian)
Medvet Hilliard
Columbus, Ohio
USA

Dennilyn Parker DVM, DABVP (Avian)
Department of Small Animal Clinical Sciences
Western College of Veterinary Medicine
University of Saskatchewan
Saskatoon
Canada

Lauren Virginia Powers DVM, DABVP (Avian Practice), DABVP (Exotic Companion Mammal Practice)
Avian and Exotic Pet Service
Carolina Veterinary Specialists
Huntersville, North Carolina
USA

Shane Raidal BVSc (Syd), PhD (Syd), FACVSc (Avian Health), DECZM (Wildlife Health)
Department of Veterinary Pathobiology
School of Animal & Veterinary Sciences
Charles Sturt University
Wagga Wagga, New South Wales
Australia

Cameron Ratliff DVM
Department of Surgical Sciences
Wisconsin School of Veterinary Medicine
University of Wisconsin-Madison
Madison, Wisconsin
USA

Christy L. Rettenmund DVM, DACZM
Milwaukee County Zoo
Milwaukee, Wisconsin
USA

Karen E. Russell DVM, PhD, DACVP (Clinical Pathology)
Department of Veterinary Pathobiology
College of Veterinary Medicine & Biomedical Sciences
Texas A&M University
College Station, Texas
USA

Melissa Smith DVM
CountryChase Veterinary
Tampa, Florida
USA

Stephen A. Smith MS, DVM, PhD
Department of Biomedical Sciences
and Pathobiology
VA/MD College of Veterinary Medicine
Blacksburg, Virginia
USA

Nadia Stegeman DVM, MPH
Animal Health Associates
Eugene, Oregon
USA

Devorah Marks Stowe DVM, DACVP (Clinical)
Clinical Pathology
North Carolina State University
Raleigh, North Carolina
USA

Tim Tristan DVM, DABVP (Reptilian and Amphibian)
Texas Sealife Center
Corpus Christi, Texas
USA

Thomas N. Tully, Jr., DVM, MS, DABVP (Avian), DECZM (Avian)
Department of Veterinary Clinical Sciences
Louisiana State University School of Veterinary Medicine
Baton Rouge, Louisiana
USA

Trevor T. Zachariah DVM, MS, DACZM
Brevard Zoo, Sea Turtle Healing Center
Melbourne, Florida
USA

Preface

This book was born of a series of lectures and labs I produced on the collection of samples and the interpretation of the clinical pathology of exotic animals. In creating these works, I was struck by not only the dearth of information for some very common species but also by the conflicting nature of some works and the lack of information in the veterinary realm which was available in the older laboratory animal and wildlife literature. Therefore, the purpose of this book became to provide the veterinarian, scientist, and biologist easier access to the basic knowledge available in the major species often seen in clinical veterinary practice.

This book was more difficult that I could have imagined. Despite the use of a prescriptive outline and thorough guidelines, many authors and I struggled with the dearth of information and the presentation of dogma for exotic animal clinical pathology, which lacks referenced support. Other authors struggled with an excessive amount of information for the species which obscured finding older publications with clinical import. Thus, a secondary goal of this text became to highlight materials which are still needed to better assess and diagnose health and illness on the basis of clinical pathology assessment for veterinarians and biologists today.

For many reasons, this work took more than double the time anticipated. Luckily, clinical pathology of exotic animals continues to advance slowly, and I hope the reader will still find this work of value in their daily practice. The text is organized in a straightforward manner on the basis of species with similar chapter organization to make data easy to find and interpret. More details on how to best use this book are provided at the end of the introductory chapter. It is my most sincere and earnest hope that this book will provide guidance to veterinarians and others interested in diagnosis and treatment in order to improve the standard of care for exotic animals.

Acknowledgment

I thank Rita Heatley and Sylvia Hester, who were both instrumental in making this first edition a reality. I gratefully acknowledge each and every author as well as the interns, residents, and veterinary technicians who have helped keep my referral veterinary practice functional while I was working on what they all refer to as "The Book." Finally, I would like to Thank Karen E. Russell and Jeffery Musser for accommodations in Port O'Connor and a new cat (Lilyfur Blaze Heatley) during the writing process.

When I agreed to help with this text, I did not realize what I was in for. This has truly been a learning experience, and I look forward to seeing the final product. First and most of all, I want to acknowledge Jill. She is a great colleague and friend and working with her has been an honor. She is the mover behind this project, and it would not have been completed had it not be for her. I also would like to thank all the contributors. Your hard work and patience are what made this happen. Finally I would like to thank my husband, Jeffrey Musser, for his contribution toward discussions about various topics, but more for the shared good fishing, blue crabs, and good times in Port O'Connor.

Key to symbols used in the Tables of this book: For many of the tables of this book, animal specific and sample specific characteristics have been indicated by symbols to allow ease of referencing the numeric values. Below is a brief key of these symbols:

Free living ⲩ	Captive Ħ	Pet ¥	Mixed population ₥
Outdoor Ϫ	Indoor ⌂		
Male ♂	Female ♀		
Adult ₪	Juvenile Ó		
Spring/ Rainy Season ☔	Summer ✪	Dry Season ➳	Fall ☘ Winter ❄
Reproductive ∞	Nonreproductive Ф		
Anesthetized ₳	Manual Restraint ☝		
[Sample size if not in header]			
Ә electrophoresis method	Buiret method Ѣ		

1

Introduction

Karen E. Russell DVM, PhD, DACVP (Clinical Pathology)[1] *and J. Jill Heatley DVM, MS, DABVP (Avian, Reptilian, Amphibian), DACZM*[2]

[1] *Department of Veterinary Pathobiology, College of Veterinary Medicine & Biomedical Sciences, Texas A&M University, College Station, Texas, USA*
[2] *Department of Small Animal Clinical Sciences, College of Veterinary Medicine & Biomedical Sciences, Texas A&M University, College Station, Texas, USA*

Introduction

Veterinary clinical pathology is a branch of laboratory medicine that focuses on the study of animal disease through the examination of blood, serum or plasma, urine, body fluids, and tissues. The discipline covers a wide range of laboratory assays and methods and is important for diagnoses, patient care, prevention of disease, and the quality and accuracy of the laboratory tests.

Obtaining the appropriate sample from exotic animals may be challenging because of widely varying physiology and anatomy. While appropriate references and excellent techniques and illustrations exist, it is difficult for the researcher, biologist, or clinician to find and access them from the literature. Hence, we review the biological, basic science, laboratory animal, and exotic animal references to create a single useful text which will serve as a quick and easy reference for the veterinarian, biologist, researcher, or technician in need of guidance regarding what is known and what is unknown in order to obtain, handle, and store diagnostic samples for exotic animals.

Interpretation of results from clinical pathologic testing of zoo, wildlife, and exotic animals may be just as challenging, if not more so, than obtaining the sample. In fact, some advocate foregoing many tests because of the challenge of interpretation. While physical examination should remain the bedrock of diagnosis in clinical exotic animal medicine, clinicopathologic testing is an extremely useful tool which should not be overlooked in the clinician's diagnostic arsenal. Additionally clinicopathologic testing may be more useful in these species than in others because of their instinctual stoicism. Many exotic animals are prey species, and occult disease is common; clinical signs may not be apparent until complete health decompensation occurs. Clinical pathological testing is one of many possibilities that offer the hope of diagnosis earlier in the disease process and the chance of a better prognosis for the animal based upon early diagnosis.

Much of the challenge of clinicopathologic interpretation of exotic animals is based on lack of data. Another issue is the availability of data from the extant literature which, for exotic animals, is found scattered among many disciplines and stretches through time back to early anatomical drawings of the late 1800s. If knowing is indeed half the battle, then this text provides what is known and what is not known in a format accessible to the busy clinician. In addition, references have been curated to those of most use and importance to the researcher and clinician. Most chapters make the assumption that the reader has standard baseline veterinary clinicopathologic knowledge and continue into detailed specifics regarding sample collection and preservation, and result interpretation for the species. For more basic information regarding standard-specific clinical pathologic methods, we recommend consultation of the basic veterinary and exotic animal clinicopathology textbooks listed in the references of this section [1–15].

Reference Intervals

An additional challenge for those faced with interpretation of clinicopathologic data in exotic animals is that few true reference intervals are available for exotic, zoo, or wildlife animals. Reference intervals are an important part of all laboratory results. They are designed to be used as guidelines for interpretation and to determine if

Exotic Animal Laboratory Diagnosis, First Edition. Edited by J. Jill Heatley and Karen E. Russell.

a result is "normal" or "abnormal." Reference intervals are often referred to as reference range, reference value, "normals," normal range, or normal value; however, these terms are incorrect, and their use is strongly discouraged for several reasons. A reference interval represents a statistical calculation from a group of results obtained from a defined population of animals. In determining this population (often referred to as a reference population), defining what normal actually means is challenging. Furthermore, sick animals may have laboratory results that fall within the reference interval. Use of terms such as "normal range" or "normal values" is not recommended, and they should not be used because of the difficulty in defining "normal." Reference intervals often vary from laboratory to laboratory depending on the instrumentation and methodology.

Reference intervals are influenced by many factors, such as the species, breed, age, and sex of the animal. Results can be affected by diet, exercise, excitement, medications, time of day, or season. Collection and processing of the sample can also influence the result. When establishing reference intervals, the criteria for inclusion of an individual needs to be defined before sample collection begins. Reference intervals are based on the measurement of an analyte in a population of clinically healthy animals that meet the inclusion criteria. Obtaining many samples from a single kennel or herd is not recommended as animals may lack sufficient variation needed for the reference interval to be representative, resulting in an overly narrow reference interval.

In general, samples from at least 120 individuals are recommended to establish a reference interval. However, this is usually quite difficult in veterinary medicine because of the lack of availability of appropriate individuals and the expense of obtaining and analyzing samples. Some veterinary guidelines suggest that a more realistic number is at least 60 qualified individuals that meet the selection criteria. Statistical guidance for the creation of reference intervals is available for researchers creating useful data sets for future reference [16]. Many of the data tables provided in this text fail to meet aforementioned criteria are therefore labeled as reference ranges, but the data may still serve as a starting point for evaluation of the patient and are meant to represent the best extant data available for the species group.

Reference intervals are typically derived from the mean ± 2 standard deviations of the mean of the values fitting a normal (Gaussian) distribution. This assumes that 95% of the healthy population will fall within the established reference interval. When data are not normally distributed, nonparametric analysis or data transformation is typically used to remove the top and bottom 2.5 percentiles, as 2.5% of "normal" animals have values outside the reference range on the basis of this statistical model. Often, the ideal reference values are previous values, often called healthy or baseline values, obtained from the individual patient. Figure 1.1 illustrates the likely minimum number needed to create a reference interval for base excess in passerine birds. By convention, for a normally distributed data set, the reference interval for a particular test include 95% of all values from the general (presumed healthy) population. Because 5% of results fall outside this interval, values that may actually be unremarkable or acceptable can therefore sometimes be outside this range. Additionally, normal distributions may be less common for many analytes in exotic animal medicine, making statistical assessment of values for the creation of reference intervals more challenging.

In human medicine, reference intervals for a single analyte are created for a single instrument and/or laboratory, and values from a sample of hundreds of apparently healthy people may be stratified on the basis of gender, age, race, size, or other factors. The results are then further statistically evaluated to create a reference interval (Figures 1.1 and 1.2). Again, seldom in zoo, exotic, or wildlife species do we have the necessary numbers to create reference intervals meeting these stringent definitions, which creates a further barrier to publication of the data which we do have, but also creates a problem in interpretation. The publication and use of data for very small numbers of animals, which are of questionable health can lead to erroneous interpretation of clinical pathology, possibly to the animal's detriment. *The wise clinician remembers that clinical pathology is used to confirm and further define a diagnosis, seldom to discover one, and this should be particularly true of nontraditional animal medicine.* This intent of this text is also to provide extant reference data and to provide guidelines for interpretation of these analytes on the basis of the species at hand. To accomplish these goals, we have asked authors to provide a relevant literature review combined with their experience in clinical medicine. Chapters are meant to provide a clinically useful overview with references available for additional in-depth consultation to the researcher and student.

Laboratory Choices: The Use of a Reference or an In-House Laboratory

The ability to perform or request various diagnostic assays is available to the clinician in a variety of settings. Choices include sending samples to diagnostic reference veterinary laboratories or laboratories at teaching universities, establishing an in-house laboratory, or utilizing a combination of both; there are advantages and disadvantages to each of these scenarios. Exotic animal

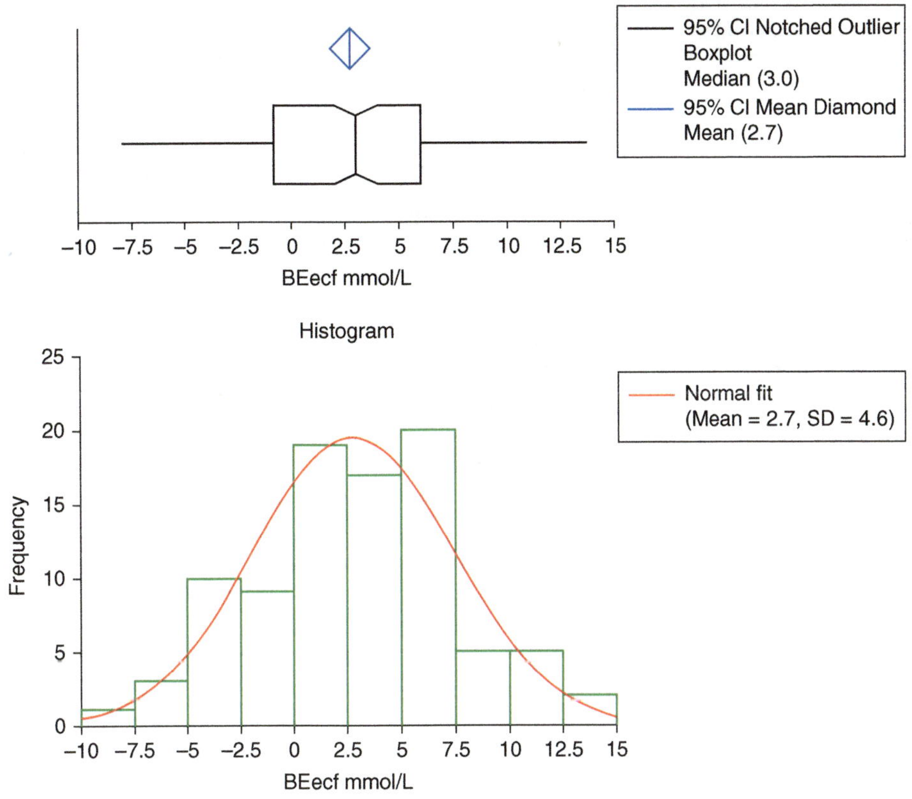

Figure 1.1 Normal distribution of base excess for passerine birds. Note that the tails (edges) of the histogram are the minimum number needed to create the shaper of a normal distribution (1–5), but the total number (because the top bars to create the parabola must be incrementally higher) for this study was 91.

practitioners face specific challenges regarding this choice, including analyte determination, sample volume, costs, client expectations, and patient health.

Diagnostic reference laboratories and laboratories at teaching universities typically process high sample numbers daily. They have trained personnel who perform laboratory tests and maintain the instrumentation by performing the required instrument maintenance and routine quality control protocols on a regular basis. These activities are extremely important to ensure that results obtained are valid. Many larger laboratories have established reference intervals for the common species (canine, feline, equine, and bovine). Some may have reference intervals for additional species or resources about some of the more uncommon species. An additional advantage of using a larger laboratory is the availability for consultations with clinical pathologists, internists, radiologists, or other specialists. Some laboratories have courier services, but many require that samples be mailed or shipped by the user. The turnaround time for routine laboratory results can be variable, but next day reporting is typical. Larger laboratories commonly offer specialized or advanced testing such as flow cytometry, specialized chemistry tests (e.g., hormone assays), molecular diagnostics for certain diseases and infectious agents, as well as histology, serology, toxicology, parasitology, and microbial culture and susceptibility testing.

Many private practices choose to invest in an in-house laboratory. Some tests such as urinalysis or cytology require minimal equipment and can be performed in the clinic at relatively low costs. In addition, smaller, relatively less expensive benchtop analyzers for complete blood counts (CBCs), clinical chemistry, blood gas analysis, and basic coagulation assays are available and are validated for certain veterinary species.

A major advantage of having an in-house laboratory is the shorter turnaround time for results, which can be crucial for critically ill patients and convenient for patient management and owners. However, there are many aspects to consider when thinking about having an in-house laboratory. One of the most important is the establishment of a quality control program and the willingness to dedicate the time and expense that is required. Additional considerations include the cost-effectiveness of not only purchasing an instrument, but the associated costs of maintenance and upkeep, upgrades and replacements, as well as disposable products and ancillary

Box 1.1 Considerations for Establishing an In-House Laboratory

- How often will the instrument be used?
  1) What is the anticipated or expected number of patient samples and corresponding tests: How many patients are there and how often will tests be run?
- Financial aspects
  2) Acquisition costs: How much does the instrument cost, and what are the costs of the accessories such as software, and disposables such as calibrators, controls and reagents, tubes, pipettes, and paper?
  3) Operating costs: What does it cost to run the instrument? This includes controls, reagents, disposables, service contracts, repair costs, and instrument and/or software upgrades. What kinds of ancillary equipment, such as computers and printers, are needed? How much does a yearly maintenance agreement cost?
  4) Revenue generated from having the instrument: Is it sufficient to cover the cost of the instrument throughout its life span and possibly use toward an upgrade later?
- How easy is a test to perform and how easy is it to maintain the instrument?
  5) Technical expertise required: How user-friendly is the instrument, is the instrument easy to run and maintain, and what training is required?
  6) Who will be responsible for routine and preventative maintenance? Who is responsible for running and recording the tests?
  7) Customer technical service: Does the manufacturer provide technical support when there are problems with the instrument? Who will troubleshoot problems?
- What else is there to think about?
  8) Establishing reference intervals, test validation, quality assurance and quality control protocols, preventative maintenance protocols and schedules, record keeping: Who will be responsible?
  9) Turnaround time: How fast are you going to generate results?
  10) How long has the instrument been on the market? What is the company's reputation? Will they be around for the next several years?
  11) Who else uses the instrument and what is their opinion and experiences? Find out!
  12) What is the average life span of the instrument? When does it become obsolete?
- Will you be committed to a quality control program?
- Should the practice just send samples to a reference laboratory? This is a viable option.

equipment that are needed. Although many instruments are relatively user-friendly, time is needed to train personnel to use the instrument, perform routine maintenance, and troubleshoot when problems arise or the instrument is not working properly. As with any piece of equipment used in a private practice, the question of how often it will be used and how many samples will be run are important to know because these factors directly impact the actual costs to the practice. Box 1.1 summarizes some of the questions to be asked when deciding whether to establish an in-house laboratory.

The Quality Control Program: What Is It and Is It Really Important?

It is imperative that laboratory testing yield correct and reliable results. Valid data are essential for making medical decisions. Inaccurate results are misleading and can prove disastrous. Every laboratory or clinical practice that analyzes samples should have a program that is designed to prevent and detect unacceptable errors in its assays and ensure that only valid results are generated and reported.

Quality control (QC) measures should be in place to minimize laboratory errors and ensure that the instrument is working properly. A QC program will help identify problems with the equipment, test methodology, operator, or potentially, multiple factors. The manufacturer should provide recommendations for the care and QC of the instrument. A QC program should not rely solely on internal, electronic quality control capabilities that are programmed into an instrument and should incorporate the use of commercially available liquid controls and calibrators specific for the instrument (Box 1.2). A summary of a basic QC program is provided in Box 1.3.

Quality Control: Record Keeping

A record of control results should be kept and reviewed regularly. The most common record keeping method is the use of Levey–Jennings plots (also referred to as QC charts) (Figures 1.2–1.5). These are graphs used to plot daily results obtained from each of the controls. Controls are typically designed to test upper limits ("high"), normal limits, and low limits. A predetermined, acceptable range for each control, usually within ±2 standard deviations, for the expected results of that particular control is

Box 1.2 Definitions: Reagents, Controls, and Calibrators

Calibrator: These are solutions designed to adjust or establish instrument settings for a particular assay.

Instruments should be recalibrated for every new reagent lot as needed, when the instrument malfunctions, or if the control results are no longer precise and accurate.

Control: Solutions designed to determine the precision and accuracy of an assay (and the instrument) on an hourly, daily, or weekly basis. These are generally available in low, normal, and high concentrations for the analyte of interest. The chemical and physical characteristics (i.e., the "matrix") of control solutions must approximate those qualities of the unknown sample.

Reagent: Reagents contain chemicals, dyes, enzyme cofactors, or other substances necessary to measure the amount, concentration, or activity of a particular substance. A reagent can be in the form of a liquid or a dry slide, depending on the instrument requirements.

Box 1.3 Basic Constituents of a Quality Control Program

1) Regular scheduled use of liquid controls to ensure that the instrument, test reagents, and operator are working properly.
2) Performance of routine maintenance to include cleaning, replacement of components that wear out or expire on the basis of the manufacturer's recommendations.
3) Routine scheduled use of calibrators to calibrate the instrument to ensure proper working order and valid test results.
4) Keep daily records, and review them regularly.

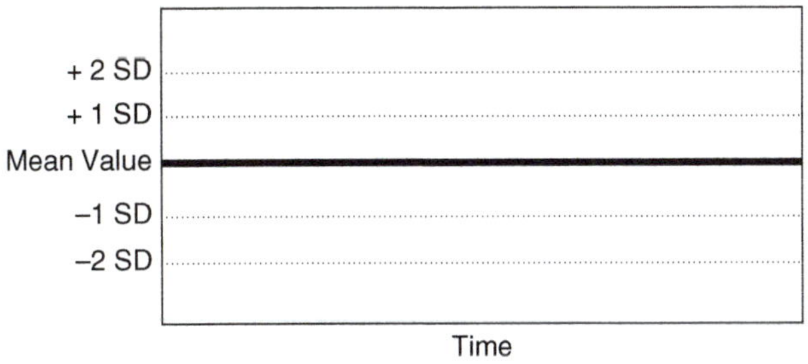

Figure 1.2 A Levey–Jennings plot (or quality control chart). The mean and standard deviations (SD) are provided for each control lot and are used to create the values for the *Y* axis. The *X* axis is typically plotted on a daily basis.

recommended. When results fall outside this acceptable range, this should alert the operator to a potential problem. There are several steps that can be taken when this occurs (Box 1.4).

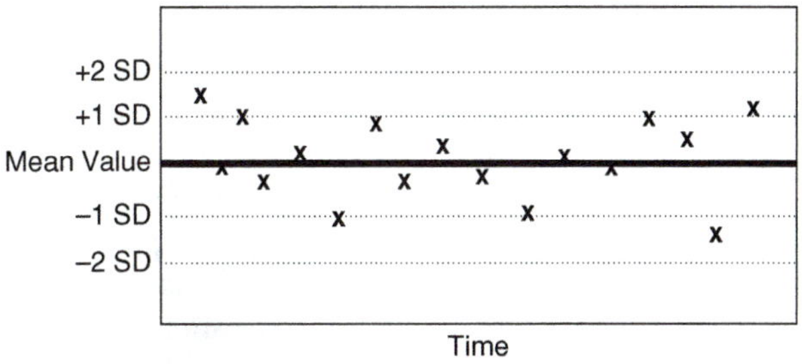

Figure 1.3 Levey–Jennings plot, acceptable. In this example the control data are within the acceptable ±2 SD of the mean for the control.

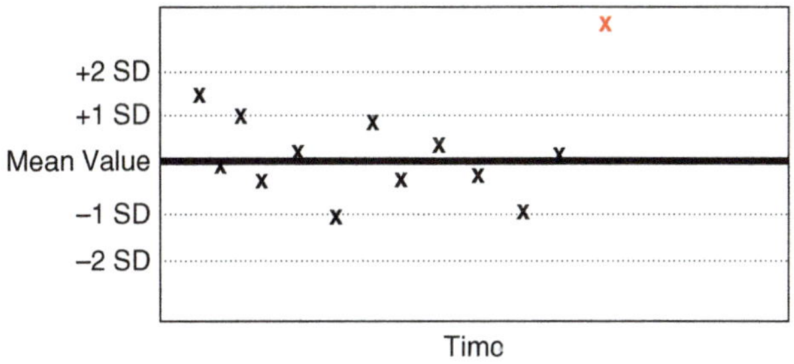

Figure 1.4 Levey–Jennings plot, error. In this example, a control result (red X) falls outside of the acceptable ±2 SD range. This error requires correction, and no patient results are reported until the problem is resolved.

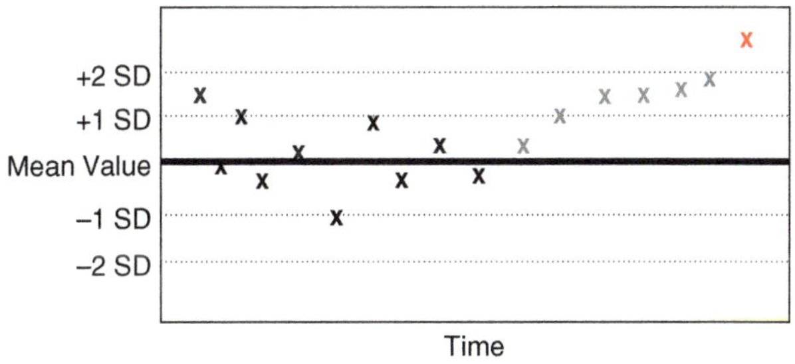

Figure 1.5 Levey–Jennings plot, drift. In this example, the control result is "drifting" upward (blue X's) and eventually is (red X) within the acceptable range. This may indicate a need to calibrate the instrument.

Box 1.4 What to Do When a Control is Out of the Acceptable Range

1) Repeat the test. If result falls within the acceptable range, patient results can be reported.
2) If result falls out of acceptable range, proceed with the following as appropriate:
3) Make sure correct control was used and the correct test was performed.
4) Check expiration dates of reagents and control.
5) Make up new reagent and repeat the test.
6) Make up new control and repeat the test.
7) Consult the troubleshooting section of the instrument operation manual.
8) Call for technical assistance.

Laboratory-Associated Error

Error can occur due to many causes. Make it a policy to call the laboratory if any results you receive do not make sense. Conversations with the clinical pathologist or laboratory technician allow you to develop an appropriate relationship with the laboratory and will improve diagnostic satisfaction as well as clinician education regarding laboratory needs to provide the best patient diagnosis. If you are unfamiliar or unsure of the appropriate samples for a desired test, always call the laboratory before obtaining samples. This policy conserves fiscal resources and time and reduces the patient stress of multiple sampling episodes. Particularly in exotic animal medicine, you may only have one chance to get the right sample. Preparation gives you the best chance of getting the correct sample. While many blame laboratory error when apparently erroneous results are obtained, *many* potential reasons may cause questionable clinical pathology analyte results. Valid test results depend on *preanalytical*, *analytical*, and *postanalytical* factors.

Preanalytical factors that can lead to an error typically occur before the sample reaches the laboratory and include factors endogenous to the patient, the sample, or a combination. Examples of common patient factors that can affect results include lipemia, hemolysis, icterus, agglutination, and drugs, which may interfere with test method.

Examples of preanalytical error associated with the sample include collection methods, anticoagulant used, sample container, and sample handling. Results of testing may be altered depending if a sample is collected from an atraumatic versus a traumatic venipuncture, forced through a needle into the collection tube, obtained from a catheter, or from different sites, which is especially important in some of our exotic species. The anticoagulant used may affect results. For example ethylenediaminetetraacetic acid (EDTA) should not be used for clinical chemistry panels because it prevents coagulation by binding divalent ions (calcium, magnesium) and contains either sodium or potassium. Furthermore, EDTA should not be used for CBCs in some species, such as corvids, because it causes increased hemolysis. Heparin samples can be used for CBCs and clinical chemistry, but it affects blood cell morphology and can cause clumping of leukocytes and thrombocytes. The sample container (plastic versus glass; colorless versus dark) may affect results. Sample handling and processing are especially critical. Storage temperature (room, ice, refrigerated, or frozen), period of time between centrifugation and separation of serum or plasma, and period of time between collection and actually performing the testing can influence results. In addition, correct sample identification with appropriate and clear labeling, completing the submission form correctly, and requesting the appropriate test are other factors that can lead to preanalytical error if not done properly. Many studies have shown that the highest incidence of laboratory-related errors occur in the preanalytical phase of laboratory testing.

Factors that can result in analytical error are those that involve the laboratory and running the test. If a test method has not been validated, questionable results may be obtained. Unfortunately validation of many tests is seldom done in less common species that exotic animal veterinarians see often because it is cost prohibitive. Quality of instrumentation and equipment as well as routine maintenance and use of in-date reagents and materials are of particular concern for in-house laboratories and can be a significant source of error in the exotic animal veterinary practice. The lack of or a poor QC program in the laboratory is especially concerning. If you or your practice or laboratory cannot provide adequate time or personnel to ensure that all of the aspects of the laboratory and instrumentation is properly maintained, this may present serious sources of error which could lead to a wrong treatment plan or diagnosis. In this case, use of a reference laboratory is highly recommended.

Post analytical error occurs after the testing, once a result is obtained as well as when the result is reported. Often, this involves human error such as reporting incorrect results due to inaccurate or incorrect manual entry, or reporting results from the wrong patient. The result delivery to the clinician may have an unreasonable turn-around-time, which can delay treatment. Data should also be reported in a manner that is clear, easy to read, and not prone to misinterpretation by the clinician.

In summary laboratory-related errors may be attributed to many sources. To avert preanalytical error, the clinician, biologist, or researcher should strive to avoid being the cause of the error and have knowledge of how to obtain, label, handle, process, store, and ship samples. A full understanding about how reference intervals are generated and the lack of appropriate reference intervals for many species as well as the potential limitations will allow the clinician to better interpret results. Finally, if an unusual or unexpected result is obtained and potential preanalytical factors have been eliminated as a cause, the clinician should contact the laboratory.

Basic Clinicopathologic Concepts

Some basic methodologies are necessary to understand more advanced concepts and to appreciate why certain tests, and their inherent bias and foibles, are more appropriate for certain species. To avoid revisiting these concepts ad infinitum throughout the text, we have outlined the major methods below from a clinician's standpoint. More in-depth methodological reviews can be found in many of the references at the end of this chapter. These selected concepts are limited to major examples which are either under the clinician's control or those that may affect clinical interpretation of results and include choice of cellular stain solutions, cell counting techniques, and last but not least, the creation of the blood smear.

Cell Staining Solutions

Options for cell staining are many and include Phloxine B (PB), Natt and Herrick (N&H), methanol-based quick stains (Diff Quick), and modified Wright's stains. In general practice, methanol-based stains are commonly used because of ease of use. These stains do not require a slide stainer, and should they become overly stained, they can be de-stained using methanol and then restained. Modified Wright's stains are commonly preferred by reference laboratories. Most of the images in this book are taken from slides stained with modified Wright's stain, but, sometimes, slides stained with Diff-Quik or other quick-based stains are included for comparison.

Phloxin B and N&H stains (Table 1.1) are preferred for counting cells in the hemocytometer. Manual cell counts remain necessary in avian, reptile, amphibian, and fish species because automated cell counts using current instrumentation are not possible due to nucleated thrombocytes and erythrocytes. However, depending on the character of each stain, inherent bias exists in cell counts performed with them. Phloxine B or an eosin-based stain is preferred in species in which the heterophil predominates in the total white blood cell count (TWBC) count because only the granulocytes (heterophils and eosinophils) are stained for counts. The TWBC is then obtained from fractions determined from the leukocyte differential (aka indirect WBC). This method is likely less accurate and less precise when used in species in which lymphocytes are the predominant leukocyte. Conversely, N&H stains stain all cells for differentiation and counting in the hemocytometer. However, depending on the increased number of cells to count and differentiate and the difficulties in doing so, this method provides vastly differing results compared to the previous method. Both methods are dependent upon adequate laboratory skills and proficiency. Most reference diagnostic laboratories choose to use only one technique depending on the expense, training, expertise, and time necessary to properly and reproducibly complete these rather cumbersome tasks in a cost-effective manner.

Table 1.1 Natt and Herrick solution and stain.

Sodium chloride (NaCl)	3.88 g	Bring to a final volume of 1000 ml with distilled water, and then filter through Whatman #10 medium filter paper
Sodium sulfate ($NaSO_4$)	2.50 g	
Sodium phosphate ($NaHPO_4$)	1.74 g	
Potassium phosphate (KH_2PO_4)	0.25 g	
Formalin (37%)	7.50 ml	
Methyl violet	0.10 g	

Cell Counting Techniques

Leukocyte counting techniques include the direct total white blood cell count (TWBC) and the indirect total white blood cell count (iTWBC), which is dependent upon the cell-differential (Boxes 1.5 and 1.6). Advantages of the TWBC method include the following: (1) total erythrocyte and thrombocyte counts can also be obtained from the same charged hemocytometer (Figure 1.6), (2) it is less differential dependent, and (3) it may be more accurate for species which have a granulocyte-poor differential. In the direct TWBC method, blood is diluted 1:200 using the N&H solution (Box 1.5) and red blood cell diluting pipettes. After mixing, the diluted blood is placed into a Neubauer-ruled hemacytometer counting

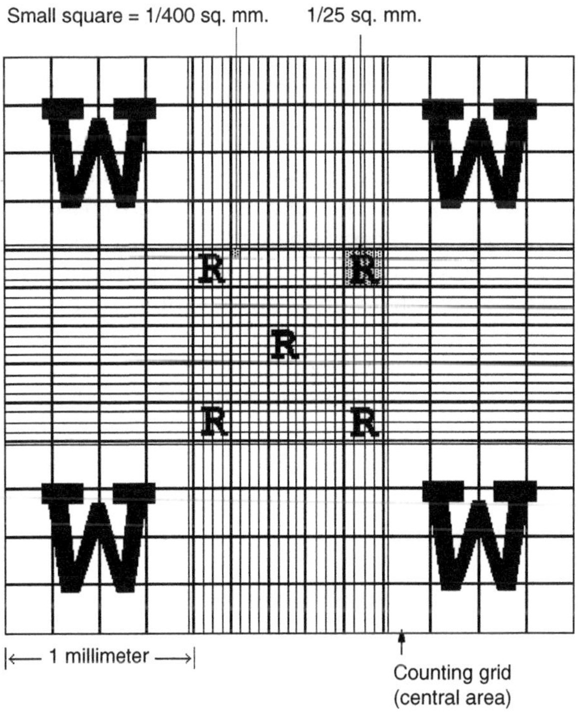

Figure 1.6 Neubauer-improved hemocytometer grid. Erythrocytes are counted based on the small cell grid in the squares denoted R, while granulocytes are counted in the larger grid within the four squares denoted W.

Box 1.5 Method for Indirect White Blood Cell Count

1) 0.01 ml (10 µl) blood (pipettor).
2) Add 0.31 ml eosinophil stain (syringe).
3) Swirl to mix.
4) Place 0.01 ml in one side of hemocytometer (1 drop fills chamber).
5) Wait 5 min for cells to settle.
6) Count total cells in 4 **(W)** large corner squares = X.
7) (X)(80) = total granulocyte count = **TG.**

Box 1.6 Method for White Blood Cell Differential Count

1) Create two direct fresh blood smears.
2) 20 DIPS in each quick stain.
3) Count 100 WBC, get percentages.
4) % Heterophils + % Eosinophils = TG.
5) Recalculate remaining cells from ratios.

chamber (Figure 1.7), and the cells are permitted to settle for 5 min. The TWBC is obtained by counting all the dark-blue staining leukocytes in the nine large squares in the ruled area of the hemacytometer chamber using the formula:

$$\text{TWBC} = \left[\left(\#\text{ cells in 9 large squares}\right) \times 1.1 \times 0.2\right] \times 10^9/\text{l}\left(\text{or} \times 10^3/\mu\text{l}\right)$$

The iTWBC procedure was simplified by using the eosinophil Unopette 5877 system (Becton Dickinson); however, this is no longer commercially available. Advantages of the indirect method are that it is easier to perform and has been shown in birds to be more precise for hematocytometer counting than the N&H method [17]. However, in cases where the heterophil/eosinophil count is low, greater inaccuracy is expected. Blood is diluted 1:32 with 0.1 Phloxine B solution. After loading, the hemacytometer counting chamber is permitted to sit for 5 min in high humidity. The eosin-stained heterophils and eosinophils are then counted in both sides of the chamber (18 large squares). A leukocyte differential is also required from a stained smear (see below) in order to calculate the TWBC indirectly using the following formula:

$$\text{iTWBC} = \frac{\left(\#\text{cells in 18 large squares} \times 1.111 \times 16 \times 0.1\right)}{\left(\text{differential \% of heterophils and eosinophils}\right)} \times 10^9/\text{l}\left(\times 10^3/\mu\text{l}\right)$$

A leukocyte differential, morphological evaluation of erythrocytes and leukocytes, and presence of any extracellular or intracellular or inclusions parasites require examination of a blood smear stained using a Romanowsky stain (e.g., Wright–Giemsa). While rapid stains (e.g., Diff-Quik, American Scientific Products, McGraw Park, Illinois) may be preferred in practice, they can produce inferior results, causing heterophils to be less distinct due to granule coalescence [18, 19]. Furthermore, if the stain is old or not changed on a regular basis, increased stain precipitate or bacterial contamination may occur.

The standard technique of using a microhematocrit capillary tube and centrifugation at 12,000 g for 5 min can be used to obtain a packed cell volume (PCV). To run a PCV for a for an exotic animal patient, blood is placed in a microhematocrit tube filled approximately to 3/4 of the tube. After a clay plug is placed at the bottom of the tube, the tube is centrifuged and then placed against a chart to determine the PCV. The PCV with the TRBC is used to determine the mean corpuscular volume (MCV). The calculation for MCV (fl) is (PCV × 10)/TRBC and expresses the average volume of individual erythrocytes [2].

The total red blood cell count (TRBC) can be determined using automated or manual methods established for mammals. Using either of the manual methods outlined below, erythrocytes located in the four corner and central squares are counted, and the TRBC is calculated as follows:

$$\text{TRBC} = \left[\left(\#\text{erythrocytes counted in 5 squares}\right) \times 10\right] \times 10^9/\text{l}\left(\text{or} \times 10^3/\mu\text{l}\right)$$

Hemoglobin concentration (Hb) is determined by the standard cyanmethemoglobin method, except that the free nuclei must be removed by centrifugation of the cyanmethemoglobin–blood mixture before obtaining the optical density value, to avoid overestimation.

The mean corpuscular hemoglobin concentration (MCHC) and the mean corpuscular hemoglobin MCH) can be calculated using the PCV and Hb and the Hb and TRBC, respectively. The MCHC represents the average Hb concentration per average erythrocyte. The MCH represents the amount of Hb in an average erythrocyte. The formula for MCHC (g/dL) is (Hb x 100)/PCV. The formula for MCH (pg) is (Hb x 10)/TRBC. Generally, MCHC is considered more accurate than MCH because it does not use the TRBC in the calculation.

Preparation of the Blood Smear

Best preparation of the blood smear is critical for accurate evaluation of the total white blood cell counts and the leukocyte differential in nonmammalian vertebrates. If a delay is expected between sample collection, submission, and processing, for example, in the case of samples shipped to the laboratory or collected after hours, always make two or three peripheral blood

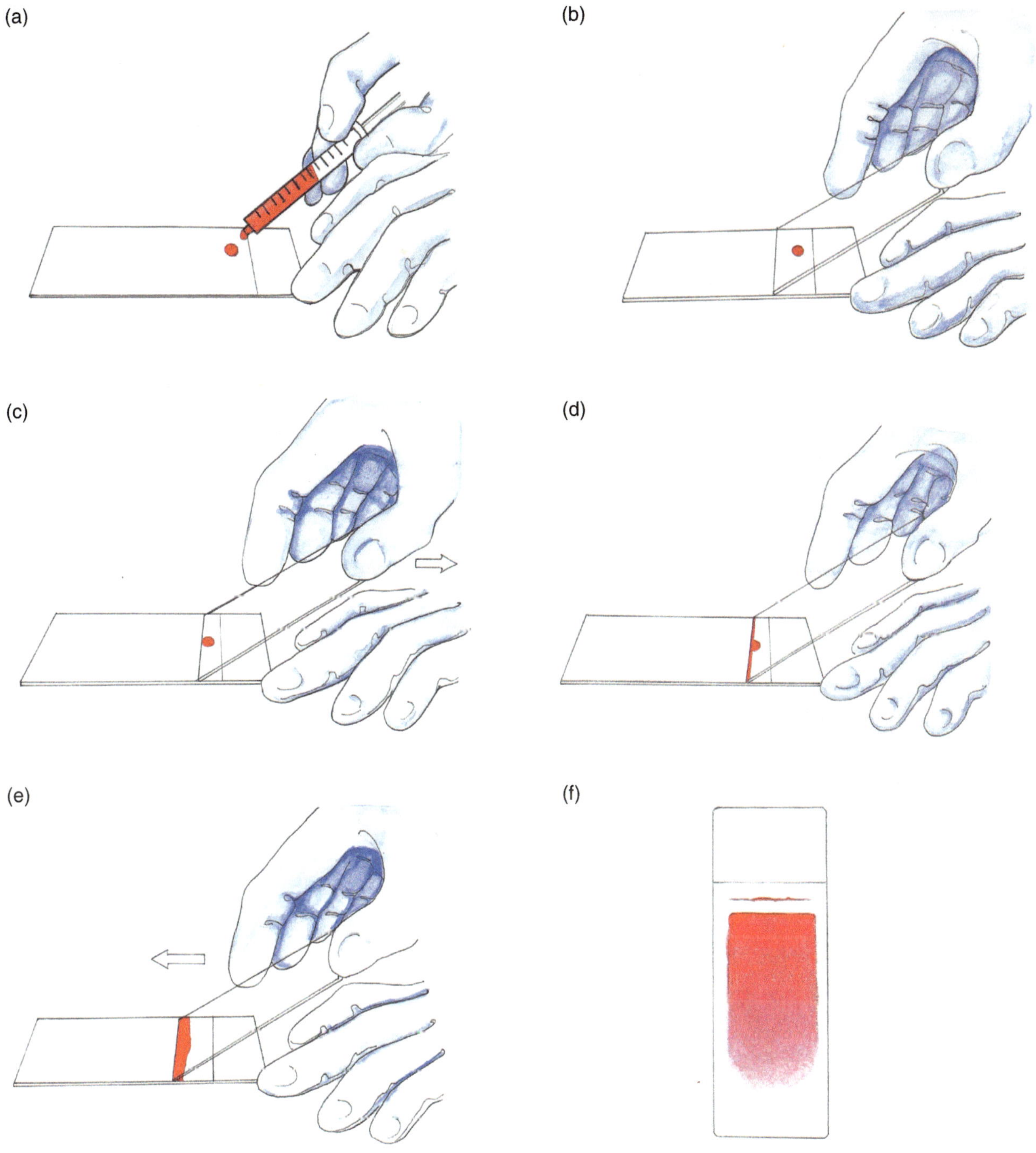

Figure 1.7 Blood smear technique: Wedge smear or slide-to-slide technique of making a peripheral blood smear. Use two clean, preferably precleaned, high-quality slides with an epoxy coated end, labeled with patient identification. (a) Place a drop of blood on the slide by touching (not dropping) the end of the venipuncture sample collection syringe. One drop of blood (2 µl) is placed at one end. Allowing blood to drop from the syringe often creates an overly large amount of blood to properly spread. Instead create a slight eversion of blood from the syringe end and by touch allow this microdrop to adhere to the slide. This provides a blood smear free from anticoagulant artifact should the smear be completed prior to clot formation. The drop of blood should measure approximately 4 mm in diameter and be placed approximately 0.5 cm from the labeled area. (b) Correct angle to hold spreader slide. Hold the spreader slide edges with your first two or three fingers and your thumb. Do not touch the spreading edge (short non-frosted end) with your hands. Use complete and even contact to the spreading end of the spreader slide at a 30°–45° angle to the blood drop slide in front of the blood droplet. Hold the blood drop slide to prevent movement during the smear process. Blood spreads across width of slide. (c) In one smooth motion, draw the spreader slide back through the entire drop of blood. (d) and (e) Once the blood spreads along the edge of the spreader slide (this occurs quickly), gently and steadily drive the spreader slide forward and push the blood forward along the length of the lower slide. Maintain a constant smooth motion and the same angle for the spreader slide when spreading the drop of blood as well as a consistently even contact (with very slight downward pressure) between the two slides. (f) Completed wedge smear: if the drop size, speed, contact, pressure, and angle of the spreader slide are correct, you will exhaust the blood before reaching the slide's end of the slide, create a feathered edge, and the smear will not extends more than three-quarters of the slide's length.

smears. Many factors may compromise the quality of the blood smear. Clean slides must be used. Ground glass dirt, oil or other materials imparted by touching either the slide surface or the spreader slide edge will result in a poor-quality smear. Inappropriate drop size is a common problem. An overly large blood drop or too much blood picked up by the spreader slider may result in a smear which extends to the slide edge, is too thick to evaluate microscopically, lacks a feathered edge, and may extend beyond the area that can be stained if an automated stainer is used. A small drop may produce a smear which is poorly representative of patient blood, and may be too thick to adequately evaluate cell morphology because of no monolayer. The speed and angle of the spreader slide across and from the smear slide determine the length and thickness of the smear. In general, 30°–45° is optimal. A short smear with most of the cells at the feathered edge may result from an overly quick motion of the spreader slider at a >40° angle, and most cells may be ruptured. A long smear which, lacks a feathered edge, may result from a lower (more acute angle) or a slow movement of the spreader slide. Continued even contact between the two slides must be maintained during smear preparation, but avoid applying excessive pressure to the spreader slider. See Figures 1.8–1.11 and Table 1.2 for examples of acceptable and unacceptable blood smears as well as methods of preparation and a brief overview of the approach to slide examination. Blood films should be actively air-dried and fixed immediately after preparation through immersion in absolute methanol for 5 minutes for fixation. Unfixed blood films should not be exposed to the elements or volatile compounds (including formalin fumes), to ensure retention of staining integrity and cellular morphology. Once fixed, blood films can be stained at a later time with Wright–Giemsa stain. Use of clean fresh materials and equipment to fix and stain blood films will reduce the incidence of artifacts.

Organization of This Book

This book is specifically designed to help the reader access information quickly. The text is organized into taxonomically based sections of commonly presented animals in private veterinary practice. Each major section heading has a unique color code on the side table to facilitate quick reference: Herbivore Mammals, Carnivore Mammals, Marsupials and Insectivores, Terrestrial Invertebrates, Primate, Reptile, Avian, and Aquatic. Author guidelines discouraged speaking in generalities and required that useful analyte values be clearly referenced *for the species determined* and that analytes of unknown value in certain species also be clearly stated. Each section's general outline is similar and includes the following topics, in order: introduction and species definition, obtaining the sample, sample handling and storage, hematology, biochemistries (to include blood gases and acid base balance), vitamins, minerals, metals and toxins, and urinalysis and

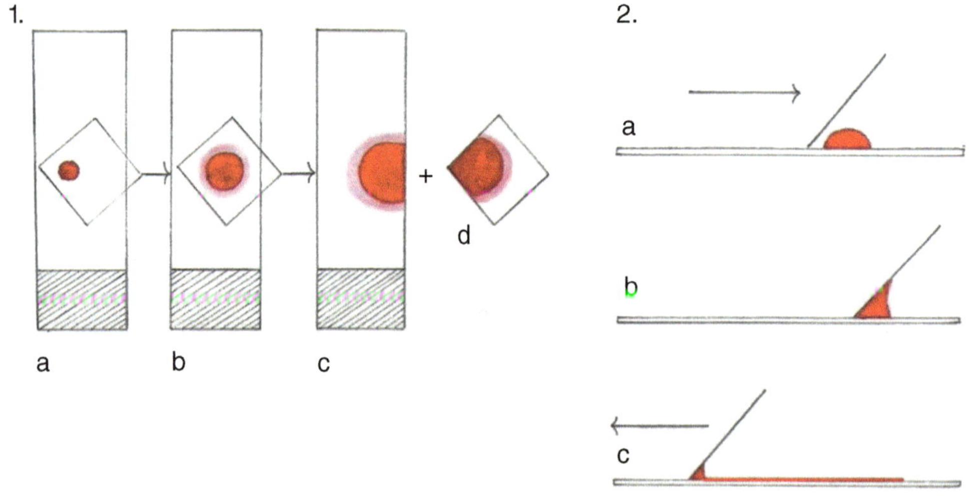

Figure 1.8 Blood smear technique: Coverslip to slide. This method is best used should you experience numerous smudge cells upon slide review (you are heavy-handed) or should you have concerns that a particular blood sample may have fragile cells on the basis of the species or suspected condition. 1. After the sample spreads between the slide and coverslip, the coverslip is slid smoothly from the glass slide in a horizontal plane at a right angle to the glass slide, and both coverslip and glass slide are air-dried. 2. the cover slip is used as a lighter version of the spreader slide in the wedge or slide to slide technique. a. approach to the blood drop b. blood drop adhesion c. blood smear creation via cover slip advancement.

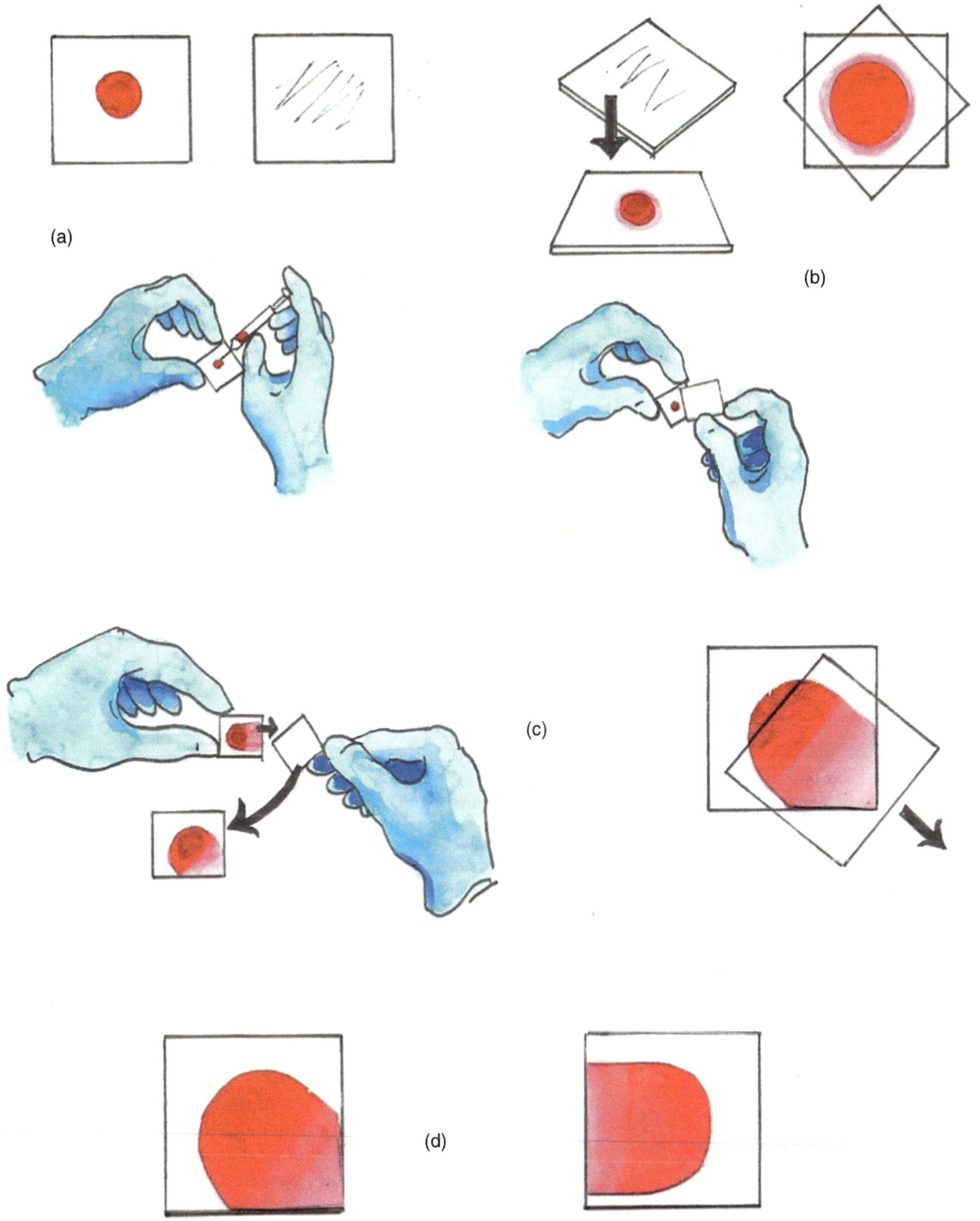

Figure 1.9 Blood smear technique: Coverslip to coverslip. Coverslip smears are made on 22 × 22 mm coverslips. The correct method will result in two quality smears that will appear similar to a thumbprint (d). To create a coverslip smear a coverslip is picked up by the corner, and the point is held between the thumb and forefinger in one hand. A small drop of blood is placed on to the center of the coverslip (a). A second coverslip is then placed over the first. The two entwined overlapping offset squares then form an octagram star shape (b). When the blood has spread almost to an edge, the coverslips are slid apart in a parallel fashion, without rotation, using the points of the star for manipulation (c). Challenging aspects of the coverslip blood smear include the excellent manual dexterity and vision necessary for manipulation and handling of the small fragile coverslip to avoid breakage. Coverslip smears are not compatible with standard automated slide stainers, and method modification is necessary. One may store many coverslips in the space required for only a few slides; however, their small size makes continuous handling, storage, and labeling problematic.

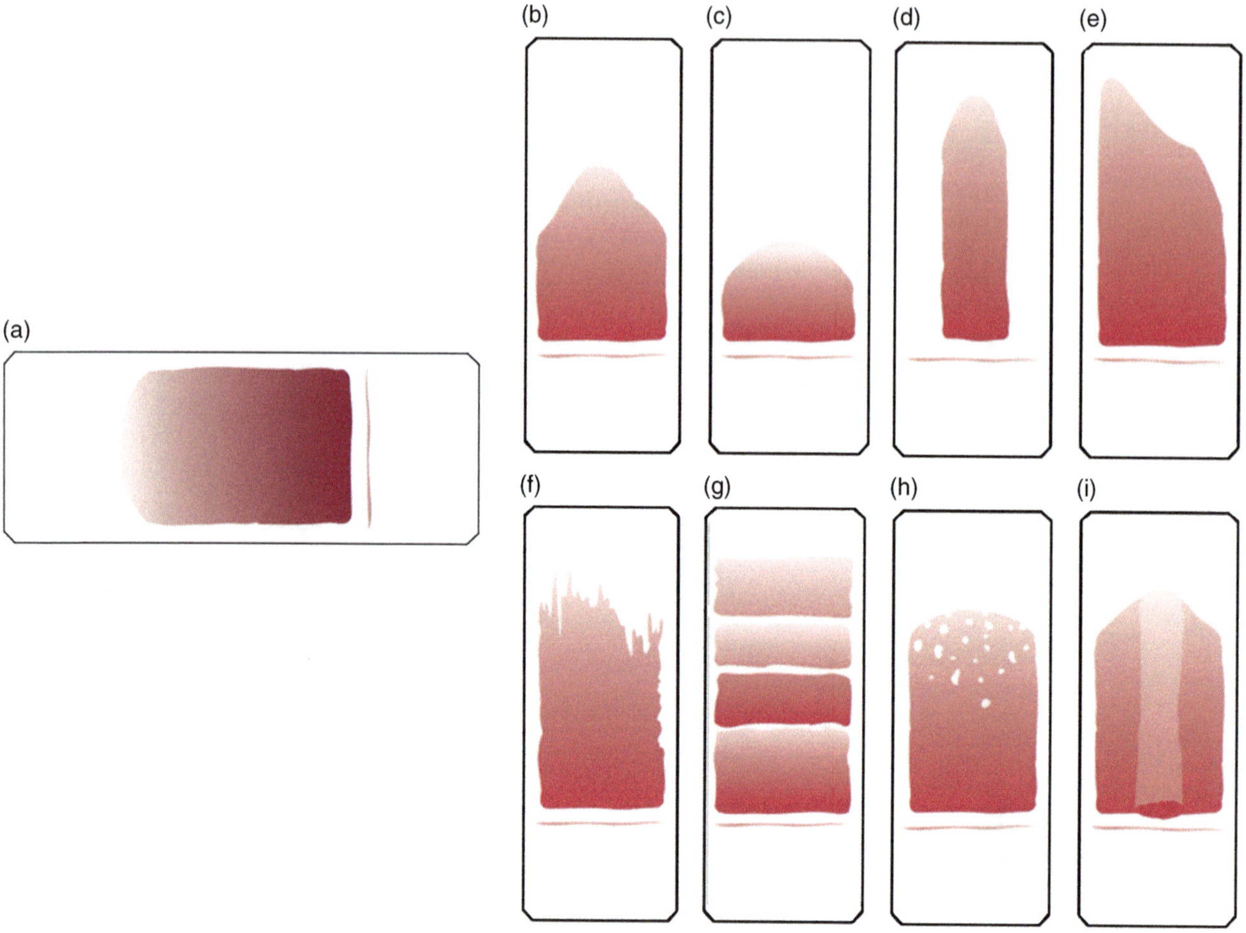

Figure 1.10 The good, the bad, and the ugly: Preferred, acceptable, and unacceptable blood smears. Appearances of optimum blood smears and those associated with the most common errors are shown. However, multiple causes may combine to result in unacceptable blood smears. In the author's experience: (a) shows the optimal shape of a peripheral blood smear. Characteristics of the best blood smear include: from two-thirds to three-fourths of the length of the slide is occupied by the smear; the thin feathered edge is slightly rounded; the entire drop is spread and the lateral edges of the smear are visible (using beveled cornered slides may help); the smear lacks irregularities, streaks, or holes, creating a smooth appearance; and the feathered edge diffracts light (has a rainbow appearance) when light is viewed through it. However, images (b–d) (passing grade) may also produce a reasonable result for cell differentials. Images (e–i) illustrate blood smears that should be remade if possible. (b) Spreader slide pushed too quickly; generally, the spreader slide should be moved through the same time as the blood takes to spread across the short edge of the spreader upon contact with the blood drop. (c) Blood drop overly small. (d) Impatience: Spreader slide moved before the blood drop spread across the width of the slide. (e) Uneven pressure applied to the spreader slide. (f) Rough, chipped, or dirty edge of spreader slide. (g) Hesitation or variable forward motion of spreader slide. (h) Dirt, grease on the slide; or increased blood lipid content. (i) Drop of blood began to dry or clot depending on time delay. *Source:* From Ref. [1].

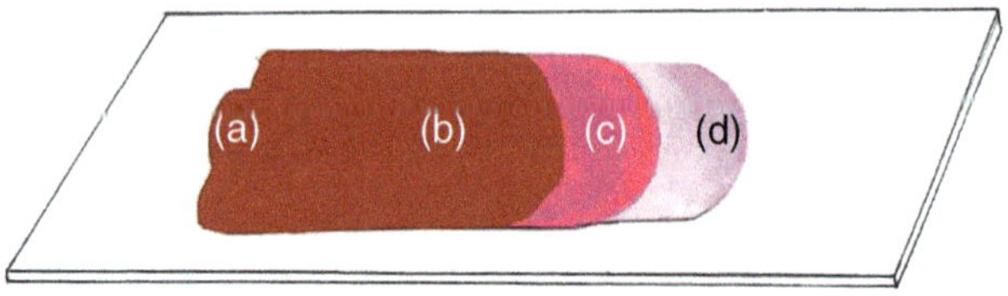

Figure 1.11 Zones of an ideal blood smear as a guide for cytological assessment. The good blood smear progresses from thick (a) to thin (d). The head application point of the blood drop is generally a nondiagnostic area. The thick region of smear is generally too thick for most things like cell morphology, but one may find some things like microfilaria. In the intermediate zone of the smear the goal is to create a **monolayer** of cells. This is the ideal or area to assess cell morphology, perform a cell differential, and estimate platelet counts. The **feathered edge**, also called the **tail** is the thinnest area of the blood smear. This is a good zone to observe large platelet clumps, very large cells and sometimes microfilaria.

serology and PCR use for the species. Tables include at least hematology and biochemistries, but may also include a variety of other diagnostics useful in the species such as blood gases, clotting times, urinalysis, laboratories familiar with diagnostic testing of the species, and so on.

Organization of Each Section

Each section will begin with an introduction and overview of the blood collection sites, techniques, appropriate sample preparation and collection techniques, and recommended anticoagulants and storage options.

Table 1.2 Common blood smear problems and suggested corrective actions.

Problem	Corrective action(s)
Small, short smear	Increase blood drop size Decrease angle and or speed of spreader slide
Long smear, no feathered edge	Decrease blood drop size Increase angle and or speed of spreader slide
Waves, ridges, or uneven smear	Decrease downward force of spreader slide Increase speed of spreader slide Maintain even contact between the two slides, and push forward with smooth motion
Drop incompletely moved by spreader slide Lopsided blood pick up	Draw spreader slide completely back through drop or wait for blood to spread the width of the slide via contact. Make complete contact of edge of the spreader slide with the stationary slide
Overly thick smear	Decrease blood drop size, decrease angle of spreader slide Increase the speed of the spreader slide
Overly thin smear	Use a larger drop of blood Increase the angle, and/or decrease the speed of the spreader slide

Sample analysis methodology will be discussed when multiple techniques are available that may affect results and interpretation. The effects of common sample abnormalities which may result in sample degradation will include the effects of hemolysis, lipemia, and increased time on sample degradation and expected changes in certain factors. Each chapter will progress in a similar format to include clinical enzymology, electrolytes, blood gases, urinalysis, coagulation testing, endocrine testing, toxicology, and finally serologic immunologic testing. Lipid analysis and appropriate gastrointestinal testing may also be included in select species where applicable. Diagrams for appropriate testing and diagnosis of certain systems may be included in each section.

Common clinical enzymes useful in each species will be reviewed in the next section on the basis of system utility. Liver, kidney, muscle, cardiac, gastrointestinal enzymes, and lipid biomarkers useful in each species will be covered. Expected changes in these enzymes in disease processes of the species will also be detailed. Electrolyte normals and abnormalities will briefly be reviewed for each species; similarly, blood gases and their possible application in this species will be covered. End-tidal Co_2 as a diagnostic modality may also be included in this section. A section on urinalysis will include expected normals for the species as well as known abnormalities which do and do not affect the urinary system of this species. Additionally, appropriate approaches for collection of urine for the species will be reviewed. Coagulation testing will be reviewed as to the coagulation factors known for each species, and the current state of testing, and the necessity of cross-matching and known blood types will also be included.

Endocrine testing will be reviewed from the perspective of the normal endocrine physiology of the species, known effects of epinephrine and other endogenous hormone on clinical hematology, and the utility of hormonal testing for diagnosis of endocrine disease. Reference ranges for common toxicants will be detailed when diagnostic testing is available. Rodenticide toxicities and the resultant necessity of coagulation testing, expected heavy metal levels for most species, and acetylcholinesterase testing will be reviewed in applicable species. Expected results for certain toxicants – example: elevation of certain enzymes in lead toxicity – will also be reviewed when these are known for each species.

Serologic, PCR, and immunologic tests are overviewed for common diseases in each species. Included within these sections are diagnostics applicable for each species and a table of available laboratories for tests. Available tests for each common disease (PCR, Elisa, or other serology), and comments on sample types, handling and shipment, and result interpretation are also provided. The individual clinician, researcher, or biologist is responsible for assessment of diagnostic laboratories with respect to experience with exotic species and test validity.

Discussion of clinical hematology in this text is limited to expected findings for healthy species, interpretation of reference ranges, and common cellular and cell count abnormalities associated with disease or dysfunction. Reference ranges for common species will be included for each species in both standard international (SI) and American (US) units. For each of the commonly seen species wherein a full hematologic profile of white and red blood cells is not given in previous texts, a color plate of cells is included. Images such as urinalysis findings, illustration of cellular inclusions or toxic change, cell staining artifacts or cells comparatively different from other species are included for each species.

Reference ranges for hematology, biochemistries, and other common analytes are provided in tabular format at the end of each species-based section. Both SI and US units are used in the text on the basis of the original source material, and both units SI and US units are provided in all tables. A conversion table and commonly used abbreviations for most analytes provided in the text are located on the back inside cover. Inside the front cover is a key for many of the tables of this book, in which animal-specific and sample-specific characteristics have been indicated by symbols to allow ease of referencing the numeric values. Listings at the ends of each section will allow the reader to flip to the end of each tabbed section to determine abnormalities and then read the significance of these abnormalities within the same section. The reader can also quickly ascertain which values currently have no references ranges and therefore may not be as useful in diagnostic testing or may require the sampling of additional apparently healthy animals at that time for test interpretation.

We certainly hope this brief introduction provides you with an overview of the goals and design of the text and the options for incorporation of clinical pathology into your daily diagnostics in the practice of exotic animal veterinary medicine. Below please find additional recommended texts for basic and advanced in-depth clinicopathologic reference.

References

1 Rodak, B.F., Fritsma, G.A., and Keohane, E.M. (2012). *Hematology: Clinical Principles and Applications*, 4e. St. Louis: Saunders.

2 Campbell, T.W. and Ellis, C.K. (2013 Jul 3). *Avian and Exotic Animal Hematology and Cytology*. Wiley.

3 Campbell, T.W. and Grant, K.R. (2011 Jun 9). *Clinical Cases in Avian and Exotic Animal Hematology and Cytology*. Wiley.

4 Clark, P., Boardman, W., and Raidal, S. (2009 Sep 8). *Atlas of Clinical Avian Hematology*. Wiley.

5 Flatland, B., Freeman, K.P., Vap, L.M., and Harr, K.E. (2013 Dec 1). ASVCP guidelines: quality assurance for point-of-care testing in veterinary medicine. *Veterinary clinical pathology* 42 (4): 405–423.

6 Flatland, B., Freeman, K.P., Friedrichs, K.R. et al. (2010 Sep 1). ASVCP quality assurance guidelines: control of general analytical factors in veterinary laboratories. *Veterinary clinical pathology* 39 (3): 264–277.

7 Gunn-Christie, R.G., Flatland, B., Friedrichs, K.R. et al. (2012 Mar 1). ASVCP quality assurance guidelines: control of preanalytical, analytical, and postanalytical factors for urinalysis, cytology, and clinical chemistry in veterinary laboratories. *Veterinary clinical pathology* 41 (1): 18–26.

8 Harr, K.E., Flatland, B., Nabity, M., and Freeman, K.P. (2013 Dec 1). ASVCP guidelines: allowable total error guidelines for biochemistry. *Veterinary clinical pathology* 42 (4): 424–436.

9 Kaneko, J.J., Harvey, J.W., and Bruss, M.L. (2008 Sep 4). *Clinical Biochemistry of Domestic Animals*. Academic press.

10 Lester, S., Harr, K.E., Rishniw, M., and Pion, P. (2013 Jan 15). Current quality assurance concepts and considerations for quality control of in-clinic biochemistry testing. *Journal of the American Veterinary Medical Association* 242 (2): 182–192.

11 Stockham, S.L. and Scott, M.A. (2013 May 31). *Fundamentals of Veterinary Clinical Pathology*. Wiley.

12 Thrall, M.A., Weiser, G., Allison, R., and Campbell, T.W. (2012 Jul 2). *Veterinary Hematology and Clinical Chemistry*. Wiley.

13 Walberg, J. (2001 Apr 1). White blood cell counting techniques in birds. *Seminars in Avian and Exotic Pet Medicine* 10 (2): 72–76. WB Saunders.

14 Weiss, D.J. and Wardrop, K.J. (2011 Jul 26). *Schalm's Veterinary Hematology*. Wiley.

15 Westgard, J.O. and Klee, G.G. (1996). Quality management. In: *Chapter 16 in Fundamentals of Clinical Chemistry*, 4e (ed. C. Burtis), 211–223. Philadelphia: WB Saunders Company.

16 Friedrichs, K.R., Harr, K.E., Freeman, K.P. et al. (2012 Dec 1). ASVCP reference interval guidelines: determination of de novo reference intervals in veterinary species and other related topics. *Veterinary Clinical Pathology* 41 (4): 441–453.

17 Dein, F.J., Wilson, A., Fischer, D., and Langenberg, P. (1994 Sep 1). Avian leucocyte counting using the

hemocytometer. *Journal of Zoo and Wildlife Medicine* 25: 432–437.

18 LeBlanc, C.J., Heatley, J.J., and Mack, E.B. (2000). A review of the morphology of lizard leukocytes with a discussion of the clinical differentiation of bearded dragon, Pogona vitticeps, leukocytes. *Journal of Herpetological Medicine and Surgery.* 10 (2): 27–30.

19 LeBlanc, C.J. (2001). Clinical Differentiation of Chinese Water Dragon, Physignathus spp., Leukocytes. *Journal of Herpetological Medicine and Surgery.* 11 (3): 31–32.

2

Ferrets

Cheryl B. Greenacre DVM, DABVP (Avian and Exotic Companion Mammal)

Department of Small Animal Clinical Sciences, College of Veterinary Medicine, University of Tennessee, Knoxville, Tennessee, USA

Introduction

Evaluation of bodily fluids such as blood and urine is commonly performed in ferrets. Compared to other exotic pet animal species, more scientific references are available in both the laboratory and pet animal literature evaluating various analytes in ferrets. Much anecdotal information, or information based on small numbers of subjects or nonspecific data, is also available. Indications for obtaining clinical pathologic data in ferrets vary but include determination of the presence of disease processes such as infection, inflammation, anemia, or organ dysfunction. The most common tests performed on ferrets include a blood glucose test to evaluate for insulinoma, an adrenal panel to evaluate for adrenal tumor, and a CBC to evaluate for infection, inflammation, or lymphoma.

Obtaining a useful sample from a ferret on the basis of size is relatively easy, but some limitations to evaluating clinical pathologic data in ferrets include lack of research pertaining to some analytes, limited samples to repeat studies, partial information gathered (evaluation of a complete blood count (CBC) could indicate infection, but not pinpoint the source of etiology of infection), or in the case of an adrenal panel, the assay is sensitive, but clinically imprecise. The analytes do not reveal which adrenal gland is affected, which may or may not be necessary information depending on the treatment chosen. Most tests have limitations when evaluating the whole animal, so that other diagnostic tests and treatment choices may be needed to direct the diagnostic path.

Sample Collection

Blood samples collected from ferrets under isoflurane anesthesia result in decreased hematological values compared to those of ferrets sampled when awake [1]. The most profound change was a 36% reduction in packed cell volume (PCV), but other values were also reduced [1].

The use of a product containing sugars (Nutrical or Laxatone), given orally to distract the ferret during phlebotomy, will change the blood glucose values rather quickly, so these products should not be used if evaluating blood glucose. Ideally sampling for blood glucose should be done after a 4 h fast to prevent causing hypoglycemia and to avoid misinterpreting a postprandial hyperglycemia. Application of a topical anesthetic cream to the phlebotomy site 30 min prior to phlebotomy may facilitate sampling [2].

Sample Handling

The jugular vein, cranial vena cava, lateral saphenous vein, and cephalic vein are common venipuncture sites in the ferret. Other sites such as the caudal artery of the tail, orbital sinus, and cardiocentesis have been described but are not recommended for general practice because of pain, toughness of tissues, or use as part of a terminal procedure [2]. The site chosen also depends on the amount of sample desired. Larger to smaller sample volumes can be obtained from the cranial vena cava, the jugular vein, and the lateral saphenous and cephalic veins in that order. If only a drop is needed for blood glucose determination using a handheld glucometer, then the easiest site for the handler and the ferret is to nick a small superficial ear pinna vein and apply the glucometer strip directly to the drop (Figure 2.1). Some veterinarians pre-heparinize the syringe prior to drawing blood to prevent clotting based on slow blood flow. Sodium heparin, but not lithium heparin, can interfere with some testing and is not recommended for use with benchtop chemical analyzers.

Exotic Animal Laboratory Diagnosis, First Edition. Edited by J. Jill Heatley and Karen E. Russell.

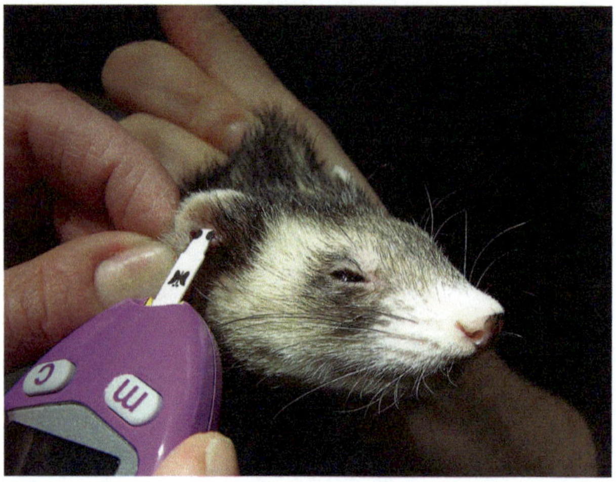

Figure 2.1 Approach for determination of glucose from a ferret ear nick.

Methods

The total blood volume in ferrets is approximately 5%–7% of body weight, so that the blood volume for an approximately 750 g female (jill) is 40 ml and for a 1000 g male (hob) is 60 ml [3–5]. Generally it is considered safe to remove up to 10% of blood volume in a healthy animal; therefore, in a healthy 750 g jill, up to 4.0 ml can be removed, and up to 6.0 ml from a healthy 1 kg hob [3, 4]. However, many ferret patients are sick, and the blood sample volume should then be reduced. Another rule is that 10% of the blood volume can be removed only every 14 days to avoid repeated sampling over a short period of time. Most hematology and biochemical parameters can be evaluated on 1–1.5 ml of blood. A differential can be performed with one drop of blood smeared on a slide with a gross estimate of the white blood cell count. Most automated counters for evaluating the CBC use about 0.3 ml of blood. An Abaxis VetScan can be used in ferrets to evaluate several biochemical parameters on 0.1–0.2 ml of blood (the company website provides reference intervals) [6]. Most commercial laboratories use either a Hitachi 911 or a COBAS, both of which use about 0.3–0.5 ml of serum or plasma to run a typical biochemical panel. An adrenal panel can be performed on as little as 0.1 ml of serum, although the laboratories prefer 0.3 ml.

Jugular Vein

Moderate venous samples typically drawn for diagnostic purposes (1–3 ml) can be obtained from the jugular vein. Successful restraint of a fully alert ferret for jugular phlebotomy requires patience and experience. To restrain an awake ferret to perform phlebotomy on the jugular vein, some phlebotomists prefer the ferret scruffed while wrapped in a towel in dorsal recumbency on the table or with the body suspended vertically [5, 7]. The vertical method of restraint is sometime referred to as the hanging jugular (Figures 2.2 and 2.3). The jugular vein is approached either cranially or caudally while the holder or the phlebotomist occludes flow of the jugular vein temporarily at the thoracic inlet (Figure 2.4). An alternate approach restrains the ferret with the neck and legs stretched over the table edge as for jugular phlebotomy in the domestic cat. One may use a 1 or 3 cm^3 syringe and a 25, 23, or 22 g. (gauge) needle for venipuncture. Venipuncture of the jugular vein is often blind as the vessel is not usually palpable or visible. The skin is surprisingly tough in ferrets, so more force is needed than expected to puncture the skin. The vein is usually superficial, and therefore a shallow angle, about 30%, is used to approach the jugular vein [7]. The vein can roll laterally if not enough force is used to puncture the vein with the needle. The method generally employed for venipuncture is to forcefully push the needle into the neck, and then slowly withdraw the needle while aspirating until almost out, then forcefully push the needle into another, hopefully more suitable position, and repeat. Blood flow is slow, and repositioning the needle typically does not increase flow, although turning the needle in place may

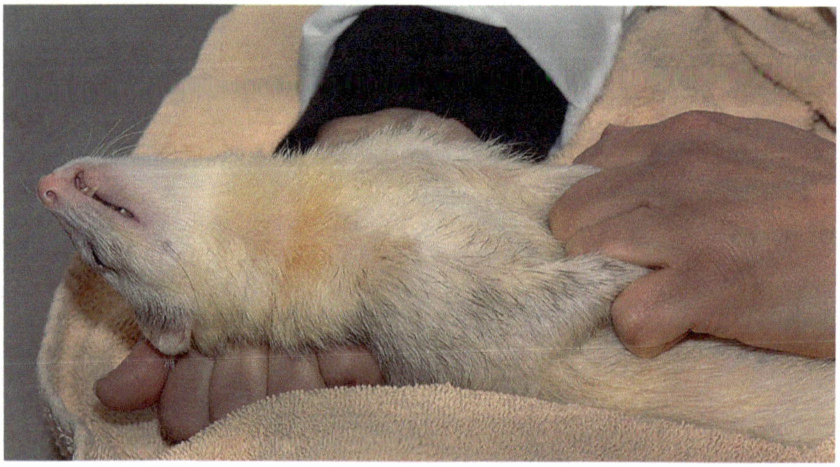

Figure 2.2 Restraint for venipuncture of the lateral jugular vein of a ferret.

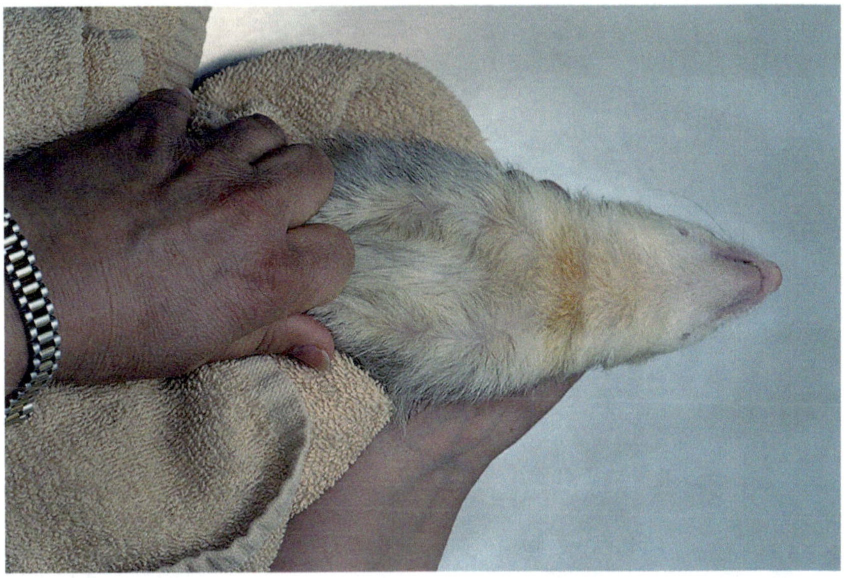

Figure 2.3 Alternate method of restraint for jugular venipuncture in the ferret.

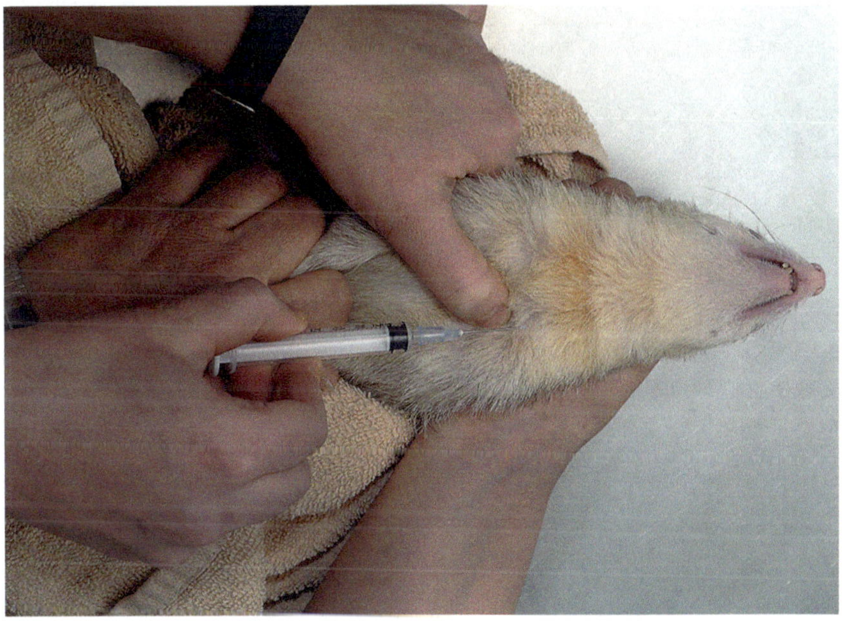

Figure 2.4 Approach for venipuncture of the ferret.

dislodge a bevel suctioned to the vein wall. Shaving the neck is generally forgone for a simple alcohol application to flatten the hair and possibly visualize the jugular vein. However, fur can be shaved if necessary for better visualization.

Lateral Saphenous Vein

The lateral saphenous vein is commonly used and can provide a usable sample, but usually the sample volumes are smaller than those obtained from the jugular, because of vein collapse. Smaller samples (<1 ml) for rechecking a blood glucose on a handheld device can be drawn from the lateral saphenous vein. Use of a 25g. needle and a 1 cm^3 syringe will help prevent collapse of the vein. The ferret can be restrained such that its rear leg hangs over the edge of the table, where the holder can temporarily occlude the vein while simultaneously holding the knee in a locked extended position. The phlebotomist can then grasp the foot to still the leg while drawing the blood. The lateral saphenous vein courses over the lateral tarsal area (Figures 2.5 and 2.6).

Cephalic Vein

The cephalic vein can be used for venipuncture, but is a small vein usually reserved for potential cephalic catheter placement or when low-volume samples will suffice. This vessel courses along the medial antebrachium as in a dog, although one typically does not roll the vein or

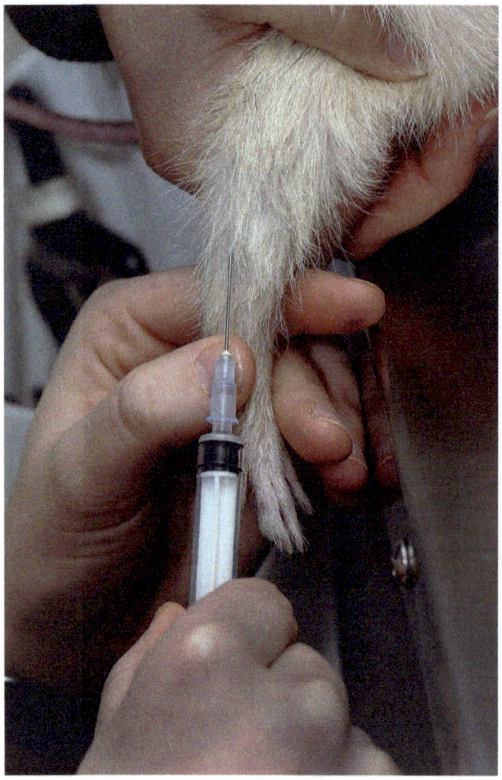

Figure 2.5 Approach for lateral saphenous venipuncture of the ferret.

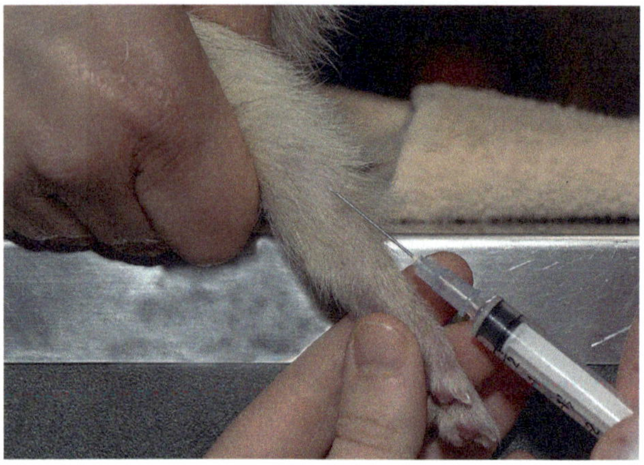

Figure 2.6 Additional view of approach for lateral saphenous venipuncture of the ferret.

otherwise move it from its normal position during phlebotomy as this may collapse the vein. Use of topical anesthetics may facilitate sampling from this vessel, as does open collection with a 25g. needle, capillary flow into the hub, and collection from the needle hub with heparinized hematocrit tubes. Samples can then be used for White blood cell count (WBC) estimation, PCV/TS determination, and blood glucose determination on a handheld analyzer [8].

Cranial Vena Cava

Blood collection from the cranial vena cava or the nearby brachiocephalic trunk has been described as a method for routine blood collection in the still awake, the sedated, or the anesthetized ferret [5]. This author does not prefer phlebotomy from the cranial vena cava, because digital pressure cannot be adequately applied after phlebotomy if needed. Large amounts (4–10ml) drawn for blood transfusion purposes are best drawn from the cranial vena cava to minimize the occurrence of clots. The author prefers to perform this method only in anesthetized ferrets if large amounts (≥4 ml) of blood are needed rapidly for blood transfusion purposes. Although this procedure can be used in the awake or sedate ferret, anesthesia is recommended to prevent unwanted movement during the procedure and damage to the great vessels. The ferret must be adequately restrained to prevent movement during this procedure. A 25g. needle is inserted at the thoracic inlet between the first rib and the manubrium and positioned toward the opposite rear leg at a 45° angle (Figures 2.7–2.9) [5]. The vessel is relatively shallow, and therefore after passing the skin, application of negative pressure usually results in excellent blood flow into the syringe. If patient movement occurs, immediately remove the needle from the thorax and abort the procedure [2].

Caudal Tail Artery

Arterial sampling can be performed on the caudal tail artery on ventral midline, but this method is painful, so perform under anesthesia or apply topical lidocaine or prilocaine cream topically 30min prior to phlebotomy [5]. Also, since it is an artery, remember to apply 2 to 3 min of digital pressure afterward to prevent hematoma or hemorrhage. Insert a 25g. needle about 3–4cm caudal to the anus along the ventral midline of the tail and about 2–3mm deep to access the caudal tail artery [5, 7].

Sampling from a Catheter

If withdrawing blood from a catheter, one should remove about 1ml of blood from the catheter using a heparinized (about 1–1.5ml of 5U/ml heparinized saline) syringe, then using a separate syringe remove the sample, and replace the first milliliter of blood taken back into the catheter to the ferret [7].

Urine Sampling

Urine samples can be obtained from either a cystocentesis, free catch, or from a urethral catheter. Gentle manual expression can be used to obtain a voided sample. Voided

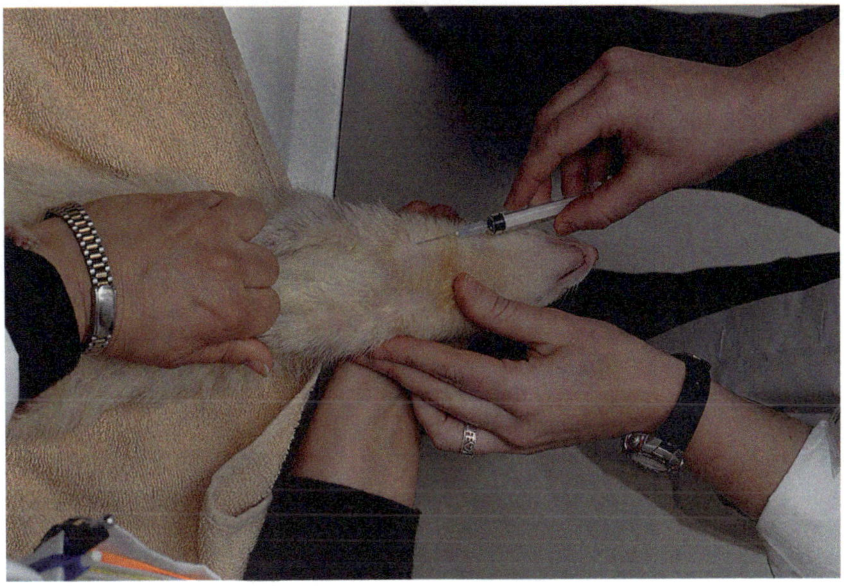

Figure 2.7 Approach for venipuncture of the vena cava in the ferret.

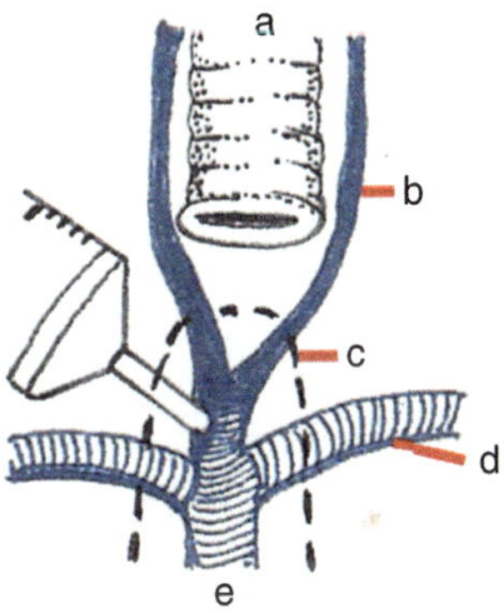

Figure 2.8 Illustration of magnified view of the approach and anatomical landmarks for ferret phlebotomy via the cranial vena cava: (a) trachea, (b) jugular vein, (c) manubrium, (d) brachiocephalic vein, (e) cranial vena cava.

samples can also be collected in a litter box with non-absorbable material, by catching with a shallow container, or by collecting off a clean surface. Cystocentesis is usually performed in an anesthetized ferret using a 25 g. or smaller needle, attached to a 1–3 ml syringe, so as not to damage the relatively thin bladder wall. The urinary bladder can usually be easily palpated a few centimeters cranial to the pelvis.

Voided samples have the disadvantage of becoming contaminated with bacteria, making culture of the urine inaccurate, but voided "clean" samples can still be used for urinalysis. Sometimes the ferret will urinate with the stress of handling due to epinephrine-mediated bladder contraction in ferrets. Urethral catheterization can be performed in the male ferret with a 3.0–3.5 French red rubber or silicone catheter (Slippery Sam Tomcat

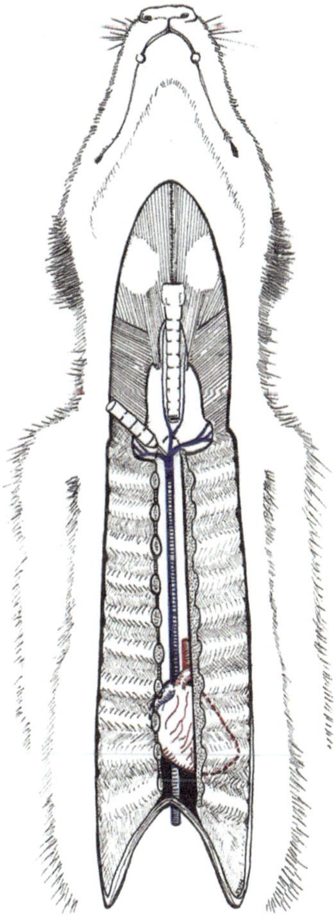

Figure 2.9 Approach for ferret phlebotomy via the cranial vena cava. Note the lack of proximity to the heart and accompanying great vessels and the landmarks of the manubrium and first rib for entry into the thorax. Heavy sedation or anesthesia is recommended for this procedure.

Urethral Catheters, Surgivet, Smith's Medical, Norwell, Massachusetts; Ferret Urinary Catheter, Mila international, Erlanger, Kentucky); however, trauma associated with urethral catheter placement can introduce blood into the urine sample. A 22 g. jugular catheter with the stylet removed can also be used, but with care because of possible trauma from this more rigid catheter. Catheterization can be challenging for the practitioner who is not familiar with ferret penile anatomy. The ventral urethral opening is at the distal end of the pink penile tissue, not at the end of the white curved os penis which extends more distally than the tissue. Further, the urethral opening is not obvious. Female ferrets can be more difficult to catheterize. Their urethral opening should be directly visualized approximately 1 cm cranial to the clitoral fossa on the ventral surface of the vestibule [9].

The area is aseptically prepared, while an assistant exposes the penis. Ferrets have an os penis that extends beyond the pink penile tissue and curves distally. The urethral opening is located on the ventral surface at the junction of the white os penis and the pink musculature of the penis distally. Carefully, use the shaft of a 25 g. needle or a blunted 25 g. nasolacrimal cannula to lift the urethral opening, since it is usually flush against the tissue and not easily pushed open by the advancing catheter. The premeasured catheter is placed retrograde in the urethra and then sutured and taped to the body [10]. The distal most part of the catheter taped to the base of the tail. Watch for chewing and twisting of the catheter [11].

Beware that urethral catheter placement may not be possible in some male ferrets with urinary tract outflow blockage due to obstruction from prostatic hypertrophy secondary to adrenal disease. Overzealous efforts at catheter placement in a diseased and or compromised urethra can result in urethral laceration and puncture. Ascending peritonitis may result; a serious and life-threatening complication associated with adrenal disease and prostatic enlargement in male ferrets.

Bone Marrow Sampling

Since collection of a bone marrow sample (aspiration or biopsy) is temporarily painful, it should be performed under general anesthesia, with anesthetics such as isoflurane or sevoflurane, and the local area should be infiltrated with lidocaine. The proximal femur is the preferred site, but samples can also be obtained from the iliac crest and the proximal humerus. After shaving the area and aseptic preparation of the skin is done, a 2–3 mm skin incision is made with a #15 or #11 scalpel blade. For bone marrow aspiration, typically a 20–22 g., 1.5 in. spinal needle (with a stylet) or an 18 g. Jamshidi-type needle is used [7]. Insert into the femur just medial to the greater trochanter, as is done in small dogs and cats, by gently pushing the needle through the cortex and simultaneously rotating (twisting in an alternating clockwise and counterclockwise fashion) the needle [5, 7, 12, 13]. Once in the bone marrow, remove the stylet and suction with a 12 cm^3 syringe just until a sample appears. Further suction can result in blood contamination. Squash cytological preparation of the sample is preferred. The gross presence of fat globules suggests a good bone marrow aspirate. If blood contamination is suspected, hold the slide vertically after expelling the sample on the slide to allow blood to run onto another slide while marrow spicules remain on the first slide.

A core biopsy of the cortex can be performed using the same tools and methods, but usually a Jamshidi-type needle is used. Upon cortex penetration, the stylet is removed and the cannula is advanced in the marrow for approximately 0.5 cm, then rotated and withdrawn by a few millimeters, then rotated again, perhaps, repeating a final time, then removed. The goal is to obtain a sample of intact bone marrow without any breaks that is about 0.5 cm long. It is best to obtain a core sample from another location than the aspirate. If an aspirate is obtained from the same site after a core biopsy is taken, the sample may clot from release of thromboplastin. Additionally, if a core biopsy is done in the same place after an aspirate is taken, the sample can mimic hypoplasia. A core biopsy allows evaluation of causes of hypocellular bone marrow and quantification of marrow iron stores. If marrow clots, or is retrieved from a postmortem specimen, it can be placed in 10% formalin and submitted for histopathologic examination as one would for a biopsy specimen [13].

Cerebrospinal Fluid Sampling

The collection of cerebrospinal fluid (CSF) has been described in a study of 42 adult (20–26 week old) intact ferrets that had CSF collected from the cisterna magna (cerebellomedullary cistern) under brief isoflurane or sevoflurane anesthesia [14]. The reference points for the procedures are similar to those of the dog or cat. Approximately 0.26 ml of CSF/kg body weight of ferret can be safely removed [14].

Sample Handling

Collect blood into EDTA tubes for hematologic evaluation and into lithium heparin tubes for biochemical analysis. Some hormone and other tests require collection into red top tubes (e.g., Adrenal Hormone Panel). Basically, sample handling is the same as for the dog and cat, but there are a few differences, usually because of the comparatively smaller size of the ferret. One generally fills whole blood tubes first, such as the EDTA tube for the CBC, or the lithium heparin tube, before the sample clots, and then the tubes for serum collection can be filled next. Small plastic tubes (Microtainer® brand by Becton-Dickinson) are available with a variety of anticoagulants, additives, and serum separators. The anticoagulant in these tubes is in a powder form (lyophilized) on the walls of these tubes. Thus, dilution of sample is generally not a concern. However, to best prevent clot formation, the sample should be quickly and repeatedly inverted immediately after placement into the tube to expose the blood to the entire inner surface and therefore all anticoagulant present.

Specific Analytes

Complete Blood Count

Hematologic reference ranges for adult domestic ferrets, the endangered black-footed ferret, and the European polecat have been published and are included in Table 2.1 [3, 5, 15–21]. There are several references for CBC ranges in adult domestic ferrets. The studies have many unreported factors and many factors which vary that could, and likely do, affect the reported results; they include coat color, age, health, fasting time, anesthetic type, amount of blood drawn, reproductive status and gender, and methods of analysis. Therefore, the clinician should be wary of direct comparison of the analytes provided for ferrets. These details, when known, are given in the key for Table 2.1. Blood cell morphology of ferrets is similar to those of other domestic companion mammals (Figures 2.10–2.15).

Hematologic results for 10–16-week-old ferrets are included in Table 2.2 [3]. Hematocrit (HCT), hemoglobin (HGB), and red blood cell (RBC) are generally lower in younger ferrets than in adult ferrets [3]. Isoflurane causes a decrease in the PCV of ferrets, but also has other effects. In six intact female ferrets at 15, 30, and 45 min post intubation with isoflurane (after mask induction), multiple hematologic parameters decreased compared to pre-anesthetic baseline [1]. Fifteen minutes post intubation, a 35% reduction in RBC count, 30% reduction in hemoglobin, 36% reduction in hematocrit, 24% reduction in WBC, and a 20% reduction in plasma protein levels were documented. Forty-five minutes after cessation of isoflurane delivery, the RBC, hemoglobin, and hematocrit reduced by 3%–5%, WBC by 14%, and plasma protein by 6% below baseline levels. Mean cell volume (MCV), mean corpuscular hemoglobin (MCH), and mean corpuscular hemoglobin concentration (MCHC) were unchanged. Similar effects occur with isoflurane or halothane in humans, nonhuman primates, dogs, pigs, and horses [1]. If ferrets are anesthetized for phlebotomy, this artifactual change must be accounted for or clinical judgments might erroneously limit chemotherapy or suggest that other disease processes were present, such as anemia or dehydration. Aplastic anemia can occur in intact female ferrets because of induced ovulation. Female ferrets will stay in heat until bred. After approximately one month of being in heat, hyperestrogenism leads to bone marrow suppression and aplastic anemia. Mortality can result in as little as three months. Other major differentials for anemia in ferrets include bone marrow effacement, usually by lymphoma dirofilariasis (destruction), anemia of chronic disease, and adrenal disease (hyperestrogenism).

A ferret with diarrhea and an absolute eosinophil count over 1700 is indicative of eosinophilic gastroenteritis (EGE). In the ferret, EGE is more common than in other species. Other causes of diarrhea in the ferret should be ruled out as treatment often includes steroids, which could worsen other infections [23].

Coagulation Panel

Coagulation times in albino ferrets (n = 28 males, 11 females) were comparable to those of the rat and dog to include a prothrombin time of 15.7 s and a kaolin-cephalin of 54.9 s [15].

Blood Types

Domestic ferrets lack detectable blood groups, and therefore cross-matching is not typically performed prior to a blood transfusion because of the minimal risk of transfusion reaction [3, 5, 24]. Naturally acquired blood group antibodies were not evident when ferret serum and erythrocytes were randomly paired from 212 ferrets of two different sources [24].

Biochemical Panel

Biochemical reference ranges have been published on adult domestic ferrets, the endangered black-footed ferret, and the European polecat (Table 2.3). The biochemical panel in ferrets is similar to that of other laboratory animals except that the concentrations of glucose and ammonia are higher, and the Blood urea nitrogen (BUN) is lower [38].

Liver Enzymes and Markers

Enzymes such as alanine aminotransferase (ALT), aspartate aminotransferase (AST), and sorbitol dehydrogenase (SDH) are released after hepatocellular injury or necrosis and can be measured to determine if damage is present. Other substances, such as alkaline phosphatase (ALP) and gamma glutamyl transferase (GGT), bilirubin, and bile acids, increase during cholestasis.

Table 2.1 Hematologic reference ranges in adult domestic ferrets (*Mustela putorius furo*), the black-footed ferret (*Mustela nigripes*), and the European polecat (*Mustela putorius putorius*).

		Fitch ferrets		Albino ferrets[e] [15]	Pet ferrets[f] [5]	Black-footed ferret [16]	European polecat [16]
Analyte (abbreviation)	**Units, SI [conventional]**	**Males[a,b,c,d] [3, 17–19] Neutered Φ[d] [19, 20]**	**Female [3, 18, 19,21]**	**Male ♂ Female ♀**	**Males & Female**	**Males & Female [16]**	**Male & Female [16]**
Animals sampled		**17–16 animals 3–22♂ 10♀ 19–3 ♂, 5♀, 5 ♂ Φ**	**6–14 animals**	**♂28 ♀ 11**	**60 animals**	**54–260 animals**	**n > 100 *[unless noted]***
White blood cell count (WBC)	$\times10^9$/l = [$\times10^3$/μl]	11.320 (7.700–15.400)[d] [19] 6.2 (1.7–11.9)[a] [17] 8.4 (4.9–13.8)[b] [3] 5.7 (2.0–9.8)[c] [18] 7.287 (5.600–10.800) Φ	5.875 (2.500–8.600)[d] [19] 7.2 (5.1–12.6)[b] [3] 5.6 (2.1–9.6)[c] [18] 5.84 ± 3.23[g] [21]	9.7 (4.4–19.1) ♂ 10.5 (4.0–18.2) ♀	4.3–10.7	3.976 (1–13.6)	6.141 (2.1–15.8)
Neutrophils absolute	$\times10^9$/l = [$\times10^3$/μl]	4.493 (2.744–8.778)[d] [19] 3.8 (1.4–7.0)[b] [3] 1.69 (0.62–3.33)[c] [18] 2.659 (0.616–7.020) Φ	1.825 (0.725–2.409)[d] [19] 4.2 (2.5–6.2)[b] [3] 1.45 (0.63–2.54)[c] [18]			2.312 (0.069–10.10)	2.810 (0.504–11.40)
Neutrophils	Proportion of 1.0 [%]	0.24–0.72[a] [17] [24–72][a] [17] 0.415 (0.240–0.766)[b] [3] [41.5 (24.0–76.6)][b] [3] 0.282 (0.127–0.478)[c] [18] [28.2 (12.7–47.8)] [18][c] 40.1 (24–78)[b] [3]	0.577 (0.488–0.710)[b] [3] [57.7 (48.8–71.0)][b] [3] 0.291 (0.065–0.435)[c] [18] [29.1 (6.5–43.5)][c] [18] 31.1 (12–41)[b] [3]	0.570 (0.11–0.82) ♂ [57.0 (11–82)] ♂ 0.595 (0.43–0.84) ♀ [59.5 (43–84)] ♀	0.18–0.47 [18–47]		
Bands absolute	$\times10^9$/l = [$\times10^3$/μl]	0.106 (0–0.256)[d] [19] 0.233 (0–0.972) Φ	0.099 (0–0.248)[d] [19]			0.076 (0.002–1.040)	0.227 (0.026–1.970) *[26]*
Bands	Proportion of 1.0 [%]	0–0.01[a] [17] [0–1][a] [17] 0.9 (0–2.2)[b] [3]	1.7 (0–4.2)[b] [3]				
Lymphocytes absolute	$\times10^9$/l = [$\times10^3$/μl]	5.626 (3.157–7.808) [19] [3.8 (2.0–6.7)] [3] 3.2 (0.83–0.611)[c] [18] 3.791 (1.728–4.704) Φ	3.426 (1.475–5.590)[d] [19] 2.5 (1.7–5.5)[b] [3] 3.4 (1.3–8.3)[c] [18]			1.457 (0.027–5.760)	2.855 (0.256–11.00)
Lymphocytes	Proportion of 1.0 [%]	0.26–0.73[a] [17] [(26–73)][a] [17] 0.474 (0.147–0.666)[b] [3] [47.4 (14.7–66.6)][b] [3] 49.7 (28–69)[b] [3] 0.538 (0.401–0.820) Φ[c] [18] [53.8 (40.1–82.0)] Φ[c] [18]	0.333 (0.227–0.433)[b] [3] [33.3 (22.7–43.3)][b] [3] 0.5776 (0.396–0.864)[c] [18] 57.76 (39.6–86.4)][c] [18] 58.0 (25–95)[b] [3]	0.356 (0.12–0.54) ♂ [35.6 (12–54)] ♂ 0.334 (0.12–0.50) ♀ [33.4 (12–50)]	0.41–0.73 [41–73]		
Monocytes absolute	$\times10^9$/l = [$\times10^3$/μl]	0.747 (0.385–0.924)[d] [19] 0.2 (0.1–0.8)[b] [3] 0.46 (0.18–0.9)[c] [18] 0.176 (0–0.432) Φ[d] [19]	0.263 (0.100–0.372)[d] [19] 0.1 (0.1–0.2)[b] [3] 0.4 (0.21–0.66)[c] [18]			0.131 (0.001–0.881)	0.216 (0.022–1.170)

Monocytes	Proportion of 1.0 [%]	0.01–0.04[a] [17] [(1–4)][a] [17] 0.017 (0.07–0.05)[b] [3] [1.7 (0.7–5)][b] [3] 0.069 (0.065–0.094)[c] [18] [6.9 (6.5–9.4)][c] [18] 6.6 (3.4–8.2)[b] [3]	0.018 (0.01–0.03)[b] [3] [1.8 (1.0–3.0)][b] [3] 0.0764 (0.041–0.107)[c] [18] [7.64 (4.1–10.7)][c] [18] 4.5 (1.7–6.3)[b] [3]	0.044 (0–0.09) ♂ [4.4 (0–9)] ♂ 0.044 (0.02–0.08) ♀ [4.4 (2–8)]	0–0.04 [0–4]		
Eosinophils absolute	$\times10^9$/l = [$\times10^3$/µl]	0.267 (0–0.768)[d] [19] 0.5 (0.2–0.9)[b] [3] 0.378 (0.112–0.768) Φ[d] [19] 0.32 (0.13–0.564) Φ[c] [18]	0.214 (0.050–0.516)[d] [19] 0.3 (0.2–0.5)[b] [3] 0.24 (0.154–0.49)[c] [18]			0.083 (0.001–0.512)	0.266 (0.022–1.768)
Eosinophils	Proportion of 1.0 [%]	0–0.03 [(0–3)][a] [17] 0.056 (0.019–0.085)[b] [3] [5.6 (1.9–8.5)][b] [3] 0.0502 (0.019–0.08)[c] [18] [5.02 (1.9–8)][c] [18] 2.3 (0–7)[b] [3]	0.043 (0.023–0.085)[b] [3] [4.3 (2.3–8.5)][b] [3] 0.046 (0.022–0.62)[c] [18] [4.6 (2.2–6.2)][c] [18] 3.6 (1–9)[b] [3]	0.024 (0–0.07) ♂ [2.4 (0–7)] ♂ 0.026 (0–0.05) ♀ [2.6 (0–5)]	0–0.04 [0–4]		
Basophils absolute	$\times10^9$/l = [$\times10^3$/µl]	0.048 (0–0.172)[d] [19] 0 (0)[b] [3] 0.054 (0.011–0.085)[c] [18] 0.050 (0–0.112) Φ[d] [19]	0.048 (0–0.172)[d] [19] 0 (0)[b] [3] 0.048 (0.10–0.082)[c] [18]			0.059 (0.000–0.246)	0.091 (0.006–0.381) [30]
Basophils	Proportion of 1.0 [%]	0.001 (0–0.003)[b] [3] [0.1 (0–0.3)][b] [3] 0.0101 (0.0035–0.0303)[c] [18] [1.01 (0.35–3.03)][c] [18] 0.7 (0–2.7)[b] [3]	0 (0–0.001)[b] [3] [0 (0–0.1)][b] [3] 0.0089 (0.003–0.0152)[c] [18] [0.89 (0.3–1.52)][c] [18] 0.8 (0–2.9)[b] [3]	0.001 (0–0.02) ♂ [0.1 (0–2)] ♂ 0.002 (0–0.01) ♀ [0.2 (0–1)] ♀	0–0.02 [0–2]		
Hematocrit	Proportion of 1.0 [%]	0.434 (0.36–0.50)[d] [19] [43.4 (36–50)][d] [19] 0.531 (0.48–0.59)[a] [17] [53.1 (48–59)][a] [17] 0.423 (0.336–0.472)[b] [3] [42.3 (33.6–47.2)][b] [3] 0.473 (0.367–0.549)[c] [18] 47.3 (36.7–54.9)][c] [18] 0.491 (0.46–0.57) Φ[d] [19] [49.1 (46–57)] Φ[d] [19]	0.484 (0.47–0.51)[d] [19] [48.4 (47–51)][d] [19] 0.391 (0.356–0.447)[b] [3] [39.1 (35.6–44.7)][b] [3] 0.47 (0.405–0.53)[c] [18] 47 (40.5–53)][c] [18] 0.456 ± 0.0297[g] [21] 45.6 ± 2.97[g] [21]	0.554 (0.44–0.61) ♂ [55.4 (44–61)] ♂ 0.492 (0.42–0.55) ♀ [49.2 (42–55)]	0.36–0.48 [36–48]	0.544 (0.357–0.802) [54.4 (35.7–80.2)]	0.42 (0.24–0.71) [41.6 (24.2–71.0)]
Hemoglobin	g/l [g/dl]	143 (120–163)[d] [19] [14.3 (12.0–16.3)][d] [19] 169 (154–185)[a] [17] [16.9 ((15.4–18.5)][a] [17] 155 (120–169)[b] [3] [15.5 (12.0–16.9)][b] [3] 149.5 (111–171)[c] [18] [14.95 (11.1–17.1)][c] [18] 161 (152–177) Φ[d] [19] [16.1 (15.2–17.7)] Φ[d] [19]	159 (152–174)[d] [19] [15.9 (15.2–17.4)][d] [19] 145 (129–159)[b] [3] [14.5 (12.9–15.9)][b] [3] 148.3 (131–166)[c] [18] [14.83 (13.1–16.6)][c] [18] 158.7 ± 16.2[g] [21] 15.87 ± 1.62[g] [21]	178 (153–182) ♂ 17.8 (16.3–18.2) ♂ 162 (148–174) ♀ 16.2 (14.8–17.4) ♀	122–165 [12.2–16.5]	174 (107–257) [17.4 (10.7–25.7)]	141 (60–53) [14.1 (6.0–52.9)]

(*Continued*)

Table 2.1 (Continued)

Analyte (abbreviation)	Units, SI [conventional]	Fitch ferrets: Males[a,b,c,d] [3, 17–19] Neutered Φ[d] [19, 20]	Fitch ferrets: Female	Albino ferrets[e] [15]: Male ♂ Female ♀	Pet ferrets[f] [5]: Males & Female	Black-footed ferret [16]: Males & Female [16]	European polecat [16]: Male & Female [16]
Animals sampled		**17–16 animals** **3–22♂ 10♀** **19–3 ♂, 5♀, 5 ♂ Φ**	**15 = 6–14 animals**	**♂28 ♀ 11**	**60 animals**	**54–260 animals**	**n > 100** ***[unless noted]***
Red blood cell (RBC) count	$\times 10^{12}$/l = [$\times 10^{6}$/μl]	11.3 (10.1–13.2)[b] [17] 9.1 (7.1–10.2)[b] [3] 9.53 (6.35–11.2)[c] [18]	8.2 (7.5–9.3)[b] [3] 9.4 (7.42–10.9)[c] [18] 12.64 ± 4.12[g] [21]	10.23 (7.30–12.18) ♂ 8.11 (6.77–9.76) ♂	7.01–9.65	9.82 (6.44–14.6)	8.12 (4.23–15.00)
Reticulocytes	Proportion of 1.0 [%]		0.1183 ± 0.0267[g] [21] [11.83 ± 2.67][g] [21]	0.04 (0.01–0.12) ♂ [4.0 (1–12)] ♂ 0.053 (0.02–0.14) ♀ [5.3 (2–14)] ♀			0.6 (0.0–2.5) [6]
Platelets	$\times 10^{9}$/l = [$\times 10^{3}$/μl]	476 (369–648)[b] [3] 553 (277–732)[g] [21]	631 (543–771)[b] [3] 627 (278–882)[c] [18] 468.3 ± 242.1[g] [21]	453 (297–730) ♂ 545 (310–910) ♀	200–459	699 (156–1500)	308 (104–500)
Mean corpuscular volume (MCV)	μm^3 = fl	47.1 (42.6–51)[a] [17] 46.6 (44.1–52.5)[b] [3] 50.0 (45.6–54.7)[c] [18]	48.4 (44.4–53.7)[b] [3] 50.28 (48.8–54.5)[g] [21] 48.33 ± 12.07[g] [21]	54 ♂ 61 ♀	50–54	55.0 (39.0–88.4)	51.5 (38.0–72.9)
Mean corpuscular hemoglobin (MCH)	pg/cell	15.0 (13.7–16)[a] [17] [17.1 (16.5–19.7)][b] [3] [15.8 (14.0–17.5)][c] [18]	17.6 (16.4–19.4)[b] [3] 15.91 (15.3–17.6)[c] [18]	17.6 ♂ 19.9 ♀	15–18	17.1 (12.3–25.2)	17.0 (12.5–25.6)
Mean corpuscular hemoglobin concentration (MCHC)	g/dl	32.0 (30.3–34.9)[a] [17] 3.7 (3.5–4.1)[b] [3] 31.7 (30.7–32.6)[c] [18]	37.0 (35.1–42.2)[b] [3] 31.2 (30.8–32.9)[c] [18]	32.2 ♂ 32.8 ♀	32–35	32.3 (18.3–43.5)	33.8 (28.0–115.0)

Source: Data presented as mean (range) unless otherwise stated.
[a] Fasted, adult, 1 kg, male ferrets suspected healthy and intact. Blood collected via cardiac puncture and unknown anesthetic [17].
[b] Marshall Farm ferrets anesthetized with acepromazine and ketamine; blood collected via cardiac puncture and placed into citrate. Females not in estrus [3].
[c] Samples collected from jugular vein via isoflurane anesthesia from unknown neuter status, age, and number of ferrets. Samples treated with EDTA and analyzed via CellDyn 3500 [18].
[d] Four- to eight-month-old ferrets with unknown fasting status, anesthetized with ketamine. Samples treated with EDTA and analyzed via Coulter electronic counter, "Channelyzer" [19].
[e] Age, fasting status, and neuter status unknown, presumed adult and intact. Anesthetized with ether and exsanguinated. Samples analyzed via Coulter electronic counter, Model D [15].
[f] Age, gender distribution, neuter status, health, and anesthesia status of animals unknown [5].
[g] Adult, intact apparently healthy ferrets anesthetized with ketamine and exsanguinated [21].

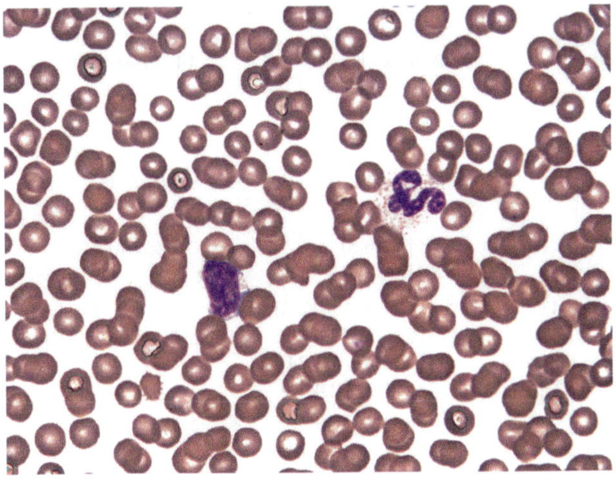

Figure 2.10 Ferret lymphocyte (lower left) and neutrophil (upper right), magnification 1000×.

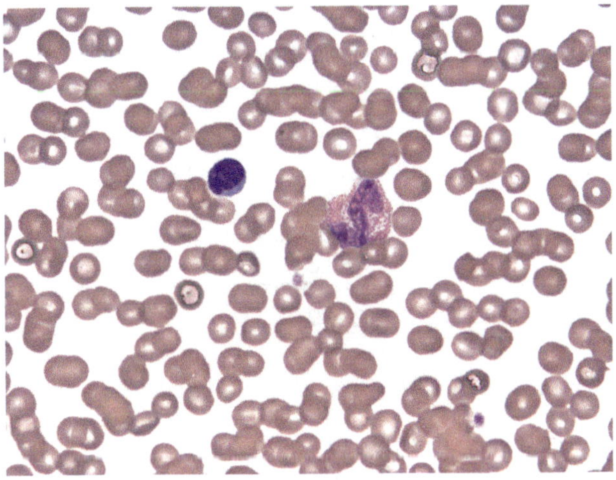

Figure 2.11 Ferret small lymphocyte (upper left) and eosinophil (lower right), magnification 1000×.

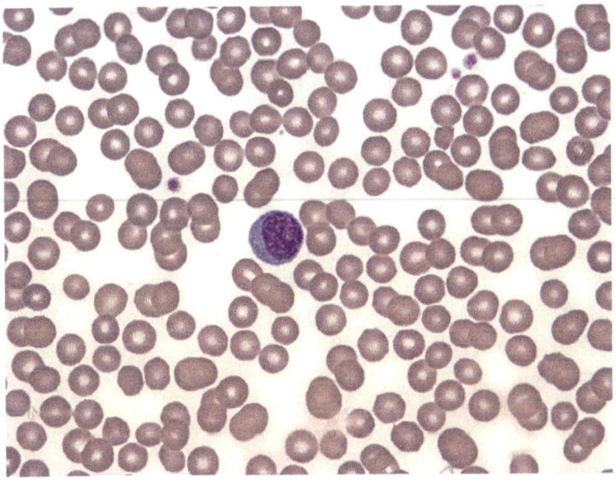

Figure 2.12 Ferret reactive lymphocyte, magnification 1000×.

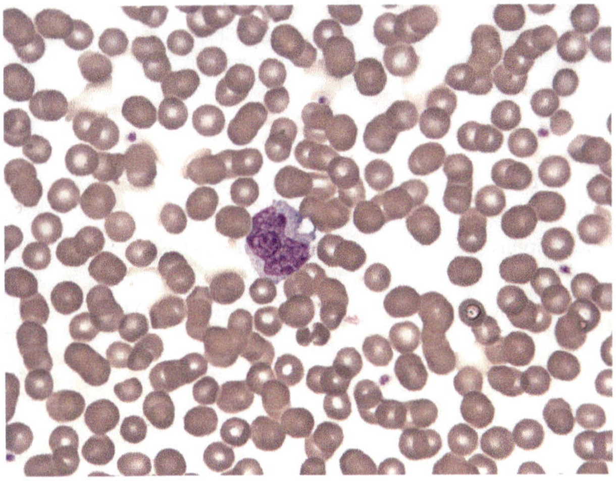

Figure 2.13 Ferret monocyte, magnification 1000×.

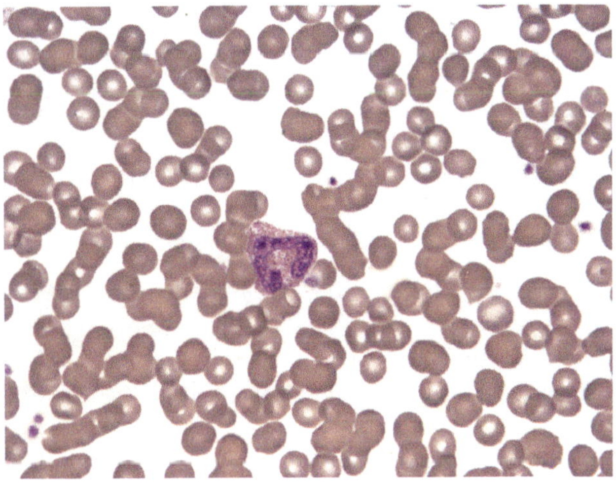

Figure 2.14 Ferret eosinophil, magnification 1000×.

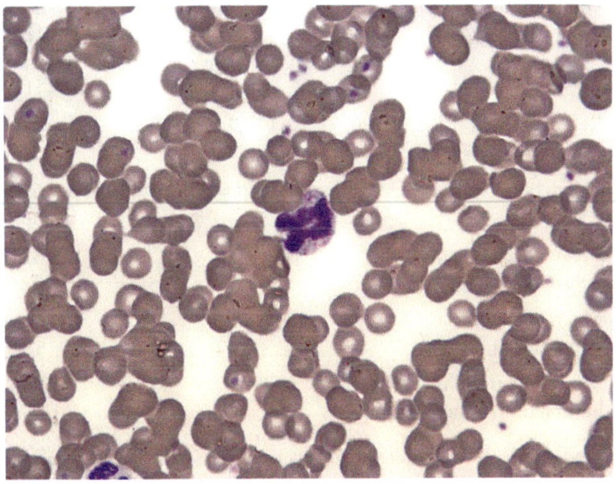

Figure 2.15 Ferret basophil, magnification 1000×.

Table 2.2 Hematologic reference ranges of young domestic Marshall Farms ferrets (*Mustela putorius furo*), unknown color [3].

Analyte (abbreviation)	Units, SI [conventional]	10 week old	12 week old	14–16 week old ♂
Animal number		♂15 ♀6	♂15 ♀8	9
White blood cell count (WBC)	$\times10^9$/l = [$\times10^3$/μl]	8.0 (5.3–12.0) ♂ 9.2 (6.7–12.6) ♀	8.4 (5.3–11.7) ♂ 6.7 (5.8–9.8) ♀	9.5 (5.2–15.0)
Neutrophils absolute	$\times10^9$/l = [$\times10^3$/μl]	2.7 (1.5–4.8) ♂ 2.6 (2.2–3.3) ♀	3.5 (1.8–6.5) ♂ 1.9 (1.5–3.0) ♀	3.5 (2.1–6.2)
Neutrophils	Proportion of 1.0 [%]	0.327 (0.243–0.451) ♂ [32.7 (24.3–45.1)] ♂ 0.286 (0.206–0.333) ♀ [28.6 (20.6–33.3)] ♀	0.433 (0.243–0.683) ♂ [43.3(24.3–68.3)] ♂ 0.279(0.217–0.324) ♀ [27.9(21.7–32.4)] ♀	0.375(0.279–0.582) [37.5(27.9–58.2)]
Lymphocytes absolute	$\times10^9$/l = [$\times10^3$/μl]	4.4 (2.8–6.3) ♂ 5.6 (3.5–8.6) ♀	3.9 (1.8–6.5) ♂ 4.1 (3.3–5.9) ♀	4.9 (1.6–7.9)
Lymphocytes	Proportion of 1.0 [%]	0.548 (0.422–0.643) ♂ [54.8 (42.2–64.3)] ♂ 0.6(0.524–0.682) ♀ [60.0 (52.4–68.2)] ♀	0.461 (0.221–0.628) ♂ [46.1 (22.1–62.8)] ♂ 0.618 (0.578–0.67) ♀ [61.8 (57.8–67.0)] ♀	0.509 (0.301–0.606) [50.9 (30.1–60.6)]
Monocytes absolute	$\times10^9$/l = [$\times10^3$/μl]	0.2 (0.1–0.5) ♂ 0.2 (0.1–0.3) ♀	0.2 (0.1–0.3) ♂ 0.1 (0.1–0.2) ♀	0.2 (0.1–0.2)
Monocytes	Proportion of 1.0 [%]	0.028 (0.017–0.043) ♂ [2.8 (1.7–4.3)] ♂ 0.025 (0.014–0.041) ♀ [2.5 (1.4–4.1)] ♀	0.021 (0.007–0.047) ♂ [2.1 (0.7–4.7)] ♂ 0.02 (0.015–0.024) ♀ [2.0(1.5–2.4)] ♀	0.017 (0.011–0.029) [1.7 (1.1.–2.9)]
Eosinophils absolute	$\times10^9$/l = [$\times10^3$/μl]	0.3 (0.1–0.6) ♂ 0.4 (0.2–0.7) ♀	0.4 (0.2–0.5) ♂ 0.2 (0.2–0.3) ♀	0.5 (0.3–0.9)
Eosinophils	Proportion of 1.0 [%]	0.044 (0.027–0.061) ♂ [4.4 (2.7–6.1)] ♂ 0.042 (0.021–0.069) ♀ [4.2 (2.1–6.9)] ♀	0.044 (0.033–0.058) ♂ [4.4 (3.3–5.8)] ♂ 0.037 (0.022–0.057) ♀ [3.7 (2.2–5.7)] ♀	0.054 (0.036–0.082) [5.4 (3.6–8.2)]
Basophils absolute	$\times10^9$/l = [$\times10^3$/μl]	0	0 (0.0–0.1)	0
Basophils	Proportion of 1.0 [%]	0.001 (0–0.002) ♂ [0.1(0–0.2)] ♂ 0.001 (0–0.001) ♀ [0.1(0–0.1)] ♀	0.001(0–0013) ♂ [0.1 (0–1.3)] ♂ 0.001(0–0.003) ♀ [0.1(0–0.3)] ♀	0.001 (0–0.002) [0.1(0–0.2)]
Hematocrit	Proportion of 1.0 [%]	0.329 (0.293–0.368) ♂ [32.9 (29.3–36.8)] ♂ 0.321 (0.27–0.348) ♀ [32.1 (27.0–34.8)] ♀	0.334 (0.309–0.381) ♂ [33.4 (30.9–38.1)] ♂ 0.341 (0.313–0.385) ♀ [34.1 (31.3–38.5)] ♀	0.391 (0.298–0.432) [39.1 (29.8–43.2)]
Hemoglobin	g/l [g/dl]	118 (104–136) ♂ [11.8 (10.4–13.6)] ♂ 115 (96–125) ♀ [11.5 (9.6–12.5) ♀]	120 (110–137) ♂ [12.0 (11.0–13.7)] ♂ 122 (112–138) ♀ [12.2 (11.2–13.8)] ♀	143 (127–159) [14.3 (12.7–15.9)]
Red blood cell (RBC) count	$\times10^{12}$/l = [$\times10^6$/μl]	6.4 (5.5–7.4) ♂ 6.1 (5.0–7.0) ♀	6.4 (4.8–7.8) ♂ 6.4 (5.7–7.8) ♀	8.2 (6.2–9.2)
Platelets	$\times10^9$/l = [$\times10^3$/μl]	696 (629–775) ♂ 665 (529–830) ♀	560 (382–745) ♂ 654 (533–769) ♀	506 (376–610)
Mean corpuscular volume (MCV)	μm^3 = fl	51.3 (47.8–54.8) ♂ 52.0 (49.6–54.5) ♀	51.4 (49.0–53.5) ♂ 52.5 (48.8–57.6) ♀	47.8 (44.9–53.6)
Mean corpuscular hemoglobin (MCH)	pg/cell	18.3 (17.5–19.1) ♂ 18.9 (17.8–19.6) ♀	18.9 (17.4–22.8) ♂ 19.1 (17.7–20.4) ♀	17.6 (16.4–20.6)
Mean corpuscular (MCHC) hemoglobin concentration	g/dl	35.7 (34.7–37.0) ♂ 35.7 (34.8–36.9) ♀	35.9 (34.7–36.7) ♂ 35.8 (35.3–37.0) ♀	36.9 (35.1–42.6)

Blood collected into citrate tubes via cardiac puncture via anesthesia with acepromazine and ketamine. Data presented as mean (range) unless otherwise stated.

Table 2.3 Biochemical reference ranges for adult domestic ferrets (*Mustela putorius furo*).

Analyte (abbreviation)	Units, SI [conventional]	Fitch ferrets Male [3, 17–19][a–d] Neutered Φ[d] [19]	Fitch ferrets Female	Albino ferrets[e] [15]	Pet ferrets[f] [5] Male & Female	Ferrets [6][g]	Black-footed ferret[h] [16]	European polecat[h] [16]
Animals sampled		16 Animals[a] [17] [b] [3] Unknown[i] [18] 3 Male, 5 MN[d] [19]	5 Animals[d] [19] 10 animals[b] [3] Unknown[i] [18] 6–14 Animals[c] [21]	Male♂ = 28 Female♀ = 11 *[except where noted]*	60	96–104	*n* = 57–236 *[except where noted]*	N = 57–127 *[except where noted]*
Alanine aminotransferase (ALT)	U/l = [IU/l]	157.6 (82–289)[d] [19] 109 (78–149)[a] [17] 121 (54–272)[b] [3] 138.1 (48–292)[i] [18] 201.3 (82–287)	150.3 (110–240)[d][19] 96 (54–280)[b] [3] 165.8 (72–338)[i] [18]		65–128	65–346	148 (0–597)	105 (19–384)
Albumin	g/l [g/dl]	37 (35–38) [3.7 (3.5–3.8)][d] [19] 39 (35–42) [3.9 (3.5–4.2)][a] [17] 37 (32–40) [3.7 (3.2–4.0)][b] [3] 39 (34–48)[i] [18] [3.94 (3.4–4.8)][i] [18] 37 (34–40) [3.7 (3.4–4.0)]	38 (33–41) [3.8 (3.3–4.1)][d] [19] 32 (29–35) [3.2 (2.9–3.5)][b] [3] 39 (34–48) [3.93 (3.4–4.8)][i] [18]	33 (28–38)♂ [3.3 (2.8–3.8)]♂ 32 (26–36)♀ [3.2 (2.6–3.6)] ♀	25–40 [2.5–4.0]	19–38 [1.9–3.8]	36 (20–53) [3.6 (2.0–5.3)]	32 (19–48) [3.2 (1.9–4.8)]
Albumin (EPH)	g/l [g/dl]				25–33 [2.50–3.31]			41 (40–41) [4.1 (4.0–4.1)] *[2]*
Albumin:globulin ratio	g/l [g/dl]	18 (13–21) [1.8 (1.3–2.1)][a] [17] 12 (8–14)[b] [3] [1.2 (0.8–1.4)][b] [3]	12 (10–16)[b] *[3]* [1.2 (1.0–1.6)][b] [3]		10.5-13.3 [1.05–1.33]			
Alkaline phosphatase (ALP)	U/l = [IU/l]	52.4 (43–67)[d] [19] 42 (31–64)[a] [17] 23 (18–32)[b] [3] 40.6 (14–144)[i] [18] 63.3 (30–120)	44.3 (30–62)[d] *[19]* 21 (3–40)[b] [3] 35 (20–106)[i] [18]	26 (11–84) ♂ 19 (9–30) ♀	25–60	8–72	132 (0–632)	48 (3–374)
Amylase	U/l	42.5 ± 6.18 [21]			26–36	4–50	23 (0–60)	29 (0–129)
AST U/l	U/l = [IU/l]	117 (74–248)[a] [17] 74 (37–121)[b] [3] 68.3 (46–118)[i] [18]	68 (42–108)[b] *[3]* 63.3 (20–130)[i] [18]	57 (28–113) ♂ 73 (40–120) ♀	70–100		177 (0–925)	64 (18–174)
Bicarbonate	mmol/l = [mEq/l]						25.6 (15.0–35.0) *[15]*	22.9 (15.0–29.0) *[17]*

(*Continued*)

Table 2.3 (Continued)

Analyte (abbreviation)	Units, SI [conventional]	Fitch ferrets Male [3, 17–19][a–d] Neutered Φ[d] [19]	Fitch ferrets Female	Albino ferrets[e] [15]	Pet ferrets[f] [5] Male & Female	Ferrets [6][g]	Black-footed ferret[h] [16]	European polecat[h] [16]
Bile acids	μmol/l	9.1 (1–28)[i] [18]	4.4 (2–14)[i] [18]			1–8		
Bilirubin, direct	μmol/l [mg/dl]	0 (0–1.7)[b] *[3]* [0 (0.0–0.1)][b] [3]	0 (0–1.7)[b] [3] [0 (0.0–0.1)][b] [3]				1.7 (0–8.6) [0.1 (0.0–0.5)]	0 (0–3.4) [0.0 (0.0–0.2)] *[21]*
Bilirubin, indirect	μmol/l [mg/dl]	5.1 (3.4–5.1)[b] [3] 0.3 (0.2–0.3) [25]	5.1 (3.4–5.1)[b] [3] 0.3 (0.2–0.3)[b] [3]				1.7 (0–8.6) [0.1 (0.0–0.5)]	3.4 (0–8.6) [0.2 (0.0–0.5)] *[20]*
Bilirubin, total	μmol/l [mg/dl]	<17.1[a] [17] [<1.0][a] [17]	4.1 ± 0.53[c] [21] [0.24 ± 0.031][c] [21]	<17.1 [<1.0] ♂ <17.1 [<1.0] ♀	3.4–8.6 [0.2–0.5]	5.1–10.3 [0.3–0.6]	6.8 (0–36) [0.4 (0.0–2.1)]	3.4 (0–17.1) [0.2 (0.0–1.0)]
Blood urea nitrogen (BUN)	μmol/l [mg/dl]	7.9 (4.3–10.0)[d] [19] [22.0 (12–28)][d] [19] 5.4 (3.0.9–8.9)[a] [17] [15 (11–25)][a] [17] 12.5 (10.7–14.3)[b] [3] [35 (30–40)][b] [3] 10.4 (0.2–16.3)[i] [18] [29.2 (0.60–45.6)][i] [18]	11.9 (5.4–15.4)[d] [19] [33.3 (15–43)][d] [19] 9.3 (5.7–15.4)[b] [3] [26 (16–43)][b] [3] 11.2 (5.3–16.1)[i] [18] [31.4 (14.82–45.00)][i] [18] 8.24 ± 0.72[c] [21] [23.075 ± 2.024][c] [21] 10.0 (7.5–15.0) [28.1 (21–42)]	8.2 (3.9–13.9) ♂ [23 (11–39)] ♂ 7.1 (3.6–16.1) ♀ [20 (10–45)] ♀	6.4–11.4 [15, 18–20, 23–33]	3.6–13.6 [10–38]	8.6 (0–21.1) [24 (0–59)]	8.2 (2.9–18.6) [23 (8–52)]
BUN:creatinine		25.2 (22.0–30.0)[b] [3]	44.5 (18.2–86.0)[b] [3]					
Calcium	mmol/l [mg/dl]	2.4 (2.3–2.6)[d] [19] [9.5 (9.0–10.5)][d] [19] 2.1 (2.2–2.4)[a] [17] [8.5 (8.7–9.4)][a] [17] 2.5 (2.3–2.5)[b] [3] [9.8 (9.3–10.1)][b] [3] 2.1 (1.9–2.4) [18] [8.31 (7.6–9.6)][i] [18]	2.3 (2.2–2.4)[d] [19] [9.0 (8.8–9.4)][d] [19] 2.3 (2.2–2.6)[b] [3] [9.2 (8.7–10.2)][b] [3] 1.9 (1.8–2.1)[i] [18] [7.65 (7.2–8.2)][i] [18] 2.86 ± 0.379[c] [21] [11.456 ± 1.516][c] [21] 2.3 (2.2–2.6) [9.3 (8.6–10.2)]	2.4 (2.1–3.0) ♂ [9.4 (8.3–11.8)] ♂ 2.2 (2.0–2.6) ♀ [8.9 (8.0–10.2)] ♀	2.0–2.4 [8.1–9.5]	2.0–2.6 [8.0–10.4]	2.3 (0–3.1) [9.2 (0.0–12.4]	2.2 (1.8–2.9) [8.9 (7.1–11.6]
Calcium, ionized	mmol/l [mg/dl]	0.616 ± 0.05[c] [21] [2.462 ± 0.20][c] [21]						

Chloride	mmol/l = [mEq/l]	112.5 (102–118)[d] [19] 121 (118–126)[a] [17] 117 (115–121)[b] [3]	117.1 (115–120)[d] [19] 119 (114–123)[b] [3] 119.83 ± 7.69[c] [21] 117.3 (114–121)	114 (106–125) ♂ *[12]* 117 (112–124) ♀ *[12]*			116 (0–133)	118 (99–135)
Cholesterol	mmol/l [mg/dl]	3.8 (3.1–5.3)[a] [17] [148 (119–201)][a] [17] 4.8 (4.3–5.7)[b] [3] [187 (165–221)][b] [3]	5.6 (4.2–7.1)[b] [3] [216 (163–272)][b] [3] 3.04 ± 0.31[c] [21] 117.25 ± 12.11[c] [21]	4.0 (1.7–5.5)♂ [156 (64–212)] ♂ 4.5 (3.2–7.7) ♀ [174 (122–296)] ♀	3.1–4.2 [119–163]	2.6–6.3 [102–245]	4.6 (0–8.9) [176 (0–340)]	4.4 (2.3–9.1) [168 (87–353)]
CO_2	mmol/l = [mEq/l]	23.4 (18–27)[d] [19] 24.9 (20–28)[a] [17] 22 (18–25)[b] [3] 18.5 (12.2–22.2)	22.1 (16.5–27.8)[d] [19] 22 (19–27)[b] [3]	[15, 17–20, 23, 24, 26, 27, 34] ♂	22–29		24.5 (0.0–36.2)	23.1 (12.0–54.4) *[27]*
Creatine (CK) Kinase	U/l = [IU/l]	245 (93–564)[c] [21] 219.6 ± 35.27[c] [21]	228 (58–494)[i] [18]		55–93		390 (0–1740)	3432 (38–2500)
Creatinine	μmol/l [mg/dl]	35.4 (17.7–53.0)[d] [19] [0.4 (0.2–0.6)][d] [19] 44.2 (35.4–61.9)[a] [17] [0.5 (0.4–0.7)][a] [17] 123.8 (114.9–141.4)[b] [3] [1.4 (1.3–1.6)][b] [3] 50.4 (8.8–106.1)[i] [18] [0.57 (0.1–1.2)][i] [18] 26.5 (22.1–30.9) [0.3 (0.25–0.35)]	35.4 (26.5–39.8)[d] [19] [0.4 (0.30–0.45)][d] [19] 61.9 (0–88.4)[b] [3] [0.7 (0–1)][b] [3] 42.4 (27.4–40.7)[i] [18] [0.48 (0.31–0.46)][i] [18] 73.0 ± 7.34[c] [21] [0.825 ± 0.083][c] [21]	53.0 (35.4–80.0) ♂ [0.6 (0.4–0.9)] ♂ 53.0 (35.4–61.9) ♀ [0.6 (0.4–0.7)] ♀	7.7–44.2 [0.2–0.5]	7.7–61.9 [0.2–0.7]	53 (0–195) [0.6 (0.0–2.2)]	44.2 (17.7–123.8) [0.5 (0.2–1.4)]
Gamma (GGT) glutamyl transferase	U/l = [IU/l]	1 (1–3)[b] [3]	3 (1–8[b]) [3]		8–34	5–15	7 (0–62)	11 (0–40) *[48]*
Globulin	g/l [g/dl]	22 (20–29)[a] [17] [2.2 (2–2.9)][a] [17] 31 (27–40)[b] [3] [3.1 (2.7–4.0)][b] [3] 16 (2–24)[i] [18] [1.6 (0.2–2.4)][i] [18]	26 (22–32)[b] [3] [2.6 (2.2–3.2)][b] [3] 12 (2.6–17.1)[i] [18] [1.2 (0.26–1.71)][i] [18]			23–45 [2.3–4.5]	27 (13–46) [2.7 (1.3–4.6)]	25 (12–46) [2.5 (1.2–4.6)]
Globulin, alpha-1 (EPH)	g/l [g/dl]				33–56 [0.33–0.56]			
Globulin, alpha-2 (EPH)	g/l [g/dl]				36–60 [0.36–0.60]			

(*Continued*)

Table 2.3 (Continued)

Analyte (abbreviation)	Units, SI [conventional]	Fitch ferrets Male [3, 17–19][a–d] Neutered Φ[d] [19]	Fitch ferrets Female	Albino ferrets[e] [15]	Pet ferrets[f] [5] Male & Female	Ferrets [6][g]	Black-footed ferret[h] [16]	European polecat[h] [16]
Globulin, beta, (EPH)	g/l [g/dl]				83–120 [0.83–1.20]			
Globulin, gamma, (EPH)	g/l [g/dl]				31–81 [0.31–0.81]			
Glucose	mmol/l [mg/dl]	5.8 (5.0)[d] [19] [104.0(90–122)][d] [19] 6.4 (5.9–7.7)[a] [17] [115 (107–138)][a] [17] 8.0 (6.8–11.0)[b] [3] [145 (122–198)][b] [3] 6.7 (5.5–8.0)[i] [18] [120.5 (100–144)][i] [18] 5.3 (3.5–6.4) [95.4 (62.5–116)]	5.8 (4.7–7.4)[d] [19] [104.0 (85–134)][d] [19] 8.3 (6.9–10.5)[b] [3] [149 (125–189)][b] [3] 6.3 (6.0–6.7)[i] [18] [114 (108–120)][i] [18] 9.12 ± 1.98[c] [21] 164.25 ± 35.58[c] [21]	7.0 (5.2–9.4)♂ [126 (94–169)] ♂ 8.0 (5.5–11.5) ♀ [145 (100–207)] ♀	4.4–6.5 [80–117]	3.6–8.0 [65–145]	6.9 (0–12.0) [124 (0–215)]	6.1 (0.9–11.0) [111(16–198)]
Iron	µmol/l [mg/dl]						38.8 (9.0–58.9) [217 (50–329)] *[29]*	33.5 (27.4–42.1) [187(153–235)] *[1]*
Lactate dehydrogenase (LDH)	U/l = [IU/l]	460 (241–752)[a] [17] 252 (168–389)[b] [3] 278 (222–344)[i] [18]	369 (161–767)[b] [3] 367 (182–544)[i] [18] 676.625 ± 61.66[c] [21]		200–1400		2986 (0–9942)	297 (71–1286) *[44]*
Lipase	U/l	266.24 ± 77.57[c] [21]					208 (105–843) *[36]*	626 (44–2279) *[23]*
Magnesium	mmol/l [mg/dl]	1.32 ± 0.17[c] [21] [3.2 ± 0.42][c] [21]						0.88 (0.35–1.15) [2.13 (0.86–2.80)] [36]
Osmolarity	mOsm/l						301 (296–306) [31]	311 (294–343) *[11]*
Phosphorus, inorganic	mmol/l [mg/dl]	2.2 (1.8–2.8)[d] [19] [6.7 (5.7–8.7)][d] [19] 1.8 (1.7–2.5)[a] [17] [5.6 (5.2–7.6)][a] [17] 2.4 (2.1–2.8)[b] [3] [7.5 (6.6–8.6)][b] [3] 2.4 (1.7–3.2)[i] [18] [7.32 (5.2–10)][i] [18] 1.95 ± 0.37[c] [21] [6.05 ± 1.13][c] [21] 2.0 (1.8–2.3) [6.1 (5.6–7.0)]	2.2 (2.0–2.4)[d] [19] [6.7 (6.3–7.5)][d] [19] 2.1 (1.5–3.3)[b] [3] [6.5 (4.5–10.1)][b] [3] 2.2 (1.1–2.7)[i] [18] [6.71 (3.4–8.4)][i] [18]	1.9 (1.3–2.6) ♂ [6.0 (4.0–7.9)] ♂ 1.8 (1.4–2.9) ♀ [5.7 (4.2–9.1)] ♀	1.7–2.1 [5.1–6.5]	1.2–2.4 [3.6–7.3]	1.8 (0–3.8) [5.6 (0.0–11.9)]	2.0 (1.1–3.6) [6.1 (3.4–11.0)]

Potassium	mmol/l [mEq/l]	4.9 (4.6–5.2)[d] [19] 4.4 (4.1–4.9)[a] [17] 5.1 (4.8–5.4)[b] [3] 5.331 ± 1.379[c] [21] 4.9 (4.7–5.2)	4.9 (4.3–5.3)[d] [19] 4.9 (4.2–6.4)[b] [3]	5.3 (4.5–7.3) ♂ 6.5 (4.8–7.7) ♀	4.5–6.1	4.1–5.5	4.7 (0.0–6.6)	4.6 (3.4–6.5)
Sodium	mmol/l [mEq/l]	154.4 (152–160)[b] [3] 154 (152–156)[d] [19] 153 (151–156) [25] 148.3 ± 4.00 [4] 150.6 (146–155)	150.4 (148–153)[b] [3] 152 (146–156) [25]	149 (137–162) ♂ 148 (142–154) ♀	142–148	146–156	150 (0–167)	152 (140–164)
Sorbitol (SDH) dehydrogenase	[μU/ml]	[5.4 (1.9–11.2)][d] [19] [3.3 (0.2–9.0)]	[2.6 (1.0–7.6)][d] [19]					
Total protein	g/l [g/dl]	59 (53–62)[d] [19] [5.9 (5.3–6.2)][d] [19] 66 (62–71)[a] [17] [6.6 (6.2–7.1)][a] [17] 68–(65–72)[b] [3] [6.8 (6.5–7.2)][b] [3] 52 (43–60)[i] [18] [5.24(4.3–6.0)][i] [18]	60 (56–72)[d] [19] [6.0 (5.6–7.2)][d] [19] 59 (54–63)[b] [3] [5.9 (5.4–6.3)][b] [3] 46–24–57)[i] [18] [4.63 (2.4–5.7)][i] [18] 52.75 ± 0.91[c] [21] [5.275 ± 0.091[c] [21] 58 (54–64) [5.8 (5.4–6.4)]	61 (53–74) ♂ [6.1 (5.3–7.4)] ♂ 58 (51–66) ♀ [5.8 (5.1–6.6)] ♀	45–62 [4.5–6.2]	50–76 [5.0–7.6]	63 (46–87) [6.3 (4.6–8.7)]	57 (44–82) [5.7 (4.4–8.2)]
Triglycerides	mmol/l [mg/dl]	0.20 (0.11–0.36)[a] [17] [18 (10–32)][a] [17]			0.34–1.6 [30–140]		0.50 (0.15–1.71) [44 (13–151)]	0.9 (0.23–4.35) [77 (20–385)] *[16]*
Uric acid	μmol/l [mg/dl]	130.9(89.2–172.5)[b] [3] [2.2 (1.5–2.9)][b] [3]	101.1 (47.6–184.4)[b] [3] [1.7 (0.8–3.1)][b] [3] 95.2 ± 34.5[c] [21] [1.6 ± 0.58][c] [21]		77.3–113.0 [1.3–1.9]		137 (0–274) [2.3 (0.0–4.6)]	65.4 (0–154–7) [1.1 (0.0–2.6)] *[37]*

Source: Data presented as mean (range).

[a] Blood collected from anesthetized, fasted, adult, 1 kg, suspected healthy and intact ferrets via cardiac puncture [17].

[b] Marshall Farm ferrets with blood collected via cardiac puncture under anesthesia with acepromazine and ketamine [3].

[c] Apparently healthy, not in season, adult, intact animals [21].

[d] Four to eight months old, unknown fasting status, anesthetized with ketamine. Most chemical values determined via automated sequential multiple analysis except SDH determined by kinetic analysis, chloride by electrometric titration, sodium and potassium by flame photometry, CO_2 by phenolphthalein dye reaction, BUN by diacetyl monoxime method, ALP with p-nitrophenylphosphate substrate, ALT by nicotinamide-adenine dinucleotide (reduced) disodium salt disappearance, TP by biuret reaction, albumin by BCG reaction, CA by complexing with cresophthalein dye, P by a phosphomolybdate method, glucose by a glucose oxidase enzymatic procedure, and creatinine by reaction with alkaline picrate [19].

[e] Unknown age, unknown fasting status, adult weight, suspect intact animals anesthetized with ether and exsanguinated. Sodium and potassium measured by flame photometry, total cholesterol manually estimated using Liebermann–Burchard reagent [15].

[f] From Cray, C Avian & Wildlife Laboratory, University of Miami, FL. Age, gender distribution, reproductive, health, and anesthetic status unknown [5].

[g] Samples collected from age, gender, coat color, health status, fasting status, venipuncture method not reported, presumed healthy ferrets. Sample analysis on Abaxis VetScan and Abaxis VetScan VS2 [6].

[h] Unknown health or anesthetic status, sexes, and ages combined. (Note: Some analyte ranges start at zero, which is incompatible with life) [16].

[i] Samples collected via jugular venipuncture under isoflurane anesthesia from age, gender, health, and neuter status unknown fitch ferrets. Samples placed in lithium heparin and analyzed via Hitachi [18].

Alanine Aminotransferase (ALT)

Alanine aminotransferase (ALT) is used to evaluate hepatic damage. The half-life of ALT in ferrets is unknown, but may be similar to dogs at approximately 60 h [4]. In cases of exocrine pancreatic tumors in ferrets, elevations in lactate dehydrogenase (LDH), ALT, and AST were observed [37]. Muscle necrosis can cause an increase in ALT.

Gamma Glutamyltransferase (GGT)

Elevations in GGT are the result of enzyme induction involving hepatocytes or biliary epithelial cells. GGT has been evaluated in the domestic ferret, the endangered black-footed ferret, and the European polecat [3, 16].

Alkaline Phosphatase (ALP)

ALPs are a group of isoenzymes known to hydrolyze monophosphates at an alkaline pH in many tissues, including bone, liver, and intestines. The placenta of pregnant animals, intestinal mucosa, kidneys, liver, and bone are tissues rich in this enzyme. Because ALP is found in higher levels in membranes bordering the bile canaliculus than the sinusoidal surface of hepatocytes, ALP levels are higher in biliary stasis than with hepatic necrosis. Increased ALP levels are the result of enzyme induction often due to cholestasis, drug, or hormonal effects. Alkaline phosphatase activities tend to be increased in younger ferrets compared to adult ferrets because of bone growth (Table 2.4). Chemistry panels conducted in 10- week-, 12-week-, and 14–16-week-old ferrets (n = 14, 15, and 10, respectively) showed a mean ALP of 184, 173, and 97 IU/l, respectively, compared to adult male (n = 9) and female (n = 11) ferrets at 23 and 21 IU/l, respectively [3]. Common causes of increased ALP activities in adult ferrets include GI foreign body, gastritis, and gastric ulceration [28].

Sorbitol Dehydrogenase (SDH)

This enzyme is considered to be liver specific in all species studied, but is more specific for hepatic disease than AST and ALT in horses, sheep, goats, and cattle. Values for ferrets have been reported [19].

Lactate Dehydrogenase (LDH)

LDH is a non-liver-specific enzyme that can increase from hepatocellular damage, muscle damage, or hemolysis. Enzyme activities for ferrets have been cited in multiple reports, and evaluation of all five isoenzymes has been delineated [21]. Exocrine pancreatic tumors have been reported in ferrets, and elevations in LDH, ALT, and AST were observed [37].

Bilirubin

Bilirubin is produced by the breakdown of the heme portion of hemoglobin by hepatocytes, metabolized to urobilinogen by bacteria in the intestine, and then reabsorbed and excreted in the urine. Increased bilirubin levels can occur with either hepatocellular damage or biliary tree dysfunction. Hyperbilirubinemia is uncommon in ferrets, but can be associated with hepatic tumors such as hepatic hemangioma, bile duct cystadenoma, biliary carcinoma, or hepatoma [28].

Bile Acids

Bile acids are created in the liver from cholesterol, resorbed in the portal circulation, and recycled via enterohepatic circulation. Elevations suggest liver dysfunction. One report measured bile acids in ferrets while anesthetized with isoflurane [28].

Ammonia

Ammonia is created by the breakdown of amino acids and urea in the GI tract and then transported to by the portal circulation to the liver. The resting serum ammonia level in the ferret is 200–400 μg/dl [38].

Muscle Enzymes

Elevations in *creatine kinase (CK)* activity are indicative of muscle damage that can occur secondary to recent or active trauma, muscle necrosis, or muscle degeneration. Although not known in ferrets, in dogs and cats serum CK activity returns to reference intervals within 48–72 h after cessation of injury, indicating recent injury. *Aspartate aminotransferase (AST)* is a non-liver-specific enzyme released during tissue damage. Common causes of increased AST activity in ferrets include gastritis, gastric ulceration, and enteritis. Epizootic catarrhal enteritis, caused by a coronavirus, affects both the liver and the intestines [28]. Exocrine pancreatic tumors of ferrets have been reported along with elevations in LDH, ALT, and AST [37]. Hemolysis can cause an increase in AST activity. Although not known specifically for ferrets, in most species serum AST increases slower than CK and LDH following muscle damage and stays increased for several days past cessation of damage.

Renal Analytes

The gold standard for evaluating kidney function, determination of glomerular filtration rate (GFR) via the clearance rate of inulin, is an impractical test. Therefore, indirect methods of evaluating kidney function are used clinically, including measuring plasma or serum urea nitrogen and creatinine levels.

Azotemia is defined as an increased *BUN* or creatinine due to decreased GFR, which can occur because of prerenal, renal, or postrenal causes. These analytes are assumed similar to dogs and cats in that prerenal azotemia occurs from decreased renal perfusion such as with shock, cardiac disease, or most commonly

Table 2.4 Biochemical reference ranges for young, male, Marshall Farms domestic ferret (*Mustela putorius furo*), unknown color [3].

Analyte (abbreviation)	Units, SI [conventional]	10 week old	12 week old	14–16 week old
Animals sampled		**14**	**15**	**10**
Alanine (ALT) aminotransferase	U/l = [IU/l]	248 (95–544)	210 (93–366)	131 (78–279)
Albumin	g/l [g/dl]	30 (26–32) [3.0 (2.6–3.2)]	29 (26–32) [2.9 (2.6–3.2)]	33 (30–36) [3.3 (3.0–3.6)]
Albumin/globulin ratio	g/l [g/dl]	15 (13–17) [1.5 (1.3–1.7)]	15 (12–19) [1.5 (1.2–1.9)]	15 (11–17) [1.5 (1.1–1.7)]
Alkaline (ALP) phosphatase	U/l = [IU/l]	184 (117–277)	173 (126–272)	97 (41–181)
AST U/l	U/l = [IU/l]	96 (63–152)	85 (70–112)	76 (47–128)
Bilirubin, direct	μmol/l [mg/dl]	0.1 (0.0–0.6) [1.7 (0–10.2)]	0 (0–0.1) [0-(0–1.7)]	0 [0]
Bilirubin, indirect	μmol/l [mg/dl]	0.5 (0–0.9) [8.5 (0–15.3)]	0.5 (0.1–1.9) [8.5 (1.7–32.3)]	0.3 (0.2–0.8) [5.1 (3.4–13.6)]
Blood urea nitrogen (BUN)	mmol/l [mg/dl]	9.6 (7.1–13.9) [27 (20–39)]	10.4 (6.8–15.4) [29 (19–43)]	10 (5–15) [28 (14–42)]
BUN:creatinine	–	25.6 (17.1–36.7)	26.6 (20.8–35.0)	24.5 (17.5–32.7)
Calcium	mmol/l [mg/dl]	2.8 (2.6–3.1) [10.8 (10.1–12.1)]	2.6 (2.4–2.7) [10.1 (9.6–10.7)]	2.6 (2.5–2.7) [10.2 (9.8–10.7)]
Chloride	mmol/l = [mEq/l]	118 (115–121)	117 (113–122)	119 (114–124)
Cholesterol	mmol/l [mg/dl]	7.1 (6.1–8.5) [278 (239–332)]	7 (5.8–8.8) [273 (227–343)]	5.4 (4.4–6.3) [212 (170–247)]
CO_2	mmol/l = [m/Eq l]	22 (13–27)	22 (17–26)	20 (16–24)
Creatinine	μmol/l [mg/dl]	97.2 (53–123.7) [1.1 (0.6–1.4)]	97.2 (61.8–141.3) [1.1 (0.7–1.6)]	106 (70.7–141.3) [1.2 (0.8–1.6)]
Gamma glutamyl transferase (GGT)	U/l = [IU/l]	7 (2–20)	4 (1–11)	1 (1–2)
Globulin	g/l [g/dl]	20 (17–24) [2.0 (1.7–2.4)]	20 (18–24) [2.0 (1.8–2.4)]	23 (19–30) [2.3 (1.9–3.0)]
Glucose	mmol/l [mg/dl]	7.8 (6.4–13.8) [140 (116–249)]	7.3 (5.8–8.3) [131 (105–149)]	7.9 (6.9–9.4) [143 (124–170)]
Lactate (LDH) dehydrogenase	U/l = [IU/l]	553 (362–920)	508 (400–711)	382 (247–577)
Phosphorus, inorganic	mmol/l [mg/dl]	3.5 (2.7–4.7) [11.0 (8.6–14.7)]	3.2 (2.6–3.7) [10.1 (8.2–11.8)]	2.8 (2–3.2) [8.7 (6.2–10.0)]
Potassium	mmol/l = [mEq/l]	5.3 (4.7–8.3)	5.1 (4.6–6.0)	5.1 (4.5–5.5)
Sodium	mmol/l = [mEq/l]	151 (146–154)	149 (145–152)	151 (148–155)
Total protein	g/l [g/dl]	50 (44–56) [5.0 (4.4–5.6)]	48 (44–52) [4.8 (4.4–5.2)]	56 (49–64) [5.6 (4.9–6.4)]
Uric acid	mmol/l [mg/dl]	160.7 (95.2–297.5) [2.7 (1.6–5.0)]	136.9 (101.2–190.4) [2.3 (1.7–3.2)]	125 (65.5–172.6) [2.1 (1.1–2.9)]

Source: All data presented as mean (range).

dehydration, but can also occur with a higher than recommended protein diet or GI hemorrhage [23]. *Creatinine* is created by the breakdown of phosphocreatine in muscle and excreted by glomerular filtration at a constant rate [23]. Although not proved in the ferret, it is assumed they are similar to dogs and cats in that an increase in creatinine is associated with a decreased GFR, and lie BUN can be due to prerenal, renal, or postrenal causes. Ferrets have a narrow normal range for creatinine compared to other species and a poor correlation of BUN with renal failure. Even with a BUN as high as 300 mg/dl, a not so impressive concomitant increase in creatinine (2–3 mg/dl with a normal range of 0.2–0.9 mg/dl) is common. Therefore, even a slight increase over normal range of creatinine in a ferret is considered a cause for concern.

Uric Acid

Although uric acid is not considered clinically useful for evaluation of urinary system in mammals, uric acid concentrations have been reported for the domestic ferret, the endangered black-footed ferret, and the European polecat [3, 16].

Pancreas

Amylase and Lipase

In most animals, amylase can be found in salivary glands, intestine, pancreas, and mostly in liver tissue. Although ferrets are likely similar, no studies have proved this theory. The half-lives of amylase and lipase in the ferret are unknown. Although these analytes are used clinically to help diagnose pancreatic disease, they are cleared from the plasma by glomerular filtration, and therefore renal disease may influence levels. Pancreatitis is uncommon, but does occur in the ferret. Amylase and lipase activities are reported in a few references for domestic ferrets and for the endangered black-footed ferret and European polecat [3, 16, 21].

Lipase values are reported in a few references for domestic ferrets and also for the endangered black-footed ferret and the European polecat [3, 16, 21].

Glucose

Common diseases causing blood glucose abnormalities in the ferret include diabetes, insulinoma, sepsis, and lymphoma. Generally, diabetes will cause hyperglycemia, while insulinoma, sepsis, and lymphoma will cause blood sugar to decrease. Clinicians should be aware of the specific calibration of the analyzer they use for glucose measurement, especially handheld analyzers. Many of these analyzers are adjusted to read 10 mg/dl lower than actual to provide a higher margin of safety for human diabetic patients. Additionally, plasma for glucose measurement, as stated above, should be separated from blood cells immediately to prevent lowering of glucose caused by cellular metabolism.

Both type 1 and type 2 diabetes mellitus (DM) have been reported in ferrets, but are uncommon. DM is associated with a profound hyperglycemia, usually greater than 400 mg/dl, but over 1000 mg/dl is possible. Glucose can be decreased by inappropriate handling of the sample. Allowing RBCs to remain in plasma will facilitate their glucose uptake from the sample before it is separated. At room temperature, plasma glucose levels decrease by approximately 7% an hour when exposed to RBCs [3]. Acute or chronic stress and administration of glucocorticoids can increase glucose levels. Epinephrine causes glycolysis of glycogen stores in the liver (glycogenolysis). Patient struggling during venipuncture may increase the blood glucose as high as 200–300 mg/dl in a ferret without DM [3].

Administration of sugar-containing products such as Nutrical (Vetoquinol, USA, Inc., Buena, New Jersey) or Laxatone (Vetoquinol USA Inc., Ft. Worth, Texas) orally to distract the ferret during phlebotomy can change the blood glucose values rather quickly. Use of these products is not recommended prior to evaluating blood glucose. Ideally, sampling for blood glucose should be done after a 4 h fast, to prevent causing hypoglycemia and to avoid misinterpreting a postprandial hyperglycemia.

Insulinoma

Insulinoma, also known as beta cell carcinoma, secretes high levels of insulin-decreasing glucose in the blood. Pancreatic beta cell tumors occur in about 30%–40% of ferrets over three years of age. Clinical signs include lethargy, posterior paresis, splenomegaly (due to extramedullary hematopoesis) syncope, seizures, and coma. In most cases, insulinoma cannot be cured, but can be treated with medical therapy ± surgery. Up to two years of resolution of clinical signs can be obtained if the disease is diagnosed early.

A highly suggestive diagnosis is a glucose of 3.9 mmol/l (70 mg/dl) or less in a ferret that has been fasted 4 h. Normal blood glucose in a fasted ferret is about 5.1–11.5 mmol/l (92–207 mg/dl). An adjusted insulin glucose ratio (AIGR) can also be performed; however this measurement may not be clinically helpful: [serum insulin (μg/ml) × 100] divided by [plasma glucose (mg/dl) – 30]; if the result is greater than 30, than it is suggestive of insulinoma.

Insulin

Insulin is secreted by the beta cells of the pancreas. In ferrets over three years of age, 43% are estimated to have insulinoma. Hypoglycemia is commonly associated with this disease, but concurrently measured insulin levels may be increased or normal. The added cost, the varying insulin levels with disease, and the approximately 1 ml of serum that is needed for this test prompt most practitioners not to evaluate the insulin level in insulinoma-suspect ferrets, but diagnose the disease on the basis of repeated or persistent hypoglycemia. The normal insulin levels of ferrets range from 35 to 250 pmol/l (4.88–34.84 μU/ml). Ferrets with insulinoma may have insulin levels over 2000 pmol/l (>279 μU/ml). Ferrets with reported insulinoma had insulin levels ranging from 772.7 to 12 470 pmol/l (107.7–1738 μU/ml) [3, 25]. If insulin levels are evaluated, then the AIGR can be used for further evaluation, but is no longer recommended because of false positive results:

$$\frac{\text{Serum insulin}\left(\mu\text{U/ml}\right)\times 100}{\text{Plasma glucose}\left(\text{mg/dl}\right)-30} => 30 \text{ is abnormal}$$

Cardiac

Serum cardiac troponin T (cTnT) levels were determined in 7 male fitch ferrets immediately after induction and after 45 minutes under anesthesia with ketamine. Blood was drawn via cardiac puncture to induce cardiac trauma. The results were highly variable (0.1–133 ng/ml). Cardiac puncture caused cardiac injury since untreated healthy ferrets had undetectable cTnT levels and those that did have cardiac puncture had increased in cTnT concentrations, but cardiac puncture was not a good model for cardiac injury based on highly variable results [29]. In dogs, the higher the cTnT levels, the more severe the cardiac damage.

Lipids: Cholesterol and Triglycerides

In general, the total serum lipoprotein values are similar to what is measured in dogs, except that the major lipoprotein fraction in ferrets is of high density: 10.63–12.1 g/l (1.063–1.21 g/ml) [38]. Cholesterol and triglycerides are plasma lipids described for ferrets [26]. Increases in plasma cholesterol typically occur secondary to endocrine, hepatic, or renal diseases. Cholesterol levels in ferrets have been described [3, 15]. In dogs and cats, a postprandial hypertriglyceridemia occurs 4 to 6 h after eating. It is unknown if postprandial hypertriglyceridemia occurs in the ferret.

Electrolytes, Osmolality, and Anion Gap

Electrolytes have been reported and appear fairly consistent across all references [3, 5, 15, 19, 25]. Iatrogenic Addison's disease has been reported anecdotally after surgically removing both neoplastic adrenal glands in ferrets. Accessory adrenal tissue occurs in ferrets, but these tissues rarely become neoplastic. Addison's disease is associated with a low sodium level (<130 mEq/l) and a high potassium level (>5 mEq/l). Hyperkalemia can occur with acute renal failure or postrenal urinary obstruction. Hypokalemia can be seen with anorexia and polyuric renal failure. Osmolality and anion gap have not been described or calculated in ferrets. Osmolarity of ferrets has been reported as 328 ± 1 mOsm/kg and 324.0 ± 10 [21, 38].

Blood Proteins

For ferrets, only total protein and albumin concentrations are described in multiple sources. Total protein is commonly measured by the biuret reaction and albumin by BCG reaction, but these methods are less accurate than using electrophoresis. Common causes of decreased total protein (TP) in ferrets occurs with loss of protein from proliferative bowel disease or enteritis, especially with a loss of albumin or seen with concurrent hypoalbuminemia. Plasma electrophoresis values for albumin, alpha-1 and -2 globulin, beta globulin and gamma globulin have been described and are included in Table 2.3 [5]. Hypergammaglobulinemia is associated with Aleutian disease in ferrets.

Blood Gases, pH, and Lactate

Baseline values for blood gases, pH, and lactate are not described for ferrets in the literature, other than CO_2 levels in several sources (Table 2.2). Ferrets under urethane anesthesia had a mean arterial blood pH of 7.283 ± 0.025 with a bicarbonate concentration of 15.7 ± 0.7 mM [38]. In another study, 18 adult fitch ferrets were anesthetized with a combination of varying doses of medetomadine, midazolam, and ketamine, and had a mean pH of 7.3 and a varying PaO_2 5 min into anesthesia of 38.5, 47.7, and 54.0 mmHg, and a $PaCO_2$ of 52.7, 45.8, and 49.6 mmHg, depending on the dose and route of ketamine [35]. Blood parameters during short-term anesthesia of mink included a pH that remained fairly constant and other parameters that varied widely, such as a pH of 168.5–169.7 nmol/l (7.25–7.3), a pCO_2 of 5.5–8.4 kPa (41.2–63.0 mmHg), a PO_2 of 5.6–12.0 pKa (42–90 mmHg), and a HCO_3 of 18.9–28 mEq/l (18.9–28 mmHg) [36].

Vitamins, Minerals and Metals, Toxins

Plasma vitamin concentrations have not been determined in ferrets. A baseline mean serum *B*-carotene level in ferrets was 0.6 μg/dl [22, 39]. A thorough evaluation of all amino acids has been delineated for ferrets [21]. Plasma calcium levels can decrease proportionally to increasing phosphorus levels. Ionized calcium has not been reported for the ferret. Hypercalcemia of malignancy has not been reported in the ferret. Phosphorus allows indirect evaluation of GFR on the basis of excretion through glomerular filtration and tubular reabsorption. Hyperphosphatemia can occur with decreased renal clearance, increased intestinal absorption, or hemolysis and increases concomitantly with BUN. Other nonrenal causes of hyperphosphatemia also include pseudohypoparathyroidism, hypervitaminosis D, soft tissue trauma, dietary mineral supplements, dehydration, and hemolysis. One case report describes suspected psuedohypoparathyroidism in a domestic ferret with hypocalcemia and hyperphosphatemia that resolved with vitamin D and calcium supplementation [40]. Many trace elements have been evaluated in female fitch ferrets including mean values for zinc via atomic absorption 15.4 ± 4.5 μmol/l (100.4 ± 29.29 μg/dl) ($n = 5$), copper at 11.5 ± 0.9 μmol/l (73.33 ± 5.73 μg/l) ($n = 3$), and iron at 31.1 ± 6.4 μmol/l (174.0 ± 35.48 mg/dl) ($n = 4$) [21].

Toxins

Blood cholinesterase via the colorimetric method was described in six normal intact female fitch ferrets as 469.5 ± 72.71 IU/l (1 IU is equivalent to a mmol of sulfhydryl groups liberated in 1 min) [21].

Hormones – Thyroid, Adrenal, and Reproductive

Hormone reference data published for ferrets are provided in Table 2.5.

Thyroid Hormones

Hypothyroidism rarely occurs in ferrets. Thyroiditis and thyroid adenocarcinoma have been described histopathologically in the ferret [31]. Normal T_4 (thyroxine) and T_3 (triiodothyronine) levels determined by radioimmunoassay (RIA) have been described for intact and neutered ferrets (Table 2.5) [31, 41]. Units of thyroid hormone levels may be reported in ng/ml or μg/ml. To convert from ng/ml to μg/dl, divide by a factor of 10. One study of 13 ferrets showed baseline T_4 levels that increased from a baseline of 32.6 ± 12.0 nmol/l (2.53 ± 0.93 μg/dl) to 51.1 ± 15.7 nmol/l (3.97 ± 1.22 μg/dl) 4 h after administration of 1 IU TSH IV. In one case of the author's, a male neutered ferret with obesity and alopecia had a baseline T_4 concentration of 8.5 nmol/l (6.6 ng/ml = 0.66 μg/dl). A TSH response test using 1 IU/kg IM human recombinant TSH (Thyrogen by Genzyme) showed a minimal increase in thyroxine to 18.7 nmol/l (14.7 ng/ml = 1.47 μg/dl). Six months after the ferret was supplemented with thyroxine at 25 μg/day, baseline T_4 levels were 36.3 nmol/l (28.2 ng/ml = 2.82 μg/dl), and 11 months later were 40.7 nmol/l (31.6 ng/ml = 3.16 μg/dl).

Endocrine Hormones Including Adrenal Hormones

Ferrets with adrenal disease usually have an adrenal tumor that does not secrete excessive cortisol. Cortisol levels, the ACTH stimulation test, and the dexamethasone suppression test are of little diagnostic value for ferrets with adrenal tumors [31]. Adrenal cortical hormone diagnostic panels for ferrets include estradiol, androstenodione, and 17-B-OH-progesterone (Table 2.5) and are available at the University of Tennessee and the University of Miami. Measuring these three hormones is about 95% accurate in diagnosing adrenal disease in the ferret [26]. Measuring only estradiol is less expensive, but only about 75% accurate in diagnosing adrenal disease in ferrets with adrenal disease.

Reproductive Hormones

Aplastic anemia occurs in intact female ferrets that are not bred while in heat, resulting in a prolonged estrus with hyperestrogenemia and subsequent bone marrow suppression [32]. Estrogen may be evaluated to confirm a diagnosis of remnant ovarian tissue if this is suspected; however, adrenal tumors are much more common than remnant ovaries as causes of disease in ferrets. Plasma progesterone levels of pregnant and pseudopregnant ferrets have been described (Table 2.5) [27].

Urinalysis

Normal urinalysis findings are summarized in Table 2.6. Ferrets with DM may have glucosuria. The bladder of a large (1.5 kg), intact male ferret can hold approximately 10 ml [23]. Urine volume is variable with a range of 8–140 ml/ferret/day, and a mean of 26–28 ml/ferret/day. Ferrets fed a diet of 30%–40% crude protein consisting of a high-quality meat-based protein have a urine pH of 6.0 to 6.5. A urine pH of >6.5 will likely cause struvite formation [9]. As in dogs, a proteinuria can indicate renal disease. Protein >1+ in urine that is not highly concentrated is considered abnormal. Renal protein loss can occur at the glomerular membrane or from failure to reabsorb. Postrenal proteinuria is usually associated with cystitis [27]. Rarely, DM is seen with concurrent glucosuria; stress glucosuria is uncommon in the ferret. Ketones in ferret urine can occur with prolonged anorexia. Bilirubin must be conjugated by the liver prior to excretion in the urine. Bilirubinuria may be seen in ferrets with intravascular hemolysis, liver disease, extrahepatic biliary obstruction, fever, and starvation [9].

Ferrets fed a diet of dog food, with a poor-quality and low level of protein causing a higher pH, had a 14% incidence of struvite (ammonium magnesium phosphate) uroliths at necropsy (Figure 2.16) [9]. Uroliths should be submitted for composition analysis. Struvite urinary calculi are uncommon unless a ferret has a diet that lowers the urine pH. Proteinaceous sludge desquamated from abnormal prostatic tissue in male ferrets with adrenal disease is common (Figures 2.17 and 2.18).

Differentials for hematuria in the ferret should include urolithiasis, cystitis, paraurethral masses or prostatic hyperplasia secondary to adrenal disease, neoplasia, specifically renal lymphosarcoma, or iatrogenic trauma from urethral catheterization or cystocentesis. One case of transitional cell carcinoma has been reported in the ferret [9]. Green urine has been associated with dirofilariasis in a ferret, likely due to intravascular hemolysis (Figure 2.19) [42].

Cerebral Spinal Fluid Evaluation

Cerebrospinal fluid analysis has been described in normal adult domestic ferrets. Numbers of WBCs and RBCs are determined using a hemocytometer, and TP concentration is obtained by an automated chemical analyzer (Table 2.7). The WBC numbers were slightly higher than

Table 2.5 Hormone reference ranges for adult domestic ferrets (*Mustela putorius furo*).

Analyte (abbreviation)	Units, SI [conventional]	Male [31, 41]	Female[a] [3, 8, 18]	Neutered ferrets [8][a]	Pregnant and pseudopregnant jills[b] [27]		
					Day	Flourimetry	Competitive binding
Animals sampled		♂27 + ♂Φ 4 [31, 41] 40♂	10♀ + 3♀Φ 35–11 fitch jills	13♂Φ + 13♀ Φ			
Thyroxine (T_4)	nmol/l [μg/dl]	41.7 (1.0–106.7) [31, 41] [3.24 (1.01–8.29)]	24.1 (9.14–44.1) [1.87 (0.71–3.43)]	19.3–43.5 nmol/l [1.5–3.38 μg/dl]			
Triiodothreonine (T_3)	nmol/l [ng/ml]	0.81 (0.63–1.1) [31, 41] [0.58 (0.45–0.78)]	0.74 (0.41–10.2) [0.53 (0.29–0.73)]				
Estradiol	pmol/l [pg/ml]	109–278[a] [8] [29.7–75.7]	165.5 (122–210)[a] [8] [45.0(33.2–57.2)][a] [8]	106 (30–180.0) [28.9 (8.17–49.0)]			
17 *B*-hydroxy progesterone	nmol/l [ng/ml]	0.24–1.54[a] [8] [0.08–0.5]	7.7 (2.3–13.1)[a] [8] [2.4(0.72–4.1)][a] [8]	0.4 (0–0.8) [0.13 (0–0.25)]	7–11	79.4 ± 9.6 [24.8 ± 3.0]	67.8 ± 5.1 [21.2 ± 1.6]
					12–16	125.4 ± 13.4 [39.2 ± 4.2]	74.9 ± 9.6 [23.4 ± 3.0]
					17–21	110.4 [34.5]	74.9 ± 8.6 [23.4 ± 2.7]
					22–26	86.4 ± 15.4 [27.0 ± 4.8]	56 ± 5.8 [17.5 ± 1.8]
					27–31	54.4 ± 12.2 [17.0 ± 3.8]	56.6 ± 10.6 [17.7 ± 3.3]
					32–36	541.6 [13.0]	35.2 ± 5.4 [11.0 ± 1.7]
					37–41	31.4 ± 11.2 [9.8 ± 3.5]	31.4 ± 7.0 [9.8 ± 2.2]
Androstenodione	nmol/l [ng/dl]	0.63–9.32[a] [8] [18.1–267.4]	58.3 (20–96)[a] [8] [1673(574–2755)][a] [8]	6.6 (0–15.00) [189.4 (0–429.8)]			

Source: Data presented as mean (range) or mean ± SD.
[a] University of Tennessee Endocrinology laboratory [8].
[b] Unknown number of ferrets, sample obtained awake or anesthetized with ether by cardiac puncture at varying days post breeding [27].

Table 2.6 Urinalysis findings typical of adult domestic ferrets (*Mustela putorius furo*) [9].

Analyte (abbreviation)	Units, SI [conventional]	Adult domestic ferret
Urine clarity	–	Clear
Urine color	–	Varying degrees of yellow depending on hydration status
Urine pH	–	6.0–7.5
Specific gravity	–	Not reported
Urine protein	mg/l [mg/dl]	0–330 (0–33) Or + 1 on Ames dipstick
Urine protein: Creatinine ratio	–	Not described
Urine glucose		Negative
Urine ketones		Negative
Urine RBCs		0–3 per high power field
White blood cells		0
Casts		0
Bacteria		0

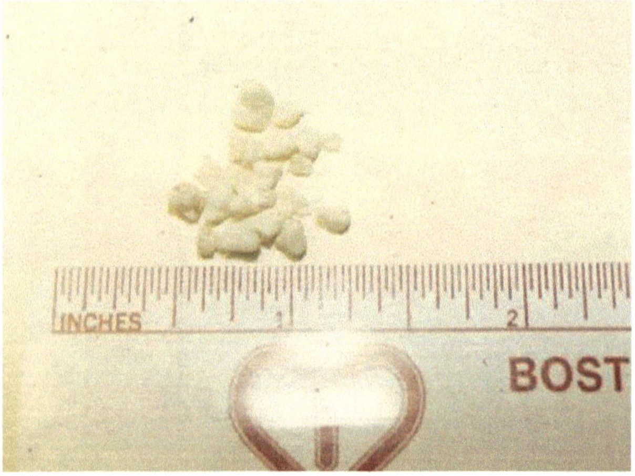

Figure 2.16 Lateral contrast urethrogram of a ferret with a prostatic cyst demonstrating urethral and ureteral dilation.

reported for in dogs and cats. Blood contamination had a small, but significant effect on WBC numbers, but not on TP concentration. TP was slightly higher than reported for dogs and cats.

Bone Marrow Examination

Evaluation of bone marrow can provide vital information for evaluating anemia, thrombocytopenia, leukopenia, pancytopenia, proliferative diseases such as plasma cell myeloma, and neoplasia of the hematopoietic system (the most common in ferrets being lymphoma) [5]. Causes of anemia include loss or lysis of RBCs, aplastic anemia of intact non-bred females, some adrenal tumors, Aleutian disease, and idiopathic. Aplastic anemia is best diagnosed by a history of prolonged

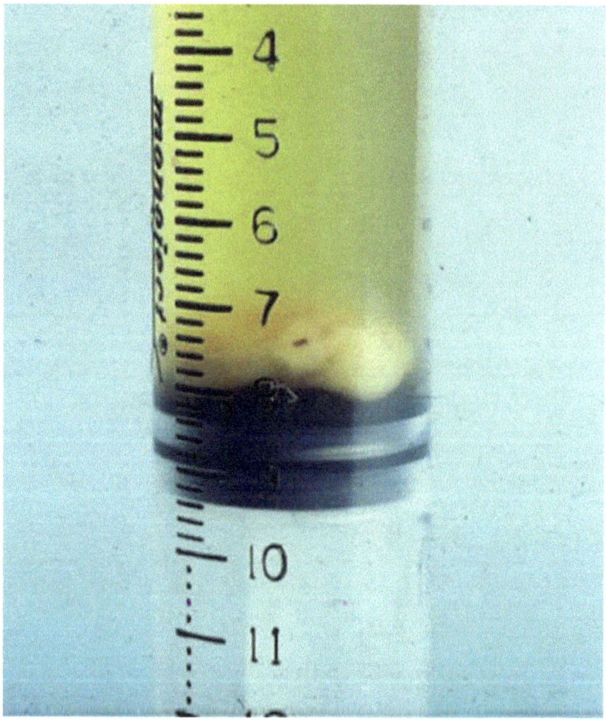

Figure 2.17 Urine collected from a ferret with a prostatic cyst showing gross cellular sludge, which can make catheterization challenging.

(>1 month) estrus in a non-bred intact female ferret in conjunction with a non-regenerative anemia. Bone marrow will exhibit pancytopenia with myeloid, erythroid, and megakaryocytic cell suppression. Aleutian disease caused by a parvovirus can cause a severe hypergammaglobulinemia and increased plasma cells (often over

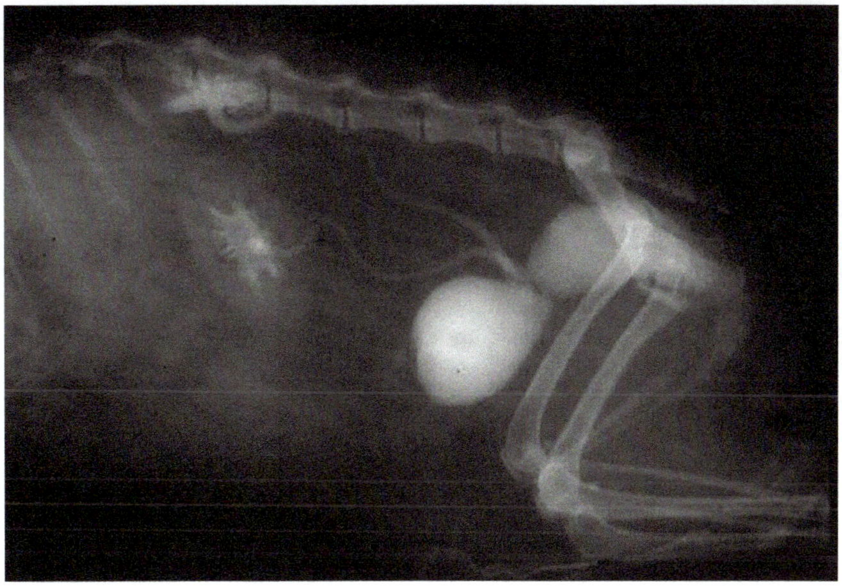

Figure 2.18 Struvite stones collected from a ferret cystotomy.

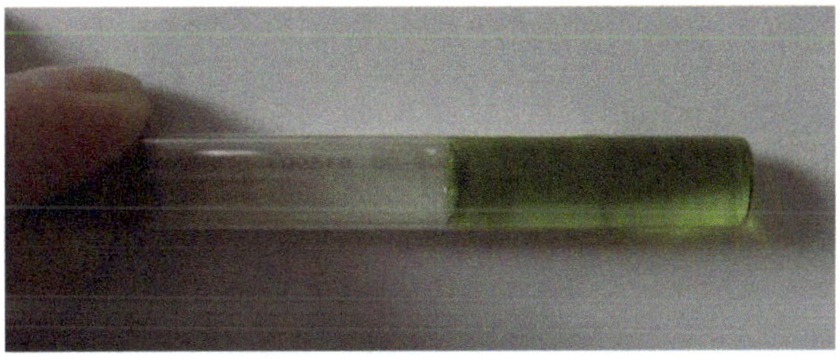

Figure 2.19 Green urine from a ferret with dirofilariasis.

Table 2.7 Cerebrospinal fluid of 42 adult (30–36 week old) domestic intact ferrets (*Mustela putorius furo*) [14].

Analyte (abbreviation)	Units, SI [conventional]	Adult domestic ferret
White blood cells	cells/μl	1.59
Total protein	mg/dl	31.4 (20.8–60.8)
Red blood cells	cells/μl	20.3

10%) on bone marrow aspirates [13]. Immune mediated red cell aplasia was successfully treated in a ferret after diagnosis from a core biopsy sample [43].

Evaluation and interpretation of bone marrow cytology in ferrets is similar to that for the dog and cat. The sample should be submitted to a veterinary pathologist for evaluation along with concurrent submission of a blood sample for CBC [13]. Despite extramedullary splenic hematopoiesis in ferrets, significant quantities of mature cells are not released into the peripheral circulation from this site [13]. In cases of regenerative anemia, the myeloid:erythroid (ME) ratio should be less than 1 : 3.

Serology and PCR

Viruses

Aleutian Disease

Ferrets can become infected with a parvovirus called the Aleutian disease virus that causes Aleutian disease in ferrets and enteritis in mink. A common finding with clinical disease is hypergammaglobulinemia >20% of the TP. A globulin level greater than 5.0 g/dl requires further testing. A PCR test can be performed on 1–5 g of tissue (intestine or spleen), 1 ml of blood, or a fecal swab at the Diagnostic Center for Population and Animal Health (DCPAH) at Michigan State University (www.ferrethealth.msu.edu), or on 0.5 ml of urine, 0.2 ml of blood, or an oral swab at the University of Georgia's Infectious Disease Laboratory (www.vet.uga.edu/SAMS/IDL). DNA in situ hybridization is also performed on tissue at both the above laboratories. The University of Miami's Comparative Pathology Laboratory (www.pathology.med.miami.edu/cpl) and Charles River Laboratory (www.criver.com/SiteCollectionDocuments/rm_d_r_ferret_health_surveillance.pdf) also run a PCR for Aleutian disease. A counterimmunoelectrophoresis (CIE or CEP) test is run on 0.2 ml of serum or plasma to detect antibody and is available from the Animal Health Laboratory at the University of Guelph (http://guelphlabservices.com). A highly sensitive and highly specific ELISA test to detect antibody in saliva, serum, or plasma is available from Avecon Diagnostics, Inc. (www.avecon.com).

Canine Distemper Virus

Although an immunofluorescent antibody IFA test can be performed on a conjunctival swab as in dogs, canine distemper is considered 100% fatal in unvaccinated ferrets. A PCR can be performed on 5g of tissue (lung, kidney, bladder, and brain), 1ml of blood or serum, or a nasal orconjunctival swab. Many laboratories perform canine distemper PCR and immunohistochemistry on tissue and serology including DCPAH, Charles River Laboratories, and Zoologix (www.zoologix.com/zoo/Datasheets). Ideally, swabs are made of synthetic material and are placed in 0.5–1.0ml of saline or PBS prior to shipment.

Epizootic Catarrhal Enteritis (ECE) (Coronavirus)

In the ferret, ECE is thought to be caused by a coronavirus since it was found in ferrets with clinical signs, but Koch's postulates have not been fulfilled. It is sometimes called enteric coronavirus to distinguish it from systemic coronavirus that is thought to cause FIP-like signs in ferrets. Electron microscopy (EM) of a ferret with diarrhea may show corona-like organisms, and this may be the cause of the diarrhea [23]. A PCR test on 1–5g of tissue (jejunum and ileum), or a swab of feces in saline or PBS, or serology can be run at DCPAH or at Charles River Laboratories. Many laboratories can provide EM or immunohistochemical testing for coronavirus.

Influenza

Influenza caused by an Orthomyxovirus occurs in ferrets with associated fever, upper respiratory disease, with or without diarrhea. The same virus occurs in people, and zoonotic and anthropozoonotic (human to animal) infections have been described. Testing is not typically performed in ferrets except under research conditions, although DCPAH and Charles River Laboratories offer a PCR and immunohistochemical testing. The ferret is used for the development of the human influenza vaccine yearly.

Rabies Virus

Rabies can occur in ferrets much the same as in dogs, and postmortem rabies testing is similarly performed. The best source of information is the Compendium of Animal Rabies Prevention and Control, 2011, by the National Association of State Public Health Veterinarians (www. nasphv.org/Documents/RabiesCompendium.pdf). According to the NASPHV Compendium, the gold standard for rabies testing in ferrets is the Direct Fluorescent Antibody (DFA) test that is run by a qualified laboratory that has been designated by the local or state health department. Imrab-3® (Merial) is the licensed rabies vaccine for ferrets. No serologic test is available for rabies exposure in this species.

Rotavirus

Rotavirus causes diarrhea in young (two- to six-week-old) ferrets and is generally not seen by the practitioner. Diagnosis based on electromicroscopy (EM) of feces demonstrating the organism can be performed at many laboratories. A PCR for rotavirus group A and C can be performed on a fecal swab or tissue (jejunum, ileum) at DCPAH.

BACTERIAL

Proliferative Bowel Disease (PBD) or Proliferative Colitis Caused by *Lawsonia intracellularis*

PBD of ferrets is similar to PDB in other animals. It has been described in ferrets and is caused by *Lawsonia intracellularis*. Diagnosis is usually based on typical clinical signs or demonstration of typical gross and histopathologic lesions consisting of firm, thickened colon and/or small intestine with mucosal surface proliferation. Histopathologically there is hypertrophy of the muscularis and monocytic and/or granulocytic infiltration [23]. A PCR test run on 0.5ml feces, rectal swab, or 0.5ml fresh, frozen, or fixed ileum is available from Zoologix (www.zoologix.com/zoo/Datasheets/Lawsonia.htm), DCPAH, or Charles River Laboratories.

Helicobacter mustelae – Associated Gastritis

Infection with *Helicobacter mustelae*, with or without clinical signs, is considered ubiquitous in ferrets, therefore making diagnosis using various tests difficult [20, 30]. Definitive diagnosis of *H. mustelae* associated gastritis in ferrets is based on histopathology of pyloric mucosal biopsy. Biopsy can be obtained via endoscopy or by surgical incision of the greater curvature of the stomach [20]. Other diagnostic tests include culture, PCR, ELISA, and urease detection. A PCR test is available from Charles River Laboratories (see http://www.criver.com/info/diagnostic_sample_submission).Culture of *H. mustelae* is not typically performed at veterinary diagnostic laboratories. A real-time PCR of a gastric biopsy, or gastric swab, can confirm the presence of the organism and provide quantification. Seventy-four percent (23/40) of histopathology confirmed that *H. mustelae* positive ferrets were positive on gastric swab PCR (Research Associates Laboratory, R.A.L. Inc., in Dallas, Texas, www.vetdna.com) [20]. Samples were obtained by snugly inserting a culture swab for attachment to the distal end of a soft red rubber feeding tube. The device was then passed orally to the stomach in a sedated ferret [20]. Measuring ammonia production produced by *H. mustelae* is impractical and reserved for use in research [34, 44]. Urease measured in a biopsy sample lacks specificity and sensitivity, based on intestinal reflux, blood contamination, or low bacteria numbers in the sample [20]. High antibody titers measured by ELISA or other methods for *H. mustelae* are often found and are not protective in the ferret. Antibody titers can determine the effect of treatment as titers decrease after eradication of *H. mustelae* in ferrets [33].

Leptospirosis

Fluorescent antibody (FA) testing can be performed on 1 g of tissue (kidney, liver, or placenta) or 10 ml of urine. Serology can be performed on 0.5 ml of plasma or serum via the microagglutination. All of these tests are available from DCPAH. All six serovars are tested: Pomona, Grippotyphosa, Hardjo, Canicola, Icterohemorrhagiae, and Bratislava.

Tyzzer's Disease (*Clostridium piliforme*)

A PCR for *Clostridium piliforme*, the causative agent of Tyzzer's disease, is available from DCPAH.

Parasites

A PCR for enteric coccidiosis of ferrets (*Eimeria furonis*) is available from DCPAH. Ferrets can become infected with heartworm and develop disease. Besides ultrasound to visualize the parasite, an ELISA test to detect antigen can be used; however, the low worm burden found in ferrets often gives only a weak positive result, and false negative results are likely common. Green urine may also be observed in some cases likely due to intravascular hemolysis [42].

References

1 Marini, R.P., Jackson, L.R., Esteves, M.I. et al. (1994). Effect of isoflurane on hematologic variables in ferrets. *Am. J. Vet. Res.* 55: 1479–1483.

2 Joslin, J.O. (2009). Blood collection techniques in exotic small mammals. *J. Exot. Pet. Med. Surg.* 18 (2): 117–139.

3 Fox, J.G. (1998). Normal clinical and biological parameters. In: *Biology and Diseases of the Ferret*, 2e, 183–210. Baltimore, MD: Williams and Wilkins.

4 Murray, M.J. (2000). Rabbit and ferret laboratory medicine. In: *Laboratory Medicine – Avian and Exotic Pets* (ed. A.M. Fudge), 265–268. Philadelphia, PA: WB Saunders Co.

5 Quesenberry, K.E. and Orcutt, C. (2012). Basic approach to veterinary care. In: *Ferrets, Rabbits and Rodents, Clinical Medicine and Surgery*, 3e (ed. K.E. Quesenberry and J.W. Carpenter), 13–26. St. Louis, MO: Saunders.

6 Abaxis Inc. website, www.abaxis.com, accessed 3-21-12.

7 Marini, R.P. and Fox, J.G. (1998). Anesthesia, surgery, and biomethodology. In: *Biology and Diseases of the Ferret*, 2e (ed. J.G. Fox), 449–484.

8 Riggs, S.M., Heatley, J.J., Nevarez, J., and Mitchell, M.A. (2002). Ferret blood collection: a quick and simple technique. *Exotic D.V.M.* 4 (6): 6–7.

9 Hoefer, H.L. (2000). Rabbit and ferret renal disease diagnosis. In: *Laboratory Medicine – Avian and Exotic Pets*, vol. 14 (ed. A.M. Fudge), 311–318. Philadelphia, PA: WB Saunders Co.

10 Tully, T; et al. Urethral Catheterization of Male Ferrets – A Novel Technique. 3.2 29 Exotic DVM.

11 Greenacre CB. Technique for urethral catheterization of the male domestic ferret (*Mustela putorius furo*). (manuscript and video). International Virtual Conference on Veterinary Medicine (IVCVM). Diseases of Exotic Animals and Wildlife at the following web site: https://www.youtube.com/watch?v=soPbN6LDqXc, accessed 12-3-18.

12 Palley, L.S., Marini, R.P., Rosenbald, W.D., and Fox, J.G. (1990). A technique for femoral bone marrow collection in the ferret. *Lab. Anim. Sci.* 40: 654.

13 Williams, B.H. (2000). Disorders of rabbit and ferret bone marrow. In: *Laboratory Medicine – Avian and Exotic Pets* (ed. A.M. Fudge), 276–284. Philadelphia, PA: WB Saunders Co.

14 Platt, S.R., Dennis, P.M., McSherry, L.J. et al. (2004). Composition of cerebral spinal fluid in clinically normal adult ferrets. *Am. J. Vet. Res.* 65 (6): 758–760.

15 Thornton, P.C., Wright, P.A., Sacra, P.J. et al. (1979). The ferret, *Mustela putorius furo*, as a new species in toxicology. *Lab. Anim.* 13: 119.

16 International Species Information System (ISIS), March 2002 data, accessed March, 2012.

17 Fox, J.G., Hotaling, L., Ackerman, J.B. et al. (1986). Serum chemistry and hematology reference values in the ferret (*Mustela putorius furo*). *Lab. Anim. Sci.* 36: 583.

18 Fudge, A.M. (2000). Ferret hematology. In: *Laboratory Medicine – Avian and Exotic Pets* (ed. A.M. Fudge), 269–275. Philadelphia, PA: WB Saunders Co.

19 Lee, E.J., Moore, W.F., Fryer, H.C. et al. (1982). Haematological and serum chemistry profiles of ferrets (*Mustela putorius furo*). *Lab. Anim.* 16: 133.

20 Johnson-Delaney, C.A. (2005). The ferret gastrointestinal tract and *Helicobacter mustelae* infection. *Vet. Clin. North Am. Exot. Anim. Pract.* 8 (2): 197–212.

21 Ohwada, K. and Katahira, K. (1993). Reference values for organ weight, hematology and serum chemistry in the female ferret (*Mustela putorius furo*). *JIkken Dobutsu* 42 (2): 135–142.

22 Fox, J.G. and McLain, D.E. (1998). Nutrition. In: *Biology and Diseases of the Ferret*, 2e, 149–172. Baltimore, MD: Williams and Wilkins.

23 Hoefer, H.L., Fox, J.G., and Bell, J.A. (2012). Gastrointestinal diseases. In: *Ferrets, Rabbits and Rodents, Clinical Medicine and Surgery*, 3e (ed. K.E. Quesenberry and J.W. Carpenter), 86–102. St. Louis, MO: Saunders.

24 Manning, D.D. and Bell, J.A. (1990). Lack of detectable blood groups in domestic ferrets: implications for transfusion. *J. Am. Vet. Med. Assoc.* 197 (1): 84–86.

25 Rosenthal, K.L. and Wyre, N.R. (2012). Endocrine diseases. In: *Ferrets, Rabbits and Rodents, Clinical Medicine and Surgery*, 3e (ed. K.E. Quesenberry and J.W. Carpenter), 86–102. St. Louis, MO: Saunders.

26 Antinoff, N. and Williams, B.H. (2012). Neoplasia. In: *Ferrets, Rabbits and Rodents, Clinical Medicine and Surgery*, 3e (ed. K.E. Quesenberry and J.W. Carpenter), 103–121. St. Louis, MO: Saunders.

27 Heap, R.B. and Hammond, J. (1974). Plasma progesterone levels in pregnant and pseudopregnant ferrets. *J. Reprod. Fertil.* 39: 149–152. Soc Reprod Fertility.

28 Jenkins, J.R. (2000). Rabbit and ferret liver and gastrointestinal testing. In: *Laboratory Medicine – Avian and Exotic Pets* (ed. A.M. Fudge), 291–304. Philadelphia, PA: WB Saunders Co.

29 O'Brien, P.J., Dameron, G.W., Beck, M.L. et al. (1997). Cardiac troponin T is a sensitive, specific biomarker of cardiac injury o in laboratory animals. *Lab. Anim. Sci.* 47 (5): 486–495.

30 Williams, B.H. (2000). Ferret microbiology and virology. In: *Laboratory Medicine – Avian and Exotic Pets* (ed. A.M. Fudge), 334–342. Philadelphia, PA: WB Saunders Co.

31 Fox, J.G. and Marini, R.P. (1998). Diseases of the endocrine system. In: *Biology and Diseases of the Ferret*, 2e, 291–305. Baltimore, MD: Williams and Wilkins.

32 Erdmann, S.E., LI, X., and Fox, J.G. (1998). Hematopoetic diseases. In: *Biology and Diseases of the Ferret*, 2e, 231–246. Baltimore, MD: Williams and Wilkins.

33 Fox, J.G. and Marini, R.P. (2001). *Helicobacter mustelae* infection in ferrets: pathogenesis, epizootiology, diagnosis and treatment. *Semin. Avian Exot. Pet. Med.* 10 (1): 36–43.

34 Fox, J.G., Correa, P., Taylor, N.S. et al. (1990). *Helicobacter mustelae* – associated gastritis in ferrets: an animal model of *Helicobacter pylori* gastritis in humans. *Gastroenterology* 99: 352.

35 Schemthaner, A., Lendl, C.E., Hartmann, K. et al. (2011). Medetomidine/midazolam/ketamine anesthesia in ferrets: effects of cardiorespiratory parameters and evaluation of plasma drug concentrations. *Vet. Anaesth. Analg.* 38 (5): 439–450.

36 Wamberg, S., Svendsen, P., and Johansen, B. (1996). Acid-base status and cardiovascular function in mink (*Mustela vison*) anaesthetized with ketamine/midazolam. *Lab. Anim.* 30 (1): 55–56.

37 Hoefer, H.L., Patnaik, A.K., and Lewis, A.D. (1992). Pancreatic adenocarcinoma with metastasis in two ferrets. *J. Am. Vet. Med. Assoc.* 201: 466–467.

38 Whary, M.T. and Andrews, P.L.R. (1998). Physiology of the ferret. In: *Biology and Diseases of the Ferret*, 2e, 103–148. Baltimore, MD: Williams and Wilkins.

39 Ribaya-Mercado, J.D., Holmgren, S.C., and Fox, J.G. (1989). Dietary *B*-carotene absorption and metabolism in ferrets and rats. *J. Nutr.* 119: 665.

40 Wilson, G.H., Greene, C.E., and Greenacre, C.B. (2003). Suspected pseudohypoparathyroidism in a domestic ferret. *J. Am. Vet. Med. Assoc.* 222 (8): 1093–1096.

41 Garibaldi, B.A., Pecquet-Goad, M.E., Fox, J.G. et al. (1988). Serum thyroxine and tri-iodothreonine radioimmunoassay values in the normal ferret. *Lab. Anim. Sci.* 38: 455.

42 Bradbury, C., Saunders, A.B., Heatley, J.J. et al. (2010). Transvenous heartworm extraction in a ferret with Caval syndrome. *JAHAA* 46 (1): 31–35.

43 Malka, S., Hawkins, M.G., Zabolotzky, S.M. et al. (2010). Immune mediated red cell aplasia in a domestic ferret. *J. Am. Vet. Med. Assoc.* 237 (6): 695–700.

44 Fox, J.G. (1998). Bacterial and Mycoplasmal diseases. In: *Biology and Diseases of the Ferret*, 2e, 321–354. Baltimore, MD: Williams and Wilkins.

3

Procyonids

Cameron Ratliff DVM[1] and J. Jill Heatley DVM, MS, DABVP (Avian, Reptilian, Amphibian), DACZM[2]

[1] Department of Surgical Sciences, Wisconsin School of Veterinary Medicine, University of Wisconsin-Madison, Madison, Wisconsin, USA
[2] Department of Small Animal Clinical Sciences, College of Veterinary Medicine & Biomedical Sciences, Texas A&M University, College Station, Texas, USA

Introduction

Procyonids are omnivores of the order Carnivora, with ranges restricted to the New World: North and Central America. The common raccoon is widely dispersed throughout the United States and frequently encountered venturing into urban settings. While raccoons are best known for their role in rabies and other infectious disease dispersal, they have also been used to study intelligence and physiology in the laboratory setting. This chapter will focus on clinicopathologic data for the raccoon and coati where available, although other Procyonidae may be referenced when data is sparse.

Species

Species in the family Procyonidae include the raccoon (*Procyon lotor*), coatimundi (*Nasua nasua*), kinkajou (*Potus flavus*), olingo (*Olingo gabbii*), and the cacomistle (*Bassariscus astutus*). Of this group, only the raccoon, coati and kinkajou are occasional exotic pets. However, as a rabies vector, private ownership of the raccoon is restricted in many states, counties, and municipalities of the United States. Many procyonids are solitary, arboreal, and nocturnal; however, the coatimundi is social and diurnal [1]. The red panda (*Ailurus fulgens*), closely allied to the Procyonidae phylogenetically but now classified as Ailuridae, is mentioned in this chapter when clinicopathologic data for other procyonids is lacking.

Sample Collection

Restraint

Procyonidae may be trained to enter tubes or kennels [2]. Manual restraint is generally only attempted with individuals which are accustomed to humans [3]. Smaller individuals may be netted and manually restrained with gloves. Reinforced gloves are required to withstand the relatively long canines of some members of this group. With manual restraint, the neck may be held in one hand while the hind limbs are stretched with the other hand. Alternatively, each forearm may be restrained by a grip close to the axillae to avoid the animal's bite radius. Longer duration of restraint requires immobilization with anesthetic drugs. Hand injection of drugs during manual restraint or use of a squeeze cage is recommended because of the relatively bulky pelage and small muscle mass of these species. Excellent references for sedation and anesthesia of these species are available [4, 5].

Collection Sites and Sample Volume

Blood may be collected from the jugular, cephalic, and lateral saphenous veins or femoral vein, which are anatomically similar to domestic companion animals. The authors recommend a minimum of heavy sedation for sampling most of these sites, but anesthesia is a requirement for sampling of the femoral vein. Needle gauges of 20–25 g. (gauge), syringes of 1–5 cm^3, Vacutainer® systems, and butterfly infusions sets are useful for obtaining samples from Procyonidae, some of which may have thick, tough skin. Exam gloves and a long-sleeved laboratory coat are the minimum recommended personal protective equipment (PPE) for these species as known rabies vectors, and because of the wide variety of infectious diseases with which they may be infected as free-living omnivores.

The blood volume of the raccoon is 8.5 ml of blood per 100 g of body weight [6]. No greater than 7.5 ml/kg (<1% body weight) is a safe volume of blood to collect in a single sampling in a healthy raccoon. The sample volume for an unhealthy raccoon or for multiple collections should be lessened accordingly.

Exotic Animal Laboratory Diagnosis, First Edition. Edited by J. Jill Heatley and Karen E. Russell.

Sample Handling

Handling of a blood sample post collection is like that of domestic small animals. EDTA anticoagulant is preferred for determination of complete blood counts. For biochemical analysis, blood may be allowed to clot in uncoated tubes for serum harvest or may be collected into lithium heparin tubes for analysis of plasma.

Specific Analytes

Complete Blood Count (CBC)

Reference hematologic values for procyonids are listed in Table 3.1. Red and white blood cell morphology is like that of the domestic canids [10]. Red blood cells are biconcave disks with central pallor. Platelets tend to clump in groups and are pale blue in color. Cytoplasm of neutrophils stained with modified Wright stain is a very light sky blue color, and faint reddish-blue granules may be observed. Eosinophils in raccoons often have an S-shaped nucleus and are large with bright red to pink staining granules. Procyonidae have a lower neutrophil/lymphocyte ratio (1.3) than that of domestic Canidae and Felidae, and often have less dramatic increases in neutrophil count based on stress or bacterial infection [11]. A coati implanted with melengesterol acetate developed pyometra, uterine adenocarcinoma, and marked leukocytosis (116 900 mm^{-3}) with 94% neutrophils [12]. Few reference images of coati blood smears are available; however, abnormalities such as immune-mediated hemolytic anemia have been observed [13]. Blood smears from an apparently healthy coati are shown in Figures 3.1 and 3.2.

Hemoparasites

Hepatozoon procyonis infection has been demonstrated in both the raccoon and coati. This blood parasite may be detected on blood smear infecting neutrophils and monocytes; the gametocyte measures approximately 10 × 4 μm and has a basophilic hyaline-like cytoplasm [14]. *Brugia spp.* microfilarid parasites [15] and *Dirofilaria tenuis* [16, 17] have been detected on blood smears and with Knott's test in raccoons and coati; however, the clinical significance of these infections is unknown. Raccoons rarely serve as aberrant hosts for *Dirofilaria immitis*, but are not considered a competent vector for heartworms, may not suffer clinical disease, and are rarely microfilaremic [18]. Flukes have been found in the lymphatics

Table 3.1 Hematological reference data for Procyonidae.

Cell parameter (abbreviation)	Units, SI (conventional)	Raccoon [7] (*Procyon lotor*)	White-nosed Coatimundi [8] (*Nasua narica*)	Kinkajou [9] (*Potus flavus*)
Sample size & attributes		♂♀ all ages, H n > 70 or *[n]*	♂♀ all ages, H n > 90 or *[n]*	♂♀ all ages, H n ≥ 59 or *[n]*
Data format		**95% CI, mean**	**95% CI, mean**	**95% CI, mean**
Red blood cell count (RBC)	10^{12}/L = (10^6/μL)	3.66–11.77, 8.4	5.42–9.82(7.57)	5.26–12.97(8.66)
Hemoglobin (Hb)	g/L (g/dl)	64–159, 119) (6.4–15.9, 11.9)	80–145, 114 (8.0–14.5, 11.4)	97–177, 134 (9.7–17.7, 13.4)
Hematocrit (HCT)	%	17.9–50.0, 35.1	26.1–46.1, 35.3	29.9–52.0, 39.6
Mean corpuscular hemoglobin (MCH)	pg/cell	11.3–17.11, 4.0	12.3–17.8, 15.1	10.7–22.8, 16.1
Mean corpuscular hemoglobin concentration (MCHC)	g/dl	27.9–41.6, 34.0	27.1–38.2, 32.7	(30.1–38.6, 34.4)
Mean corpuscular volume (MCV)	fl	30.7–56.4, 41.0	37.5–58.4, 46.5	31.4–64.7, 46.8
White blood cell count (WBC)	10^9/l = (10^3/μl)	3.67–18.57, 8.94	4.01–17.54(8.81)	2.48–20.07, 8.74
Segmented neutrophils	10^9/l = 10^3/μl)	1.23–9.16(3.88)	1.71–13.1(5.52)	0.91–8.77, 3.84
Band neutrophils	10^9/l = (10^3/μl)	0.02–0.09(0.04)	0.02–0.1(0.04)	0.01–0.1, 0.04
Lymphocytes	10^9/l = (10^3/μl)	1.05–7.44(3.71)	0.54–6.38(2.48)	0.42–8.45, 3.13
Monocytes	10^9/l = (10^3/μl)	0.05–1.0(0.33)	0.05–0.85(0.3)	0.05–0.68, 0.26
Eosinophils	10^9/l = (10^3/μl)	0.08–2.1(0.67)	0.05–1.2(0.4)	0.05–4.8, 1.2
Basophils	10^9/l = (10^3/μl)	0.0–0.18(0.08) *[10]*	0.0–0.2, 0.1 *[9]*	0.04–0.16, 0.1
Platelets	10^9/l = (10^3/μl)	75–895(491) *[54]*	213–832, 526 *[56]*	59–815, 467 *[11]*

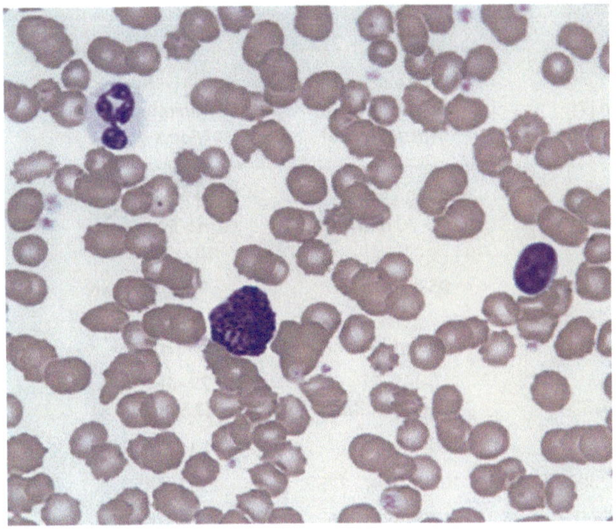

Figure 3.1 Blood smear of a juvenile male coati (*Nasua nasua*). Red blood cells are distributing typical central pallor and occasional crenation of cells. From left to right, a neutrophil, basophil, and lymphocyte are present. 1000× magnification.

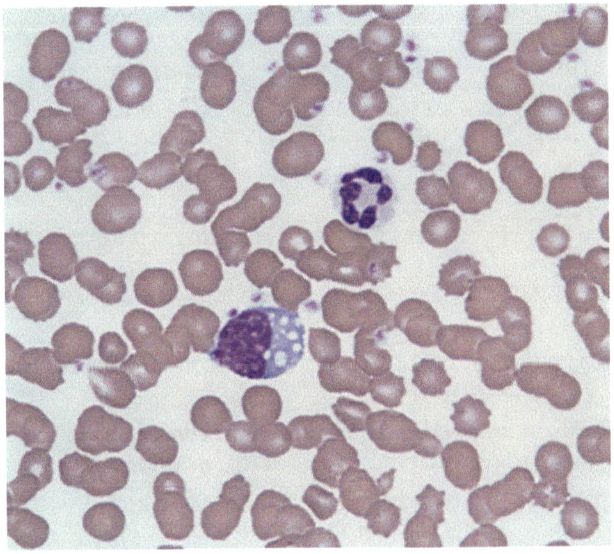

Figure 3.2 Blood smear from the coati in Figure 3.1. A monocyte and neutrophil are present. 1000× magnification.

and lungs of procyonids, and no life stage has yet been seen in peripheral blood [19]. Free-ranging coatis naturally infected with *Trypanosoma evansi* demonstrated moderately decreased hematocrit, hemoglobin, and red blood cell count [20].

Hemostasis and Coagulation Testing

Reference data for coagulation testing in raccoons is available, and hemostasis values in procyonids are comparable to those of domestic canids. Coagulation assay values are relatively conserved throughout Carnivora [11]. The activated partial thromboplastin time (APTT) mean time for raccoons was 26.2 s, which is longer than some other Carnivora [21]. In one male raccoon, the prothrombin time (PT) ranged from 10.2 to 49.9 s depending on the reagents used, and total whole blood clotting time was 8.1 min [22]. To the best of the authors' knowledge, blood-typing in procyonids has not been investigated.

Biochemical Panel

Liver Enzymes

To the best of our knowledge, the specificity or sensitivity of liver enzymes, or other liver biomarkers, in the Procyonidae has not specifically been investigated; the literature suggests they are similar to those of the domestic canid. Hyperbilirubinemia (6.5 mg/dl; normal 0.0–0.06 mg/dl) and mildly increased activities of alanine aminotransferase (ALT) and aspartate aminotransferase (AST) occurred in a red panda diagnosed with Tyzzer's disease [23]. Tyzzer's disease has also been reported in the raccoon [24]. A kinkajou with cholelithiasis and gallbladder necrosis had significantly increased ALT, AST, and ALP activities [25]. A coati infected with *Trypanosoma evansi* experienced increased activities of ALT and AST, with decreased blood glucose, albumin, and activity of ALP [20, 26].

Muscle Enzymes

Reference ranges of creatine kinase (CK) and AST are in Table 3.2. A raccoon with eosinophilic myositis had an increased CK activity of 2170 IU/l [27]. Serum CK and AST may have increased activities depending on capture or restraint of Procyonidae.

Renal Analytes

Uric acid has been measured in populations of coati (1.15 ± 0.9 mg/dl) [28], raccoon (0.9 ± 0.2 mg/dl) [2], and the kinkajou (0.8 ± 0.4 mg/dl) [2]. However, the utility of this analyte for disease diagnoses in these species is doubtful. Reference intervals for blood urea nitrogen and creatinine are provided in Table 3.2.

Pancreas (Endocrine and Exocrine)

A coati with pyometra and uterine adenocarcinoma experienced severely hypoglycemia (26.7 mg/dl) [12]. A raccoon with glucosuria and hyperglycemia (484 mg/dl) and increased fructosamine (514 mmol/l) concentrations was diagnosed with Type 2 diabetes mellitus that was managed with insulin and diet modification [29]. A functional endocrine pancreatic carcinoma capable of producing insulin, glucagon, and somatostatin has been documented in the raccoon [30]. Lipase has been measured in the coati (95% CI = 0–1065 IU/l, mean = 572 IU/l) [8] and the kinkajou (mean = 35 IU/l) [9].

Table 3.2 Biochemical reference data for Procyonidae.

Analyte (abbreviation)	Units, SI (conventional)	Raccoon [7] (*Procyon lotor*)	White-nosed Coatimundi [8] (*Nasua narica*)	Kinkajou [9] (*Potus flavus*)
Sample attributes		**Ħ ♂♀ all ages** ***n* > 70 or *[n]***	**Ħ ♂♀ all ages** ***n* > 70 or *[n]***	**Ħ ♂♀ all ages** ***n* > 60 or *[n]***
Data format		**95% CI, mean**	**95% CI, mean**	**95% CI, mean**
Alanine transferase (ALT)	IU/l	53–203, 111	105–456, 233	18–107, 51
Albumin (Alb)	g/l (g/dl)	14–45, 33 (1.4–4.5, 3.3)	16–41, 31 (1.6–4.1, 3.1)	29–46, 38 (2.9–4.6, 3.8)
Alkaline phosphatase (ALP)	IU/l	21–140, 63	10–94(34)	14–124, 52
Amylase	IU/l	0–6143, 3013 *[28]*	659–5346, 2259	383–5450, 3074 *[17]*
Aspartate (AST) aminotransferase	IU/l	43–170(84)	120–438, 265	90–316, 186
Blood urea nitrogen (BUN)	mmol/l (mg/dl)	2.9–12.5(6.8) (8–35, 19)	2.9–8.9(5.4) (8–25, 15)	1.1–11.8(4.3) (3–33, 12)
Calcium	mmol/l (mg/dl)	1.9–2.7, 2.3 (7.6–10.6, 9.0)	2.0–2.6, 2.3 (8.0–10.2, 9.0)	2.1–2.7, 2.3 (8.2–10.8, 9.3)
Carbon dioxide (tCO_2)	mmol/l = (mEq/l)	12.2–28.9, 20.3 *[21]*	7.2–24.3, 15.8 *[11]*	13.9–30.9, 22.6 *[24]*
Chloride	mmol/l = (mEq/l)	104–117 110	99–120, 110	96–116,105 *[56]*
Cholesterol	mmol/l (mg/dl)	2.93–10.3, 5.3 (113–398, 206)	2.69–11.8, 6.3 (104–455, 243)	1.6–3.9, 2.5 (62–152, 97) *[57]*
Creatine kinase (CK)	IU/l	22–1184, 358 *[67]*	490–4045, 1464	0–673, 317 *[8]*
Creatinine (Crea)	mmol/l (mg/dl)	27–124, 71 (0.3–1.4, 0.8)	44–150, 97 (0.5–1.7, 1.1)	18–88, 53 (0.2–1.0, 0.6)
Gamma (GGT) glutamyltransferase	IU/l	0–9, 4 *[29]*	8–53, 24	0–14, 6 *[21]*
Globulin (Glob)	g/l (g/dl)	25–62, 39 (2.5–6.2, 3.9)	26–57, 40) (2.6–5.7, 4.0)	27–54, 38 (2.7–5.4, 3.8)
Glucose (Glu)	Mmol/l (mg/dl)	1.8–8.3, 4.3 (32–149, 78)	2.28–9.44, 5.3 (41–170, 96)	2.8–10.9(5.7) (51–196[102])
Lactate (LDH) dehydrogenase	IU/l	0–1664, 966 *[11]*	—	0–370(168) *[4]*
Phosphorus	mmol/l (mg/dl)	1.0–2.5(1.6) (3.1–7.7[4.9])	0.9–2.8(1.6) (2.8–8.7[4.9])	1.0–2.6(1.7) (3.2–8.1[5.3])
Potassium	mmol/l = (mEq/l)	3.5–5.2(4.3)	3.4–5.7(4.3)	2.7–5.9(4.5) *[58]*
Sodium	mmol/l = (mEq/l)	138–154(145)	137–154(144)	133–152(141) *[58]*
Total bilirubin (Tbil)	mmol/l (mg/dl)	0.0–10.3, 3.42 (0.0–0.6, 0.2)	1.71–15.4, 6.8 (0.1–0.9, 0.4)	0.0–8.55, 3.42 (0.0–0.5, 0.2)
Total protein (TP)	g/l (g/dl)	59–86, 72 (5.9–8.6, 7.2)	55–83, 71 (5.5–8.3, 7.1)	61–91, 76) (6.1–9.1, 7.6)
Triglycerides	mmol/l (mg/dl)	0–0.6, 0.3 (0–54, 29) *[25]*	0–1.0, 0.5 (0–91, 44) *[51]*	0.1–0.6, 0.3 (4–54, 30) *[22]*

Gastrointestinal and Cardiac Biomarkers, Lipids, and Electrolytes

Published clinicopathologic data concerning gastrointestinal and cardiac analytes in procyonids does not appear extant. Reference data for lipids and electrolytes of procyonids are provided in Table 3.2.

Blood Proteins

A coati with pyometra and uterine adenocarcinoma experienced hyperglobulinemia of 5.63 mg/dl (reference data 4.49–5.05) [12]. Fibrinogen of a raccoon with eosinophilic myositis was 163 mg/dl [27]. Serum total protein is typically higher in males, and fluctuates seasonally with higher concentrations in autumn than in spring, correlating with body mass [31].

Blood Gases

Coatimundi lack collateral ventilation between pulmonary lobules, resulting in pulmonary arterial hypertension during hypoxia [32]. In the coati, ranges of various blood gas parameters have been measured, with blood pH of 7.29–7.4, venous PO_2 of 38–44 mmHg, and venous PCO_2 of 35–41 mmHg [33]. Bicarbonate values (mean ± SE) in the raccoon and kinkajou are 21 ± 0 mEq/l and 25 ± 4.2 mEq/l, respectively [2]. The bicarbonate range and mean mEq/l values of the white-nosed coati are 11.9–22.9 and 17.3 [8].

Vitamins, Minerals and Metals, Toxins

Vitamin D concentrations in procyonids are expected to fall within the normal range for mammalian species (24.96–74.88 nmol/l [10–30 mg/l]); in the red panda, serum 25-hydroxy vitamin D concentrations were increased (53.66–130.04 nmol/l [21.5–52.1 mg/l]) in animals affected by severe hyperostosis but with unchanged calcium and phosphorus concentrations [34]. Serum magnesium (mean ± SD mg/dl) was measured in the coati (2.01 ± 0.05) [28], raccoon (3.05 ± 0.07), and kinkajou (2.95 ± 0.35) [2].

Zinc and copper concentrations (range µl/dl) of three coatimundi were 11.8–16.6 and 1.7–2.08, respectively [35]. Reference iron concentrations in the raccoon are 71–231 µg/dl (mean 158) [7], and in the kinkajou animals sampled had average iron concentrations of 278 µg/dl [2]. Raccoons are relatively resistant to lead toxicosis, with experimental lead administration resulting in blood lead levels as high as 77.5 g/dl with no clinical signs or clinicopathologic alterations [36]. Lead sampling of wild raccoons showed exposure at levels as high as 17 µg/dl [37].

Hormones – Thyroid and Adrenal and Reproductive

In male raccoons, plasma testosterone concentration is higher (7.57 ± 3.42 ng/ml) in the winter compared to the summer (0.76 ± 0.13 ng/ml), coincident with the winter breeding season [38]. Raccoons have a low thyroxine secretion rate compared to other species [39]. Total thyroxine concentrations for the raccoon are 2.4 ± 0.4 µg/dl [2]. A raccoon with a functional thyroid adenoma had an increased total T4 of greater than 156 nmol/l, well above the canine reference interval of 11–60 nmol/l. Free T4 measured by equilibrium dialysis was 128 nmol/l, also well beyond the upper limit of the canine reference interval of 6–23 nmol/l [40]. Fecal glucocorticoid metabolites, validated by adrenocorticotropic hormone (ACTH) challenge in the raccoon, can measure physiological stress in raccoons, and increase after capture and other stressful stimuli [41]. Serum leptin concentrations, measured using canine leptin ELISA, were increased in autumn (3.46 ± 0.45 ng/ml) from the spring (0.71 ± 0.07 ng/ml), correlating with body condition [42].

Urinalysis

There is a paucity of published reference values of urine parameters in procyonids. A study performed on a small population of 24 wild raccoons used urine dipsticks to obtain qualitative urine values on free-caught samples [43]. All raccoon samples had proteinuria, and 33% had ketonuria. Urine pH was low (5.0–7.0) with most animals having a pH of 6.0. No glucosuria was detected in healthy wild-caught raccoons; however, glucosuria has been reported in a diabetic raccoon [29].

Bone Marrow

Bone marrow samples may be obtained from the femur immediately postmortem in raccoons [44]. Bone marrow collection from the procyonid patient should be similar to the approach for dogs. Bone marrow differentials of raccoons are similar to those of domestic Carnivora, although raccoons may have increased numbers of eosinophil progenitors, attributed to the higher parasite burden of free-living animals.

Cerebrospinal Fluid

Cerebrospinal fluid from a raccoon with eosinophilic myositis and *Sarcocystis* infection had nucleated cell counts and a lymphocytic and eosinophilic pleocytosis [27]. The cerebrospinal fluid sample discussed in this report was obtained postmortem within 15 min of euthanasia.

Serology and PCR

As members of the Carnivora, many assays designed for infectious disease detection or diagnosis in domestic animals may be useful in Procyonidae. However, most of these assays have not been validated for procyonids. In species of public health significance, such as raccoons, it is highly recommended to contact the laboratory prior to collecting and sending samples to obtain valid and appropriate results for the species and the owner, caretaker, or person who may have inadvertently contacted the animal. Assay results in these species may have serious public health consequences; thus, sample collection, handling, and shipping should be treated with appropriate care and attention.

Free-living raccoons in the United States are rabies vectors, therefore postmortem rabies testing is routinely performed in this species for public health purposes. Kansas State University Veterinary Diagnostic Laboratory offers antemortem rabies serum neutralization assays (rapid fluorescent foci inhibition test [RFFIT]); however, lack of antibody detection does not guarantee a rabies negative individual. Immunostaining on various tissues to detect rabies antigen is only 60% sensitive, and therefore direct immunofluorescence assay on fresh brain section postmortem remains the gold standard for diagnosis [45].

Serologic survey of free-ranging urban raccoons near a zoological garden found exposure for canine distemper virus in 54.1%, canine adenovirus-1 in 6.9%, feline parvovirus in 49.7%, and *Leptospira interrogans* in 15.2% of the population. Results varied by year as animals seroconverted. Hemagglutination inhibition was used for feline parvovirus, serum neutralization for canine distemper and adenovirus, and microagglutination assay titers for *Leptospira spp.* detection [46]. Immunohistochemistry staining can identify *Sarcocystis neurona* [47], and indirect immunofluorescent antibodies for *Trypanosoma cruzi* can identify Chagas disease in raccoons [48].

References

1 Beisiegel, B.M. (2001). Notes on the coati, *Nasua nasua* (Carnivora:Procyonidae) in an Atlantic forest area. *Brazilian Journal of Biology* 61 (4): 689–692.

2 Ramsay, E. (2015). Procyonids and viverids. In: *Fowler's Zoo and Wild Animal Medicine*, vol. 8 (ed. R.E. Miller and M.E. Fowler), 491–497. Elsevier Saunders.

3 Association of Zoos & Aquariums Small Carnivore Taxon Advisory Group (2010). *Procyonid (Procyonidae) Care Manual*, 114. Silver Spring, MD: Association of Zoos and Aquariums.

4 Kollias, G.V. and Abou-Madi, N. (2007). Procyonids and mustelids. In: *Zoo Animal and Wildlife Immobilization and Anesthesia*, 2e, vol. 9 (ed. G. West, D. Heard and N. Caulkett), 607–617.

5 Kreeger, T.J., Raath, J.P., and Arnemo, J.M. (2002). *Handbook of Wildlife Chemical Immobilization*. Wildlife Pharmaceuticals.

6 Burke, J.D. (1954). Blood volume in mammals. *Physiological zoology* 27 (1): 1–21.

7 Teare JA. 2013. *Procyon lotor* No selection by gender All ages combined Conventional American units 2013 CD. html in: ISIS Physiological Physiological Reference Intervals for Captive Wildlife: A CD-ROM Resource. International Species Information System, Eagan, MN. Accessed 8 February 2016.

8 Teare JA. 2013. *Nasua narica* No selection by gender All ages combined Conventional American units 2013 CD. html in: ISIS Physiological Physiological Reference Intervals for Captive Wildlife: A CD-ROM Resource. International Species Information System, Eagan, MN. Accessed 8 February 2016.

9 Teare JA. 2013. Potus flavus No selection by gender All ages combined Conventional American units 2013 CD. html in: ISIS Physiological Physiological Reference Intervals for Captive Wildlife: A CD-ROM Resource. International Species Information System, Eagan, MN. Accessed 8 February 2016.

10 Kennedy, A.H. (1935). Cytology of the blood of normal mink and raccoon: iii. Morphology and numbers of the blood elements in raccoon. *Canadian Journal of Research* 12 (4): 495–507.

11 Hawkey, C. (1977). The haematology of exotic mammals. In: *Comparative Clinical Haematology* (ed. R.K. Archer and L.B. Jeffcott), 103–160. Oxford: Blackwell Scientific Publications.

12 Chittick, E., Rotstein, D., Brown, T., and Wolfe, B. (2001). Pyometra and uterine adenocarcinoma in a melengestrol acetate–implanted captive coati (*Nasua nasua*). *Journal of Zoo and Wildlife Medicine* 32 (2): 245–251.

13 Hawkey, C.M. and Denett, T.B. (1989). *Color Atlas of Comparative Veterinary Hematology*, 192. Ames, IA: Iowa State University Press.

14 Rodrigues, A.F., Daemon, E., and Massard, C.L. (2007). Morphological and morphometrical characterization of gametocytes of *Hepatozoon procyonis* (Protista, Apicomplexa) from a Brazilian wild procionid *Nasua nasua* and *Procyon cancrivorus* (Carnivora, Procyonidae). *Parasitology Research* 100: 347–350.

15 Orihel, T.C. (1964). *Brugia guyanensis sp. n.* (Nematoda: Filarioidea) from the coatimundi (*Nasua nasua vittata*) in British Guiana. *Journal of Parasitology* 50 (1): 115–118.

16 Pung, O.J., Davis, P.H., and Richardson, D.J. (1996). Filariae of raccoons from Southeast Georgia. *Journal of Parasitic Diseases* 82 (5): 849–851.

17 Sauerman, D.M. Jr. and Nayar, J.K. (1985). Prevalence of presumed *Dirofilaria tenuis* microfilariae in raccoons near Vero Beach, Florida. *Journal of Parasitic Diseases* 71 (1): 130–132.

18 Snyder, D.E., Hamir, A.N., Hanlon, C.A., and Rupprecht, C.E. (1989). Dirofilaria immitis in a raccoon (Procyon lotor). *Journal of Wildlife Diseases* 25 (1): 130–131.

19 Olson, E.J., Conboy, G.A., Stromberg, B.E., and Hayden, D.W. (2011). Pulmonary trematodosis (Pharyngostomoides sp.) in a juvenile raccoon (Procyon lotor). *Journal of Veterinary Diagnostic Investigation* 23 (3): 560–564.

20 Silva, R.A., Victorio, A.M., Ramirez, L. et al. (1999). Hematological and blood chemistry alterations in coatis (*Nasua nasua*) naturally infected by *Trypanosoma evansi* in the Pantanal. *Brazil Revue Élev Méd vét Pays trop* 52 (2): 119–122.

21 Lewis, J.H. (1996). *Comparative Hemostasis in Vertebrates*. Springer Science & Business Media.

22 Jacobs, G.J. (1957). Blood values of two American carnivores. *Journal of Mammalogy* 38 (2): 261–262.

23 Langan, J., Bemis, D., Harbo, S. et al. (2000). Tyzzer's disease in a red panda (*Ailurus fulgens fulgens*). *Journal of Zoo and Wildlife Medicine* 31 (4): 558–562.

24 Wojcinski, Z.W. and Barker, I.K. (1986). Tyzzer's disease as a complication of canine distemper in a raccoon. *Journal of Wildlife Diseases* 22 (1): 55–59.

25 Potier, R. and Reineau, O. (2015). Obstructive cholelithiasis in a kinkajou (Potus flavus). *Journal of Zoo and Wildlife Medicine* 46 (1): 175–178.

26 Herrera, H.M., Alessi, A.C., Marques, L.C. et al. (2002). Experimental *Trypanosoma evansi* infection in South American coati (*Nasua nasua*): hematological, biochemical and histopathological changes. *Acta Tropica* 81: 203–210.

27 Hamir, A.N., Rupprecht, C.E., and Ziemer, E.L. (1989). Generalized eosinophilic myositis with eosinophilia of blood and cerebrospinal fluid in a raccoon (*Procyon lotor*). *Journal of Veterinary Diagnostic Investigation* 1: 192–194.

28 Rovirosa-Hernandez, M.J., Garcia-Orduna, F., Morales-Mavil, J.E. et al. (2012). Hematological and blood chemistry values in the semi-free population of white-nosed coatis (Nasua narica) in La Venta Tabasco, Mexico. *Acta Zoológica Mexicana* 28 (2): 391–400.

29 McCain, S., Kirk, C., and Ramsay, E. (2009). Transient type 2 diabetes mellitus in a raccoon (*Procyon lotor*). *Journal of Zoo and Wildlife Medicine* 39 (4): 622–625.

30 Yoshikawa, M.S., Tsuchiya, T., and Kadota, K. (1999). Pancreatic endocrine carcinoma with multiple hormone production in a raccoon (*Procyon lotor*). *Journal of Comparative Pathology* 120: 301–306.

31 Doyle, T.J., Hoff, G.L., and Bigler, W.J. (1975). Seasonal variations in total serum protein concentration in an estuarine raccoon population. *Journal of Wildlife Diseases* 11 (1): 58–61.

32 Hanson, W.L., Boggs, D.F., Kay, J.M. et al. (1993). Collateral ventilation and pulmonary arterial smooth muscle in the coati. *Journal of Applied Physiology* 74 (5): 2219–2224.

33 Grant, B.J., Davies, E.E., Jones, H.A., and Hughes, J.M. (1976). Local regulation of pulmonary blood flow and ventilation-perfusion ratios in the coatimundi. *Journal of Applied Physiology* 40 (2): 216–228.

34 Lynch, M., McCracken, H., and Slocombe, R. (2002). Hyperostotic bone disease in red pandas (*Ailurus fulgens*). *Journal of Zoo and Wildlife Medicine* 33 (3): 263–271.

35 Nicolier, A., Welle, M., Walzer, C., and Robert, N. (2005). Congenital follicular dysplasia in five related coatimundis (*Nasua nasua*). *Veterinary Dermatology* 16: 420–424.

36 Hamir, A.N., Lehmann, B., Raju, N. et al. (1999). Experimental lead toxicosis of raccoons (*Procyon lotor*). *Journal of Comparative Pathology* 120 (2): 147–154.

37 Hamir, A.N., Galligan, D.T., Ebel, J.G. et al. (1994). Blood lead levels of wild raccoons (*Procyon lotor*) from the eastern United States. *Journal of Wildlife Diseases* 30 (1): 115–118.

38 Okuyama, M.W., Shimozuru, M., Yanagawa, Y., and Tsubota, T. (2014). Changes in the immunolocalization of steroidogenic enzymes and the androgen receptor in raccoon (*Procyon lotor*) testes in association with the seasons and spermatogenesis. *Journal of Reproduction and Development* 60: 155–161.

39 Bauman, T.R., Clayton, F.W., and Turner, C.W. (1965). The l-thyroxine secretion rate, l-triiodothyronine equivalent, and biological half-life (t12) of l-thyroxine-I131 in the raccoon (*Procyon lotor*). *General and Comparative Endocrinology* 5 (3): 261–266.

40 Gardhouse, S., Eshar, D., Meindel, M.J. et al. (2014). Thyroid neoplasia in a raccoon (*Procyon lotor*). *Israel Journal of Veterinary Medicine* 69 (2): 102–106.

41 Monello, R.J., Millspaugh, J.J., Woods, R.J., and Gompper, M.E. (2010). The influence of parasites on faecal glucocorticoid metabolite concentrations in raccoons: an experimental assessment in a natural setting. *Journal of Zoology* 282: 100–108.

42 Shibata, H., Akahane, R., Honjoh, T. et al. (2005). Seasonal changes in serum leptin of the feral raccoon (*Procyon lotor*) determined by canine-leptin-specific ELISA. *Journal of Experimental Zoology Part A: Comparative Experimental Biology* 303 (7): 527–533.

43 Lotze, J.H. and Fleischman, A.I. (1978). The raccoon (*Procyon lotor*) on St. Catherine's island, Georgia. 1. Biochemical parameters of urine and blood serum. *American Museum Novitates* 2644: 1–5.

44 Strolle, L.A., Nielsen, S.W., and Diters, R.W. (1978). Bone marrow and hematologic values of wild raccoons. *Journal of Wildlife Diseases* 14: 409–415.

45 Dunbar, M.R. and MacCarthy, K.A. (2006). Use of infrared thermography to detect signs of rabies infection in raccoons (*Procyon lotor*). *Journal of Zoo and Wildlife Medicine* 37 (4): 518–523.

46 Junge, R.E., Bauman, K., King, M., and Gompper, M.E. (2007). A serologic assessment of exposure to viral pathogens and *Leptospira* in an urban raccoon (*Procyon lotor*) population inhabiting a large zoological park. *Journal of Zoo and Wildlife Medicine* 38 (1): 18–26.

47 Hamir, A.N. and Dubey, J.P. (2001). Myocarditis and encephalitis associated with *Sarcocystis neurona* in a raccoon (*Procyon lotor*). *Veterinary Parasitology* 95: 335–340.

48 Yabsley, M.J. and Noblet, G.P. (2002). Seroprevalence of Trypanosoma cruzi in raccoons from South Carolina and Georgia. *Journal of Wildlife Diseases* 38 (1): 75–83.

4

Skunks

Dennilyn Parker DVM, DABVP (Avian)[1], Frank J. Krupka DVM[2] and J. Jill Heatley DVM, MS, DABVP (Avian, Reptilian, Amphibian), DACZM[3]

[1] *Department of Small Animal Clinical Sciences, Western College of Veterinary Medicine, University of Saskatchewan, Saskatoon, Canada*
[2] *Avon Lake Animal Clinic, Avon Lake, Ohio, USA*
[3] *Department of Small Animal Clinical Sciences, College of Veterinary Medicine & Biomedical Sciences, Texas A&M University, College Station, Texas, USA*

Introduction

Striped skunks *(Mephitis mephitis)* are becoming popular exotic pets in some areas of North America. Free-living skunks of various species are used as sentinel species for disease surveillance in urban regions, as well as in other areas of research. The baseline data for clinical pathology in skunks is a useful starting point, for health assessment, although there is variation in the data between wild and socialized skunks. The use of chemical restraint may also lead to variations when compared to manual restraint. Most of the information in the literature is based on a small number of animals, and there is little data on how analytes change in disease conditions. Skunks belong to the family Mephitidae, and multiple species are found in North America (Table 4.1).

Restraint

Pet skunks are descented at a young age, which facilitates handling without sedation. Free-living skunks with intact scent glands should be captured in a trap or net. The handler should use a protective barrier as well as wearing goggles and protective clothing. During handling, the tail should be held ventrally against the body to help prevent the release of liquid from the anal sacs. Although immobilization is often necessary for sample collection from skunks, few published protocols exist. Tiletamine-zolazepam at 10 mg per skunk given intramuscularly (IM; average dose of 4.91 mg/kg) provided approximately 20 min of immobilization in wild striped skunks after preliminary immobilization with halothane [1]. Another source recommends Tiletamine-zolazepam IM at 10 mg/kg plus an additional 10 mg/kg ketamine IM if necessary [2]. An alternative protocol is 15 mg/kg ketamine IM plus 0.2 mg/kg acepromazine IM [2]. Isoflurane inhaled anesthesia administered via a face mask or in combination with an induction chamber is common practice in the clinic setting and has also been used with success in the field [3]. Use of sedation and muscle relaxant in drugs (alpha 2 agonists and benzodiazepines) in skunk species may lessen the chance of scent gland expulsion [4].

Sample Collection

The most common site for blood collection is the jugular vein (Figure 4.1). The skunk can be restrained with the forelimbs outstretched, the body stretched out, and the head slightly raised similar to cat positioning. The cranial vena cava can also be used. For this site, the skunk should be in dorsal recumbency with the forelimbs pulled caudally (Figure 4.2). At the point where the first rib meets the manubrium just to the left or right of midline, the needle should be directed toward the opposite hip at a 45° angle. Other sites for blood collection include the cephalic vein (Figure 4.3), the medial saphenous or femoral vein (Figure 4.4), and the lateral saphenous vein. Equipment used for venipuncture will vary depending on the animal size and weight as well as the venipuncture site, but 1–3 cm^3 syringe and 25–22 gauge (g.) needles are recommended.

The total blood volume of skunk remains uninvestigated, but it is presumed to be similar to or less than the domestic house cat. Thus, removal of less than 10–12 ml blood/kg of skunk is the maximum amount to be considered as a single sample in a healthy adult skunk. A lower sample volume amount (50% or less) is recommended in skunks which are debilitated, injured, or ill.

Exotic Animal Laboratory Diagnosis, First Edition. Edited by J. Jill Heatley and Karen E. Russell.

Table 4.1 North American skunk species.

Common name	Scientific name	Range, additional information
American hog-nosed skunk	*Conepatus leuconotus*	Southwest United States to Central America, largest North American species.
Hooded skunk	*Mephitis macroura*	Scrub and dry grasslands of SW United States and Central America, 4 subspecies
Striped skunk	*M. mephitis*	Southern Canada, most of the United States and parts of Northern Mexico, 13 subspecies
Eastern spotted skunk	*Spilogale putorius*	Eastern United States, small parts of Canada and Mexico
Plains spotted skunk	*S.p. interrupta*	Subspecies within ranges above
Appalachian spotted skunk	*S.p. putorius*	
Florida spotted skunk	*S.p. ambivarlis*	
Western spotted skunk	*Spilogale gracilis*	Western United States, Northern Mexico, and SW British Columbia, 7 subspecies
Island spotted skunk	*S. g. amphiala*	Subspecies of Western spotted skunk on the Channel Islands
Southern spotted skunk	*S. angustifrons*	Central America and Mexico
Pygmy spotted skunk	*S. pygmaea*	Mexico

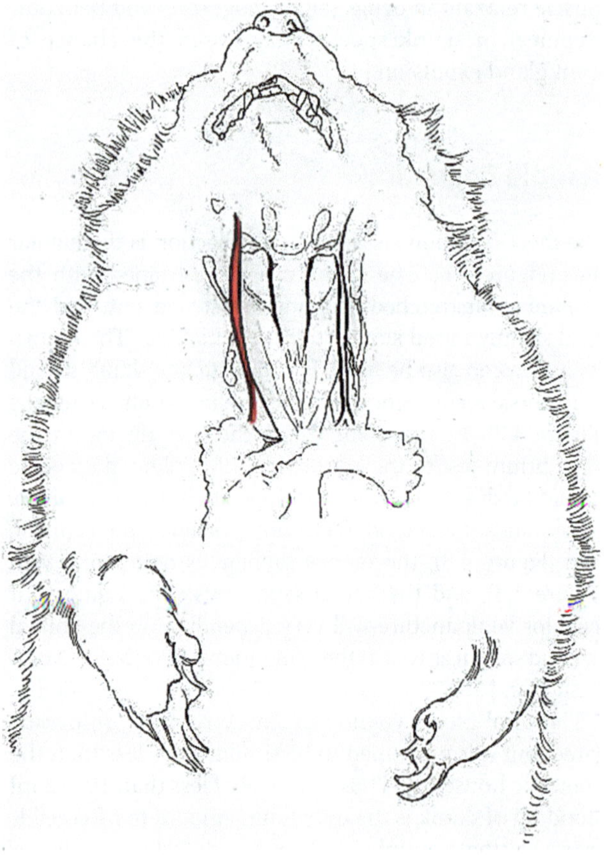

Figure 4.1 Location of the jugular vein in a striped skunk (*M. mephitis*). *Source:* Drawn from dissection courtesy of the Wildlife Center of Virginia.

Sample Handling

Sample handling is generally thought to be similar to that employed for small domestic mammals. Blood for a complete blood count should be submitted in EDTA, and blood for serum chemistries should be submitted without anticoagulant. Most of the chemistry reference intervals in this chapter are based on serum, although some references [5, 6] do not indicate whether the samples were serum or plasma. With small exotic pet mammals, we often use heparin as an anticoagulant and run chemistries on plasma to increase the yield in small samples. This is an option; however, there have been no studies on the differences in values between plasma and serum in skunks.

Specific Analytes

Complete Blood Count (CBC) is used to evaluate the blood cells in skunks as it is in other species. The results are similar to those in other small mammals. Variation between animals that are manually restrained and chemically restrained occurs; however, statistical analysis was not performed based on differing group methodology [7]. Blood cell morphology and presumed function in skunks are similar to those of domesticated mammals such as the cat (Figures 4.5–4.8). Hemoparasites of skunks include *Trypanosoma cruzii* and *Dirofilaria immitis* [8, 9].

Figure 4.2 Positioning of a striped skunk *(M. mephitis)* for blood collection from the cranial vena cava. *Source:* Dissection and photo courtesy of the Wildlife Center of Virginia.

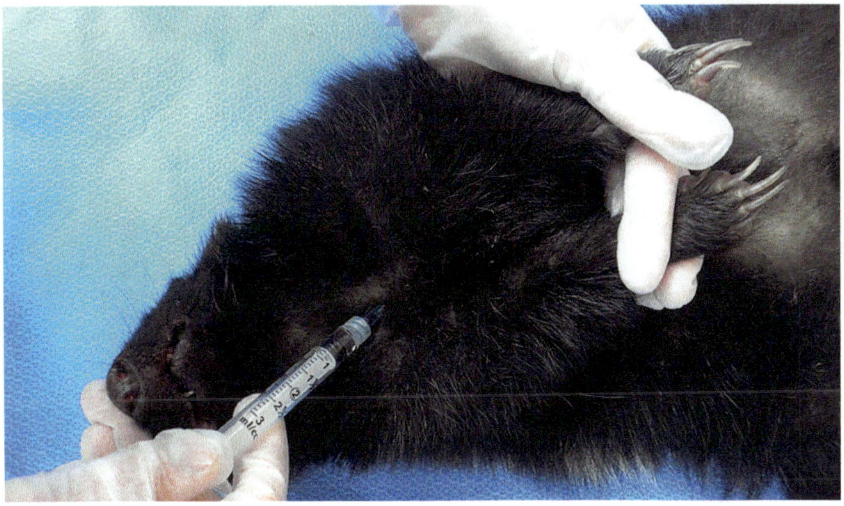

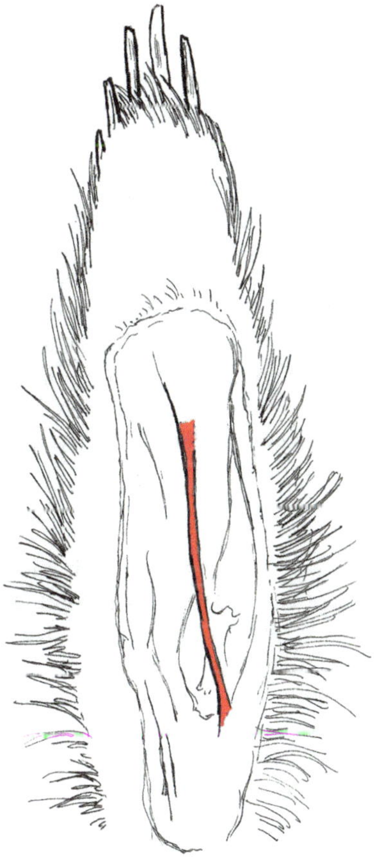

Figure 4.3 Course of the cephalic vein on the forelimb of a striped skunk *(M. mephitis)*. *Source:* Drawn from dissection courtesy of Wildlife Center of Virginia.

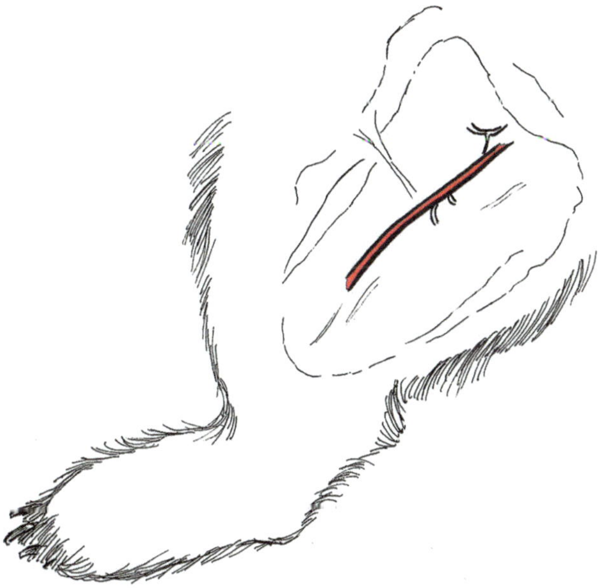

Figure 4.4 Course of the medial saphenous vein of a striped skunk *(M. mephitis)*. *Source:* Drawn from dissection courtesy of Wildlife Center of Virginia.

No information specific to hemostasis, blood types, or clotting factors for skunks is available in the literature. Anecdotally, skunk blood transfusions have been performed [10]. Hemoconcentration occurred in one skunk with Aleutian's disease on the basis of findings of increased hemoglobin 168 g/l (16.8 g/dl, 10.43 mmol/l) and mean corpuscular hemoglobin (21.01 pg) concentrations [9].

Biochemical Panel

The information on serum chemistry values in skunks is limited, and what is available is based on small numbers of animals (Table 4.2). Skunks with Aleutian disease can have a variety hematologic and biochemical abnormalities; however, animals may also have normal hematologic assessment and relatively unremarkable biochemical profiles [9].

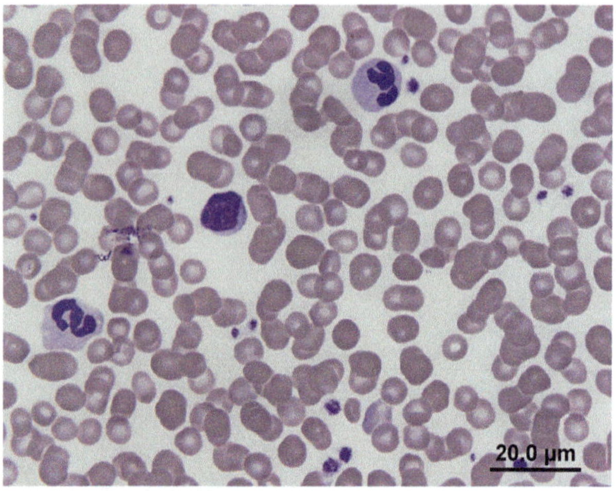

Figure 4.5 Photomicrograph of normal lymphocyte with two normal segmented neutrophils of a striped skunk *(M. mephitis)*. *Source:* Courtesy of Dr. M. Kerr (H&E, 100×).

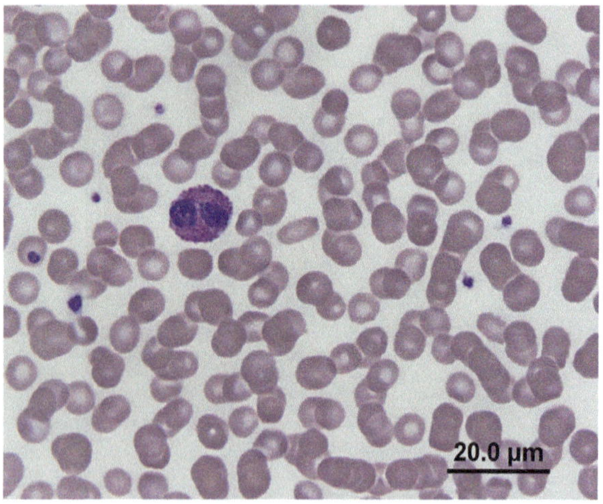

Figure 4.6 Photomicrograph of normal eosinophil of a striped skunk *(M. mephitis)*. *Source:* Courtesy of Dr. M. Kerr (H&E, 100×).

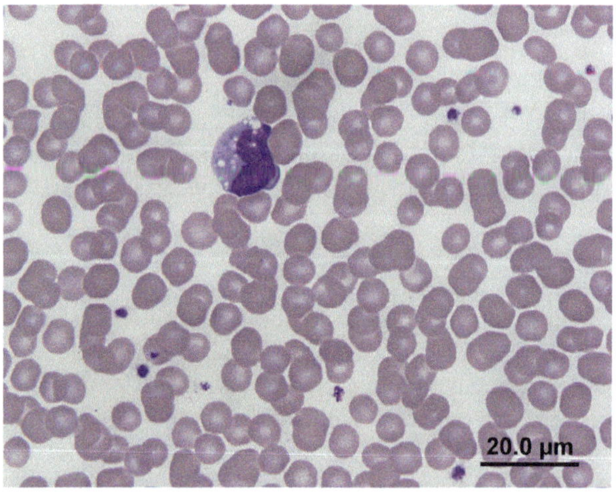

Figure 4.7 Photomicrograph of normal monocyte of a striped skunk *(M. mephitis)*. *Source:* Courtesy of Dr. M. Kerr (H&E, 100×).

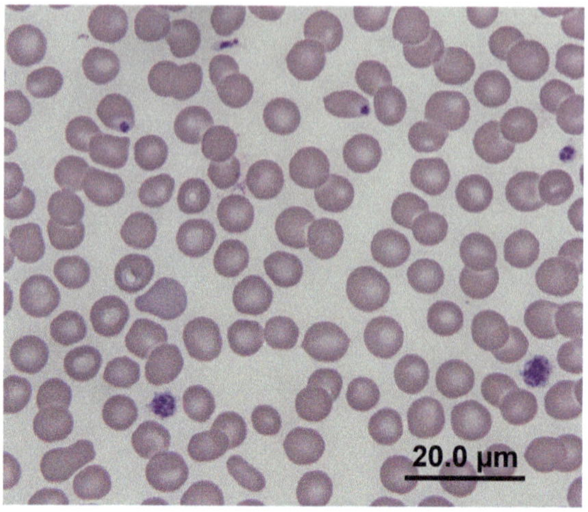

Figure 4.8 Normal blood smear of a striped skunk *(M. mephitis)* showing red blood cell morphology variation as well as variable sized platelets. *Source:* Courtesy of Dr. M. Kerr (H&E, 100×) *(polychromasia demonstrated in cell in lower middle part of the slide – looks like an ice cream cone)*.

Liver Enzymes

Increased aspartate aminotransferase (AST) activity (134 IU/l; reference interval: 47–124 IU/l) in one skunk and increased alkaline phosphatase (ALKP) activity (159 IU/l) in another skunk with Aleutian disease was suggestive of increased hepatocellular permeability and cholestasis, respectively [9]. In two cases of nutritional secondary hyperparathyroidism (NSHP) in captive skunks, biochemical abnormalities included increased plasma activities of the enzymes alanine amino transferase (ALT) and aspartate aminotransferase (AST) [12].

Muscle Enzymes

Wild animals tend to have higher stress levels, and increased struggling at capture, or longer trap confinement, may result in higher creatine kinase (CK) activity. Intramuscular injections can also increase CK activities compared to animals without injections that are more accustomed to handling. Increased AST activity has been reported in skunks afflicted with Aleutian's disease and nutritional secondary hyperparathyroidism [9, 12].

Renal Analytes

Azotemia has been associated with histologic renal lesions, likely due to leptospirosis, in free-living skunks [4]. In a report of a skunk with renal fibrous osteodystrophy, the blood urea nitrogen (BUN) was elevated at 37.8–40.3 mmol/l (106–113 mg/dl), as was the phosphorus 3.0 mmol/l (9.3 mg/dl) and creatinine 212 μmol/l (2.4 mg/dl), while the protein and calcium were 48 g/l (4.8 g/dl) and 2.02 mmol/l (8.1 mg/dl), respectively [13]. In another case report, typical kidney values increased with confirmed renal disease: urea nitrogen

Table 4.2 Hematological reference ranges for skunks.

Analyte (abbreviation)	Units, SI (US)	Striped skunk [5] (*M. mephitis*)	Spotted skunk [5] (*S. putorius*)	Eastern spotted skunk [11] (*Spilogale putorius interrupta*)[a]	Island spotted skunk [7] (*Spilogale gracilis amphiala*) [Free-living]		
Sample size, Attributes		**Variable Ħ**	**Variable Ħ**	**6**	**8–10 ₳ [Dry Season]**	**2–6 [Manual Restraint] [Spring/Rainy Season]**	**5–18 [Manual Restraint] [Dry Season]**
White blood cell count	$\times 10^9$/l ($\times 10^3$/µl)	6.939 ± 2.981	6.808 ± 3.915	10.03 [8.58–11.47]	8.54 ± 2.10	8.52 ± 2.84	8.82 ± 2.44
Absolute neutrophil	$\times 10^9$/l ($\times 10^3$/µl)	3.513 ± 1.928	2.121 ± 1.202		5.041 ± 1.850	5.788 ± 3.019	5.824 ± 2.146
Absolute bands	$\times 10^9$/l ($\times 10^3$/µl)	0.216 ± 0.315	0.043 ± 0.049				
Absolute lymphocytes	$\times 10^9$/l ($\times 10^3$/µl)	2.631 ± 1.499	3.965 ± 2.893		2.733 ± 0.951	1.874 ± 1.726	2.245 ± 1.434
Absolute monocytes	$\times 10^9$/l ($\times 10^3$/µl)	0.241 ± 0.167	0.166 ± 0.130		0.185 ± 0.112	0.311 ± 0.214	0.272 ± 0.199
Absolute eosinophil	$\times 10^9$/l($\times 10^3$/µl)	0.382 ± 0.442	0.561 ± 0.383		0.484 ± 0.419	0.414 ± 0.377	0.493 ± 0.337
Absolute basophil	$\times 10^9$/l($\times 10^3$/µl)	0.069 ± 0.050	0.075 ± 0.073			0.092 ± 0.031	0.134 ± 0.102
Relative neutrophil	%				58.22 ± 12.29	69.50 ± 26.38	63.72 ± 17.43
Relative lymphocytes	%				33.33 ± 11.42	22.17 ± 21.68	27.94 ± 15.11
Relative monocytes	%				2.38 ± 1.51	3.67 ± 2.50	3.06 ± 1.95
Relative eosinophil	%				5.13 ± 3.39	5.20 ± 4.92	5.35 ± 3.32
Relative basophil	%					1.00 ± 0.00	1.40 ± 0.89
Hematocrit	l/l (%)	0.380 ± 0.063 (38.0 ± 6.3)	0.393 ± 0.049 (39.3 ± 4.9)	0.4507 [0.4315–0.4699] (45.1 [43.2–47.0])	0.334 ± 0.045 (33.4 ± 4.58)	0.4615 ± 0.0228 (46.2 ± 2.2)	0.4376 ± 0.0370) (43.2 ± 3.7)
Hemoglobin	g/l g/dl	120 ± 17 (12.0 ± 1.7)	111 ± 12 (11.1 ± 1.2)	151.5 [144.7–158.3] (15.15 [14.47–15.83])	100.40 ± 8.5 (10.40 ± 0.85)	141.5 ± 9.9 (14.15 ± 0.99)	133.9 ± 10.7 (13.39 ± 1.07)
MCH	pg	15.7 ± 1.9			13.87 ± 0.56	13.87 ± 0.37	13.27 ± 0.58
MCHC	g/l g/dl	315 ± 28 (31.5 ± 2.8)	273 ± 27 (27.3 ± 2.7)		315.0 ± 28.4 31.50 ± 2.84	306.2 ± 11.3 30.62 ± 1.13	306.3 ± 9.5 30.63 ± 0.95
MCV	fl	50.0 ± 5.4			44.20 ± 4.57	45.50 ± 1.87	43.40 ± 1.92
RBC	$\times 10^{12}$/l ($\times 10^6$/µl)	7.70 ± 1.23		8.93 [8.88–8.93]	7.54 ± 0.78	10.20 ± 0.78	10.14 ± 1.05
Platelet count	$\times 10^9$/l($\times 10^3$/µl)	312.0 ± 120.0					

Animals were wild in origin but housed in a laboratory for several months [11].

Key: Free-living [Free-living], Captive Ħ, Pet ¥, Dry Season [Dry Season], Spring/Rainy Season [Spring/Rainy Season], Anesthetized ₳, Manual Restraint [Manual Restraint].

[a] All data presented as mean ± SD unless presented as mean [95% confidence interval].

38.6–66.8 mmol/l (108–220 mg/dl), creatinine 469–522 µmol/l (5.3–5.9 mg/dl), and total protein 87–88 g/l (8.7–8.8 g/dl) [14]. One skunk with Aleutian's disease suffered hyperphosphatemia, 2.81 mmol/l (8.7 mg/dl), possibly due to decreased glomerular filtration [9]. In two cases of secondary nutritional hyperparathyroidism in captive skunks, biochemical abnormalities included hyper- or hypoalbuminemia, hyperphosphatemia, and hypokalemia [12].

Pancreas

Derangements of glucose in captive pet skunks are anecdotally common and include hypoglycemic and diabetic syndromes likely associated with obesity, inappropriate diet, and limited exercise. Hypoglycemia, 2.05 mmol/l (37 mg/dl), was reported in one skunk with Aleutian's disease, possibly secondary to excess insulin release following pancreatic inflammation [9]. Mild hyperglycemia, 8.82 mmol/l (158 mg/dl), was described in one skunk with Nutritional Secondary Hyperparathyroidism (NSHP) and Vitamin D deficiency [9, 12].

Gastrointestinal, and Cardiac Biomarkers, Lipids, and Electrolytes

Few analytes have been reported specific to the gastrointestinal or cardiac systems of the skunk. Values reported or lipids and electrolytes are given in Table 4.3. Hypokalemia has been reported in one case of nutritional secondary hyperparathyroidism and Vitamin D deficiency [12].

Plasma proteins have been documented for apparently healthy and diseased skunks (Table 4.3). Skunks affected by Aleutian disease may have normoalbuminemia, hyperglobulinemia with 52, 74 g/l (5.2, 7.4 mg/dl) suggestive of antigenic stimulation, and a decreased A: G ratio (0.48, 0.51). Hyperproteinemia was also present in one case: 112 g/l (11.2 g/dl) [9]. In a report of a skunk with renal fibrous osteodystrophy, plasma protein was decreased to 48 g/l (4.8 g/dl) [13]. In another case report with confirmed renal disease in a skunk, total protein was 87–88 g/l (8.7–8.8 g/dl) [14]. In two cases of NSHP in captive skunks, biochemical abnormalities included hyper- or hypoalbuminemia [12].

Vitamins Mineral Metals and Toxins

Plasma vitamins, blood gases, and toxins have received little investigation in skunks. In NSHP in two skunks, Vitamin D deficiency was reported as 8 nmol/l (3.21 ng / ml) of 25-hydroxyvitamin D (25OHD$_3$). Ionized and non-ionized calcium were considered low in these cases and ranged from 0.55 to 0.83 mmol/l (2.2 to 3.32 mg/dl) and 1.12–1.60 mmol/l (4.48–6.4 mg/dl), respectively [12].

Hormones

Thyroid hormones have been investigated in a small number of captive pet skunks (Table 4.4). In two skunks with NSHP, parathyroid hormone (PTH3) levels were reported as 22.0 pmol/l and 30.1 pmol/l [12]. The striped skunk exhibits variable gestation periods with brief periods of delayed implantation occurring if females are mated early in the season, while the spotted skunk always exhibit a prolonged period of delayed implantation lasting several months [16]. Prolactin is the primary pituitary hormone causing increased luteal activity and blastocyst implantation in the spotted skunk, but the levels are correlated with progesterone [16, 17]. Mean plasma progesterone concentrations of pregnant spotted skunks given diluent or left untreated ranged from 0.47 to 2.52 nmol/l (1.5 to 8 ng/ml) over three months of gestation [18]. Prolactin trends seasonally in the western spotted skunk during preimplantation, with mean concentrations ranging from 5 ng/ml (5 µg/l, 217.4 pmol/l) during the period of short day length in January to 17.1 ng/ml (17.1 µg/l, 743.5 pmol/l) during the long day photoperiod in early May [17]. Melatonin administration delays the seasonal rise of prolactin and implantation [17].

Urinalysis

Urine specific gravity for the skunk has been reported for a skunk with renal fibrous osteodystrophy as 1.009 and in another skunk with confirmed renal disease as 1.030 but prior to treatment [13, 14]. Skunk urine pH is approximately 6.0 [19].

Serology and PCR

Skunks species may serve as vectors or sentinels for several infectious disease of public health importance [20–27]. Several serology tests have been used in skunks (Table 4.5). Skunks have been experimentally infected with *T. cruzii* and became serologically positive 24 days post inoculation by both direct and latex agglutination tests [20]. Infectious canine hepatitis can cause hepatitis in skunks as identified by virus neutralization [21]. Rotaviral diarrhea in skunks has been detected with commercial ELISA kits and confirmed with electron microscopy [22]. Free-living skunks have shown serological exposure to *D. immitis* and canine parovirus [8].

Table 4.3 Biochemical reference ranges for skunks.

Analyte (abbreviation)	Units, SI (US)	Striped skunk [5, 6, 15] (*M. mephitis*) Ħ			Spotted skunk [5] (*S. putorius*)	Eastern spotted skunk [11] (*Spilogale putorius interrupta*)		Island spotted skunk [7] (*Spilogale gracilis amphiala*)	
Sample size, attributes		**Variable**	**12**	**39 ¥**	**Variable Ħ**	**6 Ħ**	**12 ₳**	**6**	**18**
Albumin: Globulin ratio								0.82 ± 0.08	1.22 ± 0.48
Albumin	g /l(g/dl)	32 ± 7 (3.2 ± 0.7)	36 ± 3.1 3.6 ± 0.31	{27–37 (2.7–3.7)}	34 ± 5 (3.4 ± 0.5)	13.7 [11.9–15.5] (1.37 [1.19–1.55])	26.3 ± 0.9 (2.63 ± 0.09)	41.8 ± 4.3 (4.18 ± 0.43)	47.9 ± 9.9 (4.79 ± 0.99)
Alkaline phosphatase (ALP)	U/l (units/l)	53 ± 48	26 ± 16	{4.0–94}	97 ± 76		13.25 ± 5.56		
Alanine aminotransferase (ALT)	U/l (units/l)	134 ± 141	16 ± 7.2	{28–266}	68 ± 33		121.08 ± 25.69	215.67 ± 260.23	178.72 ± 115.67
Aspartate aminotransferase (AST)	U/l (units/l)	83 ± 42	30.0 ± 9.1	{55–155}	131 ± 23		333.00 ± 134.19	600.17 ± 295.87	611.06 ± 183.88
Amylase	U/l (units/l)	36.82 ± 20.35	430 ± 120		22.39 ± 7.215				
Calcium	mmol/l (mg/dl)	2.40 ± 0.25 (9.6 ± 1.0)	2.3 ± 0.1 9.2 ± 0.4	{2.16–2.63 (8.65–10.55)}	2.58 ± 0.18 (10.3 ± 0.7)	2.59 [2.48–2.71] (10.4 [9.94–10.86])	2.35 ± 0.11 9.43 ± 0.43	1.41 ± 0.29 5.65 ± 1.16	1.60 ± 0.32 6.42 ± 1.30
Chloride	mmol/l (mEq/l)	113 ± 5		{107–125}	114 ± 4	109.0 [103.81–114.19]	109.92 ± 2.23		
Cholesterol	mmol/l (mg/dl)	4.29 ± 1.81 (166 ± 70)	3.7 ± 0.9 (143 ± 35)	{2.72–4.42 (105–171)}	6.03 ± 1.37 (233 ± 53)	4.66 [4.06–5.26] (180.17 [156.81–203.53])	4.39 ± 0.70 (169.58 ± 26.98)	5.31 ± 0.59 (205.17 ± 22.87)	5.43 ± 0.75 (210.00 ± 28.90)
Creatine kinase (CK)	U/l (units/l)	481 ± 309	242 ± 111		218 ± 99		4883.42 ± 5994.71	8150.17 ± 13 961.59	3058.06 ± 3326.06
Creatinine	µmol/l (mg/dl)	71 ± 35 (0.8 ± 0.4)	59 ± 10 0.7 ± 0.1	{41–72 (0.46–0.82)}	27 ± 9 (0.3 ± 0.1)		21 ± 11 (0.24 ± 0.12)	86 ± 14 (0.97 ± 0.16)	68 ± 12 (0.77 ± 0.14)
Gamma glutamyltransferase	U/l (units/l)	4 ± 4			5 ± 3				
Globulin	g/l (g/dl)	35 ± 10 (3.5 ± 0.1)		{28.7–46.7 (2.87–4.67)}	41 ± 6 (4.1 ± 0.6)	62.1 [60.0–64.2] (6.21 [6.00–6.42])	50.0 ± 4.0 (5.00 ± 0.40)	51.5 ± 4.5 (5.15 ± 0.45)	42.2 ± 8.6 (4.22 ± 0.86)
Glucose	mmol/l (mg/dl)	5.88 ± 2.16 (106 ± 39)	4.5 ± 0.4 81 ± 7	{4.44–6.55 (80–118)}	6.77 ± 1.22 (122 ± 22)	10.56 [9.48–11.63] (190.2 [170.8–209.6])	3.59 ± 1.47 (64.75 ± 26.53)	3.27 ± 2.01 (58.83 ± 36.20)	7.54 ± 3.41 (135.89 ± 61.35)
Lactate dehydrogenase	U/l (units/l)	870 ± 810			240 ± 19				
Lipase	U/l (units/l)	144.6 ± 121.8							
Magnesium	mmol/l (mg/dl)	0.8 ± 0.2 (1.9 ± 0.5)			0.8 ± 0.1 (1.9 ± 0.3)				
Phosphorus	mmol/l (mg/dl)	1.81 ± 0.78 (5.6 ± 2.4)	1.4 ± 0.9 (4.3 ± 2.8)	{1.16–2.26 (3.6–7.0)}	1.49 ± 0.32 (4.6 ± 1.0)	1.97 [1.64–2.30] (6.09 [5.07–7.11])	1.12 ± 0.26 (3.46 ± 0.81)	2.61 ± 0.35 (8.07 ± 1.07)	2.14 ± 0.48 (6.64 ± 1.48)

(*Continued*)

Table 4.3 (Continued)

Analyte (abbreviation)	Units, SI (US)	Striped skunk [5, 6, 15] *(M. mephitis)* Ħ			Spotted skunk [5] *(S. putorius)*	Eastern spotted skunk [11] *(Spilogale putorius interrupta)*	Island spotted skunk [7] *(Spilogale gracilis amphiala)*		
Sample size, attributes		**Variable**	**12**	**39 ¥**	**Variable Ħ**	**6 Ħ**	**12 ₳**	**6 ✋ 🌧**	**18 ✋**
Potassium	mmol/l (mEq/l)	5.0 ± 0.5	4.4 ± 0.3	{4.5–5.5}	4.1 ± 0.3	5.8 [4.99–6.61]	4.18 ± 0.31	7.75 ± 0.69	7.12 ± 1.05
Sodium	mmol/l (mEq/l)	151 ± 6	143.1 ± 1.4	{147–157}	149 ± 3	146.32 [144.14–148.50]	146.75 ± 2.90	144.17 ± 2.40	145.06 ± 7.02
Bilirubin, total	µmol/l (mg/dl)	3 ± 3 (0.2 ± 0.2)	3.7 ± 1.4 0.2 ± 0.1	{1–4 (0.05–0.21)}	7 ± 5 (0.4 ± 0.3)	1 [0–4] (0.08 [0.0–0.22])	2 ± 1 (0.11 ± 0.03)	5 ± 2 (0.27 ± 0.12)	2 ± 2 (0.11 ± 0.12)
Protein, total	g/l(g/dl)	66 ± 11 (6.6 ± 1.1)	58 ± 1.8 5.8 ± 0.18	{59–80 (5.9–8.0)}	76 ± 6 (7.6 ± 0.6)		76.3 ± 4.1 (7.63 ± 0.41)	93.3 ± 7.9 (9.33 ± 0.79)	90.2 ± 8.4 (9.02 ± 0.84)
Triglyceride	mmol/l (mg/dl)	0.93 ± 0.67 (82 ± 59)			0.90 ± 0.44 (80 ± 39)				
Urea	mmol/l (mg/dl)	8.9 ± 5.4 (25 ± 15)	6.9 ± 2.3 (19 ± 6)	{5.2–10.4 (14.5–29.0)}	8.9 ± 3.9 25 ± 11)	6.6 [6.0–7.3] (18.5 [16.67–20.33])	9.0 ± 1.6 (25.08 ± 4.44)	15.3 ± 4.4 (42.83 ± 12.21)	10.6 ± 3.1 (29.67 ± 8.76)

Data presented as mean ± SD except when presented as {Range} or mean [95% confidence interval].
Free-living origin animals, laboratory housed for several months [11].
Key: Free-living, Captive Ħ, Spring/Rainy Season 🌧, Anesthetized ₳, Manual Restraint ✋, Pet ¥, Dry Season.

Table 4.4 Thyroid values for apparently healthy pet skunks (*M. mephitis*).

Analyte (abbreviation)	Units, SI (US)	Mean	95% CI	Sample number
Thyroxine, free (FT4) dialysis	pmol/l (ng/dl)	18.13 (1.4)	14.2–22.0 (1.1–1.7)	27
Thyroxine, total (TT4)	nmol/l (μg/dl)	50.3 (3.91)	40.7–59.9 (3.17–4.65)	28
Free triiodothyronine (FT3)	pmol/l (pg/dl)	5.9 (383)	5.2–6.7 (337–435)	22
Triiodothyronine, total (TT3)	nmol/l (ng/dl)	0.5 (32.5)	0.42–0.59 (27.27–38.31)	24

Data provided by Frank Krupka, DVM, via the diagnostic laboratory at Michigan State University Diagnostic Center for Population and Animal Health.

Table 4.5 Serologic and PCR tests used in skunks.

Serology	Samples and test information	Laboratory
Canine distemper	Antibodies detected with serum neutralization	Cornell University, College of Veterinary Medicine, Animal Health Diagnostic Center. Ithaca, New York 14853–6401 Phone: (607) 253–3900 Fax: (607) 253–3943 Email: diagcenter@cornell.edu Website: http://ahdc.vet.cornell.edu/sects/serol/
Canine parvovirus	Antibodies detected with hemagglutination inhibition	
Leptospira interrogans	Microscopic agglutination microtiter	Illinois College of Veterinary Medicine Veterinary Diagnostic Laboratory, 2001S Lincoln Ave. PO Box U, Urbana IL 61802 6199 Phone: 217–333-1620 Fax: 217–244-2439 Texas A&M Veterinary Medical Diagnostic Laboratory Website: http://tvmdl.tamu.edu/
Sarcocystis neurona	Agglutination (SAT)	Center for Molecular Medicine and Infectious Diseases, Virginia–Maryland Regional College of Veterinary Medicine, Virginia Tech (0342)1410 Prices Fork Rd. Blacksburg, Virginia 24061 (540) 231–6377 Website: http://www.vetmed.vt.edu/research/cmmid/index.asp
Rotavirus	ELISA, confirmed EM	Commercial ELISA test kit (Rotazyme, Abbott Laboratories, North Chicago, Illinois 60664, USA)
Toxoplasma gondii	Modified direct agglutination	Illinois College of Veterinary Medicine Veterinary Diagnostic Laboratory, 2001S Lincoln Ave. PO Box U, Urbana IL 61802 6199 Phone: 217–333-1620 Fax: 217–244-2439
Tularemia (*Francisella tularensis*)	Microagglutination	
PCR	**Samples**	**Lab**
Aleutian disease virus	DNA extract from the heart, liver, lungs, and spleen	Research Technology Support Facility of Michigan State University. Plant Biology Laboratories, 612 Wilson Road, Genomics Core, Rm S-18 East Lansing, MI 48824. Phone: 517–432-9814 Email: gtsf@msu.edu Website: http://rtsf.msu.edu/contact.html

Source: From Refs. [4, 6, 8, 14, 20].

References

1 Lariviere, S. and Messier, F. (1996). Immobilization of striped skunks with Telazol. *Wildlife Society Bulletin* 24 (4): 713–716.
2 Kreeger, T. (1996). *Handbook of Wildlife Chemical Immobilization*, 219. Laramie, Wyoming: International Wildlife Veterinary Services Inc.
3 Kocer, C.J. and Powell, L.A. (2009). A field system for Isoflurane anesthesia of multiple species of Mesopredators. *The American Midland Naturalist* 161 (2): 406–412.
4 Crowell, W.A., Stuart, B.P., and Adams, W.V. (1977). Renal lesions in striped skunks (*Mephitis mephitis*) from Louisiana. *Journal of Wildlife Disease* 13: 300–303.
5 Species 360 (Previously ISIS (International Species Information Systems)) Reference Ranges for Physiological Values in Captive Wildlife CD-ROM, 2002 ed.
6 Kramer, M.H. and Lennox, A. (2003). What veterinarians need to know about skunks. *Exotic DVM* 5 (1): 36–39.
7 Crooks, K.R., Garcelon, D.K., Scott, C.A. et al. (2003). Hematology and serum chemistry of the Island spotted skunk on Santa Cruz Island. *Journal of Wildlife Diseases* 39 (2): 460–466.
8 Bakker, V.J., Van Vuren, D.H., Crooks, K.R. et al. (2006). Serologic survey of the ISLAND spotted skunk on Santa Cruz Island. *Western North American Naturalist* 66 (4): 456–461.
9 Pennick, K.E., Lattimer, K.S., Brown, C.A. et al. (2007). Aleutian disease in two domestic striped skunks (*Mephitis mephitis*). *Veterinary Pathology* 44 (5): 687–690.
10 Skunk Haven web page http://www.skunkhaven.net/VetCare4.htm. Accessed Dec 17, 2012.
11 Heidt, G.A. and Hargraves, J. (1974). Blood chemistry and hematology of the spotted skunk, Spilogale putorius. *Journal of Mammalogy* 55 (1): 206–208.
12 Hanley, C.S., Wilson, G.H., and Divers, S. (2004). Secondary nutritional hyperparathyroidism associated with vitamin D deficiency in two domestic skunks *(Mephitis mephitis). Veterinary Record* 155: 233–237.
13 Heard, D.J., Cantor, G.H., and Hager, D. (1986). Osteosclerosis in a skunk with renal fibrous Osteodystrophy. *JAVMA* 189 (9): 1162–1163.
14 Allender, M.C., Schumacher, J., Thomas, K.V. et al. (2008). Infection with Aleutian disease virus-like virus in a captive striped skunk. *JAVMA* 232 (5): 742–746.
15 Smart, N.L. (1990). Serum biochemical values in the skunk. *Canadian Veterinary Journal* 31 (3): 223.
16 Mead, R.A. (1981). Delayed implantation in mustelids, with special emphasis on the spotted skunk. *Journal of Reproduction and Fertility* 29: 11–24. Supplement.
17 Kaplan, J.B., Berria, M., and Mead, R.A. (1991). Prolactin levels in the western spotted skunk: changes during pre- and Periimplantation and effects of melatonin and lesions to the anterior hypothalamus. *Biology of Reproduction* 44: 991–997.
18 Berria, M., Joseph, M.M., and Mead, R.A. (1989). Role of prolactin and luteinizing hormone in regulating timing of implantation in the spotted skunk. *Biology of Reproduction* 40: 232–238.
19 Rivera, S. (2010). Chapter 17: Skunks. In: *Exotic Animal Medicine for the Veterinary Technician*, 2e (ed. B. Ballard and R. Cheek), 263. Hoboken, NJ: Wiley-Blackwell.
20 Davis, D.S., Russell, L.H., Adams, L.G. et al. (1980). An experimental infection of *Trypanosoma cruzi* in striped skunks *(Mephitis mephitis). Journal of Wildlife Diseases* 16 (3): 403–406.
21 Karstad, L., Ramsden, R., Berry, T.J., and Binn, L.N. (1975). Hepatitis in skunks caused by the virus of infectious canine hepatitis. *Journal of Wildlife Diseases* 11: 494–496.
22 Evans, R.H. (1984). Rotavirus-associated diarrhea in young raccoons *(Procyon lotor)*, striped skunks *(Mephitis mephitis)* and red foxes *(Vulpes vulpes). Journal of Wildlife Disease* 20 (2): 79–85.
23 Berrada, Z.L., Goethert, H.K., and Telford, S.R. (2006). Raccoons and skunks as sentinels for enzootic tularemia. *Emerging Infectious Diseases* 12 (6): 1019–1021.
24 Cheadle, M.A., Yowel, C.A., Sellon, D.C. et al. (2001). The striped skunk *(Mephitis mephitis)* is an intermediate host for Sarcocystis neurona. *International Journal for Parasitology* 31: 843–849.
25 Gehrt, S.D., Kinsel, M.J., and Anchor, C. (2010). Pathogen dynamics and morbidity of striped skunks in the absence of rabies. *Journal of Wildlife Diseases* 46 (2): 335–347.
26 Mitchell, S.M., Richardson, D.J., Cheadle, A.M. et al. (2002). Prevalence of agglutinating antibodies to Sarcocystis neurona in skunks *(Mephitis mephitis)*, raccoons *(Procyon lotor)*, and opossums *(Didelphis virginiana)* from Connecticut. *Journal of Parasito* 88 (5): 1027–1029.
27 Norman, L., Brooke, M.M., Allain, D.S., and Gorman, G.W. (1959). Morphology and Virulence of Trypanosoma cruzi-Like Hemoflagellates isolated from Wild Mammals in Georgia and Florida. *Journal of Parasitology* 45 (4): 457–463.

5

Rabbits

Barbara L. Oglesbee DVM, DABVP (Avian)

Medvet Hilliard, Columbus, Ohio, USA

Introduction

Rabbits have become increasingly popular as companion animals. With this popularity, pet owners demand the same level of diagnostic investigation and medical treatment as they would for cats and dogs. As prey species, rabbits instinctively hide signs of illness. Therefore, clinical pathology is especially important in diagnosing disease. Collection of diagnostic samples and interpretation of results differ in rabbits as compared to other companion species, as discussed within this chapter. Although many commercial laboratories accept samples from rabbits, there is little published data for companion rabbits. Rabbits have long been used in laboratory research, and most reference values are based on results collected from laboratory species. Laboratory animal populations used in the development of reference intervals were of the same breed, often the same gender, and kept under identical housing conditions and diet. Husbandry and breed may affect analyte values in pet rabbits differently than in laboratory animals. Most published reference intervals for rabbit blood parameters are based on laboratory or production animals, where groups are maintained under identical conditions. Husbandry practices vary widely for pet rabbits, and thus far, how husbandry affects blood parameters remains largely undocumented.

Species

Laboratory and companion rabbits are lagomorphs of the species *Oryctolagus cuniculus* and descendants of the European wild rabbit. Breed differences in size, conformation of the face, and pinnae can be pronounced. The American Rabbit Breeders Association recognizes more than 50 breeds. Large breeds, which range in weight from 7 to 10 kg, include the giant chinchilla and the Flemish giant. Medium breeds, ranging from 2 to 6 kg, include species commonly used as laboratory animals, such as the New Zealand white and Californian. Small breeds are popular as pets and range from 1 to 2 kg, and include the lop-eared and miniature breeds. There are many other species of lagomorphs, worldwide, but this chapter will concentrate on the domestic rabbit.

Sample Collection

Restraint

In rabbits, the level of stress inflicted during restraint is a uniquely important consideration. As a prey species, rabbits are easily frightened in unfamiliar settings such as a veterinary clinic, and may respond with an exaggerated catecholamine response. Under severely stressful circumstances, the release of catecholamines can result in cardiac arrest [1]. Proper restraint is essential, as rabbits have a lightweight skeleton but powerful rear limbs that predispose to spinal injury. Injury is most likely to occur if the front half of the body is firmly restrained, but the rear limbs are able to kick. Covering the eyes may relax the animal. In the fractious or painful rabbit, sedation or anesthesia should be considered to facilitate venipuncture and other sample collection. A combination of midazolam and buprenorphine is usually sufficient, but some particularly fractious animals, or for more invasive sample collection such as urethral catheterization, some rabbits may require additional administration of isoflurane or sevoflurane gas. Fasting prior to anesthesia or sedation to avoid vomiting and or aspiration is not necessary in the rabbit, but withholding food and water to decrease materials in the mouth and oropharynx and increase the likelihood of a clear respiratory pathway is recommended.

Exotic Animal Laboratory Diagnosis, First Edition. Edited by J. Jill Heatley and Karen E. Russell.

Venipuncture Sites and Positioning

Preferred venipuncture sites include the lateral saphenous vein, the cephalic vein, and jugular vein. Because of the small size of many popular pet breeds, venipuncture can be challenging. The author prefers the lateral saphenous vein, as it is easy to locate and can be accessed with minimal stress and discomfort to the patient. To access the lateral saphenous vein, the rabbit is restrained in sternal recumbency with its head tucked between the restrainer's elbow and body. The rear leg is extended and the vessel occluded by encircling the leg proximal to the stifle joint (Figure 5.1). Alternatively, the rabbit can be restrained in ventral recumbency, with the leg extended over the back of a table. The vein is superficial and can be visualized after wetting the fur with alcohol. If necessary, the fur overlying the vein can be plucked or clipped. The vein is most visible running approximately midline over the mid-tibial region, and then curving caudally at the level of the stifle joint (Figure 5.2). Avoid collapsing the vein by collecting blood slowly using a 1 or 3 ml syringe and 25 gauge (g.) needle. Hematoma formation is common following collection, and can be minimized by applying a temporary pressure wrap.

The cephalic vein is less preferable, as hematoma formation is common, and this vein is usually reserved for indwelling catheter placement. To access the cephalic vein, restraint is similar to that in other small mammals. Hold the rabbit in sternal recumbency, and occlude the vessel by encircling the limb at the elbow. In small breed rabbits, the short antebrachium may make occlusion of the vein difficult. Visualize by moistening with alcohol, plucking, or shaving as needed.

The jugular vein may be used if larger blood samples are needed. However, restraint in the nonsedated patient requires extending the head upward. This positioning of the head may cause dyspnea, or result in respiratory arrest in rabbits with preexisting respiratory disease or those that are severely stressed. Rabbits are obligate nasal breathers with the epiglottis normally positioned dorsal to the soft palate. Extending the head upward can alter the position of the epiglottis, leading to respiratory distress. Additionally, a large dewlap in female rabbits, or subcutaneous fat in obese rabbits, may make locating the vein difficult. However, based on vessel anatomy and the small size of the rabbit internal jugular vein, the external jugular vein is quite large compared to that of similar sized cat. Blood collection from the jugular vein of the nonsedated rabbit is performed in a manner similar to that of the cat, with the rabbit restrained at the edge of a table, head extended upward and front legs pulled down (Figure 5.3). Alternatively, the sedated rabbit may be restrained in dorsal recumbency at the edge of a table with its front legs pulled caudally and head tipped slightly toward the floor.

The marginal ear veins and central ear artery may be used to collect blood in large-breed pet rabbits, and is commonly used in laboratory settings. For small breeds, short-eared breeds or other pet rabbits, avoid this technique, which may result in bruising of the ear, thrombosis of the vessel with subsequent avascular necrosis, and skin sloughing. Laboratory rabbits, especially the New Zealand white, have large ears and vessels that are easily visualized, and cosmetic aspects of bruising are of less concern, making this technique more appropriate in a laboratory setting. Numerous techniques for collection from the ear have been described. Application of a topical anesthetic cream to the area 30 min prior to venipuncture aids collection by minimizing patient movement and resultant laceration of the vein. The

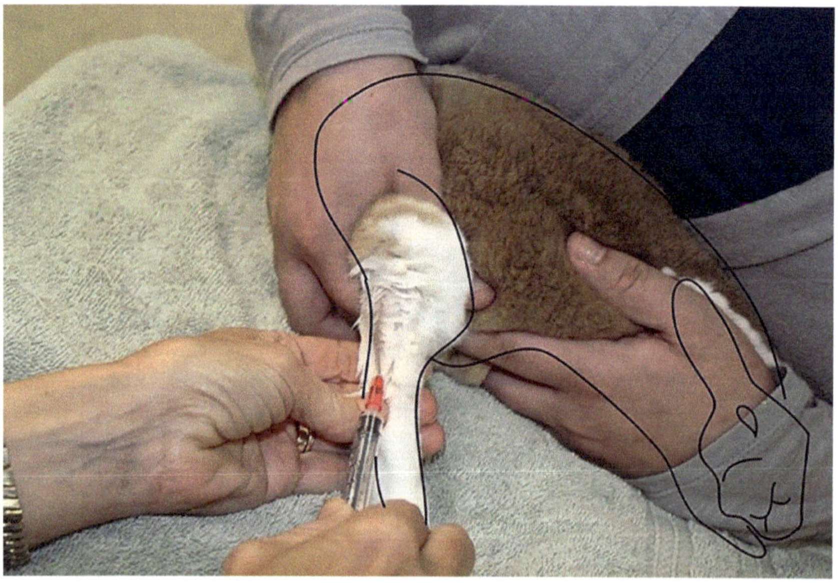

Figure 5.1 Restraint method for lateral saphenous venipuncture in the rabbit.

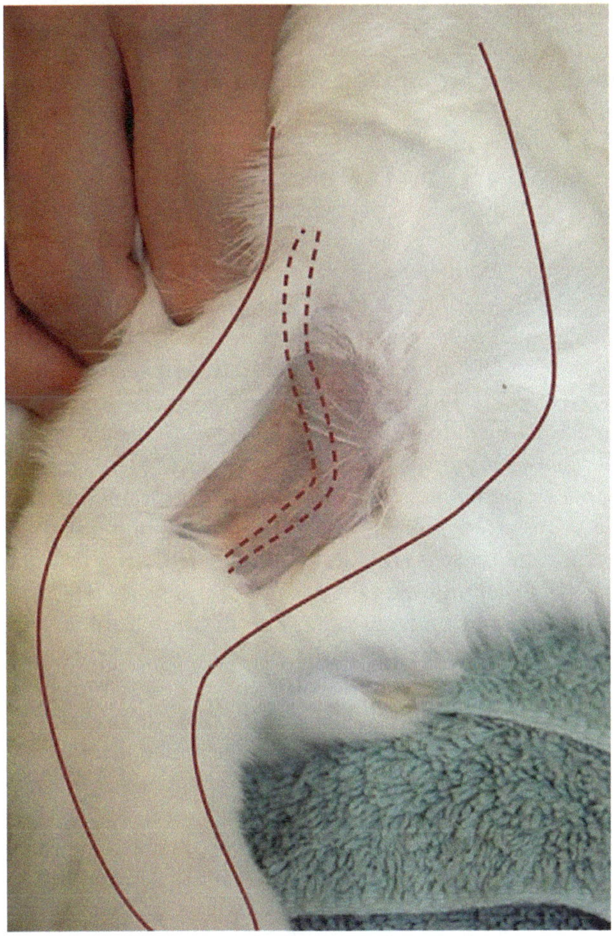

Figure 5.2 Lateral saphenous vein of the rabbit.

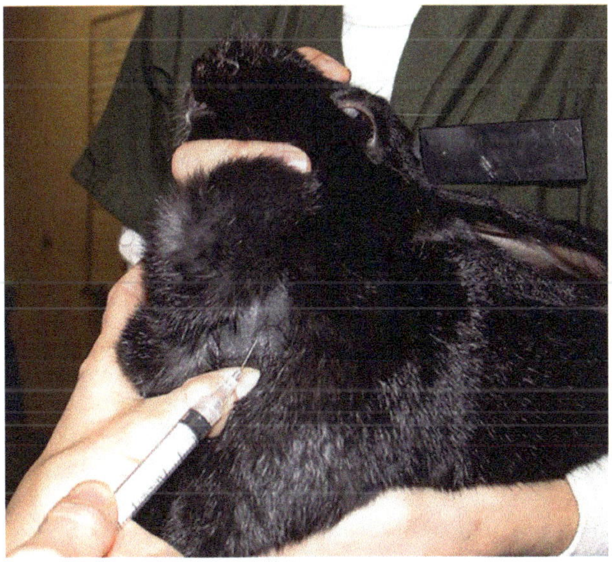

Figure 5.3 Jugular venipuncture of the rabbit.

patient should be securely restrained, wrapped in a towel. Avoid application of alcohol to the ear, which will cause peripheral vasoconstriction, making access difficult. If needed, the fur can be plucked or shaved. Warming the ear prior to collection with warmed towels, rice socks, or warm water bags fashioned from exam gloves dilates the vessels. Position the warming device under the pinna to stabilize the ear. To access the marginal veins, which run along the periphery of the pinna, insert a 25–26 g. needle through the skin next to the vein, then into the vein itself to minimize hematoma formation. Depending on the size of the rabbit, 0.5–5 ml can be collected from these veins.

The central ear artery is easier to access, but more prone to hematoma formation. Sedation or anesthesia is recommended for this technique. In large or giant breeds, a 21 to 22 g. butterfly catheter can be used to collect up to 30–40 ml of blood. The artery is superficial, and gentle traction on the pinna will aid in stabilization of the vessel. Insert the needle in a distal to proximal direction into the artery. After withdrawing the needle, apply firm pressure to the venipuncture site for several minutes to avoid hematoma formation.

Maximum Safe Sample Volume

Rabbits vary in size from 1 to 2 kg in dwarf breeds to over 10 kg in large breeds such as the Flemish giant. The total blood volume is 4.5%–8.1% of the total body weight, or approximately 57–78 ml/kg. Up to 6–10% of the blood volume, or 3.3–6.5 ml/kg, may be safely collected from healthy rabbits. Rabbits regenerate red blood cells quickly, and laboratory New Zealand white rabbits have been bled repeatedly as much as 6–8 ml/kg/week without adverse effects [2].

Sample Handling

Rabbit erythrocytes lyse easily, and rabbit blood clots quickly at room temperature. To avoid sample collection artifacts, use 23–25 g. needles with an attached 1–3 ml syringe, as larger syringes may collapse the vein. To avoid hemolysis during transfer to the collection tube, remove the needle used for collection prior to adding the sample to the tube. Hemolysis may increase serum potassium, and phosphorus concentrations can be artifactually increased because of erythrocyte release [3, 4]. Clotting may artifactually increase lactate dehydrogenase (LDH), aspartate transaminase (AST), creatinine kinase, total protein, potassium, and may affect hematology results. To prevent clotting, the needle and syringe may be coated with heparin by drawing a small amount into the needle and syringe, then expelling it back into the bottle. Detach the needle, fill the syringe with air, and then forcefully expel the residual heparin from the needle. The remaining small amount of heparin will not alter hematologic parameters [5]. To avoid artifactual changes in cell morphology due to contact with anticoagulants, make several air-dried blood smears at the time of venipuncture for manual cell counts. Rabbit erythrocytes are small in size, and variable diameters may cause problems with some automated flow cytometers; manual cell counts may be more accurate. Place the remaining blood in ethylenediaminetetraacetic acid (EDTA) tubes for complete blood cell (CBC) counts and red top or lithium heparin tubes for biochemical analysis. If only a small volume of blood is collected, one lithium heparin tube can be used for both CBC and biochemical evaluation. Prevent dilution by using tubes appropriate for the sample size, such as BD Microtainer collection tubes (BD, Franklin Lakes, New Jersey). Adequate data can be obtained for CBC from EDTA-preserved blood samples if stored at ambient temperature for up to 48 h [6].

Complete Blood Count

Erythrocytes

The rabbit erythron is anucleate, round, and biconcave, with an average diameter of 6.7–6.9 μm. The life span of the rabbit red blood cell (RBC) is short, ranging from 45 to 70 days (average 57 days) [3, 7]. Because of this short life span, findings that would indicate regenerative anemia in other mammalian species, such as anisocytosis, polychromasia, and occasional nucleated RBCs or Howell–Jolly bodies, occur in healthy rabbits (Table 5.1). Anisocytosis of 1%–2% is seen, and RBCs vary in diameter from 5.0 to 7.8 μm. Polychromasia ranging from 2% to 4% or reticulocyte counts between 1.4% and 3.9% are also common in healthy rabbits [1, 3, 4]. Although occasional nucleated RBCs occur in the blood of healthy rabbits, large numbers may indicate endothelial damage, as with acute infectious processes and septicemia [10, 11]. Rouleaux formation, platelet clumping, RBC fragments, and poikilocytes often result from poor sample preparation and generally do not indicate a pathologic process in the rabbit patient.

Rabbit age, gender, and reproductive status may cause variation in erythrocyte numbers. Young or newborn rabbits have lower PCV and RBC counts, with a higher mean corpuscular volume (MCV) and mean corpuscular hemoglobin (MCH) as compared to adults, while healthy pregnant does show no differences in erythrocytes as compared to non-pregnant rabbits [12]. Males have a significantly higher hemoglobin concentration and PCV values than do females [13]. Rabbits housed outdoors with natural diets have higher PCV, RBC counts, hemoglobin values, and lymphocyte counts, as compared to those that are caged, on commercial diets, and those with dental disease [14]. Cold stress may also cause increased RBC counts and PCV, along with increased total plasma protein, platelets, and decreased in serum albumin [15].

A PCV greater than 45%–50% is seen with dehydration [5, 6]. Although the PCV reference range for laboratory rabbits is 30%–50%, pet rabbits' PCV is approximately 10% lower [3]. Regenerative anemia due to blood loss is characterized by a rapid, marked reticulocytic response [3]. Common causes include trauma and uterine hemorrhage due to endometrial disease. Chronic blood loss may be seen with heavy flea infestation or urinary tract disease [3, 5]. Other types of internal bleeding, such as intestinal bleeding, are rare in rabbits [3]. Intravascular hemolysis is rare, but has occurred due to Solanaceae (potato, night shade) ingestion. Heinz body anemia has been reported following ingestion of *Alliums* (onions, garlic, and chives) [16]. Autoimmune hemolytic anemia occurs in laboratory rabbits with lymphosarcoma [17] and following endocarditis [18]. Lead poisoning can cause regenerative anemia, characterized by nucleated RBCs, hypochromasia, poikilocytosis, and cytoplasmic basophilic stippling [3].

Nonregenerative anemia is characterized by insufficient bone marrow production of erythrocytes, resulting in circulation of RBCs that are normal in appearance, and is associated with chronic disease processes. Common causes in rabbits include uterine disease (adenocarcinoma, endometrial hyperplasia, pyometra), dental disease, neoplasia, chronic renal failure, or other chronic metabolic disease [5, 10, 19]. Bacterial infections, such as osteomyelitis, dental, or other abscesses, pododermatitis, otitis media, sinusitis, pneumonia, mastitis, and bacterial cellulitis are common chronic diseases in pet rabbits which tend to result in nonregenerative anemia [20]. Additionally, lymphoscarcoma, experimentally induced septicemia, and streptococcal endocarditis can also cause nonregenerative anemias [11, 21, 22].

Leukocytes

Heterophils

The most common granulocyte in rabbits is the heterophil (Table 5.1) (Figure 5.4) [23–25]. The function of the heterophil is primarily phagocytic, and the cells contain acidophilic or eosinophilic cytoplasmic granules. Because of this, novices may misidentify them as eosinophils, and they are sometimes referred to as "pseudoeosinophils" or "amphophils" in the literature. Heterophils are slightly smaller than eosinophils, ranging from 10 to 15 μm in diameter, as compared to eosinophils, which measure 12–16 μm. Cytoplasmic granules of heterophils are smaller than those of eosinophils, vary in size and staining characteristics, and may incompletely occupy the cytoplasm. Heterophil cytoplasmic granules vary in size

Table 5.1 Hematologic reference ranges of lagomorphs.

Analyte (abbreviation)	Units, SI [conventional]	Domestic rabbits [2]	New Zealand white rabbits [8]		European brown hares [9]	
Data format		**Range**	**Range**	**Range**	**Mean ± SD (Range)**	**Mean ± SD (Range)**
Animals sampled			**12 ♂**	**14 ♀**	**21 Ó**	**27 ₪**
White blood cell (WBC) count	$\times 10^9$/l = [$\times 10^3$/µl]	5.2–12.5	4.2–12.3	4.4–13.2	3.49 ± 1.24	3.19 ± 1.46 (0.59–6.06)
Heterophils	Proportion of 1.0 [%] $\times 10^9$/l = [$\times 10^3$/µl]	20–75 —	27–94 —	27–79 —	— 1.11 ± 0.76	— 0.74 ± 0.85 (0–2.56)
Lymphocytes	Proportion of 1.0 [%] $\times 10^9$/l = [$\times 10^3$/µl]	30–85 —	16–70 —	20–69 —	— 1.92 ± 1.21	— 2.11 ± 0.96 (0–4.11)
Monocytes	Proportion of 1.0 [%] $\times 10^9$/l = [$\times 10^3$/µl]	1–4 —	0–3 —	0–3 —	— 0.23 ± 0.13	— 0.21 ± 0.15 (0–0.51)
Eosinophils	Proportion of 1.0 [%] $\times 10^9$/l = [$\times 10^3$/µl]	1–4 —	0–2 —	0–2 —	— 0.03 ± 0.03	— 0.01 ± 0.02 (0–0.19)
Basophils	Proportion of 1.0 [%] $\times 10^9$/l = [$\times 10^3$/µl]	1–7 —	0–1 —	0–1 —	— 0.06 ± 0.07	— 0.08 ± 0.15 (0–0.27)
Hematocrit (HCT)	Proportion of 1.0 [%]	0.33–0.50 [33–50]	0.29–0.44 [29–44]	0.36–0.44 [36–44]	0.55 ± 0.03 (0.49–0.61) [55 ± 3.0 (49–61)]	0.60 ± 0.03 (0.54–0.66) [60 ± 3.0 (54–66)]
Hemoglobin (Hgb)	g/l [g/dl]	100–174 10.0–17.4	104–140 10.4–14.0	123–151 12.3–15.1	187.4 ± 16.4 (154.6–220.2) 18.7 ± 16 (15.4–22.0)	208.1 ± 12.2 (183.7–232.5) 20.8 ± 1.2 (18.4 ± 23.30)
Red blood cell (RBC) count	$\times 10^{12}$/l = [$\times 10^6$/µl]	5.1–7.9	4.08–6.96	4.98–6.85	9.26 ± 0.70 (7.86–10.66)	10.00 ± 0.71 (8.58–11.42)
Platelets	$\times 10^9$/l = [$\times 10^3$/µl]	250–650	390–821	353–703	385 ± 132	343 ± 124 (105–618)
Mean corpuscular volume (MCV)	µm^3 = fl	57.8–66.5	61.4–70.3	60.2–72.8	59.41 ± 2.08	60.50 ± 4.13 (53.20–66.85)
Mean corpuscular hemoglobin (MCH)	pg/cell	17.1–23.5	19.7–26	19.2–25.2	20.21 ± 0.78	20.87 ± 0.98 (18.68–22.49)
Mean Corpuscular hemoglobin concentration (MCHC)	g/dl	29–37	309–371	316–346	338.1 ± 17.6	345.6 ± 16.2 (308.2–376.5)

depending on the presence of two distinct populations of granules, which differ in size, staining characteristics, function, and timing of formation from the golgi. Small, pink granules are most numerous, and typically constitute from 80% to 90% of the granules [2, 26]. These granules contain peroxidase, alkaline phosphatase, and other bactericidal substances, most of which are released extracellularly [27]. The less numerous granules are larger, more darkly staining, and formed earlier. These granules contain primarily lysozymes and acid hydrolases and function as lysosomes during phagocytosis [26–28]. The mature heterophil nucleus is usually segmented. An increase in the number of band heterophils, as identified by unsegmented nuclei, can occur because of a severe inflammatory response. This increased number of bands, called a left shift, is uncommon in rabbits. Absence of band heterophils does not rule out infection. Toxic changes in heterophils, with vacuolated bluish cytoplasm, can occur along with premature heterophil release. Toxic change must be differentiated from stain-induced degranulation

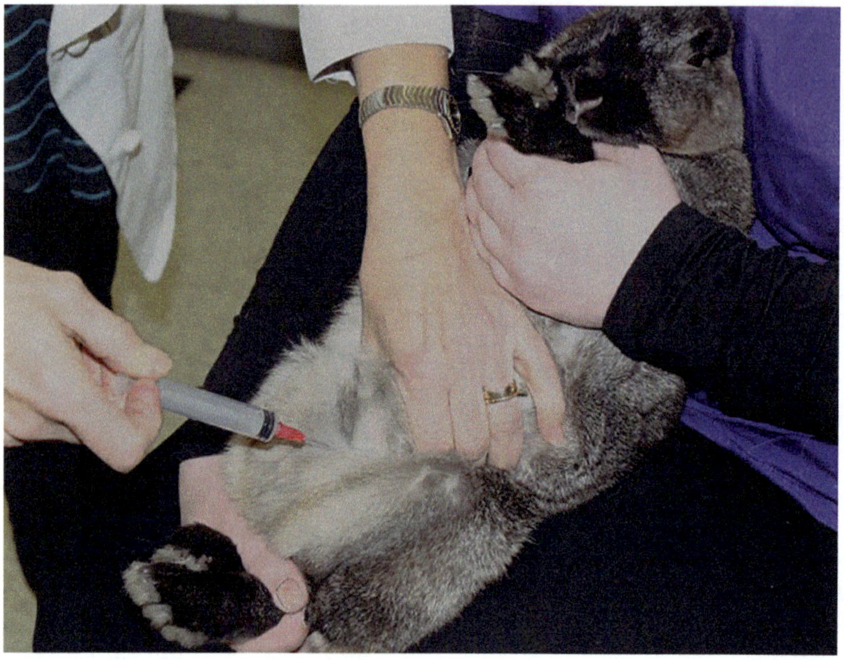

Figure 5.4 Cystocentesis of the rabbit.

as seen with the use of rapid methanol-based stains such as Diff-Quik (American Scientific Products, McGraw Park, Illinois) [23].

A relative heterophilia is the most common response to inflammation. However, in rabbits, the total leukocyte count does not typically increase. Instead, the ratio of heterophils:lymphocytes (H:L) is inverted. In healthy rabbits, the lymphocyte is the dominant leukocyte in peripheral circulation, typically ranging from 50% to 60% of the total white blood cell (WBC) count [4, 10, 23]. Acute infections often result in a heterophil count of 60% or more, and a decrease in lymphocytes to 30% or less, inverting the ratio [2, 23]. Despite the differential cell count, the total leukocyte count rarely increases to more than 2–3× the reference range, if at all [3, 11]. However, a relative heterophilia alone should not be used to diagnose acute infections, since rabbits with acute infection may have a low leukocyte count or a normal distribution [2, 3, 15]. Acute stress or exogenous steroid administration can also result in this inverse H:L ratio. Stress-induced catecholamine release, such as may occur with travel to a veterinary clinic, can result in an elevation of total WBC count with a relative heterophilia, lymphopenia, and eosinopenia [3, 7, 29]. These changes may last for 24–48 h [10]. Alternatively, chronic stress, such as occurs with chronic disease processes or poor husbandry conditions, causes depression of all cell lines, resulting in both leukopenia and lymphopenia [2, 5, 30].

Lymphocytes

The lymphocyte is the most common cell in peripheral circulation and functions in immune response (Table 5.1) (Figure 5.5) [2, 3, 31]. Both large and small lymphocytes occur, and are morphologically similar to those of other species [32]. Although lymphocytes typically lack granules, large lymphocytes occasionally contain azurophilic granules near the nuclear indentation. Small lymphocytes, the most abundant cell type, are approximately the size of the rabbit erythrocyte, whereas large lymphocytes are approximately the size of heterophils [3, 33, 34]. When reactive, lymphocyte cytoplasm becomes intensely blue.

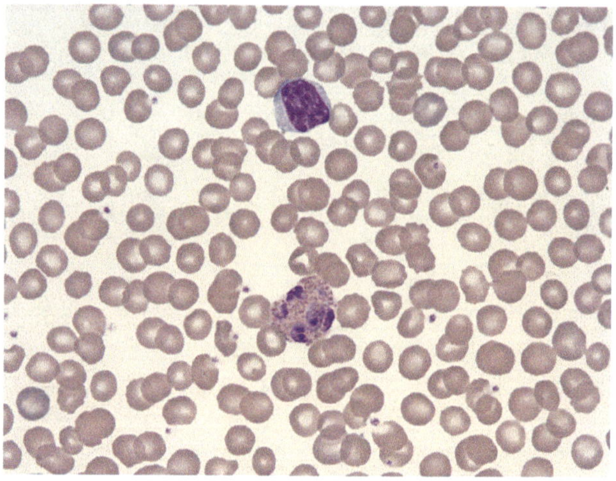

Figure 5.5 Heterophil (below) and lymphocyte (above) of the rabbit.

Lymphopenia is a common response to disease in rabbits [8, 10, 23]. Bacterial infections typically cause a lymphopenia and a total WBC count within reference intervals, based on a relative heterophilia [11, 23]. With chronic infections, such as dental disease, a marked lymphopenia with a low total WBC count [14] is common, along with a nonregenerative anemia as all production of cell lines is depressed. Experimentally induced viral infections may result in an increased relative lymphocyte count, or the lymphocyte count may remain within the reference interval [35].

Lymphocytosis is an unusual finding in rabbits. A relative lymphocytosis may occur in rabbits with lymphoma. In strains of rabbits with hereditary lymphosarcoma, a consistent hematologic pattern occurs as the bone marrow of affected rabbits is gradually replaced with lymphocytic precursors. Granulocyte (heterophils, eosinophils, and basophils) numbers diminish with progression of disease. Total WBC counts remain within the reference interval based on increased lymphocyte numbers. Immature and atypical lymphocytes are sometimes found in peripheral circulation. Erythrocytes also often decrease with PCVs of 30% or less [21, 22]. In domestic rabbits with lymphosarcoma, lymphoblastic leukemia is occasional but causes severe leukocytosis, with WBC counts ranging from 30 000 to greater than 100 000, and most circulating cells are lymphocytes [19, 36, 37].

Monocytes

The largest rabbit leukocyte is the monocyte, measuring 15–18 μm in diameter (Figure 5.6) [32]. They are distinguished from large lymphocytes by a large, amoeboid-shaped nucleus with loosely packed chromatin, abundant blue-gray staining cytoplasm, and the lack of a non-staining perinuclear area. Occasionally, a small number of cytoplasmic vacuoles may be observed. Large, dark red intracytoplasmic granules are associated with nonspecific toxicity. Monocytosis occurs in rabbits with chronic inflammatory diseases, such as abscesses, labyrinthitis, and mastitis [30]. However, monocytosis is not present in all rabbits with chronic bacterial infections. For example, rabbits with chronic osteomyelitis due to dental disease, an extremely common condition in pet rabbits, often have a WBC count within the reference interval [5].

Eosinophils

Rabbit eosinophils are distinguished from heterophils by their size and the appearance of cytoplasmic granules (Figure 5.4). They are slightly larger (12–16 μm in diameter) than heterophils [32]. Granules are more abundant and completely fill the cytoplasm. Compared to primary and secondary granules of heterophils, granules in eosinophils are 3–4 times larger, with a consistent size and more intense acidophilic staining. The nucleus is bi-lobed or horseshoe shaped and stains purple. Rabbit eosinophils are active in immune function, wound healing, and phagocytosis [3, 15, 17, 38]. Eosinophils are often low in number, or are absent from circulation [3, 4, 28]. Eosinophilia may be seen in rabbits with chronic diseases of tissues that contain mast cells such as the skin, GI tract, lungs, and uterus, or during wound healing, and in rabbits with parasitism (excepting *Encephalitozoon cuniculi*) [1, 5, 23, 39]. Exogenous steroid administration and chronic disease may cause eosinopenia (Table 5.3).

Basophils

Rabbit basophils are morphologically similar to those of other species, and similar in size to the heterophil [32]. Basophils are a commonly encountered cell in the rabbit and may account for 5%–30% of the leukocyte differential count in healthy animals (Figure 5.7) [2, 23]. The function of the basophil is not clear, but increased basophil counts have been reported in rabbits with chronic skin diseases, along with eosinophilia [16].

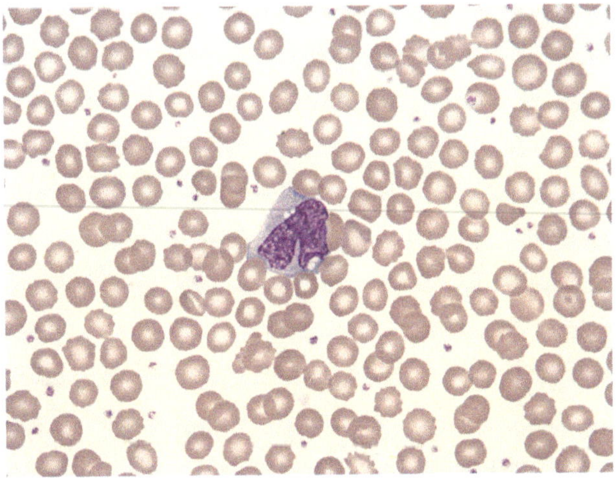

Figure 5.6 Monocyte of the rabbit, and the relatively small platelets of the rabbit. Modified Wrights stain, 1000×.

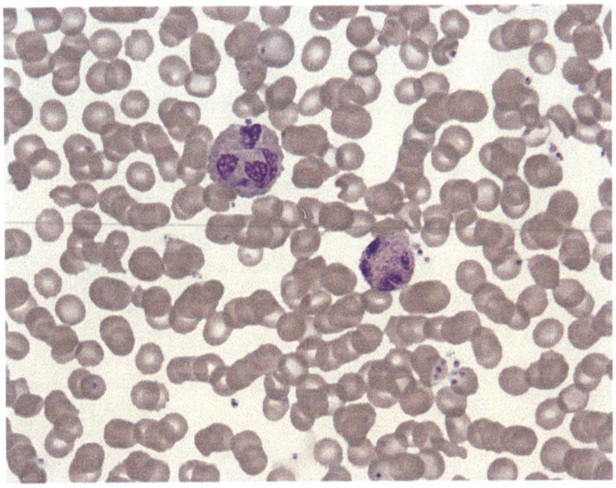

Figure 5.7 Eosinophil (upper left) and heterophil (lower right) of the rabbit. Modified Wrights stain, 1000×.

Hemostasis, Platelets, and Blood Types

Rabbit platelets are morphologically similar to those of other mammals, and participate in hemostasis [32]. They are often clumped on blood films. Rabbit hemostasis is similar to that in other mammals (Table 5.2) [31, 40, 41]. New Zealand white rabbits have demonstrated higher concentrations of factors II, V, V, VIII, X XI, and XIII compared to other mammals, with factor V being exceptionally high [40]. Thus, rabbits may have a more active intrinsic system of coagulation [31]. The rabbit extrinsic coagulation system is similar to that of other mammals. However, platelet aggregation does not occur in the presence of epinephrine [42]. Some rabbits have a genetic resistance to warfarin, and may be less susceptible to anticoagulant rodenticide toxicosis [3, 42]. Despite a lack of recognized rabbit blood groups, cross-matching is recommended before transfusions. Anecdotally in practice, and on the basis of the author's experience, blood transfusions are well tolerated [1].

Biochemical Panel Liver Enzymes

No single commercial assay is liver specific for the rabbit. Elevations of serum alanine transaminase (ALT), AST, serum alkaline phosphatase (SAP), LDH, and gamma-glutamyl transpeptidase (GGT), bilirubin, and bile acids may each indicate hepatobiliary disease. Trends useful in the diagnosis of hepatic disease in rabbits are given in Table 5.3. Other findings, such as hypoglycemia and decreased albumin, also occur with severe liver disease [43, 44].

AST is found in liver, skeletal muscle, cardiac muscle, kidney, and pancreas. The highest activity is found in liver and skeletal muscle, and increased serum concentrations indicate cellular damage and leakage. AST appears a consistent indicator of liver damage in the rabbit [15]. Elevations occur with damage to liver mitochondria, as more than half of AST is associated with mitochondrial membranes. Rabbits experimentally infected with rabbit hemorrhagic disease virus (RHDV), a calicivirus, suffer fulminant liver failure and demonstrate changes in several liver enzymes commensurate with the degree of liver pathology [43–45]. Increases in serum AST most precisely correlated with the degree of hepatocellular degeneration. AST elevations are characterized as mild (up to 20-fold increase), moderate (150–200-fold increase), and severe (more than 1000-fold increase). AST activity greater than 6000 IU/l is associated with imminent death. Proportionately lower increases were observed in ALT (Table 5.1).

ALT has little tissue specificity and is not as useful in evaluation of liver disease in rabbits [5, 15]. Although the highest concentrations of ALT are found in liver and cardiac muscle, ALT activity is lower and the half-life is shorter in rabbits (5 h) than in dogs or ferrets (45–60 h) [46]. ALT may differentiate liver from muscle as a source of plasma enzyme abnormalities, as AST and LDH may both increase as a result of struggling during restraint, whereas restraint does not affect ALT concentrations [46].

Table 5.3 Trends useful in the interpretation of selected analytes for common liver disorders in rabbits.

Analyte	Liver			Muscle/ handling
	Hepatocellular Injury	Lipidosis	Cholestasis	
AST	+++	+++	+/–	++
ALT	++	+/–	–	–
GGT	++	++	+++	–
ALP	+	+	++	–
Bilirubin	++	+/–	+++	–
LDH	+/–	+/–	+/–	++
CK	–	–	–	+++

Note: – not increased, + mild increase, ++ moderate increase, +++ substantial increase.

Table 5.2 Reference intervals for coagulation tests of lagomorphs [31, 40, 41].

Analyte (abbreviation)	Units, SI [conventional]	New Zealand white rabbits	European brown hares
	Sample *[n]*	*12 or [6]*	*30*
Prothombin time [PT]	s	7.5 ± 1.5 – 14.6 ± 4.3	13.32 ± 2.15
Russell's viper venom Time [RVVT]	s	14.3 ± 3.3	
Activated partial thromboplastin time [APTT]	s	32.8 ± 4.5	16.73 ± 1.86
Thrombin time [TT]	s	22.9 ± 5.9	13.97 ± 1.37
Bleeding Time	min	3.87 ± 0.41 *[6] Template, posterior ear surface* 2.91± 0.85 *[6] Marginal ear vein*	

Increases in ALT alone have been documented in asymptomatic rabbits with exposure to aflatoxins or those housed on aromatic wood shavings [47].

Along with AST and ALT, an increase in GGT activity is common in rabbits with liver disease caused by *Eimeria stiedae* [48], some hepatic neoplasms [28], and liver lobe torsion [49–51]. The combination of these enzymes may also be useful for the diagnosis of hepatic lipidosis, a common condition in pet rabbits. In rabbits with experimentally induced hepatic lipidosis, serum AST and GGT activity, but not ALT, were consistently elevated [24, 52–54]. GGT increases in rabbits with these and other hepatic disorders such as Eimeria and liver lobe torsions were likely because of cholestasis [51, 55, 56]. GGT occurs in the liver and kidney, with the greatest concentration found in renal tubular epithelium. However, renal GGT is expelled in the urine, and therefore elevations in serum GGT are liver specific [57]. Hepatic GGT concentrations are highest in the bile duct epithelial cells. Thus, conditions that cause biliary obstruction result in increased serum activity [7, 57].

Alkaline phosphatase (ALP) is an induced liver enzyme, and may increase with many types of liver disease, especially those that result in cholestasis such as neoplasia, lipidosis, hepatic coccidiosis, or abscesses [5, 15, 49]. Large increases in serum ALP occur in rabbits with experimental ligation of common bile duct [7]. However, ALP is not specific for liver disease, as it also originates from bone, liver, intestinal and renal tubular epithelium, and placenta [3]. Most circulating ALP is a combination of three different isoenzymes, one intestinal isoenzyme, and two which originate from the liver or kidney [5, 7, 57]. In cases of liver disease, concurrent elevations in other liver analytes are generally present. High concentrations of ALP alone may occur in asymptomatic rabbits housed on aromatic bedding, in growing animals, and rabbits with bone lesions such as neoplasia, osteomyelitis, or fractures (Table 5.4).

The principal bile pigment excreted by the rabbit liver is biliverdin, for which there is no commercially available assay [57]. On the basis of low biliverdin reductase activity, only approximately 30% of total biliverdin is converted to bilirubin [58]. In rabbits with healthy hepatobiliary function, circulating concentrations of bilirubin range from 0.0 to 0.75 mg/dl [3]. Conditions that result in cholestasis, such as neoplasia, hepatic coccidiosis, and fulminant liver failure caused by RVHD, cause clinical jaundice and increased serum bilirubin. Usually, other liver enzyme activities also increase [5, 57]. Bile acids and LDH have limited diagnostic use in rabbits. Although LDH may also increase in hepatic disease, it is nonspecific and not generally diagnostically useful [15]. Because of the practice of ceocotrophy in rabbits, fasting is not possible, and the measurement of pre- and postprandial circulating bile acids is not commonly used for assessment of liver function).

Muscle Enzymes

Creatinine kinase (CK) isoenzymes have been identified from the rabbit brain, cardiac, skeletal, and smooth muscle [57]. Increased CK activities are associated with myocyte damage in the rabbit. AST and LDH may also originate from skeletal muscle. These enzymes will often increase with restraint and handling, although ALT, GGT, and ALP will not. These differing activities may help to distinguish hepatic from muscular or restraint-induced change in liver and muscle enzymes.

Renal Analytes

In rabbits, blood urea nitrogen concentration is influenced by a variety of physiologic functions, especially the concentration and quality of proteins in the diet, and liver function. Published reference values are based on findings in laboratory rabbits, maintained on a standard diet. Because of the wide variation in diets fed to pet rabbits, blood urea nitrogen (BUN) is often higher and more variable than published values [5]. BUN concentration can also fluctuate depending on varying use of urea by cecal microflora, making interpretation of small deviations challenging [5]. Diurnal variation causes a late afternoon to evening peak in BUN which may be related to cecotrophy [57]. Creatinine is a more sensitive indicator of renal function, as it is not influenced by extrarenal factors such as protein intake. Creatinine is filtered through the glomerulus but is not reabsorbed by renal tubules. Compared with other companion mammals, the reference interval for creatinine in rabbits is broad: 50–190 mmol/l or 0.5–2.0 mg/dl.

With dehydration, the degree of prerenal azotemia can be pronounced, and both BUN and creatinine can be elevated to such a degree that a diagnosis of renal failure would be assumed if comparable values were noted in a cat or dog. These changes may occur within hours in rabbits with anorexia from GI stasis, or dental disease, or with fluid loss caused by diarrhea. These relatively rapidly induced clinicopathologic signs of dehydration occur because of the limited capacity of the lapine kidney to concentrate urine [59]. BUN and creatinine should decline to within the reference interval once the rabbit patient is rehydrated. If azotemia is due to renal disease, increases in BUN and creatinine are usually accompanied by hyper- or hypokalemia, hyperphosphatemia, nonregenerative anemia, and isothenuric urine. Hypercalcemia has also been reported to indicate renal insufficiency in the rabbit [5, 15, 60]. As with other mammals, a loss of 50%–70% of functional nephrons is needed before BUN and creatinine increase, making the diagnosis of early disease challenging. Causes of renal insufficiency in rabbits include nephrolithiasis, severe *E. cuniculi* infection,

Table 5.4 Biochemical reference ranges of lagomorphs.

Analyte (abbreviation)	Units, SI [conventional]	Domestic rabbits [2]	New Zealand white rabbits [8]	European brown hare [9]	
Data Format		**Range**	**Range**	**Mean ± SD (Range)**	**Mean ± SD (Range)**
Animals sampled			**60–110**	**21 Ó**	**27 ₪**
Alanine (ALT) aminotransferase	U/l = [IU/l]	48–80	—	20.37 ± 8.80 (2.77–367.97)	48.88 ± 29.15 (0–107.18)
Gamma (GGT) glutamyl transferase	U/l = [IU/l]	0–14	0–14	7.07 ± 1.69	8.31 ± 1.53 (4.20–11.07)
Alkaline (ALP) phosphatase	U/l = [IU/l]	4–16	17–192	203.32 ± 67.10 (69.12–337.52)	60.81 ± 27.25 (6.31–115.31)
Lactate (LDH) dehydrogenase	U/l = [IU/l]	34–129	59–389	—	—
Bilirubin, total	μmol/l [mg/dl]	0.0–0.7	—	1.71 ± 0.86 (0–3.43)	1.03 ± 0.34 (0.35–1.17)
CK U/l	U/l = [IU/l]	—	218–2705	—	—
AST U/l	U/l = [IU/l]	14–113	—	85.91 ± 34.20	94.82 ± 41.93 (14.77–165.41)
Blood urea nitrogen (BUN)	μmol/l [mg/dl]	13–29	81–250	11.47 ± 3.33 (4.81–18.13)	16.25 ± 2.47 (11.31–21.19)
Creatinine	μmol/l [mg/dl]	0.5–2.5	0.14–1.6	11.1 ± 2.1	12.9 ± 3.0 (3.54–18.81)
Calcium	mmol/l [mg/dl]	5.6–12.5	12.9–15.0	—	—
Phosphorus	mmol/l [mg/dl]	4.0–6.9	2.7–7.3	—	—
Magnesium	mmol/l Mg/dl	—	15.8–32.4	—	—
Amylase	U/l	166.5–314.5	—	—	—
Glucose	mmol/l [mg/dl]	75–155	81–183	95.5 ± 17.7 (60.1–131.9)	114.0 ± 13.3 (87.4–140.6)
Cholesterol	mmol/l [mg/dl]	10–80	—	0.58 ± 0.10 ()	0.50 ± 0.11 (0.33–0.77)
Sodium	mmol/l = [mEq/l]	131–155	138–148	—	—
Potassium	mmol/l = [mEq/l]	3.6–6.9	3.4–5.1	—	—
Chloride	mmol/l = [mEq/l]	92–112	96–109	—	—
Protein, total	g/l [g/dl]	5.4–8.3	—	40.6 ± 6.6 (27.4–53.8)	52.5 ± 7.1 (38.3–66.7)
Albumin	g/l [g/dl]	2.4–4.6	—	25.7 ± 5.5 (14.7–36.7)	36.0 ± 4.9 (25.2–45.8)
Globulin	g/l [g/dl]	1.5–2.8	—	14.5 ± 4.3	16.3 ± 7.5 (3.1–28.0)
Alpha 1 globulins	g/l	—	—	2.4 ± 1.2	2.5 ± 2.3 (0–6.3)
Alpha 2 globulins	g/l	—	—	2.7 ± 1.1	2.3 ± 1.4 (0–5.1)
Beta 1 globulins	g/l	—	—	4.8 ± 2.5	5.2 ± 3.5 (0–11.2)
Beta 2 globulins	g/l	—	—	2.3 ± 1.2	2.8 ± 1.3 (0–5.2)
Gamma globulins	g/l	—	—	2.2 ± 1.3 (0–4.8)	3.4 ± 2.1 (0–6.7)
Albumin: globulin		—	—	1.97 ± 0.92	2.65 ± 1.57 (0–5.14)

chronic interstitial nephritis, pyelonephritis, glomerulonephropathy, and neoplasia [15]. Postrenal uremia may be caused by calculi, masses, tumor, or abscesses which obstruct urine flow. Decreased BUN occurs in rabbits with severely impaired liver function, low dietary protein intake (anorexia, decreased cecotrophy), or after administration of anabolic steroids [2, 46].

Pancreas

Increased activity of serum amylase may occur in rabbits with pancreatitis, pancreatic duct obstruction, peritonitis, or abdominal trauma. In rabbits, amylase is found exclusively in the pancreas; little to none is present in the salivary glands, intestines, or liver [5]. Because amylase is cleared by the kidneys, elevated serum activity may occur in rabbits with renal failure. Corticosteroid administration may also cause increased amylase [46]. The function or diagnostic value of lipase in rabbits is largely unknown.

Glucose

Herbivore carbohydrate metabolism differs from that of carnivores. Even when not consuming food, rabbits continuously absorb nutrients. Bacterial fermentation within the cecum produces volatile fatty acids, which are continually absorbed as a primary energy source. Rabbits subjected to four days of starvation had no reduction in blood glucose concentration [61]. Withholding food is not equivalent to fasting, because of consumption of night feces or cecotrophs. Hypoglycemia can occur with extreme starvation, in young rabbits, in late stages of chronic disease, or cases of fulminant liver failure, acute renal failure, or sepsis [5, 16, 44, 62].

The most common cause of hyperglycemia is stress. Rabbits that have been transported, handled, or restrained for diagnostic procedures may suffer hyperglycemia and glucosuria [2, 7, 57, 63]. Hepatic lipidosis, acute intestinal obstruction, mucoid enteropathy, hyperthermia, and hypovolemic shock can also cause hyperglycemia. Administration of exogenous glucocorticoids and certain anesthetic agents such as halothane and xylazine may also cause hyperglycemia [15, 57, 64]. Naturally occurring diabetes mellitus is an uncommon cause of hyperglycemia in rabbits [65]. Rabbits selectively bred for the study of diabetes had clinical signs such as polyphagia, weight loss, polyuria, polydipsia, elevated blood glucose (>500 mg/dl), and glycosuria. Ketoacidosis was mild or not observed [65, 66].

Lipids

Information on lipids in pet rabbits is limited. Cholesterol and triglycerides are influenced by a variety of physiologic factors, and wide variations can exist with an individual rabbit, or depending on gender or breed [57, 67]. In the individual, diurnal variation exists, with the highest concentrations of cholesterol found later in the day [57]. Males have lower cholesterol levels than females, and familial hypercholesterolemia has been reported in some breeds, such as the Wantanabe [57, 68]. Cholesterol and triglyceride concentrations can be affected by dietary fat, and cholesterol-fed rabbits are used as a model of atherosclerosis [69]. In other species, fasting samples are required to assay cholesterol and triglycerides, but gastrointestinal physiology and cecotrophy in rabbits prevents a true fast. Increased concentrations of circulating cholesterol and triglycerides were observed in rabbits fed a high-fat diet, obese rabbits, and those suffering liver disease, pancreatitis, diabetes mellitus, and chronic renal failure [4, 15, 16].

Electrolytes

Most electrolyte abnormalities in rabbits follow similar patterns as in other mammals. Phosphorus, potassium, sodium, and chloride may be helpful in the diagnosis of renal disease in rabbits; increased plasma concentrations of phosphorus generally parallel azotemia [5, 15, 57]. Rabbits with experimentally induced renal failure developed hyperkalemia, and hypernatremia, but exhibited minimal change in chloride concentrations [62]. Potassium and phosphorus may be artifactually increased as a result of hemolysis during sample collection or storage [3]. Hyperproteinemia and lipemia can cause an artifactual decrease.

Blood Proteins

In rabbits, as with other mammalian species, the most common cause of increased total protein and albumin is dehydration. The albumin fraction of protein is approximately 60%, which is much higher than that of other mammals [57]. Hypoalbuminemia can be seen with severe liver disease, as the liver is the site of albumin synthesis [44, 45]. Cecotrophy is a significant source of dietary protein. Conditions that prevent cecotrophy, such as dental disease, gastrointestinal disease, or obesity, may also be associated with low serum albumin concentration. Poor-quality diets and diets that are low in fiber may also contribute, as dietary fiber is important in the manufacture of protein within cecotrophs [4, 15]. If both albumin and globulin are low, protein loss, such as may occur with blood loss or exudative skin lesions, is the likely cause. Changes in plasma globulin concentrations follow those of other mammals, with increases most commonly the result of inflammation or immune stimulation.

Vitamins Minerals Metals and Toxins

Calcium and Vitamin D3

Plasma concentration, range, and urinary excretion of calcium are higher in rabbits than in other mammals. Total serum calcium is 30%–50% higher in rabbits in parallel to intestinal absorption [70–72]. Vitamin D3 does not play major role in regulating intestinal calcium absorption, which is absorbed in direct proportion to dietary amounts rather than metabolic need [72–74]. Fluctuations in serum concentration of calcium may occur depending on diet, age, and gender. Young, growing rabbits and pregnant does both have increased calcium needs. Serum concentrations in these animals rarely exceed 3.5 mmol/l (14 mg/dl), as compared to 4.25 mmol/l 917 mg/dl) in non-pregnant adults [5, 74]. Hypocalcemia can cause seizures in late pregnant and lactating does [33]. Other potential causes of hypocalcemia include hypoalbuminemia, losses through diarrhea, renal hyperparathyroidism, and halothane anesthesia [2, 64].

The most common cause of hypercalcemia in the rabbit is excessive dietary calcium. Hypercalcemia also occurs rabbits with renal failure, as the kidneys play a vital role in calcium excretion (45%–60% fractional excretion of calcium vs. 2% in most mammals) [5, 15, 60]. Excretion can be impaired in rabbits with severe renal disease, while absorption continues unabated. Severe hypercalcemia can cause mineralization of the kidneys and aorta [15, 74–76]. Hypercalcemia can also occur with paraneoplastic syndrome as reported in one rabbit with thymoma [77].

Lead toxicosis has been reported in rabbits, with an associated anemia [1]. Some rabbits have a genetic resistance to warfarin, and may be less susceptible to anticoagulant rodenticide toxicosis [3, 42].

Hormones – Adrenal and Reproductive

Reported clinical adrenal and thyroid disease in rabbits is limited to a single report of behavioral changes in two rabbits with adrenal hyperplasia and neoplasia associated with increased blood testosterone [78]. Serum concentrations of steroid hormones determined for 29 neutered rabbits were progesterone 0.25 ± 0.02 ng/ml, 17-hydroxyprogesterone 6.40 ± 1.35 ng/ml, androstenedione 2.47 ± 0.22 ng/ml, testosterone 0.02 ± 0.00 ng/ml, and cortisol 7.28 ± 0.40 ng/ml. No differences in hormone concentrations between neutered male and female rabbits were reported [34].

Urinalysis

Urine Collection

Urine may be collected by free catch, cystocentesis, or catheterization. If a sterile sample is not required, free catch is adequate. Application of gentle pressure on the bladder in a cranial to caudal direction usually results in

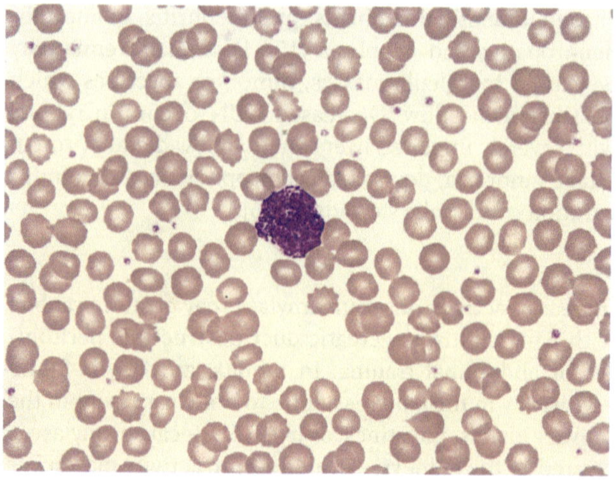

Figure 5.8 Basophil of the rabbit. Modified Wrights stain, 1000×.

expression of urine. Pet rabbits are usually litter box trained, and urine can often be obtained by caging these animals with an empty litter box or one containing a nonabsorbent material. In a laboratory setting, commercially available metabolic cages can be used for quantitative urine collection.

Cystocentesis is preferred for collection of a sterile sample needed for bacterial culture. The bladder rests just rostral to the pelvic brim. "Blind" cystocentesis should be avoided, as one must avoid the large, thin-walled cecum, which is located slightly dorsal to the urinary bladder. Inadvertent laceration or puncture of the cecum will likely occur if the patient moves suddenly, or if the bladder is not clearly identified prior to cystocentesis. Depending on the volume of urine present, the bladder can be flaccid and difficult to palpate. Ultrasound should be used if the bladder cannot be definitively identified and immobilized via palpation.

To obtain the sample, wrap the rabbit securely in a towel, place in dorsal recumbency, and pull back the towel to expose the ventral abdomen (Figure 5.8). Once the bladder is identified by palpation, immobilize it by grasping between the thumb and forefinger. Use a 25 g., 1 in. needle to aspirate urine from the bladder, with an attached 3–6 ml syringe.

Collection of urine via urethral catheterization is less preferable as the urethral opening is not sterile in male or female rabbits. Further, introduction of the catheter risks bacterial urinary tract infection and may result in contamination of samples for bacterial culture. The rabbit must be sedated and may require anesthesia for this procedure. A sterile, well-lubricated 9-French catheter is adequate for most rabbits. Males are usually restrained in a sitting position to extrude the penis. The female urethra is located on the floor of the vagina, and can be accessed while the rabbit is maintained in sternal recumbency.

Urinalysis

The average volume of urine produced daily by a rabbit is 130 ml/kg/day (range 20–350 ml/kg/day) [15]. The color can vary from pale yellow to shades of orange or red-brown depending on the diet (Table 5.5). Plant porphyrin pigments are responsible for red coloration of healthy rabbit urine, and the color can vary from day to day. Red urine should be distinguished from hematuria by means of urine dipstick for blood, or sediment examination for red blood cells (normally <3 RBC/hpf). The most common cause of hematuria in intact female rabbits is uterine disease, as blood from the uterus mixes with urine during micturition. Other causes include cystitis, bladder neoplasia, or occasionally, cystic calculi.

Urine turbidity varies from clear to extremely thick and turbid. The cloudy appearance is due to normal calcium excretion. The mean fractional excretion of calcium in rabbits is extremely high, averaging 45%–60% as compared to 2% in most other mammals, and appears in the urine as calcium carbonate or calcium oxalate crystals. Hypercalciuria, or sludgy urine, is a common disorder in pet rabbits. In these rabbits, calcium crystal formation is excessive, and retention within the bladder can form calculi, calcium sand, or thick sludge. This sludge may be voided, producing urine the consistency of paste. Some rabbits with sand or sludge in the bladder will void clear urine as calcium crystals precipitate out into the bladder lumen. Therefore, the absence of crystals or cloudy urine cannot be used to rule out hypercalciuria.

Dipstick testing can assess rabbit urine for the presence of blood, glucose, ketones, and pH, but is not considered reliable for determination of WBC or other parameters [5]. Rabbit urine is alkaline, with an average pH of 8 (range: 7.5–9). Acidic urine has been anecdotally associated in rabbits with acidosis based on fever, pregnancy toxemia, or hepatic lipidosis [15]. Although glucosuria is common based on stress hyperglycemia, diabetes is rare in rabbits. Ketones in the urine are always abnormal, and have been associated with anorexia, hepatic lipidosis, or pregnancy toxemia [1].

Measuring of specific gravity (SG) with a refractometer is more reliable than with a urine dipstick. Healthy rabbits typically produce dilute urine, with an average SG of 1.015 (range 1.003–1.036). In azotemic rabbits, SG <1.015 is suggestive of renal failure. Measuring urine protein along with the SG is also useful in the diagnosis of renal failure. Healthy rabbits, especially young rabbits or adults with concentrated urine, may have a trace of protein in the urine. Dilute urine (SG <1.020) with protein suggests renal disease, as proteinuria may occur early in the course of renal disease [5]. A urine protein/creatine ratio of >0.6 may also indicate renal disease [2, 15, 46].

Crystalluria is a common finding during examination of healthy rabbit urine sediment. Crystals usually consist of calcium oxalate, but calcium carbonate, ammonium phosphate, or monohydrate crystals are also commonly found. The presence of white blood cells, erythrocytes, bacteria, and casts are interpreted as in other mammals.

Table 5.5 Urinalysis data for rabbits [2].

Quantitative values	Rabbits
Sample size	Unknown
Data format	Range
Specific gravity	1.003–1.035
Semiquantitative values	
Protein multistix	Trace
Glucose	Negative
Ketones	Negative
Bilirubin	Negative
Urobilinogen	Negative
Occult blood	Negative
pH	8–9
Appearance	Cloudy to clear, yellow to orange/tan
Microscopic analysis	
Red blood cells	0–3/hpf
White blood cells	occasional
Epithelial cells	Absent to rare
Casts	Absent to rare
Crystals	Many calcium carbonate, moderate phosphate
Bacteria	Absent to rare

Serology and PCR

Pasteurella multocida

Bacterial respiratory disease is extremely common in rabbits, and *Pasteurella multocida* is frequently implicated. Serologic testing for *Pasteurella multocida* is widely available. However, testing is of limited usefulness in clinical practice. A positive titer indicates only exposure, and results cannot differentiate previous exposure from active infection. Many rabbits harbor the agent in the nasal cavities without developing clinical disease, making a single positive titer nondiagnostic. Demonstration of a fourfold rise in titer within a two- to four-week interval is suggestive of active infection. Rabbits younger than two months may have a positive titer based on the presence maternal antibodies, rather than exposure. A high antibody titer is not protective but may indicate subclinical disease.

Encephalitozoon cuniculi

The rabbit is the primary host for the obligate intracellular microsporidian parasite *E. cuniculi* [79]. Infection may be asymptomatic, or can result in nephritis, encephalitis, or phacoclastic uveitis. There is a high incidence of infection worldwide; however, most infected rabbits remain asymptomatic, and diagnosis *in vivo* is difficult. A positive antibody titer demonstrates only exposure, and does not confirm *E. cuniculi* as the causative agent for clinical disease [80]. In rabbits experimentally infected with *E. cuniculi*, serum antibodies develop within three weeks [81]. Seroconversion occurs as early as two weeks before organisms are detected on histologic examination, four weeks prior to onset of renal lesions or the appearance of spores in the urine, and eight weeks prior to the development of brain lesions [82, 83]. Once seroconversion occurs, antibody titers remain high for several months, followed by a small decrease, and then persist for years [84]. Although several studies demonstrate a correlation between serologic results and histologic lesions in the brain and kidneys, many infected rabbits with high titers and histologic lesions at necropsy are asymptomatic [80, 85–88]. Because the rate of seroconversion does not differ between symptomatic and asymptomatic animals, serology is most useful to rule out *E. cuniculi* as a cause of neurologic disease. In general, a negative titer indicates the absence of infection [86]. However, a small number of seronegative rabbits have been shown to have histologic lesions. This should not add confusion when differentiating the cause of neurologic signs, since this is most likely to occur in early infection, when rabbits are asymptomatic [82, 84, 86].

Various antibody tests are available to detect antibodies to *E. cuniculi* in rabbits. ELISA and indirect fluorescent antibody (IFA) testing correlate and are generally available [89]. Both conventional and nested PCR testing has been investigated as a diagnostic tool for *E. cuniculi*. In rabbits with phacoclastic uveitis, conventional PCR of the lens is an excellent diagnostic tool. However, neither conventional nor nested PCR of urine or CSF is reliable. On postmortem examination, nested PCR may be effective in diagnosing *E. cuniculi* in brain tissue. However, histologic examination appears to be the most sensitive method of detection [86].

Treponema cuniculi

T. cuniculi, or rabbit syphilis, is a sexually transmitted disease causing characteristic facial and perineal dermatitis. Serology is most useful as a screening tool for groups of rabbits, prior to acceptance into breeding colonies or laboratories. Usefulness in companion rabbits is limited, since rabbits do not seroconvert for at least three months following infection. Dermatologic signs occur prior to the development of a positive titer. Titers decline and symptoms resolve rapidly once treatment is initiated [5, 82].

References

1 Marshall, K.L. (2008). Rabbit hematology. *Vet Clin North Am Exot Anim Pract* 11 (3): 551–567.

2 Benson, K.G. and Paul-Murphy, J. (1999). Clinical pathology of the domestic rabbit: acquisition and interpretation of samples. *Vet Clin North Am Exot Anim Pract* 2 (3): 539–551.

3 Fudge, A.M. (2000). Rabbit hematology. In: *Laboratory Medicine: Avian and Exotic Pets* (ed. A.M. Fudge), 273–275. Philadelphia, PA: WB Saunders.

4 Harcourt-Brown, F. and Harcourt-Brown, N.H. (2002). Clinical pathology. In: *Textbook of Rabbit Medicine*, 140–165. Oxford, UK: Butterworth-Heinemann.

5 Melillo, A. (2007). Rabbit clinical pathology. *J Exot Pet Med: Rabbits* 16 (3): 135–145.

6 O'donoghue, J.M., Strong, M.A., and Detolla, L.J. (1998). Effects of varying storage time and temperature on stability of complete blood count measurements. *J Am Assoc Lab Anim Sci* 37 (6): 52–54.

7 McLaughlin, R. and Fish, R. (1994). Clinical biochemistry and hematology. In: *The Biology of the Laboratory Rabbit*, 2e (ed. P.J. Manning, D.H. Ringler and C.E. Newcomer), 111–127. San Diego: Academic Press.

8 Hewitt, C.D., Innes, D.J., Savory, J. et al. Normal biochemical and hematological values in New Zealand white rabbits. *Clin Chem* 35 (8): 1777–1779.

9 Marco, I., Cuenca, R., Pastor, J. et al. (2003). Hematology and serum chemistry values of the European Brown hare. *Vet Clin Path* 32 (4): 195–198.

10 Toth, L. and January, B. (1990). Physiological stabilization of rabbits after shipping. *Lab Anim Sci* 40 (4): 384–387.

11 Toth, L. and Krueger, J. (1989). Hematologic effects of exposure to three infective agents in rabbits. *J Am Vet Med Assoc* 195 (7): 981–986.

12 Bortolotti, A., Castelli, D., and Bonati, M. (1989). Hematology and serum chemistry values of adult, pregnant and newborn New Zealand rabbits (*Oryctolagus cuniculus*). *Lab Anim Sci* 39 (5): 437–439.

13 Poljičak-Milas, N., Kardum-Skelin, I., Vuđan, M. et al. (2009). Blood cell count analyses and erythrocyte morphometry in New Zealand white rabbits. *Veterinarski arhiv* 79 (6): 561–567.

14 Harcourt-Brown, F. and Baker, S. (2001). Parathyroid hormone, haematological and biochemical parameters

in relation to dental disease and husbandry in rabbits. *J Small Anim Pract* 42 (3): 130–136.

15 Harkness, J. and Wagner, J. (1995). Hematology, clinical chemistry and urinalysis. In: *The Biology and Medicine of Rabbits and Rodents*, 5e, 117–122. Williams & Wilkins.

16 Saunders, R.A. and Davies, R.R. (2005). *Notes on Rabbit Internal Medicine*. Wiley-Blackwell.

17 Weisbroth, S.H., Flatt, R.E., and Kraus, A.L. (1974). *The Biology of the Laboratory Rabbit*. San Diego: Academic Press.

18 Allison, S.O., Artwohl, J.E., Fortman, J.D. et al. (2007). Iatrogenic hemolytic anemia and endocarditis in New Zealand white rabbits secondary to Achromobacter xylosoxidans infection. *J Am Assoc Lab Anim Sci* 46 (6): 58–62.

19 Toth, L., Olson, G., Wilson, E. et al. (1990). Lymphocytic leukemia and lymphosarcoma in a rabbit. *J Am Vet Med Assoc* 197 (5): 627–629.

20 Harrenstien, L. (1994). Critical care of ferrets, rabbits, and rodents. *Semin Av Exot Pet Med.* 3 (4): 217–228.

21 Fox, R.R., Meier, H., Crary, D.D. et al. (1970). Lymphosarcoma in the rabbit: genetics and pathology. *J Natl Cancer Inst* 45 (4): 719–729.

22 Fox, R.R., Norberg, R.F., and Meier, H. (1976). Clinical hematological progression of hereditary lymphosarcoma in rabbits. *J Hered* 67 (6): 376–380.

23 Campbell, T.W. and Ellis, C.K. (2007). Hematology of small mammals. In: *Avian and Exotic Animal Hematology and Cytology*, 113–138. Blackwell Publishing.

24 Fang, Y., Liang, L., and Fu, J. (2008). Establishment of rabbit model of juvenile non-alcoholic steatohepatitis. *Zhejiang Da Xue Xue Bao Yi Xue Ban* 37 (3): 240–244.

25 Shanklin, W.M., Sheppard, L.B., and Burke, G.W. (1977). Staining of rabbit eosinophil and pseudoeosinophil leukocytes. *Acta Anat* 97 (2): 147–150.

26 Nachman, R., Hirsch, J.G., and Baggiolini, M. (1972). Studies on isolated membranes of azurophil and specific granules from rabbit polymorphonuclear leukocytes. *J Cell Biol* 54 (1): 133–140.

27 Zarember, K., Elsbach, P., Shin-Kim, K., and Weiss, J. (1997). p15s (15-kD antimicrobial proteins) are stored in the secondary granules of rabbit granulocytes: implications for antibacterial synergy with the bactericidal/permeability-increasing protein in inflammatory fluids. *Blood* 89 (2): 672–679.

28 Baggiolini, M., Hirsch, J.G., and De Duve, C. (1969). Resolution of granules from rabbit heterophil leukocytes into distinct populations by zonal sedimentation. *J Cell Biol* 40 (2): 529–541.

29 Harkness, J. (1987). Rabbit husbandry and medicine. *Vet Clin North Am Sm Amin Pract* 17 (5): 1019–1044.

30 Hinton, M., Jones, D., and Festing, M. (1982). Haematological findings in healthy and diseased rabbits, a multivariate analysis. *Lab Anim.* 16 (2): 123–129.

31 Dodds, W.J. (2000). Rabbit and ferret hemostasis. In: *Laboratory Medicine: Avian and Exotic Pets* (ed. A.M. Fudge), 285–290. Philadelphia, PA: WB Saunders.

32 Schermer, S. and van Winsen, T. (1967). *The Blood Morphology of Laboratory Animals*, 3e, 5–24. Philadelphia: F.A. Davis.

33 Barlet, J.P. (1980). Plasma calcium, inorganic phosphorus and magnesium levels in pregnant and lactating rabbits. *Reprod Nutr Develop* 20 (3): 647–651.

34 Fecteau, K.A., Deeb, B.J., Rickel, J.M. et al. (2007). Diagnostic endocrinology: blood steroid concentrations in neutered male and female rabbits. *J Exot Pet Med* 16 (4): 256–259.

35 Schock, A. and Reid, H. (1995). Characterization of the lymphoproliferation in rabbits experimentally affected with malignant catarrhal fever. *Vet Microbiol* 53 (1): 111–119.

36 Cloyd, G.G. and Johnson, G.R. (1978). Lymphosarcoma with lymphoblastic leukemia in a New Zealand white rabbit. *Lab Anim Sci* 28 (1): 66–69.

37 Finnie, J., Bostock, W.D.E., and Walden, N. (1980). Lymphoblastic leukemia in a rabbit: a case report. *Lab Anim* 14 (1): 49–51.

38 Song, B.Z., Donoff, R.B., Tsuji, T. et al. (1993). Identification of rabbit eosinophils and heterophils in cutaneous healing wounds. *Histochem J* 25 (10): 762–771.

39 Gupta, S. and Trivedi, K. (1981). Ascaris suum infection on blood picture of rabbits in relation to the production of immunity. *Zool Anez* 06 (3-4): 246–251.

40 Lewis, J.H. (1996). Rabbits. In: *Comparative Hemostasis in Vertebrates* (ed. J.H. Lewis), 182–193. New York: Springer Publishing.

41 Pikula, J., Adam, V., Bandouchova, H. et al. (2007). Blood coagulation times in the european brown hare (Lepus europaeus). *Vet Clin Path* 36 (4): 361–363.

42 Dodds, W.J. (1978). Platelet function in animals: species specificities. In: *Platelets: A Multidisciplinary Approach* (ed. G. de Gaetano and S. Garattini), 45–59. New York: Raven Press.

43 Ferreira, P., Costa-e-Silva, A., Monteiro, E. et al. (2006). Liver enzymes and ultrastructure in rabbit haemorrhagic disease. *Vet Res Commun* 30 (4): 393–401.

44 Tunon, M.J., Sanchez-Campos, S., Garcia-Ferreras, J. et al. (2003). Rabbit hemorrhagic viral disease: characterization of a new animal model of fulminant liver failure. *J Lab Clin Med* 141 (4): 272–278.

45 Ferreira, P., Costa-e-Silva, A., Oliveira, M. et al. (2006). Severe leukopenia and liver biochemistry changes in

adult rabbits after calicivirus infection. *Res Vet Sci* 80 (2): 218–225.
46 Jenkins, J.R. (2000). Rabbit and ferret liver and gastrointestinal testing. In: *Laboratory Medicine: Avian and Exotic Pets* (ed. A.M. Fudge), 291–304. Philadelphia: WB Saunders.
47 Fekete, S. and Huszenicza, G. (1993). Effects of T-2 toxin on ovarian activity and some metabolic variables of rabbits. *Lab Anim Sci* 43 (6): 646–649.
48 Çam, Y., Atasever, A., Eraslan, G. et al. (2008). *Eimeria stiedae*: experimental infection in rabbits and the effect of treatment with toltrazuril and ivermectin. *Exp Parasitol* 119 (1): 164–172.
49 Stanke, N.J., Graham, J.E., Orcutt, C.J. et al. (2011). Successful outcome of hepatectomy as treatment for liver lobe torsion in four domestic rabbits. *J Am Vet Med Assoc* 238 (9): 1176–1183.
50 Taylor, H.R. and Staff, C.D. (2007). Clinical techniques: successful management of liver lobe torsion in a domestic rabbit (*Oryctolagus cuniculus*) by surgical lobectomy. *J Exot Pet Med* 16 (3): 175–178.
51 Wenger, S., Barrett, E., Pearson, G. et al. (2009). Liver lobe torsion in three adult rabbits. *J Sm Anim Pract* 50 (6): 301–305.
52 Fu, J.F., Fang, Y.L., Liang, L. et al. (2009). A rabbit model of pediatric nonalcoholic steatohepatitis: the role of adiponectin. *World J Gastroenterol* 15 (8): 912–918.
53 Kainuma, M., Fujimoto, M., Sekiya, N. et al. (2004). Cholesterol-fed rabbit as a unique model of nonalcoholic, nonobese, non-insulin-resistant fatty liver disease with characteristic fibrosis. *J Gastroenterol* 41 (10): 971–980.
54 Yanni, A.E., Agrogiannis, G., Nomikos, T. et al. (2010). Oral supplementation with l-aspartate and l-glutamate inhibits atherogenesis and fatty liver disease in cholesterol-fed rabbit. *Amino Acids* 38 (5): 1323–1323.
55 Hein, B. and Lammler, G. (1978). Alteration of enzyme activities in serum of *Eimeria stiedae* infected rabbits. *Z Parasitenkd* 57 (3): 199–211.
56 Joyner, L.P., Catchpole, J., and Berrett, S. (1983). Eimeria stiedae in rabbits: the demonstration of responses to chemotherapy. *Res Vet Sci* 34 (1): 64–67.
57 Campbell, T.W. (2012). Clinical chemistry of mammals: laboratory animals and miscellaneous species. In: *Veterinary Hematology and Clinical Chemistry*, 2e (ed. M.A. Thrall, G. Veiser, R. Allison and T.W. Campbell), 571–581. Ames, IA: Wiley.
58 Fekete, S. (1989). Recent findings and future perspectives of digestive physiology in rabbits: a review. *Acta Vet Hung* 37 (3): 265–279.
59 Brewer, L.R. and Cruise, L.J. (1994). Physiology. In: *The Biology of the Laboratory Rabbit* (ed. P.J. Manning, D.H. Ringler and C.E. Newcomer), 63. Academic Press.
60 Tvedegaard, E. (1987). Arterial disease in chronic renal failure—an experimental study in the rabbit. *Acta Pathol Microbiol Immunol Scand A* 290: 1–28.
61 Kozma, C., Macklin, W., Cummins, L. et al. (1974). Anatomy, physiology and biochemistry of the rabbit. In: *The Biology of the Laboratory Rabbit* (ed. S.H. Weisbroth, R.E. Flatt and A.L. Kraus), 59–64. San Diego: Academic Press.
62 Chen, S.Y., Chou, C.C., Liu, C.I. et al. (2008). Impairment of renal function and electrolyte balance in rabbit hemorrhagic disease. *J Vet Med Sci* 70 (9): 951.
63 Knudtzon, J. (1984). Plasma levels of glucagon, insulin, glucose and free fatty acids in rabbits during laboratory handling procedures. *Z Versuchstierkd* 26 (3): 123–133.
64 Bito, L.Z. and Eakins, K.E. (1969). The effect of general anesthesia on the chemical composition of blood plasma of normal rabbits. *J Pharmacol Exp Ther* 169 (2): 277–286.
65 Conaway, H.H., Faas, F.H., Smith, S.D. et al. (1981). Spontaneous diabetes mellitus in the New Zealand white rabbit: physiologic characteristics. *Metab Clin Exp* 30 (1): 50–56.
66 Roth, S. and Conaway, H. (1982). Animal model of human disease. Spontaneous diabetes mellitus in the New Zealand white rabbit. *Amer J Pathol* 109 (3): 359–362.
67 Yu, L., Pragay, D., Chang, D. et al. (1979). Biochemical parameters of normal rabbit serum. *Clin Biochem* 12 (3): 83–87.
68 Atkinson, J.B., Hoover, R.L., Berry, K.K. et al. (1989). Cholesterol-fed heterozygous Watanabe heritable hyperlipidemic rabbits: a new model for atherosclerosis. *Atherosclerosis* 78 (2): 123–136.
69 Daley, S., Herderick, E., Cornhill, J. et al. (1994). Cholesterol-fed and casein-fed rabbit models of atherosclerosis. Part 1: differing lesion area and volume despite equal plasma cholesterol levels. *Arterioscler Thromb Vasc Biol* 14 (1): 95–104.
70 Eckermann-Ross, C. (2008). Hormonal regulation and calcium metabolism in the rabbit. *Vet Clin Exot Anim Pract* 11 (1): 139–152.
71 Redrobe, S. (2002). Calcium metabolism in rabbits. *Semin Av Exot Pet Med* 1 (23): 94–101.
72 Warren, H.B., Lausen, N.C.C., Segre, G.V. et al. (1989). Regulation of calciotropic hormones in vivo in the New Zealand white rabbit. *Endocrinology* 25 (5): 2683–2690.
73 Bourdeau, J.E., Schwer-Dymerski, D.A., Stern, P.H. et al. (1986). Calcium and phosphorus metabolism in chronically vitamin D-deficient laboratory rabbits. *Miner Electrolyte Metab* 12 (3): 176–185.
74 Kamphues, V., Carstensen, P., Schroeder, D. et al. (1986). Effects of increasing calcium and vitamin D supply on calcium metabolism of rabbits. *J Physiol Anim Nutrit* 56: 191–208.

75 Garibaldi, B.A. and Goad, M.E. (1988). Hypercalcemia with secondary nephrolithiasis in a rabbit. *Lab Anim Sci* 38 (3): 331–333.

76 Quimby, F., Foote, R., Profit-Olstad, M. et al. (1982). Hypercalcemia, hypercalcitonism and arterial calcification in rabbits fed a diet containing excessive vitamin D and calcium. *Lab Anim Sci* 32: 415.

77 Vernau, K.M., Grahn, B.H., Clarke-Scott, H.A. et al. (1995). Thymoma in a geriatric rabbit with hypercalcemia and periodic exophthalmos. *J Am Vet Med Assoc* 206 (6): 820–822.

78 Lennox, A.M. and Chitty, J. (2006). Adrenal neoplasia and hyperplasia as a cause of hypertestosteronism in two rabbits. *J Exot Pet Medicine* 15 (1): 56–58.

79 Künzel, F. and Joachim, A. (2010). Encephalitozoonosis in rabbits. *Parasitol Res* 106 (2): 299–230.

80 Künzel, F., Gruber, A., Tichy, A. et al. (2008). Clinical symptoms and diagnosis of encephalitozoonosis in pet rabbits. *Vet Parasitol* 151 (2): 115–124.

81 Cox, J.C., Hamilton, R.C., and Attwood, H.D. (1979). An investigation of the route and progression of *Encephalitozoon cuniculi* infection in adult rabbits. *J Eukaryot Microbiol* 26 (2): 260–265.

82 Cox, J. and Gallichio, H. (1978). Serological and histological studies on adult rabbits with recent, naturally acquired encephalitozoonosis. *Res Vet Sci* 24 (2): 260–261.

83 Fisher, P.G. and Carpenter, J.W. (2012). Neurologic and musculoskeletal diseases. In: *Ferrets, Rabbits and Rodents. Clinical Medicine and Surgery*, 2e (ed. K. Quesenberry and J. Carpenter), 245–255. WB Saunders.

84 Waller, T., Morein, B., and Fabiansson, E. (1978). Humoral immune response to infection with *Encephalitozoon cuniculi* in rabbits. *Lab Anim* 12 (3): 145–148.

85 Csokai, J., Gruber, A., Künzel, F. et al. (2009). Encephalitozoonosis in pet rabbits (*oryctolagus cuniculus*): Pathohistological findings in animals with latent infection versus clinical manifestation. *Parasitol Res* 104 (3): 629–635.

86 Csokai, J., Joachim, A., Gruber, A. et al. (2009). Diagnostic markers for encephalitozoonosis in pet rabbits. *Vet Parasitol* 163 (1): 18–26.

87 Dipineto, L., Rinaldi, L., Santaniello, A. et al. (2008). Serological survey for antibodies to *Encephalitozoon cuniculi* in pet rabbits in Italy. *Zoonoses Publ Health* 55 (3): 173–175.

88 Harcourt-Brown, F.M. (2004). *Encephalitozoon cuniculi* infection in rabbits. *Semin Av Exot Pet Medicine* 13 (2): 86–93.

89 Boot, R., Hansen, A., Hansen, C. et al. (2000). Comparison of assays for antibodies to *Encephalitozoon cuniculi* in rabbits. *Lab Anim* 34 (3): 281–289.

6

Rats and Mice

James Kusmeirczyk VMD[1]*, Melissa Kling DVM*[2]*, Ann B. Kier DVM, PhD, DACLAM*[3]*, Sherrelle M. Milligan DVM*[3] *and J. Jill Heatley DVM, MS, DABVP (Avian, Reptilian, Amphibian), DACZM*[4]

[1] *Cameron Park Zoo, Waco, Texas, USA*
[2] *Mercer University School of Medicine, Macon, Georgia, USA*
[3] *Department of Veterinary Pathobiology, College of Veterinary Medicine & Biomedical Sciences, Texas A&M University, College Station, Texas, USA*
[4] *Department of Small Animal Clinical Sciences, College of Veterinary Medicine & Biomedical Sciences, Texas A&M University, College Station, Texas, USA*

Introduction

Knowledge and technology of clinical pathology in rats and mice have been transformed over the past two decades based on the increasing use of these animals in biomedical research. The development of techniques and instrumentation has allowed for a wider variety of biomarkers to become available. These advances have allowed clinically useful information to become accessible from laboratory animal resources to the companion pet community. Standards of care for these pets continue to rise, and armed with more information than ever, owners of rats and mice expect better veterinary medical and surgical care. Higher expectations of owners coupled with refinement of blood collection techniques have compelled private practitioners to become proficient at safely collecting samples and interpreting results of exotic companion rodents. The development of monoclonal antibodies and their use as reagents in immunoassays has been a major influence in the field of rodent clinical pathology. Many of the analytes historically measured by colorimetric and end point assays are now measured by enzymatic tests with better specificity and sensitivity. Commercial companies now measure analytes and biomarkers in rodent blood using a combination of colorimetric, enzymatic, electrochemical, and immunologic methods. The use of laboratories that offer validated assays specifically for rodent blood is imperative to ensure accurate and precise results. A comprehensive understanding of the pathophysiology of the rat and mouse combined with a wide variety of readily measureable analytes allows interpretation of alterations in hematology, clinical chemistry, special chemistries, endocrinology, urinalysis, and blood coagulation. The investigation of transgenic and spontaneous genetic mutations of the rat has contributed to the discipline of comparative pathophysiology but is limited as compared with the mouse. The Mouse Genome Database manages this emerging data and includes phenotypic and clinical chemistry information. Extreme variations in hematology and clinical biochemistry of rats and mice occur depending on various factors, including age, sex, strain, hydration status, diet, fasting/fed status, cyclic biorhythms, husbandry (noise exposure, degree of confinement, environmental temperature), restraint/handling, venipuncture site, shipment, sedation/anesthesia, pathogens, and exposure to drugs. Corticosteroid-mediated stress and fasting are also common adjuncts of illness in the rat and mouse. On the basis of these confounding factors, reference intervals may be broad and misleading when applied to a specific population of animals or to an individual. Most reference values should be interpreted as approximations as they are gathered from a number of sources and do not represent specific populations or strains of rodents. Moreover, the laboratory processing the samples should be considered when selecting reference values and ranges to be used for interpretation of test results.

Species

This chapter will focus on the domestic brown rat *(Rattus norvegicus)* and the domestic house mouse *(Mus musculus)* as species which belong to the order Rodentia, suborder Myomorpha, family Muridae, and subfamily Murinae. Because of their use in biomedical research, thousands of outbred stocks and inbred strains exist. Fancy varieties developed by breeders for the show and pet industry are commonly presented to the private practitioner; little

Exotic Animal Laboratory Diagnosis, First Edition. Edited by J. Jill Heatley and Karen E. Russell.

information is available on what changes in clinical pathology, if any, can be expected in fancy varieties of pet rats or mice. The spiny mouse *(Acomys cahirunus)* is a precocial, nocturnal arid-adapted, human commensal species, which in the wild subsists on a mixed diet including insects, snails, and seeds [1, 2]. In the laboratory, this species serves as a model of insulin resistance and diabetes, wound healing, development, and behavior.

Sample Collection

Restraint and Site Preparation

Restraint methods for mice and rats are many and could easily be a chapter unto itself; our comments are limited to those useful for pet rats and mice based on sample collection. Because of the small size of these species, manual restraint specific to each venipuncture technique is often necessary and are therefore detailed, depending on each vascular access technique below. Patient stabilization should be attempted in these diminutive patients and should be made prior to considering sample collection, especially prior to manual restraint. Topical anesthesia, local anesthesia, general sedation, or general anesthesia should be used alone or in combination when necessary and appropriate, especially when dealing with pet rodents. Sedation, local or systemic analgesia, or anesthesia are recommended in these patients in exotic pet practice to facilitate venipuncture. Midazolam, buprenorphine, sevoflurane, and isoflurane are common drug choices in these patients. Rodents need not be fasted prior to anesthesia as, because of their strong pyloric sphincter, they cannot readily vomit and aspirate. However, adequate ventilation and venous return also deserve consideration. Excellent reviews of rodent restraint and anesthesia are available.

Patient warming and administration of warmed fluids will facilitate peripheral blood flow and sample collection, but may affect the analytes of interest. Warming options include placing the patient's tail in warm water (<104°F), applying warm packs or compresses to the appendage to be sampled, placing the entire patient in a warmed chamber, near a heat lamp, or on a heating pad [3]. In all cases, the patient should be monitored during the process to avoid overheating. A variety of commercially available and homemade restraint devices are used for blood collection in the awake patient, including acrylic tubes, syringe cases, plastic bags, socks, and cloth jackets and cocoons. Personnel involved with sample collection from these species should wear appropriate personal protection equipment as zoonotic potential for many diseases exists in laboratory-housed and privately owned animals.

Blood collection sites should be prepared by clipping or plucking the fur, or by application of a lubricating jelly and by cleaning with warmed disinfectant. Topical application of petroleum jelly, silicone gel, or alcohol to flatten and smooth the fur against the skin can also facilitate open blood collection by minimizing clot formation and facilitating drop formation. Topical anesthetic creams such as lidocaine jelly may be applied to reduce the pain of venipuncture. Wintergreen gel application or application of warm water or compress to the area of venipuncture can facilitate venous distension. Blood sample collection in rodents may be hindered by thick skin, small patient size, and small easily collapsible relatively deep vessels. Blood should be withdrawn slowly to avoid vessel collapse or suction attachment of the needle bevel to the vessel wall. Fine movements of the needle and needle bevel, such as rotation or application of slight pressure to the needle above, below or to the side of the puncture site, may facilitate blood collection [3].

Equipment

For the small rodent, right-sized, purpose-made equipment is available. Because the vessels of mice and rats are small, minimal aspiration pressure can result in vessel collapse. Appropriate microcollection equipment will facilitate sample collection, minimize patient harm, and increase sample volume for analysis. Proper needle size, minimizing force when transferring blood into a sample tube, and immediately separating blood cells from plasma or serum will reduce artifacts caused by hemolysis; plasma separator tubes are available for use in these species. Clinically useful information may be obtained from a single microhematocrit tube of blood and a well-prepared blood smear. Some diagnostic laboratories can perform a hematocrit, complete blood count with differential, and several plasma chemistries with as little as 150 µl of whole blood, affording this level of diagnostic medicine available to patients weighing as little as 15 g. Currently, for a typical blood chemistry test, 20–50 µl of serum or plasma are required. Insulin syringes with a swaged 27–29 gauge (g.) needle and the plunger removed are introduced into the vessel. Blood is collected from the hub of the needle into hematocrit tubes placed inside the syringe barrel. Small-gauge hypodermic needles can also be introduced into the vessel and blood collected in the same manner, but the use of the syringe barrel technique often provides greater needle stability during blood collection.

Blood and Sample Collection Volume

Table 6.1 provides physiologic parameters of rats and mice, including blood volumes and amounts of blood that may be safely removed. The circulating blood volume

Table 6.1 Physiologic and sample collection data for mice and rats [4–8].

Species	Adult body weight (g)	Average blood volume ml/100 g	Sample Volume 1% Body weight	10% blood volume ml/100 g	Exsanguination ml/100 g
Mouse (*Mus musculus*)	♂ 20–40 ♀ 18–35	5.85	♂ 0.2–0.4 ♀ 0.18–0.35	0.585	2.93
Spiny mouse (*Acomys cahirinus*)	Range: 39–85 Mean: 48.6	4.0 ± 0.162	~0.5	0.3–0.5	~3
Rat (*Rattus norvegicus*)	♂ 267–520 ♀ 250–325	6.4 (5.8–7.0)*	♂2.67–5.2 ♀2.5–3.25	0.6	3

of rodents is typically 6.3–8 ml/100 g of body weight [9]. The maximum blood volume that can be safely removed from a healthy mouse or rat patient in a single collection is 10%–15% of total blood volume or less than or equal to 1% of body weight [9]. Maximal blood draw volumes are restricted to once every 14–28 days. Removal of blood volume up to 20% is only permissible (as in the case of blood donor) if warmed replacement fluids of twice the volume are immediately provided to the patient. A four-week period may be necessary for recovery of all hematologic parameters. The effect of daily blood collection of a small amount of blood may be marked in the mouse. Blood volume is restored in 24 h, but red blood cells and reticulocytes take up to two weeks to return to normal concentrations. No more than 15% every four weeks may be obtained in order to facilitate total recovery of hematologic values [9]. Exsanguination is typically equal to half of the total blood volume in rodents. The average blood volume of rodents is dependent upon the body weight. The maximum blood volume recommend to be obtained for a single sample from a rat is 5 ml/kg of body weight [5]. The plasma volume of the laboratory rat ranges from 15.3–40.4 ml/kg [5].

Sample Handling and Storage

Proper handling and collection of blood in mice and rats is essential for minimizing hemolysis and reducing artifacts. Ethylenediaminetetraacetic acid (EDTA) is the anticoagulant of choice for a complete blood count, as the blood has better staining characteristics with Romanowsky-type stains than blood anticoagulated with heparin. EDTA tubes should be filled with the amount of blood volume recommended by the manufacturer. Excessive blood volume may result in clot formation, and too little may result in cellular artifacts and inaccurate cell counts. After collection, samples for hematologic analysis should be transported to the laboratory within a few hours, without freezing or excessive heat. If analysis is delayed, blood smears should be prepared within 4 h of collection. Smears that cannot be stained within 24 h may be fixed in absolute methanol for 10 min and stored at room temperature to ensure good cellular morphology. Whole blood is more stable for evaluation when stored between 2 °C and 8 °C than at room temperature. The stability of parameters over time is dependent on instrumentation and species. Rat samples have increased mean corpuscular volume (MCV) and decreased mean corpuscular hemoglobin concentration (MCHC), cell hemoglobin concentration mean (CHCM), and monocyte count at 24 h using the Bayer Advia 120 hematology analyzer, while mouse samples have increased MCV, red cell distribution width (RDW), and mean platelet volume (MPV) and decreased MCHC, CHCM, and monocyte counts at 24 h [4]. Refrigerated blood should be warmed to room temperature prior to analysis. Hemolysis due to collection technique results in errors in several red cell measurements. A fresh blood smear should be made at the time of sampling, especially with very small samples, to enable manual hematologic counts in-house and observation of blood cell morphology.

Anticoagulant

Plain, uncoated microtubes are available for serum collection. Microtubes treated with an anticoagulant such as lithium heparin or EDTA for plasma collection are also available. Use of collection tubes with gel separators may improve the serum or plasma volume recovery from a blood sample and minimize metabolite changes in plasma associated with storage time. If sample size is a concern, collection of blood for hematology and plasma chemistry into a single lithium heparin tube is a viable option to maximize usable sample volume [10]. Cellular morphology is preserved longer in a heparinized sample, and liquid EDTA-containing tubes may artificially dilute small samples as well as cause crenation of the red blood cells. Use of EDTA for plasma chemistry determinations will result in chelation of potassium and calcium, yielding artifactually lower concentrations of these analytes. Freezing of serum or plasma may affect the determination of certain analytes.

Anticoagulant coating of microhematocrit tubes may result in sample hemolysis. However, plasma collection has greater yield than serum if the volume is critical. Proper handling of the samples is essential. Serum or plasma should be separated from the cellular components, as glucose, potassium, and phosphorus are unstable in whole blood. Depending on the collection tube, the sample can be stored after centrifugation and gel separation for two to three days before decantation into an untreated sample tube.

Venipuncture Sites of Rats and Mice

The choice of venipuncture procedure and preferred venipuncture site depends upon the species, the animal's use (pet or laboratory subject), volume of blood required, intended frequency of bleeding, analytes desired, and whether or not sedation or anesthesia is used. Quality control of sample collection and handling is mandatory to ensure the most accurate values for analytes. This QC is particularly important for these animals, as venipuncture of smaller vessels is technically more challenging. Overnight fasting, consistent sample collection times, and attention to the quality of procedure for blood collection are all critical to the integrity of the clinical pathology results. Limitations obviously exist in the volume of sample that is obtained and the size of the collection devices. However, development of ultramicroanalytical techniques and microcollection equipment has overcome many of these restrictions. As compared to most other exotic animals, where the collection methods are primarily closed, rodent sample collection differs as historical methods of blood collection are used which do not require closed collection. Thus, blood collection includes open methods (blood collection from a lacerated or punctured vessel) and semi-open methods (blood collection into a device introduced into the vessel to facilitate blood flow via patient blood pressure and capillary action, not by human aspiration). While these methods may appear daunting, if performed by experienced phlebotomists, open collection techniques may be more humane, resulting in decreased patient morbidity, less likelihood of venous collapse, increased sample integrity, and increased sample volume, particularly in the diminutive patient. Many vessels are used for sample collection rats and mice, owing to their extensive use in research. Below we present venipuncture sites based on anatomical areas: vessels of the head and neck, central vessels (cardiac and cranial vena cava), and then the more peripheral sampling sites of the legs and tail. Within these groups, sampling sites are ordered from cranial to caudal. Unacceptable sites for use in exotic pet practice are provided last. Most information presented here is derived from the laboratory animal medicine literature for the hooded rat, *R. norvegicus*, and the mouse, *M. musculus*. However, many genera and species of rat and mouse exist for which these sites may or may not be applicable. For example, techniques for blood collection from the hispid cotton rat *(Sigmodon hispidus)* will also be included (Figure 6.1).

Superficial Temporal Vein

This technique is predominantly used in the mouse, often without sedation or anesthesia. The mouse may be held in a vertical position (upright posture) to modulate the force of the puncture, or laterally on a flat surface in lateral recumbency during venipuncture. Mice may be manually restrained by scruffing, extending the head and neck, or anesthesia. Judicious restraint is necessary to avoid respiratory distress in the conscious mouse. The loose skin of the dorsal neck between the mouse's ears is held with the thumb and forefingers, to draw the skin firmly against the face without causing the mouse's eyes to bulge. Because the sebaceous gland is a landmark, restraint must maintain the gland close to its natural location. The palpable cranial edge of the sebaceous gland is a landmark to locate the superficial temporal vein. A smooth, controlled, and swift stab with a lancet or needle is inserted into the superficial temporal vein, found one eye length caudal and one eye width dorsal to

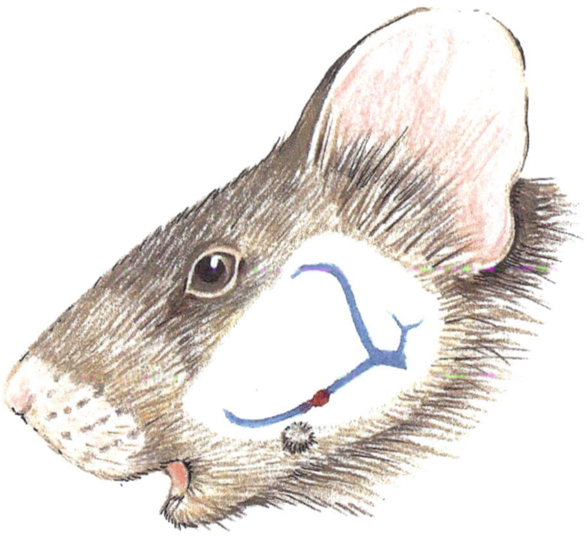

Figure 6.1 Rodent facial veins with anatomic landmarks for venipuncture are shown in a mouse. The facial vein and the submandibular vein conjoin at the caudal aspect of the mandible and become the jugular vein. The superficial temporal vein is also shown as it course lateral to the eye and below the ear. The sebaceous gland, shown as a fur-covered protrusion past midway along the jawline, is a helpful local anatomic landmark.

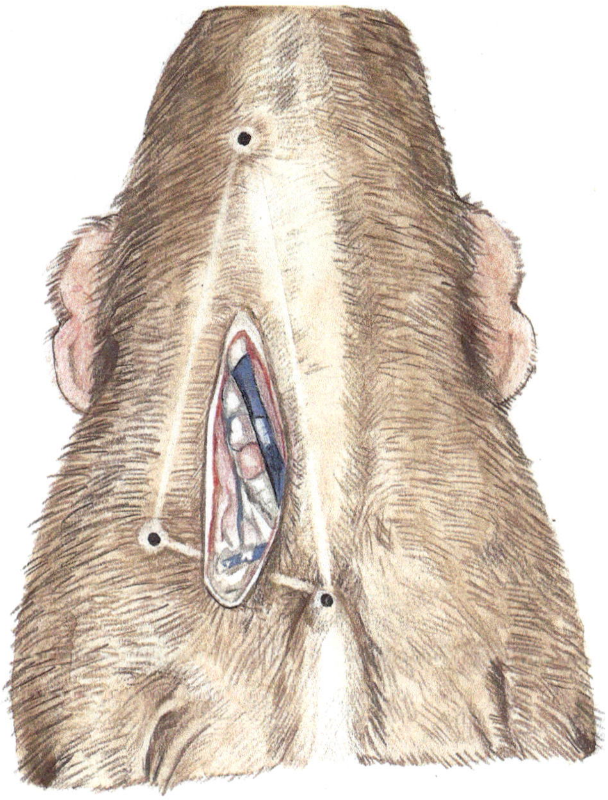

Figure 6.2 Rodent jugular vein is here drawn from the rat. Landmarks for jugular venipuncture of the rat are the three points of the caudal ramus of the mandible, the manubrium, and the greater tubercle. The triangulation of these three points (bisection of the angles when the three points are joined) provides a small window which is centered over the cranial aspect of the jugular vein for venipuncture.

the sebaceous gland (Figure 6.2). Avoid damage to the facial muscles or nerves by parallel insertion of the flat edge of the lance to the masticatory muscle [11]. Controlled puncture and appropriate mouse position allow for open blood collection into a microtube. Avoid overbleeding and shock with this method, which may occur if greater than 10–12 drops of blood are collected from the mouse. After completion, compress the site with sterile gauze for 15–20 s to facilitate hemostasis. The mouse can then be returned to its enclosure. Possible complications include damage to the adjacent facial muscles or nerves. Mortality rate in one study was approximately 1% [11]. A mild leukocytosis occurred in mice after two or three samples obtained with this method, from 5000 white blood cells per microliter of blood to 10 000 white blood cells per microliter of blood [11].

Submandibular Vein/Facial Vein/Angle of the Jaw Vein

Sampling of the veins of the head is mainly used on the mouse and does not require the use of anesthesia [12]. This method has replaced most tail clipping in mice as it causes less permanent damage, and pain and distress to the patient [13]. This method has largely been replaced by the superficial temporal vein method (above) and is similar (Figure 6.2). The anatomic site for venipuncture targets the retroorbital and submandibular veins draining the face of the mouse as they join to become the jugular vein [12]. The animal is restrained by holding the skin between the scapulae but not the ears, to lessen facial distortion during venipuncture. The optimal puncture point is slightly behind the hinge of the jaw toward the ear. For this open technique, a 23–18 g. needle or a mouse size specific lancet is quickly inserted into the vein, and blood is allowed to drip into the blood collection tube. One may obtain up to 0.7 ml from a single mouse. Blood flows rapidly after lancet or needle introduction; may quickly clot within the needle, reducing sample size; and flow often slows shortly after puncture. In the hispid cotton rat (*S. hispidus*), this method yielded only one to two drops in one out of five attempts [13]. Complications of this blind method may include damage to the submandibular vascular or glandular structures, insufficient application of lancet pressure resulting in no or minimal sample, penetration of the cheek resulting in blood accumulation in the oral cavity, possible aspiration and death, or penetration of the ear canal resulting in bleeding from the ear [12, 13].

Subzygomatic Sinus

This phlebotomy technique has been described for use in the hispid cotton rat (*S. hispidus*) and generally provides 0.3–0.5 ml of blood [13]. The venous sinus located below the zygomatic arch of the maxilla and deep to the masseter muscle. The subzygomatic sinus may be unique to this species and is suspected to connect to the retroorbital sinus [13]. The landmarks are easily palpable, and the vein may be visualized as a slight bulge when the area is shaved. The rat was anesthetized and held in the nondominant hand by gathering the dorsal skin from the base of the tail with the fourth and fifth fingers and rolling the hand forward to grasp the neck over the skin with the thumb and forefinger. This scruff method encourages venous congestion of the head and holds the skin taught over the cheek. The ventral aspect of the caudal rim of the zygomatic arch and the ramus of the mandible where it meets the zygomatic bone are used as landmarks. The angle formed rostral to the intersection of these bones, just below the lateral canthus of the eye, is the preferred puncture site. Vascular puncture was made in a controlled manner to a depth of 2–4 mm with the patient in lateral recumbency. Upon blood flow, the rat was then held above the collection tube so that blood flowed into the tube, generally with the hindquarters held more elevated than the head. An 18 g. 3/4′ needle facilitated large drop formation and blood flow, and lessened clot formation. After sample collection, hemostasis is achieved by releasing the scruff hold and applying gentle pressure to the venipuncture site with a gauze pad. Histologic examination of acute puncture sites showed hemorrhage, edema, and inflammation similar to findings from submandibular puncture in mice, while older puncture sites showed evidence of healing and regeneration [13].

Sublingual Vein

Sublingual venipuncture is an alternative venipuncture site for use in the anesthetized rat [14]. An assistant holds the unconscious animal in a supine position and scruffs the skin at the nape of the neck to temporarily occlude venous return from the head. A second person extends the tongue forward with a cotton-tipped applicator stick to grasp it with thumb and forefinger. Forceps should not be used, to avoid blunt trauma to the tongue. The two sublingual veins are visible at the base of the tongue as they course to left and right of the tongue midline. Puncture the vein with a 23 g., 0.60 × 25 mm hypodermic needle as far peripherally as possible to allow sufficient blood flow for collection of 0.5–1.0 ml of blood. Careful puncture is necessary to avoid sticking the needle through the vein. For later blood samples, the sublingual veins can be punctured alternately and more proximal to the tongue base. After venipuncture, the rat is returned to a prone position, and the blood allowed to drip into the collection tube. As the required volume of blood is collected, scruffing is halted to release neck compression. The rat is replaced in a supine position, to re-extend the tongue and apply a solution of antiseptic to the venipuncture site with a cotton-tipped applicator. Red blood cell counts do not change, but white blood cell counts are decreased for 2 h after collection, but return to baseline within 8 h of sampling via this method. This method allows for serial blood collection, but decreased feed consumption is a potential complication [15]. In the hispid cotton rat *(S. hispidus)*, this was the only classical phlebotomy technique to yield measureable amounts of blood, from 0 to approximately 0.25 ml [13]. In the cotton rat, less prominent sublingual veins and a shorter tongue attached more caudally in the oral cavity contributed to difficulty in sample collection [13]. Larger bore 22 g. needles better facilitated blood flow and increased the sample volume collected in this species. Hemostasis was achieved with application of light pressure to the tongue base with a gauze square [13].

Jugular Vein

The jugular vein is a preferred sampling site for rodents because of the vessel size, which allows for collection of maximal volumes [3]. This method does not require patient warming [16]. However, this site may be more challenging in mice because of their small size. The short neck of rats and mice, their relatively deep jugular vein, ample mobile rodent neck skin, the relatively large salivary gland which may partially cover the jugular vein, and the fat bodies which may cover the jugular groove all make accessing this vessel challenging for the inexperienced [17]. The vein may be visualized as it courses from just below the angle of the jaw to the manubrium; in the mouse, the blue color of the vessel may often be visualized 2–4 mm lateral to the sternoclavicular junction [17, 18].

Mice and rats should be anesthetized for this technique, and local anesthetic cream may be applied prior to the procedure to facilitate a lighter plan of anesthesia during phlebotomy and a pain-free recovery [16, 18]. The patient may be positioned in dorsal, lateral, or supine recumbency. Hyperextension of the head is necessary and may be accomplished via traction on the upper incisors as facilitated by a gauze square, string, or suture [3]. After aseptic preparation of the area, the vessel is occluded at the thoracic inlet. The vein may be entered from the cranial or caudal aspect, from above the well-developed clavicle of these species. In the mouse, the vein may be visualized and accessed 2–4 mm lateral to the sternoclavicular junction with a 25 g. and/or smaller needle and a 0.3–1.0 ml syringe directed cranially. Insertion should be shallow, at 30°, with only 1–4 mm of the needle inserted into the blood vessel [16, 18]. Advancement of the needle through a small amount of the sternal musculature is recommended to stabilize the approach in the mouse [18]. As the needle is advanced with intermittent aspiration, blood withdrawal confirms placement into the jugular vein [3].

Cranial Vena Cava

Some practitioners consider phlebotomy of the cranial vena cava as the preferred approach in pet rats and mice [19]. However, cranial vena cava sampling may present more risk to smaller rodent species [20]. Possible complications of cranial vena caval puncture include hemorrhage into the thoracic cavity or pericardial sac, laceration of the great vessels or atria, and cardiac, thymic, or lung puncture [21]. Anatomic knowledge, use of short, small-gauge needles, patient anesthesia for immobilization, and a steady hand may reduce the risk of patient morbidity or mortality associated with this technique [19]. Rats and mice have well-developed clavicles; placement of the needle dorsal to the clavicle may hinder phlebotomy of the cranial vena cava [21]. To further minimize risks associated with sampling, 25–27 g. needles < 0.5 in. (12 mm) and a 0.3–1.0 ml syringe are used in rats and mice. Cranial vena cava blood collection is a closed technique. The patient is anesthetized and placed in dorsal recumbency, and the area of insertion is aseptically prepared. Hair removal is generally unnecessary. The manubrium, clavicle, and first ribs are identified as palpable landmarks for this technique. The needle is inserted between the clavicle and the first rib at an angle of 45°. Introduce the needle into the thoracic inlet on the right or left side of the neck. The needle is advanced slowly caudally and medially and as shallowly as allowed by local anatomy toward the rat's opposite elbow. A slight negative pressure is maintained on the syringe plunger until the appearance of a flash of blood in the needle hub signals a halt to advancement and the beginning of the process of sample collection. Failure of blood to flow after the initial flash of blood may mean that the needle was advanced thought the vessel, the bevel is obstructed by the vessel wall, or the vein has collapsed owing to excessive aspirative pressure. Fine needle adjustments, such as withdrawal, rotation, or redirection, may alleviate lack of blood flow [19]. However, excessive motion of the needle may lacerate the vessels or other thoracic tissues, resulting in patient mortality (Figure 6.3).

Cardiac Puncture

Cardiac puncture is only acceptable as a terminal procedure and requires anesthesia, but allows for maximum blood collection [18]. This technique's inclusion here for use in pet rodents is based on the precepts of herd health management. Thus, a terminal blood sample collection from an ill animal prior to diagnostic necropsy may be necessary and increase the likelihood and timeliness of herd diagnosis. During cardiocentesis, the animal should be in at least the surgical plane of anesthesia if not deeper. Blood may be obtained from an approach to the ventricle through the ventral or left lateral chest wall [18]. For the ventral approach, the animal is placed in dorsal recumbency, and the heart impulse is palpated. In the mouse, a 1 in 22 g. needle is introduced in the notch slightly to the left or right of and under the xiphoid, directed cranially toward the cardiac contractions. Negative pressure is applied after the needle is introduced underneath the skin. Reflux of blood confirms correct needle placement into the heart. Blood should be aspirated slowly to avoid ventricular collapse [18]. In the normal rat, a small left lung exposes the heart to the left thoracic wall and allows visualization of the cardiac impulse (heat beat) in rib spaces three to five [22]. For the left lateral approach to cardiac puncture, place the animal in right lateral recumbency and palpate the cardiac contractions emanating from beneath the left lateral thoracic wall, located at approximately the point of flexed elbow. Insert the needle slowly between ribs five and six and into the ventricle of the heart (Figure 6.4).

Saphenous Vein

Saphenous venipuncture may be accomplished in the mouse and rat without anesthesia or a restraint device [15]. The animal is positioned in ventral recumbency via manual restraint. Adequate peripheral perfusion is required for successful phlebotomy of this site [23]. Appropriate restraint facilitates success of this technique, as the location of the vein varies. Area preparation may include application of antiseptics or alcohol to wet down the fur, or clipping or otherwise removing the fur, application of local anesthetic cream, and then application of

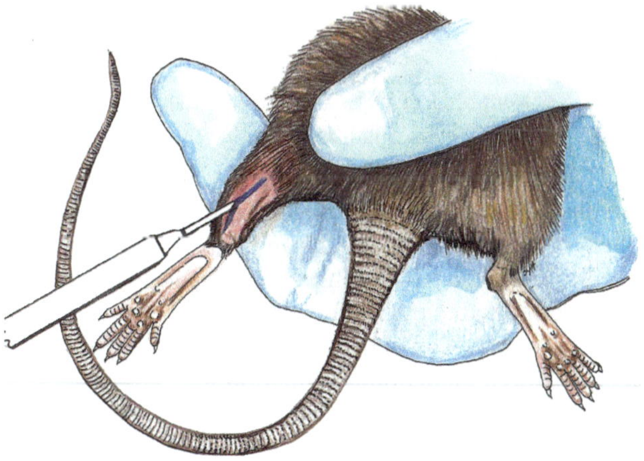

Figure 6.3 Caudal saphenous venipuncture for rodents is depicted in the mouse. Restraint and extension of the hind limb is accomplished by application of gentle downward pressure above the knee joint. This restraint method should also stretch the skin to facilitate hair removal and immobilization of the saphenous vein. The method facilitates open collection of blood from the saphenous vein with collection into a capillary tube. To stop blood flow, relaxation of restraint and gentle pressure applied to the venipuncture site is generally sufficient.

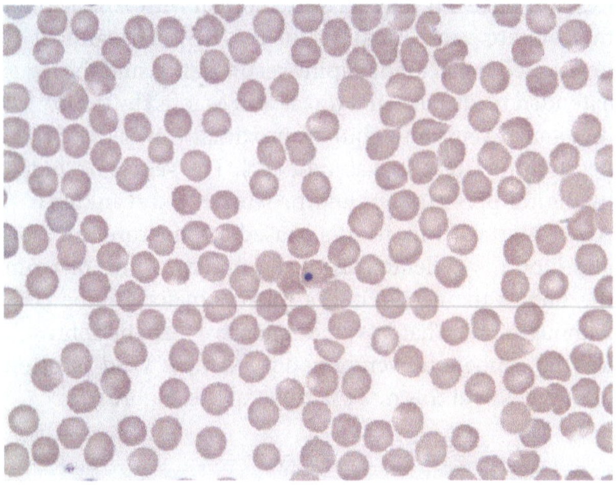

Figure 6.4 Nucleated erythrocytes are not uncommon in the blood smears of normal rodents, owing to the relatively short rodent erythrocyte life span. Mouse nucleated red blood cell (nRBC), 1000× magnification, modified Wright's stain, EDTA anticoagulant.

a thin coat of silicone grease. At this point, the vein can usually be visualized as it courses along the caudal surface of the thigh. The leg must be held in extension by applying gentle downward pressure above the knee [15]. This hold stretches and holds taut the skin over the ankle, which stabilizes the somewhat mobile saphenous vein. The vein may be punctured above or below the ankle, as it becomes the pedal vein (see below). An appropriately sized lancet or needle (23–25 g.) is used to puncture (not lance) the vein to allow blood flow. In mice, a 25 g. 0.6 mm needle is usually sufficient to allow adequate blood flow [15]. Up to 100 μl of blood may then be collected into a microhematocrit tube or blood capillary collection device. Should closed collection be attempted from the saphenous vein, small-volume syringes may reduce the risk of venous collapse. After collection, apply pressure to the site until hemostasis is achieved. The scab that forms may be removed and additional samples collected over a 24 h period [15]. Criticisms of this method include that it is time and labor intensive and often yields less than 0.3 ml [12].

Lateral Vein of Tarsus (Vena Plantaris Lateralis)

Distal to the saphenous vein, blood may be sampled from the lateral marginal vein of the tarsus, also called the pedal vein. Because of the small vein size, this method is more commonly used in larger rodents such as the rat but has been described for use in the mouse [16, 19]. Because adequate peripheral perfusion is required for blood collection at this site, patient warmth and hydration should be optimized prior to venipuncture [23]. The animal may be sedated, anesthetized, or held in a restraint device; local anesthetic cream should be applied to the site prior to phlebotomy. Hair may not need removal in rats and mice but may be wetted down with 70% alcohol to facilitate vein visualization [15, 16]. The animal is positioned in lateral or supine recumbency, and the leg is extended to visualize the tarsal vein as it fed by the dorsal metatarsal veins and courses proximally over the dorsal pes and the lateral tarsal joint [17]. The vein is occluded by digital pressure applied proximal to the ankle [16]. A 22–27 g. × 5/8-in. needle is used to puncture the vein, and blood is collected from the puncture site or from the hub of the needle into a microhematocrit tube [16]. Although somewhat less labor intensive than the approach for the saphenous venipuncture, sample yield is often relatively less at this more peripheral site (Figure 6.5).

Femoral Vein

Sampling of the femoral vein requires anesthetized rodents and practice, but may yield a reasonable sample volume from rats [21]. For this closed collection, the rodent is positioned in dorsal recumbency and a 27–25 g.

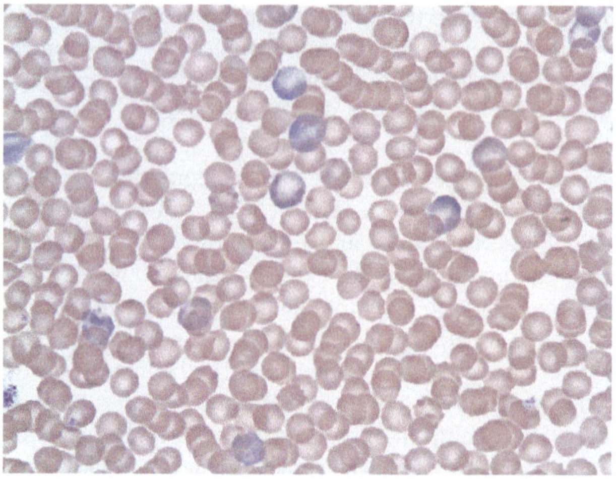

Figure 6.5 Mild to moderate polychromasia is an expected finding in healthy rodent blood smears owing to the rapid turnover of these cells in these species. Cells shown at 1000× magnification, modified Wright's stain, EDTA anticoagulant.

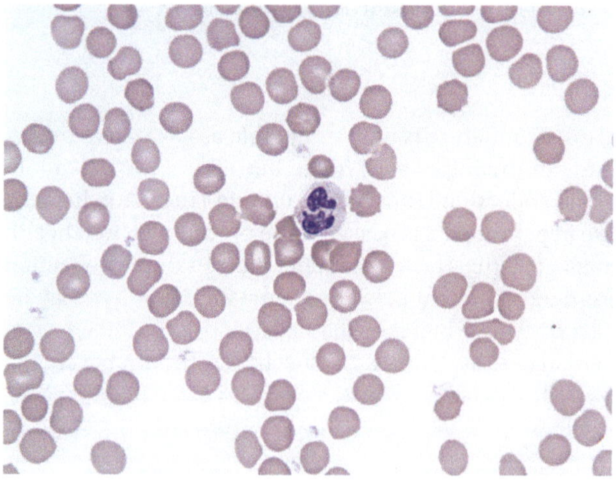

Figure 6.6 Neutrophil of a rat. Cells shown at 1000× magnification, modified Wright's stain, EDTA anticoagulant.

needle and a 0.3–1 ml syringe are used. The arterial pulse is palpated deep in the inguinal region, and the needle is inserted parallel and medial to this site. Pressure must be applied to the venipuncture site for several minutes after collection should the artery be inadvertently sampled [21]. Hematoma formation and arteriovenous fistula are possible complications with this sampling technique (Figure 6.6).

Tail Veins

Two lateral tail veins and the ventral caudal artery are available for venipuncture in mice and rats. In the exotic pet setting, this venipuncture technique is more commonly used in rats because of their larger tail. Warming the animal for 5–10 min (24 °C–27 °C) or placing the tail in warm water (≤40 °C) may promote vasodilation and therefore improve the volume of sample collected. Tail flicking or massage may also facilitate blood flow toward the tail and therefore its successful phlebotomy [3]. However, the tail should not be rubbed directionally from base to tip, which may result in leukocytosis of tail vein samples [18]. The patient is restrained in dorsal recumbency for these techniques [3]. If manual restraint rather than anesthesia is chosen for tail vein sampling, the animal should receive heavy sedation and systemic analgesics as well as application of topical anesthetic cream. Anesthesia is preferred for phlebotomy of the artery of the tail. In general, tail vein phlebotomy usually results in less sample volume than tail artery phlebotomy, but up to 2 ml may be collected from the tail vein of rats [16, 23]. Tail phlebotomy attempts should be limited to three and proceed distally to proximally along the tail, to minimize the likelihood of hematoma formation and vessel collapse, which could further hinder phlebotomy attempts or arterial obstruction and result in tail necrosis. In the hispid cotton rat (*S. hispidus*), this method is not recommended because of the dark tail pigmentation, which hinders vein visualization and the potential for tail slip or tail loss in this species [13] (Figure 6.7).

The paired tail veins course along the lateroventral aspect of the tail. Veins are occluded at the tail base with digital pressure or a tourniquet. Blood may be collected from the hub of a 22–25 g. needle into a capillary tube, with a needle and syringe, from a 22 to 23 g. butterfly catheter with most of the tubing removed, or via open collection of puncture made by a lancet or needle [16]. In general, tail vein phlebotomy usually results in less sample volume than tail artery phlebotomy [23]. Should multiple collections be anticipated to assess patient health, aseptic placement of an intravenous catheter is indicated. However, multiple samples may be obtained by entering the same site or moving proximally along the tail (Figure 6.8).

Tail Artery

Phlebotomy of the tail artery can yield an adequate sample, but the technique requires practice and experience [24]. To sample the ventral tail artery, rats are sedated or anesthetized and placed in dorsal recumbency. Application of a topical anesthetic cream is recommended to prevent discomfort from this procedure. The central tail artery courses slightly off the central midline deep to the ventral aspect of the tail. Materials which may be used to access the artery for blood collection include 27–25 g. needles attached to a 1 cm^3 tuberculin syringe with the plunger removed, a 23–25 g. butterfly infusion set modified as for lateral tail vein access, or a 25–22 g. needle and syringe [3, 23]. The tail is held with gentle traction as the needle, with proximal facing bevel, is inserted at a 30°–45° angle, at a point approximately one third the length of the tail from the base of the tail or more distally, and the needle is advanced until blood appears within the bevel of the needle [3, 20]. Once the artery is entered, blood is allowed to enter the syringe barrel or tubing depending on the arterial pressure. Blood collection proceeds in a semi-closed (blood drips into the collection tube or is collected from the syringe barrel with hematocrit tubes) or closed manner depending on the equipment used. After sample collection, application of gentle pressure to the venipuncture site to ensure hemostasis is required. Packed cell volume (PCV) and hemoglobin measurements from samples collected from the tail vein may be higher than those collected from other sites [25]. Possible complications of tail artery

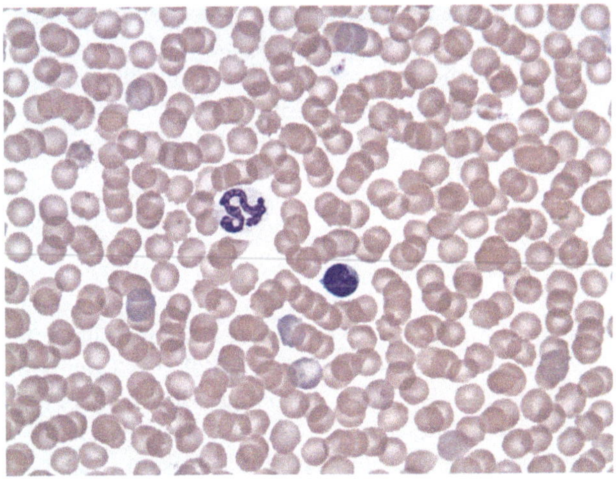

Figure 6.7 Mouse neutrophil (left), lymphocyte (right), and a small platelet clump shown uppermost, right of center. Cells shown at 1000× magnification, modified Wright's stain, EDTA anticoagulant.

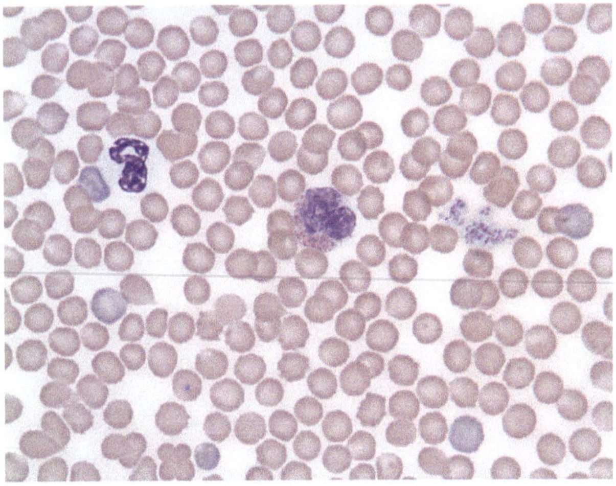

Figure 6.8 Mouse nucleated erythrocyte (nRBC, lower left), neutrophil (upper left), eosinophil (center), and platelet raft (upper right). Cells shown at 1000× magnification, modified Wright's stain, EDTA anticoagulant.

venipuncture are few, but include tail necrosis. Sampling attempts should be limited to three and progress down the tail to avoid this complication (Figures 6.9 and 6.10).

Unacceptable Phlebotomy Sites

Unacceptable techniques for phlebotomy of the pet mouse or rat include the retroorbital or ophthalmic venous plexus or sinus puncture, tail snip or sectioning the tail, clipping the nail bed, surgical approaches that require sample collection from the inferior vena cava or abdominal aorta, severing the brachial plexus or the carotid artery, and phlebotomy of the penile vein or the marginal ear vein or artery [23]. Specific approaches to these sites will not be given; rather, the discussion will be limited to humane considerations and sample quality

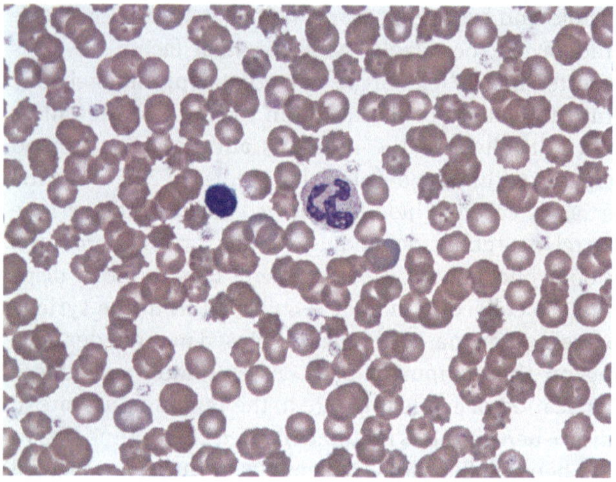

Figure 6.9 Rat lymphocyte (left) and eosinophil (right) as well as numerous platelets. Cells shown at 1000× magnification, modified Wright's stain, EDTA anticoagulant.

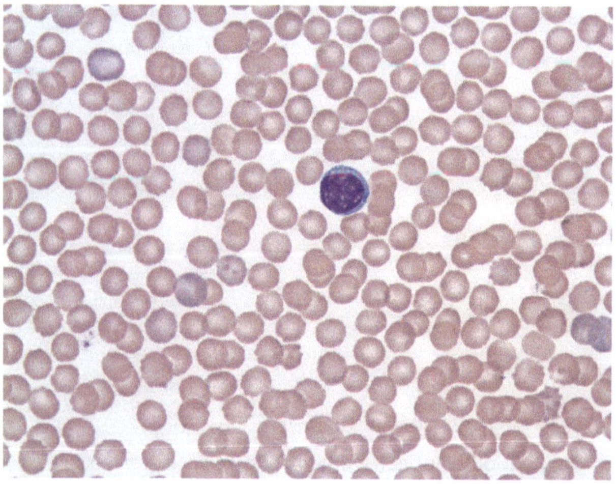

Figure 6.10 Mouse large lymphocyte at 1000× magnification, modified Wright's stain, EDTA anticoagulant.

associated with these techniques. Although commonly mentioned in older texts, retroorbital collection of blood is no longer considered humane or acceptable for use in pet or laboratory animals. Special dispensation must be given by animal care committees for this procedure, which is now relegated to part of a terminal procedure that includes anesthesia. Samples collected from this site are often small, not representative of cell percentages in peripheral circulation, shown to have higher serum glucose concentrations, and prone to clot formation [26]. Both acute and chronic adverse effects of this technique are described for rats and include corneal damage, ocular discharge, orbital bone fractures, abnormal eye positions, intraocular alterations, keratitis, enophthalmia, loss of vitreous humor, infection, microophthalmia, abscessation, and blindness [13, 18]. Further, histological damage to bone and soft tissue structures secondary to this sampling method have been documented in mice and rats [27]. Therefore, the approach and materials necessary for blood collection from these sites are not provided here. Similarly, the method of sample collection from sniping or sectioning the tail or clipping a nail bed causes pain both during and after the procedure. These techniques create an open wound that may increase the likelihood of focal or systemic infection of the patient. Similar to samples collected from orbital sinus, nail or tail blood samples are mixed with tissue fluids, prone to clot formation, and compromised for clinical chemistries based on artifactually increased creatine kinase, calcium, and total protein [23].

Arterial Sampling

Arterial samples are most commonly obtained from the caudal artery, but femoral artery, aorta, and heart may also be used. The latter more invasive sites are generally restricted to the research setting. Collection of multiple samples to serially monitor blood gases is often impractical because of the necessary sample volume. Noninvasive methods such as transcutaneous blood gas monitoring in the mouse and the rat have limited clinical application at this time [28].

Clinical Hematology

In rats and mice, hematologic values may vary depending on the site of blood withdrawal [29–33]. Counts of red blood cells (RBCs), white blood cells (WBCs), and platelets in the mouse are lower in central veins or cardiac blood compared with peripheral sites. In rats, PCV, hemoglobin (Hb), and WBC are higher in tail vein blood compared with blood obtained by cardiac puncture because of decreased flow rates and sludging of blood through small vessels of the tail [34]. Hemoglobin and

PCV are increased in samples from the rat's tail, compared to those from the abdominal aorta or heart. Variations can also occur because of the effects of anesthesia such as lower PCV due to splenic sequestration. The basic morphology of the blood cell types of mice and rats is given in Table 6.2. Discussion is limited to interpretation of cell counts (normal and abnormal) and abnormal cell morphology. Mild leukocytosis secondary to repeated phlebotomy of the tail and facial vein may occur in mice [11].

Table 6.2 Blood cell morphology of rats and mice [9, 30, 35–37] with cells ordered by frequency in the healthy animal cell count, color, and shapes described on the basis of morphology of blood smear monolayer cells with modified Wright's stain.

Cell	Species	Size	Cytoplasm	Nucleus	Comments
Erythrocyte	Rat	Diameter 5.7–7 um, Volume 55.1–61.5 fl	Round biconcave disk with central pallor	Anucleate	Moderate anisocytosis common, diameters 1/3 of cell average
	Mouse	Diameter 5–7 um, thickness 2.1–2.13 um, volume 40–50 fl			Howell–Jolly bodies, nucleated RBC (nRBC) occasional, both species
Platelet	Rat, mouse	1–4 um, round to oval to elongate	Margins indistinct, pink to gray, blue angular granules centrally,± red granules	Anucleate	Round, RBC-sized platelets and platelet clumps common
Lymphocyte	Rat	Small: diameter ~6 um,~ size of normal neutrophil Large: diameter to 15 um	Small: scant cytoplasm, occasional granules Large: variable amount, deep to pale blue, ± large dark azurophilic granules; according to [36] this applies to both small and large	Nucleus of large lymphocyte is slightly larger than the erythrocyte	
	Mouse	Small and large	Small: scant cytoplasm Large: extensive cytoplasm. Occasional purple granules	Small: eccentric with smudged, indistinct chromatin Large: stippled chromatin	
Neutrophil	Rat	11 μm	Pale cytoplasm, fine diffuse granule, pale to clear, small faint pink granules	Highly segmented, coiled or ribbon-like with numerous indentations, ring forms not uncommon, Figure of 8 forms occasional	
	Mouse		Pale to clear, small faint pink granules	Segments connected by threads. Chromatin variable clear or condensed	
Monocyte	Rat	Largest leukocyte	Basophilic, vaculolated, ±azurophilic granules	pleomorphic: Round, indented or lobular	
	Mouse	Largest leukocyte, 3 × RBC diameter	Extensive, pale gray-blue, vacuoles, occasional acidophilic granules	Pleomorphic: round indented or lobular	
Eosinophil	Rat	Generally larger than neutrophils	Small round, strongly acidophilic, reddish granules fill the cytoplasm	Less segmentation than neutrophil, occasional ring form. Immature nuclei commonly doughnut shaped	
	Mouse		Abundant ruddy orange to red large round granules with indistinct borders	Band or ring shaped, partially obscured by granules	
Basophil	Rat, mouse		Rat: few granules, as if partly degranulated, variable Romanowksi stain uptake Both: few to many large round purple granules	lobulated, may be obscured by granules	Rarely observed on peripheral blood smear. Differentiate from mast cells if cardiac puncture is used for blood collection

Erythrocytes

The erythrocytes of mice and rats are more numerous and generally smaller than in other rodents. The short erythrocyte life span in mice and rats (40–68 days) results in increased basophilic stippling and numbers of reticulocytes, polychromatophils, and polychromasia (Table 6.2). Thus, anisocytosis and polychromasia are prominent in the normal animal [37]. Rouleaux formation is rare in mice and rats. Erythropoiesis occurs predominately in the bone marrow, but also within the healthy mouse spleen. Hemoglobin, erythrocyte, and hematocrit values are lower in the newborn mouse and rat than in the adult. Neonates have larger red cells, and increased numbers of circulating reticulocytes that reach adult values at about three weeks [37]. Aged mice and rats typically have a decreased hematocrit, secondary to plasma expansion rather than a decrease in red cell production, and have lower numbers of circulating reticulocytes. Erythrocyte numbers, amount of hemoglobin, and PCV tend to be higher in males compared to females (Figure 6.11).

Polycythemia is uncommon in the pet rodent, but may occur depending on both pathologic and physiologic processes such as acclimatization to altitude [38]. In mice and rats, a relative increase in red blood cell mass (relative polycythemia) occurs with decreased plasma volume owing to increased water loss (secondary to disease) or decreased water intake. Absolute increases in red blood cell mass (absolute polycythemia) are classified as appropriate or inappropriate responses. An appropriate response occurs because of decreased tissue oxygenation and from an abnormal hemoglobin (methemoglobinemia) or respiratory pathology (i.e., murine respiratory mycoplasmosis).

Anemia, an absolute decrease in red cell mass, may be regenerative or non-regenerative. Causes of regenerative anemia include increased red cell loss (hemorrhage or repeated phlebotomy) or increased destruction/hemolysis (immune-mediated processes, blood parasites such as *Plasmodium berghei* in rats, oxidative damage secondary to toxins, or mechanical damage). In mice, hemolysis is commonly extravascular. Immune-mediated hemolytic anemia is uncommon in the pet mouse but occurs in some laboratory strains. Primary immune-mediated hemolytic anemia is rare in the rat. Non-regenerative causes of anemia include disease processes affecting the bone marrow chemically such as drugs that are toxic or suppressive to hematopoietic stem cells or physically such as myelophthisis secondary to neoplasia. Other causes include renal disease as a result of decreases in erythropoietin and anemia of chronic disease. Anemia of chronic disease develops quickly in mice and rats because of the short life span of their erythrocytes. Decreased erythrocyte production in mice dramatically affects red blood cell parameters (higher mean corpuscular hemoglobin and lower MCV and RDW) as there is a decrease in reticulocytes, which are normally present in high numbers.

Relative decreases (lower PCV) are seen with plasma expansion in aged rats and pregnant females. RBC, reticulocyte counts, MCV, MCH, and plateletcrit, of both sexes and HCT and hemoglobin concentration of female rats may vary depending solely on rat origin [39]. Pregnant rats may have lower RBC, hemoglobin, and hematocrit and higher MCHC and reticulocyte percentages than nonmated rats of the same strain [40].

Causes of falsely decreased erythrocytes include clotted samples, improper analyzer gate settings for the small size of mice and rat erythrocytes, and dilution from excess anticoagulant. Lipemia or the presence of Heinz bodies artificially increases the amount of hemoglobin measured. As a result, indices which rely on hemoglobin, such as mean cell hemoglobin (MCH) and MCHC, may also be artifactually increased by lipemia. Fasting rats for 16 h may increase HCT and Hgb in males, while 48 h fasts increase RBC in males and females.

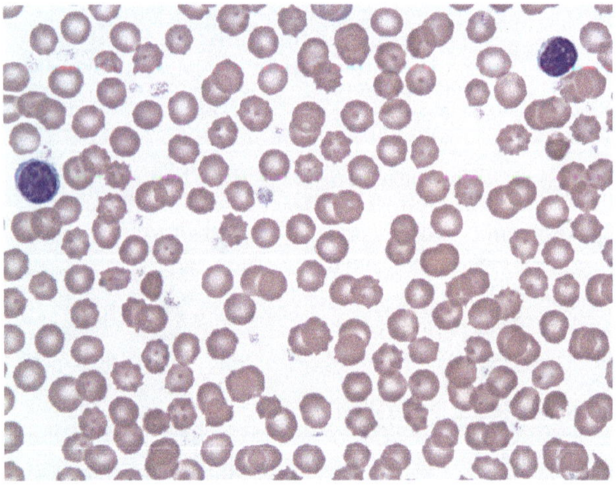

Figure 6.11 Rat large lymphocytes, some RBC crenated, shown at 1000× magnification, modified Wright's stain, EDTA anticoagulant.

Platelets

Rat and mouse platelet counts are high compared to other domestic animals and highly variable [35, 37]. Platelet activation, degranulation, aggregation, and clumping or partial clot formation in samples may lead to falsely decreased platelet counts, and increased eosinophil counts by automated analyzer. Some analyzers are unable to accurately count mouse and rat platelets because of their size. Therefore, automated platelet count validity should be considered in combination with microscopic examination of the blood smear [37]. Neonatal mouse platelet counts are low, but reach adult concentrations just after weaning. Mouse and rat platelet counts do not differ on the basis of sex or strain, but may be higher in pregnant compared to nonmated rats, or vary depending on rat origin [39, 40]. Platelet-deficient models of both mice and rat exist, but these genetic abnormalities appear rare to nonexistent in pet rat and mice. Higher platelet numbers in peripheral blood are associated with higher platelet production secondary to certain inflammatory conditions, increased erythropoiesis, or iron deficiency [35]. Giant platelets may be seen in peripheral blood during increased thrombopoiesis. Lower platelet numbers in peripheral blood are most commonly based on artifactual changes, but true thrombocytopenia may be due to decreased production or shortened platelet half-life [35]. Decreased production is usually due to damaged progenitor cells or megakaryocytes from immune-mediated, neoplastic, or toxic causes. Shortened platelet half-life is due to destruction via immune-mediated disease or consumption, usually from hemorrhage. A common cause of true thrombocytopenia is activation and consumption due to hemorrhage or DIC. Thrombocytopenia may occur secondary to bone marrow progenitor cell damage, but usually only after notable reductions in neutrophil, eosinophil, and monocyte numbers [35].

Leukocytes

WBC count may be estimated using a blood smear of fresh blood as in other species. However, this method provides only a very rough estimate and findings should be confirmed by an actual hemocytometer or automated count. Morphological changes to cells observed are likely of more clinical import than WBC counts estimated with this method. The importance of sending rodent samples to a laboratory properly equipped for and familiar with assessment of rodent blood samples cannot be overstated.

Total WBC

Table 6.5 provides hematologic reference data for rats and mice. Causes of leukocytosis in the mouse and rat are similar to those in other mammals; leukogram changes can occur in seconds to minutes because of the release or administration of catecholamines or glucocorticoids. Excitement and resultant catecholamine release causes leukocyte release from the marginated pool and increased circulating leukocytes, neutrophils, lymphocytes, and monocytes. Stress from handling, restraint, or transportation, and glucocorticoids increase circulating neutrophils and decrease lymphocytes and eosinophils (Table 6.4). Other causes of leukocytosis include inflammation, neoplasia, leukocyte adhesion deficiencies in certain laboratory strains, and allergies or hypersensitivity reactions. As inflammation becomes more chronic, neutrophil, lymphocyte, and monocyte counts increase. Changes in absolute numbers of leukocytes may be more meaningful than relative changes. Platelet clumps, young reticulocytes that are lyse-resistant, and nucleated erythrocytes can artifactually increase the total WBC. Comparing automated counts with a blood smear may elucidate sources of error. The collection site also affects leukocyte concentrations.

Leukocyte counts are low at birth, further decrease during the postnatal period, and then increase to adult counts by six to seven weeks of age. As mice and rats age, lymphocyte counts decrease and neutrophils increase. In addition, their response to inflammation differs. Young mice may have a mild leukocytosis or normal total leukocytes, whereas older mice will show a mild to marked leukocytosis. Sex and strain differences affecting WBC vary [44].

Table 6.3 Coagulation parameters of rats and mice [9, 35, 41, 42].

Analyte	Unit	Mouse [9]	Rat [35, 41, 42]
Sample population			*Strain Sex*
Prothrombin time (PT)	s	7–19*	4–8 *Norway* ♂♀ 15–19 *Wistar* ♂♀ 13.6–16.6 *Sprague Dawley* 28.8 *Non-Sprague Dawley*
Activated prothrombin time (APTT)		16–110*	17–25 *Norway* ♂♀ 12–20 *Wistar* ♂♀ 10.4–16.3 *Sprague Dawley* 19.3 *Non-Sprague Dawley*
Bleeding time	min	<1*	**2–5***
Clotting time		2–10	
Fibrinogen	mmol/l (mg/dl)	6.17–7.85 (210–267) 114–324*	150–230 *Norway* ♂♀

Table 6.4 Clinicopathologic responses of rats to stress, fasting, and catabolic diet [41, 43].

Analyte change	Stress	Fasting	Two-week catabolic feed restriction
Increase	Neutrophil count Monocyte count Lymphocyte count, immediate response [41] Cholesterol Potassium Glucose Adrenaline Corticosterone Adrenocorticotrophic hormone Arginine vasopressin	Unconjugated bilirubin Erythrocytes Hemoglobin PCV	Glucose Bilirubin Urea Sodium Chloride
Decrease	Eosinophil count Basophil count Lymphocyte count, chronic response [41] Testosterone Prolactin Triglycerides	Free fatty acids Triglycerides T4, T3, TSH Transthyretin Glucose Alkaline phosphatase	Total protein Globulin Potassium Calcium

The animal's circadian rhythm can influence peripheral leukocyte concentration such that cell counts increase during the light phase and decrease in the dark phase [45]. Breeder or origin-specific differences in rats of the same strain may occur in WBC, lymphocytes, monocytes, and eosinophils of both sexes. Pregnant rats may have increased WBC, segmented neutrophils, lymphocytes, and monocytes compared to nonmated rats of the same strain [40].

Hematopoietic neoplasms are uncommon but can cause a leukocytosis. Certain rat strains are prone to lymphoblastic lymphoma and large granular cell leukemia. However, myelogenous leukemias are rare. Nonhematopoietic neoplasms may also cause a leukocytosis. Alternatively, any neoplasm as well as toxic compounds or infections that affect the bone marrow can cause a leukopenia. Leukocyte adhesion defects will cause increases in circulation of the leukocyte(s) affected.

Lymphocytes

The predominant cell of the mouse and rat leukogram is the lymphocyte. These cells account for 70%–80% in the mouse and 60%–75% of the differential leukocyte count in the rat [35]. Mouse and rat lymphocytes are heterogeneous in size and range from the size of an erythrocyte to a neutrophil. Ovariohysterectomized females may have increased lymphocyte counts. In young healthy mice, 80% of the differential may be lymphocytes. In mice, lymphocytes decrease with age, causing total leukocytes to increase with aging [37]. As rodents age, lymphocytes decrease and neutrophils increase, resulting in a higher neutrophil:lymphocyte ratio [35]. Lymphocyte numbers may be increased by excitement and decreased by chronic stress in rats and mice [35, 41]. The inflammatory response in rats and mice is associated with increased lymphocytes [35]. Deer mice, *Peromyscus maniculatus*, experimentally infected with *Trypanosoma brucei* suffered leukocytosis associated with lymphocytosis [46].

Neutrophils

Neutrophils are the second most common white blood cell of rats and mice, accounting for 12%–38% and 20%–30% of the total WBC count respectively [35]; counts are variable in the mouse and higher in the male than in the female [35, 37]. Increased neutrophil counts are among the many cellular and biochemical changes induced in the rat by stress, and may also be markedly increased in the leukogram of aged mice with chronic inflammation (Table 6.4) [35, 41]. The inflammatory response in rats and mice is associated with increased neutrophils, but the absolute increase is generally less than that of dogs or primates [35]. Thus small changes in the neutrophil count of these species may still reflect significant inflammation. The relatively short life span of the rodent neutrophil suggests that neutropenia may occur relative to decreases of other leukocytes when neoplasia or other agents damage progenitor cells in the bone marrow [35]. In the mouse, acute severe inflammation may cause a neutropenia [47]. Immature neutrophils (band cells) are not typically seen in peripheral circulation unless there is severe inflammation; normal multiple indentations, segmentation, and ring or figure 8 form of the nuclei of these species should not be interpreted as band forms [35, 37]. Transient neutropenia occurs in the rat 2 h after blood collection but resolves within 8 h.

Eosinophils

Eosinophils are present in low numbers in the normal rat (1%–4%) and mouse (0%–7%) [35]. Platelet clumps may be mistaken for eosinophils, and a manual differential count should be performed when the relative eosinophil count is greater than 4%. Allergies or hypersensitivity are typically associated with eosinophilia. Helminth parasitism is associated with peripheral eosinophilia in the rat and mouse [48, 49]. However, deer mice, *P. maniculatus*, experimentally infected with the blood parasite *T. brucei* suffered eosinopenia [13]. Corticosteroid-mediated stress (stress leukogram) may reduce the number of circulating eosinophils in the rat and mouse [35]. The relatively short life span of the rodent neutrophil, monocyte, and eosinophil suggests that lower counts of these cell types may occur before decreases in other leukocytes when neoplasia or other agents damage progenitor cells in the bone marrow [35].

Basophils

Basophils are rare but do exist in the rat and mouse [37]. Basophils may be artifactually increased in the mouse sample obtained from the tail, because of massage or "milking," which may cause expression of tissue basophils [37]. Similarly, blood samples collected via cardiac puncture may contain mast cells, which should be differentiated from basophils [35]. Mouse basophilia may occur secondary to antigenic stimulation, but increased basophil counts in response to delayed hypersensitivity reactions instigated by contact allergens, soluble proteins, allografts, viruses, and tumors appear nonexistent [50]. However, parasitic infection is associated with basophilia of mice and rats. Nematode infection *(Nippostrongylus brasiliensis* and *Trichinella spiralis)* stimulates basophilia in the blood of inbred and outbred rats and deer mice, *P. maniculatus*. Deer mice, *P. maniculatus*, experimentally infected with *T. brucei* also suffered basophilia [13, 49].

Monocytes

Monocytes are uncommon cells comprising 0%–2% and 1%–6% of the differential leukocyte count in rats and mice, respectively [35]. Unlike other mammals, glucocorticoids may decrease the amount of circulating monocytes in the mouse. The relatively short circulatory life span of the mouse monocyte (24–60 h) suggests that decreased counts of this cell type may occur before decreases in other leukocytes, owing to damage to progenitor cells in the bone marrow from neoplastic or other causes [35]. Deer mice, *P. maniculatus*, experimentally infected with *T. brucei* had monocytosis [13].

Blood Parasites

A number of erythrocyte parasites occur in free-living rats and mice but are rare in laboratory and pet rodents [9, 51–53]. These include malarial parasites such as *P. berghei* and mycoplasmas such as *Mycoplasma coccoides* (previously *Eperythrozoon coccoides*) and *Mycoplasma haemomuris* (previously *Haemobartonella muris*) [54]. Parasitism is most often asymptomatic but can cause anemia in immunosuppressed or splenectomized individuals [53]. Some hemoparasites are vector-borne, such as *M. haemomuris*, which is spread by the louse *Polyplax spinulosa* [55]. Similarly, a rodent malaria, *P. berghei*, may be transmitted to mice via the mosquito, *Anopheles stephensi* [56]. On peripheral blood smears, hemoplasma genera appear as centrally or peripherally located basophilic inclusions in the erythrocytes, which must be differentiated from other basophilic inclusions such as Heinz bodies.

The protozoal hemoparasite *Trypanosoma musculi*, endemic in wild mice found in Central America, West Africa, and the Mediterranean, may cause a transient anemia [57, 58]. Natural infection in laboratory or pet mice has not been reported [58]. Rats may be infected with a host-specific trypanosome, *Trypanosoma lewisi*, as well as *Trypanosome cruzi*, the causative agent of Chagas disease [59]. Trypanosomes on peripheral blood smears appear as elongated, leaf-like nucleated flagellates [60]. Diagnosis may be made on the basis of blood smear review or polymerase chain reaction (PCR). *Hepatozoon muris*, an apicomplexan protozoal parasite of rats, causes mainly asymptomatic infections, although rats with a heavy burden can suffer morbidity and mortality [59]. The gametocytes are seen in leukocytes of peripheral blood as ellipsoid intracytoplasmic inclusions with a distinct nucleus. The parasitized leukocyte's nucleus is often disrupted or pushed to the periphery of the cell. *Babesia microti* strains infecting the free-living cotton rat *S. hispidus*, resemble those pathogenic to humans [61]. PCR testing for rodent hemoplasma, trypanosoma, and babesia genera, with the exception of *T. cruzi*, are generally limited to research purposes and are not commercially available [54, 61, 62].

Hemostasis, Coagulation Panel, and Blood Types

Coagulation factors and function in pet mice and rats are similar to those in other animals [63, 64]. In rats and mice, models of factor deficiencies and disseminated intravascular coagulation have been created for research purposes [63, 64]. Thus, coagulation and hemostasis data for rats and mice abound but provide minimal clinically applicable information (Table 6.3) [35]. Causes of altered coagulation times of mice and rats are similar to those for other animals. Prolonged coagulation times may occur as a result of consumption secondary to massive hemorrhage, DIC as occurs with sepsis, sudden inflammatory response syndrome (SIRS), neoplasia, warfarin-based rodenticides, and genetic defects. The most common causes of increased coagulation times are an improper blood preparation or analysis: lack or incorrect anticoagulant ratio, difficulty in obtaining sample, collection of samples from animals in ill-health, and inexperience in sample analysis [35]. Shortened coagulation times in mice appear to have little biologic consequence. In general, coagulation tests are insensitive; small but consistent changes in assay results may indicate a significant biological in vivo change [35]. Measurement of individual coagulation factors is possible in rats and mice, but generally unnecessary as factor deficiencies are rare in outbred (pet) strains [63]. In general, bleeding or clotting times, activated partial thromboplastin time (APTT), prothrombin time (PT), and fibrinogen determinations appear most useful to assess hemostasis of rodents. D-dimers, antithrombin, thrombin time, fibrin degradation products (FDP), and thromboelastography (TEG) may be measured in the rat or mouse, but normative data for comparison remains minimal, and the clinical value of these tests is unclear [35, 63, 65]. Standard human assays of FDP do not accurately cross-react with rat plasma to provide diagnostic information. The sampling site affects measurements of coagulation parameters; rat PT and PTT are increased and have increased variability collected from the orbital venous plexus rather than the vena cava [35]. Trisodium citrate (3.8%) is the preferred anticoagulant for determination of coagulation parameters [65]. Samples for analysis of coagulation parameters should be processed immediately or frozen if immediate analysis cannot be performed.

Bleeding time (BT) (similar to a buccal mucosal bleeding time, BMBT) may be measured by making a small incision in the tail or by needle prick to the mesenteric veins [66, 67]. The bleeding site is then blotted with filter paper, or submerged in warm isotonic saline until clot formation is evident. BT primarily assesses the quality of the initial hemostatic plug. Therefore, platelet numbers, function, and factors of primary hemostasis affect BT [67]. BTs may vary greatly depending on methodology.

APTT measures the intrinsic (Factors XII, XI, IX, and VIII) and common pathways (Factors X, V, and II) [68]. Although relatively easy to assay using commercially available kits, APTT is strain dependent [35, 69]. Therefore, in the lab or exotic animal practice, comparable healthy mice should be assessed for reference values. In the rat sample, hemolysis and freezing of the sample as well as anticoagulant rodenticides may increase APTT times. With the exception of the orbital sinus, most venipuncture sites appear to have predictable and acceptable agreement for this analyte [69].

PT is used to measure the extrinsic pathway, Factor VII, and the common pathway [70]. Mouse plasma reacts similarly with human thromboplastin [tissue factor (TF) plus phospholipids] and crude mouse thromboplastin, so that commercially available human kits are used to measure PT. For rats, rabbit brain is also a viable source for TF used in coagulation testing. Although PT is less strain specific than APTT, laboratories must develop their own reference intervals. On the basis of the short half-life and vitamin K dependency of murine Factor VII, anticoagulant rodenticides cause a prolongation in PT before APTT. In the rat, hemolysis may increase PT and clotting time and decrease clotting factors. Freezing causes slight increases in PT but decreases in clotting time and clotting factors.

Fibrinogen is measured in plasma by enzyme-linked immunosorbent assay (ELISA), Western blotting, or protein electrophoresis [70, 71]. Fibrinogen is an acute phase protein and increase indicates inflammation [72, 73]. Causes of hypofibrinogenemia include decreased liver production or increased consumption secondary to hemorrhage or DIC. Fibrinogen concentrations decrease with hemolysis but are unaffected by freezing rat samples.

Blood Groups

Genes and gene products analogous to the ABO antigen system and Rh antigen system exist in the mouse [74–76]. Translation of this finding into functional blood typing and implications for transfusion medicine are yet to be done. Rats have blood groups, but their clinical relevance is unknown as transfusions have been given experimentally without determining the blood type [77]. Nevertheless, cross-matching is recommended in rodents prior to transfusion in a clinical setting. Transfusion of fresh or recently stored (<24h) RBC is recommended [78].

Biochemical Panel

Biochemical reference data for rats and mice are provided in Table 6.6.

Markers of Liver Disease

Alanine Aminotransferase (ALT)

In mice and rats, ALT is a cytosolic and mitochondrial leakage enzyme with a wide tissue distribution to include intestine, kidney, heart, muscle, skin, pancreas, spleen, erythrocytes, and brain, but the greatest concentrations occur in the liver [87]. Serum ALT activity is not influenced by age or sex. Increases in serum activity of ALT occur in mice and rats primarily by liver damage of any etiology. Additional causes for increased ALT in mice include mouse hepatitis virus (MHV) and *Helicobacter hepaticus* [87]. The spiny mouse (*Acomys cahirinus*) has

Table 6.5 Hematological reference data for rats and mice [5, 42].

Analyte (abbreviation)	Units, SI (conventional)	Sprague Dawley rat [42] *Rattus norvegicus*	Non-Sprague Dawley rat [42] *R. norvegicus*	Mouse [42] *Mus musculus*	Spiny mice [79] *Acomys cahirinus*
	Data format	Range	Range	Range	Mean (SD)
Hematocrit (HCT)	Proportion of 1.0 (%)	0.37–0.69 (37–69)	0.44–0.062 (44–62)	0.42–0.44 (42%–44%)	47(3) 46.8(3.5)
Hemoglobin (Hg)	g/l (g/dl)	130–230 (13–23)	130–190 (13–19)	122–162 (12.2–16.2)	14.6(1.0) 14.8(0.9)
Red blood cell (RBC) count	$\times 10^{12}$/l ($\times 10^6$/μl)	5.8–10.0 (5.8–10.0)	6.6–9.7 (6.6–9.7)	8.7–10.5 (8.7–10.5)	7.87(0.68) 7.84(0.57)
Reticulocytes (RET)	Proportion of RBC (%)	0.013–0.049 (1.3–4.94) [5]	0–0.2 (0–2) [80]	0.01–0.05 (1–5) [81]	
Mean corpuscular hemoglobin (MCH)	pg/cell	17–25	17–22	15–18 [81]	18.68(1.05) 18.9(1.25)
Mean corpuscular hemoglobin MCHC concentration	g/l (g/dl)	270–380 (27–38)	260–340 (26–34)	300–380 (30–38) [81]	30.99(1.11) 31.72(1.39)
Mean corpuscular volume (MCV)	μm^3 = fl	58–77	60–70	45–55 [81]	60.3(3.7) 59.7(3.2)
White blood cell count (WBC)	K/ul	2.4–18 (2.4–18)	1.9–12 (1.9–12)	5.1–11.6 (5.1–11.6)	9.03(3.49) 13.21(5.57)
Lymphocytes	Proportion of 1.0 (%)	1.5–12 (15–120)	1.0–7.5 (10–75)	0.63–0.95 (63–75)	85.5(8.1) 89.4 (4.8)
Neutrophils		0.014–0.055 (14–55)	0.019–0.053 (19–53)	0.067–0.372 (6.7–37.2)	9.46 (6.72) 6.37(4.4)
Eosinophils		0.0–0.5 (0–5)	0.0–0.5 (0–5)	0.009–0.038 (0.9–3.8)	3.05(3.11) 1.87 (2.29)
Basophils		0.0–0.017 (0–1.7)	0.0–0.013 (0–1.3)	0–0.015 (0–1.5)	0.029(0.17) 0.00(0.00)
Monocytes		0.001–0.014 (0.1–1.4)	0.0–0.010 (0.1–1.0)	0.007–0.026 (0.7–2.6)	1.67(1.71) 2.13(1.45)
Platelets	$\times 10^9$/l ($\times 10^3$/μl)	800–2600 (800–2600)	700–1600 (700–1600)	100–1000 (100–1100)	
Fibrinogen	Mmol/l (mg/dl)	6.17–7.85 (210–267) [81]		3.35–9.53 (114–324) [81]	

similar levels of aminotransferases as mice [4]. In rats, increases twofold above the upper limit of the reference interval can occur without histologic liver lesions, and handling can cause fivefold increases in ALT activity. Hepatocellular hyperplasia (not uncommon in older rats) is hypothesized to increase hepatic enzyme activities because of increased turnover of hepatic cells. ALT is a stable analyte, which is measured in serum or plasma with little associated difference. Fasting may cause increased or decreased activities of ALT in Wistar rats. Hepatocellular necrosis in rats is associated with increased serum activity of ALT, which is liver specific in this species [41].

Alkaline Phosphatase (AP)

AP is a membrane-bound enzyme involved with membrane transport in many tissues. In mice and rats, AP is classified as intestinal AP (IAP) or tissue nonspecific AP. Both IAP and AP may contribute to serum AP activity in these species. Non-intestinal forms of AP occur in bone, teeth, cartilage, liver, kidneys, and placenta in the mouse. In rats, AP is highly sensitive but lacks specificity for liver disease, as isoforms exist in several tissues [41]. The predominant AP isoenzyme of the rat is of intestinal origin, and activity is therefore increased after feeding a fatty meal and decreased by food deprivation [87]. Increased activity of AP is nonspecific for but may be

Table 6.6 Biochemical parameters of rats and mice [5, 42, 81]

Analyte (abbreviation)	Units, SI (conventional)	Sprague Dawley rat [5, 42] *(Rattus norvegicus)*	Non-Sprague Dawley rat [42] *(R. norvegicus)*	Mouse [42] *(Mus musculus)*
Alanine (ALT) aminotransferase	IU/l (units/l)	24.1–113.9 (24.1–113.9)	41–89 (41–89)	26–185.3 (26–185.3)
Albumin (ALB)	gl (g/dl)	32–42.5 (3.2–4.25)	38.8–46.3 (3.88–4.63)	31.5–53.4 (3.15–5.34)
Alkaline (AP) phosphatase	IU/l (units/l)	75.3–173.7 (7.53–17.37)	40.3–58.8 (4.03–5.88)	13.3–78.3 (13.3–78.3)
Amylase (AMY)	IU/l (units/l)	766–1850 (766–1850) [5]	128–313 [82] (128–313)	512.6–744.2 (512.6–744.2) [83]
Aspartate (AST) aminotransferase	IU/l (units/l)	44.5–153.5 (44.6–153.5)	4–688 (4–688) [80]	63.4–328.6 (63.4–328.6)
Bile acids	μmol/l (mg/dl)	30–50 (1.18–1.96)	20–40 (0.79–1.57)	23–79 (0.9–2.9) [84]
Bilirubin, total (TBIL)	μmol/l (mg/dl)	2.22–11.45 (0.13–0.67)	3.42–6.84 (0.2–0.4)	2.56–14.54 (0.15–0.85)
Calcium (CA)	mmol/l (mg/dl)	2.77–3.24 (11.06–12.94)	2.50–2.27 (10–11)	1.71–2.97 (6.84–11.88)
Chloride (Cl)	mmol/l (meq/l)	101.1–106.4 (101.1–106.4)	103–109 (103–109)	117.8–133.9 (117.8–133.9)
Cholesterol (CHOL)	mmol/l (mg/dl)	1.75–4.41 (67.7–170.3)	2.13–3.63 (82.3–140.0)	1.34–4.41 (51.9–170.3)
Corticotropin (ACTH)	pmol/l (pg/ml)		6.6–22 (30–100)	572–1188 (2600–5400)
Creatinine (CR)	μmol/l (mg/dl)	50–73 (0.57–0.83)	8.84–114.92 (0.1–1.3) [80]	57–137 (0.65–1.55)
Creatine kinase (CK)	IU/l (units/l)	162.5–387.5 (162.5–387.5)	350–450 (350–450)	155 (155) [85]
gamma-glutamyl transpeptidase (GGT)	IU/l = (units/l)	0–3.8 (0–3.8)		None detected [85]
Globulin (GLB)	g/l (g/dl)	12–20 [5] (1.2–2.0)	13–36 1.3–3.6 [80]	21.3–23.3 (2.13–2.33) [73]
Glucose (GLC)	mmol/l (mg/dl)	5.21–7.32 (93.8–131.9)	5.69–7.08 (102.5–127.5)	3.17–8.33 (57.1–150.1)
Lactic (LDH) dehydrogenase	IU/l (units/l)	163–387 (163–387)	575–725 (575–725)	102–701 (102–701)
Phosphorous (P)	mmol/l (mg/dl)	1.44–2.84 (4.7–8.8)	1.87–5.20 (5.8–16.1) [80]	(3.0–6.0) [86]
Potassium (K)	mmol/l = (meq/l)	5.43–7.75 (5.43–7.65)	4.45–5.15 (4.45–5.15)	7.1–8.9 (7.1–8.9)
Protein, total (TP)	g/l(g/dl)	65–80 (6.5–8.0)	65.8–75.2 (6.58–7.52)	33–56.5 (3.3–5.65)
Sodium (Na)	mmol/l = (mEq/l)	144.5–153.4 (144.5–153.4)	146–152 (146–152)	157.4–174.6 (157.4–174.6)
Thyroid-stimulating hormone (TSH)	ng/ml	0.57–3.4 ng ml^{-1}[a]		300
Thyroxine (T_4)	μg/dl	4.7–5.5[a]		6.9–7.9
Triglyceride (TG)	mmol/l (mg/dl)	2.3–10.6 (89.3–408.7)	1.3–3.7 (51.25–143.25)	0.8–3.9 (29.4–149.5)
Triiodothyronine (T_3)	ng/dl	62.5–69.5 Strain not specified in text		65–85 [81]
Urea nitrogen (BUN)	mmol/l (mg/dl)	6.0–8.7 (16.8–24.4)	4.46–6.25 (12.5–17.5)	6.39–20.75 (17.9–58.1)

[a] Strain not specified.

due to cholestasis in the mouse and rat. Increased AP activity may also occur because of isoforms present in bone, teeth, kidneys, and intestine in mice. AP activity may change, depending on age, sex, strain, sample quality, and assay [88]. Increased AP activity in juveniles is associated with the bone isoform. Increased AP activity also occurs in the geriatric mouse or rat, male rats, and female mice. In samples, AP is relatively stable and unaffected by freezing. However, hemolysis and fasting can falsely decrease serum AP activity in the rat. Assay methodology may greatly affect measured AP activity. In mice, the Hausamen technique measures only nonhepatic isoforms of AP [89].

Aspartate Aminotransferase (AST)

AST is found in many tissues including liver, brain, intestine, kidney, skeletal muscle, cardiac muscle, erythrocytes, blood vessels, and testes. AST is commonly included in biochemical profiles aimed at assessing hepatocellular damage. In the mouse, AST concentrations are low, poorly specific, and therefore of questionable diagnostic value; Spiny mice are likely similar. Increased AST activity may occur in mice infected with MHV, and mice suffering cardiac muscle and testicular injury. In contrast to the mouse, the rat has high concentrations of AST. Hepatocellular necrosis of rats is associated with increased serum activity of AST [41]. However, activities of twice the upper limit of the normal reference interval may occur in the rat without histologic lesions. Thus, in rats, AST is considered a sensitive but poorly specific indicator of liver disease [41, 87]. No age, sex, or strain differences are reported in AST. AST is a stable analyte which is unchanged by freezing, but may be increased from hemolysis because of the presence of this enzyme in erythrocytes.

Bile Acids

Mice have two main types of bile acids, cholic and chenodeoxycholic, which are conjugated to taurine before secretion into the intestines via the hepatobiliary tract. In mice, increased bile acids generally indicate decreased uptake from portal circulation secondary to decreased hepatic functional mass or cholestasis. In rats, bile acids are highly variable. Compounds that alter bile acid excretion or conjugation limit the use of bile acids in assessing hepatobiliary function. In the rat, bile acids concentrations peak at 7× control values after removal of 70%–80% of the liver. Bile acid concentrations normalize by 21 days, and liver mass returned to 80% of presurgical mass in about five days [87]. Increased concentrations of bile acids have been associated with cholestatic disease and impaired hepatic function of rats [41, 87].

Total Bilirubin

Total bilirubin measures unconjugated and conjugated bilirubin and is used to assess the excretory capacity of the liver. Bilirubin may be sensitive, but is poorly specific for hepatic disease in the mouse and rat as it may be artifactually increased because of in vivo or in vitro hemolysis [41].

Gamma-Glutamyl Transferase (GGT)

As a membrane-bound enzyme of the liver and renal tubules, renal GGT is lost in the urine, and therefore increased serum activity of GGT is specific but insensitive for liver disease and cholestatic disease in the rat [41, 87]. Healthy rats have low plasmas activities of GGT that may markedly increase in cholestasis [87].

Iditol Dehydrogenase (ID)

ID is a cytosolic and mitochondrial membrane enzyme that may leak across damaged membranes. Most ID occurs in the liver, followed by the kidneys and seminal vesicles [87]. ID has excellent sensitivity and specificity for hepatic injury and is frequently the most sensitive and specific indicator of hepatocellular toxicity in rats [41, 87]. Hepatocellular necrosis of rats is associated with increased ID serum activity [41]. However, ID is extremely unstable and requires analysis soon after collection. Concentrations of ID increase with hemolysis and decrease with freezing. No sex, age, or strain differences are reported.

Other Enzymes

Lactate dehydrogenase (LDH) is less sensitive and specific for liver damage in rats than AST and is not recommended as a diagnostic marker of liver injury or disease in rats [87].Ornithine transcarbamylase (OTC), 5′-nucleotidase (5′NT), and arginase are additional biomarkers of liver injury which are not commonly available for serum biochemical panels [41, 87]. In particular, glutamate dehydrogenase (GLDH) shows promise as a potential liver biomarker for assessing hepatocellular injury in the rat [41, 87]. Arginase and OTC are specific but insensitive biomarkers, which may help quantify hepatocellular necrosis [87].

Muscle and Cardiac Biomarkers

Cardiac Biomarkers

Cardiomyopathy in male Sprague–Dawley rats is a relatively common naturally occurring disease [77]. Primary muscular disorders in outbred or pet mice and rats appear rare. Numerous enzymes are often assessed in

simultaneously to assess skeletal and cardiac muscle health. Mouse AST is high in cardiac muscle and lowest in skeletal muscle [87]. An increase in AST and creatine kinase (CK) without a concomitant increase in ALT and ID should increase suspicion of skeletal or cardiac muscle damage in the rat [41]. Increased plasma troponin T enzymes are specific to cardiac injury of the rat [41]. Isoenzyme determinations of CK or LDH are not useful in the diagnosis or assessment of cardiac pathology in the rat [41].

Creatine Kinase (CK)

CK is a cytosolic and mitochondrial membrane-associated leakage enzyme of skeletal and cardiac muscle. Age, sex, collection method, and anesthesia can each impact CK measurement. Mouse CK activities are greatest in skeletal muscle and much less in heart and brain [87]. Thus, increased CK activities commonly occur with skeletal muscle injury; this biomarker is less useful for detection of cardiac muscle damage in mice and rats. Brain CK does not contribute to serum concentrations because of the blood brain barrier. Increased concentrations of CK and AST have increased specificity for muscle injury. CK activity alone is less specific, as the enzyme increases with hemolysis and decreases with freezing of the sample.

Lactate Dehydrogenase (LDH)

LDH isoenzymes one to five are cytosolic and increase with cell membrane damage [87]. In the mouse and the rat, LDH activity is greatest in muscle (skeletal or cardiac) followed by liver, kidney, and intestines [87]. LDH activities are increased in male mice and increase with age in both sexes [87]. Increased LDH activity can occur with muscle injury (skeletal and cardiac) and is often assessed in conjunction with CK and AST. In the rat, bacterial infection, cardiac hypertrophy, and exercise can increase LDH activity. In the mouse, causes for increased LDH include ectromelia virus (mousepox), MHV, and lactate dehydrogenase-elevating virus (LDV), a virus which causes lifelong increases of LDH in infected mice without clinical signs. LDH activity increases with hemolysis and decreases with freezing of the sample [87].

Renal Biomarkers

Blood urea nitrogen (BUN) and creatinine (CR) are generally the most useful analytes to assess renal diseases or dysfunction in mice and rats [87]. However, in comparison to biomarkers of liver injury, analytes for the detection of renal injury are relatively insensitive; increases in these analytes occur only after 70%–75% of kidney function is impaired [41, 87]. Measuring fractional excretion of sodium, chloride, or potassium to assess kidney function is possible but limited by the challenge of collecting serum and urine [41]. Uric acid is not a diagnostic urinary analyte in rats [41]. Changes in BUN and CR occur for the same prerenal, renal, and postrenal causes in rats and mice as in larger mammals [87]. Rat- and mouse-specific causes of renal pathology include renal amyloidosis, glomerular immune complex disease, polycystic kidney disease, *Encephalitozoon cuniculi* infection, and parasitism in rats with the bladder nematode, *Trichosomoides crassicauda* [87, 90]. Because of the renal tubular secretion of α-2 urinary globulin, the kidney is an organ predisposed to age-related deterioration and renal carcinoma in male rats [41]. In the rat, GGT, NAG (β-N-acetylglucosaminidase), and alanine amino peptide (AAP) are useful determinants of renal injury when measured in urine, rather than in serum or plasma [87].

Blood Urea Nitrogen (BUN)

Causes of increased BUN secondary to renal pathology (renal azotemia) are similar to those in other mammals [87]. Prerenal causes include dehydration and protein catabolism (inflammation, starvation, high-protein diet, and gastrointestinal bleeding). A postrenal cause of increased BUN is obstruction. Decreased BUN may occur because of decreased hepatic production or low dietary protein. While rats exhibit age-related reductions in BUN, mouse BUN concentrations increase from 3 to 12 months but age-related decreases are seen in some strains [87].

Creatinine

Prerenal, renal, and postrenal causes of increased CR are the same as those for BUN. Increased serum CR is more specific and more consistently elevated in glomerular disease in rats [41]. Slightly higher basal concentrations of CR have also been associated with increased muscle mass, and in juvenile (<8 m) male rats [87]. Decreased CR may occur with impaired hepatic function and low dietary protein. Assay methods influence CR concentrations; some automated analyzers used picric-acid-based tests, which may overestimate CR concentrations of rodents. Other assays such as high-performance liquid chromatography may offer more accurate determinations.

Exocrine Pancreas

Amylase, Lipase, and Other Assays

In the mouse, amylase is produced from the parotid salivary gland and the exocrine pancreas. Pancreatic amylase is filtered through the glomerulus, but in the mouse, is not reabsorbed by tubular epithelium and is excreted into the urine [87]. Thus, basal plasma amylase in mice is primarily salivary, not pancreatic in origin. Male mice may have higher basal amylase concentrations. Lipase has two isoenzymes in the mouse [87]. Amylase and lipase are useful biomarkers for rat and mouse pancreatitis, but lack specificity because of salivary-gland-origin amylase [41]. In mice and rats with experimentally induced pancreatitis, amylase and lipase concentrations increase [87, 91–94]. Exocrine pancreatic disease has been extensively studied in the rat [41]. Pancreatic injury in the rat results in increased immunoreactive trypsin-associated proteins. Fecal chymotrypsin is a sensitive indicator of exocrine pancreatic insufficiency in the rat [41].

Endocrine Pancreas

Primary biomarkers for endocrine pancreatic function in the rat include serum and urinary glucose, the two isoforms of insulin, and as biomarkers of chronic hyperglycemia, IGF-1, glycated hemoglobin, and glycated albumin [41].

Glucose

Glucose concentration for rats and mice is determined using plasma, serum, or whole blood. In mice, blood glucose is commonly assessed using hexokinase or glucose oxidase (a coating on urine test strips). Glucose measurements are subject to artifactual change based on numerous factors, both intrinsic and extrinsic to the rat or mouse, including fasting, stress, anesthetic agent, and delay of serum or plasma separation from blood cells [87] While freezing does not affect glucose concentrations of the sample, hemolyzed blood samples from the rat have relatively increased glucose. Glucose concentrations will be falsely decreased in plasma or serum left in contact with whole blood because of cellular consumption. Patient fasting also decreases glucose levels. Collection site and anesthesia can also affect glucose concentrations. Blood glucose concentrations are often increased in blood samples collected from cardiac or retroorbital sinus sites compared to those collected from jugular or tail veins. Radioimmunoassay of glycosylated hemoglobin or fructosamine assesses long-term average blood glucose concentrations in rats and mice [87].

In mice and rats, females tend to have lower baseline glucose concentrations, and concentrations decrease slightly with increasing age [41, 87]. Some mice strains show decreased baseline serum glucose concentrations from 3 to 12 months of age and increased baseline concentrations after 24 months. Circadian rhythms can significantly affect blood sugar concentrations. Causes of hyperglycemia in the mouse and the rat include the stress of handling (which can significantly and quickly increase glucose concentrations), diabetes mellitus, and administration of exogenous compounds such as glucocorticoids. Diabetes mellitus has been studied extensively in mice and rats, and several strains develop the disease [83, 90]. These strains are not common outside of the laboratory, and diabetes mellitus is uncommon in the pet mouse or rat [95]. Hypoglycemia may be secondary to sepsis, liver failure, starvation, or malabsorption.

Compared with other laboratory or pet rodents, spiny mice exhibit a variety of differences in glucose-regulating enzymes. The activity of the glycolytic enzymes glucokinase, pyruvate kinase, aldolase, glucose-6-phosphate dehydrogenase, and 6-phosphogluconate dehydrogenase is generally decreased, while the activity of the gluconeogenic enzymes glucose-6-phosphatase and pyruvate carboxylase is increased [1]. In addition, this species shows a unique liver response to starvation and a different dietary threshold that changes enzyme activities [1].

Insulin and Glucagon

In the mouse and the rat, two isoforms of insulin occur [87]. Liver glucose production may be more sensitive to insulin in *Acomys* than in other rodents, to offset their decreased insulin production [79]. Assays for insulin should be validated for the species, as insulin molecules may have species-specific differences. Insulin and glucagon can be determined via a commercially available assay, but it is uncommonly done in pet mice and rats.

Some strains of the spiny mouse, *Acomys cahirinis*, have a propensity for obesity, glycosuria, and hypertrophy of the islets of Langerhans [79]. This species fails to rapidly secrete insulin in response to glucose challenge [79]. Diabetes in this species has been associated with high-fat diets and a slower insulin response [79].

Lipids and Cholesterol

Serum is preferred for the measurement of plasma lipids, and can be stored at 4 °C for five to seven days with no adverse analyte effect. Lipemic samples have increased turbidity and interfere with assays for albumin or calcium. Ultracentrifugation or the addition of polyethylene glycol 600 is used to precipitate lipids from the sample.

In the rat and mouse, lipids occur in plasma as free cholesterol, esterified cholesterol, triglycerides, and phospholipids, and are usually complexed with proteins to form apoproteins or apolipoproteins. In rat and mouse serum, high-density lipoproteins (HDL) concentrations are greatest followed by very low-density lipoproteins (VLDL) [87]. Because of low concentrations of low-density lipoproteins (LDL) and deficiency of cholesteryl ester transfer protein (CETP) in these species, spontaneous atherosclerosis does not occur [87]. Concentrations of triglycerides and cholesterol vary widely among strains and also differ on the basis of age and sex. Male mice have increased concentrations of cholesterol and triglycerides [87]. Female rats of the same strain have increased cholesterol and triglycerides when pregnant compared to nonmated rats [40]. Cholesterol and triglyceride levels decrease as mice and rats age [87]. Causes of hyperlipidemia include a recent meal (transient postprandial hyperlipidemia), diabetes mellitus, high-fat diets, and nephrotic syndrome. In Wistar rats, fasting decreases triglycerides in males and females, whereas cholesterol decreases only in females [96]. Hyperlipemia occurs in 30% of overnight fasted rats, but cholesterol concentrations are not affected [77]. Cholesterol increased in rats fed a high cholesterol (1%), fructose (68%), or wheat bran diet [87].

Electrolytes

In mice and rats, electrolyte concentrations are measured with standard assays, and they behave similarly in disease states as they do in larger mammals. In the mouse, sodium concentrations are slightly higher than in other mammals [87]. Sodium concentrations may be falsely increased if anticoagulants such as sodium citrate are used. Artifactual increases in potassium occur in hemolyzed samples. Stress may increase potassium concentrations in mice. Fasting has little to no effect on electrolytes in Wistar rats [97].

Blood Proteins

Albumin

Albumin is the most abundant blood protein in mice and rats, accounting for approximately 46%–58% of total serum protein in these species [73]. In mice and rats, albumin and total protein values increase in the first few weeks of life [73]. The albumin:globulin ratio increases as mice age, but decreases with age in rats attaining their adult plateau at about 45 days [73]. Adult concentrations of α1 and α2 globulins of rats (8%–20%, 7%–9%) and mice (6%–10%, 12%–17%) attain adult values by 45 days. β-globulin concentrations of the rat (19%–27%) increase into adulthood, while those of the two-week-old mouse are similar (16%–28%), but decrease as the mouse nears adulthood [73]. Gamma-globulin concentrations of healthy rats and mice are low and variable (2%–5.5%) [73]. Outbred mice may have increased total protein, albumin, and α-globulins, and differing ϒ-globulins than inbred strains [73]. In rats and mice, increased albumin is often an artifact of dehydration and or hemolysis. Samples inadequately mixed after thawing may show falsely decreased albumin concentrations. Differentials for decreased albumin concentrations for disease in rats and mice are similar to those of other mammals, and include decreased albumin due to decreased hepatic production secondary to liver disease, inflammation, or malabsorption, or increased loss from hemorrhage, protein-losing enteropathy, or protein-losing nephropathy.

Acute Phase Proteins

Acute phase proteins are valuable in diagnosis, prognosis, and monitoring of health status in exotic pets. These molecular thermometers are part of the early defense or innate immune system, and are useful in research-purposed rats and mice to assess stress and pain [41, 72, 98, 99]. Inflammation, trauma, infection, neoplasia, and/or stress can incite an acute phase response and may alter the protein patterns. However, these molecular thermometers rarely diagnose specific diseases. Acute phase response indicators differ between rats and mice (Table 6.7). Radioimmunoassay, ELISA, nephelometry, and immunoturbidimetry, Western blotting, and mRNA analyses have each been used to measure individual acute phase

Table 6.7 Acute phase responses of the rat and mouse [41, 72, 98, 99].

	Rat	Mouse
Increased	Platelets	
	Fibrinogen[a]	Fibrinogen
	α2 macroglobulins[a]	Haptoglobin[a]
	C-reactive protein[a]	C-reactive protein[a]
	α-1 acidoglycoprotein[a]	Serum amyloid P[a]
	Haptoglobin	Serum amyloid A[a]
	Transferrin	
	α-1 proteinase inhibitor	
	Ceruloplasmin	Ceruloplasmin
	Total α and β globulins[a]	
Decreased	Erythrocyte count[a]	
	Reticulocyte count	
	Albumin[a]	Albumin
	Serum Fe[a]	

[a] Major or most consistently changed analytes in the acute phase responses of the mouse and rat.

proteins [71]. Measurement of protein fractions (albumin, α1, α2, β, and γ) by gel electrophoresis has also proved useful and is commonly employed. However, capillary electrophoresis may be a preferred alternative because of the small samples available (2 μl of serum) [100].

Blood Gases [41, 45, 101–104]

Arterial blood gases are challenging to obtain in mice and rats because of the anesthetic and sedative effects on these analytes and sampling difficulties. One should interpret samples obtained from sedated or anesthetized animals with caution. In the rat, and to a lesser extent the mouse, many studies employ blood gases as a part of their experimental design. However, minimal literature elucidates blood gas reference intervals for these species. In the awake rat, blood pH is more alkaline than in man or dog. The rat may have an increased buffering ability with increases in P_aCO_2 causing smaller increases in $[H^+]$ compared to humans and dogs. In the rat, acid base abnormalities induced by toxicity are rare [41]. Abnormalities most commonly encountered that could affect blood gas and acid base status include severe systemic disease or toxicity, alterations or sequestration of gastric acid, changes in renal function, and lactic acidosis. In addition, severe pulmonary pathology, as occurs in late stage murine respiratory mycoplasmosis, may also be expected to cause blood gas alterations. Diseases in the rat which could cause acid base abnormalities relating to severe systemic disease or toxicity include those with altered or sequestered gastric acid or alterations in renal function, followed by lactic acidosis (in severe diabetes mellitus, mitochondrial, and other metabolic intoxications) [41]. The expected plasma pH for the laboratory rat is 7.4 ± 0.06 with CO_2, and the partial pressure of CO_2 is recorded as 22.5 ± 4.5 mm 1 and 40 ± 5.4 mm Hg, respectively [5].

Vitamins, Minerals, Metals, and Toxins

Most literature addressing vitamins, metals, and trace minerals in rodents often concerns experimental models, genetic manipulation, cell cultures, specific nutrient deficient diets, and so on. Minimal literature addresses the measurement, concentrations, and pathology of deficiencies or excesses from a clinical standpoint.

Calcium

Calcium homeostasis in mice and rats is similar to that in larger mammals and is measured by similar means. Sex differences in calcium have been reported and appear to be strain dependent. Serum calcium concentrations naturally decrease in both specific strains and outbred laboratory mice from 3 to 12 months of age, as does phosphorous from 1 to 12 months [87]. Hypercalcemia may result from increased concentrations of parathyroid hormone. Neoplasms such as multiple myeloma can secrete parathyroid hormone-related protein. Hypocalcemia is due to hypoalbuminemia, renal disease, pancreatitis, and hypomagnesemia. Calcium concentrations are increased in samples collected via orbital puncture versus cardiac [87].

Vitamin K

Coagulation and the effects of rodenticides on vitamin K, a fat-soluble vitamin, have been studied extensively in the rat and the mouse. Rats are relatively resistant to the effects of vitamin K-antagonizing rodenticides because of a mutation in the vitamin K 2, 3-epoxide reductase enzyme complex [87]. Vitamin K concentrations may also be reduced in hepatic disease due to cholestasis or malabsorptive enteric disease.

Endocrine Testing

Corticosterone and Adrenocorticotropic Hormone

Corticosteroid-mediated stress and fasting are also common adjuncts of illness in the rat and mouse. In mice and rats, the major circulating glucocorticoid is corticosterone. Cortisol-binding globulin (CBG) and albumin bind more than 99% of circulating corticosterone in the mouse [87]. Mouse corticosterone and CBG concentrations, and rat ACTH and corticosterone change depending upon the circadian rhythm. The concentrations of these molecules reach their zenith near dusk and their nadir at dawn [87]. In the mouse, ACTH secretion does not involve steroid feedback, occurs at irregular intervals, and is influenced by the light cycle, with peaks occurring in the early spring [87]. The circadian cycle of ACTH in mice cannot be changed by manipulation of the light cycle [87]. In mice and rats, females have increased concentrations of circulating corticosterone. In sexually mature cycling female rats, corticosterone concentrations are approximately threefold higher than those of males. Concentrations are highest in late proestrus and lowest in early diestrus [87]. Increased secretion of ACTH results in a more marked corticosterone response in intact female rats [87]. Corticosterone concentrations are lower in aged rats (23 m) [87].

Corticosteroid-mediated stress and fasting are common adjuncts of illness in the rat and mouse, and may confound clinical pathology results when not measured under controlled conditions. Reported changes to multiple parameters are presented in Table 6.4 [41]. Corticosterone concentrations of rats and mice are affected by food restriction, obesity, overcrowding, handling, and drugs. Because changes can occur rapidly in response to stress, obtaining true baseline concentrations is challenging. Measuring urinary excretion over a 24 h period may be a reasonable alternative [41]. Corticosterone is measured by radioimmunoassay (RIA), ELISA, or fluorometric assays on serum or plasma [71].

Thyroxine (T4) and Triiodothyronine (T3)

Circulating concentrations of T4 in mice and rats are increased compared to T3. In the mouse, T4 is primarily transported bound to albumin or α-globulin. Albumin binds most of T4 and all of T3 in the rat [87]. Rats use transthyretin for T4 transport, but mouse transthyretin does not bind T4. Rats lack thyroid binding globulin, the principle T4 transport molecule of humans [87]. Concentrations of T3 and T4 vary, depending on age and strain. In rats, T3 and T4 hormone concentrations decrease with age [87]. Sex affects thyroid hormones in the rat. Female intact rats have relatively increased concentrations of thyroid-stimulating hormone (TSH) and T3, while males have increased T4 [87]. In sexually mature females, TSH peaks during proestrus [87]. In contrast to other mammals, rats often have hypothyroidism rather than hypertriglyceridemia, but still suffer hypercholesterolemia [41]. Non-regenerative anemia is not clearly linked to hypothyroidism in the rat as in other mammals [41]. Radioimmunoassay may be used to measure T3 and T4. Thyroid hormone concentrations are influenced by increased clearance due to increased liver mass or drugs that affect the liver, such as phenobarbital. Other factors, like autoantibodies, may also influence assays.

Sex Hormones

In mice, albumin binds approximately 98% of circulating testosterone. Like ACTH and TSH, testosterone is secreted in a pulsatile pattern related to the circadian rhythm in the mouse [87]. Age-related decreases in testosterone may occur in some mouse and rat strains. In older female mice, a delayed and reduced increase in estradiol just prior to parturition occurs. Older females also have a slower decline in progesterone prior to parturition, which may prolong gestation. In rats, release of luteinizing hormone (LH) is suppressed by lactation [87]. In older rats, prolonged estrous cycles are associated with increased estradiol concentrations [87]. Testosterone, estradiol, and progesterone may be measured by ELISA or RIA, but are seldom used for clinical diagnosis of pet mice and rats.

Urinalysis

In the scientific realm, assessment of renal injury caused by specific organisms or compounds via routine qualitative and quantitative urinalysis is considered of limited value in the mouse and rat [87]. Rather, specific urinary enzymes or proteins (NAG, ϒGT, AAP, β2 microglobulin, $\alpha_2$globulin) are used for the determination, quantitation, and localization of injury to the urinary system in the rat and mouse [87]. These assays are not readily available to the veterinary practitioner. Urine collection and interpretation in the rat and mouse is challenging because of small-volume collections, sample contamination, and normal proteinuria of these species [105]. However, in the clinical exotic animal practice, valuable diagnostic information may be obtained from rat and mouse urinalysis with minimal expense, staff expertise, or time investment [3]. Small quantities of urine can provide valuable qualitative information for veterinary diagnosis, such as measurement of urinary pH, protein, glucose, bilirubin, hemoglobin, ketone, urobilinogen, and CR concentrations.

Sample Collection

Urine may be collected from rats and mice by free-catch, collection from a clean surface, manual bladder expression, urethral catheterization, or cystocentesis [19, 21, 34, 41, 106, 107]. The methods are listed in increasing order of expense, invasiveness of procedures, or likelihood of patient pain, but also increasing sample quality and quantity [105]. For all methods, materials for sample collection should be prepared to collect fresh samples.

Free-catch, also known as voluntary voiding or micturition, is the most commonly employed method of urine collection in rats and mice in exotic pet practice. These species may reflexively urinate when handled. In mice, the collection device is placed under the prepuce or vulva as the animal is picked up [108]. Devices for urine collection include plastic petri dishes, weigh boats, capillary tubes, or polystyrene beakers. Some authors recommend avoidance of the first part of the urine stream which may contain exudate flushed from the urethra, but small sample size may preclude this precaution [3]. In rats, lifting the tail and scratching the dorsal haunches may allow for collection of urine into a small container (polystyrene beaker) placed so as to enclose the urethra (Figure 6.12) [105]. Preparation of the perineum via clipping and local disinfection reduces the contamination of urine collected in this manner. Hand holding of the beaker produces urine more quickly, but tape attachment of the beaker is less prone to sample loss and fecal contamination [105]. Collection from a surface is commonly used in laboratory settings in the form of metabolic cages. In the clinical environment, placing the mouse or rat on a cold surface may stimulate urination. The urine can then be aspirated into a syringe and transferred to a collection tube. To further facilitate urine collection from a surface, mice or rats may be placed in an enclosure with a non-absorbent substrate, without substrate, or in a plastic,

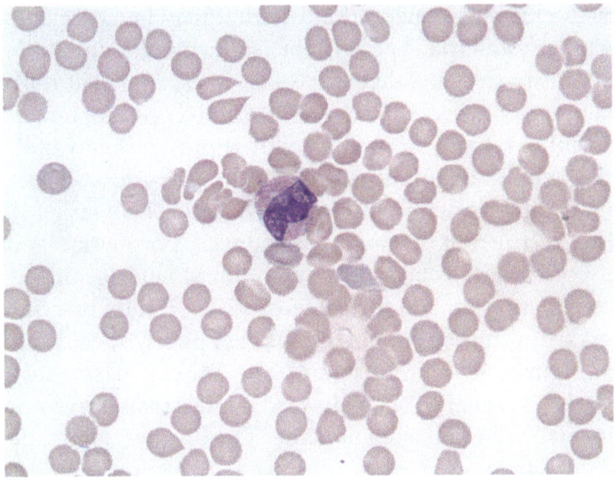

Figure 6.12 Mouse eosinophil at 1000× magnification, modified Wright's stain, EDTA anticoagulant.

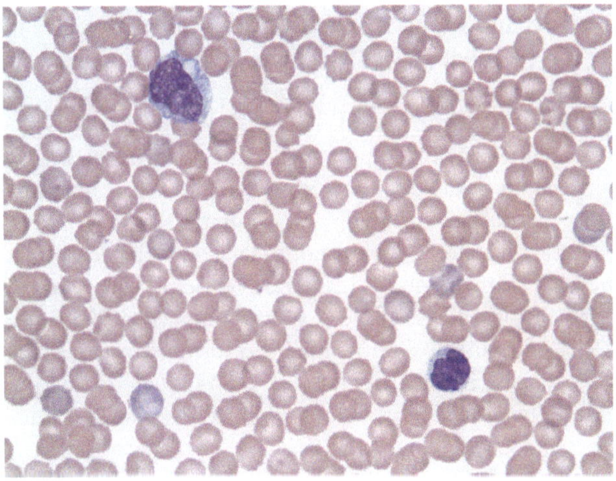

Figure 6.13 Mouse monocyte (upper right) and lymphocyte (lower right) shown at 1000× magnification, modified Wright's stain, EDTA anticoagulant.

ventilated, cooled bag [34, 105]. Urine collected from a surface is often contaminated with feces (Figure 6.13).

Manual bladder expression may also be used in the rat and mouse. This method may be performed as an adjunct after the mouse has voided when picked up. Light digital pressure is applied to the caudal abdomen to encourage further voiding of the bladder. Avoid use of excessive force which may cause blood contamination of the urine or bladder rupture [3]. Bladder expression for sample collection is contraindicated in cases of recent bladder trauma, complete or partial urethral obstruction, recent cystotomy, or suspected primary bladder diseases such as bladder neoplasia [21]. Hematocrit tube collection may be used for male mice and rats who are stimulated to urinate in this manner; urine is collected by placing the capillary tube at the urethral orifice as urine is excreted based on manual bladder expression [105] (Figure 6.14).

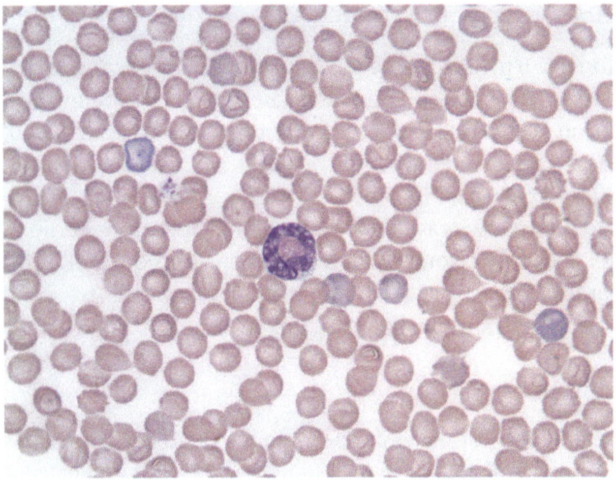

Figure 6.14 Ring form of mouse eosinophil (center), platelets clump (upper left), and acceptable polychromasia for this species. Cells shown at 1000× magnification, modified Wright's stain, EDTA anticoagulant.

Urethral catheterization and cystocentesis require heavy sedation or anesthesia of rodent patients. Catheterization for urine collection is most commonly performed in female rats, but may also be performed in female mice. Catheterization of male mice and rats or female mice <4 months of age is difficult and therefore uncommonly performed, because of the small urethral diameter [109]. Materials should include a sterile urinary catheter, sterile water-soluble lubricant, 2% xylocaine (lidocaine–HCl) jelly, 2% lidocaine, sterile gloves, and an aseptic solution [8]. The choice of catheter depends on patient size, but the largest size that can easily be introduced is preferred to avoid urine leakage outside the catheter [8]. For mice, 24 g. or smaller intravenous catheters with the stylet removed may be used. For rats, a 3.5 French tomcat catheter and or flexible intravenous catheters with the stylet removed, 18–22 g. may suffice [109]. This sterile, atraumatic technique begins with cleansing of the external urethral orifice with a disinfectant solution. For insertion, the animal is held in ventral recumbency with the head directed down and the tail lifted to access the urethral papilla. Anatomical landmarks for this procedure are given in Figure 6.10 [8]. Resistance upon urethral catheterization may be more a more common occurrence in rats than in mice; application of topical anesthetics to the outside or through the catheter during placement may alleviate urethral spasm [109].

Cystocentesis is the preferred method for collection of samples for urine culture. This technique is similar to that used in small companion mammals and is performed using a ventral midline approach; ultrasound guidance is recommended in these species as cecal penetration is a potential procedural complication [21].

Sample Handling and Storage

Rodent urine samples should be immediately transferred into a capped tube to prevent sample loss due to evaporation [105]. Urine samples of rodents are best analyzed soon after collection, particularly for examination of urine sediment. However, refrigeration is recommended and may allow reasonable sample interpretation within 2 to 3 h of collection [3]. Rodent urine at stored room temperature may become more alkaline, owing to urea decomposition [3] (Figure 6.15).

Sample Assessment

Parameters for assessment of mouse and rat urine are given in Tables 6.8 and 6.9. Rodent urine color and clarity should be evaluated upon collection of the sample. Porphyrins may impart a red or orange color, and myoglobin or methemoglobin may impart a brown color [3].

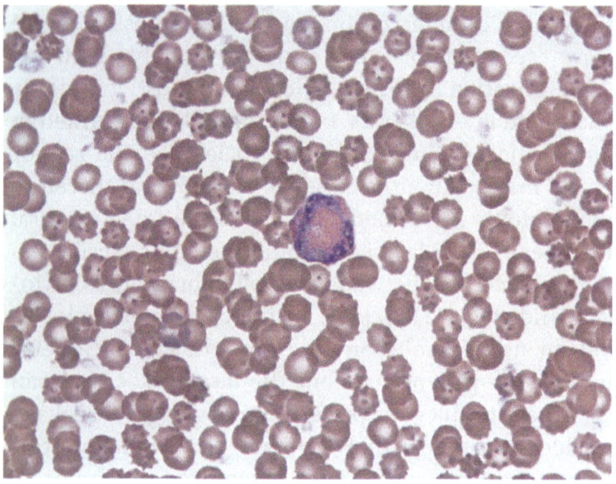

Figure 6.15 Ring form of rat eosinophil (center) shown at 1000× magnification, modified Wright's stain, EDTA anticoagulant.

In the rat and mouse, cloudy urine may be associated with crystalluria because of sulfonamide antibiotic administration or calciuria, WBC, RBC, epithelial cells, bacteria, or casts [3]. Red or white blood cells are rare to absent in rat and mouse urine; their presence may indicate trauma or inflammation of the urinary or reproductive tracts due to infection, calculi, or neoplasia [3]. The distinction between hematuria, porphyria, and myoglobinuria is best made with microscopic sediment examination for the presence of RBC. Results of urine test strips may be supportive, but are poorly specific for hematuria of the mouse and rat. Tubular casts, suggestive of renal tubular disease, and parasites are not normally found in rodent urine. The bladder nematode *Trichosomoides crassicauda* has a pigmented double-operculated egg and not uncommonly occurs in urine of infected rats. Rat and mouse urine pH tends to be alkaline, but varies depending on the diet and circadian rhythm. In the absence of contamination, the high pH of rat urine may result in a false positive protein depending on the methodology [87]. Low urinary pH may result from high-protein diets, catabolic states or starvation, and fever [3] (Figure 6.16).

Proteinuria is normal in mice and rats and increases with age in both sexes; males have increased concentrations of protein in their urine compared to females. In diabetic mice, females, but not males, typically exhibit an increase in proteinuria. Increased urine protein, clinical dehydration, increased PCV, increased plasma BUN, and CR, along with low urine specific gravity may indicate renal disease in mice and rats [3]. Urine specific gravity is best determined by refractometry, as the test strip is relatively inaccurate (Figure 6.17).

Glucosuria is abnormal for the mouse and rat, but a trace to moderate amounts may be present because of acute pain or chronic stress [3]. In diabetic mice, females, but not males typically exhibit an increase in proteinuria.

Table 6.8 Urinalysis parameters for rats and mice [5, 41, 42, 86, 110].

Parameter	Rat *(Rattus norvegicus)*	Mouse *(Mus musculus)*
Description	Turbid yellow to milky	Turbid yellow to milky
Volume	11–21 ml/24 h	0.5–2.5 ml/24 h
Specific gravity	1.022–1.070	1.034–1.058
pH	7.3–8.5	5.0–8.5
Leukocytes	Negative	Negative
Erythrocytes	Negative	Negative
Protein	Proteinuria normal	Proteinuria normal
Bilirubin	Negative	Negative
Glucose	Negative, 9.9 ± 3.9 ♂ 5.5 ±2.3 ♀	Negative, 0.53 ± 0.19
Ketones	Negative	Small amounts normal

Table 6.9 Select laboratories offering rat and mouse health testing.[a]

Diagnostic laboratory	Mailing address	Phone number/ fax number	Website address Email address	Services provided
Bioreliance Laboratory Animal Diagnostic Services (LADS)	14 920 Broschart Road Rockville, MD 20 850–3349	(p) 800-804-3586 (f) 301-610-2587	www.bioreliance.com lads@bioreliance.com	Clinical Pathology, Microbiology, Parasitology, Serology (ELISA, IFA, HAI, WIB), PCR, Cell Line Testing, Molecular Antigen PCR Identification Test (MAP-IT), Reagents for in-house testing, Health Assessment Panels, Necropsy, Histopathology, Environmental Monitoring, Custom Profiles, Consultations
Charles River	251 Ballardvale Street Wilmington, VA 01887	(p) 800-338-9680	www.crvier.com comments@crl.com askcharlesriver@crl.com	Clinical Pathology, Microbiology, Serology(MFIA™, ELISA, IFA, WIB, HAI), PCR, Prevalent Rodent Infectious Agent (PRIA) Panel (alternative to Mouse and Rat Antibody Production), Necropsy, Histopathology, Environmental Screening, Custom Testing, Technical Services/Consultations
Comparative Pathology Lab, University of California, Davis	UCD Comparative Pathology Laboratory 1000 Old Davis Road, Building R-1 Davis, CA 95 616–8520	(p) 530-752-2832	www.vetmed.ucdavis.edu cpl@ucdavis.edu	Clinical Pathology, Microbiology, Parasitology, Serology (MFIA™, ELISA, IFA), PCR, Necropsy, Histopathology, Environmental Testing, Custom Testing, Consultation
Molecular Diagnostic Services, Inc.	204 Sorrento Valley Blvd., Suite G San Diego, CA 92 121	(p) 858-450-9990 (f) 858-450-0619	www.mds-usa.com services@mds-usa.com	Clinical Pathology, Microbiology, Serology (ELISA), Necropsy, Histopathology, Environmental Monitoring
Northwest Zoo Path	654 W. Main Street Monroe, WA 98272	(p) 360-794-0630 (f) 360-794-4312	www.zoopath.com zoopath@aol.com	Histopathology
Research Animal Diagnostic Laboratory	Discovery Ridge Research Park 4011 Discovery Drive Columbia, MO 65201	(p) 800-669-0825 (f) 573-882-5983	www.radil.missouri.edu RADIL@missouri.edu	Clinical Pathology, Microbiology, Parasitology, Serology (MFI™, IFA, WIB), PCR, Necropsy, Histopathology
Research Associates Laboratory	14 556 Midway Road Dallas, TX 75 244	(p) 972-960-2221 (f) 972-960-1997	www.vetdna.com	DNA Based Testing, Microbiology
University of Georgia, Veterinary Diagnostic Lab, Georgia Laboratory Animal Diagnostic Services	AVDL, College of Veterinary Medicine, University of GA Athens, GA 30 602	(p) 706-542-5568 (f) 706-542-5977	www.vet.uga.edu/dlab	Clinical Pathology, Microbiology, Parasitology, Serology (ELISA, confirmatory testing using MFIA and IFA), PCR, Necropsy, Histopathology, Custom Testing, Consultation
University of Miami, Leonard M. Miller School of Medicine, Department of Pathology	1611 NW 12th Avenue Miami, FL 33 136	(p) 305-585-6303 (f) 305-326-9363	www.cpl.med.miami.edu compathlab@med.miami.edu	Clinical Pathology, Microbiology, Parasitology, Serology (ELISA), Histopathology. Custom Testing
Veterinary Molecular Diagnostics, Inc.	5989 Meijer Drive, Suite 5 Milford, OH 45 150	(p) 513-576-1080 (f) 513-576-6177	www.VMDLABS.com	PCR
Zoo/Exotic Pathology Service	2825 KOVR Drive West Sacramento, CA 95 605	(p) 916-725-5100 (f) 916-725-6155	www.zooexotic.com mail@zooexotic.com	Nucleic Acid-based Diagnostics, Toxicology, Necropsy, Histopathology, Consultations
Zoologix	9811 Owensmouth Avenue, Suite 4 Chatsworth, CA 91 311–3800	(p) 818-717-8880 (f) 818-717-8881	www.zoologix.com info@zoologix.com	PCR

[a] This is not a complete listing of all laboratories providing diagnostic testing of rodents, but those with which the authors have experience.

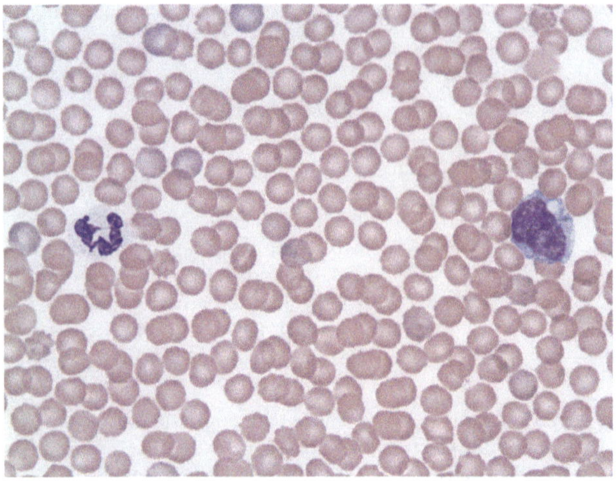

Figure 6.16 Mouse monocyte (right) and neutrophil (left) at 1000× magnification, modified Wright's stain, EDTA anticoagulant.

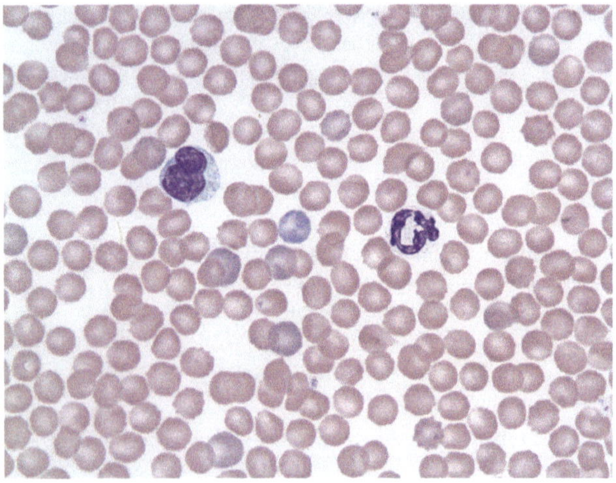

Figure 6.17 Mouse monocyte (left) and ring form of neutrophil (right) shown at 1000× magnification, modified Wright's stain, EDTA anticoagulant.

Measuring urine glucose by the glucose oxide method (common on many test strips) may yield false negative results owing to the ascorbic acid concentration in mouse urine. Ketone presence in rodent urine is associated with prolonged inanition or starvation [3]. Increased urinary bilirubin in rodents may indicate damage to

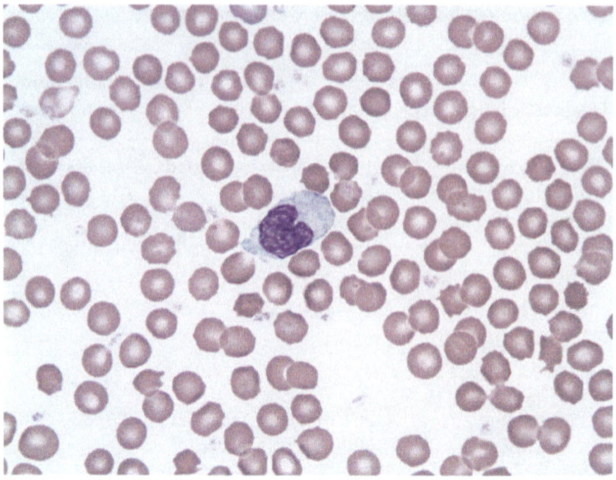

Figure 6.18 Rat monocyte shown at 1000× magnification, modified Wright's stain, EDTA anticoagulant.

RBCs or muscle cells leading to heme destruction, or diseases of the biliary tree [3] (Figure 6.18).

Serology and PCR

Because of the extensive use of the rat and mouse in biomedical research, numerous serology (ELISA, indirect fluorescent antibody testing, Western blotting, and multiplex fluorescent immunoassay) and PCR tests have been developed for health surveillance. The numerous diseases affecting free-living and captive rats and mice are far beyond the scope of this chapter, but many excellent reviews are available [3, 53, 62, 102, 111]. While these assays are the foundation for the creation of disease-free laboratory colonies of rodents, they are not often pursued in clinical exotic pet practice. Table 6.9 lists laboratories that offer diagnostics for common rat and mouse pathogens such Cilia Associated Respiratory (CAR) bacillus, *Mycoplasma pulmonis*, *E. cuniculi*, *Clostridium piliforme*, MHV, and sialodacryoadenitis virus (SDAV). PCR testing for rodent hemoparasites, with the exception of *T. cruzi*, is generally limited to research purposes and is not generally commercially available [54, 61, 62].

References

1 Brunjes, P.C. (1990). The precocial mouse, *Acomys cahirinus*. *Psychobiology* 18 (3): 339–350.

2 Horowitz, M. and Borut, A. (1970). Effect of acute dehydration on body fluid compartments in three rodent species, *Rattus norvegicus*, *Acomys cahirinus* and *Meriones crassus*. *Comp. Biochem. Physiol.* 35: 283–290.

3 Jenkins, J.R. (2008). Rodent diagnostic testing. *J. Educ. Perioper. Med.* 17 (1): 16–25.

4 Ameri, M., Schnaars, H.A., Sibley, J.R., and Honor, D.J. (2011 Jun 1). Stability of hematologic analytes in monkey, rabbit, rat, and mouse blood stored at 4 C in EDTA using the ADVIA 120 hematology analyzer. *Vet. Clin. Pathol.* 40 (2): 188–193.

5 Baker, H.J., Lindsey, J.R., and Weisbroth, S.H. (2006). *Appendix 1 – Selected Normative Data. The Laboratory Rat*, 2e, 883–884. ACLAM, Academic Press.

6 Bannerman, R.M. (1983). *Ch 12 Hematology in: The Mouse in Biomedical Research*, 293–312. American College of Labroartory Animal Medicine Series.

7 Beeton, C., Garcia, A., and Chandy, K.G. (2007 Aug). Drawing blood from rats through the saphenous vein and by cardiac puncture. *J. Vis. Exp.* 23: 266.

8 Brown, C. (2011 Apr). Urethral catheterization of the female rat. *Lab. Anim.* 40 (4): 111–112.

9 Everds, N.E. (2007). Hematology of the laboratory mouse. In: *The Mouse in Biomedical Research, Normative Biology, Husbandry, and Models*, 2e, vol. 3 (ed. J.G. Fox, S.W. Barthold, M.T. Davisson, et al.), 133–170. Academic Press.

10 Wiedmeyer, C.E., Ruben, D., and Franklin, C. (2007 Mar 1). Complete blood count, clinical chemistry, and serology profile by using a single tube of whole blood from mice. *J. Am. Assoc. Lab. Anim. Sci.* 46 (2): 59–64.

11 Forbes, N., Brayton, C., Grindle, S. et al. (2010 Aug). Morbidity and mortality rates associated with serial bleeding from the superficial temporal vein in mice. *Lab. Anim.* 39 (8): 236–240.

12 Golde, W.T., Gollobin, P., and Rodriguez, L.L. (2005 Oct). A rapid, simple, and humane method for submandibular bleeding of mice using a lancet. *Lab. Anim.* 34 (9): 39–43.

13 Ayers, J.D., Rota, P.A., Collins, M.L., and Drew, C.P. (2012 Mar 15). Alternatives to retroorbital blood collection in hispid cotton rats *(Sigmodon hispidus). J. Am. Assoc. Lab. Anim. Sci.* 51 (2): 239–245.

14 Zeller, W., Weber, H., Panoussis, B. et al. (1998 Oct 1). Refinement of blood sampling from the sublingual vein of rats. *Lab. Anim.* 32 (4): 369–376.

15 Hem, A., Smith, A.J., and Solberg, P. (1998 Oct 1). Saphenous vein puncture for blood sampling of the mouse, rat, hamster, gerbil, Guinea pig, ferret and mink. *Lab. Anim.* 32 (4): 364–368.

16 Parasuraman, S., Raveendran, R., and Kesavan, R. (2010 Jul 1). Blood sample collection in small laboratory animals. *J. Pharmacol. Pharmacother.* 1 (2): 87.

17 Cook, M.J. (1965). *The Anatomy of the Laboratory Mouse*. New York: Academic Press.

18 Hoff, J. (2000). TECHNIQUE: methods of blood collection in the mouse. *Lab. Anim.* 29 (10): 47–53.

19 Lennox AM, Venipuncture in Small exotic Companion Mammals Clinician's Brief. October 2007 pp 23–26.

20 Pilny, A. (2008). Clinical hematology of rodent species. *Vet. Clin. North Am. Exot. Anim. Pract.* 11 (3): 523–528.

21 Lichtenberger, M. and Hawkins, M. (2009). Rodents: physical examination and emergency care. In: *BSAVA Manual of Rodents and Ferrets*, 5e (ed. E. Keeble and A. Meridith), 20–22. BSAVA.

22 Popesko, P., Rajitová, V., and Horák, J. (1992). *A Colour Atlas of the Anatomy of Small Laboratory Animals*. CRC Press.

23 McClure, D. (1999). Clinical pathology and sample collection in the laboratory rodent. In). Clinical pathology and sample collection. Reavill D, ed. *Vet. Clin. NorthAm. Exot Anim. Pract.* 2 (3): 565–590.

24 Bober R. Technical review: drawing blood from the tail artery of a rat. Lab animal (USA). 1988.

25 Sakaki, K. (1961). Hematological comparison of the mouse blood taken from the eye and the tail. *Exp. Anim.* 10: 14–19.

26 Fernández, I., Peña, A., Del Teso, N. et al. (2010 Mar 15). Clinical biochemistry parameters in C57BL/6J mice after blood collection from the submandibular vein and retroorbital plexus. *J. Am. Assoc. Lab. Anim. Sci.* 49 (2): 202–206.

27 Van Herck, H., Baumans, V., Van der Craats, N.R. et al. (1992 Jan 1). Histological changes in the orbital region of rats after orbital puncture. *Lab. Anim.* 26 (1): 53–58.

28 Stout, R.W., Cho, D.Y., Gaunt, S.D. et al. (2001 Dec 1). Transcutaneous blood gas monitoring in the rat. *Comp. Medicine.* 51 (6): 524–533.

29 Bernardi, C., Monetal, D., Brughera, M. et al. (1996). Haematology and clinical chemistry in rats: comparison of different blood collection sites. *Comp. Haematol. Int.* 6 (3): 160–166.

30 Nemzek, J.A., Bolgos, G.L., Williams, B.A. et al. (2001 Oct 1). Differences in normal values for murine white blood cell counts and other hematological parameters based on sampling site. *Inflamm. Res.* 50 (10): 523–527.

31 Schnell, M.A., Hardy, C., Hawley, M. et al. (2002). Effect of blood collection technique in mice on clinical pathology parameters. *Hum. Gene Ther.* 13: 155–162.

32 Seibel, J., Bodié, K., Weber, S. et al. (2010 Oct 1). Comparison of haematology, coagulation and clinical chemistry parameters in blood samples from the sublingual vein and vena cava in Sprague–Dawley rats. *Lab. Anim.* 44 (4): 344–351.

33 Van Herck, H., Baumans, V., Brandt, C.J. et al. (2001 Apr 1). Blood sampling from the retro-orbital plexus, the saphenous vein and the tail vein in rats: comparative effects on selected behavioural and blood variables. *Lab. Anim.* 35 (2): 131–139.

34 Harkness, J.E., Turner, P.V., VandeWoude, S., and Wheler, C.L. (2010). *Harkness and Wagner's Biology and Medicine of Rabbits and Rodents*, 5e, 107–131. Blackwell Publishing.

35 Bollinger, A., Everds, N.E., and Zimmerman, K.L. (2010). Chapter 110: hematology of lab animals. In: *Schalm's Veterinary Hematology*, 6e (ed. D.J. Weiss and K.J. Waldrop). Wiley Blackwell.

36 Lindstrom, N.M., Moore, D.M., Zimmerman, K., and Smith, S.A. (2015 Sep 30). Hematologic assessment in pet rats, mice, hamsters, and gerbils: blood sample

collection and blood cell identification. *Clin. Lab. Med.* 35 (3): 629–640.

37 Smith, C. and Jarecki, A. (2011). *Atlas of Comparative Diagnostic and Experimental Hematology*. Wiley.

38 Bullard, R.W., Broumand, C.Y., and Meyer, F.R. (1966 May 1). Blood characteristics and volume in two rodents native to high altitude. *J. Appl. Physiol.* 21 (3): 994–998.

39 Kampfmann, I., Bauer, N., Johannes, S., and Moritz, A. (2012). Differences in hematologic variables in rats of the same strain but different origin. *Vet. Clin. Pathol.* 41 (2): 228–234.

40 Liberati, T.A., Sansone, S.R., and Feuston, M.H. (2004). Hematology and clinical chemistry values in pregnant Wistar Hannover rats compared with nonmated controls. *Vet. Clin. Pathol.* 33 (2): 68–73.

41 Car, B.D., Eng, V.M., Everds, N.E., and Bounous, D.I. (2006). Clinical pathology of the rat. In: *The Laboratory Rat*, 2e (ed. M.A. Suckow, S.H. Weisbroth and C.L. Franklin), 128–143. Academic Press.

42 Fox, J.G. (2015 Jul 4). Biology and diseases of mice; Biology and diseases of rats. In: *Laboratory Animal Medicine* (ed. L.C. Anderson, G. Otto, K.R. Pritchett-Corning and M.T. Whary), 57–59. Elsevier 159–162.

43 Levin, S., Semler, D., and Ruben, Z. (1993 Jan 1). Effects of two weeks of feed restriction on some common toxicologic parameters in Sprague-Dawley rats. *Toxicol. Pathol.* 21 (1): 1–4.

44 Doeing, D.C., Borowicz, J.L., and Crockett, E.T. (2003 Sep 12). Gender dimorphism in differential peripheral blood leukocyte counts in mice using cardiac, tail, foot, and saphenous vein puncture methods. *BMC Clin. Pathol.* 3 (1): 3.

45 Quimby, F.M. (1999). The mouse. In: *The Clinical Chemistry of Laboratory Animals* (ed. W. Loeb and F.M. Quimby), 3–24. Philadelphia: Taylor and Francis.

46 Anosa, V.O. and Kaneko, J.J. (1983 Apr). Pathogenesis of *Trypanosoma brucei* infection in deer mice (*Peromyscus maniculatus*): hematologic, erythrocyte biochemical, and iron metabolic aspects. *Am. J. Vet. Res.* 44 (4): 639–644.

47 Koh, A.Y., Priebe, G.P., and Pier, G.B. (2005 Apr 1). Virulence of Pseudomonas aeruginosa in a murine model of gastrointestinal colonization and dissemination in neutropenia. *Infect. Immun.* 73 (4): 2262–2272.

48 Behm, C.A. and Ovington, K.S. (2000 May 1). The role of eosinophils in parasitic helminth infections: insights from genetically modified mice. *Parasitol. Today* 16 (5): 202–209.

49 Ogilvie, B.M., Askenase, P.W., and Rose, M.E. (1980). Basophils and eosinophils in three strains of rats and in athymic (nude) rats following infection with the nematodes *Nippostrongylus brasiliensis* or *Trichinella spiralis*. *Immunology* 39 (3): 385.

50 Dvorak, A.M., Nabel, G., Pyne, K. et al. (1982 Jun 1). Ultrastructural identification of the mouse basophil. *Blood* 59 (6): 1279–1285.

51 Ajayi, O.O., Ogwurike, B.A., and Ajayi, J.A. (2007 Aug 3). Blood protozoan parasites of rodents in Jos, plateau state, Nigerai. *Animal Production Research Advances.* 2 (4).

52 Fichet-Calvet, E., Jomaa, I., Ismail, R.B., and Ashford, R.W. (2000 Jan 1). Patterns of infection of haemoparasites in the fat sand rat, Psammomys obesus, in Tunisia, and effect on the host. *Ann. Trop. Med. Parasitol.* 94 (1): 55–68.

53 Kohn, D.F. and Clifford, C.B. (2002). Biology and diseases of rats. In: *Laboratory Animal Medicine*, 2e (ed. J.G. Fox, L.C. Anderson, F.M. Loew and F.W. Quimb), 127–129. New York: Academic Press.

54 Conrado, F.O., do Nascimento, N.C., dos Santos, A.P. et al. (2015 Nov 23). Occurrence and identification of hemotropic mycoplasmas (Hemoplasmas) in free ranging and laboratory rats (Rattus norvegicus) from two Brazilian zoos. *BMC Vet. Res.* 11 (1): 286.

55 Berkenkamp, S.D. and Wescott, R.B. (1988 Aug). Arthropod transmission of *Eperythrozoon coccoides* in mice. *Lab. Anim. Sci.* 38 (4): 398–401.

56 Matsuoka, H., Yoshida, S., Hirai, M., and Ishii, A. (2002 Mar 31). A rodent malaria, plasmodium berghei, is experimentally transmitted to mice by merely probing of infective mosquito, Anopheles stephensi. *Parasitol. Int.* 51 (1): 17–23.

57 Johanning, L.P., Guterman, V.K., Campos, I.V., and Carmona, M.C. (2013). Immunosuppressor effect of *Trypanosoma musculi* (Mastigophora: Trypanosomatidae) on experimental toxoplasmosis. *Intn. J. Trop. Biol. Conserv.* 61 (2).

58 Wasson, K. (2007). Protozoa. In: *The Mouse in Biomedical Research, Normative Biology, Husbandry, and Models*, 2e, vol. 3 (ed. J.G. Fox, S.W. Barthold, M.T. Davisson, et al.), 135–162. Academic Press.

59 Eyles, D.E. (1952 Jun 1). Incidence of *Trypanosoma lewisi* and *Hepatozoon muris* in the Norway rat. *J. Parasitol.* 38 (3): 222–225.

60 Schmidt, R.E. (1995). Protozoal diseases of rabbits and rodents. *Seminars in Avian and Exotic Pet Medicine* 4 (3): 126–130.

61 Clark, K., Savick, K., and Butler, J. (2012 Dec). Babesia microti in rodents and raccoons from Northeast Florida. *J. Parasitol.* 98 (6): 1117–1121.

62 Zhang, C. and Rikihisa, Y. (2002). Evaluation of sensitivity and specificity of a mycoplasma haemomuris-specific polymerase chain reaction test. *Comp. Med.* 52 (4): 313–315.

63 Emeis, J.J., Jirouskova, M., Muchitsch, E.M. et al. (2007). A guide to murine coagulation factor structure, function, assays, and genetic alterations. *J. Thromb. Haemost.* 5 (4): 670–679.

64 Gentry, P.A. (2004 Nov 30). Comparative aspects of blood coagulation. *The Vet. Journal.* 168 (3): 238–251.

65 Wohlauer, M.V., Moore, E.E., Harr, J. et al. (2011 Nov). A standardized technique for performing thrombelastography in rodents. *Shock* 36 (5): 524.

66 Schumacher, W.A., Heran, C.L., and Steinbacher, T.E. (1996 Jul 1). Low-molecular-weight heparin (fragmin) and thrombin active-site inhibitor (argatroban) compared in experimental arterial and venous thrombosis and bleeding time. *J. Cardiovasc. Pharmacol.* 28 (1): 19–25.

67 Swank, R.T., Reddington, M., and Novak, E.K. (1996 Feb). Inherited prolonged bleeding time and platelet storage pool deficiency in the subtle gray (sut) mouse. *Lab. Anim. Sci.* 46 (1): 56–60.

68 Takahashi, S., Hirai, N., Shirai, M. et al. (2011). Comparison of the blood coagulation profiles of ferrets and rats. *J. Vet. Med. Sci.* 73 (7): 953–956.

69 Saleminkt, P.J., Korsten, J., and De Leeuw, P. (1994 Sep 1). Prothrombin times and activated partial thromboplastin times in toxicology: a comparison of different blood withdrawal sites for Wistar rats. *Comp. Haematol. Int.* 4 (3): 173–176.

70 Lemini, C., Jaimez, R., and Franco, Y. (2007 Dec 31). Gender and inter-species influence on coagulation tests of rats and mice. *Thromb. Res.* 120 (3): 415–419.

71 Quimby, F.W. and Luong, R.H. (2007). Clinical chemistry of the laboratory mouse. In: *The Mouse in Biomedical Research: Normative Biology, Husbandry, and Models*, 2e, vol. 3 (ed. J.G. Fox, S.W. Barthold, M.T. Davisson, et al.), 173–208. Academic Press.

72 Cray, C., Besselsen, D.G., Hart, J.L. et al. (2010 Aug). Quantitation of acute phase proteins and protein electrophoresis in monitoring the acute inflammatory process in experimentally and naturally infected mice. *Comp. Med.* 60 (4): 263.

73 Zaias, J., Mineau, M., Cray, C. et al. (2009 Jul 15). Reference values for serum proteins of common laboratory rodent strains. *J. Am. Assoc. Lab. Anim. Sci.* 48 (4): 387–390.

74 Yamamoto, M., Lin, X.H., Kominato, Y. et al. (2001). Murine equivalent of the human histo-blood group ABO gene is a cis-AB gene and encodes a glycosyltransferase with both A and B transferase activity. *J. Biol. Chem.* 276 (17): 13701–13708.

75 Kitano, T., Sumiyama, K., Shiroishi, T., and Saitou, N. (1998). Conserved evolution of the Rh50 gene compared to its homologous Rh blood group gene. *Biochem. Biophysl. Res. Comm.* 249: 78–85.

76 Palm, J. (1962). Current status of blood groups in rats. *Ann. N. Y. Acad. Sci.* 97: 57–68.

77 Castañeda, B., Morales, J., Lionetti, R. et al. (2001 Apr 1). Effects of blood volume restitution following a portal hypertensive – related bleeding in anesthetized cirrhotic rats. *Hepatology* 33 (4): 821–825.

78 Straat, M., Klei, T.R., de Korte, D. et al. (2015 Sep 18). Accelerated clearance of human red blood cells in a rat transfusion model. *Intensive Care Med. Exp.* 3 (1): 1.

79 Keller, G.L. and Burns, K.A. (1989). Husbandry and hematology of captive spiny mice (*Acomys cahirinus*). *Lab. Anim. Sci.* 39 (6): 625.

80 Charles River Laboratories: Baseline Hematology and Clinical Chemistry Values for Charles River Fischer344 Rats-CDF® (F344)CrIBR as a Function of Sex and Age [Internet]. Criver.com. 1984 [cited 22 September 2016]. http://www.criver.com/files/pdfs/rms/f344/rm_td_baselinehematologyf344ratw.asp

81 Foster, H., Small, J., and Fox, J. (2014). *The Mouse in Biomedical Research*, 2e, 133–170. San Diego, Ca.: Elsevier Science, 173–208.

82 Gad, S. (2015). Chapter 3 "The rat". In: *Animal Models in Toxicology* (ed. M.D. Johnson, S.C. Gad and J. Christopher), 203. Boca Raton: CRS Press.

83 Otto, G.M., Franklin, C.L., and Clifford, C.B. (2015). Biology and diseases of rats. In: *Laboratory Animal Medicine*, 3e (ed. J.G. Fox, L.C. Anderson, G.M. Otto, et al.), 151–207. Academic Press.

84 Zhang, Y., Guo, G., and Klaassen, C. (2011). Diurnal variations of mouse plasma and hepatic bile acid concentrations as well as expression of biosynthetic enzymes and transporters. *PLoS One* 6 (2): e16683.

85 Caisey, J.D. (1980). Clinical chemical values for some common laboratory animals. *Clin. Chem.* 26 (13): 1877–1879.

86 Bihune, C. and Bauck, L. (2004). Basic anatomy physiology, husbandry and clinical techniques. In: *Ferrets, Rabbits and Rodents: Clinical Medicine and Surgery*, 2e (ed. K.E. Quesenberry and J.W. Carpenter). St. louis: WB Saunders.

87 Loeb, W.F. and Quimby, F.W. (1999). *The Clinical Chemistry of Laboratory Animals*, 2e, 1–49. Taylor & Francis.

88 Otto, G., Rathkolb, B., Manuela, O. et al. (2016). Clinical chemistry reference intervals for C57BL/6J, C57BL/6N, and C3HeB/FeJ mice (*Mus musculus*). *J. Am. Assoc. Lab. Anim. Sci.* 55 (4): 375–386.

89 Hausamen, T.U., Helger, R., Rick, W., and Gross, W. (1967). Optimal conditions for the determination of serum alkaline phosphatase by a new kinetic method. *Clin. Chim. Acta.* 15 (2): 241–245.

90 Whary, M.T., Baumgarth, N., Fox, J.G., and Barthold, S.W. (2015). Biology and diseases of mice. In: *Laboratory Animal Medicine*, 3e (ed. J.G. Fox, L.C. Anderson, G.M. Otto, et al.), 43–149. Academic Press.

91 Cuzzocrea, S., Mazzon, E., Dugo, L. et al. (2002). Inducible nitric oxide synthase-deficient mice exhibit resistance to the acute pancreatitis induced by cerulein. *Shock* 17 (5): 416–422.

92 Cuzzocrea, S., Tiziana, G., Mazzon, E. et al. (2004). Reduction in the development of cerulein-induced acute pancreatitis by treatment with M40401, a new selective superoxide dismutase mimetic. *Shock* 22 (3): 254–261.

93 Ding, S.P., Li, J.C., and Jin, C. (2003). Mouse model of severe acute pancreatitis induced with cerulein and lipopolysaccharide. *World J. Gastroenterol.* 9 (3): 584–589.

94 Schoenberg, M.H., Büchler, M., Gaspar, M. et al. (1990). Oxygen free radicals in acute pancreatitis of the rat. *Gut* 31: 1138–1143.

95 Collins, B.R. (2008). Endocrine diseases of rodents. In veterinary clinics of North America: exotic animal practice. *Endocrine* 11 (1): 153–162.

96 Lichtenberger, M. (2007). Shock and cardiopulmonary-cerebral resuscitation in small mammals and birds. *Vet. Clin. North Am. Exot. Anim. Pract.* 10 (2): 275–291.

97 Kale, V.P., Joshi, G.S., Gohil, P.B., and Jain, M.R. (2009). Effect of fasting duration on clinical pathology results in Wistar rats. *Vet. Clin. Pathol.* 38 (3): 361–366.

98 Cray, C. (2013 Jul 31). Biomarkers of inflammation in exotic pets. *J. Exotic Pet. Med.* 22 (3): 245–250.

99 Cray, C., Zaias, J., and Altman, N.H. (2009). Acute phase response in animals: a review. *Comp. Med.* 59 (6): 517–526.

100 Crivellente, F., Bonato, M., and Cristofori, P. (2008). Analysis of mouse, rat, dog, marmoset, and human serum proteins by capillary electrophoresis: comparison with agarose gel electrophoresis. *Vet. Clin. Pathol.* 37 (1): 73–78.

101 Brun-Pascaud, M., Gaudebont, C., Blayo, M.C., and Pocidalo, J.J. (1982). Arterial blood gases and Acid-Base status in awake rats. *Respir. Physiol.* 48: 45–57.

102 Jacoby, R.O., Fox, J.G., and Davisson, M. (2002). Biology and diseases of mice. In: *Laboratory Animal Medicine*, 2nde (ed. J.G. Fox, L.C. Anderson, F.M. Loew and F.W. Quimby), 35–53. New York: Academic Press.

103 Pepelko, W.E. and Dixon, G.A. (1975). Arterial blood gases in conscious rats exposed to hypoxia, hypercapnia, or both. *J. Appl. Physiol.* 38 (4): 581–587.

104 Sahbaie, P., Modanlou, S., Gharagozlou, P. et al. (2006). Transcutaneous blood gas CO2 monitoring of induced ventilatory depression in mice. *Anesth. Analg.* 103 (3): 620–625.

105 Kurien, B.T., Everds, N.E., and Scofield, R.H. (2004 Oct 1). Experimental animal urine collection: a review. *Lab. Anim.* 38 (4): 333–361.

106 Hrapkiewicz, K. and Medina, L. (2007). Mice. In: *Clinical Laboratory Animal Medicine, an Introduction*, 3e (ed. K. Hrapkiewicz and L. Medina), 48–50. Blackwell Publishing 86–88.

107 Sayers, I. and Smith, S. (2010). Mice, rats, hamsters, and gerbils. In: *BSAVA Manual of Exotic Pets*, 5e (ed. A. Meredith and C. Johnson-Delaney), 8–9. BSAVA.

108 Fukuta, K. (2004). *Collection of Body Fluids. In the Laboratory Mouse* (ed. H. Hedrich and G. Bullock), 543–554. Elsevier.

109 St. Clair, M.B., Sowers, A.L., Davis, J.A., and Rhodes, A.L. (1999 May 1). Urinary bladder catheterization of female mice and rats. *J. Am. Assoc. Lab. Anim. Sci.* 38 (3): 78–79.

110 Suckow M, Danneman P, Brayton C. 2001. The Laboratory Mouse. The Laboratory Pocket Animal Series. Boca Raton: CRC Press: 8-10

111 Brown, D.R., May, M., Bradbury, J.M. et al. (2010). Mycoplasma. In: *Bergey's Manual of Systematic Bacteriology*, 2e, vol. 4 (ed. N.R. Krieg, L. Ludwig, W.B. Whitman, et al.), 583. New York: Springer.

7

Hamsters and Gerbils

Gabriel P. McKeon DVM, DACLAM[1], *Claude M. Nagamine DVM, PhD*[2] *and Stephen A. Felt DVM, MPH, DACVPM, DACLAM*[2]

[1] *North Carolina State College of Veterinary Medicine, Raleigh, North Carolina, USA*
[2] *Department of Comparative Medicine, Stanford University School of Medicine, Stanford, California, USA*

Introduction

Hamsters and gerbils are a diverse group of rodents belonging to the superfamily Muroidea that includes the families Cricetidae (hamsters) and Muridae (gerbils) [1]. There are a variety of species within the families that have varying physical and behavioral characteristics; however, basic physiology remains consistent throughout the group. Representative species tend to be nocturnal, fossorial creatures which will variably hibernate during seasonal photoperiod abridgment depending on the species [2]. Unlike some of the other members of the rodent order, hamsters and gerbils tend to live in arid conditions where there is a constant threat of dehydration. This is exacerbated by a small body size and consequently a large surface area to volume ratio, predisposing the animals to excessive water loss. As a group, they cope with this challenge through a variety of behavioral and metabolic adaptations that are predicated on maximizing intake and minimizing loss of water. The clinical pathologic implications of this, although largely uncharacterized, are likely quite significant.

Species

The species contained in this section are outlined in Table 7.1.

Hamsters

Like most members of the Cricetidae family, Syrian hamsters (*Mesocricetus auratus*) have thick bodies, short tails, large cheek pouches, and abundant loose skin. Adult Syrian hamsters have a smooth coat that is grayish white ventrally with a reddish to golden brown dorsum (hence the other commonly used name – the golden hamster), and measure approximately 15–17 cm from the tip of the nose to the base of the tail [7]. The average adult hamster weight is generally between 114 and 140 g with females usually being larger. Males have a more rounded posterior end with prominent flank glands and, like other rodents, a longer anogenital distance. Conversely, females demonstrate a pointed posterior, reduced flank glands, and a shorter anogenital distance with a separate urethral opening. Life span estimates vary, but typical reports go up to three years [8].

Adult European hamsters (*Cricetus cricetus*) characteristically have brown to red dorsal fur, a dark gray to black ventrum, and white patches of fur along the lateral aspect of the body as well as the snout and paws [9]. *C. cricetus* is the largest extant member of the hamster family, measuring approximately 22–32 cm from the tip of the nose to the tail base with an average body weight of 450 g for males and 350 g for females. The typical life span for captive bred European hamsters averages three to five years; however, individuals observed in their natural habitat have been reported to live for up to 10 years [10].

Adult Chinese hamsters (*Cricetulus griseus*), also known as striped hamsters, are a relatively small rodent with an average body length of 9 cm and an average body weight of 39–46 g [10]. Females are in general approximately 10% smaller than males, and while they tend to be more aggressive than their male counterparts, members of both sexes demonstrate very high levels of conspecific belligerence [11]. The fur is light gray to white ventrally and dark gray laterally and dorsally with a narrow black strip along the spine. Life span typically ranges between 2.5 and 3 years. In one colony, the median survival time was 1180 days (3.2 years) for males and 950 days (2.6 years) for females with the oldest hamster dying at 1567 days (4.2 years) [12].

Adult Siberian hamsters (*Phodopus sungorus*) are small, nocturnal rodents measuring approximately

Exotic Animal Laboratory Diagnosis, First Edition. Edited by J. Jill Heatley and Karen E. Russell.

Table 7.1 Common species of hamsters and gerbils.

Common name	Scientific name	Common spontaneous conditions affecting chemistry
Golden (Syrian) hamster	*Mesocricetus auratus*	Renal amyloidosis [3]
European hamster	*Cricetus cricetus*	
Chinese hamster	*Cricetulus griseus*	Diabetes mellitus [3]
Siberian hamster	*Phodopus sungorus*	Chronic glomerulonephropathy [4]
Mongolian gerbil	*Meriones unguiculatus*	Chronic interstitial nephritis, seizures, tail-slip [5, 6]
Fat-tailed gerbil	*Pachyuromys duprasi*	
Fat sand rat	*Psammomys obesus*	Diabetes mellitus [6]

9–11 cm from the tip of the nose to the tail base [13]. Body weights range from 30 to 50 g with males being significantly larger. The dorsal fur is gray with a midline strip of dark brown to black extending from the nape of the neck to the tail base, while the ventrum, limbs, and tail are white. Unique to this group of hamsters is the presence of fur covering the dorsal aspect of all 4 feet. Mean survival has been described as ranging from nine months to two years; however, longer survival of up to 27 months (2.3 years) has been reported [14].

Gerbils

Adult Mongolian gerbils (*Meriones unguiculatus*) are similar to rats in overall appearance and have an average body length of 9.5–18 cm and a tail length of 10–19.3 cm. Captive males (60 g) tend to be heavier than females (50–55 g) [15]. Adults have a whitish ventrum and the upper body coloration varies from yellow, sandy, and gray with the sides generally being lighter than the dorsum. The entire tail is furred with longer fur being distributed around the tip, creating a brush-like appearance. This species displays pair-bonding tendencies and is capable of delaying implantation (extending gestation up to 48 days) when bred in the postpartum period [16]. Animals typically live three to five years in captivity [17].

Adult fat-tailed gerbils (*Pachyuromys duprasi*), aka "fat-tailed duprasi" or "duprasi," have a rounded body with a length of 14.8–18.3 cm and a tail length of 5.5–6.2 cm. Greek roots of the name of the genus *Pachyuromys* ("Pachy" ("thick") + "uro" ("tail") + "mys" ("mouse") point out one of its most distinctive features – a blunt, sparsely haired, club-shaped tail. Captive adult males (80–82 g) are approximately 25% heavier than adult non-gravid females [18]. They have long fluffy agouti-colored fur on the dorsum and white fur on the ventrum. They typically live between two and four years in captivity and are known for their tractable disposition when being handled.

Adult fat sand rats (*Psammomys obesus*) are heavy-bodied, measuring 13–19 cm from nose to tail base, with a tail length of 11–15 cm. The tail is fully furred with a black tuft on its tip. Unlike many other species of gerbilline rodents, size dimorphism has not been identified in fat sand rats with both male and female adults ranging from 125 to 208 g [4, 19]. The upper parts of the body are reddish-brown, reddish, yellowish, or sandy color, whereas the ventrum is lighter – yellowish, buffy, or whitish. Another unusual characteristic of this species is that it is predominately day-active [20].

Sample Collection

Saphenous Vein

In general, venipuncture sites in hamster and gerbil species are similar to those used for blood collection in mice and rats. In the case of hamsters (Syrian, European, Chinese, and Siberian), when smaller volumes are needed, the lateral saphenous vein can be used with manual restraint alone or with an appropriately sized restraining tube [21, 22]. For this technique, an open collection is appropriate using a capillary tube. Lateral saphenous venipuncture has also been attempted in fat-tailed gerbils, but has been found to inconsistently yield small volumes (5 μl) and proved technically challenging [23].

Jugular Vein/Cranial Vena Cava

Jugular venipuncture can be a safe and effective technique in the fat-tailed gerbil; however, general anesthesia is necessary [23]. Inhalation anesthesia generally allows for rapid induction and recovery, thus making blood collection more practical for most settings. When conditions preclude inhalant anesthesia, injectable anesthesia such as ketamine with an alpha-2 agonist is commonly used [24]. This technique is performed blindly using a 1 ml syringe with a 25 gauge (g.) needle at a 30°–45° angle at the level of the clavicle and 2–4 mm medial to the shoulder. The needle is advanced cranially 2–3 mm under the skin, the desired volume of blood withdrawn,

Figure 7.1 Percutaneous jugular venipuncture under injectable general anesthesia in a fat-tailed gerbil (*Pachyuromys duprasi*). *Source:* Picture reprinted with permission [23].

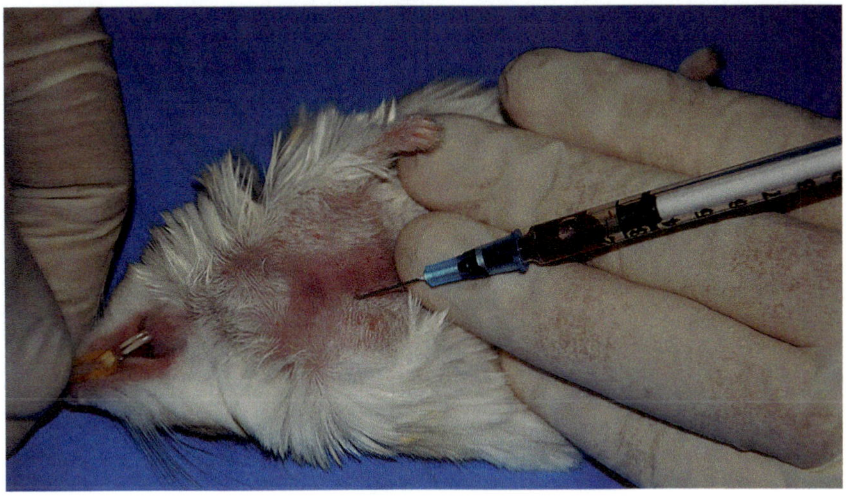

and the needle removed (see Figure 7.1). As with all species, application of gentle pressure with sterile gauze will ensure minimal hematoma formation.

Blood may also be obtained blindly from the cranial vena cava of Syrian hamsters [25]. General anesthesia is again used, and a 25 g. needle attached to a 1 ml syringe is inserted at a 30° angle between 2 and 6 mm lateral to the manubrium just cranial to the third rib. The needle is advanced caudally in the direction of the contralateral femoral head with gentle negative pressure until blood flows into the syringe. Both of the above techniques may reliably yield greater than 200 μl.

Femoral

The larger body size of Syrian and European hamsters allows potential percutaneous access to femoral veins. This technique is similar to other species within this size range and may present technical challenges for inexperienced veterinary phlebotomists. As outlined above, general anesthesia is necessary. Briefly, the animal's leg is extended gently while a 1 ml syringe with a 25 g. or 27 g. needle is inserted into the area of the femoral triangle at an angle between 10° and 30° above the horizontal plane of the leg and directed parallel to the upper hind limb as viewed from above. Gentle negative pressure is applied to the plunger of the syringe until blood is obtained. Application of gentle pressure with sterile gauze will ensure minimal hematoma formation.

Orbital Venous Plexus

Blood collection from the orbital venous sinus also allows for collection of relatively large volumes in all species. For this technique, general anesthesia is required. A heparinized, glass microhematocrit capillary tube is broken off, and the intact end is inserted behind the globe via the medial canthus and used to puncture the venous blood network behind and medial to the eye. Blood can then be collected through the broken capillary tube and into an appropriately sized collection vial. Using a piece of gauze to hold the eyelids closed after collection will ensure proper hemostasis and prevent retroorbital hematoma formation. Applying sterile ophthalmic lubricants or antibiotics during the procedure may also be beneficial. Due to the potential for serious adverse effects, other techniques should preferentially be used in order to minimize the risk of undue complications.

Blood Volumes

Blood collection for hematology and/or clinical chemistry is limited primarily by the volume that can be safely obtained at one time from an individual without compromising general welfare. For larger-bodied species such as the golden or European hamsters, samples in excess of 1 ml may be safely taken at a single time point. For smaller species such as Chinese hamsters, dwarf hamsters, and gerbils, significantly smaller volumes must be considered due to reduced circulating blood volume. When multiple samples are required, more stringent limitations for sample volume should be followed. Additionally, care should be taken when performing venipuncture on debilitated, obese, dehydrated, or geriatric animals as they may have significantly reduced circulating blood volumes [26]. Table 7.2 provides a brief summary of suggested blood sampling volumes based on current literature [21, 28].

Sample Handling

As with other mammalian species, the ideal anticoagulant for hematology remains ethylenediaminetetraacetic acid (EDTA) due to its ability to preserve the cellular components of the blood. Use of EDTA is largely inappropriate

Table 7.2 Blood volumes of common laboratory rodent species.

Species	Assumed weight (g)	Estimated circulating blood volume (ml/Kg) [1]	Recommended safe single blood draw volume (ml)
Syrian hamster (*Mesocricetus auratus*)	120	78	0.94
Mongolian gerbil (*Meriones unguiculata*)	60	67	0.40
Laboratory mouse (*Mus musculus*) [28]	25	78–80	0.20
Laboratory rat (*Rattus norvegicus*) [28]	300	50–70	1.5–2.1

Source: Data adapted from the UFAW Joint Working Group on Refinement, 1993. Laboratory mouse and rat data shown for comparison purposes only.

for clinical biochemical analyses due to indirect enzyme cofactor or direct analyte chelation reactions [29].

Serum is most commonly used for clinical chemical analysis since many anticoagulants will interfere with analyte measurements. For serum analysis, samples should be allowed to clot for 30 min at room temperature and promptly separated via centrifugation and aspiration. Specialized serum separator tubes may improve serum yield efficiency from whole blood samples. If serum is not immediately separated, placing the samples at 4–8 °C will delay enzyme degradation and hemolysis. Storage of frozen samples may degrade specific enzymes of interest; therefore, care must be taken to plan ahead if serum is to be banked for future assays. As can often be the case with small rodents, the tests to be run may be limited by the volume one can reasonably be expected to obtain at one time. When this is the case, heparin may be preferred since it interferes least with most clinical chemical analyses [29].

Sodium citrate is most often used for coagulation panels because its effects are easily reversed by adding Ca^{2+}. For this same reason, sodium citrate is unsuitable for assays looking at calcium, as well as aminotranferases and alkaline phosphatatase [29].

Analyte Interpretation

Tables 7.3–7.6 summarize the hematologic, coagulation, and biochemical parameters for the commonly characterized species addressed in this chapter. Details regarding clinical interpretation of these parameters are summarized below.

Complete Blood Count

Erythrocytes: Erythrocytes measure approximately 5–7 μm and display low levels of polychromasia. Nucleated RBSs are rare, but reticulocytes may be present at levels up to 4% under non-pathogenic conditions [40]. Under anemic conditions due to causes other than decreased production, reticulocytes commonly comprise 25% of the total red blood cell count. In these cases, maximum reticulocytosis is reached approximately four days after the inciting cause [40]. Erythrocyte life span typically ranges between 50 and 80 days, while hibernation can greatly increase erythrocyte longevity [5].

Hematocrit: Given the ability of the hamsters to hibernate, water deprivation is tolerated relatively well compared to mice and rats with little to no increase in hematocrit for a given decrease in measured blood volume [41]. Considerations when confronting an anemic patient are the same as those for other species (e.g., blood loss, increased erythrocyte destruction, decreased erythrocyte production, or a combination thereof).

Platelets: Platelet counts among hamsters and gerbils are similar to other mammalian values (Table 7.3). Changes in platelet numbers have not been well characterized in the literature; however, counts are likely useful in clinical cases where bleeding disorders are suspected.

Leukocytes: Like other rodents, lymphocytes predominate within the leukogram of hamsters, comprising some 60%–75% of the total white blood cell (WBC) count. Lymphocytes appear in the peripheral blood as relatively small, round cells with a large prominent nucleus and scant cytoplasm (Figures 7.2–7.4). Neutrophils (often referred to as heterophils) are 10–12 um in diameter with lobulated nuclei which may be segmented or non-segmented and contain dense, pinkish granules (Figure 7.5). Conditions affecting WBC differential counts have not been well characterized; however, as with other parameters, hibernation may have dramatic effects on leukocyte numbers [8]. The morphology of monocytes and eosinophils in these species is comparable to that of many other mammals (Figures 7.6 and 7.7). Thrombocytes and leukocytes, but not erythrocytes, markedly decline during hibernation but return to normal levels 24 h after arousal [30].

Table 7.3 Hematologic values for hamsters and gerbils

Cell parameter (abbreviation)	Units, SI (conventional)	European hamster [30, 31] (*Cricetus cricetus*)	Syrian hamster[a] (*Mesocricetus auratus*)	Chinese hamster [32] (*Cricetulus griseus*)	Siberian hamster [14] (*Phodopus sungorus*)	Mongolian gerbil [33] (*Meriones unguiculatas*)	Fat-tailed gerbil [34] (*Pachyuromys duprasi*)
Data type		**Range**	**95% Confidence interval**	**Mean ± SD**	**95% Confidence interval**	**Range**	**Range**
Animals sampled		**8–12**	**54–63**	**40**	**18**	**24–50**	**35–39**
Red blood cell count	10^{12}/l (10^6/μl)	7.12–8.42 (7.12–8.42)	6.6–10.0 (6.6–10.0)	7.1 ± 1.0 (7.1 ± 1.0)	8.0–8.7 (8.0–8.7)	7.0–10.0	4.39–7.37
Hemoglobin	g/l (g/dl)	169–190 (16.9–19.0)	143–173 (14.3–17.3)	124 ± 17 (12.4 ± 1.7)	130–140 (13.0–14.0)	121–169 (12.1–16.9)	64–112 (6.4–11.2)
MCV	fl		59.8–62.0	59.4 ± 5.8 fl	50.7–52.3		55.4–70.1
MCH	pg		19.5–22.1	17.5 pg	15.9–16.3		13.8–16.7
MCHC	Proportion of 1.0 (%)		0.33–0.34 (32.5–34.3)	0.295 (29.5%)	0.31–0.32 (31.0–31.5)		0.23–0.26 (22.7–26.1)
Hct/PCV	Proportion of 1.0 (%)	0.47–0.52 (47.0–52.4)	0.44–0.47 (44–47)	0.42 ± 0.056 (42.1 ± 5.6)	0.41–0.45 (41.2–44.8)		0.26–0.47 (26.0–46.7)
Platelets	10^9/l (10^3/μl)	198–408 (198–408)	282–350 (282–360)		373–481 (373–481)		75.0–736 (75.0–736)
White blood cell (WBC) count	10^9/l (10^3/μl)	4.0–12.8 (4.8–12.8)	4.4–8.3) (4.4–8.3)	5.48 ± 2.81 (5.48 ± 2.81)	1.8–3.8 (1.8–3.8)	4.3–21.6 (4.3–21.6)	2.0–13.5 (2.0–13.5)
Neutrophils	Proportion of 1.0 (%)	0.20–0.28 (20.2–28.4)	0.20–0.28 (20–28)	0.19 ± 0.02 (19.2 ± 2.2)	0.20–0.28 (20–28)	0.03–0.41 (3.0–41.0)	0.02–0.33 (1.95–32.8)
Lymphocytes	Proportion of 1.0 (%)	0.698–0.775 (69.8–77.5)	0.65–0.73 (65–73)	0.718 ± 0.07 (71.8 ± 7.2)	0.59–0.61 (59–61)	0.32–0.97 (32.0–97.0)	0.62–0.95 (62.0–95.4)
Monocytes	Proportion of 1.0 (%)	0.018–0.034 (1.8–3.4)	0.04–0.08 (4–8)	0.02 ± 0.003 (2.1 ± 0.32)	0.05–0.11 (5–11)	0.0–0.09 (0.0–9.0)	0.02–0.06 (1.56–5.57)
Eosinophils	Proportion of 1.0 (%)	0.0–0.002 (0–0.2)	0.02–0.06 (2–6)	0.017 ± 0.007 (1.7 ± 0.7)	0.02–0.04 (2–4)	0.0–0.04 (0.0–4.0)	0.0–0.03 (0.07–2.89)
Basophils	Proportion of 1.0 (%)	0.0–0.002 (0–0.2)		0.002 ± 0.004 (0.15 ± 0.04)		0.0–0.02 (0.0–2.0)	0.0–0.01 (0–0.94)

[a] Data obtained from the Stanford University Veterinary Service Center Diagnostic Laboratory using an automated Cell-Dyn 3500 hematology analyzer (Abbott Laboratories, Abbot Park, Illinois).

Table 7.4 Coagulation values for hamster species [35].

Hemostasis parameter (abbreviation)	Units, SI (conventional)	Syrian hamster (*Mesocricetus auratus*)		
		12♂	10♀	22♂,♀
One-stage prothrombin time (OSPT)	seconds	20.4 ± 7.5	18.5 ± 5.0	19.6 ± 6.4
Partial thromboplastin time (PTT)	seconds	51.5 ± 24.6	50.1 ± 29.2	50.9 ± 26.1
Factor II	Proportion of 1.0 (%)			1.00 ± 0.34 (100.0 ± 33.6)
Factor VII	Proportion of 1.0 (%)			1.13 ± 0.42 (112.8 ± 41.6)
Factor VIII	Proportion of 1.0 (%)	0.62 ± 0.2 (61.9 ± 19.9)	0.59 ± 0.13 (58.9 ± 13.4)	0.61 ± 0.17 (60.5 ± 17.0)
Factor X	Proportion of 1.0 (%)			1.05 ± 0.32 (105.2 ± 31.6)
Plasminogen	CTA U/ml	1.47 ± 0.58	1.64 ± 0.58	1.54 ± 0.58
Fibrinogen	mg/dl	276 ± 163	281 ± 125	278 ± 143
globulins				
α_1	Proportion of 1.0 (% of total)			0.12 ± 0.02 (11.6 ± 1.7)
α_2	Proportion of 1.0 (% of total)			0.09 ± 0.03 (8.6 ± 2.6)
β	Proportion of 1.0 (% of total)			0.10 ± 0.04 (9.6 ± 4.4)
γ	Proportion of 1.0 (% of total)			0.04 ± 0.02 (4.0 ± 1.8)

Data given as mean ± SD.

Hemostasis (Coagulation Panel)

Hemostasis indices have been studied previously by Dodds et al. [35] and are fairly similar to those seen in mice (Table 7.4) [41]. Aged Syrian hamsters show a marked predisposition to spontaneous atrial thrombosis secondary to renal amyloidosis [3] which may manifest biochemically as increased one-step prothrombin time (OSPT), partial thromboplastin time (PTT), fibrinogen, α_1, β, and γ globulins [35]. Additionally, platelets, plasminogen, and factors II, VII, VIII, and X are decreased.

Biochemical Panel

Liver Analytes

Multiple enzymes and other biomarkers have been used in hamsters and gerbils in an attempt to evaluate liver health and function. The enzymes alanine amino transferase (ALT), alkaline phosphatase (ALP), and gamma-glutamyl transferase (GGT) have all been implicated in assessing liver function with varying specificity. Historically, ALT has been used most consistently and has proved useful in cases of infectious hepatitis and various drug-induced hepatotoxicities [42–45]. ALP has been suggested as specific for liver damage in adult hamsters [8]; however, evidence is inconclusive, and caution should be used in interpreting data from juvenile animals due to non-liver-specific isoenzymes in growing animals. GGT shows a relatively low sensitivity for liver disease [44]. As in other mammalian species, elevated total bilirubin levels indicate cholangitis, cholangiohepatitis, or other conditions underlying cholestatic states [6, 46]. Bile acids also can serve as a useful marker for chronic hepatitis in Syrian hamsters, showing significant elevation both pre- and postprandially in affected animals [46].

Muscle Enzymes

Lactate dehydrogenase (LDH) and creatine kinase (CK) are seen to be significantly elevated in Syrian hamsters with hereditary cardiomyopathy; however, several isoenzymes exist for both, and care should be taken concerning interpretation [47, 48].

Renal Analytes

Analytes which have been evaluated for the assessment of renal health and function in hamsters and gerbils include creatinine, blood urea nitrogen (BUN), and total

Table 7.5 Serum biochemical values for hamster species.

Analyte (abbreviation)	Units, SI (conventional)	European hamster [31, 36] (*Cricetus cricetus*)	Syrian hamster[a] (*Mesocricetus auratus*)	Chinese hamster [37, 38] (*Cricetulus griseus*)	Siberian hamster [14] (*Phodopus sungorus*)
Data type		**Mean ± SD**	**95% CI**	**Mean ± SEM**	**95% CI**
Animals sampled		**7–8**	**34–69**	**10–15**	**7–18**
Bilirubin, total	μmol/l (mg/dl)	3.42–13.7 (0.2–0.8)	3.08–4.10 (0.18–0.24)		1.88–3.59 (0.11–0.21)
Blood pH	pH units	7.40 ± 0.02			
Carbon dioxide (CO_2)	mmol/l (mEq/dl)		32–36 (32–36)		32–35 (32–35)
Blood urea nitrogen (BUN)	mmol/l (mg/dl)	6.78–15.7 (19–44)	7.85–9.28 (22–26)		11.4–18.6 (32–52)
Creatinine	mmol/l (mg/dl)		28.3–33.6 (0.32–0.38)		42.4–51.3 (0.48–0.58)
Alanine aminotransferase (ALT)	U/l (units/l)	20–56 (20–56)	81–112 (81–112)		76–96 (76–96)
Aspartate aminotransferase (AST)	U/l (units/l)		40–51 (40–51)		21–34 (21–34)
Alkaline phosphatase (ALP)	U/l (units/l)		107–127 (107–127)		70–87 (70–87)
γ-Glutamyl transferase (GGT)	U/l (units/l)		4.2–7.0 (4.2–7.0)		2.5–5.0 (2.5–5.0)
Creatine phosphokinase (CPK)	U/l (units/l)		467–1281 (467–1281)		90–186 (90–186)
Lactate dehydrogenase (LDH)	U/l (units/l)		136–167 (137–167)		44–162 (44–162)
Cholesterol	mmol/l (mg/dl, mg %)	2.1–3.6 (80–140)	2.9–3.4 (111–131)	3.5 ± 0.23 (136 ± 9)	3.5–4.2 (135–161)
Glucagon	ng/l (pg/ml)			49.9 ± 10.3 (49.9 ± 10.3)	
Glucose	mmol/l (mg/dl, mg %)	0.83–6.4 (15–115)	9.1–11.3 (164–204)	6.4 ± 0.28 (116 ± 5.0)	5.6–8.5 (100–154)
Insulin	pmol/l (μIU/ml)			571.5 ± 41.7 (82.3 ± 6.0)	
Lipase	U/l (units/l)	0.0–1.0	256–285 (256–285)		339–429 (339–429)

(*Continued*)

Table 7.5 (Continued)

Analyte (abbreviation)	Units, SI (conventional)	European hamster [31, 36] (*Cricetus cricetus*)	Syrian hamster[a] (*Mesocricetus auratus*)	Chinese hamster [37, 38] (*Cricetulus griseus*)	Siberian hamster [14] (*Phodopus sungorus*)
Data type		**Mean ± SD**	**95% CI**	**Mean ± SEM**	**95% CI**
Animals sampled		**7–8**	**34–69**	**10–15**	**7–18**
Amylase	U/l (units/l)		1012–1512 (1012–1512)		262–442 (262–442)
Protein, total	g/l (g/dl)	60–73 (6.0–7.3)	65–68 (6.5–6.8)	64.2 ± 2.1	50–56 (5.0–5.6)
Albumin	g/l (g/dl)		39–42 (3.9–4.2)		30–34 (3.0–3.4)
Globulin	g/l (g/dl)		14–34 (1.4–3.4)		20–23 (2.0–2.3)
Calcium (Ca)	mmol/l (mg/dl)		3.1–3.5 (12.5–13.9)		2.4–2.6 (9.8–10.4)
Phosphorous (Phosp)	mmol/l (mg/dl)		2.4–2.7 (7.4–8.4)		2.1–2.5 (6.4–7.6)
Sodium (Na)	mmol/l (mEq/dl)		147–149 (147–149)		157–159 (157–159)
Chloride (Cl)	mmol/l (mEq/dl)		104–106 (104–106)		110–112 (110–112)
Potsasium (K)	mmol/l (mEq/l)		9.8–10.8 (9.8–10.8)		6.5–7.3 (6.5–7.3)
Thyroxine (T4)	nmol/l (μg/dl)	29.6–42.5 (1.6–3.3)			
Triglycerides	mmol/l (mg/dl)		2.2–3.1 (197–275)	2.2 ± 0.5 (195 ± 42)	1.4–2.9 (125–257)

[a] Data obtained from the Stanford University Veterinary Service Center Diagnostic Laboratory using an automated Cell-Dyn 3500 hematology analyzer (Abbott Laboratories, Abbot Park, Illinois).

Table 7.6 Serum biochemical values for gerbil species.

Analyte (abbreviation)	Units, SI (conventional)	Fat-tailed gerbil [23] (*Pachyuromys duprasi*)	Fat sand rat [39] (*Psammomys obesus*)
Data type		**Range**	**Mean ± SD**
Animals sampled		**39**	**6**
Bilirubin, total	μmol/l (mg/dl)	0.0–17.0 (0–1.0)	
Blood urea nitrogen (BUN)	mmol/l (mg/dl)	4.64–13.2 (13.0–37.0)	
Creatinine	mmol/l (mg/dl)	17.7–53.0 (0.20–0.60)	
Alanine aminotransferase (ALT)	U/l (units/l)	70.0–631 (70.0–631)	86 ± 26 (86 ± 26)
Cholesterol	mmol/l (mg/dl, mg %)		2.12 ± 0.46 (82 ± 18)
Glucose	mmol/l (mg/dl, mg %)	6.27–25.4 (113–457)	4.33 ± 0.50 (78 ± 9)
Insulin	pmol/l (μIU/ml)		55.6 ± 48.6 (8 ± 7)
Amylase	U/l (units/l)	869–1893 (869–1893)	
Protein, total	g/l (g/dl)	49–62 (4.9–6.2)	
Albumin	g/l (g/dl)	17–24 (1.7–2.4)	
Globulin	g/l (g/dl)	31–39 (3.1–3.9)	
Calcium (Ca)	mmol/l (mg/dl)	2.25–2.63 (9.0–10.5)	
Phosphorous (Phosp)	mmol/l (mg/dl)	0.78–2.23 (2.4–6.9)	
Sodium (Na)	mmol/l (mEq/dl)	140–160 (140–160)	
Potassium (K)	mmol/l (mEq/l)	3.0–5.2 (3.0–5.2)	

protein and albumin. Although elevated serum creatinine is generally considered to be a reliable indicator of impaired glomerular function in mammalian species, data supporting its utility in Syrian and Siberian hamsters with chronic renal disease is questionable [14, 27, 49]. The assessment of BUN in hamsters is similar to that of most other mammalian species. Although elevations in BUN may indicate changes in age-related tissue catabolism, gastrointestinal bleeding, or food protein content, it is generally indicative of ongoing renal disease such as renal-specific mycotoxicosis in Syrian hamsters or chronic glomerulonephropathy reported in Siberian hamsters [6, 14]. Decreased total protein and albumin levels may indicate protein-losing nephropathy in Syrian hamsters with renal amyloidosis [49]. In animals with severe hypoalbuminemia, generalized edema may be appreciated clinically [3].

Pancreatic Markers

Glucose, Enzymes, and Insulin

Although prior research has shown that food consumption significantly affects blood glucose values in hamsters [27], excessive fasting periods may have marked effects on hematologic and serum chemistry values, and as such, fasting periods exceeding 16 h are not recommended [50]. Chinese hamsters with spontaneous diabetes show marked hyperglycemia [51]. Other factors that may affect serum glucose levels include hibernation, restraint, and anesthesia [7, 27, 52]. There is little to no data related to the normal values for, and clinical

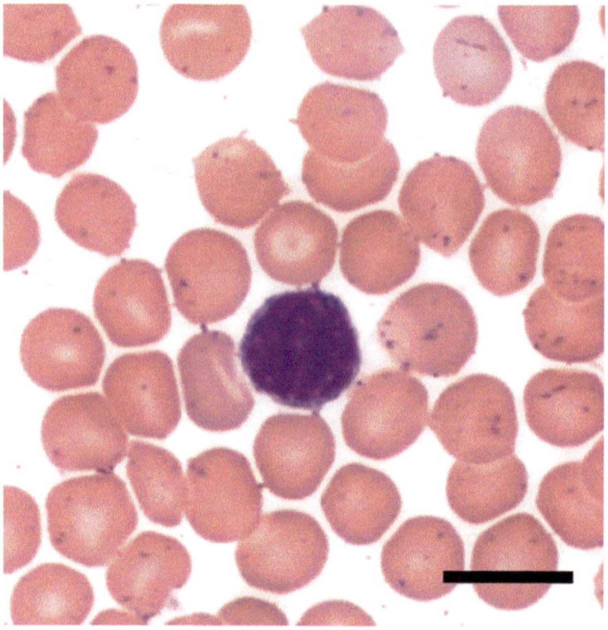

Figure 7.2 Wright–Giemsa-stained blood smear from a Syrian hamster demonstrating a typical small lymphocyte with scant basophilic cytoplasm.

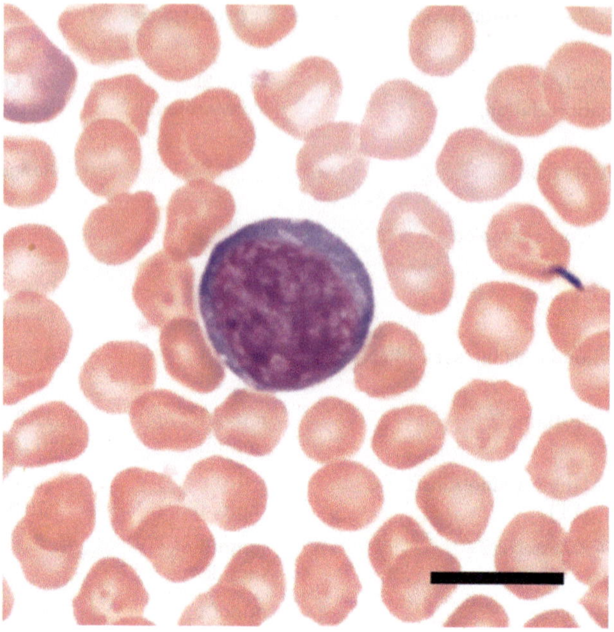

Figure 7.4 Wright–Giemsa-stained blood smear from a Syrian hamster demonstrating a reactive lymphocyte with increased basophilic cytoplasm and a prominent nucleolus. The scale bar is 10 μm.

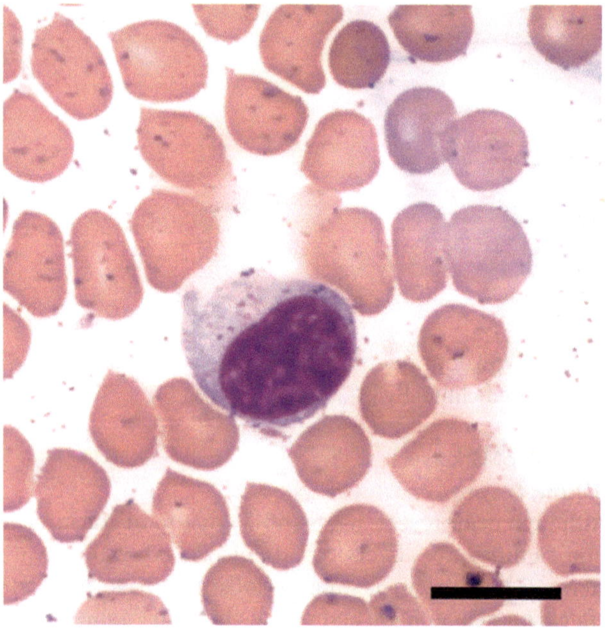

Figure 7.3 Wright–Giemsa-stained blood smear from a Syrian hamster demonstrating a large granular lymphocyte with abundant, pale blue cytoplasm containing numerous pink inclusions.

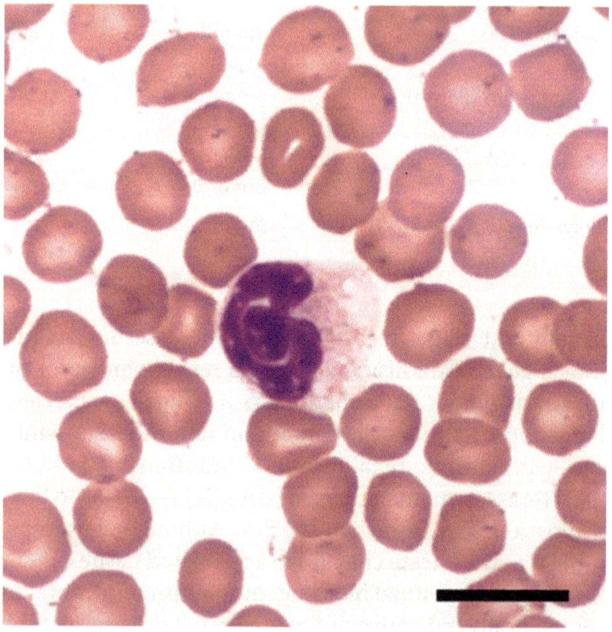

Figure 7.5 Wright–Giemsa-stained blood smear from a Syrian hamster demonstrating a typical neutrophil with abundant heterophilic cytoplasmic granules.

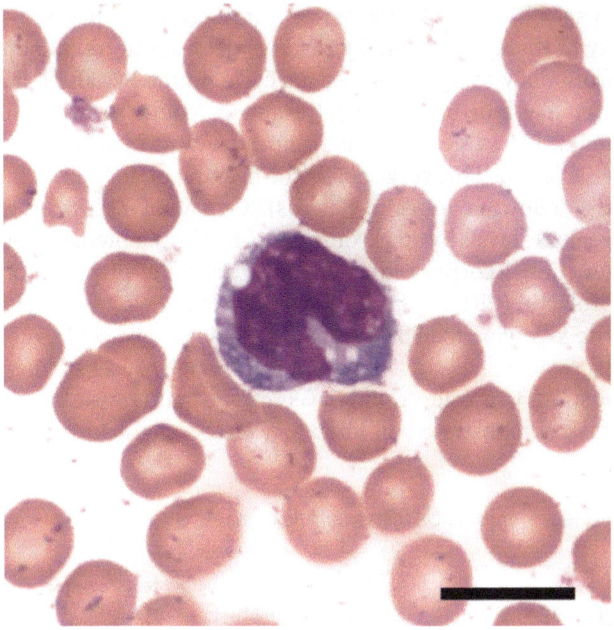

Figure 7.6 Wright–Giemsa-stained blood smear from a Syrian hamster demonstrating a typical monocyte with a bilobed nucleus and abundant pale blue, vacuolated cytoplasm.

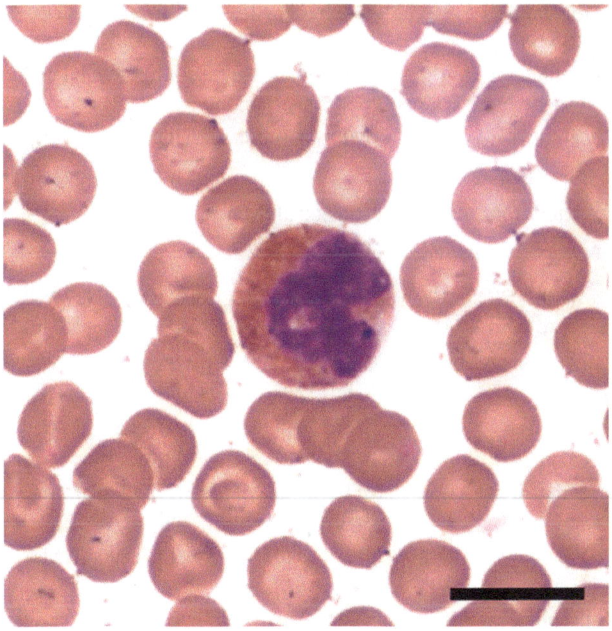

Figure 7.7 Wright–Giemsa-stained blood smear from a Syrian hamster demonstrating a typical eosinophil with a multilobulated nucleus and pinkish-orange cytoplasmic granules. The scale bar is 10 μm.

significance of, changes in serum levels of amylase, lipase, and other related pancreatic enzymes.

Insulin has been substantially characterized in the Chinese hamster due to the high prevalence of spontaneous diabetes mellitus. Affected animals display variable levels depending on disease status [51, 53]. Prediabetic animals derived from affected parents may have normal insulin, while newly diagnosed diabetic hamsters show normal to increased levels. Established diabetic animals consistently show decreased plasma insulin levels, with ketotic individuals showing a more extreme depression. While glucagon levels within pancreatic tissue tend to be higher in diabetic Chinese hamsters, it is a less reliable indicator of diabetic status in the species [11, 53].

Lipids and Lipoproteins

Cholesterol, triglycerides, and lipoprotein levels vary among species, and even among strains. Causes for variability among these values are multifactorial and include genetics, environment, and nutrition [54, 55].

Electrolytes

Reported values for Na^+, K^+, and Cl^- are all similar to those seen in other rodents (Tables 7.5 and 7.6). Changes in these values associated with pathology in hamsters are not well characterized; however, erythrocyte hemolysis has been noted to falsely elevate K^+ [56].

Blood Gases

Arterial blood gas values have been established for Syrian hamsters (Table 7.7) and closely associate with values seen in other rodents [41]. Potential causes for changes in arterial blood gases are multifactorial and can include exercise (increased PaO_2 and decreased $PaCO_2$) or general anesthesia (increased $PaCO_2$ with decreased pH and PaO_2) [41]. The extent to which various spontaneous and infectious diseases affect blood gases in these species has not been extensively studied.

Table 7.7 Blood gas values for the Syrian hamster [57].

Arterial blood gas parameter	Units, SI (conventional)	Syrian hamster [58] (*Mesocricetus auratus*)
PaO_2	mm Hg	71.8 ± 4.9
$PaCO_2$	mm Hg	41.1 ± 2.4
pH		7.48 ± 0.03
HCO_3^-	mEq/l	29.9 ± 2.9

All values given as mean ± SD; 21 animals were sampled.

Minerals, Vitamins, and Toxins

Calcium Homeostasis

Reported values for calcium, phosphorus, and magnesium in hamsters and gerbils are similar to those of other species [41]. As in other species, parathyroid hormone (PTH) tightly regulates the balance for these three minerals, promoting phospaturia, and increased renal tubular calcium and magnesium absorption [59]. Additionally, dietary vitamin D intake will antagonize these effects, leading to P_i resorption, and excretion of calcium and magnesium [60].

Vitamin deficiencies: Chronic (greater than six- to seven-week) vitamin A deficiency in Syrian hamsters can cause squamous metaplasia within the tracheal epithelial cells. Supplementation with dietary retinoic acid (3 μg/g diet) reverses these changes and normalizes blood and liver retinol levels [61]. Vitamin E deficiency can exacerbate cardiomyopathy in aged Syrian hamsters of the substrain BIO14.6. This pathologic change was reversed after 10 days of dl-α-tocopherol supplementation (10 mg/kg) [62].

Toxicoses: Although evidence of naturally occurring heavy metal intoxication is vanishingly rare in rodents, experimental exposure to lead at levels as low as 25 ppm has demonstrated accelerated development of intra-male aggression [63, 64].

Hormones

Thyroid Hormones

Triiodothyronine (T3) and thyroxine (T4) levels demonstrate circadian fluctuation in Syrian hamsters [65]. A shortened photoperiod causes a decrease in thyroid stimulating hormone (TSH) as well as concomitant drops in serum T3 and T4 [66]. Additional influences may be age (as in other species), strain, and exposure to lower environmental temperatures, with the latter leading to an increase in T3 and a corresponding drop in T4 levels [67].

Adrenal Hormones

Plasma cortisol and corticosterone are both readily measurable in the serum of Syrian hamsters with corticosterone predominating in the basal condition [58, 68]. ACTH administration and acute stress induced by restraint causes an increase in both of these hormones, while chronic stress results in only cortisol increase [68, 69]. Additionally, circadian periodicity affects levels of both of these hormones, with peak levels achieved at the onset of the dark daily phase [58, 68].

Reproductive Hormones

Beginning at about 16 days of age, the female Syrian hamster experiences daily surges of leutenizing hormone (LH) and follicular stimulating hormone (FSH), thus initiating daily surges of progesterone (P_4) and estradiol after 20 days of age [70]. Once sexual maturity is reached, the periodicity of these hormonal fluctuations decrease in frequency from daily to a four-day estrus cycle. In the Syrian hamster, day four of the cycle (proestrus) coincides with an initial LH surge in the afternoon followed by a spike in FSH levels. This surge spans the evening of day four and the following morning (estrus). Ovulation follows the peak LH levels by approximately 10 h. The maintenance of functional corpora lutea depends upon the presence of prolactin (PRL), FSH, and low levels of LH [71]. P4 levels rise following the FSH surges and gradually give way to an increase in estradiol on day four. Although causes of fluctuations in gonadotropins levels can be numerous, studies have demonstrated an inhibitory effect on gonadotropin

Table 7.8 Serological tests available for hamsters and gerbils.

Pathogen	IDEXX RADIL tests: sample volume (sp.)	CRL tests: sample volume (sp.)
Clostridium piliforme	MFIA: 20 μl (Ma)	MFIA: 200 μl (Mu)
Encephalitozoon cuniculi	MFIA: 20 μl (Ma)	MFIA: 200 μl (Ma)
Hamster parvovirus	PCR: 500 μl (Ma)	
Hantaan virus	PCR: 500 μl (Ma)	MFIA: 200 μl (Mu)
Helicobater spp.	PCR: fecal pellet (Ma, Mu)	PCR: fecal pellet (Ma, Mu)
Kilham's rat virus	PCR: 500 μl (Ma)	
Lawsonia intracellularis	PCR: fecal pellet (Ma, Mu)	PCR: fecal pellet (Ma, Mu)
Lymphocytic choriomeningitis virus	MFIA: 20 μl (Ma) PCR: 500 μl (Ma)	MFIA: 200 μl (Ma, Mu)
Minute virus of mice	PCR: 500 μl (Ma)	MFIA: 200 μl (Mu)
Mouse hepatitis virus		MFIA: 200 μl (Mu)
Mycoplasma spp.	PCR: 500 μl (Ma)	
Mycoplasma pulmonis	PCR: 500 μl (Ma)	
Parainfluenza-2 virus		MFIA: 200 μl (Mu)
Parainfluenza-3 virus		MFIA: 200 μl (Mu)
Pneumonia virus of mice	MFIA: 20 μl (Ma) PCR: 500 μl (Ma)	MFIA: 200 μl (Ma, Mu)
Reovirus 3	MFIA: 20 μl (Ma) PCR: 500 μl (Ma)	MFIA: 200 μl (Ma, Mu)
Sendai virus	MFIA: 20 μl (Ma) PCR: 500 μl (Ma)	MFIA: 200 μl (Ma, Mu)
SV5	MFIA: 20 μl (Ma)	MFIA: 200 μl (Ma)
Theiler's murine encephalomyelitis virus	MFIA: 20 μl (Ma) PCR: 500 μl (Ma)	
Toolan's H1 virus	MFIA: 20 μl (Ma) PCR: 500 μl (Ma)	

Undiluted serum and should be shipped frozen. CRL = Charles River Laboratories. Ma = Mesocricetus auratus, Mu = Meriones unguiculatus.

release when the photoperiod is decreased in length for both Syrian [2] and Siberian hamsters [72–74]

Urinalysis

The Syrian hamster will produce an average of 7 ml of urine per day with a pH range of 5.1–8.4. Grossly, the urine is cloudy due in part to the high level of protein excretion [75]. Both calcium carbonate and triple phosphate crystals are not uncommonly seen in healthy animals [76]. Diabetic Chinese hamsters consistently demonstrate glucosuria to varying degrees [51]. Further information is limited regarding urinalysis of any common hamster or gerbil species.

Serology, PCR, and Other Diagnostic Testing Options

There are a variety of diagnostic testing options for common rodent pathogens using samples from Syrian hamsters. A summary of serological and microbiological tests is given in Tables 7.8 and 7.9, respectively. Caution should be exercised when interpreting results from samples derived from other hamster or gerbil species without validation performed by the receiving diagnostic laboratory. Charles River laboratories are commonly used for rodent serology and PCR testing; additional contact information for this laboratory is found in the rat and mouse chapter (Chapter 6).

Table 7.9 Summary of microbiological testing options for hamsters and gerbils.

Pathogen	IDEXX RADIL test sample source	CRL test sample source
Bordetella bronchiseptica	Or/Np	Or/Np
Campylobacter spp.		Gi/Fe
Campylobacter coli		Gi/Fe
Campylobacter jejuni		Gi/Fe
Citrobacter rodentium	Gi/Fe	
Corynebacterium kutscheri	Or/Np	Gi/Fe
Klebsiella oxytoca	Gi/Fe	Gi/Fe
Klebsiella pneumoniae	Gi/Fe	Gi/Fe
Pasteurella multocida	Or/Np	Or/Np
Pasteurella pneumotropica	Or/Np	Or/Np
Proteus mirablis	Gi/Fe	
Proteus spp.	Gi/Fe	
Pseudomonas aeruginosa	Gi/Fe	Gi/Fe, Or/Np
Salmonella spp.	Gi/Fe	Gi/Fe
Staphylococcus aureus	Or/Np	Gi/Fe, Or/Np
Streptococcus (β-hemolytic)	Or/Np	Gi/Fe, Or/Np
Streptococcus pneumoniae	Or/Np	Gi/Fe, Or/Np

CRL = Charles River Laboratories. Or/Np = Oral or nasopharyngeal swab, Gi/Fe = Gastrointestinal swab and/or fecal pellet.

References

1 McKenna, M.C. and Bell, S.K. (1997). Part II. A classification of mammals. In: *Classification of Mammals above the Species Level* (ed. M.K. MC and S.K. Bell). New York: Columbia University Press.

2 Bartness, T.J. and Wade, G.N. (1985). Photoperiodic control of seasonal body weight cycles in hamsters. *Neuroscience and Behavioral Review* 9 (4): 599–612.

3 Percy, D.H. and Barthold, S.W. (2007). Hamster. In: *Pathology of Laboratory Rodents and Rabbits*, 3e (ed. D.H. Percy and S.W. Barthold), 179–205. Ames: Blackwell Publishing.

4 Mendelssohn, H. and Yom-Tov, Y. A report of birds and mammals which have increased their distribution and abundance in Israel due to human activity. *Israel Journal of Zoology* 45 (1): 35–47.

5 Brock, M.A. (1960). Production and life span of erythrocytes during hibernation in the golden hamster. *American Journal of Physiology* 198: 1181–1186.

6 Engelhardt, J.A., Carlton, W.W., Rebar, A.H., and Hayes, A.W. (1987). Rubratoxin B mycotoxicosis in the Syrian hamster. *Food and Chemical Toxicology* 25 (9): 685–695.

7 Biven, S.W., Olsen, G.H., and Murray, K.A. (1987). Morphophysiology. In: *Laboratory Hamsters* (ed. G.L. Van Hoosier and C.W. McPherson), 9–41. Orlando: Academic Press.

8 Gad, S.C. and Hess, F.G. (2006). The hamster. In: *Animal Models in Toxicology*, 2e (ed. S.C. Gad), 277–331. Boca Raton: CRC Press.

9 Mohr, U. and Ernst, H. (1987). The European hamster – biology, care, and use in research. In: *Laboratory Hamsters* (ed. J.R. Van Hoosier and C.W. McPherson), 351–366. Orlando: Academic Press.

10 Hankenson, F.C. and Van Hoosier, J.R. (2002). Biology and diseases of hamsters. In: *Laboratory Animal Medicine*, 2e (ed. J.G. Fox, L.C. Anderson, F.M. Loew and F.W. Quimby), 167–202. San Diego: Academice Press.

11 Chang, A., Diani, A., and Connell, M. (1987). The Chinese hamster–biology and care. In: *Laboratory Hamsters* (ed. G.L. Van Hoosier and M.P. CW). Orlando: Academic Press.

12 Benjamin, S.A. and Brooks, A.L. (1977). Spontaneous lesions in Chinese hamsters. *Veterinary Pathology* 14 (5): 449–462.

13 Cantrell, C.A. and Padovan, D. (2011). Other hamsters – biology, care, and use in research. In: *Laboratory Hamsters* (ed. G.L. Van Hoosier and C.W. McPherson), 396–387. Orlando: Academic Press.

14 McKeon, G.P., Nagamine, C.N., Ruby, N.F., and Luong, R.H. (2011). Hematologic, serologic, and histologic profile of aged Siberian hamsters (*Phodopus sungorus*). *Journal of the American Association for Laboratory Animal Science* 50 (3): 308–316.

15 Norris, M.L. and Adams, C.E. (1972). Aggressive behaviour and reproduction in the mongolian gerbil, *Meriones unguiculatus*, relative to age and sexual experience at pairing. *Journal of Reproduction and Fertility* 31 (3): 447–450.

16 Norris, M.L. and Adams, C.E. (1972). Incidence of cystic ovaries and reproductive performance in the Mongolian gerbil, Meriones unguiculatus. *Laboratory Animal* 6 (3): 337–342.

17 Norris, M.L. and Adams, C.E. (1972). Mortality from birth to weaning in the Mongolian gerbil, Meriones unguiculatus. *Laboratory Animal* 6 (1): 49–53.

18 Felt, S.A., Hussein, H.I., and Mohamed Helmy, I.H. (2008). Biology, breeding, husbandry and diseases of the captive Egyptian fat-tailed jird (Pachyuromys duprasi natronensis). *Lab Animal (NY)* 37 (6): 256–261.

19 Nowak, R.M. (1999). *Walker's Mammals of the World*, 6e. Baltimore: Johns Hopkins University Press.

20 Neuman, A., Gothilf, Y., Haim, A. et al. (2005). Nocturnal patterns and up-regulated excretion of the melatonin metabolite 6-sulfatoxymelatonin in the diurnal rodent Psammomys obesus post-weaning under a short photoperiod. *Comparative Biochemistry and Physiology – Part A: Molecular & Integrative Physiology* 142 (3): 297–307.

21 Morton, D.B., Abbot, D., Barclay, R. et al. (1993). Removal of blood from laboratory mammals and birds. First report of the BVA/FRAME/RSPCA/UFAW joint working group on refinement. *Laboratory Animal* 27 (1): 1–22.

22 Hem, A., Smith, A.J., and Solberg, P. (1998). Saphenous vein puncture for blood sampling of the mouse, rat, hamster, gerbil, Guinea pig, ferret and mink. *Laboratory Animal* 32 (4): 364–368.

23 Felt, S.A., Guirguis, F.I., Wasfy, M.O. et al. (2009). An effective venipuncture technique and normal serum biochemistry parameters of the captive fat-tailed jird (Pachyuromys duprasi). *Journal of the American Association for Laboratory Animal Science* 48 (1): 57–60.

24 Gaertner, D.J., Hallman, T.M., Hankenson, F.C., and Batchelder, M.A. (2008). Anesthesia and analgesia for laboratory rodents. In: *Anesthesia and Analgesia in Laboratory Animals* (ed. D.F. Kohn, S.K. Wixson, W.J. White and G.J. Benson). San Diego: Academic Press.

25 Picazo, M.G., Benito, P.J., and Garcia-Olmo, D.C. (2009). Efficiency and safety of a technique for drawing blood from the hamster cranial vena cava. *Lab Animal (NY)* 38 (6): 211–216.

26 Kutscher, C. (1968). Plasma volume change during water-deprivation in gerbils, hamsters, Guinea pigs and rats. *Comparative Biochemistry and Physiology* 25 (3): 929–936.

27 Bannon, P.D. and Friedell, G.H. (1966). Values for plasma constituents in normal and tumor bearing golden hamsters. *Laboratory Animal Care* 16 (5): 417–420.

28 Diehl, K.H., Hull, R., Morton, D. et al. (2001). A good practice guide to the administration of substances and removal of blood, including routes and volumes. *Journal of Applied Toxicology* 21 (1): 15–23.

29 Young, D.S., Bermes, E.W., and Haverstick, D.M. (2011). Specimen collection and processing. In: *Tietz Texbook of Clinical Chemistry and Molecular Diagnostics*, 4e (ed. C.A. Burtis, E.R. Ashwood and D.E. Bruns), 41–57. St. Louis: Saunders Publishing.

30 Reznik, G., Reznik-Schuller, H., Emminger, A., and Mohr, U. (1975). Comparative studies of blood from hibernating and nonhibernating European hamsters (*Cricetus cricetus L*). *Laboratory Animal Science* 25 (2): 210–215.

31 Silverman, J. and Chavannes, J.M. (1977). Biological values of the European hamster (*Cricetus cricetus*). *Laboratory Animal Science* 27 (5 Pt 1): 641–645.

32 Moore, W. Jr. (1966). Hemogram of the Chinese hamster. *American Journal of Veterinary Research* 27 (117): 608–610.

33 Donnelly, T.M. and Quimby, F.W. (2002). Biology and diseases of other rodents. In: *Laboratory Animal Medicine*, 2e (ed. J.G. Fox, L.C. Anderson, F.M. Loew and F.W. Quimby), 247–307. San Diego: Academice Press.

34 Felt, S.A., Merrill, N.L., Guirguis, F.I., and Hussein, H.I. (2012). Egyptian fat-tailed Jird. In: *The Laboratory Rabbit, Guinea Pig, Hamster, and Other Rodents* (ed. M. Suckow, K. Stevens and R. Wilson), 1157–1170. San Diego: Academic Press.

35 Dodds, W.J., Raymond, S.L., Moynihan, A.C., and McMartin, D.N. (1977). Spontaneous atrial thrombosis in aged Syrian hamsters II. Hemostasis. *Thrombosis and Haemostasis* 38 (2): 457–464.

36 Malan, A., Arens, H., and Waechter, A. (1973). Pulmonary respiration and acid-base balance state in hibernating marmots and hamsters. *Respiratory Physiology* 17 (1): 45–61.

37 Chang, A., Noble, R.E., and Wyse, B.M. (1977). Comparison of highly inbred and nondiabetic lines in the Upjohn colony of Chinese hamsters. *Diabetes* 26 (11): 1063–1071.

38 Chobanian, A.V., Gerritsen, G.C., Brecher, P.I., and Kessler, M. (1974). Cholesterol metabolism in the diabetic Chinese hamster. *Diabetologia* (10 Suppl): 595–600.

39 Maislos, M., Medvedovskv, V., Sztarkier, I. et al. (2006). *Psammomys obesus* (sand rat), a new animal model of non-alcoholic fatty liver disease. *Diabetes Research and Clinical Practice* 72 (1): 1–5.

40 Desai, R.G. (1968). Hematology and microcirculation. In: *The Golden Hamster; its Biology and Use in Medical Research* (ed. R.A. Hoffman, P.F. Robinson and H. Magalhaes), 185–191. Ames: Iowa State University Press.

41 Buetow, B.S., Treuting, P.M., and Van Hoosier, G.L. (1999). The hamster. In: *The Clinical Chemistry of Laboratory Animals* (ed. W.F. Loeb and F.W. Quimby), 49–64. Philadelphia: Taylor and Francis Publishing.

42 Iwaki, T., Ishizaki, K., Kinoshita, S. et al. (2007). Protective effects of ursodeoxycholic acid on chenodeoxycholic acid-induced liver injury in hamsters. *World Journal of Gastroenterology* 13 (37): 5003–5008.

43 Lupo, S., Yodis, L.A., Mico, B.A., and Rush, G.F. (1987). In vivo and in vitro hepatotoxicity and metabolism of acetaminophen in Syrian hamsters. *Toxicology* 44 (2): 229–239.

44 Pinlaor, S., Sripa, B., Sithithaworn, P., and Yongvanit, P. (2004). Hepatobiliary changes, antibody response, and alteration of liver enzymes in hamsters re-infected with *Opsthorchis viverrini*. *Experimental Parasitology* 108 (1–2): 32–39.

45 Sbrana, E., Xiao, S.Y., Popov, V.L. et al. (2006). Experimental yellow fever virus infection in the golden hamster (*Mesocricetus auratus*)III. Clinical laboratory values. *The American Journal of Tropical Medicine and Hygeine* 74 (6): 1084–1089.

46 Brunnert, S.R. and Altman, N.H. (1991). Laboratory assessment of chronic hepatitis in Syrian hamsters. *Laboratory Animal Science* 41 (6): 559–562.

47 Bulien, D. and Hughes, B. (1976). The effect of indomethacin on serum and skeletal muscle enzyme activities of dystrophic hamsters. *Biochemical Pharmacology* 25 (8): 981–983.

48 Yasuda, J., Tateyama, K., Syuto, B., and Too, K. (1990). Lactate dehydrogenase and creatine phosphokinase isoenzymes in tissues of laboratory animals. *Japanese Journal of Veterinary Research* 38 (1): 19–29.

49 Murphy, J.C., Fox, J.G., and Niemi, S.M. (1984). Nephrotic syndrome associated with renal amyloidosis in a colony of Syrian hamsters. *Journal of the American Veterinary Medical Association* 185 (11): 1359–1362.

50 Matsuzawa, T. and Sakazume, M. (1994). Effects of fasting on Haematology and clinical chemistry values in the rat and dog. *Comparative Haematology International* 4 (3): 152–156.

51 Gerritsen, G.C. and Blanks, M.C. (1974). Characterization of Chinese hamsters by metabolic balance, glucose tolerance and insulin secretion. *Diabetologia* (10 Suppl): 493–499.

52 Tomson, F.N. and Wardrop, K.J. (1987). Clinical chemistry and hematology. In: *Laboratory Hamsters* (ed. G.L. Van Hoosier and C.W. McPherson), 43–59. Orlando: Academic Press.

53 Bell, R.H. Jr. and Hye, R.J. (1983). Animal models of diabetes mellitus: physiology and pathology. *Journal of Surgical Research* 35 (5): 433–460.

54 Sicart, R., Sable-Amplis, R., and Guiro, A. (1984). Comparative studies of the circulating lipoproteins in hamster (*Mesocricetus auratus*) with a normal or spontaneous high level of cholesterol in the plasma. *Comparative Biochemistry and Physiology – Part A: Molecular and Integrative Physiology* 78 (3): 511–514.

55 Trautwein, E.A., Liang, J., and Hayes, K.C. (1993). Plasma lipoproteins, biliary lipids and bile acid profile differ in various strains of Syrian hamsters Mesocricetus auratus. *Comparative Biochemistry and Physiology – Part A: Comparative Physiology* 104 (4): 829–835.

56 Mitruka, B.M. and Rawnsley, H.M. (1981). *In Clinical Biochemical and Hematological Reference Values in Normal Experimental Animals and Normal Humans*, 2e. New York: Masson Publishing.

57 O'Brien, J.J., Lucey, E.C., and Snider, G.L. (1979). Arterial blood gases in notmal hamsters at rest and during exercise. *Journal of Applied Physiology* 46 (4): 806–810.

58 Albers, H.E., Yogev, L., Todd, R.B., and Goldman, B.D. (1985). Adrenal corticoids in hamsters: role in circadian timing. *American Journal of Physiology* 248 (4 Pt 2): R434–R438.

59 Burnatowska, M.A., Harris, C.A., Sutton, R.A., and Dirks, J.D. (1977). Effects of PTH and cAMP on renal handling of calcium, magnesium, and phosphate in the hamster. *American Journal of Physiology* 233: F514–F518.

60 Burnatowska, M.A., Harris, C.A., Sutton, R.A., and Seely, J.F. (1985). Effects of vitamin D on renal handling of calcium, magnesium, and phosphate in the hamster. *Kidney International* 27: 864–870.

61 Shankar, S. and De Luca, L.M. (1988). Retinoic acid supplemetation of a vitamin A-deficient diet inhibits retinol loss from hamster liver and serum pools. *Journal of Nutrition* 118 (6): 675–680.

62 Sakanashi, T., Sako, S., Nozuhara, A. et al. (1991). Vitamin E deficiency has a pathological role in myocytolysis in cardiomyopathic Syrian hamster (BIO 14.6). *Biochemical and Biophysical Research Communications* 181 (1): 145–150.

63 Cervantes, M.C., David, J.T., Loyd, D.R. et al. (2005). Lead exposure alters the development of agonistic behavior in golden hamsters. *Developmental Phychobiology* 47 (2): 158–165.

64 Delville, Y. (1999). Exposure to lead during development alters aggressive behaviors in golden hamsters. *Neurotoxicology and Teratology* 21 (4): 445–449.

65 Vaughan, M.K., Brainard, G.C., and Reiter, R.J. (1984). The influence of short photoperiod and temperature conditions on plasma thyroid hormones and cholesterol in male Syrian hamsters. *International Journal of Biometeorology* 28 (3): 201–210.

66 Vaughan, M.K., Powanda, M.C., Richardson, B.A. et al. (1982). Chronic exposure to short photoperiod inhibits free thyroxine index and plasma levels of TSH, T_4, triiodothyronine (T_3) and cholesterol in female Syrian hamsters. *Comparative Biochemistry and Physiology – Part A: Comparative Physiology* 71 (4): 615–618.

67 Hoffman, R.A., Johnson, L.B., Vaughn, M.K., and Reiter, R.J. (1989). Interaction of hardarian glands, illumination, and temperature on thyroid hormones in golden hamsters. *Journal of Comparative Physiology B* 158 (6): 697–702.

68 Ottenweller, J.E., Tapp, W.N., Burke, J.M., and Natelson, B.H. (1985). Plasma cortisol and corticosterone concentrations in the golden hamster (*Mesocricetus auratus*). *Life Sciences* 37: 1551–1558.

69 Gebhardt-Heinrich, S.G., Fischer, K., Hauzenberger, A.R. et al. (2007). The duration of capture and restraint during anesthesia and euthanasia influences glucocorticoid levels in male golden hamsters. *Lab Animal (NY)* 36 (4): 41–46.

70 Donham, R.S., DiPinto, M.N., and Stetson, M.H. (1984). Twenty four-hour rhythm of gonadotropin release induces cyclic progesterone secretion by the ovary of prepubertal and adult golden hamsters. *Endocrinology* 114 (3): 821–826.

71 Siegel, H.I. and Greenwald, G.S. (1978). The temporal pattern of LH, FSH, and ovulatory responsiveness to luteinizing hormone releasing hormone in the cycling hamster. *Proceeding of the Society for Experimental Biology and Medicine* 158 (3): 313–317.

72 Kenny, H.A., Bernard, D.J., Horton, T.H., and Woodruff, T.K. (2002). Photoperiod-dependent regulation of inhibin in Siberian hamsters: I. Ovarian inhibin production and secretion. *Journal of Endocrinology* 174: 71–83.

73 Simpson, S.M., Follett, B.K., and Ellis, D.H. (1982). Modulation by photoperiod of gonadotropin secretion in intact and castrated Djungarian hamsters. *Journal of Reproduction and Fertility* 66: 243–250.

74 Bartke, A., Klemcke, H.G., Amador, A. et al. (1983). Relationship of the length of exposure to short photoperiod to the effect of prolactin on pituitary and testicular function in the golden hamster. *Journal of Reproduction and Fertility* 69 (2): 587–595.

75 Cox, R.A. and Gokcen, M. (1974). Circulating lipids in the golden hamster (*Mesocricetus auratus*). *Comparative Biochemistry and Physiology – Part B: Biochemistry and Molecular Biology* 49B: 655–661.

76 Schuchman, S.M. (1980). Individual care and treatment of rabbits, mice, rats, Guinea pigs, hamsters, and gerbils. In: *Current Veterinary Therapy VII, Small Animal Practice* (ed. R.W. Kirk), 741–767. Philadelphia: Saunders Publishing.

8

Hystricomorph Rodents

Guinea Pigs, Chinchillas, Degus, and Viscachas

Christy L. Rettenmund DVM, DACZM[1] *and J. Jill Heatley DVM, MS, DABVP (Avian, Reptilian, Amphibian), DACZM*[2]

[1] *Milwaukee County Zoo, Milwaukee, Wisconsin, USA*
[2] *Department of Small Animal Clinical Sciences, College of Veterinary Medicine & Biomedical Sciences, Texas A&M University, College Station, Texas, USA*

Introduction

General indications for blood collection for clinicopathologic evaluation of hystricomorph rodents include illness or general health assessment. Clinical pathology is helpful in ill animals to better define differentials for illness and to evaluate the general health of an animal. Blood samples can be difficult to obtain in these species because of small patient size and challenging restraint. Patient size and temperament can make obtaining adequate sample volume difficult, which limits the analytes that can be assessed. Laboratory reference ranges exist for guinea pigs as they are extensively used in research, but reference ranges for chinchillas, viscachas, and degus are less common. This chapter will review known analytes for these four herbivorous South American species, as well as sample collection and handling.

Species

The four small South American hystricomorph species are the guinea pig, chinchilla, viscacha, and degu. Guinea pigs (*Cavia porcellus*), also known as cavies, are hystricomorph rodents commonly kept as pets and used for research models of infectious disease, diabetes, and cardiovascular and pulmonary physiology. Many breeds of guinea pigs are recognized, the most common of which are the American, the Abyssinian, and the Peruvian. Guinea pigs require a dietary source of vitamin C and are a food source for people in parts of South America. Chinchillas (*Chinchilla laniger*) are native to the Andes Mountains and are commonly kept as pets, but are also a model for auditory research and are raised for the fur trade. Chinchillas can be found in a variety of colors including standard gray, white, black velvet, beige, ebony, violet, sapphire, and blends of these colors. The viscacha (*Lagostomus maximus*) is closely related to the chinchilla but has an appearance similar to a rabbit. The five species of viscacha are native to South America and are rarely kept in captivity; they are not commonly used in research. Degus (*Octodon degus*), also known as the brush-tailed rat or common degu, are endemic to Chile and have been used to study diabetes, behavior, circadian rhythms, development, and aging and are becoming more popular as pets.

Sample Collection

Restraint

Guinea pigs are easily frightened and can become stressed during restraint for sample collection. Their stocky bodies, short necks, and delicate, short limbs, as well as the fact that they are obligate nasal breathers, make sample collection difficult. Chinchillas are also easily frightened, and if not properly restrained can shed patches of fur (but not skin). This "fur slip" can be concerning to owners as the dense fur of the chinchilla may take several weeks to regrow. They are also agile jumpers, and if not properly restrained, can easily escape. Their long legs and delicate hair coat can make them difficult to restrain for blood collection, but they tend to be more amenable to restraint than guinea pigs. Restraining degus can be difficult because of their small size and aggression toward humans. Degus may bite. The degu's long, haired tails should not be handled distally for restraint as the degu will spin and deglove the tail. The degu will then amputate the degloved tail by severing the tendons and vertebrae with its teeth. The stump usually heals well but tail regeneration does not occur. Degus are

Exotic Animal Laboratory Diagnosis, First Edition. Edited by J. Jill Heatley and Karen E. Russell.

best scooped up with one hand while holding the base of the tail and allowing them to cling to a coat sleeve or cloth with their tiny, sharp claws. Viscachas have powerful hind legs with large claws and large sharp incisors to scratch and bite. Tractable animals can be picked up by the base of the tail for examination but holding the tail distally results in fracture. Animals can be netted or pinned down quickly by holding the neck, the base of the tail, and the hind feet [1]. Most degus and viscachas require sedation or anesthesia for sample collection [1].

Midazolam (0.5–2 mg/kg IM), isoflurane, or sevoflurane gas anesthesia is recommended for adequate sedation and restraint for blood collection in each of these species. As these are small rodents, short fasting times should clear the mouth of food and reduce stomach volume to facilitate adequate ventilation. Vomiting in the healthy rodent would be unexpected based on their well-developed cardiac gastric sphincter. If the animal becomes unduly stressed or dyspneic during restraint for attempted sampling, sedation with midazolam or anesthesia with isoflurane or sevoflurane may be indicated for blood sample collection.

Blood Collection

The blood volume of guinea pigs averages 7 mls per 100 grams, and approximately 7%–10% of the total blood volume can be safely collected in a healthy guinea pig, or approximately 0.5–0.7 mls per 100 grams [2, 3]. The blood volume and plasma volume of guinea pigs decrease with age. Blood and plasma volumes at birth are 11.5% and 5.75% of body weight respectively, whereas at maturity, the blood and plasma volumes are 5.9% and 3% of the body weight, respectively, in 900 g guinea pigs [4]. Blood volume has not been determined for chinchillas, degus, or viscachas. In hystricomorph patients, sample volume collected should be reduced or forgone until patient stabilization is achieved. Venipuncture in hystricomorph rodents is challenging. A variety of blood collection sites are described including the jugular vein, cranial vena cava, lateral saphenous vein, cephalic vein, medial saphenous/femoral vein, submandibular vein (Figure 8.1), and ventral tail artery; approaches for more commonly used sites are detailed below [5].

The jugular vein can be used for blood collection in guinea pigs, chinchillas, and possibly viscachas [5]. Restraint for jugular venipuncture is similar to restraint of cats, wherein the forelegs are extended down over the table edge and the head and neck are held in extension. Guinea pigs have short thick necks, and shaving may facilitate jugular vein visualization. Restraint for jugular venipuncture can be stressful for guinea pigs, causing dyspnea or collapse in the ill patient. This sampling option is not recommended for use in the dyspneic guinea pig. Chinchillas may better tolerate restraint for jugular

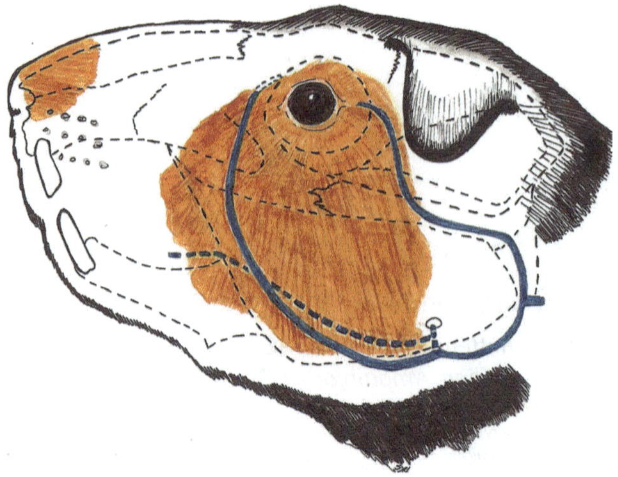

Figure 8.1 Illustration of the lateral view of the submandibular vein in a guinea pig. This vein can be used to obtain small volumes of blood, and is generally approached from the ventromedial aspect of the mandible with the guinea pig in ventrodorsal recumbency.

venipuncture. The major advantage of the jugular vein is that a relatively large sample can be collected quickly. A jugular venous sample is usually collected using a 1 or 3 ml syringe with a 27 or 25 g. (gauge) needle.

Blood can be collected from the cranial vena cava in guinea pigs, degus, and chinchillas. The animal is placed in dorsal recumbency and the needle inserted into the "notch" where the first rib meets the manubrium. The needle is then directed across the midline of the body toward the opposite leg. A 25 g. needle with a 1 or 3 ml syringe is most often used for sample collection. This technique should only be performed under anesthesia, as the associated risks include laceration of the great vessels, iatrogenic bleeding into the thoracic cavity or pericardial sac, and cardiac tamponade.

The lateral saphenous vein (Figures 8.2 and 8.3) can be used in guinea pigs, chinchillas, and viscachas for blood collection. The cephalic vein can be used in guinea pigs and chinchillas and likely the viscacha. The medial saphenous/femoral vein can be used for blood collection in chinchillas, degus, guinea pigs, and viscachas. In degus, only a small volume of blood can be collected from the medial saphenous vein [6]. Some form of sedation or anesthesia is often needed when collecting blood from the medial saphenous vein in chinchillas, but the collection method is the same as for cats. Use of insulin syringes or a 1 ml syringe with 25 or 27 g. needle is recommended for blood collection from these sites which although readily accessible, generally yield only small amounts (~0.2–0.5 ml).

The ventral tail artery is the most useful blood collection site in the degu and can also be used in the chinchilla. The ventral tail artery courses along the ventral midline of the tail. Anesthesia is recommended for this

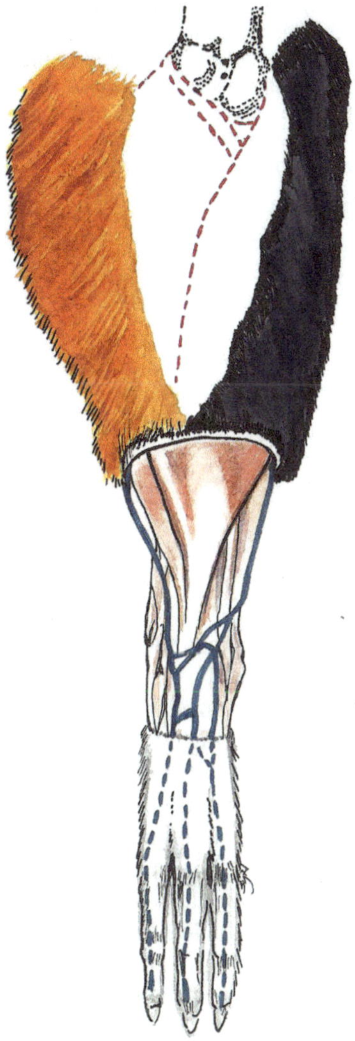

Figure 8.2 Illustration of the dorsal view of the veins in a guinea pig hind limb.

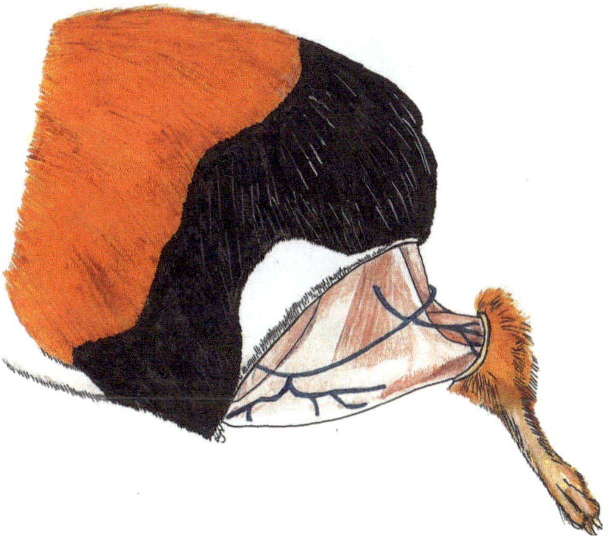

Figure 8.3 The lateral saphenous vein of the guinea pig is most easily accessed for venipuncture just proximal to the ankle joint extending laterally along the thigh.

method to allow placement of the animal in dorsal recumbency for best sample collection. Insert a small-gauge needle (25 or 27 g.) attached to a 1 ml syringe at a 30° angle on the ventral midline of the tail for best results. Drawbacks of this method include degloving injury to the tail from excessive restraint and damage to arterial supply of the tail and subsequent necrosis. Avoid application of excessive force to the tail during collection and restraint, and apply pressure after collection for a minimum of 2 min to avoid continued bleeding, hematoma formation, or vascular damage [6].

Several other blood collection sites have been described in the chinchilla, which include the lateral abdominal vein, dorsal penis, auricular veins, and transverse sinus. The lateral abdominal vein and the dorsal vein of the penis are difficult to locate visually and are not used for routine venipuncture. Small volumes of blood can be collected from the auricular veins using a 27 g. needle, insulin syringe, or microcapillary tubes [7, 8]. The transverse sinus circles the auditory bulla and can be accessed by removing the hair from the dorsal aspect of the skull and inserting a needle 1 mm medial to the border of the auditory bulla to a depth of 1–2 mm (Figure 8.4). This can be done with a 25 g. butterfly catheter attached to a 1 ml syringe and allows for collection of larger blood volumes as compared to some of the other venipuncture sites in chinchillas [9].

Urine Collection and Handling

Owing to the small size and fragility of these animals, urine is often collected as a free catch sample or by manual expression of the bladder. Catheterization techniques for both the male and female guinea pig have also been described [10, 11]. Cystocentesis can be performed with a small 25 g. needle in a similar fashion as performed in other species. Anesthesia may be necessary for adequate restraint. Ultrasound can help visualize the bladder and avoid the cecum for sample collection. If a urine culture is desired, cystocentesis should be performed. Urinalysis is best performed within 2 h of collection. Analysis of refrigerated samples can be performed within 48 h, but urine should warmed to room temperature prior to testing and examination [12]. Urinary electrolytes have been reported in chinchillas and have been shown to vary with gender and time of day [7].

Bone Marrow Collection and Composition

Bone marrow can be collected from the ileum, femur, and humerus utilizing techniques described for canine and feline patients [13], although smaller-gauge needles

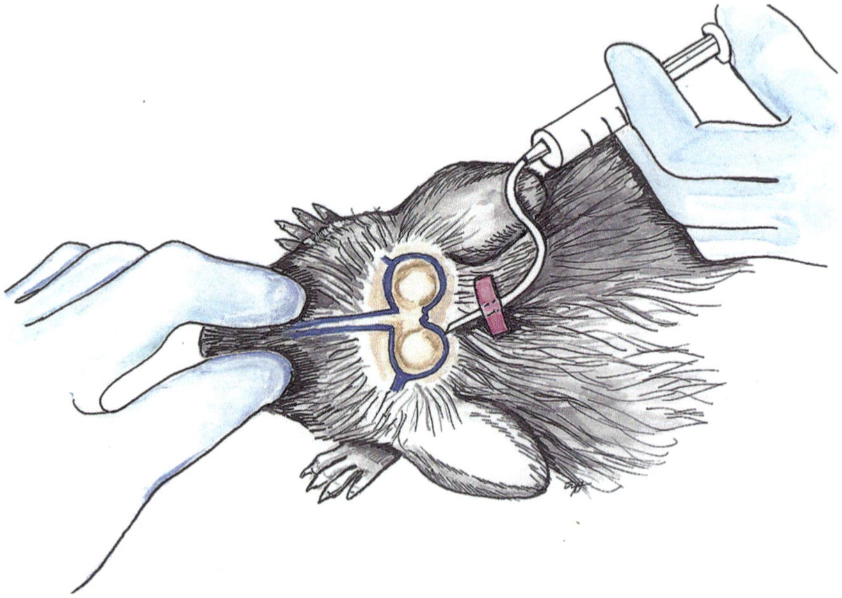

Figure 8.4 This illustration demonstrates blood collection from the transverse sinus in the chinchilla, which is located on the dorsal caudal aspect of the head. A butterfly catheter is used for venipuncture at this site, and insertion of the needle is only 1–2 mm through the skin.

and syringes will be used in these exotic species. Care should be taken during bone marrow aspiration, as these species, especially guinea pigs, chinchillas, and degus, have small delicate bones which can fracture with aggressive handling. Techniques for bone marrow aspiration from the ilium, sternum, femur, tibia, and bones of the proximal third of the tail in exotic pet species have been described [14]. Preparation and handling of samples is consistent with that for other domestic species. Bone marrow of guinea pigs is composed of 26.7% erythroblasts, 63.3% myeloid, 4.6% lymphocytes, and 5.4% reticulum cells with a myeloid ratio varying from 1.5:1 to 1.9:1 and does not vary with strain [3]. The bone marrow cellularity of large guinea pigs is less that than of smaller guinea pigs. The mean total bone marrow volume of guinea pigs is 7.014 ± 0.348 ml with about 50% of volume found in the limb bones. Bone marrow accounts for about 2.5% of body weight in the one-week-old guinea pig and about 1% of body weight in the adult guinea pig [3]. In chinchillas, femoral bone marrow sample analysis has been reported and found no significant differences in bone marrow composition between males and females, and bone marrow cellularity remained constant throughout the life of the chinchilla [15].

Blood Sample Handling

After sample collection, blood is typically placed in microcollection tubes containing anticoagulants such as EDTA or heparin [16]. Excessive volumes of liquid anticoagulants can dilute the blood sample, resulting in decreased hematocrit, enzyme, or cell concentrations. In contrast, excessive amounts of dry anticoagulants can create artifacts such as red blood cell shrinkage, which will affect hematocrit. Therefore, using the smallest amount of anticoagulant that will keep the sample from clotting is recommended [16]. Blood collected for a biochemical panel is typically heparinized plasma, which yields a larger sample volume for analysis and avoids hemolysis, which is common in serum samples. Timely separation of serum or plasma prevents consumption of glucose by cells. Hemolysis can increase analyte concentrations such as potassium, phosphorus, lactate dehydrogenase, and bilirubin as well as decreasing glucose [12]. Potassium concentrations are less in guinea pig serum stored in plastic rather than in glass [17]. Hematologic analysis should be performed as soon as possible after blood collection [16]. Ideally, blood smears are prepared using fresh whole blood as prolonged exposure to anticoagulant can increase cell smudging.

Complete Blood Count (Table 8.1)

Red Blood Cell Parameters and Platelets

The erythrocytes of hystricomorph rodents have a shorter half-life than dogs and cats, which results in increased polychromasia on blood smears (Figure 8.5) [16]. Guinea pigs also have larger erythrocytes than other rodent species [23]. In male guinea pigs, the reticulocyte count decreases with age [24]. The erythrocyte sedimentation rate of guinea pigs averages 1.06–1.20 mm per hour, which is longer than in the mouse, rat, and ruminant but shorter than in the rabbit, chicken, dog, pig, man, cat, or horse [3]. The guinea pig is unique in the development of acute hemolytic anemia in response to excess dietary cholesterol [3]. Hairless guinea pigs have smaller red blood cells (lower mean corpuscular volume (MCV)) which contain more hemoglobin (higher mean corpuscular hemoglobin concentration (MCHC)) and a higher packed cell volume than haired guinea pigs [25].

Table 8.1 Hematologic reference ranges for hystricomorph rodents.

Analyte (abbreviation)	Units, SI (conventional)	Guinea pig (*Cavia porcellus*)[a,b] [18, 19]	Chinchilla (*Chinchilla laniger*)[a] [18, 20]	Degu (*Octodon degus*) [21]	Viscacha (*Lagostomus maximus*) [22] ξ
Data format		**Unknown**	**95% Confidence interval [20] or unknown**	**95% Confidence interval**	**5–95th Percentile**
Animal number		**101[b] [19] or unknown**	**16 ◊ [20] or unknown**	**35 Á 35 Ó**	**44**
Hematocrit (HCT)	Proportion of 1.0 (%)	0.37–0.48 (37–48)	0.27–0.54 (27–54)	0.42–0.44 (42–44) Ó 0.44–0.46 (44–46) Á	0.34–0.42 (35–43)
Hemoglobin (Hb)	g /l (g/dl)	110–115 (11–15)	80–154 (8–15.4)	110.4–117 (11.04–11.7) Ó 114.9–120.3 (11.49–12.03)	107–132 (10.7–13.2)
Red blood cells (RBCs)	$\times 10^{12}$/l ($\times 10^6$/μl)	4.5–7 (4.5–7)	5.2–10.7 (5.2–10.7)	6.89–7.64 (6.89–7.64) Ó 8.35–9.06 (8.35–9.06) Á	4.44–5.64 (4.44–5.64)
Mean (MCV) corpuscular volume	fl	80.3–89.1[b] [19]	86.5–116.1 [20]	58.01–61.78 Ó 50.26–52.45 Á	71–81
Mean (MCH) corpuscular hemoglobin	pg	1.5–1.7 fmol/l[b] [19]	2.8–4.4 [20]	15.31–16.37 Ó 13.16–13.59 Á	22–25
Mean (MCHC) corpuscular hemoglobin concentration	g/l (g/dl)	18.1–19.7 mmol/l[b] [19]	325–382 (32.5–38.2) [20]	260.8–268.1 (26.08–26.81) Ó 257–264.9 (25.7–26.49) Á	0.3–0.32 (30–32)
White blood cells (WBCs)	$\times 10^9$/l ($\times 10^3$/μl)	7–18 (7–18)	4–11.5 (4–11.5)	6.1–8.22 (6.1–8.22) Ó 6.55–8.23 (6.55–8.23) Á	8.2–17.8 (8.2–17.8)
Neutrophils	$\times 10^9$ /l ($\times 10^3$/μl)	0.899–5.097 (0.899–5.097)[b] [19]		1.82–2.63 (1.82–2.63) Ó 2.53–3.58 (2.53–3.58) Á	6.384–13.667 (6.384–13.667)
Neutrophils, bands	$\times 10^9$/l ($\times 10^3$/μl)	0–0.072 (0–0.072)[b] [19]		0.03–0.17 (0.03–0.17) Ó 0.06–0.1 (0.06–0.1) Á	0–0.173 (0–0.173)
Lymphocytes	$\times 10^9$/l ($\times 10^3$/μl)	1.401–10.665 (1.401–10.665)[b] [19]		3.76–5.43 (3.76–5.43) Ó 3.53–4.52 (3.53–4.52) Á	0.532–4.049 (0.532–4.049)
Monocytes	$\times 10^9$/l ($\times 10^3$/μl)	0–0.657 (0–0.657)[b] [19]		0.09–0.17 (0.09–0.17) Ó 0.06–0.20 (0.06–0.20) Á	0.196–0.865 (0.196–0.865)
Eosinophils	$\times 10^9$/l ($\times 10^3$/μl)	0–1.563 (0–1.563)[b] [19]		0.07–0.15 (0.07–0.15) Ó 0.12–0.3 (0.12–0.3) Á	0.104–0.910 (0.104–0.910)
Basophils	$\times 10^9$/l ($\times 10^3$/μl)	0–0.106 (0–0.106)[b] [19]		0.0–0.02 (0.0–0.02) Ó 0.0–0.03 (0.0–0.03) Á	0–0.304 (0–0.304)
Platelets	$\times 10^9$/l ($\times 10^3$/μl)	250–850 (250–850)	254–740 (254–740)	403.9–503 (403.9–503) Ó 233.7–410.2 (233.7–410.2) Á	

[a] Animal number and reference range data format not given [18].
[b] Clinically healthy guinea pigs age 6 weeks to 5.5 years [19].
Key: Free living ξ, Male ◊, Adult Á, Juvenile Ó.

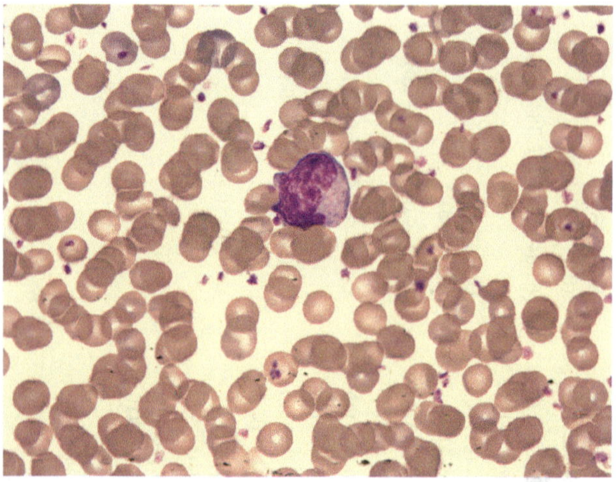

Figure 8.5 Monocytes, red blood cells, and platelets of a guinea pig (*Cavia porcellus*), magnification 1000×.

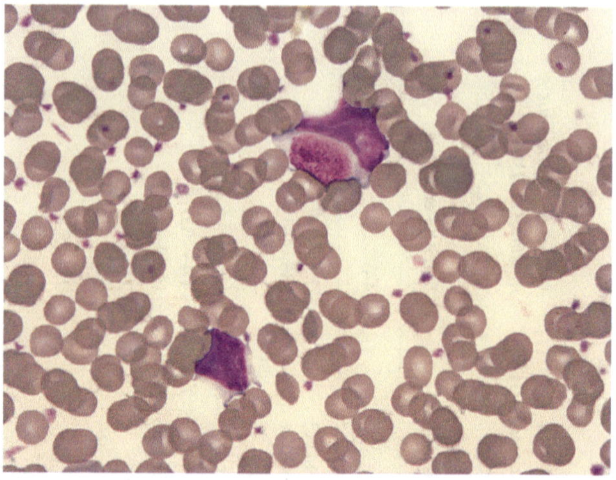

Figure 8.6 Lymphocytes of a guinea pig (*Cavia porcellus*), with (upper right) and without (lower left) a Kurloff body, magnification 1000×.

Adult degus have a higher red blood cell count and hematocrit than juveniles but a lower reticulocyte count, MCV, and mean corpuscular hemoglobin (MCH) [21]. In chinchillas, seasonal fluctuations in red blood cell parameters occur. In winter, chinchillas have a higher red blood cell (RBC) count, MCH, hemoglobin concentration (Hb), and MCHC, while in summer hematocrit (HCT) and MCV are higher. Pet chinchillas maintained in a climate-controlled environment are unlikely to experience these fluctuations [26]. Anemia (RBC 3.29, 5.55×10^{12}/l, hemoglobin 5.1, 8.6 g /dl, hematocrit 14.2, 27.4%) has been documented in two cases of renal disease in a degus [27, 28].

Guinea pig platelets are an irregular oval shape with a dark staining inner zone surrounded by a paler zone (Figure 8.5) [23]. The platelet count in male guinea pigs decreases between 100 and 200 days of age, but then increases with age after 200 days [24]. Hairless guinea pigs have an increased number of platelets compared to haired guinea pigs [25]. The platelet count is lower in adult degus than in juveniles [21].

White Blood Cell Parameters

Hystricomorph leukocytes include neutrophils, eosinophils, basophils, lymphocytes, and monocytes. Most white blood cell morphology of hystricomorph rodents is similar to that of companion mammals. Guinea pigs and other hystricomorph rodents tend to be lymphocytic (having predominantly lymphocytes) [9] with the exception of the viscacha, in which the neutrophil is predominant [22]. Age-related changes occur in leukocyte parameters of multiple hystricomorph rodents. In both guinea pig genders, the white blood cell and neutrophil counts increase with age, whereas the lymphocyte count gradually decreases with age [24]. The basophil count in female guinea pigs decreases with age, whereas the monocyte count gradually increases with age in male guinea pigs [24]. In degus, the percentage of neutrophils is higher in adults than in juveniles [21].

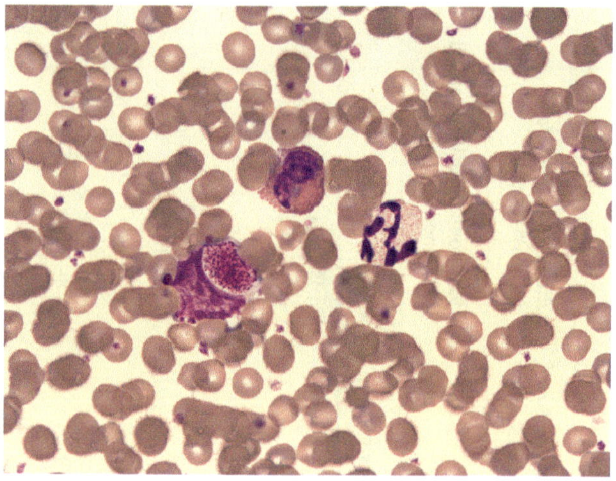

Figure 8.7 Kurloff cell (left), eosinophil (middle), and heterophil (right) of a guinea pig (*Cavia porcellus*), magnification 1000×.

Lymphocytes and Monocytes

Mononuclear cells include the monocyte and the lymphocyte, which are similar in appearance and function to those of companion mammals. The appearance of the monocyte is similar in all hystricomorph rodents (Figure 8.5) [16]. A monocytosis can be seen with acute or chronic inflammation or stress (corticosteroid response) [16]. Monocytosis occurs in guinea pigs experimentally infected with *Trixacarus caviae* [29]. The large lymphocytes of guinea pigs can contain a large intracytoplasmic inclusion called a Kurloff body (Figure 8.6 and 8.7). Kurloff bodies are likely influenced by the presence of sex hormones and are more abundant in pregnant females or guinea pigs treated with estrogen, but exist in low numbers in immature, non-pregnant, and non-estrogen-treated guinea pigs [30]. Although the function of the Kurloff body is unknown, these cells are thought to function as natural killer cells. Kurloff cells may comprise as much as 3%–4% of the leukocyte count [23]. Lymphocytosis can be associated with excitement or lymphocytic leukemia. Lymphopenia is generally associated with stress (corticosteroid response) [16]. When hairless guinea pigs were compared to their haired counterparts, the hairless guinea pigs were found to have 40% fewer leukocytes with lower numbers of lymphocytes, causing a reversal of the lymphocyte to neutrophil ratio from 1.75:1 in haired guinea pigs to 0.74:1 in hairless guinea pigs [25]. Lymphocytes were lower in adult degus as compared to juveniles [21]. Chinchillas exposed to seasonal temperature fluctuations have decreased white blood cell counts (WBC) and total lymphocyte counts in the summer and increased counts in the autumn and spring [26]. The lymphocyte count of diurnal degus is lower than that in nocturnal degus [32]. Lymphopenia (2.64×10^9 cells/l) and leukopenia (3.7×10^9 WBC/l) occurred in a young degu suffering polycystic, chronic kidney disease [28].

Granulocytes

Chinchillas have neutrophils with segmented nuclei and acidophilic cytoplasmic granules, whereas the neutrophilic equivalents in guinea pigs are heterophils which have eosinophilic granules (Figure 8.7 and 8.8). Heterophilia occurs in guinea pigs experimentally infected with *T. caviae* [29]. Basophils are rarely observed in guinea pigs and have a lobed nucleus with basophilic cytoplasmic granules which may stain black to reddish purple [23]. Basophilia has been documented in guinea pigs experimentally infested with *T. caviae, Rhipicephalus sanguineus*, or *Amblyomma americanum* [29, 32, 33]. Basophilia often occurs in conjunction with eosinophilia. Eosinophilia in guinea pigs may occur in response to experimental infestation with *T. caviae* or infection with *Treponema pallidum* [29, 34]. Leukocytosis (16.8 cells $\times 10^9$/L) with neutrophilia (14.0 cells $\times 10^9$/L) was reported in a case of renal transitional cell carcinoma and choristoma in a degu which also had a staphylococcal cystitis [27].

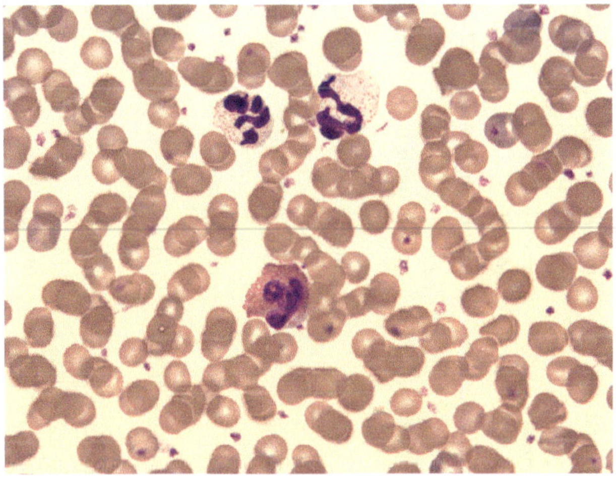

Figure 8.8 Heterophils (above) and eosinophil (below) of a guinea pig (*Cavia porcellus*) magnification, 1000×.

Coagulation Panel and Blood Types

Guinea pigs have about 50% of the plasma prothrombin of the rat or dog, resulting in a relatively slow bleeding time of about 4 min and slower coagulations times than in most rodents (Table 8.2)[3, 35]. Guinea pigs also have the least factor VII and low amounts of factor V compared to other laboratory rodents, as well as low concentrations of factor X compared to humans [3, 35, 36, 37]. Coagulation parameters have not been evaluated in other hystricomorph rodents. Thus, for evaluation of a coagulopathy in most hystricomorph rodents, collection of a sample from a healthy animal to compare with an ill animal is recommended. Collecting blood for accurate determination of coagulation can be challenging as errors in coagulation determination can occur with traumatic venipuncture, prolonged vessel occlusion, inappropriate anticoagulant use (EDTA and heparin invalidate results), incomplete blood draw, and air-contaminated syringes. Blood is typically collected in tubes containing sodium citrate so as not to interfere with coagulation values. Blood collected for coagulation testing must be analyzed immediately for accurate results [38]. Blood types for hystricomorph rodents are unknown; cross-matching is not typically performed when blood transfusions are administered.

Biochemical Panel (Table 8.3)

Liver

Blood tests to evaluate the liver include alanine aminotransferase (ALT), aspartate aminotransferase (AST), alkaline phosphatase (ALP), gamma-glutamyl transferase (GGT), lactate dehydrogenase (LDH), and bilirubin. Decreases in ALT or ALP in hystricomorph rodents do

Table 8.2 Coagulation parameters of guinea pigs (*Cavia porcellus*) [24, 36].

Seconds	Prothombin time	Activated partial thromboplastin time
Male	27.2–30	17.9–21.2
Female	26.4–29	20.3–23.8
Both	20–37	11–28

Table 8.3 Biochemical reference ranges for hystricomorph rodents.

Analyte (abbreviation)	Units, SI (conventional)	Guinea pig (*Cavia porcellus*)[a,b] [18, 19]	Chinchilla[a] [18, 20] (*Chinchilla laniger*)	Degu (*Octodon degus*) [21]	Viscacha (*Lagostomus maximus*) [22] ξ
Data format		**Unknown**	**95% Confidence interval [20] or unknown**	**95% Confidence interval**	**5–95th Percentile**
Animal number		**101[b] [19] or unknown**	**16 ◊ [20] or unknown**	**35 Á, 35 Ó**	**44**
Alanine (ALT) Aminotransferase	U/l (units/l)	10–25 (10–25)	10–35 (10–35)	27.55–40.12 (27.55–40.12) Ó 16.17–22.16 (16.17–22.16) Á	29–62 (29–62)
Albumin	g/l (g /dl)	21–39 (2.1–3.9)	24–42 (2.4–4.2)	32.97–34.97 (3.297–3.497) Ó 31.21–35.07 (3.121–3.507) Á	29–37 (2.9–3.7)
Albumin: globulin ratio				1.55–1.85 Ó 1.03–1.29 Á	
Alkaline (ALP/AP) Phosphatase	U /l (units/l)	18–28 (18–28)	3–47 (3–47)	299.4–471.86 (229.4–471.86) Ó 62.87–74.25 (62.87–74.25) Á	20–316 (20–316)
Amylase	U/l (units/l	0–159 (0–159)[a] [18]		788.62–996.41 (788.62–996.41) Ó 733.53–908.38 (733.53–908.38) Á	377–5091 (377–5091)
Aspartate (AST) Aminotransferase	U/l (units/l)	0–90 (0–90)[a] [18]	96 (96)	48.5–73.65 (48.5–73.65) Ó 37.72–56.29 (37.72–56.29) Á	86–215 (86–215)
Bile acids, total	mmol/l (μg/ml)	0–84.5 (0–34.52)[a] [18]		8.94–18.04 Á (no range for juveniles)	
Bilirubin, total	mmol/l (mg/dl)	5–15 (0.3–0.9)	7 (0.4)	1.91–2.86 (0.11–0.17) Ó 1.4–2.33 (0.08–0.14) Á	
Blood urea nitrogen (BUN)	mmol/l (mg/dl)	3.2–11.2 (9.0–31.5)	3.6–8.9 (10–25)	14.16–15.96 (39.66–44.71) Ó 9.41–10.73 (26.36–30.06) Á	10.1–23.7 (28.29–66.39)
Calcium	mmol/l (mEq/l)	1.32–3 (5.3–12)	1.4–3.02 (5.6–12.1)	3.075–3.26 (6.15–6.52) Ó 2.42–2.64 (4.84–5.28) Á	1.99–2.6 (3.98–5.2)
Chloride	mmol/l (mEq/l)	98–115 (98–115)	105–115 (105–115)	102.9–106.8 (102.9–106.8) Ó 101.3–105.4 (101.3–105.4) Á	109–117 (109–117)
Cholesterol	mmol/l (mg/dl)	0.52–1.11 (20–43)	1.03–2.59 (40–100)	2.27–2.76 (87.64–106.56) Ó 1.85–2.15 (71.43–83.01) Á	0.5–2.1 (19.3–81.08)
Creatinine	mmol/l (mg/dl)	53–194 (0.6–2.2)		51.94–60.96 (0.59–0.69) Ó 47.91–54.99 (0.54–0.62) Á	94–219 (1.06–2.48)
Creatinine kinase (CK)	U/l (units/l)	0–2143 (0–2143)[a] [18]		752.69–2627.55 (752.69–2627.55) Ó 643.71–1274.25 (643.71–1274.25) Á	4620–48 600 (4620–48 600)
Fructosamine	Mmol/l	134–271[a] [18]			161–297
γ-glutamyl transferase (GGT)	U/l (units/l)	0–13 (0–13)[a] [18]		1.8–3 (1.8–3) Ó 1.8–2.4 (1.8–2.4) Á	1–3 (1–3)

Globulin	g/l (g/dl)	17–26 (1.7–2.6)		19.05–24.36 (1.905–2436) Ó 27.71–32.26 (2.771–3.226) Á	
Glucose	mmol/l (mg/dl)	3.3–6.9 (60–125)	3.3–6.7 (60–120)	8.79–9.97 (158.38–179.64) Ó 8.27–9.52 (149.01–171.53) Á	4.7–11.2 (84.7–201.8)
Iron	mmol/l (μg/dl)	26–76 (145.3–424.6)[a] [18]			16.8–39.1 (93.9–218.44)
Lactate (LDH) dehydrogenase	U/l (units/l)	0–515 (0–515)[a] [18]		562.87–795.21 (562.87–795.21) Ó 522.16–604.79 (522.16–604.79) Á	801–2530 (801–2530)
Lipase	U/ l (units/l)	0–152 (0–152)[a] [18]		35.93–50.9 (35.93–50.9) Ó 23.95–29.34 (23.95–29.34) Á	161–397 (161–397)
Magnesium	mmol/l (mEq/l)	0.99–2.56 (1.98–5.12)[a] [18]	1.36–1.73 (2.72–3.46) [22]		0.85–1.68 (1.7–3.36)
Phosphorus	mmol/l (mg/dl)	0.97–3.87 (3–12)	1.29–2.58 (4–8)	1.97–2.37 (6.1–7.34) Ó 1.32–1.6 (4.09–4.95) Á	2.15–4.48 (6.66–13.87)
Potassium	mmol/l (mEq/l)	4.5–8.9 (4.5–8.9)	5–6.5 (5–6.5)	4.1–4.8 (4.1–4.8) Ó 3.69–4 (3.69–4) Á	3.3–5.7 (3.3–5.7)
Sodium	mmol/l (mEq/l)	132–156 (132–156)	130–155 (130–155)	140.4–144.2 (140.4–144.2) Ó 139.8–144.5 (139.8–144.5) Á	158–174 (158–174)
Total protein	g/l (g/dl)	46–62 (4.6–6.2)	50–60 (5–6)	52.68–56.74 (5.268–5.674) Ó 60.35–65.91 (6.035–6.591) Á	61–77 (6.1–7.7)
Triglycerides	g/l (mg/ dl)	0–1.4 (0–145)	1.17–2.29 (117–229.5) [22]	1.47–2.16 (130.09–191.15) Ó 1.46–2.34 (129.2–207.08) Á	0.177–2.12 (17.7–212.4)
Uric acid	μmol/l (mg/dl)				33.9–115.0 (0.57–1.93)

[a] Animal number and reference range data format not given [18].
[b] Clinically healthy guinea pigs age 6 weeks to 5.5 years [19].
Key: Free living, ξ, Male, ◊, Adult, Á, Juvenile, Ó.

not indicate disease, and concentrations of these enzymes are increased in younger degus [21]. In guinea pigs, ALT is not specific or sensitive for hepatocellular disease. Quantities are low in hepatocytes, and ALT activity in the heart is equal to that of the liver [16, 17]. Activities of AST are increased in hairless as compared to haired guinea pigs [25]. Aspartate aminotransferase activity occurs in multiple tissues including liver, heart, skeletal muscle, and red blood cells and is less specific for liver damage then ALT. Causes of increased AST activities in plasma include hepatic disease, muscle disease, or hemolysis. Activity of AST is relatively increased in hairless as compared to haired guinea pigs [25]. Guinea pig AST activities are low and have limited diagnostic value [17]. Alkaline phosphatase (ALP or AP) is found in osteoblasts, biliary epithelium, and epithelial cells of kidneys and intestines. The guinea pig also has ALP in its lymphocytes and granulocytes, unlike the rabbit, rat, hamster, or dog [3]. Juvenile degus and guinea pigs have higher ALP than adults [21, 24]. Some causes of increased ALP in juvenile/growing animals are osteoblastic activity, hepatic cholestasis, biliary tract disease, and hepatic parenchymal disease (toxin, hepatitis, neoplasia). Guinea pigs with a deficiency in magnesium or zinc can also have increased ALP [16]. ALP is lower in hairless as compared to haired guinea pigs [25]. Increased ALT (126 IU/l), AST (232 IU/l) and ALP (86 IU/l) occurred in a single case of renal transitional cell carcinoma and choristoma in a degu [27].

Gamma-glutamyl transferase (GGT) is increased in animals with hepatic injury, resulting in cholestasis. Serum GGT activity in guinea pigs can increase after blood clot formation based on leakage of GGT from erythrocytes. This artifactual increase can be avoided with use of plasma samples [16]. Lactate dehydrogenase occurs in a variety of tissues including skeletal muscle, cardiac muscle, liver, kidney, and intestines. Activity of GGT may increase in rodents with liver disease but is poorly specific based on its presence in other tissues. Lactate dehydrogenase occurs in a variety of tissues including skeletal muscle, cardiac muscle, liver, kidney, and intestines. Normal values are variable and depend on the analytic methodology [16]. Bilirubin concentrations increase with hemolysis, extrahepatic biliary obstruction, and primary hepatobiliary disease. Evaluation of the hemogram and other liver or biliary specific tests is necessary in conjunction with this test. Bile acids are a sensitive and specific test for liver disease in hystricomorph rodents [16].

Muscle

Muscle enzyme activities for which reference ranges have been determined include AST and creatinine kinase (CK). Aspartate aminotransferase occurs in liver and red blood cells and is not specific to muscle. Increased activity in both enzymes is associated with muscle disease such as trauma, inflammation, or necrosis. Hairless guinea pigs have higher CK than haired guinea pigs [25]. Increased AST activity occurred in a case of renal transitional cell carcinoma and choristoma in a degu [27].

Kidney

Renal analytes evaluated for hystricomorph rodents include blood urea nitrogen (BUN) and creatinine. Abnormally increased BUN and creatinine are referred to as azotemia. Laboratory evaluation of kidney disease in rodents is similar to that of dogs and cats. Increases in BUN concentration may be based on dehydration, renal disease, high-protein diet, gastrointestinal hemorrhage, or urinary outflow obstruction in hystricomorph rodents as in dogs and cats. Decreased BUN may occur with dietary protein restriction, hepatic insufficiency, or increased excretion (polyuria). Creatinine is more specific for renal disease then BUN. Causes of increased creatinine include dehydration, renal disease, and urinary obstruction, while decreased creatinine may occur with severe cachexia. Increased age in guinea pigs is associated with increased BUN and creatinine, but these analyte concentrations decrease with age in degus [21, 23]. Both creatinine and BUN were higher in hairless as compared to haired guinea pigs [25]. Lifestyle may also affect these analytes as BUN was higher in diurnal when compared to nocturnal degus [31]. Two cases of degus with renal disease documented hyperphosphatemia, increased BUN, and creatinine (azotemia) [27, 28].

Pancreas

Laboratory analytes associated with pancreatic assessment include amylase and lipase, although neither is sensitive or specific for pancreatic disease. Amylase occurs in a variety of tissues in the body. Causes of increased amylase values include pancreatitis and azotemia because of decreased glomerular filtration, as well as intestinal and hepatic disease. Concentrations of amylase are higher in hairless guinea pigs as compared to haired guinea pigs [25]. Lipase concentrations can also increase based on decreased glomerular filtration or pancreatitis. To the best of the author's knowledge, there is no pancreatic lipase-like assay available for hystricomorph rodents, and pancreatitis is uncommonly diagnosed in these species.

Determination of glucose concentrations is a valuable diagnostic test in hystricomorph rodents. Causes of hypoglycemia include inadequate dietary intake, hepatic insufficiency, neoplasia (beta cell tumors, other neoplasia), and sepsis. Causes of hyperglycemia include diabetes mellitus, stress, and postprandial status. Hyperglycemia (glucose 276 mg/dl) occurred in a single case of renal transitional cell carcinoma and choristoma in a degu [27]. Immunoassays for rats to measure insulin and glucagon are invalid for use in guinea pigs. Therefore, insulin and glucagon are not routinely measured in hystricomorph rodents, and no reference intervals are extant [16]. Fructosamine testing can diagnose diabetes and monitor diabetic therapy. Fructosamine indicates blood glucose concentrations over the previous one to two weeks and provides information about long-term blood glucose control. Increased fructosamine concentrations indicate increased blood glucose for the last one to two weeks. Hypoalbuminemia can falsely decrease fructosamine since albumin frequently binds to fructosamine. Reference values for fructosamine in guinea pigs and viscachas have been determined (Table 8.3).

Lipids

Lipids commonly evaluated include cholesterol and triglycerides. In the guinea pig, the intestine, not the liver, is the primary site of cholesterol synthesis [16]. Cholesterol concentrations in degus were lower in adults than juveniles, whereas in guinea pigs, total cholesterol in males increases with age [21, 24]. Hypercholesterolemia is common in guinea pigs and associated with fatty infiltration of many tissues including the liver [16, 17]. In hystricomorph rodents, cholesterol may increase with extrahepatic biliary obstruction. Triglycerides are the major storage form of fat in these species and are synthesized by intestines, adipose tissue, the liver, and the mammary gland. Triglyceride concentrations in guinea pigs increase slowly with age [24].

Electrolytes (Table 8.3)

Hystricomorph electrolyte concentrations can be interpreted as done for dogs and cats. Sodium [Na] concentrations in female guinea pigs increase with age, whereas chloride (Cl) concentrations in males decrease with age [24]. Hairless guinea pigs exhibit increased potassium and decreased sodium concentrations compared to haired guinea pigs [25]. Sodium and chloride concentrations of the pregnant guinea pig in the last half of gestation were Na [145 ± 4] and Cl [92 ± 2] in plasma and Na [134 ± 8] and Cl [140 ± 15] in amniotic fluid (all values given as mEq/l ± SD), respectively [3]. Adult degu exhibit decreased potassium concentrations compared to juveniles, and hyperkalemia (potassium 4.4 mmol/l) occurred in a single case of renal transitional cell carcinoma and choristoma in a degu [21, 27].

Blood Proteins (Table 8.3)

Total protein is a combination of albumin, globulins, and other proteins. Total protein is often estimated using a refractometer. Causes of falsely increased total protein on a refractometer include lipemia, hemolysis, hyperbilirubinemia, and increased concentrations of sodium, glucose, and chloride. Total protein concentration measured with spectrophotometric methods via chemistry analyzers is more accurate. Albumin, a carrier protein synthesized by the liver, provides most of the blood's oncotic pressure. Major causes of hyperalbuminemia are dehydration and laboratory error. Causes of hypoalbuminemia include decreased production (hepatic insufficiency, inadequate protein intake, maldigestion/malabsorption), loss (protein-losing enteropathy, protein-losing nephropathy, blood loss, cutaneous), or sequestration (vasculopathy, effusion). Low albumin concentrations (≤2.0 g dL) may be associated with body fluid shifts leading to effusion. Total protein and serum concentrations of albumin were higher in hairless guinea pigs compared to haired guinea pigs [25]. In chinchillas that experience seasonal temperature fluctuations, plasma albumin concentrations were seasonal: higher in the summer and autumn and lower in the spring and winter [39]. Hyperproteinemia (3.2 g dL) and hypoalbuminemia (1.8 g dL) were documented in a single case of renal transitional cell carcinoma and choristoma in a degu [27].

Globulins are a group of proteins that vary in size and function. Alpha globulins are produced in the liver, beta globulins are produced in the liver and lymphoid tissue and include fibrinogen, and gamma globulins are composed of immunoglobulins produced in the lymphoid tissues. Globulin concentration is not typically directly measured in biochemical profiles but is calculated by subtracting the albumin from the total protein. Hypoglobulinemia can be caused by blood loss, failure of passive transfer in neonates, immune deficiency, protein-losing enteropathy, cutaneous loss, and effusion. Hyperglobulinemia can result from dehydration (concurrent hyperalbuminemia is common), immune-mediated disease, infection (bacterial, viral, fungal, parasitic), or neoplasia. The significance of hyperglobulinemia depends on the globulin type that is increased. Total protein and globulin concentrations of adult degus are higher than in juveniles [25]. In chinchillas, the alpha-1 and gamma globulin concentrations increase in the spring, while beta-1 globulin concentrations decrease in winter and increase in summer. In female chinchillas, the alpha-2 and beta-2 globulin concentrations are higher in the winter and summer [39].

Blood Gases

Blood gas analysis is not commonly performed in hystricomorph rodents but is indicated for evaluation of gas exchange and alterations in total carbon dioxide concentration in animals with respiratory disorders. Sampling artifacts are common. In guinea pigs, blood pH values are closely controlled by the body, and good agreement of pH values exists across multiple studies. Danger values for blood pH are <7 or >7.7; these fluctuations may

Table 8.4 Blood gas parameters in guinea pigs (*Cavia porcellus*) [40].

Analyte	Units, SI (conventional)	Short Hair English	Dunkin-Hartley
Bicarbonate (HCO3)	mEq/l (mmol/l)	24.66 ± 1.01 (24.66 + 1.01)	27.22 ± 0.76 (27.22 + 0.76)
Carbon dioxide partial pressure (PCO2)	mm Hg (mm Hg)	34.25 ± 1.11	38.3 ± 0.6
Carbon dioxide total (tCO2)	mEq/l (mmol/l)	25.73 ± 1.03 (25.73 ± 1.03)	28.39 ± 0.77 (28.39 ± 0.77)
Lactate	mmol/l (mg/dl)	0.295 ± 0.028 (2.66 ± 0.25)	0.21 ± 0.047 (1.86 ± 0.42)
Oxygen partial pressure (PO2)	mm Hg (mm Hg)	47.75 ± 4.34	37.8 ± 2.23
Oxygen saturation (sO2)	% (%)	74.85 ± 5.49	71.3 ± 3.31
pH	pH units (pH units)	7.46 ± 0.01	7.45 ± 0.01

Data shown as mean ± one standard deviation for 20 animals [40].

cause death in guinea pigs [40]. Other blood gas analyte values reported vary, likely reflecting differing anesthesia protocols, blood collection techniques, and time from sample collection to analysis. Reference intervals for blood gases exist only for guinea pigs (Table 8.4), not for other hystricomorph rodents.

Vitamins, Minerals and Metals, Toxins

Hairless guinea pigs have higher inorganic phosphorus, calcium, and magnesium compared to haired guinea pigs [25]. In degus, the total calcium and inorganic phosphorus are lower in adults than in juveniles [21]. In wild viscachas, reference ranges for 17 trace elements were determined including aluminum (Al), arsenic (As), boron (B), beryllium (Be), cadmium (Cd), cobalt (Co), copper (Cu), iron (Fe), lead (Pb), lithium (Li), manganese (Mn), molybdenum (Mo), nickel (Ni), rubidium (Rb), selenium (Se), strontium (Sr), and zinc (Zn). Clinically significant elements for disease diagnosis include copper (511± 76 μg/l), iron (4327 ± 1344 μg/l), lead (0.67± 0.23 μg/l), selenium (179 ± 68 μg/l), and zinc (1387 ± 201 μg/l). When these reference ranges were compared to trace element values determined in a group of captive viscachas, captive viscachas had higher Cd, Co, Cu, Ni, Pb, Rb, Se, and Zn but lower Al, As, Li, Mo, and Sr than wild viscachas. Differences were postulated to result from dietary and environmental factors [41]. Hypocalcemia and hyperphosphatemia have been documented in a single case of renal transitional cell carcinoma and choristoma in a degu which also suffered concurrent hypoalbuminemia [27].

Lead toxicosis has been reported in chinchillas with clinical signs of seizures and blindness [42, 43]. Blood lead concentrations of 15 μg/dl are suspicious for lead toxicity, and concentrations of 25 μg/dl are definitive [44]. While no reports of lead toxicity in the other hystricomorph rodents are extant, these rodents are also likely susceptible to lead toxicity.

Hormones

Thyroid Hormones

Hyperthyroidism is commonly reported in the guinea pig and has also been reported in the chinchilla. Hypothyroidism is uncommonly reported in guinea pigs. Thyroxine (T4) and triiodothyronine (T3) determinations appear unreliable for disease diagnosis and monitoring in guinea pigs, as patients with severe clinical signs of hyperthyroidism may not have increased T3 or T4 concentrations [45]. Reference intervals for T3 and T4 concentrations in a few guinea pigs were free T4 1.26–2.03 ng/dl (16.22–26.13 nmol/l), total T3 39–44 ng/dl (0.60–0.68 nmol/l), and free T3 0.221–0.260 ng/dl (0.0034–0.004 nmol/l) [46]. Thyroxine concentrations appear more useful for diagnosing thyroid disease in guinea pigs. Serum thyroxine concentrations in healthy guinea pigs range from 14.2 to 66.9 mmol/dl (1.1–5.2 mg/dl) [47]. Thyroxine concentrations can be determined and a thyroid stimulating hormone (TSH) stimulation test can be done by injecting 100 μg of thyrogen, a recombinant human TSH (rhTSH), intramuscularly and measuring T4 concentrations before and 4 h injection. An expected result from a healthy guinea pig would be an increase in T4 to at least 1.5 times the prestimulation value by 4 h [45]. Hyperthyroidism has been documented in a chinchilla based on T4 values (T4 reference range 34–64 μg/l) [48, 49].

Adrenal Hormones

Cushing's disease is reported infrequently in the guinea pig, with diagnosis mainly based on clinical signs and response to therapy [50, 51]. In one case, salivary cortisol concentrations increased, and a marked response to adrenocorticotropic hormone (ACTH) administration occurred [51]. The primary glucocorticoid in guinea pig plasma is cortisol (reference interval 5–30 μg/dl (137.95–827.7 nmol/l)). Salivary and plasma cortisol have been investigated in guinea pigs. The concentration of plasma cortisol of guinea pigs is highest late in the dark and light periods, and lowest in the mid-dark period and early light period [12]. Post ACTH injection, plasma cortisol concentrations are higher than salivary cortisol concentrations; however, a marked response to ACTH administration in concentrations of both salivary and plasma cortisol occurs. Thus, salivary cortisol can be used to monitor cortisol in guinea pigs with suspected Cushing's disease [52]. Four hours post injection with 20 IU ACTH, mean basal saliva cortisol concentrations in guinea pigs are 6.6 ± 3.4 ng/ml and 157 ± 53 ng/ml [52, 53]. Plasma cortisol concentrations increase in guinea pigs caged singly or subjected to restraint [53].

Reproductive Hormones

Both progesterone and plasma estrogen have been studied in the guinea pig [3]. Progesterone concentrations peak in the guinea pig post ovulation at 2.8 ± 0.33 ng/ml. In the pregnant guinea pig, progesterone concentrations increase beginning 15 days post coitus and peak at 329 ± 14 ng/ml at day 30–45 of pregnancy. Progesterone concentration then drops below 200 ng/ml at day 45–60 of pregnancy, with another increase just before parturition. Plasma estrogen is detectable starting at about 20 days of pregnancy. At days 31–35, concentrations reach 12.8 ± 1.95 pg/ml, and concentrations peak at days 56–60 at 31.05 ± 5.21 pg/ml. Estrogen concentrations fall below 5 pg/ml within 2 d post parturition. Although hystricomorph rodents do develop reproductive disease, a reproductive hormone panel is not available commercially for these species.

Urinalysis

Urinalysis values have been described for viscachas, chinchillas, and guinea pigs, but not for degus (Table 8.5) [7, 22]. In guinea pigs and chinchillas, urine is often yellow to amber in color but can be orange or a darker color depending on the diet. Porphyrins (red pigments) in the urine can be mistaken for hematuria; thus, urine samples

Table 8.5 Urinalysis data for hystricomorph rodents [8, 29, 54].

Quantitative values	Guinea pig (*Cavia porcellus*) [54]	Chinchilla (*Chinchilla laniger*)	Viscacha (*Lagostomus maximus*) [22]
Sample size	50		44
Data format	Range		Range
Specific gravity	1.005–1.050	>1.045	1.012–1.060
Semiquantitative values			
Protein multistix	Trace to 2000 mg/dl	Negative to trace	Moderate (30–100 mg/dl)
Glucose	Negative	Negative	Negative
Ketones	Negative	Negative	Negative
Bilirubin	Negative	Negative	Negative
Urobilinogen	Negative	0.1–1 ng/dl	Negative
Occult blood	Negative to trace	Negative	Positive if obtained via cystocentesis
pH	8–9	8–9	7–9
Appearance	Cloudy to clear, yellow to orange/tan	Cloudy to clear, yellow to orange/tan	
Microscopic analysis			
Red blood cells	0–3/hpf	Absent	
White blood cells	0–4/hpf	Absent	
Epithelial cells	0–5/hpf	Common	
Casts	0–2/hpf	Rare	
Crystals	Many calcium carbonate, moderate phosphate, rare calcium oxalate		
Miscellaneous	Occasional renal tubular epithelial cells	Occasional squamous epithelial cells	
Bacteria	Moderate number – mostly cocci	Minimal to absent	

Table 8.6 Laboratories providing serological and PCR diagnostic tests for guinea pigs.

Lab	Address	Phone/website
Taconic	One Discovery Drive, Rensselaer, NY 12144 USA	888.TACONIC(822-6642) www.taconic.com Fax: 518-697-3910
Molecular Diagnostic Services	4204 Sorrento Valley Blvd., Suite G San Diego, CA 92121, USA	(858) 450-9990 rrda@mds-usa.com www.mds-usa.com/guineapigssero.html
Charles River	Charles River RADS, Serology Laboratory 261 Ballardvale Street, Building 22 Loading Dock Wilmington, MA 01887 USA	1-877-274-8371 www.criver.com askcharlesriver@crl.com

should immediately be examined for the presence of RBC. Urinary pH is dietary related. As hystricomorph rodents are herbivores, they tend to have alkaline urine (pH 8–9) because of the bacterial conversion of urea to ammonia. Causes of acidic urine in rodents include catabolic conditions such as starvation, fever, or ketosis [12]. Crystals in guinea pig urine are common. In one study, large numbers of calcium carbonate crystals were found in all guinea pig urine samples, large numbers of phosphate crystals were common, and calcium oxalate crystals were rare and few [54]. Crystals in the urine of other hystricomorph rodents was considered abnormal with interpretation based on that in other domestic animals [7]. However, a recent study of normal chinchilla urine found that 68% of the urine samples contained crystals, most of which were amorphous crystals, although calcium carbonate and calcium phosphate crystals were also seen in rare cases [55]. Protein, glucose, or other metabolites not usually found in urine can cause refractometer error in the determination of specific gravity. In chinchillas, urine protein concentration should be determined by quantitative protein analysis as dipstick analysis and the sulfosalicylic acid precipitation test can be inaccurate in this species [55]. Urine sediment from the healthy rodents should contain fewer than five leukocytes and erythrocytes per high power field. Increased numbers of these cells suggests neoplasia, urinary tract infection/inflammation, or urinary calculi. Urinary casts also suggest renal disease and are interpreted as for domestic animals. Uroliths occur in guinea pigs and chinchillas. In guinea pigs, most urinary calculi are composed of 100% calcium carbonate, while combinations of calcium carbonate and struvite, apatite, and calcium oxalate dehydrate are less common [56]. In chinchillas, most urinary calculi are composed of calcium carbonate [57]. When possible, uroliths should be submitted to the Minnesota Urolith Center Quantitative Urolith Analysis for further testing (www.cvm.umn.edu/depts/MinnesotaUrolithCenter). Values of urinalysis for degus with renal disease have been limited to hematuria, pyuria, occasional squamous and transitional epithelial cells, and a urine specific gravity of 1.016 [27, 28].

Serology and PCR

A variety of serologic and PCR tests, developed for use in laboratory guinea pigs, are available for use in pet guinea pigs, but have not been validated for use in other hystricomorph species [34]. Common serological assays available for guinea pigs include tests for viral (guinea pig adenovirus, guinea pig cytomegalovirus virus, lymphocytic choriomeningitis virus, parainfluenza virus 3, pneumonia virus of mice, reovirus, respiratory enteric virus, Sendai virus, and Simian virus 5) and bacterial (Encephalitozoon cuniculi, Tyzzer's disease (*Clostridium piliforme*), *Mycoplasma pulmonis*) diseases (Table 8.6).

A PCR test for lung tissue is available for guinea pig adenovirus, and a PCR for nasal swabs or transtracheal washes is available for *Bordetella bronchiseptica* testing. An ELISA for *Streptococcus pneumoniae* is described but is not commercially available [58]. For each test, be sure to contact the providing laboratory for appropriate shipment, labeling, handling, and submission form instructions.

References

1 Weir, B.J. (1970). The management and breeding of some more Hystricomorph rodents. *Laboratory Animals* 4: 83–97.

2 Ancill, R.J. (1956). The blood volume of the normal Guinea pig. *Journal of Physiology* 132: 469–475.

3 Sisk, D.B. (1976). Physiology. In: *The Biology of the Guinea Pig* (ed. J.E. Wagner and P.J. Manning), 63–92. New York: Academic Press.

4 Constable, B.J. (1963). Changes in blood volume and blood picture during the life of the rat and Guinea-pig

from birth to maturity. *Journal of Physiology* 167: 229–238.
5 Joslin, J.O. (2009). Blood collection techniques in exotic small mammals. *Journal of Exotic Pet Medicine* 18 (2): 117–139.
6 SjØberg, J.G. and Odberg, E. (2003). One perspective on selected blood collection sites in exotic species. *Exotic DVM* 5 (2): 19–23.
7 Ness, R.D. (1999 Sep.). Clinical pathology and sample collection of exotic small mammals. *Veterinary Clinics of North America: Exotic Animal Practice* 2 (3): 591–620.
8 Tappa, B., Amao, H., and Takahashi, K.W. (1989). A simple method for intravenous injection and blood collection in the chinchilla (*Chinchilla laniger*). *Laboratory Animals* 23: 73–75.
9 McClure, D.E. (1999). Clinical pathology and sample collection in the laboratory rodent. *Veterinary Clinics of North America: Exotic Animal Practice* 2 (3): 565–590.
10 Brown, C. (2011). Urethral catheterization in the female Guinea pig (*Cavia* porcellus). *Lab Animal* 40: 42–43.
11 Mans, C. (2007). Urethral catheterization of the male Guinea pig (*Cavia porcellus*). *Lab Animal* 36: 20–21.
12 Campbell, T. (2006). Clinical chemistry of mammals: laboratory animals and miscellaneous species. In: *Veterinary Hematology and Clinical Chemistry* (ed. M.A. Thrall, G. Weiser, R. Allison and T. Campbell), 464–468. Ames: Wiley.
13 Davis, H., Riel, D.L., Pappagianis, M., and Miguel, K. (2010). Diagnostic sampling and therapeutic techniques. In: *Clinical Textbook for Veterinary Technicians*, 7e (ed. J.M. Bassert and D.M. McCurnin), 603–606. St Louis: Saunders Elsevier.
14 Tully, T.N. and Mitchell, M.A. (2001). *A Technicians Guide to Exotic Animal Care*. Lakewood, CO: American Animal Hospital Association Press.
15 Strike, T.A. (1970). Hemogram and bone marrow differential of the chinchilla. *Laboratory Animal Care* 20: 33–38.
16 Campbell, T.W. and Ellis, C.K. (2007). Hematology of small mammals. In: *Avian and Exotic Animal Hematology and Cytology*, 3e (ed. T.W. Campbell and C.K. Ellis), 119–131. Ames: Blackwell Publishing.
17 White, E.J. and Lang, C.M. (1989). The Guinea pig. In: *The Clinical Chemistry of Laboratory Animals* (ed. W.F. Loeb and F.W. Quimby), 27–30. St. Louis: CV Mosby.
18 Harkness, J.E., Turner, P.V., VandeWoude, S., and Wheler, C.L. (2010). *Harkness and Wagner's Biology and Medicine of Rabbits and Rodents*, 5e. Ames: Wiley-Blackwell.
19 Hein, J. and Hartmann, K. (2003). Reference ranges for laboratory parameters in Guinea pigs. *Tierarztiche Praxis Ausgabe K Kleintiere Heimtiere.* 31 (6): 383–389.
20 Silva T de, O., Dreutz, L.C., Barcellos, L.J.G. et al. (2005). Reference values for chinchilla (*Chinchilla laniger*) blood cells and serum biochemical parameters. Ciência rural. *Santa Maria* 35 (3): 602–606.
21 Jekl, V., Hauptman, K., Jeklova, E., and Knotek, Z. (2011). Selected haematological and plasma chemistry parameters in juvenile and adult degus (*Octodon degus*). *Veterinary Record* 169: 71.
22 Wenker, C.J., Hunziker, D., Lopez, J. et al. (2007). Haematology, blood chemistry and urine parameters of free Ranging Plains Viscachas (*Lagostomus maximus*) in Argentina determined by use of a portable blood Analyser (i-STAT®) and conventional laboratory methods. *Journal of Veterinary Medicine* 54: 260–264.
23 Moore, D.M. (2004). Hematology of Guinea pigs. In: *Schalm's Veterinary Hematology* (ed. B. Feldman, J. Zinkl and N. Jain). Philadelphia: Lippincott Williams and Wilkins.
24 Kitagaki, M., Yamaguchi, M., Nakamura, M. et al. (2005). Age-related changes in haematology and serum chemistry of Weiser-maples Guinea pigs (*Cavia porcellus*). *Laboratory Animals* 39: 321–330.
25 Waner, T., Avidar, Y., Peh, H.-C. et al. (1996). Haematology and clinical chemistry values of normal and euthymic hairless adult male Dunkin-Hartley Guinea pigs (*Cavia porcellus*). *Veterinary Clinical Pathology* 25 (2): 61–64.
26 Jakubow, K., Glromadzka-Ostrowska, J., and Zalewska, B. (1984). Seasonal changes in the haematological indices in peripheral blood of chinchilla (*Chinchilla laniger*). *Comparative Biochemistry and Physiology* 78A: 845–853.
27 Lester, P.A., Rush, H.G., and Sigler, R.E. (2005). Renal Transitional Cell Carcinoma and Choristoma in a Degu (*Octodon degus*). *American Association for Laboratory Animal Science* 44 (3) May): 41–44.
28 Cadillacc, J.M., Rush, H.G., and Sigler, R.E. (2003). Polycystic and chronic kidney disease in a young Degu (Octodon degus). *American Association for Laboratory Animal Science* 42 (2): 43–45.
29 Rothwell, T.L.W., Pope, S.E., Rajczyk, Z.K., and Collins, G.H. (1991). Haematological and pathological responses to experimental *Trixacarus caviae* infection in Guinea pigs. *Journal of Comparative Pathology* 104: 179–185.
30 Revell, P.A., Vernon-Robets, B., and Gray, A. (1971). The distribution and ultrastructure of the Kurloff cell in the Guinea-pig. *Journal of Anatomy* 109 (2): 187–199.
31 Otalora, B.B., Vivanco, P., Madariaga, A.M. et al. (2010). Internal temporal order in the circadian system of a dual-phasing rodent, the *Octodon degus. Chronobiology International* 27 (8): 1564–1579.
32 Brown, S.J. and Askenase, P.W. (1982). Blood eosinophil and basophil responses in Guinea pigs parasitized by *Amblyomma americanum* ticks. *The American Journal of Tropical Medicine and Hygiene* 31: 593–598.

33 Szabo, M.P., Aoki, V.L., Sanches, F.P. et al. (2003). Antibody and blood leukocyte response in *Rhipicephalus sanguineus* tick-infested dogs and Guinea pigs. *Veterinary Parasitology* 115: 49–59.

34 Wicher, V., Scarozza, A.M., Ramsingh, A.I., and Wicher, K. (1998). Cytokine gene expression in skin of susceptible Guinea-pig infected with *Treponema pallidum*. *Immunology* 95: 242–247.

35 Lewis, J.H. (1992). Comparative hematology: studies on Guinea-pigs (*Cavia* porcellus). *Comparative Biochemistry and Physiology* 102A (3): 507–512.

36 Leitao, D.P.S., Polizello, A.C.M., and Rothschild, Z. (2000). Coagulation and fibrinolysis in capybara (*Hydrochaeris hydrochaeris*), a close relative of the Guinea pig (*Cavia porcellus*). *Comparative Biochemistry and Physiology. Part A, Molecular & Integrative Physiology* 125: 113–120.

37 Kaspareit, J., Messow, C., and Edel, J. (1988). Blood coagulation studies in guinea pigs (*Cavia porcellus*). *Laboratory Animals* 22: 206–211.

38 Coagulation Sampling Guidelines for Venipuncturists. Web. Accessed 11 Aug 2012. http://www.asvcp.org/pubs/pdf/CoagSampGuide.pdf

39 Gromadzka-Ostrowska, J. and Zalewska, B. (1985). Seasonal fluctuations of plasma protein concentrations in chinchillas (*Chinchilla langier,* M.). *Comparative Biochemistry and Physiology Part A: Physiology* 80 (2): 215–224.

40 Sanchez-Aparicio, P., Mota-Rojas, D., Verduzco-Mendoza, A. et al. (2009). Reference values for blood gas analysis, electrolytes, and critical biochemical variables for short-hair English and Duncan-Hartley Guinea pigs anesthetized with Xylazine-ketamine. *Journal of Animal and Veterinary Advances* 8 (10): 1893–1899.

41 Forrer, R., Wenker, C.H., Gautschi, K., and Lutz, H. (2001). Concentration of 17 trace elements in serum and whole blood of plains Viscachas (*Lagostomus maxiumus*) by ICP-MS, their reference ranges, and their relation to cataract. *Biological Trace Element Research* 81: 47–62.

42 Hoefer, H.L. (1994). Chinchillas. *Veterinary Clinics of Normal America Small Animal Practice* 24 (1): 113–120.

43 Morgan, R.V., Moore, F.M., Pearce, L.K., and Rossi, T. (1991). Clinical and laboratory findings in small companion animals with lead poisoning: 347 cases (1977-1986). *Journal of the American Veterinary Medical Association* 199: 93–97.

44 Donnelly, T.M. (2003). Disease problems of chinchillas. In: *Ferrets, Rabbits and Rodents: Clinical Medicine and Surgery*, 2e (ed. K.E. Quesenberry and J.W. Carpenter), 259. St. Louis: WB Saunders.

45 Mayer, J., Wagner, R., and Taeymans, O. (2010). Advanced diagnostic approaches and current Management of Thyroid Pathologies in Guinea pigs. *Veterinary Clinics of North American Exotic Animals* 13: 509–523.

46 Castro, M.I., Alex, S., Young, R.A. et al. (1986). Total and free serum thyroid hormone concentrations in fetal and adult pregnant and nonpregnant Guinea pigs. *Endocrinology* 118 (2): 533–537.

47 Müller, K., Müller, E., Klein, R., and Brunnberg, L. (2009). Serum thyroxine concentrations in clinically healthy pet Guinea pigs (*Cavia porcellus*). *Veterinary Clinical Pathology* 38: 507–510.

48 Fritsche, R., Simova-Curd, S., Clauss, M., and Hatt, J.-M. (2008). Hyperthyroidism in connection with suspected diabetes mellitus in a chinchilla (*Chinchilla laniger*). *Veterinary Record* 163: 454–456.

49 Martin, L.B., Chidambaram, R.M., Schroeder, K.E., and Mcfadden, S.L. (2005). Thyroparathyroidectomy procedures and thyroxine concentrations in the chinchilla. *Contemporary Topics in Laboratory Animal Science* 44: 31–36.

50 Gashen, L., Ketz, C., Lang, J. et al. (1998). Ultrasonographic detection of adrenal gland tumor and ureterolithiasis in a Guinea pig. *Veterinary Radiology and Ultrasound* 39 (1): 43–46.

51 Zeugswetter, F., Fenske, M., Hasan, J., and Kunzel, F. (2007). Cushing's syndrome in a Guinea pig. *Veterinary Record* 160: 878–880.

52 Fenske, M. (1996). Saliva cortisol and testosterone in the Guinea pig: measures for the endocrine function of adrenals and testes? *Steroids* 61 (11): 647–650.

53 Fenske, M. (1997). The use of salivary cortisol measurements for the noninvasive assessment of adrenal cortical functions in Guinea pigs. *Experimental and Clinical Endocrinology & diabetes* 105 (3): 163–168.

54 Bishop CR, Fischer J, Brossoit A, and Pierson C. 2010. Standardization of Renal Physiology Parameters in Guinea Pigs via Urinalysis. In Proceedings Association of Avian Veterinarians pp. 49–52.

55 Doss, G.A., Mans, C., Houseright, R.A., and Webb, J.L. (2016). Urinalysis in chinchillas (*Chinchilla lanigera*). *Journal of the American Veterinary Medical Association* 248 (8): 901–907.

56 Hawkins, M.G., Ruby, A., Drazenovich, T.L., and Westropp, J. (2009). Composition and characteristics of urinary calculi from Guinea pigs. *Journal of the American Veterinary Medical Association* 234 (2): 214–220.

57 Osborne, C.A., Albasan, H., Lulich, J.P. et al. (2009). Quantitative analysis of 4468 Uroliths retrieved from farm animals, exotic species, and wildlife submitted to the Minnesota Urolith center: 1981 to 2007. *Veterinary Clinics of North America: Small Animal Practice* 39 (1): 65–78.

58 Matsubara, J., Kamiyama, T., Miyoshi, H. et al. (1988). Serodiagnosis of *Streptococcus pneumoniae* infection in Guinea pigs by an enzyme-linked immunosorbent assay. *Laboratory Animals* 37 (2): 304–308.

9

Capybaras (*Hydrochoerus hydrochaeris*)

Jessica Hokamp DVM, PhD, DACVP (Clinical Pathology)[1,2], *Rosely Gioia-Di Chiacchio PhD*[3] *and Eliana Reiko Matushima FMVZ, USP*[4]

[1] *College of Veterinary Medicine & Biomedical Sciences, Texas A&M University, College Station, Texas, USA*
[2] *Clinical Department of Veterinary Biosciences, International Veterinary Renal Pathology Service, The Ohio State University, Columbus, Ohio, USA*
[3] *Department of Animal Pathology, Universidade Paulista, São Paulo, Brazil*
[4] *Pathology Department, São Paulo University, São Paulo, Brazil*

Introduction

The capybara, *Hydrochoerus hydrochaeris* (Linnaeus, 1766 – Rodentia: Caviidae), is the world's largest living rodent [1, 2]. It is in the order *Rodentia* and suborder *Hystricomorpha*, which also includes Brazilian porcupines (*Coendou prehensilis*), Brazilian guinea pigs (*Cavia aperea*), guinea pigs (*Cavia porcellus*), chinchillas (*Chinchilla* spp.), lowland pacas (*Agouti paca*), and agoutis (*Dasyprocta azarae*) [1]. Capybaras are native to South America, occurring from the Atlantic coast of South America to east of the Andes [3]. With the exception of the northeastern region of Brazil, the species is broadly distributed, particularly in the Pantanal biome [4], and occurs in a variety of environments ranging from areas of riparian vegetation to open fields, especially in areas that flood during rainy periods [Figure 9.1] [5]. The body mass of adult individuals ranges from 35 to 65 kg, with a mean body length of 1–1.3 m and a body height of 0.5 m [1, 6]. The tail is vestigial, the limbs are short, and the digits are united by membranes, with four digits in the forelimbs and three digits in the hind limbs. The hair is thick, measuring 30–120 mm in length, and ranges from dark brown or reddish to bright brown or yellowish gray [1, 6]. Adult males mark their territories with sebaceous secretions produced by the morillo, an ellipsoid, androgen-dependent gland that develops during puberty and is located on the snout [7]. There is a strong correlation between the volume of this gland and daily spermatic production, testosterone levels, and the mass of the testes [7, 8]. The volume of the morillo is calculated with the equation $(1/2) \times (4/3)\pi \times ABC$, where A is half the length of the gland, B is half of the width of the gland, and C is the nasal gland thickness [8]. Furthermore, the size of the morillo may be used to ascertain the hierarchical position of dominant males. This gland, although less developed, is also present in females [4].

Capybaras are herbivores, feeding on grass, aquatic plants, and readily adapt to other food items such as corn, sugarcane, and pumpkins [5]. Taxonomically, capybaras are related to guinea pigs (*C. porcellus*) and share many aspects of their physiology. As occurs in guinea pigs, coprophagy is normal in capybaras and allows the ingestion and absorption of nutrients produced in the cecum (particularly vitamins B and K) [1]. Guinea pigs and capybaras require dietary sources of vitamin C (ascorbic acid), and low dietary vitamin C levels may adversely affect reproduction in captivity [9, 10].

Capybaras are often considered a concern for public health. They are associated with the transmission of Rocky Mountain spotted fever, caused by *Rickettsia rickettsii* bacteria, which is transmitted through cayenne ticks (*Amblyomma cajennense*) [11, 12]. Other potentially zoonotic diseases may occur in capybaras, including leptospirosis, leishmaniasis, bovine tuberculosis, rabies, Chagas disease, Enterobacteriaceae infection, and other fungal, parasitic, bacterial, and viral diseases [13–15]. Because capybaras live within increasing proximity to humans, it is important to evaluate their health, both in the wild and in captivity, particularly in some South American countries where they may be used as protein sources [1]. Understanding hematological and biochemical data will, therefore, be important for the clinical diagnosis and health evaluation of this species. However, clinical pathology data for this species is limited as few complete studies on the species have been performed. Compared to many domestic species, capybaras are difficult to restrain and sample, which further decreases opportunities for sample collection and data evaluation. Limited information is currently available for this species.

Exotic Animal Laboratory Diagnosis, First Edition. Edited by J. Jill Heatley and Karen E. Russell.

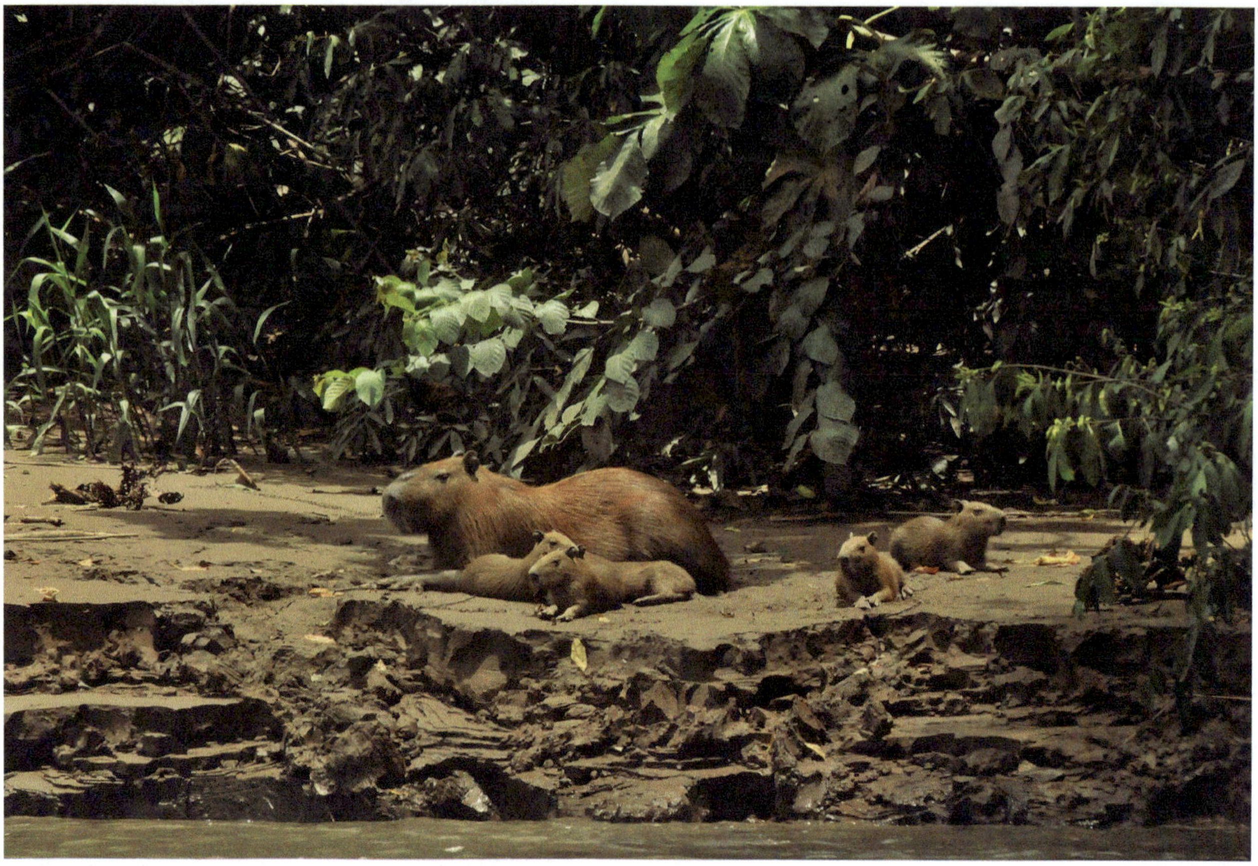

Figure 9.1 Free-living capybara.

Chemical Restraint

Capybaras may react aggressively to attempts to be captured and chemically restrained. Although restraint is generally recognized as one of the most limiting factors for the husbandry and medical care of wild animals, literature on anesthetic procedures involving wild South American rodents is scarce [1]. Chemical restraint or anesthesia is necessary to collect biological samples or to perform surgical procedures in wild animals such as capybaras [16]. Although many drugs can be used to produce chemical restraint in capybaras, the capture of free ranging capybaras frequently imposes the need for remote drug administration, which in turn requires anesthetic agents that are rapidly and completely absorbed following intramuscular injection. Ketamine is the anesthetic agent most frequently used for wild animals because of its broad margin of safety and its flexibility to be administered intramuscularly or subcutaneously. It produces unconsciousness and mild somatic analgesia and may cause muscular hypertonia, drooling, respiratory depression, and prolonged recovery [17]. To alleviate these effects, ketamine should be combined with myorelaxant and analgesic drugs. Alpha-2 adrenergic agonists produce sedation, analgesia, and muscle relaxation [18]. Xylazine, which is often combined with ketamine, has a broad margin of safety, and increases in dosage do not deepen sedation but provide more prolonged effects [19]. Midazolam, a benzodiazepine, is also commonly combined with ketamine and provides sedative, hypnotic, anticonvulsant, amnesic, and myorelaxant effects with minimal cardiorespiratory interference [20]. Several published anesthetic protocols are available (Table 9.1). For exact dosages and methods of anesthesia, refer to the *Handbook of Wildlife Chemical Immobilization* [24].

Venipuncture and Sample Handling

As with all hystricomorphs, capybaras lack readily accessible superficial veins, so intravascular injections, venipuncture, and other sample collection is challenging. Recommended blood collection sites include the femoral, cephalic, saphenous, or jugular veins [1] (Figure 9.2). For a complete blood count (CBC), blood should be collected in tubes containing an anticoagulant such as EDTA or heparin, while blood obtained for

Table 9.1 Drug protocols for restraint of capybaras *(Hydrochoerus hydrochaeris)* [1, 21–23].

Drug/dosage	Comments
Step one: Ketamine 5 mg/kg IM Xylazine 0.5 mg/kg IM *Step two:* Ketamine 3 mg/kg IM Midazolam 0.7 mg/kg IM	Initial sedation step is performed via remote anesthesia procedures (such as with a blow dart) without knowledge of patient's exact weight. Second step is performed after weighing patient to allow for more accurate dosing.
Ketamine 14–16 mg/kg Acetylpromazine 0.14–0.16 mg /kg IM	
Tiletamine HCl 0.8 mg/kg IM Zolazepam HCl 0.8 mg/kg IM Medetomidine HCl 0.008 mg/kg IM	Atipamazole is used for reversal of medetomidine.
Tiletamine HCl 2.3 mg/kg IM Zolazepam HCl 2.3 mg/kg IM	

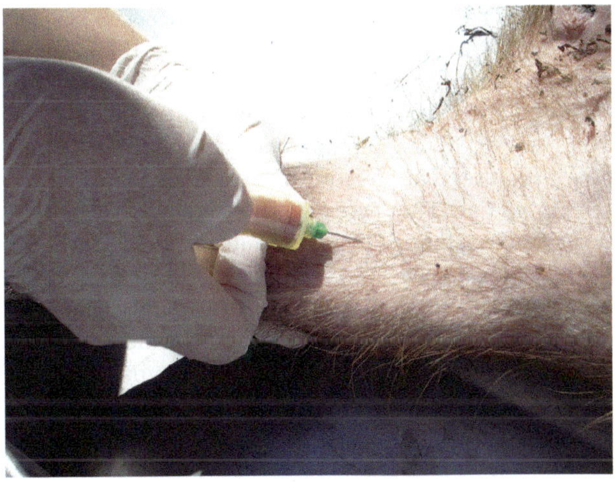

Figure 9.2 Venipuncture from the medial saphenous vein of a capybara.

serum biochemical analysis should be collected in a tube containing heparin or no anticoagulant [25]. Blood smears should be prepared directly from collected blood with no added anticoagulant for better evaluation of erythrocyte and leukocyte morphology, which can be altered by prolonged storage in an anticoagulant. Blood smears should be dried and stored at room temperature (not refrigeration as this can cause condensation and water artifact on smears). For evaluation of blood smears, slides should be stained using Wright stain or Wright-Giemsa modified stains such as quick stains (i.e., Diff-Quik [26]). Blood should be analyzed as soon as possible. If blood cannot be analyzed within 30 min, blood tubes for CBC and biochemistry should be stored in refrigeration until they can be evaluated.

Complete Blood Count (CBC)

Evaluation of a CBC is an essential part of a diagnostic evaluation as it helps to determine the presence or lack of anemia, regeneration, and indications of inflammation. Reference intervals for capybaras are in Table 9.2.

Erythrocytes

Erythrocytes of capybaras are anucleate, round, and biconcave. There is little specific published information regarding normal or abnormal erythrocyte parameters and morphology in capybaras, except that their erythrocytes have a greater mean corpuscular volume (MCV) than many domestic species (Figure 9.3 and Table 9.2). Furthermore, a "sickle" form of intracellular crystallization of hemoglobin has been reported to occur as a normal finding in capybaras [29]. Given their similarities with other hystricomorphs, capybaras may have similar erythrocyte parameters and morphologies. Evaluation of the erythron is often done to determine the presence of and characterize an anemia, a reduction in the total mass of hemoglobin-bearing erythrocytes. Anemias are classified as regenerative or non-regenerative. Regenerative anemias are caused by blood loss or hemolysis, while non-regenerative anemias are generally

Table 9.2 Hematological values for capybaras *(Hydrochoerus hydrochaeris)* [27, 28].

Analyte	27	28
PCV (%)	35.5 (33–37)	40.4 ± 2
Hgb (g/dl)	10.6 (10.2–11.1)	13.5 ± 0.7
RBC (× 10^6/μl)	3.15 (3.1–3.2)	4.5 ± 0.2
MCV (um^3; fl)	113.5 (102–125)	90.2 ± 0.9
MCH (pg)	33.8 (31.6–36.0)	30.1 ± 0.7
MCHC (%)	30.5 (30–31)	33.3 ± 1
WBC (× 10^3/μl)	7.0 (6.1–7.9)	5.3 ± 2
Segmented neutrophils/heterophils (%)	62 (55–69)	36.6 ± 19.9
Band neutrophils/heterophils (%)		1 ± 2.1
Lymphocytes (%)	34.5 (25–44)	58.9 ± 19.6
Monocytes (%)	3 (1–5)	1.5 ± 2.1
Eosinophils (%)	0	3.5 ± 11.7
Basophils (%)	0.5 (0–1)	0

Values given as mean and range or mean ± SD.

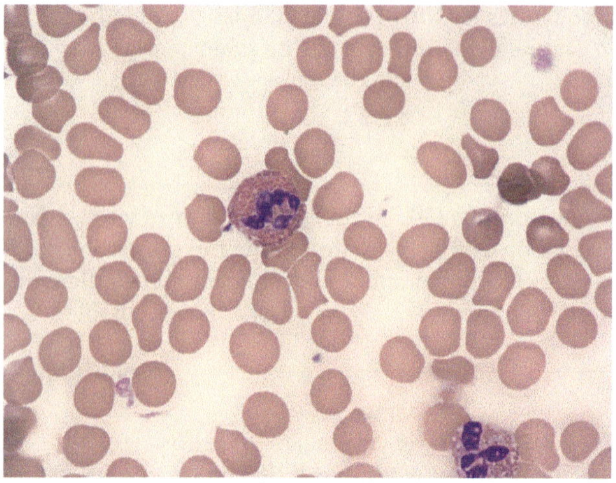

Figure 9.3 Many erythrocytes, two heterophils, and a few platelets. Blood smear from a capybara.

caused by decreased or impaired erythrocyte production secondary to a number of pathologic processes [25, 30].

Evaluating erythrocyte parameters on a CBC may elucidate some pathologic causes of abnormal erythrocyte findings. MCV is the average volume of erythrocytes in blood. Decreased MCV indicates microcytic erythrocytes and is usually associated with iron deficiency anemia. Increased MCV indicates macrocytic erythrocytes and is generally due to the presence of polychromatophils in a regenerative process. Mean corpuscular hemoglobin concentration (MCHC) is the average hemoglobin concentration in a given volume of packed red blood cells. Decreased MCHC indicates hypochromatic erythrocytes which occur with the presence of increased polychromatophils in regenerative responses or hypochromic erythrocytes because of iron deficiency anemia. Increased MCHC is an artifact and may be a secondary result of the presence of Heinz bodies, hemolysis, agglutination, lipemia, or administration of Oxyglobin®. A microcytic, hypochromic anemia is most consistent with iron deficiency, while a macrocytic, hypochromic anemia indicates a regenerative response. A normocytic, normochromic anemia indicates a lack of a regenerative response. Evaluation of erythrocyte morphology may also provide more information about the underlying cause of a patient's disease [25, 30].

Polychromatophils are young, anucleated erythrocytes that have been released into circulation early. They are larger than mature red blood cells and are more basophilic in color. These cells correlate with the presence of reticulocytes when a blood smear is stained with new methylene blue. Increased numbers of polychromatophils and elevated reticulocyte percentages or absolute reticulocyte counts occur with a regenerative response. Hypochromatic erythrocytes are pale staining red blood cells with an increased area of central pallor. These generally indicate iron deficiency [25, 30]. Nucleated red blood cells (usually metarubricytes, occasionally rubricytes, and rarely prorubricytes) are immature erythrocytes. These may be released early from the bone marrow because of regenerative anemia or hypoxia (appropriate rubricytosis) or due to lead poisoning or myelodysplasia (inappropriate rubricytosis) [30]. Inappropriate rubricytosis has been reported to occur in dogs with heatstroke [31], and although there are no published reports of heatstroke in capybaras, this should be considered as a differential for increased peripheral nucleated red blood cells.

Howell-Jolly bodies are small, round, dark blue inclusions that represent nuclear remnants and may be present because of a regenerative response or impaired splenic function [25, 30]. Acanthocytes are red blood cells with randomly spaced and variably sized projections and are usually associated with abnormal lipid content of the cell membrane. They have also reported to be associated with hemangiosarcoma in some mammals [25, 30]. Echinocytes are red blood cells with short, evenly spaced projections. These often occur because of smear preparation or a storage artifact, but they can also occur in some pathologic states (renal disease, lymphoma, drug toxicities, and snake envenomization in other species) [25, 30]. Schistocytes are red blood cell fragments that may be seen with hemangiosarcomas, disseminated intravascular coagulation, iron deficiency, glomerulonephritis, and liver disease [25, 30]. Heinz bodies are small round pale pink structures that protrude from or sit on top of the red cell membrane. These are caused by oxidative denaturation of hemoglobin [25, 30]. Rouleaux is the term for linear stacking of erythrocytes that usually occurs because of increased plasma proteins (immunoglobulins or fibrinogen) during inflammation or some neoplastic processes (lymphoma, plasma cell myeloma) [25, 30]. Agglutination is seen as clumping of erythrocytes due to abnormal antigen–antibody reactions. This is often associated with immune-mediated hemolysis but can also occur with incompatible blood transfusions [25, 30].

Leukocytes

Like erythrocytes, little information is available regarding normal leukocyte morphology and abnormalities in capybaras. However, a few morphological differences between capybara leukocytes and those of domestic species are known. The equivalent of the neutrophil in capybaras is the heterophil (Figure 9.3), which is identified from the presence of rod-shaped granules that stain eosinophilic with Romanowsky stains. However, some sources may refer to these cells as neutrophils. Although heterophils stain differently from neutrophils of most domestic animals, they are believed to have similar functions [25]. Eosinophils are also similar in appearance to those of most other mammals and contain round granules that distinguish them from heterophils (Figure 9.4).

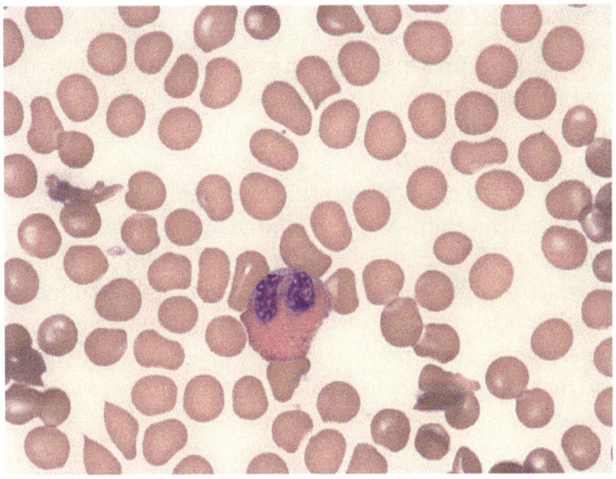

Figure 9.4 An eosinophil in a blood smear from a capybara.

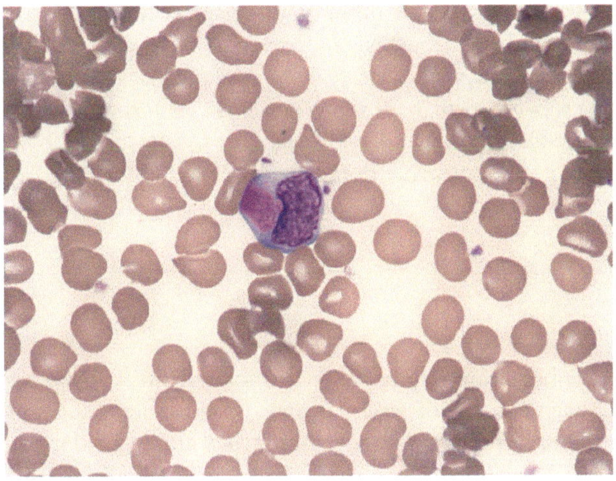

Figure 9.5 A Kurloff cell containing a Kurloff body. Blood smear from a capybara.

Small lymphocytes appear similar to those from other mammalian species. However, capybaras have a unique leukocyte known as the Kurloff cell [29, 32]. This is a large mononuclear cell with lymphocyte and monocyte properties. They are large, round-to-ovoid cells that contain an oval-to-round, blue-to-purple cytoplasmic inclusion body (Figure 9.5). These have been identified in peripheral blood and tissues of capybaras, and, as in guinea pigs, the proportions of Kurloff cells increase with pregnancy. The exact function of the cells in capybaras has not been extensively studied; however, it is presumed that they function in a similar manner to those in guinea pigs [32].

Most mammals respond similarly to disease with regard to changes in the leukon. Specific or unique characteristic changes in the capybara are not available. Neutrophil/heterophil concentrations increase when inflammation occurs, especially if caused by a bacterial infection or an infection caused by other microorganisms. A left shift occurs when there is an increased number of immature heterophils in the blood. These usually consist of band heterophils; however, earlier forms (metamyelocytes, myelocytes) may occur with severe disease. A heterophilia with a left shift indicates marked inflammation, while heteropenia with a left shift indicates severe consumption of heterophils and is usually seen with overwhelming infections. Toxic changes in heterophils are morphologic changes in the cytoplasm associated with accelerated heterophil production in the bone marrow as a response to inflammatory disease. Toxic change is characterized by heterophils that contain one or more of the following features: Döhle bodies (gray-blue cytoplasmic aggregates of endoplasmic reticulum), increased cytoplasmic basophilia, and/or cytoplasmic vacuolation [25].

Changes in neutrophil (or heterophil) to lymphocyte ratios (N:L or H:L ratios) can be evaluated in various species to further characterize changes to the CBC. The normal H:L ratio for capybaras, however, is not currently available. There are also some discrepancies in the literature regarding normal percentages of heterophils and lymphocytes in capybaras. Fowler reports reference values with the heterophil percentage slightly greater than the lymphocyte percentage, while Madella reports a higher percentage of lymphocytes compared to heterophils (Table 9.2) [27, 28]. If capybaras are assumed to be similar to other hystricomorph rodents, it is likely that capybaras tend to have a lower H:L ratio. Inflammation and/or cortisol release may cause the H:L ratio to be inverted. Stress leukograms, left shifts, and other cellular changes which occur in hystricomorph rodents are presumed to occur in capybaras [25].

Hemoparasites

Parasites have been identified in the peripheral blood of capybaras. *Trypanosoma evansi* in peripheral blood smears in capybaras are recognized by their long flagellum, undulating membrane, and subterminal kinetoplast [33, 34]. Capybaras can act as reservoirs of infection without demonstrating clinical signs; however, the parasite may cause clinical disease in other animals and people. *Plasmodium* spp. (the causative agent of malaria) has also been detected in peripheral blood smears of capybaras [35]. No information regarding clinical disease in capybaras infected with these hemoparasites has been reported.

Hemostasis

Few studies have evaluated hemostasis in capybaras, and blood types of capybaras are unknown (Table 9.3). The capybara has a prothrombin time (PT) that is shorter than the activated partial thromboplastin time (aPTT) [36]. It was also found that PT, aPTT, and thrombin time (TT) were all longer in capybaras than in humans. In both capybaras and in guinea pigs, levels of factors XII and X were very low compared to human factors, which

Table 9.3 Coagulation tests and clotting factors for capybaras (*Hydrochoerus hydrochaeris)* [36].

Assay	Clotting time (seconds)	Sample size
Activated partial thromboplastin time (aPTT)	35.5 ± 2.6	12
Factor VII	36.9 ± 0.54	13
Factor X	52.6 ± 1.07	13
Prothrombin time (PT)	24.0 ± 1.24 (18–38)	18
Thrombin time (TT)	28.75 ± 0.72 (25–33)	12

Values given as mean ± SD (range).

may explain the prolonged PT and aPTT [36]. Normal platelet morphology and abnormalities of platelet structure and function in capybaras has not been described. However, as with most mammals, it may be assumed that a thrombocytopenia can result from decreased production, increased destruction, or increased utilization or consumption.

Serum Biochemistry

Minimal data exists regarding evaluation of clinical chemistries in capybaras. The International Species Information System (ISIS) provides analyte ranges submitted from various institutions (Table 9.4) [37]. No published studies focusing on specific chemistry analytes and the causes of biochemical abnormalities are available for capybaras. Thus, causes for altered analyte values can only be extrapolated from other species of rodents, including guinea pigs.

Evaluation of Liver

Serum or plasma enzymes commonly used to detect liver disease (damage, injury, necrosis, cholestasis) in rodents include alkaline phosphatase (AP), gamma-glutamyl transferase (GGT), aspartate aminotransferase (AST), alanine aminotransferase, lactate dehydrogenase (LD), glutamate dehydrogenase (GLDH), and sorbitol dehydrogenase (SD) (also known as iditol dehydrogenase [ID]). Liver function can be evaluated by measuring the total bilirubin concentration, bile acids, and ammonia. Elevations in any of these analytes can be caused by increased production, increased release, or decreased clearance. General causes of increased serum bilirubin concentration include primary hepatobiliary disease, extrahepatic biliary obstruction, or hemolysis [38]. No published studies regarding liver enzyme activity or liver function tests are available for capybaras. Limited information is available for its close relative, the guinea pig.

Evaluation of Kidneys

Serum/blood urea nitrogen, creatinine, and electrolytes are often used to evaluate renal function. In addition to altered renal function, blood urea nitrogen (BUN) can be influenced by diet (increased BUN due to high-protein diets), liver function (decreased production of urea nitrogen with liver damage), gastrointestinal absorption, and hydration. BUN and creatinine are generally increased when there is loss of 50 to 75% of functional renal mass. Renal disease can also result in hyperphosphatemia and hypermagnesemia from decreased glomerular filtration and hypoproteinemia from urinary protein loss [38].

Glucose, Electrolytes, Acid-Base, and Osmolarity

Evaluation of glucose concentrations and significance is likely similar to that in other mammals. It is important that serum and erythrocytes be separated quickly from collection tubes to avoid a falsely decreased glucose concentration secondary to in vitro glycolysis [38]. Interpretation of serum electrolytes and acid/base status is presumed to be similar to that in other domestic mammals (Table 9.4).

Thyroid, Adrenal, and Reproductive Hormones

Few hormones have been evaluated in capybaras. Concentrations of testosterone, androstenedione, and cortisol have been measured in serum and testicular tissues in male capybaras at slaughter in Brazil (Table 9.5). Knowledge of hormones in male capybaras may be beneficial for breeders. Androgens secreted by the testes are responsible for development of internal and external genitalia, appearance of secondary sexual characteristics, development of the musculoskeletal system, and stimulation of spermatogenesis. Testosterone is the most important of the androgen hormones, while androstenedione, which is also secreted from the testes, has a lower degree of androgenicity. A negative correlation was seen between testosterone and cortisol levels but was explained by acute stress on the animals before blood sampling [39]. Values for progesterone, total triiodothyronine (T3), and total thyroxine (T4) have been listed by the International Veterinary Species Information System (Table 9.5).

Urinalysis

Currently, no studies or references regarding urine collection and urinalysis exist for capybaras, probably partially caused by the difficulty of collecting urine samples from hystricomorphs. Catheterization of guinea pigs is a

Table 9.4 Clinical chemistry and electrolyte values for capybaras *(Hydrochoerus hydrochaeris)* [37].

Analyte (abbreviation)	SI Units (conventional)	Mean	Standard deviation	Range	Sample size
Calcium	mmol/l (mg/dl)	2.85 (11.4)	0.275 (1.1)	2.375–3.85 (9.5–15.4)	48
Phosphorous	mmol/l (mg/dl)	2.003 (6.2)	1.001 (3.1)	0.646–5.911 (2.0–18.3)	40
Sodium	mmol/l and mEq/l	136	6.0	127–155	46
Potassium	mmol/l and mEq/l	5.2	1.0	3.8–8.2	49
Chloride	mmol/l and mEq/l	97	5	89–108	40
Bicarbonate	mmol/l and mEq/l	19.6	5.1	9.0–26.0	11
Carbon dioxide	mmol/l and mEq/l	20.1	3.6	14.0–28.0	10
Osmolarity	μmol/l and mOsmol/l	295	0	n/a	1
Iron	μmol/l (μg/dl)	29.2 (163)	11.6 (65)	18.4–42.4 (103–237)	4
Blood urea nitrogen (BUN)	mmol/l (mg/dl)	5 (14)	2.5 (7)	1.4–12.9 (4–36)	60
Creatinine	μmol/l (mg/dl)	159.1(1.8)	44.2 (0.5)	88.4–265.4 (1.0–2.9)	61
Uric Acid	μmol/l (mg/dl)	95.2 (1.6)	59.5 (1.0)	17.8–208.2 (0.3–3.5)	18
Total bilirubin	μmol/l (mg/dl)	3.4 (0.2)	3.4 (0.2)	0.0–17.1 (0.0–1.0)	46
Direct bilirubin	μmol/l (mg/dl)	0.0 (0.0)	17.1 (1.0)	0.0–5.13 (0.0–0.3)	15
Indirect bilirubin	μmol/l (mg/dl)	1.7 (0.1)	1.7 (0.1)	0.0–5.13 (0.0–0.3)	15
Glucose	mmol/l (mg/dl)	6.8 (122)	2.7 (48)	1.4–16.5 (25–297)	62
Cholesterol	mmol/l (mg/dl)	2.1 (83)	0.8 (30)	1.2–4.5 (48–175)	48
Triglyceride	mmol/l (mg/dl)	1.6 (146)	1.2 (107)	0.6–4.5 (51–398)	17
Creatine phosphokinase (CK)	IU/l	647	1301	30–5584	18
Lactate dehydrogenase (LDH)	IU/l	546	570	57–1718	18
Alkaline phosphatase (ALP)	IU/l	340	253	30–1130	55
Alanine aminotransferase (ALT)	IU/l	38	28	5–174	53
Aspartate aminotransferase (AST)	IU/l	37	22	7–110	56
Gamma glutamyltransferase (GGT)	IU/l	3	2	0–7	16
Amylase	U/l	3802	2350	74–8730	17
Lipase	U/l	55	41	16–138	9
Total protein (TP) (colorimetry)	g/l (g/dl)	63 (6.3)	8 (0.8)	44–79 (4.4–7.9)	54
Globulin (colorimetry)	g/l (g/dl)	32 (3.2)	9 (0.9)	16–48 (1.6–4.8)	39
Albumin (colorimetry)	g/l (g/dl)	32 (3.2)	5 (0.5)	25–48 (2.5–4.8)	39
Fibrinogen	μmol (mg/dl)	7.1 (240)	2.6 (89)	2.9–8.8 (100–300)	5

Table 9.5 Hormone levels for capybaras *(Hydrochoerus hydrochaeris)* [39].

Analyte (abbreviation)	SI Units (conventional)	Mean	Standard deviation	Range	Sample size
Progesterone	nmol/l (ng/dl)	17.4 (5.460)	n/a	n/a	1
Total triiodothyronine (T3)	nmol/l (ng/ml)	2 (128.0)	n/a	n/a	1
Total thyroxine (T4)	nmol/l (μg/dl)	16.7 (1.3)	12.87 (1.0)	2.6–24.5 (0.2–1.9)	3
Cortisol (serum)	nmol/l (μg/dl)	1203.2 (43.61)	1123.2 (40.71)	Not established	15
Cortisol (testis)	nmol/l (μg/dl)	582.1 (21.10)	246.1 (8.92)	Not established	15
Testosterone (serum)	nmol/l (ng/dl)	4.27 (123.00)	8.33 (240.04)	Not established	15
Testosterone (testis)	nmol/l (ng/dl)	541.79 (15613.6)	460.27 (13264.42)	Not established	15
Androstenedione (serum)	nmol/l (ng/dl)	0.06 (1.69)	0.03 (0.89)	Not established	15
Androstenedione (testis)	nmol/l (ng/dl)	0.34 (9.83)	0.07 (13.97)	Not established	15

successful means of urine collection, and a similar procedure may be possible in capybaras; however, use of sedation or anesthesia may be required.

Serology and Polymerase Chain Reaction (PCR)

Several infectious agents have been identified and studied in capybaras. Infection by the protozoan *Toxoplasma gondii* has been reported in feral capybaras in Sao Paulo, Brazil. Indirect immunofluorescent antibody tests (IFATs) and the modified agglutination tests (MAT) have been used to determine the seroprevalence of *T. gondii*. In one study, an IFAT detected antibodies in 69.8% of 149 capybaras evaluated, while with MAT, antibodies were found in 42.3% of the capybaras [40]. A similar study identified antibodies to *T. gondii* in 75% of 64 capybaras on the basis of MAT and in 76.6% of the capybaras on the basis of IFAT [41]. These findings demonstrate that capybaras in their native environment are frequently exposed to *T. gondii* and may be a source of infection if consumed as undercooked meat, or they may serve as a source of infection for cats, which shed oocysts after eating tissues and disseminate the oocysts in the environment via fecal contamination [40, 41]. Antibodies against *Brucella* spp. have been found in capybaras in Venezuela using immunodiffusion gel tests. In a study of 201 wild capybaras in Venezuela, 58% of sera were positive for *Brucella* spp. Organisms were identified as *B. abortus* and *B. suis* [42]. This suggests that capybaras may be an important host of *Brucella* spp. Blood sera from 73 wild capybaras in Sao Paulo, Brazil, were found to be positive for *Rickettsia rickettsia* (26%), *R. parkeri* (34.2%), and *Rickettsia belli* (68.5%) on the basis of an IFAT assay against rickettsial antigens [43]. Testing of capybara spleens by PCR did not detect rickettsial DNA. The sources of these infectious agents are Amblyomma ticks, *Amblyomma dubitatum* and *A. cajennense*, which were collected from these capybaras. *R. parkeri* can infect and cause disease in humans [43].

References

1 Pachaly, J.R. et al. (2001). Order Rodentia (Rodents). In: *Biology, Medicine, and Surgery of South American Wild Animals* (ed. E. Murray and A. Fowler), 225–237. Iowa: Iowa State University Press.

2 Paula, T.A.R.C. and Matta, S.L.P. (2002). *Avaliação histológica quantitativa do testículo de apivaras (Hydrochoerus hydrochaeris) adultas. Journal of Biosciences* 18 (1): 121–136.

3 Pinto, G.R.M. et al. (2006). *Detectability of capybaras in forested habitats. Biota Neotropica* 6 (1). http://dx.doi.org/10.1590/S1676-06032006000100008

4 Costa, D.S.P., Fonseca, C.C., and Neves, M.T.D. (2002). *Reprodução de Capivaras. Vet Zool* 5 (1): 111–118.

5 Ferraz, K.P.M.B.V. (2001). *Ecologia comportamental da capivara: bases biológicas para o manejo da espécie.* In: *A Produção Animal na Visão dos Brasileiros* (ed. W.R.S.

Mattos), 589–595. Piracicaba: SP, Brasil: Sociedade Brasileira de Zootecnia.

6 Araujo, RA, et al. 2007. Monitoramento de Um Grupo de Capivaras, *Hydrochoerus hydrochaeris*, (Mammalia: Rodentia) Em Um Parque Urbano Na Região da Pampulha, Belo Horizonte, Brasil. Anais do VIII Congresso de Ecologia do Brasil, Caxambu – MG.

7 Herrera, E.A. (1992). *Size of testes and scent glands in capybaras (Hydrochoerus hydrochaeris Rodentia: Caviomorpha). Journal of Mammology* 73: 871–975.

8 Costa, D.S. and Paula, T.A.R. (2006). Testosterone level, nasal gland volume and Leydig cell morphometry in capybaras (*Hydrochoerus hydrochaeris*). *Arquivo Brasileiro de Medicina Veterinária e Zootecnia* 58 (6): 1086–1091.

9 Alvarez, M.R. and Kravetz, F.O. (2009). *Effect of ascorbic acid on food preference and consumption in captive capybaras (Hydrochoerus hydrochaeris). Brazilian Archives of Biology and Technology* 52 (3): 563–600.

10 Cueto, G.R., Allekotte, R., and Kravetz, F.O. (2000). *Scurvy in capybaras bred in captivity in argentine. Journal of Wildlife Diseases* 36 (1): 97–101.

11 Pereira, HFA and MR Eston. 2007. Biologia e manejo de capivaras (*Hydrochoerus hydrochaeris*) no parque estadual Alberto Lofgren, Sao Paulo, Brasil. Ver. Inst. Flor., Sao Paulo. 19(1):55–64.

12 Sinkoc, AL, et al. 1997. Ocorrencia de Ixodidae parasitos de capivara (*Hydrochoerus hydrochaeris* Linnaeus, 1766) na estacao ecologica do Taim, Rio Grande - RS, Brasil. Ciencias Rural, Santa Maria. 27(1): 119–122.

13 Albuquerque, GR, et al. 2008. Eimerid coccidia from capybaras (*Hydrochoerus hydrochaeris*) in Southern Bahia, Brasil. Pesquisa Veterinária Brasileira. 28(7):323–328.

14 Salas, V and EA Herrera. 2004. Intestinal helminths of capybaras, *Hydrochoerus hydrochaeris*, from Venezuela. Memórias do Instituto Oswaldo Cruz. 99(6):563–566.

15 Silva, EF, et al. 2009. Soroprevalencia da infeccao leptopiral em capivaras (*Hydrochoerus hydrochaeris*) abatidas em um frigorifico do Rio Grande do Sul. Pesquisa Veterinária Brasileira. 29(2):174–176.

16 Szabuniewicz, M. et al. (1977-1978). *Sedacion Y Anestesia del Chiguire (Hydrochoerus Hydrochoeris, Linne)*, vol. XXVII. Universidad Central de Venezuela: Revista de la Facultada de Ciencias Veterinarias.

17 Wright, M. (1982). *Pharmacologic effects of ketamine and its use in veterinary medicine. Journal of the American Veterinary Medical Association* 180 (12): 1462–1471.

18 Klide, A.M., Calderwood, H.W., and Soma, L.R. (1992). *Cardiopulmonary effects of xylazine in dogs. American Journal of Veterinary Research* 22: 931–935.

19 Thurmon, JC, WJ Tranquilli, and GJ Benson. 1996. *Preanesthetics and anesthetic adjuncts.* Lumb & Jones' Veterinary Anesthesia. Ed. JC Thurmon, WJ Tranquilli, and GJ Benson. Baltimore: Lea & Febiger.

20 Cruz, ML, et al. 1998. Tecnicas anestesicas injetaveis em capivaras (Hydrochoerus hydrochaeruis, Linne). Ciencia Rural. 28(3).

21 King, J.D., Congdon, E., and Tosta, C. (2010). *Evaluation of three immobilization combinations in the capybara (Hydrochoerus hydrochaeris). Zoo Biology* 29 (1): 59–67.

22 Rego, M.A.F. et al. (2010). *Contencao quimica em capivaras (Hydrochoerus hydrochaeris): Proposta de protocolo anestesico em duas fases para realizacao de biometria e colheita de materiais biologicos in XIII Congresso e XIX Encontro da Associacao Brasileira de Veterinarios de Animais Selvagens*, 2010. Brasil: Campos de Jordao, SP.

23 West, G., Heard, D.J., and Caulkett, N. *Zoo Animal and Wildlife Immobilization and Anesthesia.* Ames, Iowa: Blackwell Pub.

24 Kreegar, T.J. and Arnemo, J.M. *Handbook of WildlifeChemical Immobilization*, 3e.

25 Campbell, T.W. and Ellis, C.K. (2007). *Avian & Exotic Animal Hematology & Cytology.* Ames: Blackwell Publishing.

26 Diff-Quik: American Scientific Products, Division of American Hosptial Supply Corporation, McGraw Park, IL.

27 Fowler, M.E. (ed.) (1986). *Rodents (Rodentia). Zoo & Wild Animal Medicine.* Philadelphia: W.B. Saunders Company.

28 Madella, DA, et al. 2006. Valores hematológicos de capivaras (*Hydrochoerus hydrochaeris*) Rodentia: Hydrochoeridae) de vida livre na região de Campinas-SP, Sao Paulo state, Brazil. Ciencia Rural. 36(4).

29 Canfield, P.J. (1998). *Comparative cell morphology in the peripheral blood film from exotic and native animals. Australian Veterinary Journal* 76 (12): 793–800.

30 Harvey, J.W. (2001). *Atlas of Veterinary Hematology.* Philadelphia: W.B. Saunders Company.

31 Aroch, I. et al. (2009). *Peripheral nucleated red blood cells as a prognostic indicator in heatstroke in dogs. Journal of veterinary internal medicine* 23 (3): 544–551.

32 Jara, L.F. et al. (2005). *Kurloff cells in peripheral blood and organs of wild capybaras. Journal of Wildlife Diseases* 41 (2): 431–434.

33 Morales, G.A., Wells, E.A., and Angel, D. (1976). *The capybara (Hydrochoerus hydrochaeris) as a reservoir host for Trypanosoma evansi. Journal of Wildlife Diseases* 12 (4): 572–574.

34 Munoz, K. and Chavez, A. (2001). *Trypanosoma evansi isolated from capybara (Hidrochaeris hidrochaeris). Memórias do Instituto Oswaldo Cruz* 96 (7): 945–946.

35 dos Santos, L.C. et al. (2009). *Detection of plasmodium sp. in capybara. Veterinary Parasitology* 163 (1–2): 148–151.

36 Leitao, DP, AC Polizello, and Z Rothschild. 2000. Coagulation and fibrinolysis in capybara (Hydrochaeris

hydrochaeris), a close relative of the guinea-pig (Cavia porcellus). Comparative Biochemistry and Physiology, Part A: Molecular and Integrative Physiology 125(1):113–120.

37 International Species Information System (ISIS). *Capybara Reference Ranges for Physiological Data Values.*

38 Thrall, M.A., Baker, D.C., and Lassen, E.D. (2004). *Veterinary Hematology and Clinical Chemistry.* Lassen: Wiley-Blackwell.

39 Batalha de Miranda Araujo, L. et al. (2011). *Testosterone, Androstenedione, and Cortisol Levels in Capybara Serum and Testis.* Brazil: Veterinary Medicine School of Goias Federal University, Goias and Sao Paulo.

40 Canon-Franco, W.A. et al. (2003). Seroprevalence of Toxoplasma gondii antibodies in the rodent capybara (Hidrochoeris hidrochoeris) from Brazil. *The Journal of Parasitology* 89 (4): 850.

41 Yai, L.E. et al. (2008). *Isolation of toxoplasma gondii from capybaras (Hydrochaeris hydrochaeris) from Sao Paulo state, Brazil. The Journal of Parasitology* 94 (5): 1060–1063.

42 Lord, V. and Flores, R. (1983). *Brucella spp. from the capybara (Hydrochaeris hydrochaeris) in Venezuela: serologic studies and metabolic characterization of isolates. Journal of Wildlife Diseases* 19 (4): 308–314.

43 Pacheco, R.C. et al. (2007). *Rickettsial infection in capybaras (Hydrochoerus hydrochaeris) from Sao Paulo, Brazil: serological evidence for infection by Rickettsia bellii and Rickettsia parkeri. Biomedica* 27 (3): 364–371.

10

Squirrels

J. Jill Heatley DVM, MS, DABVP (Avian, Reptilian, Amphibian), DACZM

Department of Small Animal Clinical Sciences, College of Veterinary Medicine & Biomedical Sciences, Texas A&M University, College Station, TX, USA

Introduction

As in other companion mammal species, hematology, plasma or serum biochemistry, and urinalysis can be used to assess health in squirrel species. Multiple studies have evaluated a variety of clinical-pathology-based diagnostic tools in squirrel species for assessment of wild species for public health issues and captive species for use as models of human health in laboratory environments. Most extensively studied in Sciuridae is the process and metabolic changes of hibernation. Many squirrel species are seasonal hibernators with an annual cycle which includes torpor and extremely low body temperature to allow life sustainment in the absence of food. Weight gain and relative dehydration occur in the fall in preparation for hibernation with rehydration and increased gluconeogenesis occurring at emergence in the spring. Heterothermy, prolonged fasting, and reliance upon stored lipids, rather than carbohydrates, for metabolism necessitates many alterations in commonly assessed biochemical analytes such as lipids, proteins, sugars, and vitamins in these species. Seasonal changes in percentages of blood cell types and immune system tissues also occur [1]. Not all squirrels species hibernate. However, those which do have received more attention in the physiology literature and will therefore be over-represented in this text.

Species

Squirrels are of the order Rodentia, family Sciuridae and are found free-living on all continents except Antarctica and Australia. There are about 50 genera and 273 species in the genus Sciuridae. The two subfamilies are the Pteromyinae, flying squirrels, and the seven tribes of Sciruinae, which includes the ground squirrels and tree squirrels. The tribe Sciurini includes the common tree squirrels of the Americas, Europe, and Northern Asia. The tribe Marmotini includes the marmots, prairie dogs, and ground squirrels of North America and Eurasia. Many other tribes of squirrels exist in India, Africa, and Asia. Some of these tribes are not phylogenetically classified with surety [2]. Commonly seen subfamilies include Cyonomys, the prairie dogs; Spermophilus, the ground squirrels; Marmota, the woodchucks and marmots; Ammospermophilus, the antelope squirrels; Tamias, the chipmunks; Tamiasciurus, the chickarees; Sciurus, the tree squirrels; and Glaucomys, New World flying squirrels (Table 10.1). Tree squirrel species in the United States include the eastern gray squirrel (*Sciurus carolinenesis*), the western gray (*Sciurus griseus*), the tassel-eared (*Sciurus aberti*), the Arizona gray (*Sciurus arizonensis*), the eastern fox (*Sciurus niger*), the Apache fox (*Sciurus apache*), the red (*Tamiasciurus hudsonicus*), and the chickaree or Douglas's squirrel (*Tamiasciurus douglasii*). Also included in tree squirrel species are the flying squirrels, which are separated into northern and southern species *(Glaucomys volans and Glaucomys sabrinus)*. The prairie dog is a ground squirrel, and species include the black-tailed prairie dog (*Cynomys ludovicianus*) of western United States prairies, the white-tailed prairie dog (*Cynomys gunnisoni*), from the high plains of Colorado, New Mexico, Utah, and Montana, and (*Cynomys mexicanus*) of northern Mexico. Some squirrel species are locally endangered and at risk of extinction, as is the case of the decline of the red squirrel (*Sciurus vulgaris*, Squirrel Nutkin) because of introduction of the gray squirrel and Parapoxvirus into Great Britain, Ireland, and Italy.

Sample Collection

Restraint

Most squirrel species have large powerful jaws, agile feet, and a pugnacious nature. Sample collection usually requires sedation or anesthesia for immobilization.

Exotic Animal Laboratory Diagnosis, First Edition. Edited by J. Jill Heatley and Karen E. Russell.

Table 10.1 Sciruidae commonly found in captivity or presented for rehabilitation.

Common name	Subfamily
Gray squirrel, Fox squirrel	Sciurus
Red squirrel	Tamiasciurus
Flying squirrels	Glaucomys
Chipmunk	Tamias, Eutamias, Neotamias
Prairie dog	Cyonomys
Woodchuck, Groundhog, Marmot	Marmota

As rodents, squirrels are amenable to inhalant anesthetics such as isoflurane and sevoflurane administered via chamber or face mask. Prolonged fasting is not necessary or recommended because of the minimal likelihood of vomiting and aspiration in these rodent species. Multiple injectable protocols including ketamine/xylazine, ketamine/medetomidine, and tiletamine/zolazepam have been used with success. Midazolam and acepromazine may also be useful adjunctive sedative drugs for these species. For analgesia, oxymorphone, morphine, buprenorphine, or butorphanol may be used [3].

Venipuncture Sites

Venipuncture sites for Sciuridae depend on the size, temperament, species, and areas of fur growth. Most temperate squirrels have a seasonal (fall, winter) weight gain of 10%–17% that may make vein visualization challenging. In addition, many squirrel species have relatively tough, thick skin, which may require incision for venous access. Venipuncture sites of the squirrel include the relatively short jugular, the cranial vena cava, and the brachiocephalic, lateral saphenous, cephalic, and femoral veins (Figure 10.1). A lateral tail vein large enough for sampling also occurs in some species but may require shaving of the tail. Submandibular vein access may also be a possibility

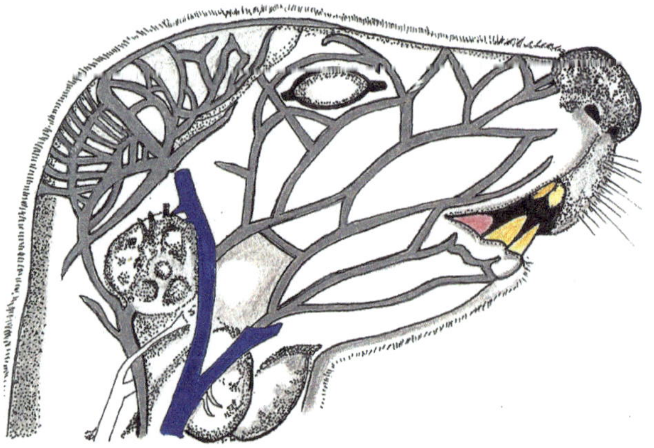

Figure 10.1 Lateral image of squirrel jugular veins, shown in blue.

for reasonable sample size collection in these species (Figure 10.2). Cardiac puncture, tail tip incision, and orbital sinus are less commonly used as sampling sites in squirrels owing to risk of morbidity or mortality and poor sample quality. Common materials for blood collection in these species include 27–23 gauge (g.) needles and 0.3–3 ml syringes. The short jugular vein can be accessed by a hanging jugular or direct approach by insertion of the needle above the clavicle and perpendicular to the skin (Figure 10.3). Aspiration is maintained until blood is visualized flowing into the syringe upon vein entry. The saphenous, cephalic, and lateral tails veins provide only small volumes of blood and are approached as for the rodentia (Figure 10.4). Approaches for collection of blood from other sites would be as for other rodents. Total blood volume of woodchucks *(Marmota morax)* averaged 6.5% but ranged from 4.8% to 8.3% of bodyweight depending on hibernation, season, weight, and fasting status [4]. Hibernation or dormancy similarly decreased blood volume of the ground squirrel *(Citellus parryi ablusis)* from 59 to 25 ml [5].

Sample Handling

As with other rodents, EDTA is the anticoagulant of choice for sciurid hematology. For biochemical analytes, lithium heparin may be used to obtain a greater volume of plasma, or tubes with no anticoagulant may be used to obtain serum after clot formation. EDTA and lithium heparin have each been used for anticoagulation of juvenile gray squirrel blood samples successfully; hemolysis was not evident at 4–6 post collection. Most parameters for the CBC can be analyzed with instruments designed for mammal use. Therefore, preparation of a blood smear without anticoagulant is recommended but is not absolutely necessary for cell differentials and morphologic evaluation. Other specifics for sample handling and storage, including the viability of samples and interferences caused by hemolysis, have not been specifically investigated or reported in Sciuridae to the author's knowledge. At this time, following those guidelines for rodents and other mammals is recommended.

Specific Analytes

Complete Blood Count

Few hematology references are published for squirrels, which are assumed to be hematologically similar to the rat. As in other small rodents, males have a higher PCV than females, and the total white blood cell count of squirrels tends to be relatively low (6000 cells/dL for the red squirrel and 2000 cells/dL for the gray squirrel). Hemoglobin, hematocrit, and erythrocyte count have been reported in a variety of squirrel species (Table 10.2) [42]. Feeding an increased-fat and reduced-lipotrope

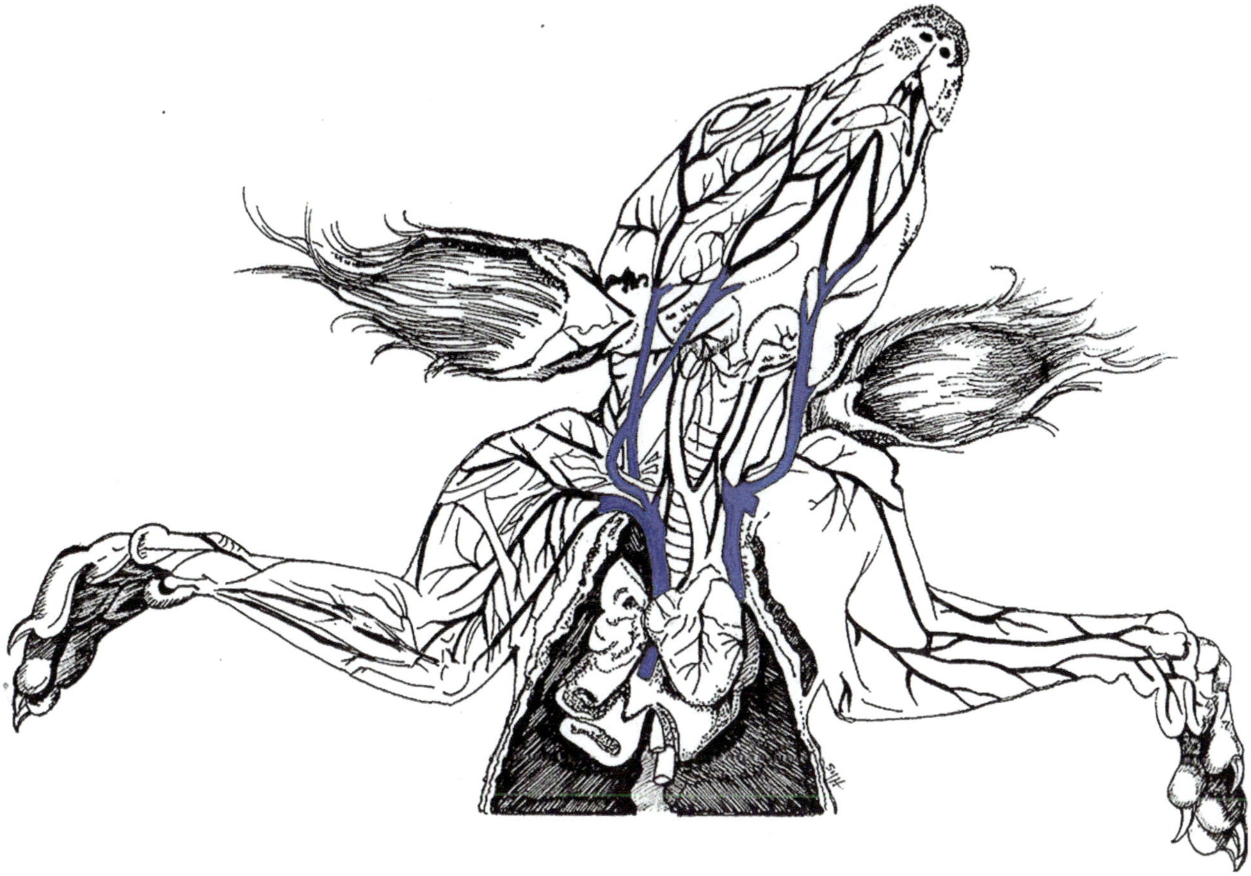

Figure 10.2 Ventral image of squirrel veins of the neck, shown in blue. The temperament, thick skin, and relatively short neck of some species may limit access to these veins without use of immobilizing drugs.

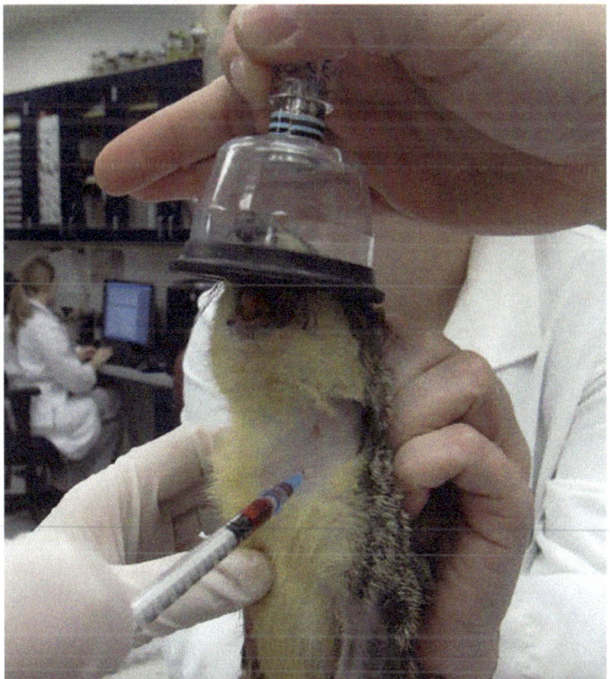

Figure 10.3 Approach for venipuncture of the squirrel jugular may be attempted with the squirrel in the upright position as the needle is advanced above the clavicle, perpendicular to the skin.

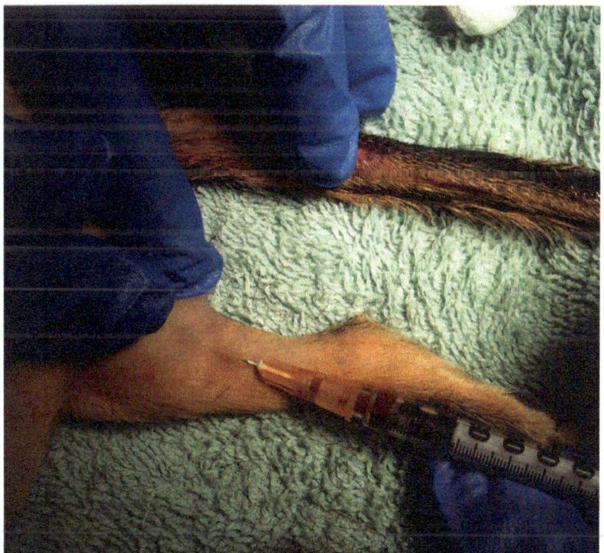

Figure 10.4 Approach to the medial saphenous vein of these species general requires anesthesia. Diagnostic volumes may be obtained from this site by a skilled venipuncturist.

Table 10.2 Hematologic data for squirrel species.

Analyte (abbreviation)	Units, SI (conventional)	Red squirrel [50] *Sciurus vulgaris*	Gray squirrel *Sciurus carolinensis*	Eastern chipmunk [50] *Tamias striatus*	Persian squirrel [6] *Sciurus anomalus*	Black-tailed prairie dog [7, 8, 12, 72] *Cynomys ludovicianus*	Yellow-bellied marmot [9] *Marmota flaviventris*	Woodchuck [40] *Marmota monax*
Data		Mean ± SD	Mean ± SD (Range)	Mean ± SD	Mean [min–max]	Mean ± SD (Range)	Mean ± SD (*n*)	Mean ± SD
Animals sampled		22♂ 28♀ⱬ heparinized suborbital sinus sample	all ⱬ ₪ 180 [10,11] 5♂7♀ [12] 7♂5♀ [50]	9♂, 10♀ ⱬ ₪ Φ ₳	30 Ħ	45 ⱬ [7] 18–20 ¥ [12] 18 wild caught Ħ [8]	≥ 122 ₪ ⱬ 76 Yearling ≥ 76ⱬ ≥ 107 Óⱬ	5 Ħ Ó
White blood cell (WBC) count	**×10^9 /l = (×10^3/μl)**	1.74 ± 0.34 ♂ 1.86 ± 0.26 ♀	5.07 ± 0.99 ♂ 6.00 ± 1.68 ♀ [50] 2.03 ± 0.78 [12] 1.1–3.9 [10] 1.5–6.7 [11]	2.50 ± 0.37 ♂ 2.48 ± 0.57 ♀	7050 [4.30–10.8]	6.30 ± 1.90 [7] 4.31 ± 1.93 (1.40–9.50) ¥ 3 ± 1.2 (1–6) [8]	9.406 ± 4.499 ₪ 9.649 ± 4.499 7.644 ± 4.306 Ó	18.64 ± 8.35
Neutrophils absolute /μl	**×10^9 l = (×10^3/μl)**	1.09 ± 0.25 ♂ 1.13 ± 0.19 ♀	3.30 ± 0.96 ♂ 4.43 ± 1.41 ♀ [50] 3.11 ± 0.67 ♂ 3.70 ± 0.75 ♀	0.47 ± 0.06 ♂ 0.44 ± 0.12 ♀	4.12 [3.06–6.26]	3900 ± 1600 [7] *2750 ± 1580* *(1040–7410)* [12]		
Neutrophil %			1–14 [12] 9–99 [11]			62.6 ± 12.7 32.0–78.0 ¥ None [7]		
Bands absolute	**×10^9 /l = (×10^3/μl)**	None reported	None reported	None reported	None reported	None reported	None reported	
Bands %			0–6 [12] 0–16 [11]					
Lymphocytes absolute	**×10^9 /l = (×10^3/μl)** **/μl**	0.65 ± 0.12 ♂ 0.73 ± 0.12 ♀	1.46 ± 0.38 ♂ 1.53 ± 0.34 ♀ [50] 1.93 ± 0.40 ♂ 2.02 ± 0.41 ♀ [10,11]	1.82 ± 0.36 ♂ 1.83 ± 0.43 ♀	2.29 [1.10–3.82]	2200 ± 900 ¥ *1240 ± 728* *(252–2960)* [7]		
Lymphocytes	**%**		75–91 [12] 4–79 [11]			28.6 ± 12.5 ¥ (14.0–58.0) [7] [1.2 ± 0.5(0.5–3)] [8]		

Monocytes	**×10^9^ /l = (×10^3^/μl)**	0	0.10 ± 0.05 ♂ 0.01 ± 0.01 ♀ [50] 0–0.4	0.06 ± 0.005 ♂ 0.05 ± 0.01 ♀	0.23 [0.19–0.30]	130 ± 110 ¥ 229 ± 161 (29.0–585) [7] [0.5 ± 0.2(0.2–0.9)] [8]		
Monocytes	**%**		2–8 [12] 0–3 [11]			6.45 ± 4.75 (1.00–14.0) [7]		
Eosinophils	**×10^9^ /l = (×10^3^/μl)**	0	0.03 ± 0.01 ♂ 0.04 ± 0.02 ♀ [50]	0.03 ± 0.01 ♂ 0.05 ± 0.01 ♀	0.090 [0.059–0.115]	100 ± 130 ¥ 73.5 ± 140 (0.00–616) [7]		
Eosinophils	**%**		0–3 [12] 0–4 [11]			1.95 ± 3.22 (0.00–14.0) [7]		
Basophils	**×10^9^/l = (×10^3^/μl)**	0	0–0.2	0.02 ± 0.004 ♂ 0.03 ± 0.01 ♀	None reported	13.5 ± 23.1 (0.00–88.0) [7]		
Basophils	**%**		0–1 [12] 0–3 [11]			0.4 ± 0.6 (0.00–2.00) [7]		
Hematocrit PCV	**Proportion of 1.0 (%)**	0.497 ±.014 ♂ 0.500 ±0.011♀ (49.7 ± 1.4 ♂ 50.0 ± 1.1 ♀)	46.3 ± 0.8 ♂ 44.6 ± 0.5 ♀ [50] 31–56 [10] 43–44 [11] 32.5–48 ♂) 28.5–36 ♀ [12]	48.4 ± 2 ♂ 51.8 ± 1.6 ♀		[36.5 ± 7.00] ¥ [38.7 ± 3.05 (33.4–45.1)] [7] [24 ± 6.7(14–36)] [8]	0.508 ± .042 ***(201)*** 0.510 ± .038 ***(150)*** 0.449 ± .031 (early) ***(128)*** 0.506 ± .026 (late) ***(103)*** (50.82 ± 4.17 ▣ 50.99 ± 3.81 44.92 ± 3.1 (early) Ó 50.64 ± 2.56 (late) Ó)	
Hemoglobin	**g /l (g/dl)**	1560 ± 30 ♂ 1530 ± 20 ♀ (156 ± 3 ♂ 153 ± 2 ♀)	1370 ± 20 ♂ 1350 ± 20 ♀ (137 ± 2 ♂ 135 ± 2 ♀) [50] 83–177 [10] [12.7–16.3♂] [9.3–12♀ [12]] [8.3–17.7]	1450 ± 60 ♂ 1600 ± 30 ♀ (145 ± 6 ♂ 160 ± 3 ♀)		12.0 ± 2.00 ¥ [12.6 ± 1.11] (10.4–15.3)] [7] 8 ± 2.1(4–11) [8]	131.2 ± 20.3 **(35)** 125.7 ± 16.0 **(34)** 104.2 ± 18.1 **(46)** 129.0 ± 26.9 **(22)** (13.12 ± 2.03] **(35)** 12.57 ± 1.6 **(34)** 10.42 ± 1.81 **(46)** 12.90 ± 2.69 **(22)**)	16.14 ± 2.60
Red blood cell (RBC) Count	**×10^12^ /l = (×10^6^/μl)** ***10^3^/μl***	8.44 ± 0.20 ♂ 7.81 ± 0.17 ♀	6.90 ± 0.22 ♂ 6.76 ± 0.15 ♀ [50] [6.51–6.85 M] [6.59–7.12♀ [12]] [4.0–10.0] [10]	9.01 ± 0.36 ♂ 9.65 ± 0.30 ♀		6.60 ± 1.10 ¥ *6.81* ± 0.61 (5.90 ± 8.10) [7] [4 ± 1.1(2–50] [8]	6160 ± 1198 **(41)** 5858 ± 1253 **(19)** 4855 ± 922**(40)** 6227 ± 1087 **(3)**	6.48 ± 0.45
Reticulocytes	**Proportion of 1.0 (%)**		None reported			None reported		
Platelets	**×10^9^ /l = (×10^3^/μl)**		Not reported			466 ± 157 ¥ [463 ± 235 (245–1190)] [7] [126 ± 67(41–239)] [8]		

(Continued)

Table 10.2 (Continued)

Analyte (abbreviation)	Units, SI (conventional)	Red squirrel [50] *Sciurus vulgaris*	Gray squirrel *Sciurus carolinensis*	Eastern chipmunk [50] *Tamias striatus*	Persian squirrel [6] *Sciurus anomalus*	Black-tailed prairie dog [7, 8, 12, 72] *Cynomys ludovicianus*	Yellow-bellied marmot [9] *Marmota flaviventris*	Woodchuck [40] *Marmota monax*
Data		Mean ± SD	Mean ± SD (Range)	Mean ± SD	Mean [min–max]	Mean ± SD (Range)	Mean ± SD (*n*)	Mean ± SD
Animals sampled		22♂ 28♀ ⍀ heparinized suborbital sinus sample	all ⍀ ⧆ 180 [10,11] 5♂7♀ [12] 7♂5♀ [50]	9♂, 10♀ ⍀ ⧆ Φ ٨	30 Ħ	45 ⍀ [7] 18–20 ¥ [12] 18 wild caught Ħ [8]	≥ 122 ⧆ ⍀ 76 Yearling ≥ 76 ⍀ ≥ 107 Ó ⍀	5 Ħ Ó
Mean corpuscular volume (MCV)	**μm^3 = fl**	63.3 ± 1.2 ♂ 66.3 ± 1 ♀	67.4 ± 1.2 ♂ 66.2 ± 0.9 ♀ [50] 40–104.3 [10]	54.0 ± 1.3 ♂ 53.9 ± 1.0 ♀		55.1 ± 5.20 ¥ 56.8 ± 3.80 (48.0–64.0) [7] 62 ± 2.5(57–66) [8]	73.26 ± 11.4 **(27)** 76.84 ± 8.4 **(26)** 80.48 ± 8.42 **(15)** 74.18 ± 6.95 **(23)**	65.60 ± 4.04
Mean corpuscular hemoglobin (MCH)	**pg/cell**	18.6 ± 0.2 ♂ 19.8 ± 0.2 ♀	19.9 ± 0.3 ♂ 20.2 ± 0.4 ♀ [50] 19.6 ± 0.3 12.6–29.7 [10]	16.4 ± 0.3 ♂ 16.6 ± 0.4 ♀		18.5 ± 1.90 ¥ 18.6 ± 1.33 (16.0–21.7) [7] 20 ± 0.8(19–22) [8]	23.71 ± 4.24 **(43)** 23.10 ± 3.61 **(19)** 24.11 ± 5.68 **(28)**	
Mean corpuscular hemoglobin concentration (MCHC)	g/L {**g/dl**}	2930± 40♂ 2980± 30♀ {293 ± 4 ♂ 298 ± 3 ♀}	296 ± 3 ♂ 304 ± 3 ♀ [50] 170–368 (28.8–40 ♂ 29.7–37.9 ♀ [12]) 17.0 – 36.8 [10,11]	300 ± 4 ♂ 309 ± 6 ♀		33.5 ± 2.20 ¥ 32.7 ± 1.43 (30.0–35.5) [7] 32 ± 1.5(29–34) [8]	26.40 ± 4.58 **(14)** 25.61 ± 2.36 **(15)** 24.32 ± 4.09 **(44)** 28.99 ± 3.71 **(9)**	38.2 ± 5.63

Key: Free living ⍀, Captive Ħ, Pet ¥, Male ♂, Female ♀, Adult ⧆, Juvenile Ó diet to woodchucks (choline, methionine, folic acid, and B12) resulted in an increased mean corpuscular volume (MCV) [40]. Woodchucks do not experience hemoconcentration during hibernation; the red blood cell count, hematocrit, and hemoglobin do not increase. The prairie dog has normochromic, microcytic blood with an increased number of red blood cells. The prairie dog also has a high concentration of small platelets [7].

The morphology of leukocytes, erythrocytes, and platelets of squirrel species is similar to that of other laboratory rodents (Figures 10.5–10.12). Gray squirrels are lymphocytic. Woodchuck white blood cell count does not increase during hibernation [43]. However, marked variation occurs in the types of white blood cells encountered throughout the year in woodchucks. Neutrophils increase during hibernation, while lymphocytes decrease; and little variation occurs in the monocytes, eosinophils, and basophils [38]. Although hemoparasitism of Sciuridae

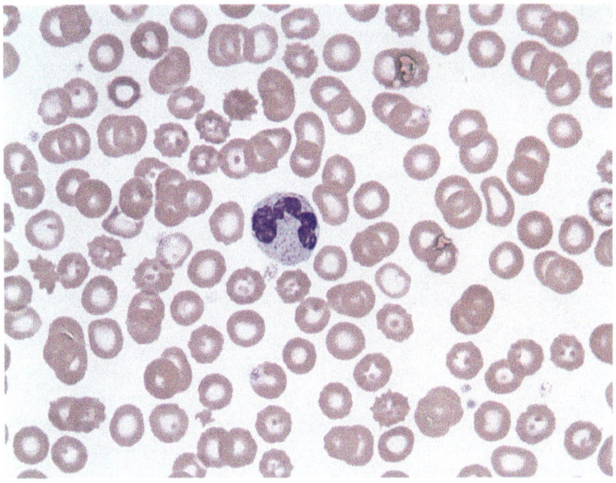

Figure 10.7 Neutrophil and platelets from a juvenile gray squirrel. Modified Wright's stain, 1000× magnification.

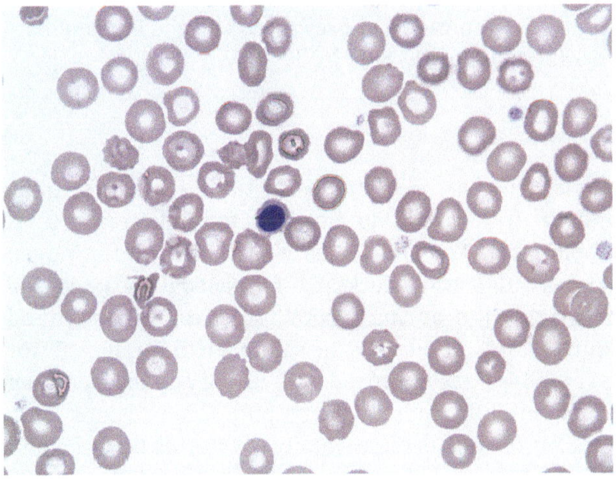

Figure 10.5 Nucleated erythrocytes and platelets from a juvenile gray squirrel. *Source:* Modified Wright's stain, 1000x magnification.

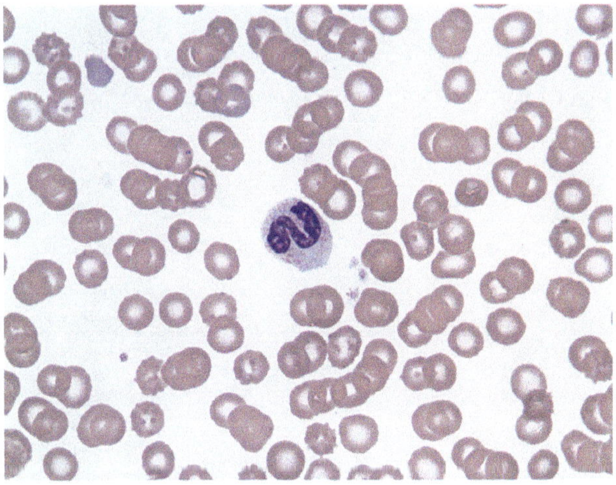

Figure 10.8 Neutrophil and platelets from a juvenile gray squirrel. Modified Wright's stain, 1000× magnification.

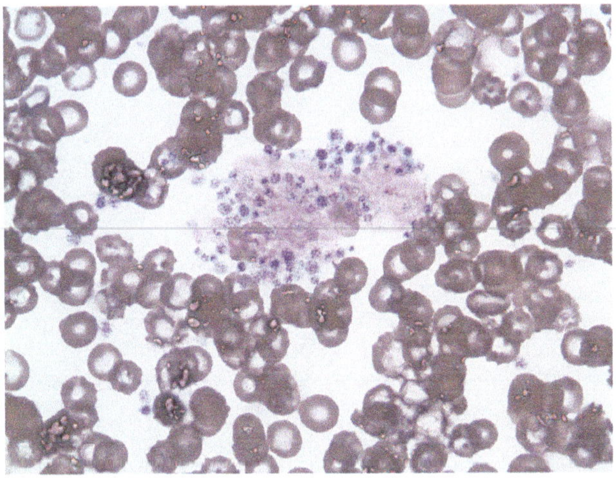

Figure 10.6 Platelet raft from a juvenile gray squirrel. Modified Wright's stain, 1000× magnification.

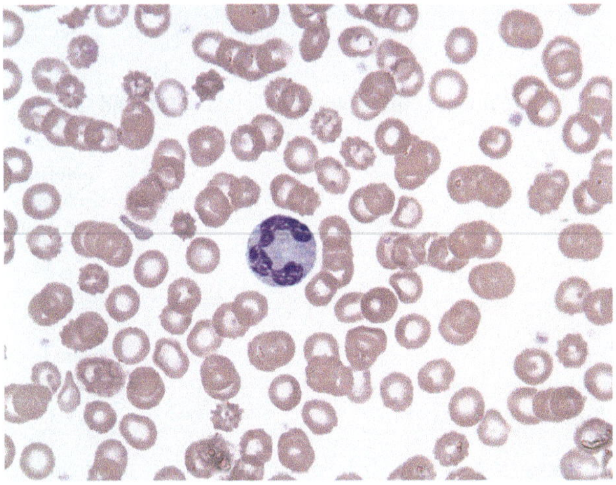

Figure 10.9 Neutrophil and platelets from a juvenile gray squirrel. Modified Wright's stain, 1000× magnification.

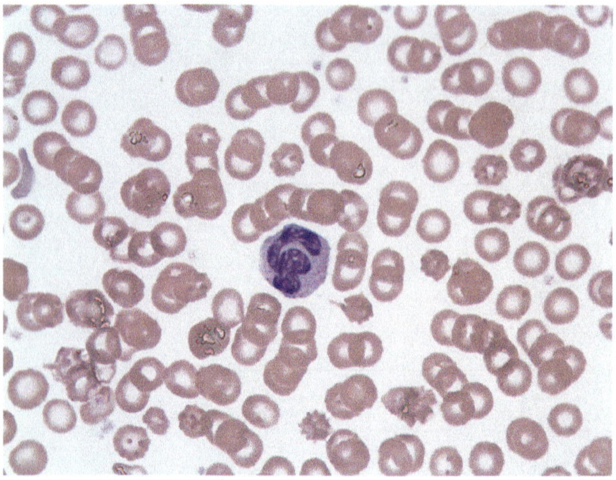

Figure 10.10 Neutrophil and platelets from a juvenile gray squirrel. Modified Wright's stain, 1000× magnification.

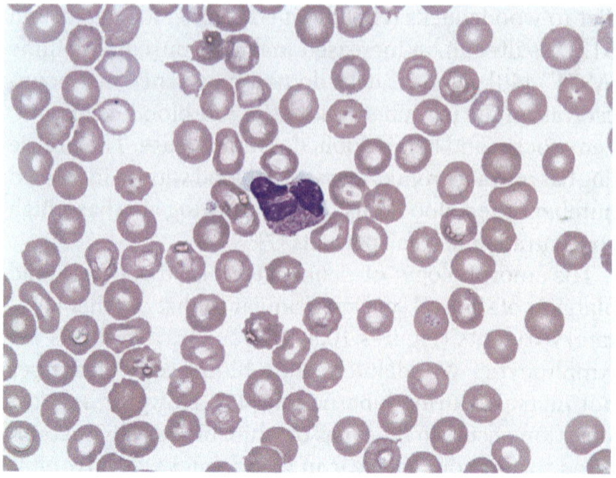

Figure 10.12 Eosinophil from a juvenile gray squirrel. Modified Wright's stain, 1000× magnification.

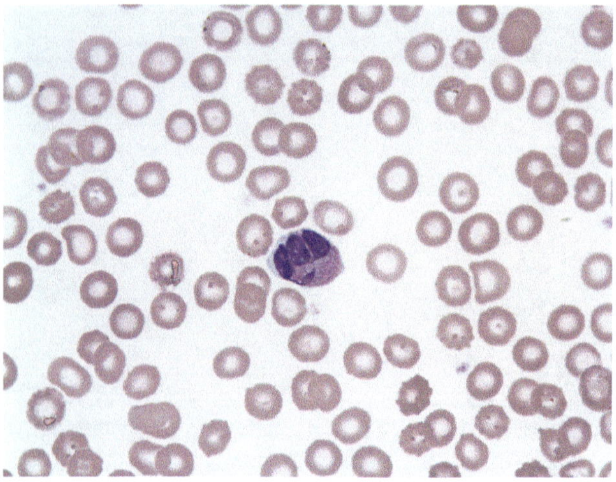

Figure 10.11 Eosinophil from a juvenile gray squirrel. Modified Wright's stain, 1000× magnification.

appears uncommon, the gray squirrel is the intermediate host for *Hepatozoon* spp. [6, 39, 44].

Hemostasis

Hemostasis has been studied in squirrels to determine optimal rodenticide applications for nuisance species (Table 10.3) [45]. The decrease or absence of fibrinogen in hibernating woodchucks may be related to the inhibition of coagulation during torpor [40]. Storage of ground squirrel red blood cells in saline medium at 5 °C for several days was improved with use of amiloride, a drug which inhibits sodium entry [46]. Transfusions have been performed experimentally in sciurids between and among species without apparent ill effect [47]; neither blood groups nor transfusion reactions have been identified in Sciuridae. However, cross-matching is still recommended prior to transfusion.

Table 10.3 Clotting times for apparently healthy ground squirrels [36, 45].

	Units	California ground squirrel *Spermophilus beecheyi*	Columbian ground squirrel *Spermophilus columbianus*		
	Seconds		Hibernating ($n = 6$)	Active ($n = 4$)	Temperature
Analyte		Average	Mean ± SD	Mean ± SD	°C
Prothrombin time (PT)		8.9	*275 ± 25*	*150 ± 75*	37
			4000 ± 500	*2600 ± 650*	5
Partial thromboplastin time (PTT)		10.1			
Protein induced by vitamin K absence or antagonists (PIVKA)		15.8			

Biochemical Panel

Overall, organ specific diagnostic assays of enzyme activity for use in squirrel species are poorly investigated or validated. Most information given here is based on physiologic studies. A recent postmortem review of 163 free-living red squirrels failed to document any associated antemortem clinicopathologic abnormalities associated with disease [35].

Liver Biomarkers

Many liver enzymes have been investigated in the Sciuridae when used as models for studies of nutrition, hibernation, or neoplasia (Table 10.4). In woodchucks on an increased-fat and reduced-lipotrope (choline, methionine, folic acid, and B12) diet, no hepatic injury or increased activities in serum markers of hepatic injury occurred unlike in rats [40]. Fasting bile acids have been determined for the prairie dog [48]. Muscle and pancreatic (endocrine and exocrine) specific enzymes have been determined only preliminarily in a few squirrel species. Their sensitivity and specificity for organ disease and dysfunction in sciurids remains largely unknown. Similarly, to our knowledge, cardiac or gastrointestinal specific biomarkers have not been investigated or reported from apparently healthy or clinical cases of sciurids experiencing illness or disease.

Renal Analytes

Blood urea nitrogen (BUN), creatinine, and uric acid in squirrel species have primarily been studied in squirrels through investigation of hydration and renal function during hibernation (Table 10.4). Their sensitivity and specificity for determination of renal dysfunction or insufficiency remains largely unknown in sciurids.

Pancreatic Biomarkers

Endocrine pancreatic function as well as sugar and fat metabolism are commonly researched topics in the many squirrel species which hibernate. Plasma insulin and body mass of females is at season minimum on emergence from hibernation (April), increases during pregnancy and lactation, further increases during fattening, and peaks in August, prior to hibernation. On emergence from hibernation, males are heavier and have about double the plasma insulin concentration. Plasma insulin decreased as did body mass during the mating period in males. Male plasma insulin concentrations increased in July and peaked in August (active, prehibernation times), coincident with the body mass maximum. Insulin acts anabolically to promote fat deposition in sciurids, to signal total body fat content, and to influence the transition from mass gain at the end of the active season to mass loss during hibernation [43].

Blood glucose concentrations are approximately 20 and 30% higher in red squirrels than in ground squirrels and chipmunks, respectively [50]. Pancreatic amylase activities decrease by about 41% in the hibernating ground squirrel (*Spermophilus tridecemlineatus*) from 41 ± 9 (mean ± SE) U/mg in active squirrels. However, plasma amylase concentrations were not determined in this study [51]. Similarly, pancreatic lipase is genetically encoded in multiple areas of the genome of this squirrel [2]. However, the utility of amylase or lipase for assessing disease or dysfunction in the pancreas or other organs of squirrel species remains uninvestigated.

Lipids

Lipids and lipoproteins have been characterized in Sciuridae based on studies of hibernation and as animal models for the study of cholesterol cholelithiasis [25, 26]. The apoproteins of prairie dog low-density lipoprotein (LDL) and high-density lipoprotein (HDL) differ structurally from those of dogs and humans. The prairie dog has lower serum values for cholesterol, VLDL, and LDL cholesterol than humans. In the prairie dog, HDL cholesterol consists of 67% of the total cholesterol concentration, and LDL:HDL is 0.3 [7]. Leptin and fatty acids have been evaluated in the free-living golden-mantled ground squirrel (*Callospermophilus lateralis*) [40, 69]. Serum values of lipid and cholesterol increased in hibernating woodchucks. Seasonal changes in plasma lipids may be more pronounced in animals at higher elevations [13]. Lactating females have the highest plasma lipids [13].

Electrolytes

Water balance studies have been performed in gray and red squirrels, prairie dogs, other ground squirrels, and the marmot regarding hibernation (Table 10.4) [53–55]. Many hibernating sciurids increase their plasma osmolality to accommodate hibernation [53–55]. The prairie dog has a higher TCO_2 concentration with a slightly increased potassium concentration than that found in humans. The anion gap is 12 with a calculated serum osmolality of 316 mOSM/L in the prairie dog (*C. ludovicianus*) [7].

Protein

In Belding's ground squirrel *(Urocitellus beldingi)*, plasma protein fractions and total plasma protein vary seasonally (Table 10.4). The lowest protein levels occur in early Spring during the first weeks of emergence from hibernation and may to relate to circulating red blood cell (RBC) regulation [13]. The prealbumin protein fraction could not be detected in all animals and varied with season and locale. When present, the prealbumin fraction constituted 5%–9% of the total protein. Hibernation-specific proteins occur in active ground squirrels (Asian chipmunks (*Tamias asiaticus*)) which hibernate, but not in nonhibernator tree squirrels [17]. The decrease or absence of fibrinogen in hibernating woodchucks *(M. morax)* could relate to blood clot inhibition during torpor [70]. Acute phase reactant proteins have been identified in Richardson's ground squirrel and include

Table 10.4 Biochemical data from healthy squirrel species.

Species		Persian squirrel (*Sciurus anomalus*) [6]	Gray squirrel *Sciurus carolinensis*	Black-tailed Prairie dog *(Cynomys ludovicianus)* [7, 8, 48] *White-tailed prairie dog* *Cynomus leucurus* [49]	Other squirrels [50] Arctic ground squirrel Thirteen-lined ground squirrel *Citellu tridecemlineatus* [15] Belding ground squirrel *Spermophilus beldingii beldingii* [13]	Woodchucks and marmots *Marmota flaviventris*
	Animals sampled	30 Ħ	7 180 [10], 5♂ 7♀ [12]	18–20¥ [8] 45 wild caught Ħ [49] 8 Ħ [7] 16 Ħ, 10♂ 16♀ 6–54 m [48]	150–159 ℷ April–July [13] 72–76 ℷ *Hibernating and active. September, November, December, February* [15]	Juvenile Ħ [25] *Adult 5* Ħ [41]
	Data Format	Median (min–max)		Mean ± SD (range) {Mean (2SEM)} *Mean (SEM)* *Mean (range)* [48]	Range [15]	Mean ± SD [25] Range of mean ± SD [41]
Analyte (abbreviation)	**Units, SI (conventional)**					
Aspartate (AST) transaminase (aminotransferase)	U/l= (IU/l)	6 [3–28]		37.5 ± 62.2 (5.00–242)¥ 35 ± 11(21–63) [49] 74.9 ± 9.3 [7]		42.0 ± 20.3 [25]
Alanine (ALT) transaminase	U/l = (IU/l)			43.9 ± 55.53 (8.00–222)¥ 39 ± 33(16–152)28 [49] 25.0 ± 16.2 [7]		3.2 ± 0.71 [25]
Gamma glutamyl transferase (GGT)	U/l = (IU/l)			1.17 ± 0.51 (0.00–2.00)¥ 10.1 ± 1.20 [7]		3.8 ± 1.68 [25]
Alkaline phosphatase (ALP)	U/l = (IU/l]	18[14–27]		125 ± 76.14 (37.0–335)¥ 153 ± 60(84–280)28 [49] 73.7 ± 22.1 [7]		33.2 ± 17.0 [25]
Bilirubin, total	μmol/l (mg/dl)			2.74 ± 1.37 (1.71–5.13) [0.16 ± 0.08 (0.1–0.3)]¥ 5.13 ± 1.71(3.42–10.3) 0.3 ± 0.1(0.2–0.6)[28] 5.82 ± 6.18 (0.34 ± 0.36) [7]		
Bile acids	μmol/l			12.5 [2–24] [48]		
Creatinine (CK) phosphokinase	IU/l = (U/l)			5150 ± 9550 (284–31 500)		
Blood urea nitrogen (BUN)	mmol/l (mg/dl)	5.58 [4.54–7.28] (15.64 [12.7–20.4])	1.43–24.99 (4–70) [10]	2.17 ± .63(1.06–3.30) (24.5 ± 7.10(12.0–37.0)¥ 2.29 ± 0.26 (1.95–2.74) 26 ± 3(22–31) [49] 2.82 ± 0.65 (32.0 ± 7.40) [7] *12.1(0.9)* (136 (10.2)) [49]		6.43–12.9 (0.18–0.36) [41]

Creatinine	μmol/l (mg/dl)	388.3 [356.8–419.9] (4.392 [4.036–4.750])		[0.7 ± 0.14(0.50–1.00)] mmol/L ¥ [0.6 ± 0.1(0.4–0.8)] mmol/L [49] 0.54 ± 0.17 mmol/L [7] *[60.4(5.6) μM]*		0.0619+/−8.93 [0.7+/−101]
Uric acid	μmol/l (mg /dl)	0.07 [0.06–0.08] (1.12 [1.009–1.34])	0.03–0.14 (0.504–2.35)			
Calcium	mmol/l (mg /dl)	1.88 [1.78–2.06] (7.53 [7.13–8.26])	1.80–3.61 (7.0–14.5) [10]	2.20 ± .11 (2.05–2.47) (8.82 ± 0.43(8.20–9.90)¥ 2.24 ± 0.17 (2.00–2.75) 9.0 ± 0.7(8–11) [49] 2.27 ± 0.10 (9.10 ± 0.40) [7]	2.70 ± 0.1 (10.8 ± 0.4) [15]	
Inorganic phosphorus	mmol/l (mg/dl)	1.76 [2.16–2.17] (5.46 [3.91–6.73])	0.99–7.00 (3.1–21.8) [10]	2.04 ± 0.40 (1.23–8.2) (6.32 ± 1.22(3.80–8.20)])¥ 2.03 ± 0.29 (6.30 ± 0.90) [7]		
Magnesium	mmol/l Mg/dl	0.62 [0.50–0.87] (1.5 [1.22–2.11])	0.22–0.91 (0.54–2.21)	0.921 ± 0.08 (0.78–1.11) *(2.24 ± 0.2 (1.90–2.70))*	1.36 ± 0.07 (3.3 ± 0.18) [15]	
Amylase	IU/l	545.2 [523.5–616.1]		133.5 ± 44.0 (75.0–214)		
Lipase	IU/l			84.6 ± 34.0 (40.0–160)		
Glucose	mmol/l (mg/dl)	5.93 [4.94–6.92] (106 [89–125])	5.8 ± 0.6 (105 ± 11) ♂ [10] 7.9 ± 0.6 (142 ± 10.8) ♀ [10] 1.39–14.15 [10] 3.83–9.82 69–177) ♂ [12] 2.22–8.05 40–145 ♀ [12]	8.44 ± 2.21 (5.55–13.1) (152.3 ± 39.8 (100–236)]¥ [50 ± 13(28–84) [49] 17.7 ± 4.97 (318 ± 89.6) [7] {9.8(0.8) (176 (14.4)) WTPD} {11.5(0.7) (207 (12.7)) BTPD} [49]	Red squirrel [50] 7.4 ± 0.9 (133 ± 16.2) ♂ 6.4 ± 0.7 (115 ± 12.6) ♀ Chipmunk [50] 5.4 ± 0.4 (97.3 ± 7.2) ♂ 5.2 ± 0.8 93.7 ± 14.4 ♀ Ground Squirrel [50] 5.1 ± 0.4 (91.9 ± 7.2) ♂ 6.0 ± 0.5 (108.1 ± 9.0) ♀ 5.66–10.8 (102–194♂)] [15]	
Cholesterol	mmol/l (mg/dl)	5.1 [4.7–5.5] (197 [182–212])	3.21–11.60 (124–448) [10] 3.10–4.6 (119.8–178) [12] ♂ 2.58–4.47 (99.8–173.0) [12] ♀	3.36 ± 0.85 (2.09–5.43) 130 ± 33.0(81.0–210))¥ 2.70 ± 0.67 (104 ± 25.8) [7]	5.79 (224) [15]	6.12+/−1.57 (236.6+/−60.8)
Triglycerides	mmol/l (mg/dl)	4.21 [4.11–4.42] (373 [364–391])	0.23–5.60 (20.4–496)	1.02 ±.74 (0.32–2.54) (990.2 ± 65.7 (28.0–225))¥ 0.67 ± 0.42 (59.6 ± 37.6) [7]		
Sodium	mmol/l = (mEq/l)			144 ± 2.80(140–150)¥ 142 ± 1.6(139–145) [49]		148–153 n = 6 [41]
Potassium	mmol/l = (mEq/l)			4.97 ± 0.75 (3.70–6.70)¥ 6 ± 0.9(5–8) [49]		4.12–7.63 [41]

(Continued)

Table 10.4 (Continued)

Species		Persian squirrel (*Sciurus anomalus*) [6]	Gray squirrel *Sciurus carolinensis*	Black-tailed Prairie dog *(Cynomys ludovicianus)* [7, 8, 48] *White-tailed prairie dog* *Cynomus leucurus* [49]	Other squirrels [50] Arctic ground squirrel Thirteen-lined ground squirrel *Citellu tridecemlineatus* [15] Belding ground squirrel *Spermophilus beldingii beldingii* [13]	Woodchucks and marmots *Marmota flaviventris*
	Animals sampled	30 Ħ	7 180 [10], 5♂ 7♀ [12]	18–20¥ [8] 45 wild caught Ħ [49] 8 Ħ [7] 16 Ħ, 10♂ 16♀ 6–54 m [48]	150–159 ϡ April–July [13] 72–76 ϡ *Hibernating and active.* *September, November, December, February* [15]	Juvenile Ħ [25] *Adult 5* Ħ [41]
	Data Format	Median (min–max)		Mean ± SD (range) {Mean (2SEM)} *Mean (SEM)* *Mean (range)* [48]	Range [15]	Mean ± SD [25] Range of mean ± SD [41]
Analyte (abbreviation)	Units, SI (conventional)					
Chloride	mmol/l = (mEq/l)		80–155 [10]	103 ± 3.30(97.0–111)¥ 84 ± 2.2(79–88) [49]		
Total CO_2	mmol/l = (mEq/l)			28 ± 2.4(23–34) [49]		
Osmolality (calculated)	mOsm/kg			304 ± 5.97 (293–315)		1.80–5.42 [41]
Total protein	g/l (g/dl)	70.2 [67.2–73.3] (7.02 [6.72–7.33])	37–66 (3.7–6.6) [10]	0.64 ± 0.05 (0.54–0.75) (6.43 ± 0.54 (5.4–7.5))¥ 0.6 ± 0.03 (0.5–0.7) (6 ± 0.3(5–7)) [49]	[0.50–0.75] 5.0–7.5 *n* = 209	0.78 ± 0.04 (7.8 ± 0.42)
Albumin	g/l (g/dl)		26 ± 10 (2.6 ± 0.1)	0.31 ± .03 (0.24–0.36) 3.07 ± 0.31 (2.40–3.60)¥ 0.24 ± 0.03 (0.2–0.3) 2.4 ± 0.3(2–3) [49]		0.44 ± .13 (4.35 ± 1.29)
Globulin	g/l (g/dl)			(0.34 ± .06 (0.25–0.46)) [3.37 ± 0.56 (2.5–4.6)]		0.45 ± 0.04 (4.55 ± 0.35)
Albumin by EPH	% of Total protein				27–50 [13]	
Alpha-1 gobulin by EPH					4–18 [13]	
Alpha-2 globulin by EPH					4–23 [13]	
Beta globulin by EPH					13–21 [13]	
Gamma globulin by EPH					6–13 [13]	
Albumin: globulin	g/l (g/dl)			[0.9 ± 0.28 (0.00–1.3)]		0.71 ± 0.04

Key: Free living ϡ, Captive Ħ, Male ♂, Female ♀

α1-antitrypsin, α2 macroglobulin, ceruloplasmin, C-reactive protein, and serum amyloid A. Only α2 macroglobulin increased during hibernation, and serum clot assay data suggest this protein may decrease blood coagulation during hibernation [36].

Blood Gases

Blood gases have been extensively studied in many squirrel species in an attempt to understand the physiological processes of hibernation. Table 10.4 summarizes blood gas values obtained from squirrels in an awakened (prehibernatory or posthibernatory arousal) state. Changes expected during hibernation include decreased hemoglobin concentrations, venous pO_2, pCO_2 and arterial pCO_2 without a significant change in pH [24]. The healthy captive prairie dog has greater blood concentrations of TCO_2 concentrations than humans [7].

Vitamins, Minerals and Metals, Toxins

Vitamins

Many vitamins are effected by hibernation in squirrels [28, 65] (Table 10.5). Plasma vitamin C (ascorbic acid) and vitamin B5 (pantothenic acid) increase during hibernation, while carnitine esters are low. Tyrosine and methionine increase upon emergence from hibernation in spring [28]. Plasma vitamin C concentrations decrease upon arousal from hibernation in ground squirrels, suggesting that this vitamin may protect from oxidant injury during hibernation and the reperfusion of arousal [65]. Hemosiderosis from excessive iron accumulation or chronic inflammatory processes has been documented in squirrel species [15, 20]. However, the total iron binding capacity (TIBC), iron plasma concentrations, or other measures of blood iron storage have not been clinically evaluated in sciurids.

Minerals

Plasma mineral concentrations have received little clinical investigation in Sciuridae. Most knowledge summarized here is derived from physiologic studies of hibernation or other physiology (Table 10.6). Significant mineral loss indicates the importance of skeletal reserves of calcium during hibernation [66]. Females may need and choose sources of greater dietary intake of calcium [60]. Hibernating animals have increased plasma magnesium concentration than active animals [15]. The increase is greater in females than males during hibernation [31]. Plasma magnesium concentrations in the golden-mantled ground squirrel (*Citellus lateralis*) ranged from 2.0 to 5.2 mg/dl. Hibernating animals had increased concentrations compared to active animals, and females exhibited a greater increase than males [31]. In a related ground squirrel species (*Citellus tridecemlineatus*), magnesium increased in hibernating animals, independent of season. However, plasma calcium was not influenced by hibernation but increased in winter [15]. Calcitonin administration resulted in hypocalcaemia, hypophosphatemia, decreased serum acid phosphatase concentrations, and growth promotion in adult Indian palm squirrels (*Funambulus pennanti*) [37, 60].

Toxins

Serum components from multiple species of squirrels have been shown to inhibit rattlesnake venom proteases by limiting tissue necrosis and lethality [56, 57]. Lead toxicosis has been diagnosed postmortem in gray squirrels inhabiting a firing range; blood levels were not determined [19]. Although strychnine, chlorophacinone, and 1080 are commonly used for control of nuisance squirrel species, toxic blood levels have not been specifically determined for squirrel species [21, 32].

Hormones

A variety of hormones have been investigated in free-living and captive squirrel species usually on the basis of the weight and hormone cycle associated hibernation. Few studies provide information directly useful to the clinician (Table 10.7). As in other rodents, both cortisol and corticosterone may be active hormones in these species [28]. In the free-living artic ground squirrel (*Spermophilus parryii*), cortisol is the primary glucocorticoid; corticosterone was below detectable levels in most animals [58]. Fecal cortisol and androgen metabolites have been measured in a number of squirrel species and may vary depending on multiple factors including diet and testicular location [61]. In free-living golden-mantled ground squirrels (*Spermophilus saturatus*),

Table 10.5 Select plasma vitamins of free-living sciurids (mean) [28, 65].

Analyte	Species	Artic ground squirrel *Spermophilus parryii*	n	Thirteen-lined ground squirrel *Spermophilus tridecemlineatus*	n
Vitamin C (Ascorbic Acid) μM	*Hibernating*	180–250	8	(150)	7
	Euthermic	43.2 ± 4.7	10	(200)	8

Table 10.6 Select hormones and steroids of squirrel species.

Analyte		Species				
		Golden-mantled ground squirrels [43] *(Spermophilus saturatus)*	Belding's ground squirrel [29] *(Spermophilus beldingi)*	Artic ground squirrel [58] *(Spermophilus parryii)*	Richardson's ground squirrels [63] *Spermophilus richardsoni*	Woodchuck [71] *Marmota monax*
Animal Info		ɣ♂♀ nonhibernating April–August	ɣÓ♂♀ July–August	ɣ☂, ☼	Ħ & ɣ Assay via RIA	Ħ
Data type	Units SI (Standard)	Mean range N = 169	Mean range *N* = 6–50	Range of graphed means N = 2–300	Range N = 5–10	
Cortisol	ng/ml	10–26		150–175 Ó ♂ ♀ 255–275 Φ ♂, Lactating ♀ 265–300 ∞ ♂, Pregnant ♀		
Corticosterone	ng/ml	6–15	28–43	8.05 +/− 1.63 n = 58 ♂ 23.8+/− 2.47 n = 13 ♂ below detectable n = 45 ♂ >100 n = 2 ♀		
Insulin	μU/ml	16–50	8–29			
Total T3 3,5,3′-triiodo-thyronine (T_3)	nmol/L (ng/dl)				1.53 -3.07 (100–200) nonhibernators 7.68–9.22 (500–600) hibernators	3.10 ± 0.34 (202 ± 22) ☂ 0.69 ± 0.41 (45 ± 27) ☼ 2.00±0.18 (130±12) 🍂 6.63 ± 0.49 (437 ± 32) ❄
Free T3	pmol/L (ng/dl)					7.83±0.61 (0.51±0.04) ☂ 2.46 ± 1.54 (0.16 ± 0.10) ☼ 3.84±0.31 (0.25±0.02) 🍂 0.52 ± 0.046 (0.034 ± 0.003) ❄
T4 L-thyroxine (T_4)	nmol/L (μg/dL)				12.9–38.6 (1.0–3.0) nonhibernators 57.9–96.5 (4.5–7.5) hibernators	5.4 ± 0.6 (5.4 ± 0.6) ☂ 2.3 ± 1.0 (2.3 ± 1.0) ☼ 3.2 ± 1.0 (3.2 ± 1.0) 🍂
Free T4	pmol/L (ng/dl)					38.62 ± 5.15 (3.0 ± 0.4) ☂ 15.45 ± 6.43 (1.2 ± 0.5) ☼ 16.73 ± 2.57 (1.3 ± 0.2) 🍂

Key: Free living ɣ, Captive Ħ, Male ♂, Female ♀
Spring ☂, Summer ☼, Fall 🍂, Winter ❄

corticosterone levels were low in both sexes upon emergence from hibernation in spring and increased throughout the active season; female levels exceeded those of males during lactation. In both sexes, cortisol concentrations decreased in the first half of the season, but increased to a maximum by season end, coincident with peak body mass. Cortisol appears to have an anabolic influence on seasonal fattening in this sciurid [43]. Live trapping of free-living artic ground squirrels elicited a strong stress response in both sexes; breeding males and females trapped in spring had free cortisol concentrations 4 and 34 times, respectively, those of baseline

Table 10.7 Urinalysis values of Sciuridae.

Parameter	Species	Gray squirrels [10] *Sciurus carolinensis*	White-tailed prairie dog *Cynomys leucurus* [49]	Black-tailed prairie dog *Cynomys ludovicianus*	Arctic ground squirrel [25] *Citellus parryi barrowensis*	Marmot [41] *Marmota flaviventris*
	Data	**Range**	**Mean ± 2 SEM**	**Mean ± 2 SEM**	**Mean ± SD**	**Range ± Range of SE**
	Animals sampled	***N* = 180** ***(comments)***	***N* = 8**	***N* = 8**	**Ħ2 wks, 1 y**	***n* = 6 (125 samples) April–Sept Ħ**
Parameter	**Units**					
pH	pH	6.0–8.0, 180				
Protein	mg/dl	Trace *(100 for 79)*				
Ketones	±	Minimal *(+ for 47)*				
Bilirubin	±	• *(+ for 1)*				
Blood hemoglobin	±	• *(+ for 2)*				
Osmolality	Mosml		2382.0 ± 224.0	13 260 ± 216.0		1978–2043 ± 473
Potassium	mmol/L = mEq/L		435 ± 42.0	214 ± 33.0		1.5–4.5
Sodium	mmol/L = mEq/L					2.8–0.4
Urea	mmolar (mg/ml)		1908 ± 173.0	1138.0 ± 164.0	mg/dl/h 52.4, 52.9	(13.63 ± 0.93–26.12 ± 1.44)
Uric acid	mg/dl/h				1.6 ± 0.8, 1.4 ± 0.5	
Urine flow	ml/day					1.068 ± 2.0–110.7 ± 18.16
	ml/kg/day					1–23
Creatinine	mg/dl/h (mg/ml)				1.7 ± 0.9, 1.9 ± 0.8	(0.75–4.31 ± 0.05–0.63)
Ammonia	mmolar		48.3 ± 2.8	71.2 ± 5.4		

Key: Free living ϡ, Captive Ħ, Male ♂, Female ♀

Table 10.8 Infectious diseases of Sciuridae [8].

Pathogen	Disease	Susceptible species
Bartonella spp.	Carrion disease, trench fever, cat-scratch disease, bacillary angiomatosis, peliosis hepatis, chronic bacteremia, endocarditis, lymphadenopathy	Prairie dog
Blastomyces dermatitidis	Blastomycosis	Prairie dog
Borrelia burgdorferi sensu lato	Lyme disease	Western gray squirrel Eastern chipmunk
Clostridium difficile	Clostridiosis	Prairie dog
Encephalomyocarditis Virus	Mengovirus, cardiovirus	Red squirrels
Francisella tularensis	Tularemia	Prairie dog, fox and gray squirrel
Leptospira spp.	Leptospirosis: multiple serovars, kirschneri, ballum, grippotyphosa	Southern flying squirrel, gray squirrel, fox squirrel
Orthopox viruses	Monkey pox, small pox, vaccinia	Prairie dog, African tree squirrels and rope squirrels
Rickettsia spp.	Spotted fever, typhus	Prairie dog, southern flying squirrel
Sporothrix schenckii	Sporotrichosis	Sciurid
Yersinia pestis	Bubonic, pneumonic, septicemic plague	Prairie dog, ground squirrels, fox squirrels

animals. Free cortisol concentrations were similar in females and juvenile males, measuring about half those in adult males [59].

Many sciurid species undergo seasonal changes in thyroid hormones during hibernation (Table 10.8) [41]. Wide seasonal alterations in thyroid hormone concentrations and plasma protein binding are likely adaptations that influence the metabolic rate and the hibernation process in the woodchuck and other sciurids [63]. To the best of the author's knowledge, neither hyperthyroidism nor hypothyroidism has been reported in captive or free-living sciurids.

Plasma dehydroepiandrosterone (DHEA) is an androgen precursor secreted by the adrenal cortex that has been examined in free-living red squirrels (*T. hudsonicus*). Plasma DHEA levels in males and females reached concentrations of 16.95 ng/ml in males and 14.6 ng/ml in females and varied with season, year, testicular mass, and population size. Increased plasma DHEA post administration of Adrenocorticotropic hormone (ACTH, also adrenocorticotropin, corticotropin) suggests that this hormone is secreted by the squirrel adrenal gland. Live trapping of free-living arctic ground squirrels increased testosterone concentrations in males over those found in samples from baseline males. Testosterone concentrations in live-trapped animals also differed among male classes: nonreproductive males had concentrations of 64% of those in breeding males and 10 times those in juveniles [59].

Urinalysis

Urine collection and urinary values from apparently healthy gray squirrels, fox squirrels, Columbian ground squirrels (*Spermophilus columbianus*), and marmots obtained by free catch and by cystocentesis have been described (Table 10.4). Many squirrel species have the ability to regulate urine and plasma osmolality via urea and sodium to facilitate hibernation [11, 30, 49, 53–55]. In marmots (*Marmota flaviventris* $n = 6$), water intake, urine excretion, sodium and potassium intake, and urinary excretion decrease as hibernation approaches [46]. The glomerular filtration rate of white-tailed and black-tailed prairie dogs is similar as is the urine urea concentration, averaging 1000 and 1500 mmol/L, respectively [67]. Urinalysis of apparently healthy free-living gray squirrels includes trace proteinuria, a pH from 6.0–8.0, and no ketones. The urine volume of the arctic ground squirrel was greater early in captivity (two weeks captivity 3.3 ± 1.7 ml/h or 79.2 ml/day) than later in captivity (2.8 ± 1.2 ml/h or 67.2 ml/day) [25].

Serology and PCR Useful in Sciurids

As rodents, sciurid species are affected by many zoonotic pathogens (Table 10.8) [22, 33, 34, 52, 64]. Testing is as for other rodents, companion animals, and wildlife species and for most diseases is available at either veterinary diagnostic laboratories or public health laboratories.

References

1 Shivatcheva, T.M. and Hadjioloff, A.I. (1987). Seasonal involution of gut-associated lymphoid tissue of the European ground squirrel. *Developmental & Comparative Immunology* 11 (4): 791–799.

2 Squire, T.L. and Andrews, M.T. (2003). Pancreatic triacylglycerol lipase in a hibernating mammal. I. Novel genomic organization. *Physiological Genomics* 16 (1): 119–130.

3 Kreeger TJ, Arnemo JM. 4th edition: Handbook of Wildlife Chemical Immobilization. Published by author. 2007 448p.

4 Rasmussen, A.T. and Rusmussen, G.B. (1917). The volume of blood during hibernation and other periods of the year in the woodchuck (*Marmota monax*). *American Journal of Physiology* 44 (2): 132–148.

5 Svihla, A. and Bowman, H.C. (1952). Oxygen carrying capacity of the blood of dormant ground squirrels. *American Journal of Physiology* 171 (2): 479–481.

6 Asadi, F., Rostami, A., Asadian, P. et al. (2007). Serum biochemistry and hematology values and hemoglobin electrophoresis in Persian squirrels (*Sciurus anomalus*). *Veterinary Clinical Pathology* 36 (2): 188.

7 Broughton, G. (1992). Hematologic and blood chemistry data for the prairie dog (*Cynomys ludovicianus*). *Comparative Biochemistry and Physiology Part A: Physiology* 101 (4): 807–812.

8 Keckler, M.S., Gallardo-Romero, N.F., Langham, G.L. et al. (2010). Reference ranges for captive black-tailed prairie dogs (*Cynomys ludovicianus*). *Journal of the American Association for Laboratory Animal Science Physiologic* 49 (3): 274.

9 Armitage, K.B. (1983). Hematological values for free-ranging yellow-bellied Marmots. *Comparative Biochemistry and Physiology Part A: Physiology* 74A (1): 89–93.

10 Hoff, G.L., LE, M.E., Bigler, W.J. et al. (1976). Blood and urinary values in the gray squirrel. *Journal of Wildlife Diseases* 12: 349–352.

11 H Hoff, G.L., Lassing, E.B., Chan, M.S. et al. (1976). Hematologic values for free-ranging urban gray squirrels (*Sciurus carolinensis*). *American Journal of Veterinary Research* 37 (1): 99–101.

12 Guthrie, D.R., Mosby, H.S., and Osborne, J.C. (1966). Hematological values for the eastern gray squirrel (*Sciurus carolinensis*). *Canadian Journal of Zoology* 44 (2): 323–327.

13 Huang, S.N.Y. and Morton, M.L. (1976). Seasonal changes in plasma proteins and lipids in the belding ground squirrel (*Spermophilus beldingi* beldingi). *Comparative Biochemistry and Physiology Part A: Physiology* 54 (2): 239–243.

14 Juan-Sallés, C., Patrício, R., Garrido, J. et al. (2009). Disseminated Mycobacterium avium subsp. avium infection in a Captive Richardson's Ground Squirrel (*Spermophilus richardsonii*). *Journal of Exotic Pet Medicine* 18 (4): 306–310.

15 Kenny, A.D. and Musacchia, X.J. (1977). Influence of season and hibernation on thyroid calcitonin content and plasma electrolytes in the ground squirrel. *Comparative Biochemistry and Physiology Part A: Physiology* 57 (4): 485–489.

16 Kirkwood, T. (1931). Tularemia from the Fox Squirrel. *Journal of the American Medical Association* 96 (12): 941–942.

17 Kondo, N. and Kondo, J. (1992). Identification of novel blood proteins specific for mammalian hibernation. *Journal of Biological Chemistry* 267 (1): 473–478.

18 Leonhard, S., Jensen, K., Salkeld, D.J. et al. (2010). Distribution of the Lyme disease spirochete *Borrelia burgdorferi* in naturally and experimentally infected western gray squirrels (*Sciurus griseus*). *Vector-Borne and Zoonotic Diseases* 10 (5): 441–446.

19 Lewis, L.A., Poppenga, R.J., Davidson, W.R. et al. (2001). Lead toxicosis and trace element levels in wild birds and mammals at a firearms training facility. *Archives of Environmental Contamination and Toxicology* 41 (2): 208–214.

20 Magee, J.S. et al. (1989). Tularemia transmitted by Squirrel Bite. *The Pediatric Infectious Diseases Journal* 8 (2): 123–125.

21 Marsh, R.E., Schmidt, R.H., and Howard, W.E. (1987). Secondary hazards to coyotes of ground squirrels poisoned with 1080 or strychnine. *Wildlife Society Bulletin* 15 (3): 380–385.

22 Masuzawa, T. (2006). Leptospirosis in squirrels imported from United States to Japan. *Emerging Infectious Diseases* 12 (7): 1153–1155.

23 Mogharabi, F. and Haines, H. (1973). Dehydration and body fluid regulation in the thirteen-lined ground squirrel and laboratory rat. *American Journal of Physiology-Legacy Content* 224 (5): 1218–1222.

24 Musacchia, X.J. and Volkert, W.A. (1971). Blood gases in hibernating and active ground squirrels: HbO_2 affinity at 6 and 38C. *American Journal of Physiology-Legacy Content* 221 (1): 128–130.

25 Musacchia, X.J. and Wilber, C.G. (1952). Studies on the biochemistry of the arctic ground squirrel. *Journal of Mammalogy* 33 (3): 356–362.

26 Naito, H.K., Holzbach, R.T., and Corbusier, C. (1977). Characterization of serum lipids and lipoproteins of prairie dogs fed a chow diet or cholesterol-supplemented diet. *Experimental and Molecular Pathology* 27 (1): 81–92.

27 Naito, H.K. and Gerrity, R.G. (1979). Unusual resistance of the ground squirrel to the development of dietary-induced hypercholesterolemia and atherosclerosis. *Experimental and Molecular Pathology* 31 (3): 452–467.

28 Nelson, C.J., Otis, J.P., and Carey, H.V. (2010). Global analysis of circulating metabolites in hibernating ground squirrels. *Comparative Biochemistry and Physiology Part D: Genomics and Proteomics* 5 (4): 265–273.

29 Nunes, S., Muecke, E.M., and Holekamp, K.E. (2002). Seasonal effects of food provisioning on body fat, insulin, and corticosterone in free-living juvenile Belding's ground squirrels (*Spermophilus beldingi*). *Canadian Journal of Zoology* 80 (2): 366–371.

30 Passmore, J.C., Pfeiffer, E.W., and Templeton, J.R. (1975). Urea excretion in the hibernating Columbian ground squirrel (*Spermophilus columbianus*). *Journal of Experimental Zoology* 192 (1): 83–86.

31 Pengelley, E.T. and Chaffee, R.R.J. (1966). Changes in plasma magnesium concentration during hibernation in the golden-mantled ground squirrel (*Citellus lateralis*). *Comparative Biochemistry and Physiology* 17 (2): 673–681.

32 Proulx G. Field evidence of non-target and secondary poisoning by strychnine and chlorophacinone used to control Richardson's ground squirrels in southwest Saskatchewan. Proceedings Ninth Prairie Conserv Endang Species C. 2011; 128–134.

33 Saravanakumar, P.S., Eslami, P., and Zar, F.A. (1996). Lymphocutaneous Sporotrichosis associated with a squirrel bite: case report and review. *Clinical Infectious Diseases* 23 (3): 647–648.

34 Shotts, E.B. Jr., Andrews, C.L., and Harvey, T.W. (1975). Leptospirosis in selected wild mammals of the Florida panhandle and southwestern Georgia. *Journal of the American Veterinary Medical Association* 167 (7): 587–589.

35 Simpson, V.R., Hargreaves, J., Butler, H.M. et al. (2013). Causes of mortality and pathological lesions observed post-mortem in red squirrels (*Sciurus vulgaris*) in Great Britain. *BMC Veterinary Research* 9 (1): 229.

36 Srere, H.K., Belke, D., Wang, L.C., and Martin, S.L. (1995). Alpha 2-macroglobulin gene expression during hibernation in ground squirrels is independent of acute phase response. *American Journal of Physiology-Regulatory, Integrative and Comparative Physiology* 268 (6): R1507–R1512.

37 Swarup, K., Tewari, N.P., and Srivastav, A.K. (1980). Response of calcitonin cells, parathyroid glands and bone to prolonged calcitonin administration in the Indian palm squirrel, *Funambulus pennanti*. *Cells Tissues Organs* 106 (2): 180–191.

38 Thorington, R.W. and Darrow, K. (2000). Anatomy of the squirrel wrist: bones, ligaments, and muscles. *Journal of Morphology* 246 (2): 85–102.

39 Watkins, Z. and BM, N.F. (2003). *Hepatozoon griseisciuri* in grey squirrel (*Sciurus carolinensis*): changes of blood leucocyte numbers resulting from infection. *Parasitology* 127 (02): 115–120.

40 Boyd, J.N., Graham, E.S., Graham, T.C. et al. (1985). A comparison of the response of woodchucks and rats to variations in dietary lipotrope and lipid content. *The Journal of Nutrition* 115 (9): 1136–1146.

41 Zatzman, M.L., Thornhill, G.V., Ray, W.J. et al. (1984). Seasonal changes of food and water consumption and urine production of the marmot, *Marmota flaviventris*. *Comparative Biochemistry and Physiology Part A: Physiology* 77 (4): 735–743.

42 Hall, F.G. (1965). Hemoglobin and oxygen: affinities in seven species of Sciuridae. *Science* 148 (3675): 1350–1351.

43 Boswell, T., Woods, S.C., and Kenagy, G.J. (1994). Seasonal changes in body mass, insulin, and glucocorticoids of free-living golden-mantled ground squirrels. *General and Comparative Endocrinology* 96 (3): 339–346.

44 Ajayi, O.O., Ogwurike, B.A., and Ajayi, J.A. (2006). Blood protozoan parasites of rodents in Jos, Plateau State, Nigeria. *Animal Production Research Advances* 2 (4): 202–207.

45 Whisson, D.A. and Salmon, T.P. (2002). Effect of diphacinone on blood coagulation in *Spermophilus beecheyi* as a basis for determining optimal timing of field bait applications. *Pest Management Science* 58 (7): 736–738.

46 Zhao, Z. and Willis, J.S. (1989). Maintenance of cation gradients in cold-stored erythrocytes of guinea pig and ground squirrel: improvement by amiloride. *Cryobiology* 26 (2): 132–137.

47 Abbotts, B., Wang, L.C.H., and Glass, J.D. (1979). Absence of evidence for a hibernation "trigger" in blood dialyzate of Richardson's ground squirrel. *Cryobiology* 16 (2): 179–183.

48 Wyre, N.R. and Eshar, D. (2015). Serum bile acids concentration in captive black-tailed prairie dogs (*Cynomys ludovicianus*). *Comparative Clinical Pathology* 25: 1–5.

49 Harlow, H.J. and Buskirk, S.W. (1991). Comparative plasma and urine chemistry of fasting white-tailed prairie dogs (*Cynomys leucurus*) and American martens (*Martes americana*): representative fat-and lean-bodied animals. *Physiological Zoology* 64 (5): 1262–1278.

50 Barker, J.M. and Boonstra, R. (2005). Preparing for winter: divergence in summer autumn hematological profiles from representative species of the squirrel family. 142: 32–42.

51 Balslev-Clausen, A., McCarthy, J.M., and Carey, H.V. (2003). Hibernation reduces pancreatic amylase levels in ground squirrels. *Comparative Biochemistry and Physiology Part A: Molecular & Integrative Physiology* 134 (3): 573–578.

52 Avashia SB, Petersen JM, Lindley CM et al. Emerging infectious diseases. First reported prairie dog–to-human tularemia transmission, Texas, 2002. 2004; 10(3):483.

53 Bakko, E.B. (1976). A field water balance study of gray squirrels (*Sciurus carolinensis*) and red squirrels (*Tamiasciurus hudsonicus*). *Comparative Biochemistry and Physiology Part A: Physiology* 51 (4): 759–768.

54 Bakko, E.B. (1977). Field water balance performance in prairie dogs (*Cynomys leucurus* and *C. ludovicianus*). *Comparative Biochemistry and Physiology Part A: Physiology* 56 (3): 443–451.

55 Bakko, E.B. (1977). Influence of collecting techniques on estimate of natural renal function in red squirrels. *American Midland Naturalist* 97 (2): 502–504.

56 Biardi, J.E. and Coss, R.G. (2011). Rock squirrel (*Spermophilus variegatus*) blood sera affects proteolytic and hemolytic activities of rattlesnake venoms. *Toxicon* 57 (2): 323–331.

57 Biardi, J.E., Coss, R.G., and Smith, D.G. (2000). California ground squirrel (*Spermophilus beecheyi*) blood sera inhibits crotalid venom proteolytic activity. *Toxicon* 38 (5): 713–721.

58 Boonstra, R., Hubbs, A.H., Lacey, E.A. et al. (2001). Seasonal changes in glucocorticoid and testosterone concentrations in free-living arctic ground squirrels from the boreal forest of the Yukon. *Canadian Journal of Zoology* 79 (1): 49–58.

59 Boonstra, R., Lane, J.E., Boutin, S. et al. (2008). Plasma DHEA levels in wild, territorial red squirrels: seasonal variation and effect of ACTH. *General and Comparative Endocrinology* 158 (1): 61–67.

60 Borges, R.M. (1990). Sexual and site differences in calcium consumption by the Malabar giant squirrel *Ratufa indica*. *Oecologia* 85 (1): 80–86.

61 Dantzer, B., McAdam, A.G., Palme, R. et al. (2011). How does diet affect fecal steroid hormone metabolite concentrations? An experimental examination in red squirrels. *General and Comparative Endocrinology* 174 (2): 124–131.

62 Dawe, A.R. and Spurrier, W.A. (1972). The blood-borne "trigger" for natural mammalian hibernation in the 13-lined ground squirrel and the woodchuck. *Cryobiology* 9 (3): 163–172.

63 Demeneix, B.A. and Henderson, N.E. (1978). Serum T4 and T3 in active and torpid ground squirrels, *Spermophilus richardsoni*. *General and Comparative Endocrinology* 35 (1): 77–85.

64 Diesch, S.L., Crawford, R.P., McCulloch, W.F. et al. (1967). Human leptospirosis acquired from squirrels. *The New England Journal of Medicine* 276 (15): 838–842.

65 Drew, K.L., Osborne, P.G., Frerichs, K.U. et al. (1999). Ascorbate and glutathione regulation in hibernating ground squirrels. *Brain Research* 851 (1): 1–8.

66 Galster, W. and Morrison, P. (1976). Seasonal changes in body composition of the arctic ground squirrel, *Citellus undulatus*. *Canadian Journal of Zoology* 54 (1): 74–78.

67 Harlow, H.J. and Braun, E.J. (1995). Kidney structure and function of obligate and facultative hibernators: the white-tailed prairie dog (*Cynomys leucurus*) and the black-tailed prairie dog (*Cynomys ludovicianus*). *Journal of Comparative Physiology B* 165 (4): 320–328.

68 Havera, S.P. and Smith, K.E. (1979). A nutritional comparison of selected fox squirrel foods. *The Journal of Wildlife Management* 43 (3): 691–704.

69 Healy, J.E. and Florant, G.L. (2012). *Living in a Seasonal World. Ghrelin, leptin, and fatty acids in free-living Callospermophilus lateralis (golden-mantled ground squirrels)*, 519–529. Berlin Heidelberg: Springer.

70 Wenberg, G.M., Holland, J.C., and Sewell, J. (1973). Some aspects of the hematology and immunology of the hibernating and non-hibernating woodchuck (*Marmota monax*). *Comparative Biochemistry and Physiology Part A: Physiology* 46 (3): 513–521.

71 Young, R.A., Danforth, E.J.R., Vagenakis, A.G. et al. (1979). Seasonal Variation and the Influence of Body Temperature on Plasma Concentrations and Binding of Thyroxine and Triiodothyronine in the Woodchuck. *Endocrinology* 104 (4): 996–999.

72 Biggs, C.D. (2007). Establishing genetic and physiological baselines for the black-tailed prairie dog (*Cynomys ludovicianus*). University of North Texas.

11

Marsupials

Rosemary J. Booth BVSc, MS

David Fleay Wildlife Park, SE Regions Terrestrial Parks, Queensland Parks & Wildlife Service Department of Environment & Resource Management (DERM), Queensland, Australia

Introduction

Clinical pathology is an essential component of a full clinical evaluation of marsupials. Care must be taken during interpretation using reference values derived from a few individuals from multiple collections using different laboratories. Consideration must also be given to differences in variables associated with sex, age, method of restraint, and season. Some species are adapted to specialized environments and will have corresponding features such as a high hematocrit in burrowing, hypoxia-adapted species. For many species of marsupials, reference values are lacking, so reliance on reference values for closely related species is required. Consequently, we encourage clinicians to take advantage of all opportunities to collect samples to develop reference values for species where none exist. Clinicopathologic responses to disorders and disease in marsupials are similar to those of other mammals. Therefore, extrapolation of clinical pathology interpretation from domestic animals is often appropriate.

Species

Marsupials are a diverse group of non-placental mammals that belong to the Infraclass Marsupialia. They are characterized by a short gestation period and prolonged lactation with young carried in a pouch, in most species. The majority of marsupial species occur in Australasia and include the orders: Dasyuromorphia (carnivorous marsupials), Peramelemorphia (bandicoots and bilbies), Notoryctemorphia (marsupial moles, *Notoryctes typhlops*, and *Notoryctes caurinus*), and the Diprotodontia (kangaroos, wallabies, wombats, koala, possums, and gliders). The remaining marsupials occur in the Americas and include the orders Didelphimorphia (opossums), Paucituberculata (shrew opossums), and the Microbiotheria (sole species: Monito del Monte, *Dromiciops gliroides*). Over 300 species of marsupial are extant; only common examples of the main orders are included in this chapter (Table 11.1).

Sample Collection

For blood collection from marsupials, the lateral tail vein, femoral vein, jugular vein, cranial vena cava, cephalic vein, radial vein, cranial tibial vein, and the medial tibial artery may be used (Table 11.2). Behavioral, physical, or chemical restraint may be required to facilitate blood collection. Restraint techniques and protocols have been reviewed [43, 49]. For all marsupials, the femoral vein is accessible in the vascular lacuna (the opening between the thigh muscles and abdomen) of most mammals (Figure 11.9 and 11.10). Clip the area if necessary and wet with alcohol. Palpate and/or visualize the femoral pulse. The femoral vein lies just anterior to the femoral artery and the saphenous nerve. Angle the syringe and needle at 45° and direct the needle just caudal to the artery, then apply gentle negative pressure. The femoral vein is very superficial at this site. If arterial puncture occurs instead of venipuncture, the blood will be bright red and rapidly fill the syringe. In this case, minimize hematoma formation by applying pressure firmly to the site post collection and for longer than required post venipuncture, generally a minimum of 2 min.

For macropods (kangaroos and wallabies), the lateral tail vein is the most common site for venipuncture and is larger at the base of the tail on the lateral aspect (Figures 11.1 and 11.2). The vein is typically easy to visualize, especially if the fur is clipped, and may branch near the tail base. In small macropods, it is more difficult to visualize, but can often be palpated. A tourniquet or

Exotic Animal Laboratory Diagnosis, First Edition. Edited by J. Jill Heatley and Karen E. Russell.

Table 11.1 Species of marsupial reviewed in this chapter.

Common name	Scientific name	Diet
Brush-tailed possum	*Trichosurus vulpecula*	Omnivore
Brush-tailed rock wallaby	*Petrogale penicillata*	Herbivore
Chuditch	*Dasyurus geoffroii*	Carnivore
Common wombat	*Vombatus ursinus*	Grazing herbivore
Eastern gray kangaroo	*Macropus giganteus*	Grazing herbivore
Gray short-tailed opossum	*Monodelphis domestica*	Omnivore
Koala	*Phascolarctos cinereus*	Folivore
Matschie's tree kangaroo	*Dendrolagus matschiei*	Arboreal herbivore
North American opossum	*Didelphis virginiana*	Omnivore
Parma wallaby	*Macropus parma*	Browsing herbivore
Red kangaroo	*Macropus rufus*	Grazing herbivore
Red-necked wallaby	*Macropus rufogriseus*	Grazing herbivore
Southern hairy-nosed wombat	*Lasiorhinus latifrons*	Grazing herbivore
Sugar glider	*Petaurus breviceps*	Exudative omnivore
Tammar wallaby	*Macropus eugenii*	Browsing herbivore
Tasmanian devil	*Sarcophilus harrisii*	Carnivore

digital pressure is used to raise the vein. This vein is particularly suited for blood collection with manual restraint. The macropod can be physically restrained in lateral recumbency or held in a heavy-duty cloth bag with the tail exteriorized. Alternative blood collection sites in chemically restrained macropods include the cranial tibial, jugular, cephalic, and femoral veins. The cranial tibial vein is found overlying the lateral aspect of the distal tibia (Figures 11.3 and 11.4).

For dasyurids, anesthesia is required for blood collection. The femoral, jugular, cephalic, and lateral saphenous veins are easily accessible in the larger dasyurids (e.g., Tasmanian devils, quolls). The ventral coccygeal vein can be useful in smaller dasyurids [25]. Insert a small-gauge needle perpendicular to the ventral surface of the tail until the ventrum of the vertebral body is reached. When the needle is slightly withdrawn, blood often fills the hub. Blood collection from the periorbital sinus is not acceptable [25].

For koalas, the cephalic vein is easily palpated when raised with a tourniquet or digital pressure (Figure 11.5). For zoo-based koalas that are frequently handled, behavioral conditioning can allow conscious blood collection while the koala sits in the fork of a tree or is gently restrained by an experienced keeper (Figure 11.8). A 23 gauge (g.) butterfly catheter allows for movement in the koala's forearm during collection. Aspiration of blood with a 3 ml syringe or smaller reduces the risk of collapsing a small vein with excess suction pressure (Figures 11.6 and 11.7). For larger volumes, the femoral vein can be used in anesthetized koalas (Figures 11.9 and 11.10).

For wombats, venipuncture typically requires sedation or anesthesia. Blood may be collected from the radial,

Table 11.2 Venipuncture sites in various marsupials.

Common name	Venipuncture site	Recommended restraint method
Kangaroos and wallabies *Macropus and Petrogale spp.*	Lateral tail vein	Manual restraint or anesthesia
	Cranial tibial vein	Anesthesia
Koala *Phascolarctos cinereus*	Cephalic	Behavioral restraint
	Femoral vein	Anesthesia
Opossum, North American *Didelphis virginiana*	Brachiocephalic vein	Anesthesia
	Jugular vein	Anesthesia
	Lateral tail vein	Manual restraint or anesthesia
	Ventral tail artery	Anesthesia
Sugar glider *Petaurus breviceps*	Cranial vena cava	Anesthesia
	Medial saphenous artery	Anesthesia
Tasmanian devil *Sarcophilus harrisii*	Cephalic or jugular vein	Anesthesia
Wombats *Vombatus* and *Lasiorhinus spp*	Radial vein	Anesthesia

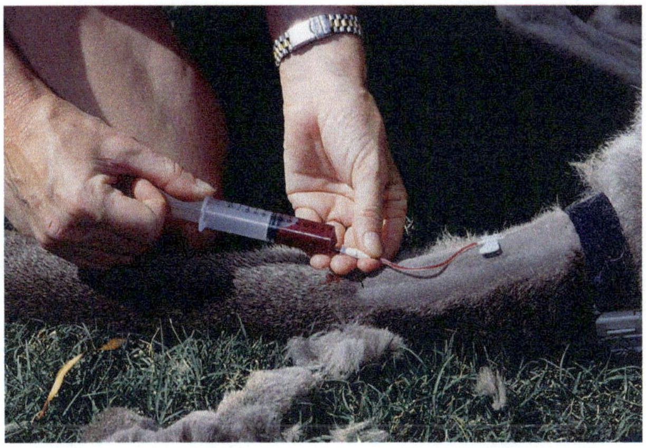

Figure 11.1 Venipuncture from the lateral tail vein of a chemically restrained eastern gray kangaroo, *Macropus giganteus*, using a 23 g. butterfly catheter and a 10 ml syringe. *Source:* Photo: R. Booth.

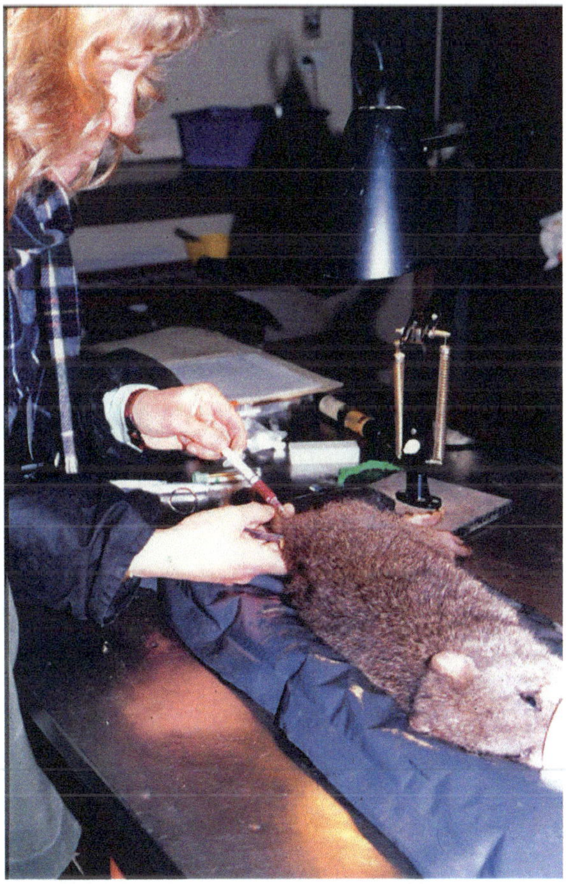

Figure 11.2 Collecting blood from the lateral tail vein of an anesthetized long-footed potoroo, *Potorous longipes*. A strategy for bleeding small-body-size animals in cold climates includes using a lamp with a 60 W bulb to warm the tail and increase peripheral circulation prior to bleeding. The use of an artery forceps and rubber band tourniquet provides better vein visibility than digital pressure alone.

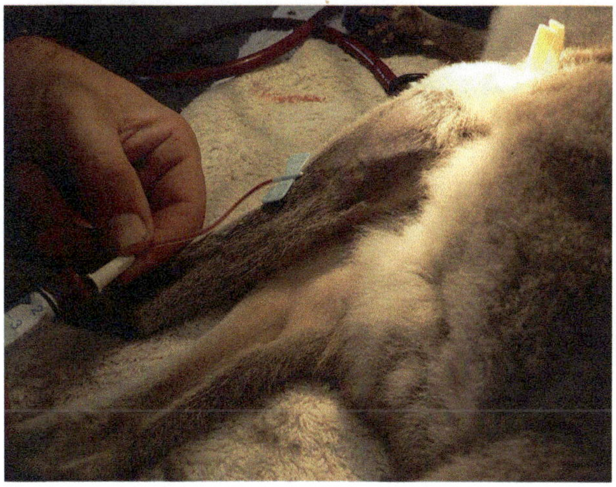

Figure 11.3 Blood collection from the cranial tibial vein of a bridled nailtail wallaby *Onychogalea fraenata* (body weight 4–8 kg). The use of 23 g. butterfly catheters facilitates gentle collection of blood to reduce the risk of hemolysis or vein collapse and allows for easier detachment and re-attachment of syringes as different blood tubes are filled. The small vein size means that blood collection takes longer than in larger species, so it is advisable to fill blood tubes with anticoagulant first, and then draw further blood for serum tubes. *Source:* Photo by R. Booth.

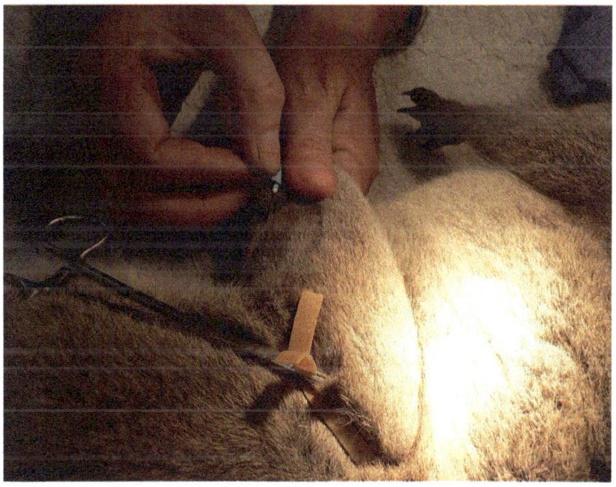

Figure 11.4 An artery forceps and rubber band tourniquet are useful to hold up the cranial tibial vein in macropods and should be positioned above the stifle joint for stability. *Source:* Photo by R. Booth.

cephalic, femoral, or jugular vein. Skin thickness can make visualization and palpation of vessels difficult. Clipping of the fur can facilitate locating the blood vessel. The radial vein on the medial aspect of the forelimb is most commonly used, though blood flow can be slow [9]. The femoral vein allows larger volumes to be collected.

For sugar gliders, the cranial vena cava is the preferred site for blood collection to ensure an adequate sample volume (Figure 11.11) [8]. Anesthesia is recommended to avoid laceration of the vessel or major organs. Similar

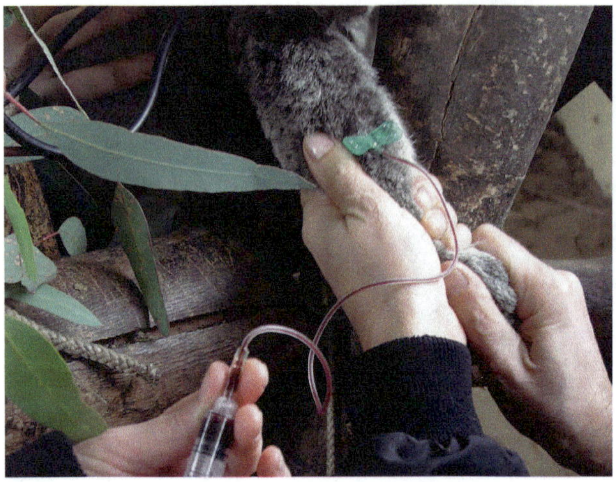

Figure 11.5 Blood collection from the cephalic vein of a koala, *Phascolarctos cinereus*. *Source:* Photo by G Pye.

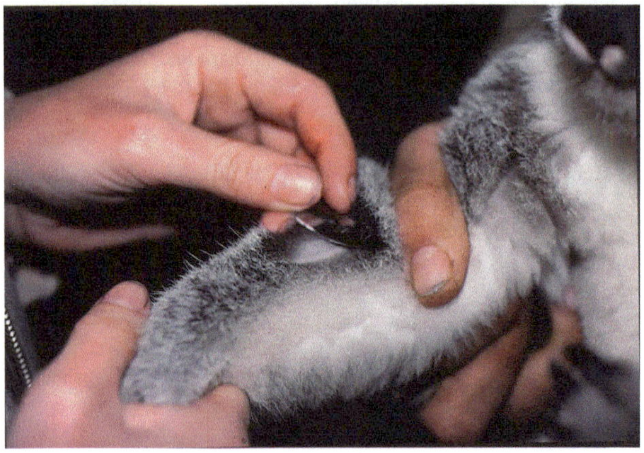

Figure 11.6 Shaving the cephalic vein of a conscious koala, *Phascolarctos cinereus*, using a scalpel blade which avoids aversive clipper noise.

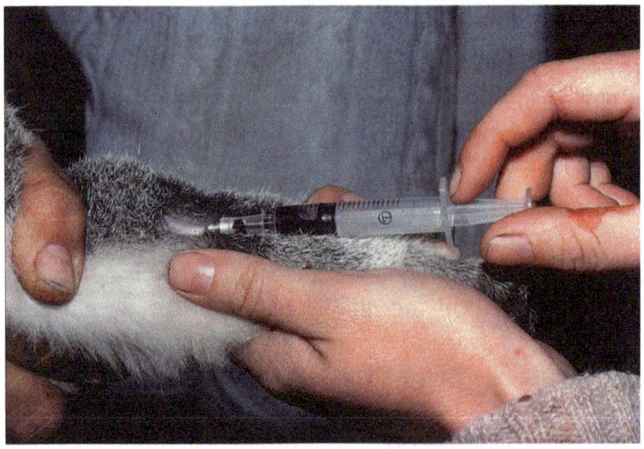

Figure 11.7 Blood collection from the cephalic vein of a koala, *Phascolarctos cinereus*.

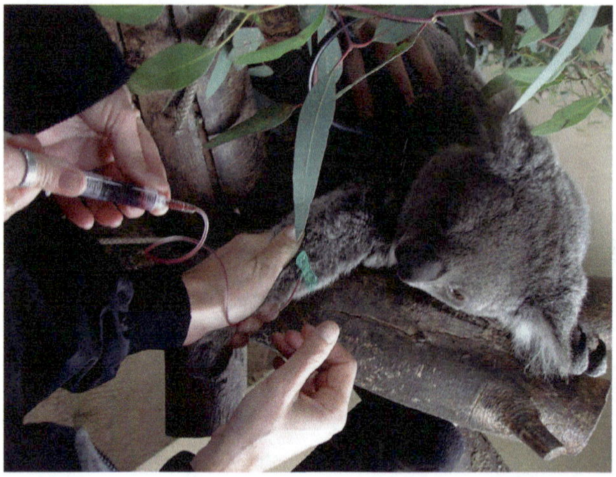

Figure 11.8 Blood collection from a conscious zoo-based koala, *Phascolarctos cinereus*.

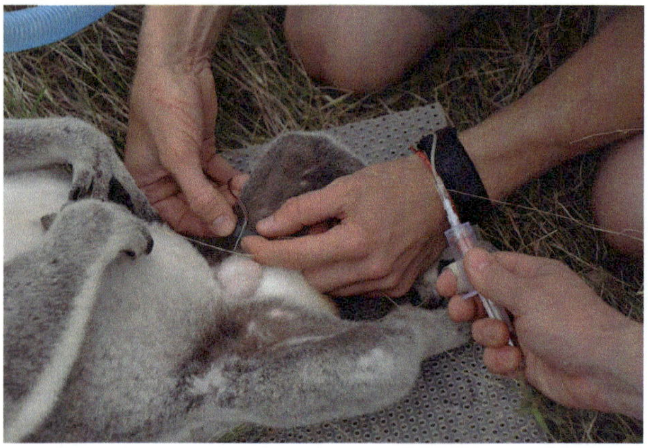

Figure 11.9 Blood collection from the femoral vein of an anesthetized free-ranging koala, *Phascolarctos cinereus*.

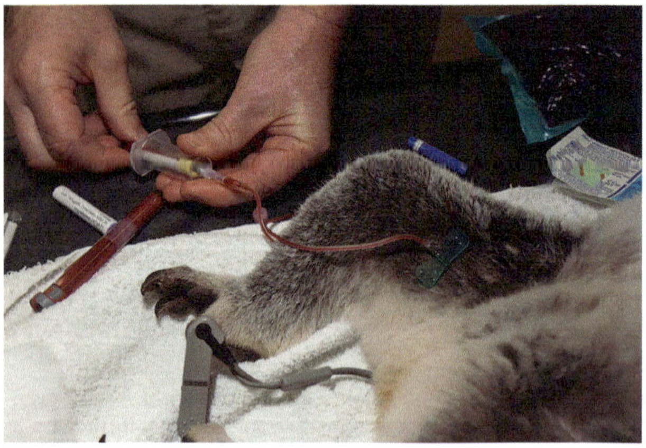

Figure 11.10 Blood collection from the femoral vein of an anesthetized zoo-based koala, *Phascolarctos cinereus*. *Source:* Photo by G Pye.

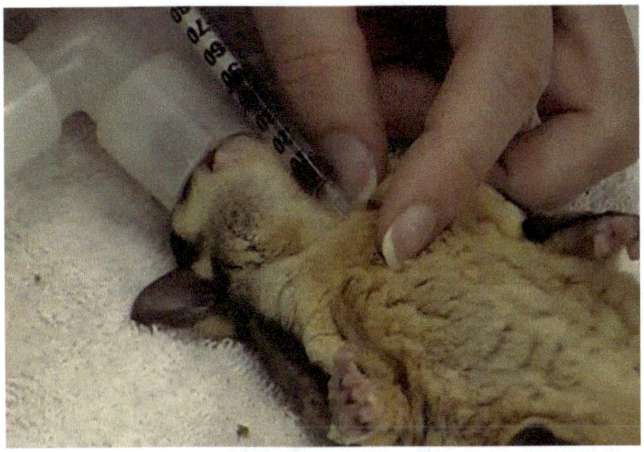

Figure 11.11 Blood collection from the cranial vena cava in a sugar glider, *Petaurus breviceps*.

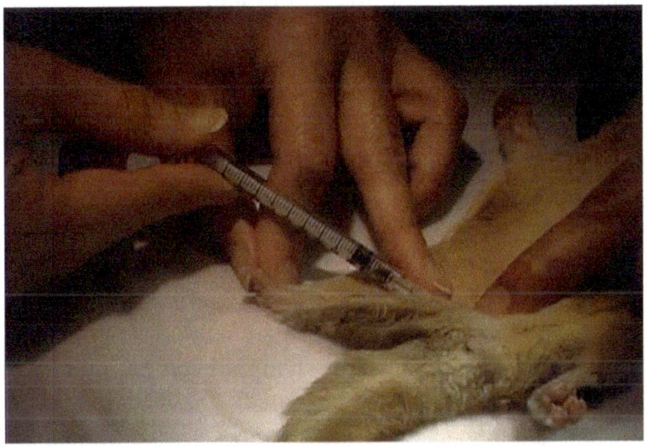

Figure 11.12 Blood collection from the femoral vein in a sugar glider, *Petaurus breviceps*.

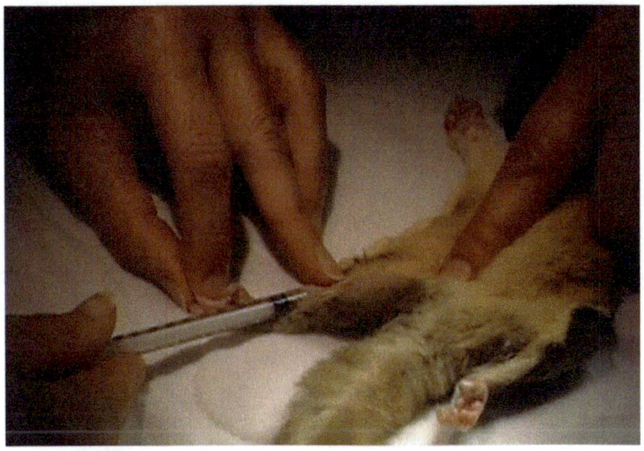

Figure 11.13 Blood collection from the medial tibial artery in a sugar glider, *Petaurus breviceps*.

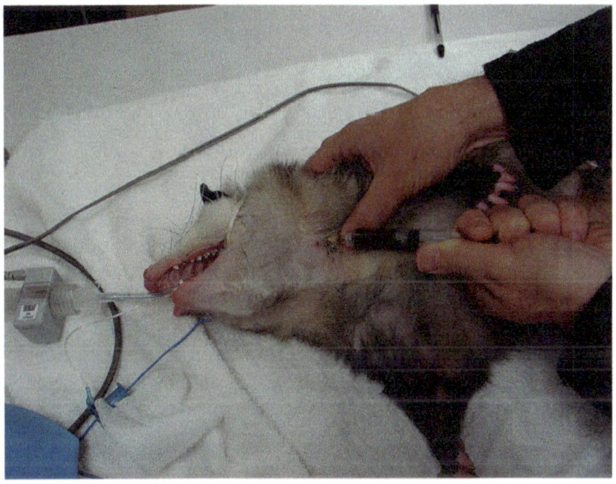

Figure 11.14 Blood collection from the jugular vein of a North American opossum, *Didelphis virginiana*. *Source:* Photo by G Pye.

to the approach used in ferrets, the needle is inserted at the thoracic inlet in the small depression in the angle created by the manubrium and the first rib. The needle is slowly and shallowly advanced toward the contralateral kidney with gentle aspiration. If there is a need to reposition, withdraw the needle to almost the skin level before adjusting the angle of insertion and slowly advancing. This cautious approach will reduce the risk of lacerating the vessel. Up to 1% of the body weight of the sugar glider in blood can be collected. Alternate vessels are the jugular and femoral veins (Figure 11.12), though these can prove difficult to access. The cranial branch of the saphenous artery coursing over the medial aspect of the tibia (Figures 11.13) is the most easily visible blood vessel to collect from, but a very fine needle is required (28 or 30 g.), and volume is often limited to 0.5 ml, though with care up to 1.0 ml may be collected.

The high incidence of obesity in captive North American opossums can make blood collection challenging. With experience, jugular (Figure 11.14), the brachiocephalic (Figure 11.15), or femoral veins can be reliably used [36]. Alternatively the lateral tail vein can be used (Figure 11.16). Blood collection from vessels in the pouch and the ventral tail, and by cardiac puncture are reported in the research literature, but are not routinely used in clinical practice [19, 27, 30, 54].

Sample Handling

Marsupials are similar to eutherian mammals in terms of sample handling. Blood should be collected into EDTA for a complete blood count and tubes with no anticoagulant for biochemical analysis. Serum separator tubes (SST) are preferred for biochemical analysis if the blood is to be transported to an off-site laboratory to avoid hemolysis en route. In some species of

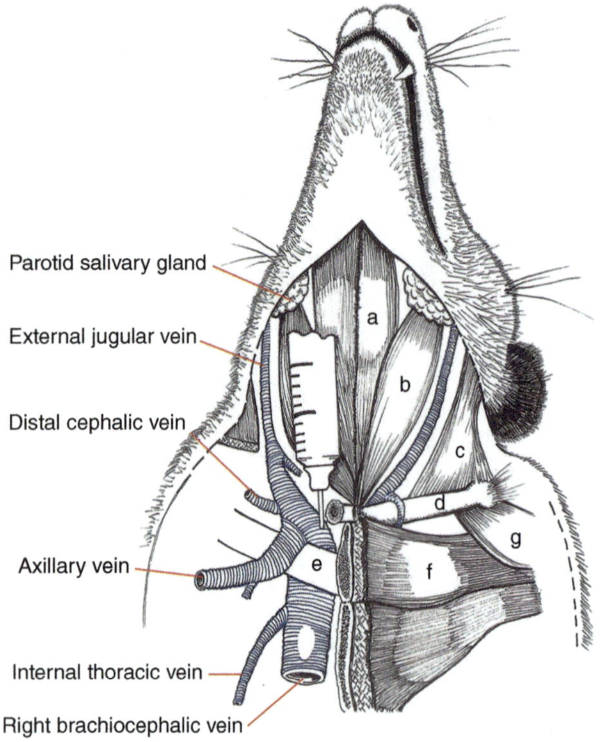

Figure 11.15 Anatomic landmarks and approach for blood collection from the brachiocephalic vein of a North American opossum (*Didelphis virginiana*) adapted [6]. A 22 g. 1.5 in. needle is inserted shallowly, 1 cm lateral to the ventral midline and dorsal to the clavicle. Key to musculoskeletal structures: a – sternohyoideus muscle, b – sternomastoideus muscle, c – cleidocervicalis muscle, d – clavicle, e – 1st rib, f – cleidobrachialis muscle, g – pectoralis superficialis muscle.

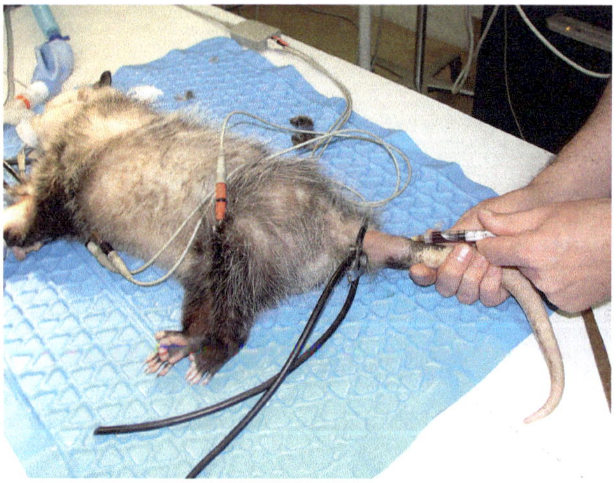

Figure 11.16 Blood collection from the lateral tail vein of a North American opossum, *Didelphis virginiana*. *Source:* Photo by G Pye.

macropods, centrifugation of the SST should be delayed for 30 min or more to allow for clot retraction to maximize serum yield.

Specific Analytes

Interpretation of marsupial blood results is similar to that in domestic animals; exceptions are discussed below.

Complete Blood Count

Reference values for hematology of representative species of Macropods are provided in Table 11.3 and for koalas, sugar gliders and opossums in Table 11.4 and for selected other marsupials in Table 11.5. A review of approximately 30 species of marsupials found that most had a hematocrit greater than 40% and a hemoglobin concentration of greater than 10 g/dl, and a third of the species had values greater than 50% for hematocrit and 15 g/dl for hemoglobin concentration [1]. In a seasonal study of 15 captive koalas, hematocrit and maximum ambient temperature were negatively correlated [12]. Anemia may occur in marsupials due to poor nutrition, chronic inflammatory diseases, lymphoid neoplasia, heavy parasite burdens, anticoagulant poisoning, and due to traumatic causes of blood loss. Nucleated red blood cells, Howell-Jolly bodies, and basophilic stippling of erythrocytes may be observed in clinically normal koalas (Figures 11.17–11.19) [16]. Circulating nucleated red blood cells have also been reported in apparently healthy sugar and yellow-bellied gliders and brush-tailed and striped possums [26].

For many marsupials, more lymphocytes compared to neutrophils are considered normal. These lymphocytic species include sugar gliders, opossums, and koalas, though normal macropods may have higher neutrophil than lymphocyte counts [48]. Neutrophilia and lymphopenia may indicate a cortisol-induced reversal of the neutrophil:lymphocyte ratio caused by the stress of chronic disease or other long-standing stress (e.g., nutritional, lactation) in marsupials as in eutherians. Lymphoid neoplasia is relatively common in koalas and possums and gliders. Leukemia (Figure 11.20), nonregenerative anemia, and thrombocytopenia have been associated with koala retrovirus [46]. Profound leukopenia may indicate septicemia in koalas [7]. Common wombats with generalized sarcoptic mange may exhibit neutrophilia with band neutrophils, lymphopenia, activated lymphocytes (increased basophilic intensity of cytoplasm), increased large lymphocytes, and monocytosis [45]. The neutrophil:lymphocyte ratio differed significantly between the sexes in the dasyurid *Sminthopsis* (males 43:50%, females 34:60%), although females were not pregnant or lactating at the time of sampling, and males and females were housed under similar conditions [22]. An unusually high percentage of reticulocytes (range 4%–13%) was also observed in two species of apparently healthy *Sminthopsis*, suggesting either a rapid rate of erythrocyte turnover or longer reticulocyte life.

Table 11.3 Hematologic reference ranges for selected macropods.

Analyte (abbreviation)	Units, SI (USA)	Brush-tailed rock wallaby [3]	Eastern gray kangaroo [43]	Red-necked wallaby [37]	Red kangaroo [48]	Matschie's tree kangaroo [6]	Parma wallaby Ħ	Tammar wallaby [34]
Data format		**95% Confidence Intervals**	**Mean ± SD**	**Mean ± SD**	**Mean ± SD**	**Min–max**	**Mean ± SD**	**Mean ± SD**
Sample size[a]		**113–115**	**45–53**	**47**	**132–216**	**121–152**	**31**	**38**
Total erythrocytes (RBC)	351000 cells/μl	4700–7500✋ *[76]* 3900–7300 ₳ *[39]*	5800 ± 800	4400–6600	5200 ± 800	3880–8280	7220 ± 660	6290 ± 80
Nucleate (nRBC) erythrocytes	per 100 WBC		1.0 ± 1.0 *[9]*	0–0.1	1.0 ± 2.0 *[63]*	0–40 *[35]*		
Mean (MCV) corpuscular volume	fl	62–75	78 ± 7	77–93	93 ± 7	66.9–119.0	65.0 ± 2.5	75.57 ± 0.49
Mean (MCH) corpuscular hemoglobin	pg	19.0–27.1	27 ± 3	27–33	33 ± 3	21.5–41.6	21.1 ± 1.9	25.85 ± 0.17
Mean (MCHC) corpuscular hemoglobin concentration	g/l (g/dl)	279–372 (27.9–37.2)	345 ± 25 (34.5 ± 2.5)	345–376 (34.5–37.6)	354 ± 23 (3.54 ± 2.3)	244–434 (24.4–43.4)	326 ± 28 (32.6 ± 2.8)	340.6 ± 1.04 *[30 ♀]* (34.1 ± 0.1) 345.74 ± 1.46 *[7♂]* (34.6 ± 0.15)
Packed cell volume (PCV)	%	34–52✋ *[76]* 28–52 ₳ *[39]*	45 ± 6	40–56	48 ± 0.07	27.5–72.9	47.0 ± 4.3	47 ± 3
Hemoglobin (Hb)	g/l (g/dl)	119–185✋ *[76]* (11.9–18.5) 93–180 ₳ *[39]* (9.3–18.0)	154 ± 21 (15.4 ± 2.1)	140–197 (14.0–19.7)	171 ± 26 (17.1 ± 2.5)	102–202 10.2–20.2	153 ± 15 (15.3 ± 1.5)	161.27 ± 1.79 *[30 ♀]* (16.1 ± 0.2) 165.86 ± 2.26 *[7♂]* (16.6 ± 0.2)
Total leukocytes (WBC)	$\times 10^6$ Cells/μl	3700–11800 ₪ *[68]* 4700–9000 Ó *[48]*	6280 ± 3040	3500–10500	4870 ± 1820	1700–15800	4356 ± 1043	6110 ± 270
Neutrophils	Cells/μl	960–5710	3570 ± 2180	1100–5000	2710 ± 1610	550–12800	1036 ± 622	1640 ± 140
Lymphocytes	Cells/μl	2050–7920 ₪ ✋ *[40]* 670–7300 ₪ ₳ *[25]* 3.12–11.77 Ó ✋ *[35]* 2.16–9.86 Ó ₳ *[13]*	2490 ± 1430	1600–5300	1950 ± 1190	350–9000	3158 ± 911	3870 ± 220

(*Continued*)

Table 11.3 (Continued)

Analyte (abbreviation)	Units, SI (USA)	Brush-tailed rock wallaby [3]	Eastern gray kangaroo [43]	Red-necked wallaby [37]	Red kangaroo [48]	Matschie's tree kangaroo [6]	Parma wallaby Ħ	Tammar wallaby [34]
Data format		**95% Confidence Intervals**	**Mean ± SD**	**Mean ± SD**	**Mean ± SD**	**Min–max**	**Mean ± SD**	**Mean ± SD**
Sample size[a]		**113–115**	**45–53**	**47**	**132–216**	**121–152**	**31**	**38**
Monocytes	Cells/μl	0–1220	170 ± 120	0–600	120 ± 110	0–1600	124 ± 76 *[24]*	200 ± 40
Eosinophils	Cells/μl	0–1750	130 ± 90	0–500	100 ± 110	0–1010	86 ± 65 *[24]*	120 ± 20
Basophils	Cells/μl	0–340	60 ± 10 *[6]*	0–200	30 ± 40 *[42]*	0–340 *[41]*	84 *[1]*	0
Platelets	Cells/μl	9000–848000 ₪ ✋ *[41]* 61000–618000 ₪ ₳ *[26]* 20000–334000 ✋ Ó *[34]* 20000–371000 ₳ Ó *[13]*	186000 ± 93000 *[28]*	136000–485000	221000 ± 108000 *[56]*	96000–171000 *[7]*	250071 ± 74120 *[28]*	254710 ± 19500
Plasma protein	g/l g/dl		60 ± 8 (6.0 ± 0.8)	62 ± 12 *[137]* (6.2 ± 1.2)	64 ± 10 (6.4 ± 1.0)	49–88 (4.9–8.8)	63 ± 5 (6.3 ± 0.5)	
Fibrinogen	μmol/l mg/dl		1.3 ± 0.5 *[17]* (44 ± 17)	1.1 ± 0.8 *[10]* (37 ± 27)	1.8 ± 1.0 [33] (61 ± 34)		5.2 ± 2.0 (177 ± 67) *[31]*	

[a] Sample sizes not within this range are given in bracketed italics next to the specific range *[xx]*.

Key: Male ♂, Female ♀, Adult ₪, Juvenile Ó, Anesthetized ₳, Manual Restraint ✋.

Table 11.4 Hematologic reference ranges for koalas (*Phascolarctos cinereus*), sugar gliders (*Petaurus breviceps*), and opossums (*Didelphis virginiana*).

Analyte (abbreviation)	Units, SI (conventional)	Koala captive Ħ	Koala free-ranging [11]	Sugar glider [8]	Opossum [38]	Opossum [50]	Opossum [32]
Data format		Mean ± SD	Range	95% confidence interval¥	Unknown	Unknown	Mean ± SD
Sample size[a]		≥100	37–43	53–62	Unknown	Unknown	21–25
Total erythrocytes (RBC)	1000 cells/μl	3350 ± 440	2700–4200	8310–8830	3400–6500	3300–5900	800 ± 765
Nucleate (nRBC) erythrocytes	/100 WBC	21 ± 9	1–20 [13]				
Mean corpuscular volume (MCV)	fl	104.9 ± 7.0	94–117	60.2–68.1	73–113	64.7–102.9	77.5 ± 9.0
Mean corpuscular hemoglobin (MCH)	Pg	35.6 ± 2.0		18.8–19.4	24.4–39.5	22.5–35.9	26.8 ± 3.3
Mean corpuscular hemoglobin concentration (MCHC)	g/l (g/dl)	340 ± 15 (34.0 ± 1.5)	298–330 (29.8–33.0)	306–310 (30.6–31.0)	327–400 (32.7–40.0)	280–430 (28–43)	347 ± 37 (34.7 ± 3.7)
Packed cell volume (PCV)	%	35 ± 5	29–44	51 – 54	33-51	28–47	37.1 ± 7.0
Hemoglobin (Hb)	g/l (g/dl)	119 ± 14 (11.9 ± 1.4)	88–140 (8.8–14.0)	158–169 (15.8–16.9)	117–179 (11.7–17.9)	83–162 (8.3–16.2)	128 ± 23 (12.8 ± 2.3)
Total leukocytes (WBC)	Cells/μl	6134 ± 1785	2800–112 000	5500–9300	3900–12 600	14 000–22 900	22 600 ± 6815
Neutrophils	Cells/μl	2165 ± 950	500–6300	1460–2200			
Lymphocytes	Cells/μl	3677 ± 1641	200–5800	3690–7160			
Monocytes	Cells/μl	188 ± 119	0–600	110–170 *[45]*			
Eosinophils	Cells/μl	151 ± 136 *[77]*	0–110	90–280 *[10]*			
Basophils	Cells/μl	64 ± 27 *[19]*	0	30–60 *[8]*			
Neutrophils %	%	36 ± 15			11–48	12–67	42.4 ± 16.4
Lymphocytes %	%	58 ± 16			26–82	13–67.5	50.0 ± 14.6
Monocytes %	%	3 ± 2			0–8	0–2	0.9 ± 1.3
Eosinophils %	%	2 ± 2 *[77]*			6–17	2–15	5.7 ± 3.8
Basophils %	%	1 ± 0 *[19]*			0–3	0–2	0.4 ± 1.0
Platelets	Cells/μl	185 000 ± 76 400	222 000–558 000 *[11]*	292 180–400 320			
Plasma protein	g/l (g/dl)	65 ± 4 (6.5 ± 0.4)					
Fibrinogen	μmol/l (mg/dl)	2.9 ± 2.9 (100 ± 100) *[97]*					

[a] Sample sizes not within this range are given in bracketed italics next to the specific range *[xx]*.
¥ With outliers removed.
Ħ San Diego Zoo in-house clinical lab values, captive animals.
Key: Male ♂, Female ♀, Adult ₪, Juvenile Ó, Anesthetized ₳, Manual Restraint 🖐.

Table 11.5 Hematologic reference ranges for select marsupials.

Analyte (abbreviation)	Units, SI (conventional)	Gray short-tailed opossum [17][a]	Brush-tailed possum [40]	Tasmanian devil [25]	Chuditch [47]	Southern hairy-nosed wombat [9]	Common wombat [9]
Sample number		**26 ♂ 20 ♀**	**79 ♂ 87 ♀**		**34–35**	**14**	**31**
Total erythrocytes (RBC)	1000 cells/µl	6800 ± 130 ♂ 6430 ± 170 ♀	7350 ± 160 ₪♂ *[25]* 6190 ± 70 ₪♀ *[23]*	6250 ± 2190	8470 ± 680	5100 ± 600	5200 ± 700
Mean corpuscular volume (MCV)	fl	53 ± 1 ♂ 53 ± 1.3 ♀	67 ± 0.5 ♂ 66 ± 0.5 ♀	64.5 ± 15.3	55.2 ± 2.1	79 ± 4	68 ± 4
Mean corpuscular hemoglobin (MCH)	Pg	20 ± 0.3 ♂ 19.7 ± 0.4 ♀	21.9 ± 0.2 ♂ 21.6 ± 0.2 ♀	23.7 ± 7.0	18.4 ± 1.1	27.8 ± 1.4	22.7 ± 1.3
Mean corpuscular hemoglobin concentration (MCHC)	g/l (g/dl)	378 ± 5 ♂ (37.8 ± 0.5) 372 ± 6 (37.2 ± 0.6) ♀	326 ± 2 ♂ (32.6 ± 0.2) 329 ± 2 (32.9 ± 0.2) ♀	366 ± 38 (36.6 ± 3.8)	334.8 ± 9.2 (33.5 ± 0.9)	350 ± 15 (35 ± 1.5)	335 ± 17 (33.5 ± 1.7)
Packed cell volume (PCV)	%	35.9 ± 0.8 ♂ 34.0 ± 1.1 ♀	50 ± 1₪♂ *[25]* 41 ± 1₪♀ *[23]*	37.3 ± 6.8	45 ± 4	40 ± 4	36 ± 6
Hemoglobin (Hb)	g/l (g/dl)	136 ± 3 ♂ (13.6 ± 0.3) 126 ± 4 (12.6 ± 0.4) ♀	167 ± 3 (16.7 ± 0.3) ₪♂ *[25]* 133 ± 3 (13.3 ± 0.3) ₪♀ *[23]*	137 ± 22 (13.7 ± 2.2)	157 ± 14 (15.7 ± 1.4)	142 ± 14 (14.2 ± 1.4)	119 ± 19 (11.9 ± 1.9)
Total leukocytes (WBC)	Cells/µl	16 840 ± 1500 ♂ 13 540 ± 1500 ♀	7820 ± 490 ♂ 8530 ± 340 ♀	6000 ± 2500	4850 ± 2490	11 400 ± 3300	8400 ± 2900
Neutrophils	Cells/µl		2220 ± 200 ♂ 2900 ± 200 ♀	3700 ± 2200	2860 ± 1890	6500 ± 2700	6100 ± 3000
Bands	Cells/µl			300 ± 200			
Lymphocytes	Cells/µl		5030 ± 410 ♂ 4880 ± 350 ♀	2200 ± 1100	1530 ± 830	4300 ± 2000	5200 ± 3000
Monocytes	Cells/µl		360 ± 30 ♂ 460 ± 40 ♀	100 ± 100	130 ± 120	400 ± 400	500 ± 500
Eosinophils	Cells/µl		220 ± 40 ♂ 260 ± 40 ♀	200 ± 300	260 ± 160	300 ± 200	150 ± 200
Basophils	Cells/µl		20 ± 60 ♂ 15 ± 40 ♀	100 ± 0	0–100	100 ± 20	10 ± 5
Neutrophils %	%	28 ± 2 ♂ 23 ± 3 ♀	28 ♂ 34 ♀		56.7 ± 13.5		

Lymphocytes %	%	52 ± 3 ♂ 48 ± 4 ♀	64 ♂ 57 ♀		33.5 ± 12.4
Monocytes %	%	14 ± 1 ♂ 19 ± 2 ♀	5 ♂ 5 ♀		2.6 ± 2.3
Eosinophils %	%	6 ± 1 ♂ 10 ± 1 ♀	3 ♂ 3 ♀		6.1 ± 3.4
Basophils %	%	0.14 ± 0.13 ♂ 0.52 ± 0.17 ♀	0 ♂ 1 ♀		0–2
Platelets	Cells/µl	312 000 ± 23 000 ♂ 334 000 ± 30 000 ♀			
Plasma protein	g/l (g/dl)		69 ± 1 ₪♂ *[25]* (6.9 ± 0.1) 70 ± 2 ₪ *[23]* (7.0 ± 0.2) ♀		66.1 ± 7.2 (6.6 ± 0.7)
Fibrinogen	µmol/l (mg/dl)			8.8 ± 0 (300 ± 0)	6.8 ± 4.4 (230 ± 150)

Data shown as Mean ± SD.

[a] Sample sizes not within this range are given in bracketed italics next to the specific range *[xx]*.

Key: Male ♂, Female ♀, Adult ₪, Juvenile Ó, Anesthetized ₳, Manual Restraint ✋.

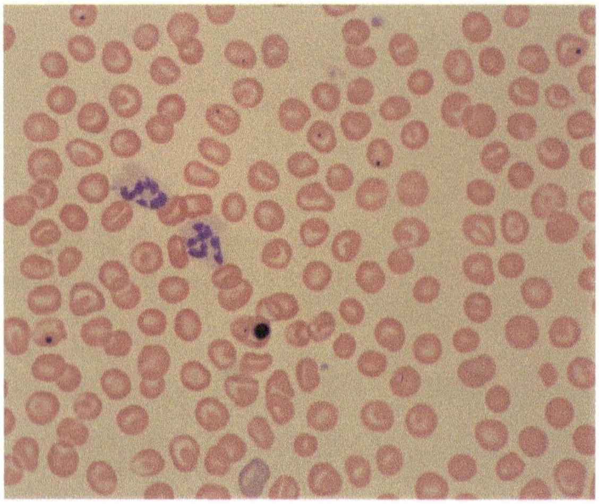

Figure 11.17 Normal blood smear from a koala (400× magnification), *Phascolarctos cinereus*. *Source:* Photo courtesy San Diego Zoo.

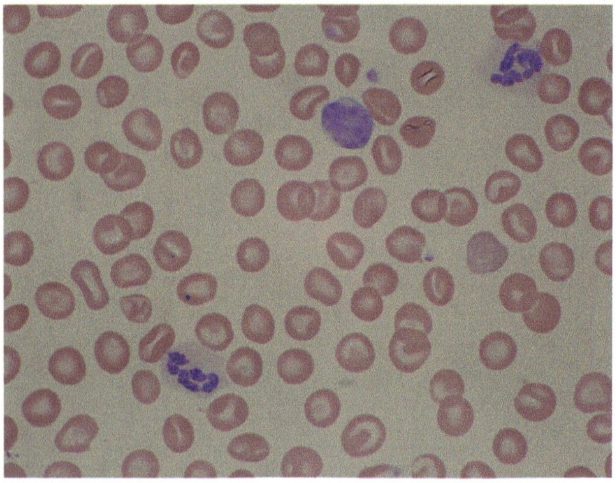

Figure 11.18 Blood smear from a normal koala, *Phascolarctos cinereus* (1000× magnification). Left to right: neutrophil, lymphocyte, neutrophil. *Source:* Photo courtesy San Diego Zoo.

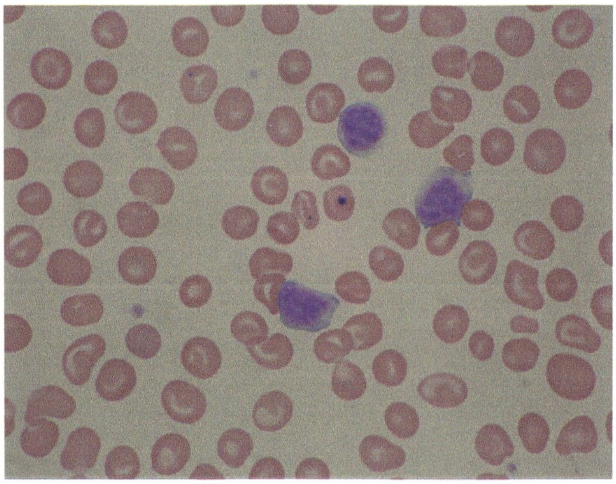

Figure 11.19 Blood smear from a normal koala, *Phascolarctos cinereus* (1000× magnification). Three lymphocytes surrounding a Howell Jolly body in an erythrocyte. *Source:* Photo courtesy San Diego Zoo.

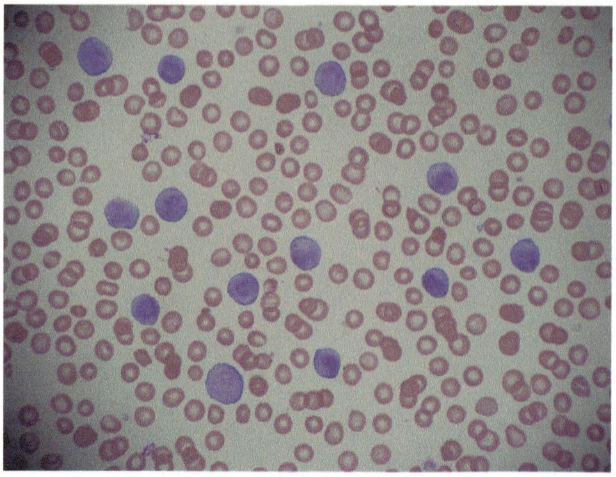

Figure 11.20 Blood smear from a koala *(Phascolarctos cinereus)* with leukemia. *Source:* Photo courtesy San Diego Zoo.

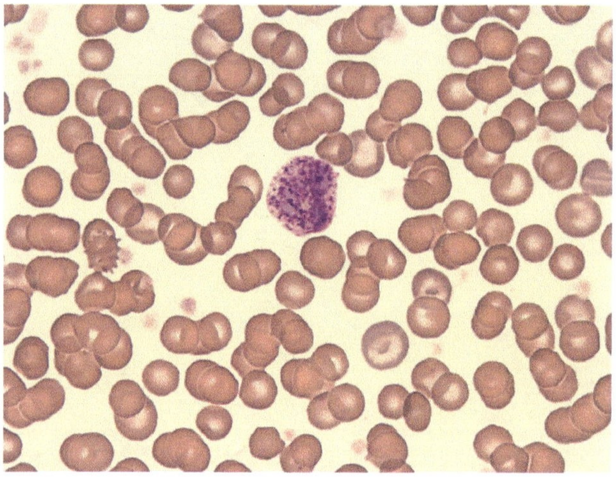

Figure 11.21 Basophil of the North American Opossum *(Didelphis virginianus)* (1000× magnification).

The total and differential white cell counts of the North American opossum change during postnatal development [15]. At birth, the few circulating leukocytes are mainly immature neutrophils. The number of leukocytes increases rapidly in the first two weeks of life, due to an accumulation of granulocytes, predominantly neutrophils. The eosinophil number then increases rapidly with their number equaling or exceeding the number of neutrophils. Eosinophils then remain a prominent, though lesser, component of the leukocytes for the remainder of development. Lymphocytes are only present in small numbers during the first 8–10 days of postnatal life, and small lymphocytes are absent during this time. Figures 11.21 and 11.22 depict erythrocytes, platelets, a neutrophil, eosinophil, and a basophil from the blood smear of a North American opossum.

An *Eperythrozoon*-like parasite has been reported in a North American opossum [35]. Its features were similar

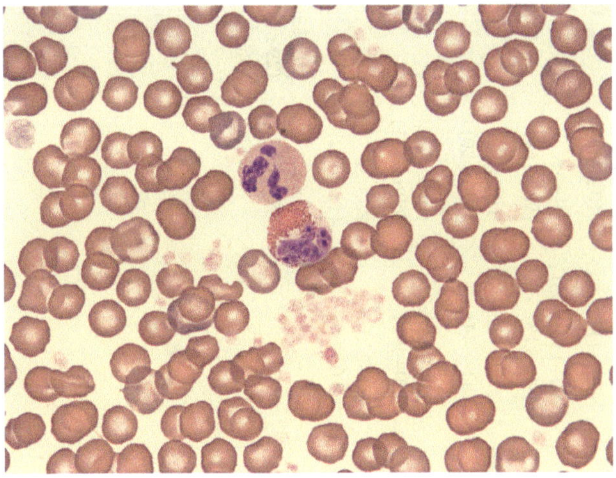

Figure 11.22 Neutrophil (upper left) and eosinophil (lower right) of the North American opossum *(Didelphis virginiana)*.

to those of *Eperythrozoon* and *Haemobartonella* species seen in other mammals. Severe anemia that was responsive to doxycycline therapy was noted.

Hemostasis and Blood Types

Coagulation parameters are available for the North American opossum (n = 11) [30]. Glass clotting times averaged 5.5 min, and clot retraction times averaged 4 min. Serum prothrombin time averaged 35 s using opossum barium-sulfate-adsorbed plasma, 53 s using human barium-sulfate-adsorbed plasma, and greater than 120 s without serum. Plasma prothrombin time averaged 32.6 s with Simplastin®, 12.3 s with opossum brain, and 16.4 s with Russell's viper venom. Partial prothrombin times averaged 23.1 s. Clinical clotting abnormality has been observed in a captive Proserpine rock wallaby with access to brodifacoum rat bait (Booth, unpublished data).

Little is known regarding the blood groups of marsupials. Six blood groups have described in the gray short-tailed opossum, *Monodelphis domestica* [13]. Blood transfusions have been performed in koalas without cross-matching without adverse effects; in some cases, multiple transfusions have been performed (A Gillett, personal communication). However, cross-matching is prudent in marsupial species as in any species prior to transfusion.

Biochemical Panel

Liver Enzymes and Analytes

Reference values for biochemistry of representative species of Macropods are provided in Table 11.6 and for koalas, sugar gliders and opossums in Table 11.7 and for selected other marsupials in Table 11.8. Analytes useful for the assessment of liver disease and or dysfunction in marsupials include the liver enzymes alanine aminotransferase (ALT), gamma-glutamyltransferase (GGT), alkaline phosphatase (ALP), sorbitol dehydrogenase (SD or SDH/also called iditol dehydrogenase (ID), glutamate dehydrogenase (GLDH), as well as bilirubin, bile acids, and ammonia. Marked elevation of aspartate aminotransferase (AST), lactate dehydrogenase (LDH), and GGT have been observed in koalas with lymphoma, though this is not a consistent finding for koalas with retrovirus-associated disease (San Diego Zoo, unpublished data) [46]. Increased ALP activities occur in healthy young koalas and are thought to be associated with bone development, as in other species [11, 16]. ALP, primarily produced in liver, bone, and intestines is also relatively high in normal macropods [48]. The cause for this "increased" ALP in some healthy marsupials is unknown; isoenzyme studies have not been published for marsupials.

Muscle Enzymes

Enzymes useful for the diagnosis of muscular disease or damage in marsupials include creatine kinase (CK) and AST. Marsupials, particularly macropods, exhibit greater lability of CK than other mammals. Elevations of CK up to 3000 U/l are rarely of clinical significance, but reflect exertion during restraint and handling. Elevations greater than 10 000 U/l are consistent with capture myopathy [48].

Renal Analytes

Prerenal and renal azotemia have been observed in koalas [4, 12, 46]. Hyperkalemia and hypercalcemia may also occur in koalas with renal insufficiency.

Pancreas, Gastrointestinal, and Cardiac

Starvation, either due to loss of food supply after bush fires or due to prolonged anorexia caused by chronic disease such as chlamydiosis can produce hypoglycemia in koalas. Hypoglycemia is also a common condition in underfed marsupial pouch young. Diabetes mellitus has been described in two koalas [23, 44]. Pancreatitis has not been reported in marsupials. Insulin and glucagon have not been reported; some levels for amylase and lipase are found in Table 11.2. Specific enzyme or biochemical markers for gastrointestinal or cardiac disease in marsupials have not been reported. Similarly, few values for cholesterol, triglycerides, or other lipids have been reported (Table 11.2).

Electrolytes

Hypokalemia is commonly associated with inanition in koalas [5]. Hyperkalemia has been observed secondary to renal failure in koalas [4]. Hypercalcemia is not common in koalas with lymphoma, though it may be an early indicator of renal disease [4, 46].

Blood Proteins

Limited information is available for serum or plasma proteins in koalas, and they are the only marsupial

Table 11.6 Biochemical reference ranges for select macropods.

Analyte (abbreviation)	Units, SI (US)	Brush-tailed rock wallaby[3]	Eastern gray kangaroo [48]	Red-necked wallaby [48]	Red kangaroo [48]	Matschie's tree kangaroo [6]	Parma wallaby Ħ	Tammar wallaby [34]
Data format		**95% Confidence Interval**	**Mean ± SD**	**Mean ± SD**	**Mean ± SD**	**Min–max**	**Mean ± SD**	**Mean ± SD**
Sample size[a]		**48–77**	**39–52**	**73–158**	**162–188**	**100–142**	**28–32**	**38**
Alkaline phosphatase (ALP)	U/l (units/l)	196–827 ₪ (196–827) 465–2775 Ó (465–2775)	1037 ± 775 (1037 ± 775)	1186 ± 1071 (1186 ± 1071)	824 ± 648 (824 ± 648)	106–5713 (106–5713)	698 ± 462 (698 ± 462)	831.26 ± 84.57 (831 ± 85)
Alanine aminotransferase (ALT)	U/l (units/l)		56 ± 32 (56 ± 32)	45 ± 26 (45 ± 26)	49 ± 28 (49 ± 28)	0–48 (0–48)	51 ± 18 (51 ± 18)	52.29 ± 1.54 (52 ± 1.5)
Amylase	U/l (units/l)		87 ± 51 *[14]* (87 ± 51)	68 ± 31 (68 ± 31)	74 ± 34 *[78]* (74 ± 34)	4–61 *[51]* (4–61)	102 ± 38 (102 ± 38)	
Aspartate aminotransferase (AST)	U/l (units/l)	20.7–61.2 ₪ (20.7–61.2) 19.9–64.8 Ó (19.9–64.8)	60 ± 25 (60 ± 25)	88 ± 71 (88 ± 71)	104 ± 65 (104 ± 65)	14–155 (14–155)	45 ± 17 (45 ± 17)	51.36 ± 2.65 (51 ± 2.7)
Bilirubin (total)	µmol/l (mg/dl)	0.63–6.59 ♀ (0.03–0.4) 0.63–6.31 ♂ (0.03–0.4)	3.0 ± 2.0 (0.2 ± 0.1)	3 ± 5 (0.2 ± 0.3)	3 ± 3 (0.2 ± 0.2)	0–8.55 0–0.5	3.4 ± 3.4 (0.2 ± 0.2)	1.9 ± 0.17 [30 ♀] 3.3 ± 1.4 [8 ♂]
Urea nitrogen (BUN)	mmol/l (mg/dl)	4.9–13.3 *[115]* (13.7–37.3)	8.6 ± 2.9 (24.2 ± 8.1)	8.9 ± 2.5 (24.9 ± 7.0)	8.6 ± 2.9 (24.2 ± 8.1)	4.3–13.9 (12–39)	9.2 ± 1.6 (25.8 ± 4.4)	
Calcium	mmol/l (mg/dl)	2.08–2.68 *[114]* (8.3–10.7)	2.48 ± 0.23 (9.9 ± 0.9)	2.58 ± 0.23 (10.3 ± 0.9)	2.65 ± 0.3 (10.6 ± 1.2)	1.9–2.75 (7.6–11)	2.55 ± 0.15 (10.2 ± 0.6)	
Chloride	mmol/l (mEq/l)		102 ± 5 (102 ± 5)	97 ± 5 (97 ± 5)	98 ± 4 *[137]* (98 ± 4)	90–113 *[105]* (90–113)	98 ± 16 (98 ± 16)	
Cholesterol	mmol/l (mg/dl)	2.1–3.7 ✋ (81–143) 1.7–3.6 ₳ (66–139) *[39]*	2.25 ± 0.67 (87 ± 26)	2.2 ± 0.67 (85 ± 26)	2.31 ± 0.67 *[144]* (89 ± 26)	2.12–11.50 (82–444)	3.3 ± 0.8 (126 ± 30)	
Creatine kinase (CK)	U/l (units/l)	293–2723♀ (293–2723) 303–9503 ♂ (303–9503)	747 ± 762 *[28]* (747 ± 762)	1371 ± 1819 *[48]* (1371 ± 1819)	638 ± 569 *[89]* (638 ± 569)	20–942 *[52]* (20–492)	636 ± 471 (636 ± 471)	
Creatinine	µmol/l (mg/dl)	₪ 65–125 (0.7–1.4) Ó 38–104 (0.4–1.2)	133 ± 53 (1.5 ± 0.6)	106 ± 35 (1.2 ± 0.4)	133 ± 44 (1.5 ± 0.5)	53–230 (0.6–2.6)	88 ± 32 (1.0 ± 0.2)	
Gamma-glutamyltransferase (GGT)	U/l (units/l)	6.1–20.0 *[41]* ₪ ✋ (6.1–20.0) 7.0–14.0 ₪ ₳ [26] (7.0–14.0) 9.0–27.0 *[35]* Ó ✋ (9.0–27.0) 6.0–18.0 [13] Ó ₳ (6.0–18.0)	18 ± 9 (18 ± 9)	46 ± 30 (46 ± 30)	6 ± 6 *[83]* (6 ± 6)		28 ± 6 (28 ± 6)	29.31 ± 1.03 (29 ± 1)

Glucose	mmol/l (mg/dl)	₪ 3.4–9.5 (61–171) Ó 4.7–9.0 (85–162)	5.9 ± 1.7 (106 ± 31)	5.9 ± 2.2 (106 ± 40)	7.0 ± 2.1 (126 ± 38)	2.4–11.0 (44–198)	10.2 ± 3.0 (184 ± 54)	
Lactate (LDH) dehydrogenase	U/l (units/l)		95 ± 52 *[17]* (95 ± 52)	578 ± 531 (578 ± 531)	155 ± 127 *[88]* (155 ± 127)	162–1142 *[71]* (162–1142)	224 ± 78 (224 ± 78)	
Magnesium	mmol/l (mg/dl)	0.62–1.21 *[115]* (1.5–2.9)				0.23–1.6 (0.57–3.90) *[9]*	0.86 ± 0.16 (2.1 ± 0.4)	
Phosphorus	mmol/l (mg/dl)	0.75–3.26 (2.3–10.1) ₪ 1.04–3.67 (3.2–11.4) Ó	2.45 ± 0.65 (7.6 ± 2.0)	2.39 ± 0.78 (7.4 ± 2.4)	2.36 ± 0.71 (7.3 ± 2.2)	0.77–3.5 2.2–10.9	1.8 ± 0.7 (5.5 ± 2.1)	
Potassium	mmol/l (mEq/l)		4.2 ± 0.8 (4.2 ± 0.8)	4.8 ± 1.2 (4.8 ± 1.2)	4.8 ± 1.0 (4.8 ± 1.0)	3.1–6.8 (3.1–6.8)	4.2 ± 0.4 (4.2 ± 0.4)	
Protein – total	g/l (g/dl)	52–75 (5.2–7.5) ✋ 42–64 ₳ *[39]* (4.2–6.4)	60 ± 8 (6.0 ± 0.8)	62 ± 3912 (6.2 ± 1.2)	64 ± 10 (6.4 ± 1.0)	49–88 (4.9–8.8)	60 ± 6 (6.0 ± 0.6)	62.05 ± 0.64 (6.2 ± 0.1)
Albumin	g/l (g/dl)	34.9–43.0 (3.5–4.3) ✋ 30.0–38.0 ₳ *[39]* (3.0–3.8)	38 ± 5 (3.8 ± 0.5)	41 ± 8 (4.1 ± 0.8)	42 ± 9 (4.2 ± 0.9)	36–62 (3.6–6.2)	49 ± 5 (4.9 ± 0.5)	46.37 ± 0.51 (4.6 ± 0.1)
Globulin	g/l (g/dl)	15.3–37.0 ₪ ✋ *[41]* (1.5–3.7) 17.0–28.0 ₪ ₳ *[26]* (1.7–2.8) 14.0–30.0 Ó ✋ *[35]* (14–30) 9.0–25.0 Ó ₳ *[13]* (0.9–2.5)	23 ± 6 (2.3 ± 0.6)	25 ± 11 (2.5 ± 1.1)	23 ± 11 (2.3 ± 1.1)	8–61 *[97]* 0.8–6.1		
Sodium	mmol/l (mEq/l)		141 ± 4 (141 ± 4)	141 ± 5 (141 ± 5)	144 ± 5 (144 ± 5)	131–149 (131–149)	142 ± 4 (142 ± 4)	
Triglycerides	mmol/l (mg/dl)	0.10–0.68 (9–60) ₪ 0.10–0.40 (9–35) Ó	0.57 ± 0.53 *[16]* (50 ± 47)	0.75 ± 0.5 (66 ± 44)	0.69 ± 0.74 *[94]* (61 ± 66)	0–3.15 (0–279) *[59]*	1.47 ± 0.72 (130 ± 64)	

[a] Sample sizes not within this range are given in bracketed italics next to the specific range *[xx]*.

Key: Male ♂, Female ♀, Adult ₪, Juvenile Ó, Anesthetized ₳, Manual Restraint ✋.

Table 11.7 Biochemical reference ranges for koalas (*Phascolarctos cinereus*), sugar gliders (*Petaurus breviceps*), and opossums (*Didelphis virginiana*).

Analyte (abbreviation)	Units, SI (conventional)	Koala Captive Ħ	Koala free-ranging [11]	Sugar glider [3]	Opossum [38]	Opossum [50]
Data format		**Mean±SD**	**Range**	**95% Confidence interval ¥**	**Range**	**Range**
Sample size[a]		**102–118**	**26–42**	**72–100**	**Unknown**	**Unknown**
Alkaline phosphatase (ALP)	U/l (units/l)	225 + 142 (225 + 142)	25–219 ₪ (25–219) 88–375 *[15]* Ó (88–375)	89–115 (89–115)	137 (137)	13.0–35.0 K-A units 92–249 (92–249)
Alanine (ALT) aminotransferase	U/l (units/l)	13 + 9 (13 + 9)	0–236 (0–236)	97–137 (97–137)	68 (68)	
Amylase	U/l (units/l)	79 + 177 (79 + 177)				
Aspartate aminotransferase (AST)	U/l (units/l)	21 + 14 (21 + 14)	0–134 (0–134)	54–99 (54–99) [38]	339 (339)	250 (250)
Bile acids	UNITS	<0.1 *[34]*				
Bilirubin (total)	μmol/l (mg/dl)	3.4 + 6.8 (0.2 + 0.4)	0–8 (0–0.5)	1.7–12.0 (0.1–0.7)	1.7–13.7 (0.1–0.8)	5.1–13.7 (0.3–0.8)
Urea nitrogen (BUN)	mmol/l (mg/dl)	2.9 + 1.4 (8 + 4)	0.2–6.6 (0.6–18.5)	5.4–6.5 (15.1–18.1)	8.2–13.6 (23–38)	8.2–21.4 (23–60)
Calcium	mmol/l (mg/dl)	2.5 + 0.1 (10.0 + 0.5)	2.3–3.0 (9.1–11.9)	2.1–2.2 (8.5–8.9)	2.4 (9.7)	2.4–2.8 (9.6–11.2)
Chloride	mmol/l (mEq/l)	102 + 3 (102 + 3)	93–107 (93–107)	106–109 (106–109)	101–129 (101–129)	80–151 (80–151)
Cholesterol	mmol/l (mg/dl)	1.7 + 0.3 (67 + 13)	1.2–3.1 (46–120)	2.9–3.2 (112–124)	2.2–5.3 (85–203)	
Creatine kinase (CK)	U/l (units/l)	306 + 312 (306 + 312)		1081–1637 (1081–1637) [47]		
Creatinine	μmol/l (mg/dl)	107 + 18 (1.2 + 0.2)	80–150 (0.9–1.8)	44–53 (0.5–0.6)	35–645 (0.4–7.3) high normal seems abnormal	
Gamma-(GGT) glutamyltransferase	U/l (units/l)	8 + 4 (8 + 4)	0–16 (0–16)			

Glucose	mmol/l (mg/dl)	7.9 + 1.9 (142 + 35)		8.5–9.5 (153–171)	3.6–7.2 (64–130)	5.5–8.0 (99–145)
Lactate (LDH) dehydrogenase	U/l (units/l)	150 + 78 (150 + 78)	79–412 (79–412)			
Magnesium	mmol/l (mg/dl)	0.9 − 0.7 (2.3 + 1.6)				
Phosphorus	mmol/l (mg/dl)	1.4 + 0.3 (4.3 + 1.0)	0.8–2.0 ₪ (2.5–6.2) 1.3–2.4 Ó [14] (3.1–7.4)	1.4–2.0 (4.4–6.1) [62]	0.6–2.7 (1.8–8.4)	1.5–2.7 (4.6–8.2)
Potassium	mmol/l (mEq/l)	5 + 1 (5 + 1)	3.5–6.8 (3.5–6.8)	4.6–5.5 (4.6–5.5)	3.1–5.1 (3.1–5.1)	4.1–6.1 (4.1–6.1)
Protein – total	g/l (g/dl)	63 − 5 (6.3 + 0.5)	58–83 ₪ (5.8–8.3) 53–78 Ó [15] (5.3–7.8)	57–70 (6.7–7.0)	38–72 (3.8–7.2)	56–80 (5.6–8.0)
Albumin	g/l (g/dl)	44 + 4 (4.4 + 0.4)	34–50 (3.4–5.0)	31–46 (3.1–4.6)	3–49 (0.3–4.9)	2–9 (0.2–0.9)
Globulin	g/l (g/dl)	17 + 4 (1.7 + 0.4)	18–39 ₪ (1.8–3.9) 13–34 Ó [13] (1.3–3.4)	39–31 (2.9–3.1)		37–71 (3.7–7.1)
Sodium	mmol/l (mEq/l)	137 + 3 (137 + 3)	132–145 (132–145)	139–143 (139–143)	131–145 (131–145)	
Triglycerides	mmol/l (mg/dl)	1.1 + 0.5 (96 + 46)	0.5–3.02 (44–267)			

[a] Sample sizes not within this range are given in bracketed italics next to the specific range *[xx]*.
Ħ San Diego Zoo in-house clinical lab values, captive animals.
¥ With outliers removed.
Key: Male ♂, Female ♀, Adult ₪, Juvenile Ó, Anesthetized ₳, Manual Restraint ✋.

Table 11.8 Biochemical reference ranges for select other marsupials.

Analyte (abbreviation)	Units, SI (conventional)	Gray short-tailed opossum [17]	Brush-tailed possum [40]	Tasmanian devil [25]	Chuditch [48]	Southern hairy-nosed wombat [9]	Common wombat [9]
Sample size[a]		**26 ♂ 20 ♀**	**3–11**	**Sample size**	**34–36**	**14**	**31**
Alkaline phosphatase (ALP)	U/l (units/l)	99 ± 7 ♂ (99 ± 7) 110 ± 10 ♀ (110 ± 10)		104 ± 66 (104 ± 66)	469 ± 231 (469 ± 231)	266 ± 125 (266 ± 125)	342 ± 214 (342 ± 214)
Alanine aminotransferase (ALT)	U/l (units/l)	134 ± 11 ♂ (134 ± 11) 132 ± 15 ♀ (132 ± 15)		26 ± 9 (26 ± 9)	47 ± 22 (47 ± 22)	69 ± 32 (69 ± 32)	24 ± 9 (24 ± 9)
Aspartate aminotransferase (AST)	U/l (units/l)	85 ± 12 ♂ (85 ± 12) 84 ± 16 ♀ (84 ± 16)		87 ± 50 (87 ± 50)	115 ± 65 (115 ± 65)	39 ± 23 (39 ± 23)	156 ± 197 (156 ± 197)
Bicarbonate	mmol/l (mEq/l)					28.3 ± 2.7 (28.3 ± 2.7)	33.6 ± 4.1 (33.6 ± 4.1)
Bilirubin (total)	μmol/l (mg/dl)	3.42 ± 0.3 ♂ (0.2 ± 0.02) 2.9 ± 0.3 ♀ (0.17 ± 0.02)		24 ± 14 (1.4 ± 0.2)	2.7 ± 1.5 (0.16 ± 0.1)	5.1 ± 3.4 (0.3 ± 0.2)	5.2 ± 3.0 (0.3 ± 0.2)
Bilirubin (direct)	μmol/l (mg/dl)			5 ± 5 (0.3 ± 0.3)			
Bilirubin (indirect)	μmol/l (mg/dl)			19 ± 21 (1.1 ± 1.2)			
Urea nitrogen (BUN)	mmol/l (mg/dl)	19.6 ± 0.5 ♂ (55 ± 1.4) 19.2 ± 0.6 ♀ (53.9 ± 1.8)	2.22 ± 0.32 ♂ (6.2 ± 0.9) 2.35 ± 0.7 ♀ (6.6 ± 2.0)	4.2 ± 1.3 (11.8 ± 3.6)	19.9 ± 2.4 (55.7 ± 6.7)	10.0 ± 3.9 (28.0 ± 10.9)	3.7 ± 5.0 (8.4 ± 14.0)
Calcium	mmol/l (mg/dl)	2.6 ± 0.03 ♂ (10.3 ± 0.1) 2.55 ± 0.05 ♀ (10.2 ± 0.2)	2.95 ± 0.1 ♂ (11.8 ± 0.4) 2.8 ± 0.3 ♀ (11.2 ± 1.2)	2.3 ± 0.2 (9.2 ± 0.8)	2.42 ± 0.14 (9.68 ± 0.56)	2.3 ± 0.13 (9.2 ± 0.5)	2.4 ± 0.4 (9.6 ± 1.6)
Chloride	mmol/l mEq/l		101 ± 1.3 ♂ (101 ± 1.3) 104 ± 8.3 ♀ (104 ± 8.3)	116 ± 4 (116 ± 4)		101 ± 4 (101 ± 4)	94 ± 5 (94 ± 5)
Cholesterol	mmol/l (mg/dl)			3.4 ± 0.8 (131 ± 31)	4.4 ± 1.1 (170 ± 42)	2.5 ± 0.6 (97 ± 23)	2.1 ± 0.7 (81 ± 27)
Creatine kinase (CK)	U/l (units/l)			1152 ± 1210 (1152 ± 1210)	1423 ± 1323 (1423 ± 1323)	641 ± 587 (641 ± 587)	233 ± 454 (233 ± 454)

Creatinine	µmol/l (mg/dl)	♂ and ♀ 15 ± 0.9 (0.17 ± 0.01)		62 ± 18 (0.7 ± 0.2)	54 ± 10 (0.6 ± 0.1)	230 ± 40 (2.6 ± 0.5)	80 ± 30 (0.9 ± 0.3)
Glucose	mmol/l (mg/dl)	7.2 ± 1.0 ♂ (129 ± 18) 6.8 ± 1.3 ♀ (122 ± 24)	7.2 ± 1.1 ♂₪ (130 ± 20) 10.6 ± 1.0 ♀₪ (191 ± 18)	6.3 ± 1.3 (114 ± 23)	6.2 ± 1.7 (112 ± 31)	5.5 ± 1.7 (99 ± 31)	5.3 ± 1.4 (95 ± 25)
Phosphorus	mmol/l (mg/dl)	2.3 ± 0.06 ♂ (7.2 ± 0.2) 1.9 ± 0.1 ♀ (6.0 ± 0.3)	2.42 ± 0.4 ♂₪ (7.5 ± 1.2) 2.26 ♀₪ *[1]* (7.0)	1.7 ± 0.5 (5.3 ± 1.5)	2.3 ± 0.6 (7.1 ± 1.9)	1.4 ± 0.4 (4.2 ± 1.2)	1.6 ± 0.4 (5.1 ± 1.4)
Potassium	mmol/l (mEq/l)		4.1 ± 0.3 ♂₪ (4.1 ± 0.3) 3.7 ± 0.4 ♀₪ (3.7 ± 0.4)	5.2 ± 2.1 (5.2 ± 2.1)		4.1 ± 0.5 (4.1 ± 0.5)	4.7 ± 1.1 (4.7 ± 1.1)
Protein – total	g/l (g/dl)	64 ± 1 ♂ (6.4 ± 0.1) 65 ± 1 ♀ (6.5 ± 0.1)	69 ± 1 ♂₪ *[25]* (6.9 ± 0.1) 70 ± 2 ♀₪ *[23]* (7.0 ± 0.2)	60 ± 6 (6.0 ± 0.6)	59.5 ± 7.1 (6.0 ± 0.7)	62 ± 5 (6.2 ± 0.5)	59 ± 11 (5.9 ± 1.1)
Albumin	g/l (g/dl)	♂ and ♀ 37 ± 1 (3.7 ± 0.1)		33 ± 3 (3.3 ± 0.3)	31.5 ± 2.1 (3.2 ± 0.2)	34 ± 3 (3.4 ± 0.3)	30 ± 6 (3.0 ± 0.6)
Globulin	g/l (g/dl)			27 ± 7 (2.7 ± 0.7)		30 ± 6 (3.0 ± 0.6)	30 ± 8 (3.0 ± 0.8)
Sodium	mmol/l (mEq/l)		153 ± 3.6 ♂₪ (153 ± 3.6) 150 ± 2.4 ♀₪ (150 ± 2.4)	148 ± 5 (148 ± 5)		142 ± 2 (142 ± 2)	134 ± 3.2 (134 ± 3.2)
Thyroid hormone (T4)	nmol/l (µg/dl)					6.3 ± 1.9 (0.49 ± 0.15)	5.7 ± 3.1 (0.44 ± 0.24)

Data Presented as Mean ± SD.
Key: Male ♂, Female ♀, Adult ₪, Juvenile Ó, Anesthetized A, Manual Restraint ✋.
[a] Sample sizes not within this range are given in bracketed italics next to the specific range *[xx]*.

Table 11.9 Reference intervals from 30 koala serum samples via the robust method [42].

Analyte/fraction	Absolute value (g/dl)	Total protein %
Total protein	4.4–7.8	N/A
A/G ratio	0.88–2.01	N/A
Albumin	2.4–4.8	50.1–68.3
Alpha 1 globulin	0.52–1.19	8.8–18.3
Alpha 2 globulin	0.28–0.65	4.2–10.7
Beta globulin	0.25–0.88	5.1–13.3
Gamma globulin	0.13–1.09	2.9–17.0
Total globulins	1.67–3.39	31.7–49.9

Total protein determined by the Biuret method by using the Ortho Vitros 250 analyzer (Ortho Clinical Diagnostics, Rochester, New York 14626, United States). Protein electrophoresis determined via Helena SPIFE 3000 electrophoresis system (Helena Laboratories, Beaumont, Texas 77704, United States) and the split b gel reagent.

species with published serum protein electrophoresis reference values [42]. Blood protein reference values for koala plasma proteins (6.0–7.5 g/dl) and serum total protein (5.8–8.3 g/dl), albumin (3.4–5.0 g/dl), and globulins (1.8–3.9 g/dl) derived from automated chemistry (non-EPH methods) analyzers correlated well with free-ranging koala serum protein electrophoresis results (Table 11.9) [4, 12, 16, 42]. Koalas normally have high plasma alpha 1 globulin concentrations [16, 40]. Immature koalas have significantly lower total protein, mainly due to reduced globulin concentrations, but no apparent sex or seasonal differences [12, 16]. Hypoproteinemia (2.2–3.2 g/dl) can occur in koalas suffering chlamydiosis, with clinical signs of conjunctivitis, urinary tract infections, and lymphoid neoplasia [12, 24, 39, 46]. Hypoproteinemia is related to the poor body condition of koalas suffering these diseases [42]. In reported koala serum electrophoresis values, differences between free-ranging and zoo-based koala results may reflect a true difference or the small sample size of the study [42]. Differences included a lower total protein in zoo-based koalas which was related to a lower albumin that could reflect different diet and/ or hydration level. Free-ranging koalas had higher beta globulin fractions, and the combined differences result in a significant difference in the albumin to globulin ratio (A:G) that may reflect an increased burden of inflammatory or infectious stimuli found in the wild versus zoo environments.

Fibrinogen concentrations may be more useful indicators of acute inflammation in macropods than the leukocyte count. Increased fibrinogen can occur in macropods with lumpy jaw (osteomyelitis of the mandible or maxilla). Ranges for red-necked wallabies were 1.3–3.6 g/l and for red kangaroos 1.2–4.5 g/l [20].

Blood Gases

Information on blood gases in marsupials is limited. Marsupials values range from 7.3–7.5 for pH, 34–72 mmHg for pCO_2, 18.9–43.9 m/ml for total CO_2, 18–42 mEq for HCO_3, and 48–160 mmHg for pO_2 [50]. These values should be interpreted in the light that the circumstances of collection are unknown (e.g., restraint method, health status, venous or arterial blood).

Vitamins, Minerals and Metals, Toxins

Many plants, including *Eucalyptus* species, contain calcium as insoluble calcium oxalate crystals in their leaves. Oxalate nephrosis is often a fatal syndrome in koalas with tubulointerstitial nephrosis and marked and progressive azotemia [7]. Dehydration of both the eucalyptus leaves and the koala may increase the risks of calcium oxalate accumulation in koala kidneys [7]. Aluminum toxicity causing renal failure has been reported in koalas, but normal or toxic blood values are not available [21]. Copper toxicity has occurred in a zoo-based southern hairy-nosed wombat. Plasma copper levels were lower in southern hairy-nosed wombats (5.2–6.5 μmol/ml) compared to common wombats (20.5–28.3 μmol/l) [2]. Hypervitaminosis D as well as calcinosis cutis has been reported in zoo-based wombats and may be related to lower vitamin D requirements of marsupials compared to eutherian mammals or dietary excesses in outdated zoo diets. Zoo-based wombats have higher levels of 25-hydroxycholecalciferol than free-ranging counterparts with both groups having lower levels than eutherian mammals [18]. Free-ranging koalas also have lower levels of vitamin D than eutherian mammals with 25-hydroxycholecalciferol levels being 7.4 ± 3.0 nmol/l (2.9 ± 1.2 ng/ml) [41]. Vitamin E deficiency is suspected to cause nutritional myopathy in macropods, particularly quokkas. Plasma Vitamin E for five normal quokkas was 2.9–3.2 mg/l, while the selenium-containing enzyme glutathione peroxidase was 537–614 U/g [48]. Serum iron levels (mg %) of 49.0 ± 4.9 (adult males, $n = 3$), 54.0 ± 2.8 (adult females, $n = 3$), and 38.0 ± 0.8 (juvenile females, $n = 3$) and serum magnesium levels (mg %) of 1.65 ± 0.09 (adult males, $n = 4$), 1.39 ± 0.25 (adult females, $n = 4$), and 1.56 ± 0.47 (juvenile females, $n = 5$) have been reported in North American opossums [19].

Thyroid Hormones

Colloid goiter occurred as an incidental finding in 4 out of 75 koalas during a disease survey [51]. Low thyroid gland activity has been proposed for koalas in the presence of normal dietary iodine, with free T4 (3.3 ± 2.1 pmol/l; 0.26 ± 0.16 ng/dl) and free T3 (1.4 ± 0.9 pmol/l; 90.9 ± 58.4 pg/dl) reported [29]. In a prospective study on parma wallabies with megaesophagus, total T4 (14–40 nmol/l; 1.1–3.1 ng/dl), free T4 (5–18 pmol/l; 0.39–1.4 ng/dl), total T3 (0.4–1.0 nmol/l; 26–65 ng/dl), and free T3 (0.8–3.8 pmol/l; 51.9–2467 pg/dl) values were considered normal [10].

Urinalysis

Normal koala urine specific gravity is usually greater than 1.060 and may need to be diluted with distilled water to read on a refractometer [4, 11]. Koala urine pH is generally 5, and false positives for ketones are common on multireagent strips [4]. Table 11.10 shows some normal urine analytes for sugar gliders [8]. Normal urine pH in macropods is 5–6 [48]. Urine from apparently healthy koalas and tree kangaroos may be deeply colored, from port wine (koalas) to almost black (tree kangaroos). Urine specific gravity in captive wombats ranges from 1.020 to 1.035 and pH ranges from 6 to 9 [9]. The arid-zone-adapted hairy-nosed wombats have a greater ability to concentrate urine than common wombats, with a urine specific gravity of 1.024–1.077 reported for free-ranging southern hairy-nosed wombats [33, 52]. Select urine analytes are given for sugar gliders in Table 11.10.

Table 11.10 Urinalysis of the sugar glider *Petaurus breviceps* [8].

Analyte	Average	95% confidence interval outliers removed	Animals sampled
Specific gravity	1.03	1.02–1.04	103
pH	6.16	6.00–6.32	98
Protein (mg/dl)	12.01	9.45–14.58	82

Serology and PCR

The serum or CSF latex cryptococcal antigen test (LCAT) is useful as a diagnostic aid when used in conjunction with a physical examination, radiographs, advanced imaging, and culture in diagnosing cryptococcosis in koalas. In other species, false positives are uncommon (*Klebsiella* spp. and *Trichosporon* spp. infections), but the occurrence of false positives in koalas is unknown [31]. No reliable cut-off for LCAT titers to differentiate subclinical from clinical disease exists, though titers ≥128 are likely associated with clinical disease and titers ≤64 likely indicate subclinical cases that will resolve spontaneously [28]. Any titer ≥2 is considered positive, and additional diagnostics should be performed. Rising or sustained titers can indicate disease, and treatment should be considered. Decreases in the LCAT titer tend to lag behind the clinical response to therapy, and treatment should continue until two negative titers one month apart are received. LCAT titers can be submitted to Texas A&M Veterinary Medical Diagnostic Laboratory (TVMDL, http://tvmdl.tamu.edu/, College Station Laboratory, PO Box Drawer 3040, College Station, TX 77841-3040, USA, Telephone: +1979-845-3414).

Chlamydiosis is a serious disease of koalas in Australia causing ocular, respiratory, urinary, and reproductive tract infections. The Clearview Chlamydia MF test is the most widely used in-house *Chlamydiaceae* antigen detection methodology used in Australia [4]. Field trials suggest a sensitivity of 91% and a specificity of 100% [53]. Reproductive tissue swabs or centrifuged urine can be used for testing [4]. PCR for koala chlamydophilosis is not commercially available.

Diagnosis of toxoplasmosis in marsupials via serology is best achieved by a direct agglutination test (DAT) to measure specific *Toxoplasma gondii* antibody (both IgG and IgM), combined with a modified agglutination test (MAT) which measures only IgG. A positive DAT with a low or negative MAT suggests acute toxoplasmosis [48]. A rising titer in sequential blood samples confirms active infection as opposed to prior exposure.

References

1 Pye, G.W. (2001). Marsupial, insectivore, and chiropteran anesthesia. *Veterinary Clinics of North America: Exotic Animal Practice: Anesthesia* 4 (1): 211–237.

2 Vogelnest, L. and Woods, R. (2008). *Medicine of Australian Mammals*. Collingwood, Australia: CSIRO Publishing.

3 Holz, P. (2008). Dasyurids. In: *Medicine of Australian Mammals* (ed. L. Vogelnest and R. Woods), 359–394. Collingwood, Australia: CSIRO Publishing.

4 Bryant, B. and Reiss, A. (2008). Wombats. In: *Medicine of Australian Mammals* (ed. L. Vogelnest and R. Woods), 329–358. Collingwood, Australia: CSIRO Publishing.

5 Brust, D. (2009). *Sugar Gliders: A Complete Veterinary Care Guide*. Veterinary Interactive Publications.

6 Moore, D.M. (1984). A simple technique for blood collection in the opossum (*Didelphis virginiana*). *Laboratory Animals* 18: 52–54.

7 Giacometti, L., Berntzen, A.K., and Bliss, M.E. (1972). Hematologic parameters of the opossum (*Didelphis virginiana*). *Comparative Biochemistry and Physiology* 43A: 287–292.
8 Jurgelski, W. Jr. (1974). The opossum (*Didelphis virginiana* Kerr) as a biomedical model. I. Research perspective, husbandry, and laboratory technics. *Laboratory Animal Science* 24 (2): 376–403.
9 Lewis, J.H. (1975). Comparative hematology: studies on opossums *Didelphis marsupialis* (*virginianus*). *Comparative Biochemistry and Physiology* 51A: 275–280.
10 Woods, H.A. II and Hellgren, E.C. (2003). Seasonal changes in the physiology of the male Virginia opossums (*Didelphis virginiana*): signs of the dasyurid semelparity syndrome? *Physiological and Biochemical Zoology* 76 (3): 406–417.
11 Agar, N.S., Reinke, N.B., Godwin, I.R. et al. (2000). Comparative biochemistry of marsupial erythrocytes: a review. *Comparative Haematology International* 10: 148–167.
12 Cleva, G.M., Stone, G.M., and Dickens, R.K. (1994). Seasonal changes in haematocrit in captive koalas (*Phascolarctos cinereus*). *Australian Journal of Zoology* 42 (2): 233–236.
13 Dickens, R.K. (1978). The koala in health and disease. In: *Fauna*, Post Graduate Committee in Veterinary Science, Proceedings, vol. 36, 105–117. Sydney: University of Sydney.
14 Johnson, R. and Hemsley, S. (2008). Gliders and possums. In: *Medicine of Australian Mammals* (ed. L. Vogelnest and R. Woods), 359–225. Collingwood, Australia: CSIRO Publishing.
15 Vogelnest, L. and Portas, T. (2008). Macropods. In: *Medicine of Australian Mammals* (ed. L. Vogelnest and R. Woods), 133–225. Collingwood, Australia: CSIRO Publishing.
16 Spencer, A.J. and Canfield, P.J. (1996). Lymphoid neoplasia in the koala *(Phascolarctos cinereus):* a review and classification of 31 cases. *Journal of Zoo and Wildlife Medicine* 27 (3): 303–314.
17 Booth, R.J. and Blanshard, W.H. (1999). Diseases of koalas. In: *Zoo and Wild Animal Medicine Current Therapy 4* (ed. M.E. Fowler and R.E. Miller), 321–333. Philadelphia: WB Saunders.
18 Skerrat, L.F. (2003). Clinical response of captive common wombats (*Vombatus ursinus*) infected with *Sarcoptes scabeii* var *wombati*. *Journal of Wildlife Diseases* 39 (1): 179–192.
19 Haynes, J.I. and Skidmore, G.W. (1991). Haematology of the dasyurid marsupials *Sminthopsis crassicaudata* and *Sminthopsis macroura*. *Australian Journal of Zoology.* 39 (2): 157–169.
20 Cutts, J.H. and Krause, W.J. (1980). Leukocytes in the peripheral blood of the developing opossum. *Journal of Anatomy* 130 (1): 113–120.
21 Messick, J.B., Berent, L.M., Ehrhart, E.J. et al. (2000). Light and electron microscopic features of *Eperythrozoon*-like parasites in a north American opossum (*Didelphis virginiana*). *Journal of Zoo and Wildlife Medicine* 31 (2): 240–243.
22 Chiscano, K.A., Hackleman, S.M., Underwood, A.R. et al. (1993). Blood groups in a marsupial (*Monodelphis domestica*). *Journal of Heredity* 84: 181–183.
23 Canfield, P.M., O'Neill, M.E., and Smith, E.F. (1989). Haematological and biochemical reference values for the koala (*Phascolarctos cinereus*). *Australian Veterinary Journal* 66 (10): 324–326.
24 Blanshard, W. and Bodley, K. (2008). Koalas. In: *Medicine of Australian Mammals* (ed. L. Vogelnest and R. Woods), 226–327. Collingwood, Australia: CSIRO Publishing.
25 Canfield, P.M., O'Neill, M.E., and Smith, E.F. (1989). Haematological and biochemical investigations of diseased koala (*Phascolarctos cinereus*). *Australian Veterinary Journal* 66 (9): 269–272.
26 Hemsley, S., Govendir, M., Canfield, P.J., and Connolly, J. (1998). Diabetes mellitus in a koala (*Phascolarctos cinereus*). *Australian Veterinary Journal* 76 (3): 203–208.
27 Shimizu, T., Yasuda, N., Kono, I. et al. (1989). Diabetes mellitus in a koala *(Phascolarctos cinereus). Veterinary Pathology* 26: 528–529.
28 Blanshard, W.H. (1994). Medicine and husbandry of koalas. In: *Wildlife.* Post Graduate Committee in Veterinary Science, Proceedings, vol. 233, 547–623. Sydney: University of Sydney.
29 Pye, G.W., Ellis, W., Fitzgibbon, S. et al. (2012). Serum protein electrophoresis values for free-ranging and zoo-based koalas *(Phascolarctos cinereus). Journal of Zoo and Wildlife Medicine* 43 (1): 183–186.
30 Presidente, P.J.A. and Correa, J. (1981). Haematology, plasma electrolytes, and serum biochemical values of *Trichosurus vulpeca* (Kerr) (Marsupialia: Phalangeridae). *Australian Journal of Zoology* 29 (4): 507–517.
31 Higgins, D.P., Hemsley, S., and Canfield, P.J. (2005). Association of uterine and salpingeal fibrosis with chlamydial Hsp60 and Hsp10 antigen-specific antibodies in *Chlamydia*-infected koalas. *Clinical Diagnostic and Laboratory Immunology* 12: 632–639.
32 Obendorf, D.L. (1983). Causes of mortality and morbidity of wild koalas, *Phascolarctos cinereus* (Goldfuss), in Victoria, Australia. *Journal of Wildlife Diseases* 19 (2): 123–131.
33 Hawkey, C.M. and Hart, M.G. (1987). Fibrinogen levels in mammals suffering from bacterial infections. *Veterinary Record* 121 (22): 519–521.
34 Wallach, J.D. and Boever, W.J. (1983). *Diseases of Exotic Animals: Medical and Surgical Management*, 575–611. Philadelphia: WB Saunders.

35 Haynes, J.I., Askew, M.J., and Leigh, C. (2004). Dietary aluminium and renal failure in the koala (*Phascolarctos cinereus*). *Histology and Histopathology* 19: 777–784.

36 Barboza PS. 1990. Copper toxicity in captive wombats (Marsupialia: Vombatidae). Proceedings of the American Association of Zoo Veterinarians Annual Conference. pp. 204–206.

37 Fowler AM and Fraser DR. 1993. Vitamin D metabolism in nocturnal marsupials. Proceedings of the Wildlife Disease Association (Australasian section) Annual Conference.

38 Pye, G.W., Ellis, W., Fitzgibbon, S. et al. (2013). Serum vitamin D levels in free-ranging koalas (*Phascolarctos cinereus*). *Journal of Zoo and Wildlife Medicine* 44 (2): 480–483.

39 Weigler, B.J., Booth, R.J., Osawa, R. et al. (1987). Causes of morbidity and mortality in 75 free ranging and captive koalas in south East Queensland, Australia. *Veterinary Record* 121 (24): 571–572.

40 Lawson, V.J., Curtis, A.J., Michelangeli, V.P. et al. (1996). Concentrations of thyroid hormones and iodothyronine binding proteins in the serum of the koala (*Phascolarctos cinereus*). *Australian Veterinary Journal* 74 (1): 55–58.

41 Burgdorf-Moisuk, A., Pye, G.W., Smith, J. et al. (2012). A retrospective and prospective study of megaesophagus in Parma wallabies (*Macropus parma*). *Journal of Zoo and Wildlife Medicine* 43 (1): 95–100.

42 McAllan, B.M., Roberts, J.R., and Barboza, P. (1995). The kidney structure of the common wombat (*Vombatus ursinus*) and the hairy-nosed wombat (*Lasiorhinus latifrons*). *Australian Journal of Zoology* 43 (2): 181–191.

43 Wells, R.T. and Green, B. (1998). Aspects of water metabolism in the southern hairy-nosed wombat, *Lasiorhinus latifrons*. In: *Wombats* (ed. R.T. Wells and P.A. Pridmore), 61–66. Chipping Norton, Australia: Surrey Beatty & Sons.

44 Malik, R., McPetrie, R., Wigney, D.I. et al. (1996). A latex cryptococcal antigen test for diagnosis and monitoring of therapy for cryptococcosis. *Australian Veterinary Journal* 74 (5): 358–364.

45 Krockenberger, M.B., Canfield, P.J., Barnes, J. et al. *Cryptococcus neoformans* var. *gatti* in the koala (*Phascolarctos cinereus*): serological evidence for subclinical cryptococcosis. *Medical Mycology* 40: 273–282.

46 Wood, M.M. and Timms, P. (1992). Comparison of nine antigen detection kits for diagnosis of urogenital infections due to *Chlamydia psittaci* in koalas. *Journal of Clinical Microbiology* 30 (12): 3200–3205.

47 Barnes, T.S., Goldizen, A.W., and Coleman, G.T. (2008). Hematology and serum biochemistry of the brush-tailed rock-wallaby (*Petrogale penicillata*). *Journal of Wildlife Diseases* 44 (2): 295–303.

48 Muir, V.Y. and Hawkey, C.M. (1991). Severe haemolytic anaemia and disseminated intravascular coagulation in a wallaby (*Macropus rufogriseus*). *Comparative Haematology International* 1 (3): 178–180.

49 Blessington, J. and Steenburg, J. (2007). Tree Kangaroo (*Dendrolagus* spp.). In: *Husbandry Manual 3rd Edition, Tree Kangaroo Species Survival Plan*. Silver Springs MD: American Association of Zoos and Aquariums.

50 McKenzie, S., Deane, E.M., and Burnett, L. (2002). Haematology and serum biochemistry of the tammar wallaby, *Macropus eugenii*. *Comparative Clinical Pathology* 11 (4): 229–237.

51 Ness, R.D. (1999). Clinical pathology and sample collection of exotic small mammals. *Veterinary Clinics of North America: Exotic Animal Practice* 2 (3): 591–620.

52 Svensson, A., Mills, J.N., Boardman, W.S.J. et al. (1998). Hematology and serum biochemistry reference values for anesthetized chuditch (*Dasyurus geoffroii*). *Journal of Zoo and Wildlife Medicine* 29 (3): 311–314.

53 Evans, K.D., Hewett, T.A., Clayton, C.J. et al. (2010). Normal organ weights, serum chemistry, hematology, and cecal and nasopharyngeal bacterial cultures in the gray short-tailed opossum (*Monodelphis domestica*). *Journal of the American Association for Laboratory Animal Science* 49 (4): 401–406.

54 Mays, A. Jr. and Loew, F.M. (1968). Hemograms of laboratory-confined opossums (*Didelphis virginiana*). *Journal of the American Veterinary Medical Association* 153 (7): 800–802.

12

Hedgehogs

Jordan Gentry DVM[1], R. Scott Larsen DVM, DACZM[2] and J. Jill Heatley DVM, MS, DABVP (Avian, Reptilian, Amphibian), DACZM[3]

[1] *Downtown Aquarium, Houston, Montgomery County Animal Shelter, Conroe, Texas, USA*
[2] *Denver Zoo, Denver, Colorado, USA*
[3] *Department of Small Animal Clinical Sciences, College of Veterinary Medicine & Biomedical Sciences, Texas A&M University, College Station, Texas, USA*

Introduction

Hedgehogs can be challenging patients because of their small size, spiny coat, and tendency to roll into a ball. Because of their short life span, their secretive and aloof nature, and their tendency to suffer from zoonotic and neoplastic diseases, clinical pathologic diagnosis via hematology, plasma biochemistry, and cytology is common in these species. Importation to the United States is strictly controlled, and captive breeding efforts have made many color varieties of the African pygmy hedgehog available.

Species

Hedgehogs are small spiny mammals of the family Erinaceidae which includes 17 species from 5 genera [1]. As primitive nocturnal mammals which share distant ancestry with shrews, the hedgehog family evolved over 58 million years ago, but has changed little over the last 15 million years [2]. There are no hedgehogs native to the Australia, and no living species native to the Americas. In Europe, the European hedgehog (*Erinaceus europaeus*) is commonly found in wildlife rehabilitation settings. Although no hedgehog species is currently considered vulnerable to extinction, CITES Appendix II lists the Cape hedgehog (*Atelerix frontalis*). In contrast, hedgehogs are introduced, invasive pests in New Zealand and on the Scottish isles. The scientific name and native range of species discussed in this chapter given in Table 12.1. The African pygmy hedgehog (*Atelerix albiventris*) is most commonly found in the US pet trade. Despite a ban on US importation of the African pygmy hedgehog in 1991 because of the potential ingress of foot-and-mouth disease, captive production continues to support the pet trade [3, 4].

Sample Collection

Restraint

Hedgehogs are typically anesthetized for blood collection because their ability to roll into a ball usually precludes adequate access for phlebotomy. While injectable anesthetics may be used, gas anesthetics, such as isoflurane and sevoflurane, are more commonly employed for rapid, safe anesthesia of hedgehogs. Isoflurane or sevoflurane can be administered by placing the awake animal in a standard canine facemask for chamber induction followed by a use of a smaller facemask; intubation is also possible [5].

Collection Sites

Vascular access points of the hedgehog include the jugular, cranial vena cava, cephalic, lateral saphenous, and femoral veins [1]. Large samples are most readily taken from the jugular vein or cranial vena cava. Smaller blood samples can be obtained from the femoral vein, lateral saphenous vein (Figure 12.1), or cephalic vein (Figure 12.2); however, samples greater than 0.5 ml are rarely obtained from these sites. Because of their small size, negative pressure on the syringe often collapses these veins, and small movements easily result in hematoma formation. The use of small needles (25 or 27 gauge (g.)) and small syringes (0.5 or 1.0 cm^3) helps to prevent vascular lumen collapse. Butterfly needles with extension tubing may be useful in providing steady small pressure, but can also be frustrating to use since a significant amount of the blood volume collected may be in the extension tubing and needs to be carefully placed into the collection tube prior to clotting or hemolysis.

Exotic Animal Laboratory Diagnosis, First Edition. Edited by J. Jill Heatley and Karen E. Russell.

Table 12.1 Select hedgehog species.

Common name	Scientific name	Range, additional information
European hedgehog	*Erinaceus europaeus*	Common to eastern Europe and United Kingdom. Frequently seen in wildlife rehabilitation.
African pygmy hedgehog/ four-toed hedgehog	*Atelerix albiventris*	Central and East Africa. Frequently kept in US pet trade.
North African hedgehog, Algerian hedgehog	*Atelerix algirus*	Endemic Mediterranean North Africa from Morocco to Libya. Its occurrence in continental Europe and on many islands may be the result of introductions by man.
Southern white-breasted hedgehog	*Erinaceus concolor*	Parts of Middle East and Mediterranean countries. Previously classified as same species as European hedgehog.
Long-eared hedgehog	*Hemiechinus auritus*	Central Asia and the Middle East

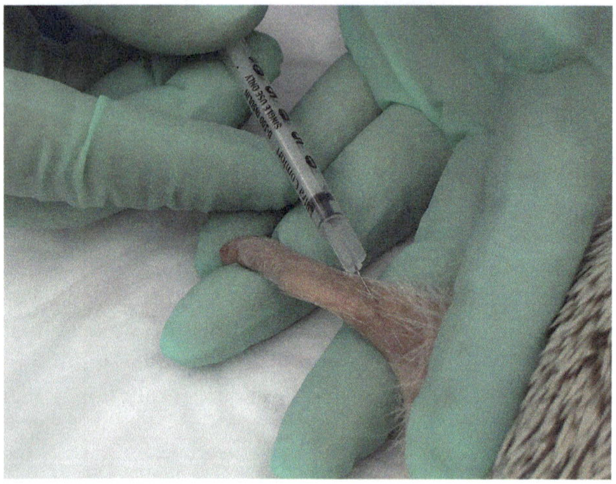

Figure 12.1 Saphenous venipuncture of the African hedgehog *(Atalerix albiventris)*.

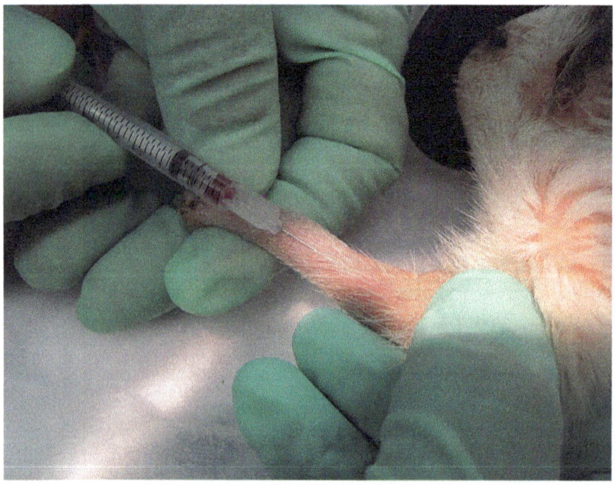

Figure 12.2 Cephalic venipuncture of the African hedgehog *(Atalerix albiventris)*.

The jugular vein is often sampled without being visualized because its location is similar to that of other mammals. The jugular is most reliably accessed by placing the anesthetized hedgehog on its back. The phlebotomist's thumb is used to gently occlude the venous outflow at or near the manubrium, and the index finger is used to extend the skin of the neck just below the chin. The remaining three fingers are used to place upward pressure on the back of the neck to stabilize the neck and help prevent the jugular vein from moving dorsally once the needle is inserted. Using this technique, the jugular vein may fill so that it can be seen or palpated; however, the jugular vein is often neither seen nor felt, particularly in hedgehogs that are overweight. The jugular vein courses in an area best described by visualizing a line between the carina and the base of the ear as it courses from the ramus of the mandible to the point of the shoulder (Figure 12.3). Alternatively, positioning the hedgehog dorsoventrally in recumbence with the legs stretched caudally over the end of a table, as for domestic cats or ferrets, may be attempted [3]. Phlebotomy of the jugular vein is usually achieved using a 23–25 g. needle and 1–3 cm^3 syringes.

Sampling from the cranial vena cava is similar to techniques described for domestic ferrets. Despite the risk of cardiac puncture because of the relatively cranial position of the heart in this species, careful attention to needle depth and angle can allow safe collection at this site. To access the cranial vena cava, the animal should be positioned in dorsal recumbency and the needle inserted at the cranial thoracic inlet at an angle toward the opposite hip (Figure 12.4). Needle depth should be superficial. Take care to avoid cardiac puncture due to over-insertion.

Blood Volume and Sample Volume

Blood volumes have been determined to change depending on hibernation in *E. europaeus*. In the summer, the

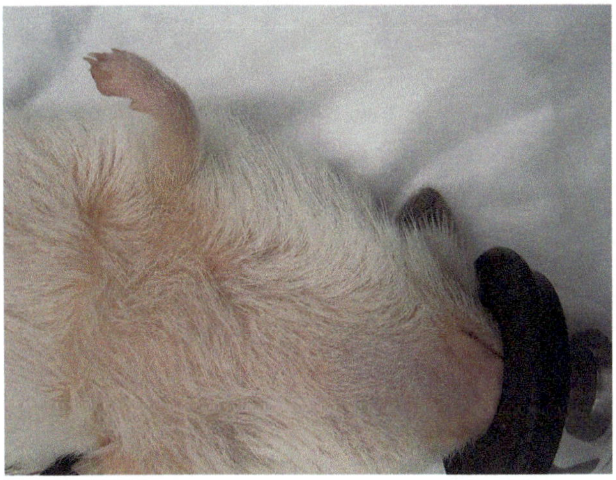

Figure 12.3 Diagrammatic representation of the area of the hedgehog jugular vein *(Atalerix albiventris)*.

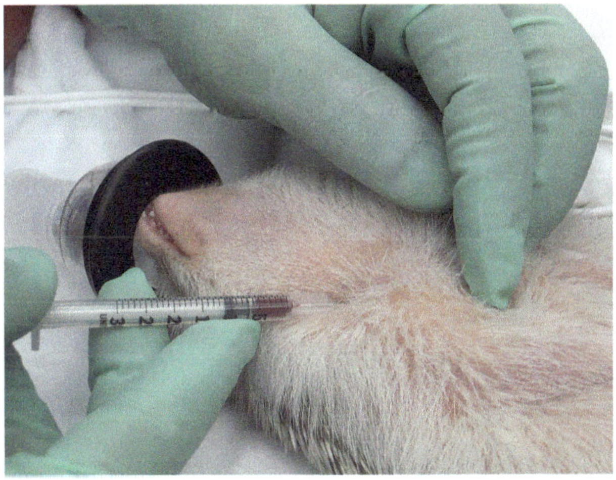

Figure 12.4 Sampling from the cranial vena cava of an African hedgehog *(Atalerix albiventris)*.

animal's blood volume was about 8% of body weight, while during hibernation the blood volume reduced to about 2%–3% of the body weight [6]. Whether other less temperate hedgehogs also undergo cyclical changes in blood volume is unknown. For most healthy small mammals, it is safe to draw 1% of the total body weight in a single blood draw [3]. If this volume is collected, further phlebotomy should not occur for at least 2 weeks.

Sample Handling

Typically, blood is placed in ethylenediaminetetraacetic acid (EDTA) anticoagulant for a complete blood count analysis. Either plasma or serum can be used for biochemistry analysis; however, plasma is usually used because more plasma can typically be obtained from a given volume of blood than serum. Further studies of appropriate anticoagulants and the effect of storage on clinical pathology of hedgehog species remain undetermined.

Specific Analytes

Interpretation of specific analytes for hedgehogs is drawn from interpretation for domestic companion carnivores such as dogs, cats, and ferrets. Reference data for blood values of the African hedgehog (*A. albiventris*), European hedgehog (*E. europaeus*), Southern white-breasted hedgehog (*E. concolor*), and long-eared hedgehog (*Hemiechinus auritus*) are given in Table 12.2 [5, 9, 11–13].

Complete Blood Count

Erythrocytes, Platelets, and Hemostasis

Evaluation of hedgehog erythrocytes includes the packed cell volume, total erythrocyte count, hemoglobin concentration, mean corpuscular volume, and erythrocyte morphology. The normal erythrocyte of the hedgehog is a biconcave disk similar to that of most other mammals (Figure 12.5). The packed cell volume in hedgehogs has been used to assess anemia and dehydration. Most hedgehogs have a PCV of 30%–40%. In apparently healthy European hedgehogs, most (>50%) platelets are large to giant (6–7 μm diameter), while the remainder are 4–6 μm in diameter [10].Tick-induced blood loss results in regenerative anemia in the European hedgehog [14] Anemia, likely of chronic disease, appears common in the captive hedgehog and has been reported in association with cases of lymphocytic-plasmacytic meningoencephalitis (cause undetermined), and as a part of paraneoplastic syndrome in cases of neoplasia [15–19]. Similarly, thrombocytopenia has been reported in a case of lacrimal duct carcinoma and in a case of mammary adenocarcinoma and a granulosa cell tumor [19, 20]. Howell-Jolly bodies have also been reported from hedgehogs suffering neoplasia [19].

Blood clotting times have been determined for the European hedgehog, and seasonal change occurs (Table 12.3) [21]. Blood groups appear unstudied in hedgehog species; transfusion reactions have not been reported, although whole blood transfusion has been reported for this species [20].

Leukocytes

Hedgehog leukocytes are similar in appearance to other mammalian leukocytes. Accurate total WBC counts can be obtained with an electronic particle counter. Neutrophils have multiple nuclear lobes separated by constrictions and contain primary and

Table 12.2 Hematologic reference data for hedgehogs.

Analyte (abbreviation)	Units, SI (US)	African pygmy hedgehog [5, 7] (*Atelerix albiventris*)			Algerian hedgehog (*Atelerix algirus*) [8]	Southern white-breasted hedgehog[a] [9] (*Erinaceus concolor*)	Long-eared hedgehog[a] [9] (*Hemiechinus auritus*)[b]	European hedgehog [8] (*Erinaceus europaeus*)		
Sample size, attributes		**Ħ [5]**	**Ħ [7]**	**1–13 Ħ [5]**	**8♂, 5♀**	**4 ↘**	**4 ↘**	**50 ♂[c] [10]**	**29 ♀[c] [10]**	**2–5 ♂♀ [5]**
White blood cell count	× 10^9/l	11 ± 6.0	9.9 ± 2.5	*11.67 ± 9.109*	19.1 [12.5–32.1]			7.19 ± 1.97	7.69 ± 1.95	15.10 ± 10.17
Neutrophil	× 10^9/l (%)	5.1 ± 5.2	5.2 ± 1.9	7.192 ± 8.632		(23.3 ± 0.5)	(23.9 ± 5.2)	3.15 ± 1.39	2.72 ± 1.38	7.979 ± 6.827
Bands	×10^9/l (%)									
Lymphocytes	×10^9/l (%)	4.0 ± 2.2	3.4 ± 0.9	3.184 ± 2.028		(65.5 ± 2.8)	(64.3 ± 4.6)	3.43 ± 1.1	4.2 ± 1.4	5.287 ± 3.353
Monocytes	×10^9/l (%)	0.3 ± 0.3	0.3 ± 0.1	0.232 ± 0.319		(2.3 ± 0.5)	(1.8 ± 0.5)	0.18 ± 0.12	0.14 ± 0.09	0.409 ± 0.213
Eosinophil	×10^9/l (%)	1.2 ± 0.9	0.7 ± 0.4	1.238 ± 1.487		(7.6 ± 1.5)	(9.0 ± 3.5)	0.35 ± 0.20	0.56 ± 0.34	1.142 ± 0.790
Basophil	×10^9/l (%)	0.4 ± 0.3	0.4 ± 0.3	0.244 ± 0.245		(1.3 ± 1.3)	(1.0 ± 0.7)	0.08 ± 0.06	0.08 ± 0.06	0.360 ± 0.230
Hematocrit	l/l (%)	0.360 ± 0.070 (36.0 ± 7.0)	0.350 ± 0.068 (35.0 ± 6.8)	0.367 ± 0.063 (36.7 ± 6.3)	39.9 [33.0–44.0]			0.33 ± 0.038 (33.0 ± 3.8)	0.33 ± 0.038 (33.0 ± 3.8)	0.342 ± 0.065 (34.2 ± 6.5)
Hemoglobin	g/l g/dl	120 ± 17 (12.0 ± 1.7)						124 ± 12.8 (12.4 ± 1.28)	126 ± 13.2 (12.6 ± 1.32)	105 ± 20 (10.5 ± 2.0)
MCH	pg	15.7 ± 1.9			13.6 [10.7–14.7]			15.3 ± 0.72	15.6 ± 0.88	17.5 ± 0.75
MCHC	g/l g/dl	315 ± 28 (31.5 ± 2.8)			20.7 [18.7–21.9]			384.0 ± 17.3 (38.4 ± 1.73)	377.0 ± 14.1 (37.7 ± 1.41)	323 ± 36 (32.3 ± 3.6)
MCV	fl	50.0 ± 5.4			34.0 [31.3–36.8]			39.9 ± 2.35	41.5 ± 2.32	53.6 ± 1.99
RBC	×10^{12}/l	7.70 ± 1.23			60.8 [59.2–62.3]			8.13 ± 0.67	8.06 ± 0.75	6.80 ± 2.69
Platelet count	× 10^9/l	312.0 ± 120.0			6.56 [5.42–7.29]			133 ± 67.8	135 ± 48.3	196 ± 120

Key: Free-living ↘; Captive Ħ; Pet ; Dry Season ; Spring/Rainy Season ; Anesthetized A; Manual Restraint .

[a] For each species: April, four years old, sexually mature, healthy, femoral vein, heparin [9].

[b] All data presented as mean ± SD unless presented as mean [95% confidence interval].

[c] Wild-caught and overwintered in an English rescue center and scheduled for release. Treated for lungworms and ectoparasites. Medial saphenous vein under general anesthesia with isoflurane anesthesia; anticoagulant was EDTA [10].

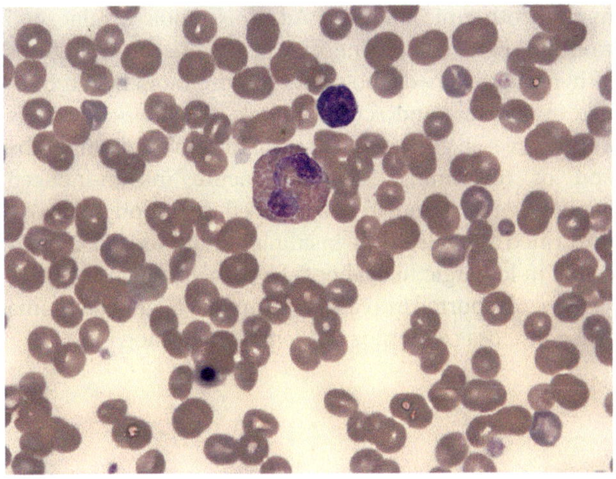

Figure 12.5 Erythrocytes, a nucleated erythrocyte, platelets, an eosinophil (€), and a lymphocyte from the peripheral blood of an African hedgehog *(Atalerix albiventris)*.

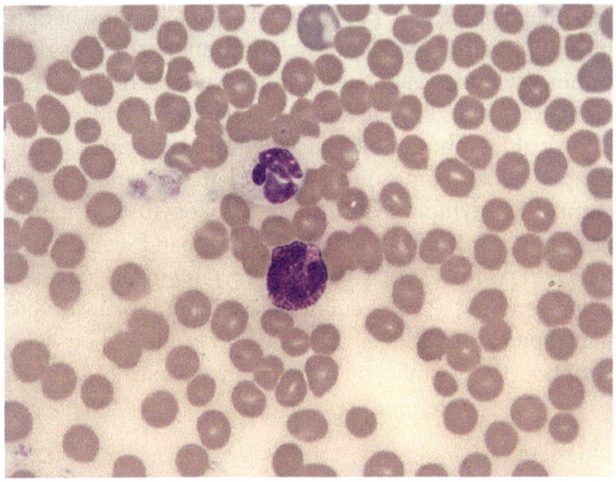

Figure 12.6 Neutrophil and basophil from the peripheral blood of an African hedgehog *(Atalerix albiventris)*.

Table 12.3 Clotting times of two healthy European hedgehogs (*Erinaceus europaeus*) [10].

Analyte (abbreviation)	Substrate/ sample type	SI units	Mean
Clotting time	Glass	Seconds	2
	Silicone		10
Partial thromboplastin time (PTT)			19.3
Prothrombin time (PT)	Serum		32.4
	Plasma		12.9
Thrombin time	Bovine thrombin		68.5

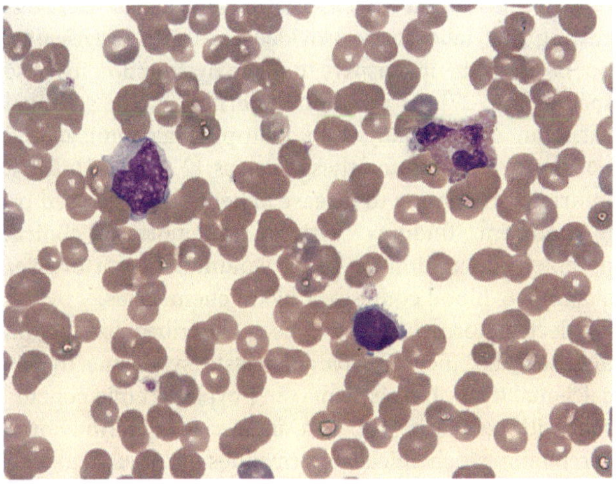

Figure 12.7 Erythrocytes, platelets, and eosinophil (€), lymphocyte (L), and a monocyte (M) from an African hedgehog *(Atalerix albiventris)*.

secondary granules (Figure 12.6). In African hedgehogs, the neutrophil appears to be the predominant white blood cell type with a neutrophil to lymphocyte ratio of approximately 2:1. The presence of band cells (immature neutrophils) at >10% indicates a left shift. Lymphocytes are small cells with scant amounts of blue cytoplasm and a round nucleus (Figure 12.7). Lymphocytes appear to be the predominant cell type in both the southern white-breasted hedgehog and the long-eared hedgehog. Hedgehog erythrocytes, leukocytes, and platelets have similar morphology to those of other mammalian species (Figure 12.8).

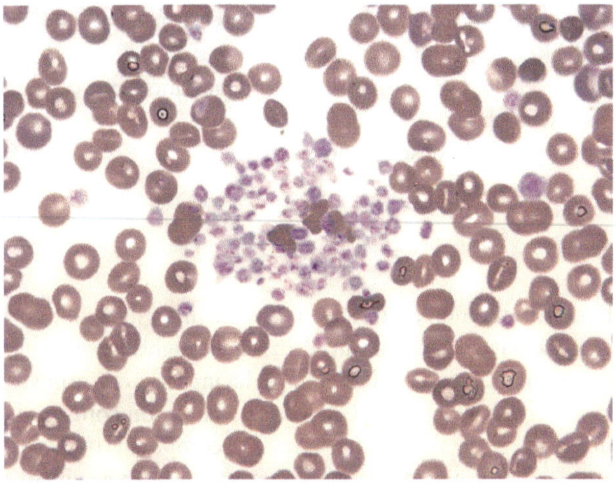

Figure 12.8 Platelet clump from the peripheral blood of an African hedgehog *(Atalerix albiventris)*.

Leukocyte Abnormalities

Leukocytosis is a common finding in diseased hedgehogs and may be due to inflammation related to infection, neoplasia, or other diseases. Paraneoplastic syndrome in hedgehogs mirrors that of other species; eosinophilia and abnormal circulating leukocytes occur [18,22]. One hedgehog suffering lacrimal duct carcinoma had leukocytosis and neutrophilia [20]. Leukocyte abnormalities in a hedgehog with mammary adenocarcinoma and a granulosa cell tumor included leukopenia with toxic neutrophils [19]. Hematologic findings in an African hedgehog with gastrointestinal lymphosarcoma included marked leukocytosis, lymphocytosis, and a regenerative left shift and atypical circulating lymphocytes [22]. Leukocytosis (mature neutrophilia and monocytosis with band cells) of a hedgehog with Chagas disease (*Trypanosoma*) has also been reported [23]. Leukocytosis, lymphocytosis, and neutropenia have been reported in a hedgehog with lymphocytic-plasmacytic meningoencephalitis [15].

Biochemistry Panel

Hedgehog blood chemistries are interpreted similarly to those of other small mammals (Table 12.4). However, lack of abnormalities in blood chemistries has been reported in numerous cases of advanced disease, suggesting that laboratory-provided reference ranges may not be accurate or sensitive to organ dysfunction in these species [22, 27]. In addition, hibernation and seasonal variation cause changes in multiple biochemical and hormonal analytes for these species [21, 28–33]. Most information relating to disease in hedgehogs is based on postmortem findings without antemortem clinical pathology data. Limited sample volume often prioritizes a complete blood count over blood chemistries.

Select abnormalities have been described for certain disease states, including paraneoplastic syndrome, hypercalcemia, hypophosphatemia, and hypoglycemia concurrent with neoplasia [18]. In a single case of lacrimal duct carcinoma, biochemical abnormalities included hypercalcemia and hypophosphatemia [20]. Biochemical abnormalities in a hedgehog with mammary adenocarcinoma and a granulosa cell tumor included hypophosphatemia, increased plasma urea and glucose concentrations, and decreased creatinine concentrations [19]. Increased creatinine kinase (CK) activity has been reported in hedgehogs with Chagas *(Trypanosoma spp.)* disease [23]. Despite the common finding of postmortem cardiac disease in hedgehogs, cardiac troponins have not been investigated in these species.

Glucose, Insulin, and Glucagon

Endocrine pancreas functionality, plasma glucagon, and glucose have been measured in wild-caught, laboratory-maintained European hedgehogs during lethargy, arousal, and active periods [34]. Glucose and glucagon concentrations were decreased in lethargic compared to active animals. A rapid increase in glucagon and then glucose concentrations occur during rewarming. Catabolism of exogenous glucagon was slower in the hypothermic than in homeothermic animals. Administration of glucagon caused a slight, delayed increase in glucose concentrations in hypothermic hedgehogs, but a more rapid hyperglycemia in arousing and active animals. This hyperglycemia only decreased glucagon secretion in active animals at the end of rewarming. Similarly, acute insulin-induced hypoglycemia stimulated alpha-cell secretion in active rewarmed animals, while insulin did not induce hypoglycemia in lethargic hedgehogs. Hyperglycemia and glucosuria were reported in a case of mammary adenocarcinoma and granulosa cell tumor in a female hedgehog [19].

Blood Gases

In the European hedgehog, hibernation is associated with increased and pO_2, pCO_2, and bicarbonate (HCO_3) and slightly decreased pH [26]. Values are comparable to those of moles and shrews (Table 12.5).

Lipids and Lipoproteins

Lipids and lipoproteins have been partially characterized from the European hedgehog in the months of April and May [35]: plasma cholesterol levels (178 + 30 mg/100 ml), triglycerides (46 of: 17 mg/100 ml), and phospholipids (252 + 35 mg/100 ml). Protein electrophoresis of hedgehogs revealed VLDL, LDL, and HDL components with HDL predominating (570 mg/100 ml). Lipoprotein band electrophoretic migration is similar to the human proteins of apolipoprotein A-I and a high-molecular-weight counterpart to apolipoprotein B. Very high-density lipoproteins transport approximately 15% of cholesterol and 20% of phospholipids. DNA encoding an apo[a]-related protein designated HaRP-1 (Hedgehog apo[a] related protein-1) has recently been characterized from the European hedgehog which may function in the regulation of lysine-dependent proteolysis [36].

Hormones

The European hedgehog has a seasonal cycle in the endocrine and exocrine hormone concentrations and function [37–40]. The recrudescence of testicular activity occurs during the period of hibernation [39, 40]. July through August, testosterone concentrations decrease and continue to remain low in autumn. Testicular function resumes in spring, and during the breeding season testosterone levels are constantly high (Figure 12.9) [41]. Plasma cortisol and thyroxine also vary seasonally in this species from approximately 10 to 130 ng/ml and from 6 to 18 ng/ml, respectively (Figures 12.10, 12.11). Adrenocortical

Table 12.4 Biochemical data for hedgehogs.

Analyte (abbreviation) sample size, attributes	**Units, SI (US)**	**African hedgehog 5, 24 *(Atelerix albiventris)* 1–12**		**European hedgehog[a] 25 *(Erinaceus europaeus)* 6♂ 6♀ ⋋ ⌂ All season mean**	**Seasonal mean fall, winter, spring, summer**
Albumin	g/l (g/dl)	29 ± 4 (2.9 ± 0.4)	26 ± 5 (2.6 ± 0.5)	36 ± 5 (3.6 ± 0.5)	
Alkaline phosphatase (ALP)	U/l	51 ± 21	42 ± 26	51	
Alanine aminotransferase (ALT)	U/l	53 ± 24	45 ± 18	69 ± 34	
Aspartate aminotransferase (AST)	U/l	34 ± 22	40 ± 25	65 ± 44	
Amylase	U/l	510 ± 170	87.69 ± 0		
Calcium	mmol/l (mg/dl)	2.2 ± 0.35 (8.8 ± 1.4)	1.9 ± 0.5 (7.6 ± 2.0)	{2.0–2.3} [11]	5.4, 5.6, 5.2, 5.7
Chloride	mmol/l	109 ± 10	114 ± 9		112, 111, 108, 118
Cholesterol	mmol/l (mg/dl)	3.39 ± 0.65 (131 ± 25)	3.471 ± 0.4144 (134 ± 16)		
Creatine kinase (CK)	U/l	863 + 413	1080 ± 536		53, 80, 40, 62
Creatinine	µmol/l (mg/dl)	35.4 ± 17.7 (0.4 ± 0.2)	35 ± 18 (0.4 ± 0.2)	27 ± 9 (0.3 ± 0.1)	(0.6, 0.9, 0.45, 0.7)
Gamma Glutamyltransferase	U/l	4 ± 1	6 ± 0		
Globulin	g/l (g/dl)	27 ± 5 (2.7 ± 0.5)	23 ± 9 (2.3 ± 0.9)	25 ± 7 (2.5 ± 0.7)	4.5, 2.1, 4.7, 3.2
Glucose	mmol/l (mg/dl)	4.94 ± 1.67 (89 ± 30)	3.386 ± 1.832 (61 ± 33)	5.828 ± 0.555 (105 ± 10)	(81, 38, 85, 57)
Lactate dehydrogenase	U/l	441 ± 258	549 ± 269		605, 670, 675, 740
Lipase	U/l		3.058 ± 0		
Magnesium	mmol/l (mg/dl)		0.946 ± 0 2.3 ± 0		
Phosphorus	mmol/l (mg dl)	1.7 ± 0.6 (5.3 ± 1.9)	1.49 ± 0.61 (4.6 ± 1.9)	{2.0–3.8} [11]	
Potassium	mmol/l	4.9 ± 1.0	5.2 ± 0.5	{3.6–5.1} [11]	5.0, 4.8, 5.2, 5.7
Sodium	mmol/l	141 ± 9	143 ± 8	{132–138} [11]	145, 144, 143, 149
Total bilirubin	µmol/l (mg/dl)	5.1 ± 5.1 (0.3 ± 0.3)	50 + 132 (0.3 ± 0.8)	5 ± 2 (0.27 ± 0.12)	
Total protein	g/l (g/dl)	58 ± 7 (5.8 ± 0.7)	51 ± 11 5.1 ± 1.1	{5.1 7 0.2} [11] 93.3 ± 7.9	90, 1254, 124, 115
Triglyceride	mmol/l (mg/dl)	0.43 ± 0.25 (38 ± 22)	0.2260 ± 0.1469 (20 ± 13)		
Urea	mmol/l (mg/dl)	4.5 ± 1.5 (27 ± 9)	7.854 ± 3.213 (47 ± 19)	{13.3–15.0} [11]	

Data presented as mean ± SD except when presented as {Range} or mean [95% confidence interval].

Key: Free-living ⋋; Captive ⌂; Spring/Rainy Season [rainy season symbol]; Anesthetized [anesthetized symbol]; Manual Restraint [manual restraint symbol]; Pet [pet symbol]; Dry Season [dry season symbol].

Free-living origin animals, laboratory housed for several months [26].

[a] Anesthesia with chloral hydrate-urethane, open thorax blood draw from aortic arch [25].

Table 12.5 Mean seasonal arterial blood gases for anesthetized, wild-caught European hedgehogs (6 males, 6 females) [25].

Analyte	Units	Fall	Winter	Spring	Summer
P02	mm Hg	28	65	34	36
pC02	mm Hg	62	122	60	52
pH		7.1	6.9	7.1	7.1
Bicarbonate	mmol/l (mEq/l)	16	20	16	15

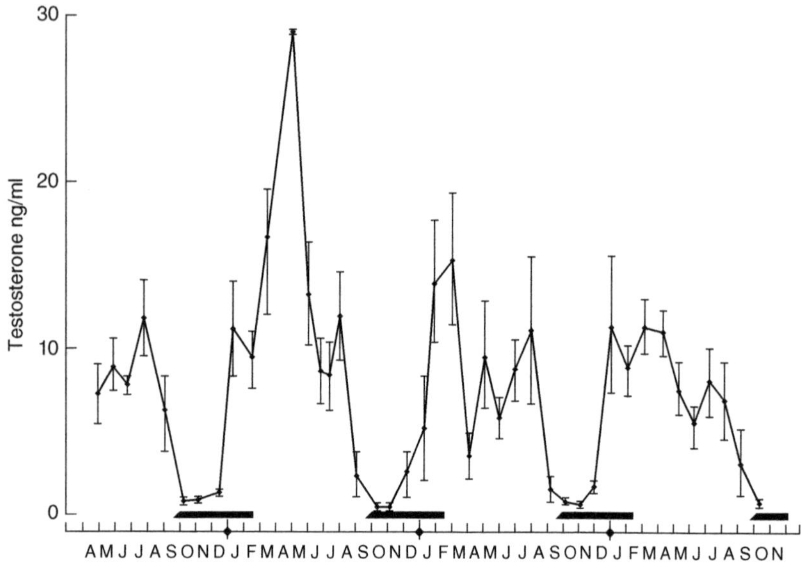

Figure 12.9 Testosterone annual cycle of the hedgehog (*Erinaceus europaeus*) [38].

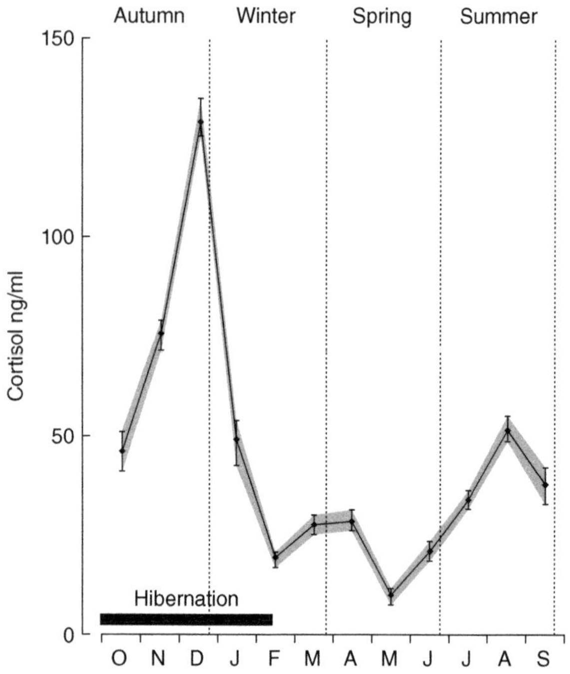

Figure 12.10 Cortisol annual cycle of the hedgehog (*Erinaceus europaeus*) [38].

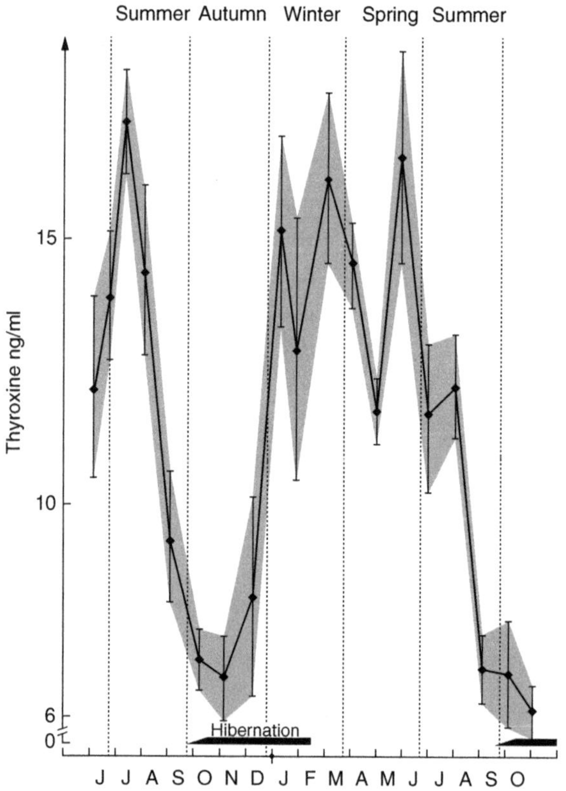

Figure 12.11 Thyroxine annual cycle of the hedgehog (*Erinaceus europaeus*) [38].

carcinoma has been reported in African hedgehogs; associated changes in concentrations of cortisol or other adrenocortical hormones have not been documented [42].

Toxins

Hedgehogs have some immunity against snake venom based on two separate mechanisms. Small amounts of the protein erinacin, an antihemorrhagic factor, are found in the muscular system [43]. A mutation of the hedgehog nicotinic acetylcholine receptor also prevents binding of alpha neurotoxins found in snake venom. [44].

Urinalysis

Sample Collection

Urine can be collected under anesthesia through gentle expression, ventral percutaneous cystocentesis or urinary catheterization [3, 24]. Expression of the urinary bladder should be performed gently to avoid trauma to the urinary bladder and abdomen. Cystocentesis should only be performed if the bladder is definitively palpated or defined during ultrasound examination. Typically, a 23–25 g. needle and a 1.0 or 3.0 cm^3 syringe are used for cystocentesis.

Urinalysis and Renal Diagnostics

Urine-concentrating ability has been evaluated in three hedgehog species: *Paraechinus aethiopicus*, *Hemiechinus auritus*, and *E. europaeus* [45] (Table 12.6). The two latter desert hedgehog species have greater concentrating ability than *E. europaeus*. More concentrated urine was observed in hedgehogs with higher-protein diets. The urine-concentrating ability of hedgehogs is approximately is 9–12 times the plasma concentration. Reference values for captive hedgehog urinalysis are not available, but their carnivorous/omnivorous diet suggests that an acidic urine pH would be normal. Urinary abnormalities have not been well documented in veterinary literature, but white blood cells, neoplastic cells, and crystals are considered abnormal findings.

Renal disease is common in hedgehogs and affected up to 50% (7/14) of hedgehogs presented for necropsy [15, 46]. 11 of 17 (73%) hedgehogs with uterine lesions had hematuria prior to ovariohysterectomy, and a hyperplastic endometrial polyp was diagnosed postmortem as the cause of antemortem red vulvar discharge [47, 48]. Proteinuria and bilirubinuria were reported in a urinalysis of a hedgehog with Chagas disease (*Trypanosoma*) [23]. Plasma biochemical and urine abnormalities in a hedgehog with mammary adenocarcinoma and a granulosa cell tumor included hypophosphatemia, elevated urea, decreased creatinine, hyperglycemia, and glucosuria [19]. A single case of congenital porphyria, resulting in pink urine, has been reported in a juvenile African hedgehog (*A. albiventris*) [49].

Serology and PCR Useful for Hedgehogs

Hedgehogs are subject to a variety of zoonotic infectious diseases, many of which are also reportable diseases [4, 50–52]. *Trichophyton erinacei* is associated with hedgehogs and zoonotic dermatophytosis. *Mycobacterium bovis* has been reported in wild hedgehogs in New Zealand [53]. Leptospirosis has been reported in African hedgehogs and European hedgehogs, and serology may be used for surveillance of disease in domestic species [54]. *Corynebacterium pseudotuberculosis* was reported in African hedgehogs [55]. *Salmonella typhimurium* is endemic in free-living hedgehogs in England, and *Salmonella* serotype *Tilene* has been carried and transmitted to humans in the United States [50, 56]. Testing for infectious disease in this species can be performed at diagnostic laboratories which accept veterinary submissions for companion or food animals.

Table 12.6 Urine-concentrating ability of hedgehogs [45].

Index	Units	European hedgehog (*E. europeaus*)	Long-eared hedgehog (*Hemichinus auritus*)	*Paranthropus aithiopicus*
Plasma osmolality	Mosmol	311.166 + 5.088	332.500 + 4.595	–
Plasma urea	mM	18.709 + 3.827	18.653 + 1.444	–
Maximal urine concentration	Mosmol/kg H_2O	3062 + 95	4010 + 195	3634 + 514
Urine urea concentration	mM	2310 + 178	2843 + 242	2334 + 152
Maximal urine/plasma ratio		9	12	

References

1 Hutterer, R., Wilson, D.F., and Reeder, D.M. *Mammal Species of the World*, 3e, 212–219. Baltimore, MD: Baltimore: Johns Hopkins University Press.

2 Eberle, J.J., Rybczynski, N., and Greenwood, D.R. (2104). Early Eocene mammals from the Driftwood Creek beds, driftwood canyon Provincial Park, northern British Columbia. *Journal of Vertebrate Paleontology* 34 (4): 739–746.

3 Evans, E.E. and Souza, M.J. (2010). Advanced diagnostic approaches and current management of internal disorders of select species (rodents, sugar gliders, hedgehogs). *Veterinary Clinics of Exotic Animal* 12/13: 453–469.

4 McLauchlan, J.D. and Henderson, W.M. (1947). The occurrence of foot-and-mouth disease in the hedgehog under natural conditions. *Journal of Hygiene* 45 (04): 474–479.

5 ISIS. (2002). Physiological Data Reference Values: International Species Information System, Apple Valley, MN.

6 Eliassen, E. (1961). Changes of blood volume in the prehibernating and deep-hibernating hedgehog. *Nature (London)* 192: 1047–1049.

7 Barbiers, R. (2003). Zoo and Wild Animal Medicine Fifth Edition: Insectivora (Hedgehogs, Tenrecs, Shrews, Moles) and Dermoptera (Flying Lemurs). In: *WILDPRO B336.35.w35. No Info on Number of Animals, Age, Sex, Reproductive Status* (ed. M.E. Fowler and R.E. Miller), 304–315. St. Louis, Missouri, USA: Saunders (Elsevier Science).

8 Günther, M. (1981). *Hämatologische Untersuchungen an winterschlafenden und nicht-winterschl fenden Igeln (Erinaceus europaeus und Aethechinus Algirus).*1981. Koln University Thesis. Trans: Hematological investigations of hedgehogs while hibernating and not hibernating. Medd Diss Koln.

9 Ozparlak, H., Celik, I., Sur, E. et al. (2011). A study of peripheral blood in hedgehogs in Turkey. *Journal of Zoo and Wildlife Medicine* 42 (3): 392–398.

10 Lewis, J.H. (1976). Comparative Hematology—studies on hedgehogs (*Erinaceus europaeus*). *Comparative Biochemistry and Physiology* 53: 237–240.

11 Bexton S, Robinson I. BSAVA manual of wildlife casualties – chapter 6: hedgehogs. WILDPRO B284.6.w6. Data from MedLab, Tarpley, Cheshire

12 Isenbugel E. (1993). Fowler Zoo and Wild Animal Medicine Current Therapy 3. Table27–1. E Isenbugel, RA Baumgartner. Chapter 27 Insectivora. 294–303. ACTUALLY from German Thesis Paper: Guenther

13 Lewis JCM, LM Frost, MR Norcott. Normal haematological values of European hedgehogs (*Erinaceus europaeus*) from an English rehabilitation Centre. Wild Pro Data Source J3.151.w2.

14 Pfäffle, M., Petney, T., Elgas, M. et al. (2009). Tick-induced blood loss leads to regenerative anaemia in the European hedgehog (*Erinaceus europaeus*). *Parasitology* 136 (04): 443–452.

15 Buergelt, C. (2002). Clinical exposures-Histopathologic findings in pet hedgehogs with nonneoplastic conditions. *Veterinary Medicine* 97 (9): 660–665.

16 Burballa, A., Martinez, J., and Martorell, J. (2012). Splenic lymphoma with cerebellar involvement in an African Hedgehog (*Atelerix albiventris*). *Journal of Exotic Pet Medicine* 21 (3): 255–259.

17 Finkelstein, A., Hoover, J.P., Caudell, D. et al. (2008). Cutaneous epithelioid variant Hemangiosarcoma in a captive African hedgehog (*Atelerix albiventris*). *Journal of Exotic Pet Medicine* 17 (1): 49–53.

18 Heatley, J.J., Mauldin, G.E., and Cho, D.Y. (2005). A review of neoplasia in the captive African hedgehog (*Atelerix albiventris*). *Seminars in Avian and Exotic Pet Medicine* 14 (3): 182–192. WB Saunders.

19 Wellehan, J.F., Southorn, E., Smith, D.A. et al. (2003). Surgical removal of a mammary adenocarcinoma and a granulosa cell tumor in an African pygmy hedgehog. *Canadian Veterinary Journal* 44 (3): 235–237.

20 Kuonen, V.J., Wilkie, D.A., Morreale, R.J. et al. (2002). Unilateral exophthalmia in a European hedgehog (*Erinaceus europeaus*) caused by lacrimal ductal carcinoma. *Veterinary Ophthalmology* 5 (3): 161–165.

21 DeWit, C.A., Persson, G., Nilsson, I.M. et al. (1985). Circannual changes in blood coagulation factors and the effect of warfarin on the hedgehog *Erinaceus europaeus. Comparative Biochemistry and Physiology Part A: Physiology* 80 (1): 43–47.

22 Helmer, P.J. (2000). Abnormal hematologic findings in an African hedgehog (*Atelerix albiventris*) with gastrointestinal lymphosarcoma. *The Canadian Veterinary Journal* 41: 489–490.

23 DeMaar, T.W., Kassell, N.L., and Blumer, E.S. (1994). Chagas's disease in an African hedgehog. *Proceedings American Association of zoo Veterinarians* 151–153.

24 Larsen, R.S. and Carpenter, J.W. (1999). Husbandry and medical management of African hedgehogs. *Veterinary Medicine* 94 (10): 877–888.

25 Johansson, B.W. and Senturia, J.B. (1972). Seasonal variations in the physiology and biochemistry of the European hedgehog (Erinaceus europaeus) including comparisons with non-hibernators, Guinea-pig and man. *Acta Physiologica Scandinavica. Supplementum* 380: 1.

26 Clausen, G. (1968). Ersland a the respiratory properties of the blood of the hibernating hedgehog *Erinaceus europaeus. Respiration Physiology* 5 (2): 221–233.

27 Black, P.A., Marshall, C., Seyfried, A.W. et al. (2011). Cardiac assessment of African hedgehogs (*Atelerix

albiventris). *Journal of Zoo and Wildlife Medicine* 42 (1): 49–53.

28 Al-Badry, K.S. and Taha, H.M. (1983). Hibernation-hypothermia and metabolism in hedgehogs. Changes in water and electrolytes. *Comparative Biochemistry and Physiology Part A: Physiology* 74 (2): 435–441.

29 Biorck, G., Johansson, B., and Veige, B. (1956). Some laboratory data on Hedgehogs, hibernating and non-hibernating. *Acta Physiologica Scandinavica* 37 (4): 281–294.

30 Edwards, B.A. and Munday, K.A. (1974). Tissue and plasma electrolyte levels in the awake state during the year, in summer cold exposure and during arousal from hibernation in the hedgehog *(Erinaceus europaeus). Comparative Biochemistry and Physiology Part A: Physiology* 49 (4): 697–705.

31 Kristoffersson RE (1965). *Hibernation of the Hedgehog (Erinaceus europaeus L.): Blood Creatinine and Creatine Levels in Relation to Seasonal and Hibernation Cycles.* Suomalainen tiedeakatemia.

32 Olsson, S.O. (1975). Comparative studies on the temperature dependence of lactic and malic dehydrogenase from a homeotherm, Guinea pig (*Cavia porcellus*); two hibernators, hedgehog (*Erinaceus europaeus*) and bat (*Nyctalus noctula*); and two poikilotherms, from (*Rana temporaria*) and cod (*Gadus callarias*). *Comparative Biochemistry and Physiology Part B: Comparative Biochemistry* 51 (1): 5–18.

33 Tähti, H. and Soivio, A. (1975). Blood gas concentrations, acid—base balance and blood pressure in hedgehogs in the active state and in hibernation with periodic respiration. *Annales Zoologici Fennici Societas Biologica Fennica Vanamo* 12: 188–192.

34 Hoo-Paris, R., Castex, C., and Sutter, B.C. (1978). Plasma glucose and insulin in the hibernating hedgehog. *Diabète & Métabolisme* 4 (1): 13–18.

35 Laplaud, P.M., Beaubatie, L., and Saboureau, M. (1983). Distribution and partial characterization of the plasma lipoproteins in the hedgehog (*Erinaceus europaeus* L.), a hibernator with potential use in the study of the hormonal regulation of lipoprotein metabolism. *Biochimica et Biophysica Acta (BBA)-Lipids and Lipid Metabolism* 752 (3): 396–406.

36 Belczewski, A.R., Laplaud, P.M., Chapman, M.J. et al. (2003). Identification of a novel Apolipoprotein (a)-related protein from the European hedgehog (*Erinaceus europaeus*). *DNA Sequence* 14 (1): 15–23.

37 Fowler, P.A. (1988). Seasonal endocrine cycles in the European hedgehog, *Erinaceus europaeus*. *Journal of Reproduction and Fertility* 84 (1): 259–272.

38 Saboureau, M. and Boissin, J. (1983). Endocrine cycles and hibernation in the hedgehog: mechanisms of adaptation to natural variations in the environment. In: *Adaptations to Terrestrial Environments*, 203–217. New York: Springer.

39 Saboureau, M. and Dutourné, B. (1981). The reproductive cycle in the male hedgehog (*Erinaceus europaeus* L.): a study of endocrine and exocrine testicular functions. *Reproduction Nutrition Dévelopement* 21 (1): 109–126.

40 Saboureau, M., Laurent, A.M., and Boissin, J. (1982). Plasma testosterone binding protein capacity in relation to the annual testicular cycle in a hibernating mammal, the hedgehog (*Erinaceus europaeus* L.). *General and Comparative Endocrinology* 47 (1): 59–63.

41 Dutourne, B. and Saboureau, M. (1983). An endocrine and histophysiological study of the testicular annual cycle in the hedgehog (*Erinaceus europaeus*). *General and Comparative Endocrinology* 50 (2): 324–332.

42 Juan-Sallés, C., Raymond, J.T., Garner, M.M. et al. (2006). Adrenocortical carcinoma in three captive African hedgehogs (*Atelerix albiventris*). *Journal of Exotic Pet Medicine* 15 (4): 278–280.

43 Omori-Satoha, T., Yamakawab, Y., and Mebs, D. (November 2000). The antihemorrhagic factor, erinacin, from the European hedgehog (*Erinaceus europaeus*), a metalloprotease inhibitor of large molecular size possessing ficolin/opsonin P35 lectin domains. *Toxicon* 38 (11): 1561–1580.

44 Drabeck, D.H., Dean, A.M., and Jansa, S.A. (2015). Why the honey badger don't care: convergent evolution of venom-targeted nicotinic acetylcholine receptors in mammals that survive venomous snake bites. *Toxicon* 99: 68.

45 Yaakobi, D.U. and Shkolnik, A.M. (1 April 1974). Structure and concentrating capacity in kidneys of three species of hedgehogs. *American Journal of Physiology - Legacy Content* 226 (4): 948–952.

46 Raymond, J.T. and White, M.R. (1999). Necropsy and histopath findings in 14 African hedgehogs (*Atelerix albiventris*): a retrospective study. *Journal of Zoo and Wildlife Medicine* 26 (2): 273–277.

47 Allison, N. (2003). A hyperplastic endometrial polyp and vascular thrombosis in a hedgehog. *Veterinary Medicine Clinical Exposures* 98 (4): 298–303.

48 Mikaelian, I. and Reavill, D.R. (2004). Spontaneous proliferative lesions and tumors of the uterus of captive African hedgehogs (*Atelerix albiventris*). *Journal of Zoo and Wildlife Medicine* 35 (2): 216–220.

49 Wolff, C.F., Corradini, P.R., and Cortes, G.L. (2005). Congenital *Erythropoietic porphyria* in an African hedgehog (*Atelerix albiventris*). *Journal of Zoo and Wildlife Medicine* 36 (2): 323–325.

50 Keymer, I.F., Gibson, E.A., and Reynolds, D.J. (1991). Zoonoses and other findings in hedgehogs (*Erinaceus europaeus*): a survey of mortality and review of the literature. *The Veterinary Record* 128: 245–249.

51 Riley, P.Y. and Chomel, B.B. (2005). Hedgehog zoonoses. *Emerging Infectious Diseases* 11: 1–5.

52 Takahashi, Y., Sano, A., Takizawa, K. et al. (2003). The epidemiology and mating behavior of *Arthroderma benhamiae* var. *erinacei* in household four-toed hedgehogs (*Atelerix albiventris*) in Japan. *Japanese Journal of Medical Mycology* 44 (1): 31–38.

53 Lugton, I.W., Johnstone, A.C., and Morris, R.S. (1995). Mycobacterium bovis infection in New Zealand hedgehogs (*Erinaceus europaeus*). *New Zealand Veterinary Journal* 43 (7): 342–344.

54 Sebeka, Z., Sixl, W., Reinthaler, F. et al. (1988). Results of serological examination for leptospirosis of domestic and wild animals in the upper Nile province (Sudan). *Journal of Hygiene, Epidemiology, Microbiology, and Immunology* 33 (3): 337–345.

55 McAllister, H.A. and Keahey, K.K. (1971). Infection of a hedgehog (*Erinaceus albiventris*) by Corynebacterium pseudotuberculosis. *The Veterinary Record* 89 (10): 280.

56 CDC. Morbidity and Mortality Weekly Report. African Pygmy Hedgehog-Associated Salmonellosis – Washington, 1994. 1995 44(24):462–464.

57 Edwards, B.A. and Munday, K.A. (1969). Electrolyte metabolism in the hibernating hedgehog *(Erinaceus europaeus). Comparative Biochemistry and Physiology* 31 (2): 329–335.

58 Lee, S.Y. and Park, H.M. (2012). Gastroesophageal intussusception with megaesophagus in a hedgehog (*Atelerix albiventris*). *Journal of Exotic Pet Medicine* 21 (2012): 168–171.

13

Callitrichids

Melissa Smith DVM[1] and J. Jill Heatley DVM, MS, DABVP (Avian, Reptilian, Amphibian), DACZM[2]

[1] CountryChase Veterinary, Tampa, Florida, USA
[2] Department of Small Animal Clinical Sciences, College of Veterinary Medicine & Biomedical Sciences, Texas A&M University, College Station, Texas, USA

Introduction

Marmosets and tamarins are small South American neotropical monkeys which range from Panama to southeastern Brazil and northern Paraguay. These small arboreal monkeys are characterized by colorful tufts, mustaches, fringes, and long nonprehensile tails. Many species serve important ecosystem roles such as seed dispersion, in their native habitat. All callitrichid species are vulnerable to, and many are in danger of, extinction. Callitrichids are maintained in captivity for display and education, as research models, and for breeding and reintroduction to the wild. Tamarins are the callitrichid most commonly seen by veterinarians and kept in captivity. Callitrichids are important research models for the study of reproduction, behavior, vision, endocrinology, psychology, aging, nephropathy, and colitis and colonic carcinoma [1–5]. Clinical pathology can be a useful tool in diagnosis of a variety of health concerns in these species, despite their diminutive size. Reference intervals for these species are limited, and most data in this chapter are summarized from laboratory study data.

Species

The main distinguishing features of species of Callitrichidae include their small size, claw-shaped nails on all digits, and their propensity to give birth to twins. Taxonomists classify callitrichids based on dental anatomy. Most callitrichids have only two molars and lack a rear inner cusp of the crown on the upper molars, called a hypocone, which is common in other primates. The incisors and canines of marmosets are the same length and enable them to gouge holes in trees for consumption of nutritive gums, saps, or exudates. The longer canine teeth of tamarins allow them to inflict a deeper bite. Goeldi's monkey (*Callimico goeldi*) is considered the most primitive of the callitrichids on the basis of singleton births and the possession of additional molars [4, 6]. The average captive life span of marmosets is 12 years and of tamarins is 17 years. The pygmy marmoset is the smallest callitrichid, with an adult weight of only 130 g. Sexual maturity is reached at 12 months for the female and 16.7 months for the male. Over 60 species of Callitrichidae occur and include marmosets (genera *Cebuella, Callibella, Mico*, and *Callithrix*), tamarins (genus *Saguinus*), lion tamarins (genus *Leontopithecus*), and Goeldi's monkey (genus *Callimico*) (Table 13.1). Marmoset species overlap in some regions results in intergrades which may be considered hybrids, subspecies, or a separate species. Examples include the black-tufted marmoset (*Callithrix penicillata*) and the common (or cotton-eared) marmoset (*Callithrix jacchus*) in southern Bahia and Geoffroy's marmoset (*Callithrix geoffroyi*) hybridization with *C. penicillata* and *C. jacchus*. Common marmosets are the most common nonhuman primates used in for research and have been used as models of teratology, periodontal disease, reproduction, immunology, endocrinology, obesity, and aging [1, 3–5, 7–9].

Sample Collection

Restraint

Area and equipment preparation is paramount prior to restraint of a callitrichid. Useful equipment includes nets, gloves, and an induction chamber if gas anesthesia is planned to facilitate a close observational exam. Leather gloves may increase the likelihood of tooth fracture in marmosets but are recommended owing to their longer upper canines. The area for restraint should be secure; very small areas may permit escape

Exotic Animal Laboratory Diagnosis, First Edition. Edited by J. Jill Heatley and Karen E. Russell.

Table 13.1 Common captive marmosets and tamarins.

Common name	Scientific name	Other names/IUCN status	IUCN status
Common marmoset	*Callithrix jacchus jacchus*	Northeastern coast of Brazil now invasive to Southeastern Brazil	Least concern
Black-tufted marmoset	*Callithrix (jacchus) penicillata*	Black tufted- marmoset	Least concern
Wied's marmoset	*Callithrix kuhlii*	Wied's black tufted marmoset, sympatric with *L.r. chrysomelas*	Near threatened
White-headed marmoset	*Callithrix (jacchus) geoffroyi*	Geoffroy's marmoset, tufted-ear marmoset	Least concern
Snethlage's marmoset	*Callithrix emiliae*	*Callithrix (Mico) emiliae*	Data insufficient
Goeldi's marmoset	*Callimico goeldii*	Goeldi's monkey	Vulnerable
Pygmy marmoset	*Cebuella pygmaea*	Two subspecies, sympatric with *S. f. fuscus*	Least concern
Black-mantled tamarin	*Saguinus nigricollis*	Sympatric with Graells's tamarin, *Saguinus graellsi*, in Columbia	Least concern
Brown-mantled tamarin	*Saguinus fuscicollis fuscus*	Saddleback tamarin, many subspecies, sympatric with pygmy marmoset	Least concern
Weddell's saddleback tamarin	*Saguinus fuscicollis weddelli*	Saddleback tamarin subspecies	Least concern
Spix's Moustached tamarin	*Saguinus mystax*	Two subspecies	Least concern
White-lipped tamarin	*Saguinus labiatus*	Three subspecies, red-bellied tamarin	Least concern
Emperor tamarin	*Saguinus imperator*	Two subspecies, Formerly *S. imperator,* Brockway monkey	Least concern
Red-handed tamarin	*Saguinus midas*	Golden-handed tamarin or Midas tamarin	Least concern
Black tamarin	*Saguinus (midas) niger*	Black-handed tamarin	Vulnerable
Pied tamarin	*Saguinus bicolor bicolor*	Near Manaus, Brazil	Endangered
White-footed tamarin	*Saguinus leucopus*	Endemic to Columbia	Endangered
Cotton-top tamarin	*Saguinus oedipus oedipus*	Endemic to Columbia	Critically endangered
Geoffroy's tamarin	*Saguinus oedipus geoffroyi*	Panamanian, red-crested or rufous-naped tamarin,	Least concern
Golden lion tamarin	*Leontopithecus rosalia rosalia*	Endemic to Atlantic coastal forests of Brazil	Endangered
Golden-headed lion tamarin	*Leontopithecus r. chrysomelas*	Endemic to Bahia, Brazil	Endangered
Black lion tamarin	*Leontopithecus r. chrysopygus*	Golden-rumped lion tamarin Endemic to Sao Paulo, Brazil	Endangered

or entrapment of these species. Callitrichids have dexterous hands and may grab at equipment or fingers, pulling them toward their mouth and teeth. Callitrichids can be restrained by holding them in the palm of the hand with the thumb and fingers encircling the body below the animal's arms and using the second hand to support the feet and body (Figure 13.1). Grasping the monkey loosely around the neck, and restraining the hind legs is an additional option. Do not restrict the patient's breathing with these restraint methods. For chemical restraint, isoflurane or sevoflurane anesthesia and injectable agents (ketamine, alpha-2 agonists, midazolam, tiletamine/zolazepam) may be used. However, the callitrichid should be fasted prior to chemical restraint [4]. Operant conditioning for medical procedures to allow venipuncture without restraint is preferred in captive species.

Collection Volume and Sites

Blood volume is small in these diminutive species, and therefore appropriate sample size is necessary. The total blood volume of these species using albumin labeled with the radioisotope Iodine-131 (I_{131}) was 82.1 ml/kg [10]. However, using the same method, the mean plasma volume of cotton-top (*Saguinus oedipus*) and white-lip

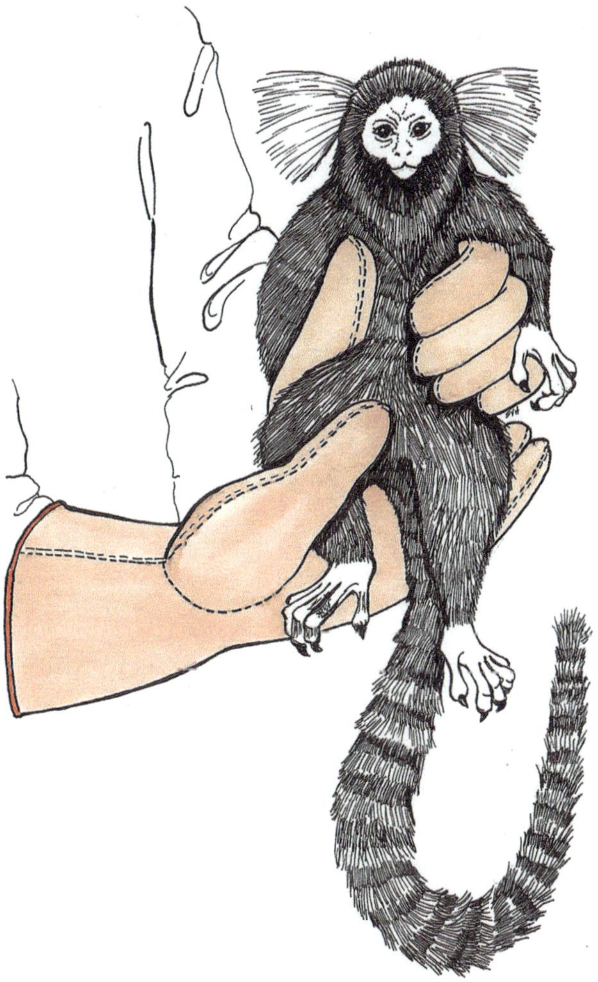

Figure 13.1 Manual restraint of a docile common marmoset.

(*Saguinus labiatus*) tamarins was 43.77 ml/kg of body weight, with a wide range [10]. A maximal one-time sample from a callitrichid should not exceed 15% of the animal's blood volume (approximately 7% of animal's body weight), and blood withdrawn should not exceed 1% of the marmoset's body weight every two to three weeks [4, 10, 11].

Phlebotomy is most commonly performed on the femoral vein in the femoral triangle (Chapter 14, Figure 14.1) in these species and generally requires heavy sedation or anesthesia. Pressure should be applied to the femoral triangle for 1 to 2 min after phlebotomy to prevent hematoma formation. The jugular vein is an additional option for collection of a larger blood sample. Other collection sites for small blood volumes (200–300 μl) include the cubital vein on the medial aspect of the elbow, the cephalic vein as it courses along the anterior surface of the forearm, and the saphenous vein on the posterior distal hind limb [11]. Small syringes (1–3 ml) and 23–27 gauge (g.) needles are typically used for blood sample collection in callitrichids.

Sample Handling

Blood samples are handled similarly to samples from other mammals. EDTA is the preferred anticoagulant for complete blood counts. Heparin is an alternative anticoagulant that may result in poor cell staining of blood smears. To avoid dilution of the sample with excess liquid anticoagulant, BD Microtainer collection tubes (BD, Franklin Lakes, New Jersey) are useful for the collection of small volumes of blood (250–500 μl). Ideally, blood smears should be made immediately after sampling and prior to mixture with an anticoagulant, and can be evaluated with a standard Wright's-type stain. For biochemical panels, blood can be placed in a red top tube for serum collection or lithium heparin tube for plasma collection. If only a small volume of blood can be obtained, it can be placed in a lithium heparin BD Microtainer tube for both hematology and biochemical panels [12, 13]. Sample analysis should occur within 24 h to avoid artifacts due to red blood cell (RBC) swelling. Refrigerate the sample (4 °C) if analysis is not performed within 2 to 3 h.

Complete Blood Count

Complete blood count data for and marmosets and tamarins can be found in Tables 13.2 and 13.3, respectively.

Erythrocytes

In the marmoset (*C. jacchus*), a small degree of anisocytosis and poikilocytosis is common, and Howell-Jolly bodies are often present. The presence of one to two nucleated RBCs per high power field is normal because of the high red-cell turnover rate of the common marmoset [15]. The average half-life of the erythrocyte in *Saguinus fuscicollis* was 15.9 days. Reticulocytes uptake stain with New Methylene Blue. Up to 5% of RBC having Heinz bodies are considered normal for the marmoset [25]. In the red-bellied tamarin (*S. labiatus*), a slight degree of anisocytosis, polychromasia, and crenation was seen along with rare nucleated RBCs, although Heinz bodies were not found [21]. For the cotton-top tamarin (*S. oedipus*), a slight degree of anisocytosis, polychromasia and poikilocytosis is seen. In a few individuals, nucleated RBCs were rarely seen, and Heinz's bodies occurred in 5% of RBCs of one clinically normal adult female. Platelets averaged 3.5 μm in diameter and contained distinctive basophilic granules [22].

Hemoparasites observed in blood smears of wild-caught callitrichids include microfilariae (multiple species which include *Mansonella*, *Dipetalonema*, etc.) and *Trypanosoma cruzi* [10]. Anemia in callitrichids may be

Table 13.2 Hematology of marmosets.

Cell parameter (abbreviation)	Units, SI (conventional)	Common marmoset [14–16] (*Callithrix jacchus*) Ħ			Goeldi's monkey [17] (*Callimico goeldii*)	White-footed tamarin [18] (*Sanguinus leucopus*)	Panamanian marmoset [19] (*Saguinus geoffroyi*)
Animal number		196	30	54	27	29	89
Data type		Range (mean) [median] {average}			Range (mean)	Range (mean) or [median]	(mean ± SD)
White blood cells (WBC)	Cells × 10^9/l = (×10^3/µl)	♂–5.5 to 16.0 (10.0) ♀–5.8 to 16.6 (10.1)	4.1–10.5 {7.3}	2.72–10.85 [5.95]	3.2–10.3 (6.3)	6.28–12.53 (9.56)	♂(10.1 ± 4.3) ♀(10.9 ± 3.8)
Segmented neutrophils	Cells × 10^9/l = (×10^3/µl)		1.0–7.0 {4.0}	1.04–15.39 [2.86]	0.4–6.3 (2.4)	2.34–7.65 (4.54)	
	Proportion of 1	♂–0.15 to 0.74 (0.364) ♀–0.14 to 0.72 (0.385)	0.26–0.84 {0.55}	0.28–0.78 [0.53]	0.13–0.61 (0.377)	0.308–0.702 (0.466)	♂(0.70 ± 0.079) ♀(0.695 ± 0.111)
	(%)	*[♂–15 to 74 (36.4) ♀–14 to 72 (38.5)]*	*[26–84 {55}]*	*[28.25–78.05 [52.50]]*	*[13.0–61.0 (37.7)]*	*[30.8–70.2 (46.6)]*	*[♂(70 ± 7.9) ♀(69.5 ± 11.1)]*
Band Neutrophils	Cells × 10^9/l = (×10^3/µl)			0–0.18 [0.00]			
	Proportion of 1 *(%)*			0.00–0.04 [0.00] *[0.00–4.00 [0.00]]*			
Lymphocytes	Cells × 10^9/l = (×10^3/µl)		1.0–5.0 {3.0}	0.49–4.4 [1.90]	0.8–7.6 (2.9)	2.97–6.80 (4.79)	
	Proportion of 1 *(%)*	♂ 0.23–0.83 (0.607) ♀ 0.25–0.84 (0.591) *[♂ 23–83 (60.7) ♀ 25–84 (59.1)]*	0.16–0.70 {0.43} *[16–70 {43}]*	0.14–0.627 [0.345] *[14.00–62.70 [34.50]]*	0.25–0.715 (0.491) *[25.0–71.5 (49.1)]*	0.309–0.671 (0.511) *[30.9–67.1 (51.5)]*	♂(0.277 ± 0.074) ♀(0.288 ± 0.101) *[♂(27.7 ± 7.4) ♀(28.8 ± 10.1)]*
Eosinophils	Cells × 10^9/l = (×10^3/µl)		0–0.3 {0.03}	0–0.71 [0.15]	0.1–3.6 (0.8)	0–0.209 [0.116]	
	Proportion of 1	♂ 0–0.04 (0.01) ♀ 0–0.03 (0.008)	0–0.06 {0.005}	0.00–0.1375 [0.0275]	0.015–0.173 (0.109)	0–0.025 [0.01]	♂(0.008 ± 0.008) ♀(0.008 ± 0.011)
	(%)	*[♂ 0–4 (1.0) ♀ 0–3 (0.8)]*	*[0–6 {0.5}]*	*[0.00–13.75 [2.75]]*	*[1.5–17.3 (10.9)]*	*[0–2.5 [1]]*	*[♂(0.8 ± 0.8) ♀(0.8 ± 1.1)]*
Monocytes	Cells × 10^9/l = (×10^3/µl)		0–0.3 {0.03}	0.07–1.63 [0.35]	0.1–0.6 (0.2)	0–0.115 [0]	
	Proportion of 1	♂ 0–0.05 (0.017) ♀ 0–0.04 (0.015)	0–0.03 {0.004}	0.02–0.171 [0.065] *[2.00–17.05 [6.50]]*	0.01–0.06 (0.029)	0–0.01 [0]	♂(0.016 ± 0.013) ♀(0.013 ± 0.013)
	(%)	*[♂ 0–5 (1.7) ♀ 0–4 (1.5)]*	*[0–3 {0.4}]*		*[1.0–6.0 (2.9)]*	*0–1 [0]*	*[♂(1.6 ± 1.3) ♀(1.3 ± 1.3)]*

Basophils	Cells × 10^9/l = *(×10^3/μl)*		0–0.5 {0.08}	[0.00]		0–0.186 [0.066]	
	Proportion of 1 *(%)*	♂ 0–0.01 (0.002) ♀ 0–0.01 (0.001) *[♂ 0–1 (0.2) ♀ 0–1 (0.1)]*	0–0.08 {0.13} *[0–8 {1.3}]*	[0.00]		0–0.02 [0.01] *[0–2 [1]]*	♂(0.004 ± 0.008) ♀(0.008 ± 0.011) *[♂(0.4 ± 0.8) ♀(0.8 ± 1.1)]*
Red blood cells (RBCs)	Cells × 10^{12}/l = *(×10^6/μl)*	♂ 5.2–7.9 (6.8) ♀ 5.4–8.1 (6.6)	6.1–7.7 {6.9}	3.47–7.88 [6.51]	5.7–6.7 (6.3)	5.6–8.0 (6.74)	♂(4.41 ± 0.90) ♀(4.39 ± 0.78)
Packed cell volume (PCV)	Proportion of 1 *(%)*	♂ 0.41–0.56 (0.48) ♀ 0.41–0.54 (0.48) *[♂ 41–56 (48) ♀ 0.41–0.54 (48)]*	0.42–0.55 {0.48} *[43–55 {48}]*	0.28–0.54 [0.45] *[28–54 [45]]*	0.38–0.505 (0.446) *[38–50.5 (44.6)]*	0.423–0.55 (0.49) *[42.3–55.0 (49)]*	♂(0.437 ± 0.076) ♀(0.417 ± 0.069) *[♂(43.7 ± 7.6) ♀(41.7 ± 6.9)]*
Hemoglobin (Hb)	g/l *(g/dl)*	♂ 123–181 (155) ♀ 127–177 (155) *[♂ 12.3–18.1 (15.5) ♀ 12.7–17.7 (15.5)]*	133–177 {155} *[13.3–17.7 {15.5}]*	34.3–106.7 [88.5] *[3.43–10.67 [8.85]]*	118–164 (143) *[11.8–16.4 (14.3)]*	140–185 (161) *[14.0–18.5 (16.1)]*	♂(129 ± 25) ♀(129 ± 20) *[♂(12.9 ± 2.5) ♀(12.9 ± 2.0)]*
Mean corpuscular volume (MCV)	μm³		62.7–74.9 {69.3}	53.32–83.45 [69.05]	65.7–75.7 (70.4)	63.5–89 (73.6)	♂(95.8 ± 12.9) ♀(95.6 ± 5.2)
Mean corpuscular hemoglobin concentration (MCHC)	g/dl *(%)*		30.3–34.3 {32.3}	18.33–21.24 [20.09]	30.0–33.5 (32.2)	26.6–38.9 (34.2)	♂(31.5 ± 6.2) ♀(30.5 ± 2.2)
Mean corpuscular hemoglobin (MCH)	fmol/cell *(Pg/cell)*		1.23–1.55 {1.39} *[19.8–25.0 {22.4}]*	1.21–1.54 [1.39] *[19.49–24.81 [22.39]]*	1.27–1.52 (1.41) *[20.5–24.5 (22.7)]*	1.18–2.11 (1.58) *[19–34 (25.4)]*	♂(1.81 ± 0.12) ♀(1.80 ± 0.099) *[♂(29.1 ± 1.9) ♀(29.0 ± 1.6)]*
Reticulocytes	Proportion of 1 *(%)*	♂ 0.025–0.10 (0.053) ♀ 0.02–0.085 (0.046) *[♂ 2.5–10.0 (5.3) ♀ 2.0–8.5 (4.6)]*	0.009–0.077 {0.017} *[0.9–7.7 {1.7}]*			0.034–0.085 (0.059) *[3.4–8.5 (5.9)]*	
Platelets	Cells × 10^9/l = *(×10^3/μl)*	♂ 183–585 (401) ♀ 215–693 (394)	298–682 {490}	17.6–788.6 [402.50]		290–560 (450)	
Fibrinogen	μmol/l *(mg/dl)*		6.32–11.73 {9.02} *[215–399 {307}]*		2.94–8.82 (5.88) *[100–300 (200)]*	2.94–11.76 [5.88] *[100–400 [200]]*	

Table 13.3 Hematology of tamarins.

Cell parameter (abbreviation)	Units, SI (conventional)	Red-bellied tamarin [20, 21] (*Saguinus labiatus*)		Cotton-top tamarin [22, 23] (*Saguinus oedipus oedipus*)		Golden lion tamarin [24] (*Leontopithecus rosalia*)
Animal number		39	25	43	35	104
Data type		Range (Mean)	Range {Average}	Range {Average}	(Mean ± SD)	95% CI (mean)
White blood cells (WBCs)	Cells × 10^9/l = (*x10^3/μl*)	♂ 4.7–20.0 (10.8) ♀ 8.3–20.9 (13.0)	4.5–11.9 {8.2}	4.2–11.1 {7.7}	♂(5.92 ± 1.85) ♀(7.41 ± 2.49)	6.70–7.56 (7.13)
Neutrophils	Cells × 10^9/l = (*×10^3/μl*)	♂ 1.4–10.044 (4.480) ♀ 1.806–15.048 (5.576)	0.42–8.14 {4.28}	2.10–8.68 {5.19}	♂(2.88 ± 1.17) ♀(3.42 ± 1.16)	4.04–4.80 (4.42)
	Proportion of 1 (*%*)		0.28–0.84 {0.56} *[28–84 {56}]*	0.53–0.78 {0.656} *[53–78 {65.6}]*	—	
Band neutrophils	Cells × 10^9/l = (*×10^3/μl*)					0.00–0.02 (0.01)
Lymphocytes	Cells × 10^9/l = (*×10^3/μl*)	♂ 2.350–15.400 (5.914) ♀ 3.984–12.075 (8.854)	1.40–5.44 {3.42}	0.91–4.28 {2.36}	♂(2.37 ± 1.09) ♀(2.96 ± 1.40)	2.00–2.34 (2.17)
	Proportion of 1 *(%)*	—	0.12–0.61 {0.37} *[12–61 {37}]*	♂ 0.10–0.56 {0.26} ♀ 0.15–0.55 {0.35} *[♂ 10–56 {26.0}* *♀ 15–55 {35.0}]*		
Eosinophils	Cells × 10^9/l = (*×10^3/μl*)	♂ 0–0.396 (0.082) ♀ 0–0.668 (0.129)	0–0.47 {0.14}	♂ 0–0.30 {0.03} ♀ 0–0.30 {0.11}	♂(0.18 ± 0.14) ♀(0.16 ± 0.14)	0.24–0.36 (0.30)
	Proportion of 1 (*%*)		0–0.05 {0.02} *[0–5 {2}]*	0–0 {0.01} *[0–0 {1.0}]*		
Monocytes	Cells × 10^9/l = (*×10^3/μl*)	♂ 0–0.610 (0.272) ♀ 0.117–0.870 (0.402)	0–0.77 {0.30}	0–0.34 {0.11}	♂(0.38 ± 0.20) ♀(0.36 ± 0.21)	0.13–0.19 (0.16)
	Proportion of 1 (*%*)		0–0.09 {0.04} *[0–9 {4}]*	0–0.05 {0.013} *[0–5 {1.3}]*		
Basophils	Cells × 10^9/l = (*×10^3/μl*)	♂ 0–0.216 (0.078) ♀ 0–0.418 (0.081)	0–0.38 {0.09}	0–0.26 {0.07}	♂(0.06 ± 0.06) ♀(0.07 ± 0.06)	0.06–0.10 (0.08)
	Proportion of 1 (*%*)		0–0.04 {0.01} *[0–4 {1}]*	0–0.04 {0.008} *[0–4 {0.8}]*		
Neutrophil:lymphocyte			0.67–3.65 {1.25}			

Red blood cells (RBCs)	Cells × 10^{12}/l = *(×10^6/μl)*	♂ 6.3–7.5 (7.0) ♀ 6.1–7.5 (6.9)	5.5–8.4 {7.0}	♂ 5.7–7.7 {6.7} ♀ 5.4–7.2 {6.3}	♂(6.42 ± 0.20) ♀(6.13 ± 0.35)	5.6–5.8 (5.7)
Nucleated red blood cells (nRBCs)	Cells × 10^9/l = *(×10^3/μl)*				♂(0.04 ± 0.05) ♀(0.02 ± 0.05)	
Packed cell volume (PCV)	Proportion of 1 *(%)*	♂ 0.48–0.56 (0.52) ♀ 0.41–0.55 (0.51) *[♂ 48–56 (52) ♀ 41–55 (51)]*	0.43–0.58 {0.51} *[43–58 {51}]*	♂ 0.5–0.58 {0.52} ♀ 0.3–0.53 {0.48} *[♂ 50–58 {52} ♀ 30–53 {48}]*	♂(0.531 ± 0.019) ♀(0.502 ± 0.03) *[♂(53.13 ± 1.92) ♀(50.22 ± 3.00)]*	0.45–0.462 (0.456) *[45.0–46.2 (45.6)]*
Hematocrit (HCT)	Proportion of 1 *(%)*				♂(0.522 ± 0.019) ♀(0.492 ± 0.03) *[♂(52.19 ± 1.94) ♀(49.21 ± 3.03)]*	
Hemoglobin (Hgb)	g/l *(g/dl)*	♂ 159–185 (174) ♀ 133–184 (166) *[♂ 15.9–18.5 (17.4) ♀ 13.3–18.4 (16.6)]*	136–205 {171} *[13.6–20.5 {17.1}]*	♂ 155–201 {175} ♀ 133–188 {160} *[♂ 15.5–20.1 {17.5} ♀ 13.3–18.8 {16.0}]*	♂(175 ± 8.5) ♀(165.1 ± 10.6) *♂(17.50 ± 0.85) ♀(16.51 ± 1.06)]*	146–152(149) *[14.6–15.2 (14.9)]*
Mean corpuscular volume (MCV)	μm^3	♂ 68–83 (74) ♀ 65–78 (73)	65.2–80.6 {72.9}	70.0–83.2 {76.8}	♂(81.33 ± 2.68) ♀(79.03 ± 4.93)	78.8–80.6 (79.7)
Mean corpuscular hemoglobin concentration (MCHC)	g/dl = *(%)*	♂ 32–35 (33) ♀ 31–35 (33)	31.7–35.7 {33.7}	♂ 31.9–36.8 34.0} ♀ 31.8–35.0 {33.3}	♂(33.31 ± 1.16) ♀(33.56 ± 0.77)	32.2–33.2 (32.7)
Mean corpuscular hemoglobin (MCH)	fmol/cell *(Pg/cell)*	♂ 1.37–1.74 (1.57) ♀ 1.30–1.61 (1.49) *[♂ 22–28 (25) ♀ 21–26 (24)]*	1.39–1.61 {1.50} *[22.4–26.0 {24.2}]*	♂ 1.48–1.78 {1.63} ♀ 1.38–1.74 {1.58} *[♂ 23.8–28.7 {26.3} ♀ 22.2–28.1{25.4}]*	♂(1.68 ± 0.083) ♀(1.67 ± 0.072) *[♂(27.08 ± 1.33) ♀(26.91 ± 1.16)]*	1.59–1.65 (1.62) *[25.6–26.6 (26.1)]*
Reticulocytes	Proportion of 1 *(%)*	♂ 0.016–0.035 (0.026) ♀ 0.014–0.066 (0.026) *[♂ 1.6–3.5 (2.6) ♀ 1.4–6.6 (2.6)]*	0.009–0.045 {0.035} *[♂ 0.9–4.5 {3.5} ♀ 1.5–7.8 {8.2}]*	♂ 0.007–0.062 {0.032} ♀ 0.004–0.115 {0.055} *[♂ 0.7–6.2 {3.2} ♀ 0.4–11.5 {5.5}]*		
Red blood cell distribution width (RDW)	Proportion of 1 *(%)*				♂(0.155 ± 0.052) ♀(0.156 ± 0.007) *[♂(15.52 ± 0.52) ♀(15.60 ± 0.70)]*	
Platelets	Cells × 10^9/l = *(×10^3/μl)*	♂ 233–532 (428) ♀ 255–510 (402)	296–564 {430}	195–607 {398}	♂(253.94 ± 57.19) ♀(267.71 ± 63.98)	
Mean platelet volume (MPV)	fl				♂13.19 ± 1.56 ♀13.28 ± 1.86	
Fibrinogen	μmol/l *(mg/dl)*		6.76–16.46 {11.47} *[230–560 {390}]*	7.35–15.29 {11.47} *[250–520 {390}]*		

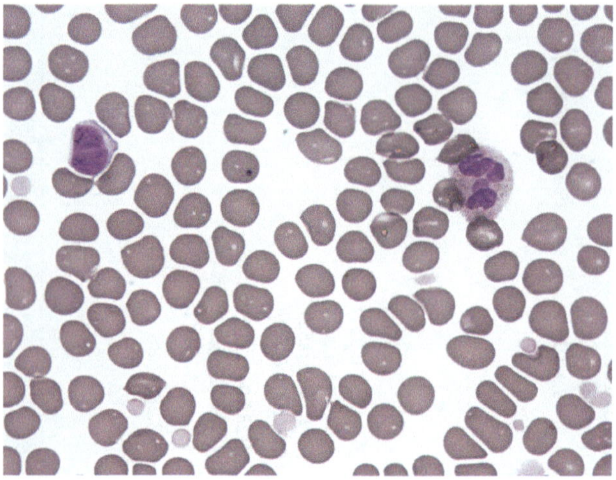

Figure 13.2 Lymphocyte (left) and neutrophil of a white-fronted marmoset.

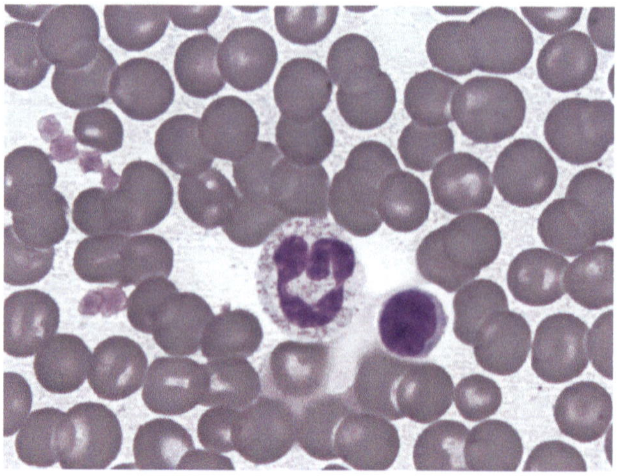

Figure 13.3 Neutrophil (left) and lymphocyte of a golden lion tamarin.

due to a number of etiologies including hemosiderosis, marmoset wasting disease, renal failure, and vitamin E deficiency [3, 9, 11, 26–29]. An increased number of Heinz's bodies and thrombocytosis has been linked with lymphoplasmacytic enteritis/colitis or wasting disease in *C. jacchus* [27].

Leukocytes

Based on the May-Grünwald Giemsa stain, neutrophils contain pink-red granules in pale pink cytoplasm with nuclear lobes ranging from three to seven, averaging four in the common marmoset [15]. In the red-bellied tamarin (*S. labiatus*), the colorless cytoplasm has small pink, red, or purple staining granules. Neutrophils are 12.5 μm in diameter, with well-lobulated nuclei ranging from two to six lobes, averaging four [21]. In the cotton-top tamarin (*S. oedipus*), the neutrophils are regular, round cells with an average diameter of 13.0 μm. The nuclear lobes are well defined and range from three to seven (averaging five) with colorless cytoplasm containing numerous small pink or red granules [22]. Examples of neutrophil morphology for callitrichids are provided in Figures 13.2 and 13.3.

Lymphocytes of the common marmoset are not easily divided into large and small forms but intermediate in size with a round or slightly indented nuclei and blue cytoplasm sometimes containing azurophilic granules [15]. In the red-bellied tamarin (*S. labiatus*), both large (10–12 μm) and small (8–10 μm) lymphocytes are seen with the cytoplasm of the larger forms sometimes containing a few small azurophilic granules [21]. In the cotton-top tamarin (*S. oedipus*), lymphocytes average 12.2 μm in diameter, with round nuclei and pale blue cytoplasm sometimes containing one or several small azurophilic granules [22]. Examples of Lymphocyte morphology for callitrichids are provided in Figures 13.2 and 13.3

Monocytes of the red-bellied tamarin (*S. labiatus*) are large (16–19 μm) with large irregularly indented pale staining nuclei containing stranded chromatin and slightly opaque gray-blue cytoplasm [21]. In the cotton-top tamarin (*S. oedipus*), monocytes are larger cells with an average diameter of 15.8 μm. They have indented nuclei and slightly opaque, blue-gray, sometimes vacuolated cytoplasm [22].

Eosinophils of the common marmoset contain irregular spherical granules which often show a bluish tinge and a trilobed nucleus within a pale blue cytoplasm [15]. In the red-bellied tamarin (*S. labiatus*), eosinophils are similar in size to the neutrophil with irregularly lobed nuclei and pale blue cytoplasm containing small spherical orange granules [21]. In the cotton-top tamarin (*S. oedipus*), eosinophils are similar in size with irregularly lobed nuclei and pale blue cytoplasm closely packed with small, spherical strongly eosinophilic granules [22].

Basophils are relatively common (approximately 7%) in the common marmoset white blood cell differential and difficult to distinguish from blue-tinged eosinophils. Basophil granules are sparse, spherical, and variable in size and stain medium blue with a nucleus that is trilobed and easily visible [15]. In the red-bellied tamarin (*S. labiatus*), basophils range from 11 to 13 μm in diameter with large irregular nuclei, and deep purple oval granules often overlaying the nucleus [21]. In the cotton-top tamarin (*S. oedipus*), basophils are smaller cells with an average diameter of 12.1 μm, with large spherical or oval purple granules completely filling the cytoplasm [22].

Hemostasis and Blood Types

Partial thromboplastin times with kaolin and prothrombin time were lower in the *C. jacchus* and *S. labiatus* than the reported values in humans (Table 13.4) [14, 20].

Table 13.4 Prothrombin and partial thromboplastin time in callitrichids.

Analyte (abbreviation)	Units, SI (conventional)	Common marmoset [14] (*Callithrix jacchus*)	Red-bellied tamarin [20] (*Saguinus labiatus*)
Animal number		**60**	**33**
Data type		**Range (mean)**	**Range (mean)**
Prothrombin time (PT)	Seconds	♂ 5.0–6.4 (5.7) ♀ 5.0–6.5 (5.6)	♂ 6.2–7.9 (7.1) ♀ 6.4–7.8 (7.1)
Partial thromboplastin time (PTT)	Seconds	♂ 30.1–43.7 (35.7) ♀ 31.9–41.0 (36.3)	♂ 26.9–37.5 (31.7) ♀ 25.7–40.4 (32.7)

Table 13.5 Blood groups in the family Callitrichidae [30].

		Blood groups			
Species	**Sample size**	**O**	**A**	**B**	**AB**
Callithrix jacchus	35	0	35	0	0
Callithrix emiliae	47	0	47	0	0
Saguinus nigricollis	14	0	14	0	0
Saguinus fuscicollis	18	0	18	0	0
Saguinus mystax	3	0	3	0	0
Saguinus oedipus	4	0	4	0	0
Saguinus midas niger	81	0	11	45	25
Saguinus fuscicollis weddelli	88	0	88	0	0

The genus *Callithrix* appears to express the A blood type. For the genus *Saguinus*, most also express A, although *Saguinus midas niger* expressed, A, B, and AB. No marmosets or tamarins have been reported with the O phenotype (Table 13.5) [30].

Biochemical Panel

Liver Enzymes

In callitrichids, alanine aminotransferase (ALT) is a sensitive indicator of hepatocellular injury but not as specific for liver cell injury as in the dog, rat, or mouse. ALT and sorbitol dehydrogenase (SDH), glutamate dehydrogenase (GLDH), and aspartate aminotransferase (AST) are markers of hepatocellular injury in callitrichids. In marmosets, most activity ALT occurs in the liver, but cardiac muscle and kidney also contain ALT. Activity of AST activity is highest in heart muscle followed by liver, skeletal muscle, kidney, and brain. The biliary and osteoblastic isoenzymes are the principle components of serum ALP activity. The biliary isoenzyme is released and activated on the basis of biliary stasis, not hepatocellular leakage. ALP is an induction enzyme associated with proliferation of endoplasmic reticulum that may be induced by xenobiotics such as phenobarbital. Young, growing animals have higher serum osteoblastic ALP activity [4]. Bilirubin metabolism in callitrichids resembles that of humans. Elevated total bilirubin may be due to hemolytic or hepatobiliary disease. A Dubin–Johnson-like syndrome with persistent conjugated hyperbilirubinemia and pigmented liver has been reported in the golden lion tamarin (*Leontopithecus rosalia)* [31].

Muscle Enzymes

Creatine kinase (CK) may be moderately increased in callitrichids because of capture and restraint, intramuscular injection, or trauma.

Renal Analytes

Increased concentrations of blood urea nitrogen (BUN) and serum creatinine (azotemia) indicate renal disease in callitrichids. A slight but progressive increase in creatinine signals progressive deterioration of renal function. An individual callitrichid's earlier creatinine value for comparison may be of greater diagnostic importance in evaluation of renal dysfunction or disease than reference values. In one population of tamarins and marmosets older than six months with proteinuria and hematuria, 91% were suspected to have an IgM-mediated mesangioproliferative glomerulonephropathy [9].

Pancreas

Serum amylase activity in callitrichids is not useful for diagnosis of pancreatitis as increased activity also occurs in association with pyometra, bone fracture, abscesses, diabetes mellitus, and diarrheic gastrointestinal conditions [32]. In addition to the amylase values given in Table 13.6, additional values have also been determined for (given as [range (mean IU/l)] the saddleback tamarin [65–1352(469.3], the white-headed marmoset [94–801(507.3)], and the black-tufted marmoset [246–659(431.3)]) [32].

Serum glucose is influenced by numerous factors, including gastrointestinal absorption, insulin, hepatic storage and release, glucagon, somatotropin, epinephrine, and cortisol. In callitrichids, stress and excitement may increase serum glucose concentrations. Fructosamine values have been reported for the cotton-top tamarin (Table 13.6) [23]. Whole glucose can be determined with a glucose meter designed for diabetic humans. Glycosylated hemoglobin (HbA1c) and fasting glucose concentrations are correlated, suggesting that both are a valid measure of hyperglycemia [5]. Glucose tolerance and insulin response curves in callitrichids are typical of most primates [10]. The use of injectable alpha-2 agonists for restraint and anesthesia may cause a transient hyperglycemia. Hyperglycemia and glycosuria also accompany islet cell hyperplasia in callitrichids [33].

Gastrointestinal and Cardiac Biomarkers, Lipids and Lipoproteins, and Electrolytes

While callitrichids are often affected by cardiac and gastrointestinal disease, antemortem clinicopathologic diagnostics specific to these diseases are few (Tables 13.6) [3, 11, 34]. Lipoprotein values have been established for obese and non-obese common marmosets (Table 13.7) [5, 16, 35], and electrolyte concentrations are similar to those of other mammals (Table 13.6).

Blood Proteins

Hyperproteinemia is an indication of dehydration or inflammation, while hypoproteinemia may be attributed to liver, gastrointestinal, or renal diseases as well as hemorrhage in callitrichid species. Reference intervals for fibrinogen and heat-precipitated protein in the marmoset were similar to those for humans; marked increases occur in sick animals [15].

Vitamins, Minerals and Metals, Toxins

Rickets and other nutritional diseases are of concern in captive callitrichids [36]. Reference intervals for free-living black-tufted marmosets (*C. penicillata*) and the common marmoset (*C. jacchus*) for PTH, iCa, and vitamin D have been determined (Table 13.8) [37, 38]. As New World primates, callitrichids require adequate sunlight exposure and may also require dietary supplementation of vitamin D to avoid osteomalacia [39]. Serum concentrations of vitamin D, 1,25-dihydroxyvitamin D_3, are approximately 10-fold higher in New World monkeys compared to Old World monkeys and apes (Table 13.8). Hepatic hemosiderosis, an inappropriate accumulation of iron leading to hepatic dysfunction, is a common postmortem finding in captive callitrichids. Ferritin and percent transferrin saturation levels correlate with hepatic iron concentration in the callitrichid [29].

Hormones

Published reference intervals for callitrichid species for thyroxine or thyroid-stimulating hormone concentrations are lacking. Iodine (I) deficiency occurred in common marmosets fed a diet composed of natural ingredients but containing only up to 12.2 ± 1.4 ug/I/kg wet weight. Plasma thyroxine concentrations declined, and plasma thyroid-stimulating hormone concentrations increased. Thyroid glands were hypertrophied and hyperplastic [40]. Cortisol determination from feces of saliva of the common marmoset provides a noninvasive method to measure stress [16]. Direct assays for conjugated urinary estrogens are used to monitor ovarian function and the reproductive cycle in callitrichids. High concentrations of conjugated estrone were measured in marmoset plasma, but estradiol 17 beta was the predominant estrogen in urine. In contrast, estrone was the most abundant estrogen measured in tamarin and callimico urine. Sulfates and glucuronides were proportionally present in urine before ovulation in the marmoset, but sulfates were predominant after ovulation. Conversely, most of the estrogens in tamarin urine appear conjugated as glucuronides [2, 7].

Table 13.6 Biochemical values of Callitrichidae.

Analyte (abbreviation)	Units, SI (conventional)	Common marmoset [14, 16, 32] (*Callithrix jacchus*)		Goeldi's monkey [17] (*Callitithrix goeldii*)	Red-bellied tamarin [20] (*Saguinus labiatus*)	Cotton-top tamarin [23] (*Saguinus oedipus oedipus*)	White-footed tamarin [18] (*Saguinus leucopus*)
Sample size		**56**	**52**	**27**	**36**	**38**	**29**
Data given as		**Range (mean)**	**Range [Median]**	**Range (mean)**	**Range (mean)**	**Mean ± SD**	**Range (Mean)**
Alkaline phosphatase (ALP)	U/l = *(IU/l)*	♂ 87–332 (203.7) ♀ 73–335 (195)	44.00–426.25 [115.50]	35.0–287.3 (230.2)	♂ 149–3790 (674) ♀ 182–1148 (519)	♂ 96.29 ± 14.76 ♀ 116.19 ± 30.89	295–1217.5 (439)
Alanine (ALT) aminotransferase	U/l = *(IU/l)*	♂ 4–22 (9.0) ♀ 5–22 (9.3)	0.79–45.33 [2.95]	20.7–47.0 (43.5)	♂ 11–62 (32) ♀ 12–60 (33)	♂ 44.71 ± 29.67 ♀ 44.43 ± 28.28	12.3–32.7 (19.3)
Lactate (LDH) dehydrogenase	U/l = *(IU/l)*		134.77–1119.69 [279.00]	5.4–58.5 (28.1)			
Asparate (AST) aminotransferase	U/l = *(IU/l)*	♂ 78–147 (134.4) ♀ 63–221 (104.9)	51.24–316.21 [155.70]	55.5–109.0 (89.8)	♂ 132–291 (184) ♀ 131–289 (179)	♂ 198.13 ± 76.41 ♀ 186.43 ± 68.16	68.4–205.6 (133.4)
Gamma-glutamyl transferase (GGT)	U/l = *(IU/l)*		0.24–13.50 [2.80]	1.0–14.0 (9.4)			
Glutamate dehydrogenase (GLDH)	U/l = *(IU/l)*		4.00–61.33 [14.15]	5.4–197.0 (28.1)			
Creatine kinase (CK)	U/l = *(IU/l)*		76.90–1801.84 [281]	110.5–251.0 (177)	♂ 116–4480 (973) ♀ 104–4290 (617)	♂ 772.47 ± 354.08 ♀ 865.25 ± 421	230.4–855.8 (508.9)
Lipase	U/l = *(IU/l)*		10.8–58.8 [27.6]	11.5–95.3 (47.3)			
Amylase	U/l = *(IU/l)*	249–880 (528)	617.4–1243.2 [924]	216.5–380.5 (308.7)	448–1276 (888.9) *n* = 22	98–952(407.7) *n* = 35	
Albumin	g/l *(g/dl)*	♂ 35–48 (41.6) ♀ 34–57 (41.6) *[♂ 3.5–4.8 (4.16) ♀ 3.4–5.7 (4.16)]*	10.77–57.88 [33.1] *[1.077–5.788 [3.31]]*	33.4–42.0 (38.3) *[3.34–4.20 (3.83)]*	♂ 28–48 (39) ♀ 34–51 (40) *[♂ 2.8–4.8 (3.9) ♀ 3.4–5.1 (4.0)]*	♂ 39.7 ± 30.0 ♀ 40.6 ± 31.0 *♂ 3.97 ± 0.30 ♀ 4.06 ± 0.31]*	24–37 (31) *(2.4–3.7 [3.1])*
Globulin	g/l *(g/dl)*					♂ 22.7 ± 34.0 ♀ 23.6 ± 27.0 *[♂ 2.27 ± 0.34 ♀ 2.36 ± 0.27]*	
Albumin: globulin						♂ 1.80 ± 0.32 ♀ 1.74 ± 0.27	

(Continued)

Table 13.6 (Continued)

Analyte (abbreviation)	Units, SI (conventional)	Common marmoset [14, 16, 32] (*Callithrix jacchus*)		Goeldi's monkey [17] (*Callitithrix goeldii*)	Red-bellied tamarin [20] (*Saguinus labiatus*)	Cotton-top tamarin [23] (*Saguinus oedipus oedipus*)	White-footed tamarin [18] (*Saguinus leucopus*)
Sample size		**56**	**52**	**27**	**36**	**38**	**29**
Data given as		**Range (mean)**	**Range [Median]**	**Range (mean)**	**Range (mean)**	**Mean ± SD**	**Range (Mean)**
Total bilirubin	µmol/l	♂ 7–21 (14.0) ♀ 3–21 (10.0)	0.03–4.24 (0.70)	0.5–1.4 (1.0)	♂ 0–19 (10) ♀ 0–22 (9)	♂ 2.57 ± 1.20 ♀ 2.45 ± 1.02	9.41–4.62 (2.05)
	(mg/dl)	*[♂ 0.4–1.2 (0.8) ♀ 0.2–1.2 (0.6)]*	*[0.002–0.25 (0.04)]*	*[0.03–0.08 (0.06)]*	*[♂ 0–1.11 (0.58) ♀ 0–1.29 (0.53)]*	*[♂ 0.15 ± 0.07 ♀ 0.143 ± 0.0598]*	0.55–0.27 [0.12]
Direct bilirubin	µmol/l						0.17–1.54 [0.86]
	(mg/dl)						*0.01–0.09 [0.05]*
Indirect bilirubin	µmol/l						0.17–2.22 [1.03]
	(mg/dl)						*0.01–0.13 [0.06]*
Urea (BUN)	mmol/l	♂ 4.1–10.6 (6.5) ♀ 2.9–9.0 (5.9)	3.37–18.67 [8.40]		♂ 4.8–13.6 (8.5) ♀ 5.0–11.5 (8.8)	♂ 5.12 ± 1.03 ♀ 5.66 ± 1.20	1.71–4.64 (2.82)
	(mg/dl)	*[♂ 11.5–29.7 (18.2) ♀ 8.1–25.2 (16.5)]*	*9.44–52.30 [23.53]*		*[♂ 13.45–38.10 (23.81) ♀ 14.00–32.21 (24.65)]*	*[♂ 14.35 ± 2.89 ♀ 15.86 ± 3.35]*	*[4.8–13 (7.9)]*
Creatinine	µmol/l		14.00–48.28 [28.00]	40.0–79.5 (51.2)	♂ 70–97 (83) ♀ 66–91 (74)	♂ 36.24 ± 13.26 ♀ 29.17 ± 7.96	26.52–57.46 (41.55)
	(mg/dl)		*0.16–0.55 [0.32]*	*[0.45–0.90 (0.58)]*	*[♂ 0.79–1.10 (0.94) ♀ 0.75–1.03 (0.84)]*	*[♂ 0.41 ± 0.15 ♀ 0.33 ± 0.09]*	*0.3–0.65 (0.47)*
Total protein	g/l	♂ 56–82 (70) ♀ 60–82 (73)	41.10–74.8 [62.05]	61.5–75.6 (66.4)	♂ 64–79 (71) ♀ 57–79 (72)	♂ 62.4 ± 40.0 ♀ 64.1 ± 35.0	54–73 (64)
	(g/dl)	*[♂ 5.6–8.2 (7.0) ♀ 6.0–8.2 (7.3)]*	*[4.11–7.48 [6.21]]*	*[6.15–7.56 (6.64)]*	*[♂ 6.4–7.9 (7.1) ♀ 5.7–7.9 (7.2)]*	*[♂ 6.24 ± 0.40 ♀ 6.41 ± 0.35]*	*5.4–7.3 (6.4)*
Glucose	mmol/l	♂ 3.4–13.1 (6.5) ♀ 4.1–17.8 (6.9)	4.01–11.89 [6.9]	5.9–13.0 (8.9)	♂ 3.9–13.4 (8.6) ♀ 4.0–11.0 (8.0)	♂ 14.63 ± 5.35 ♀ 14.59 ± 5.31	4.62–14.71 (9.44)
	(mg/dl)	*[♂ 61.3–236.0 (117.1) ♀ 73.9–320.7 (124.3)]*	*[72.25–214.23 [124.32]]*	*[106.3–234.2 (160.4)]*	*[♂ 70.3–241.4 (155.0) ♀ 72.1–198.2 (144.1)]*	*[♂ 266 ± 96.43 ♀ 262.95 ± 95.67]*	*83.3–265 (170.1)*
Fructosamine	µmol/l					♂ 255.79 ± 53.62 ♀ 255.58 ± 47.62	
	(mg/dl)					*[♂ 4.61 ± 0.97 ♀ 4.61 ± 0.86]*	
CO_2	mmol/l = (mEq/l)					♂ 24.75 ± 3.38 ♀ 26.37 ± 2.67	

Sodium	mmol/l = (mEq/l)	♂ 149–160 (153.8) ♀ 145–160 (153.8)	155.5–174 [163]	152.3–163.5 (159.5)	♂ 153–170 (159) ♀ 141–168 (156)	♂ 150.06 ± 2.54 ♀ 150.50 ± 2.12	128.1–165.5 (148.3)
Potassium	mmol/l = (mEq/l)	♂ 3.3–7.5 (5.3) ♀ 3.7–6.4 (5.3)	2.30–4.65 [3.40]	2.9–4.2 (3.7)	♂ 3.2–6.7 (4.0) ♀ 3.5–6.0 (4.5)	♂ 4.25 ± 0.64 ♀ 4.04 ± 0.44	3.7–6.1 (4.9)
Chloride	mmol/l = (mEq/l)		101.85–119.9 [109.4]	114–125 (118.6)		♂ 104.40 ± 2.35 ♀ 106 ± 2.79	90–104.1 (96.1)
Calcium	mmol/l		1.78–2.96 [2.34]	2.1–2.4 (2.3)	♂ 2.2–2.8 (2.5) ♀ 2.3–2.8 (2.6)	♂ 2.17 ± 0.15 ♀ 2.26 ± 0.13	1.83–2.55 (2.18)
	(mg/dl)		*[7.12–11.84 [9.36]]*	*[8.4–9.6 (9.2)]*	*[♂ 8.8–11.2 (10)* *♀ 9.2–11.2 (10.4)]*	*[♂ 8.69 ± 0.59* *♀ 9.02 ± 0.50]*	*[7.3–10.2 (8.7)]*
Magnesium	mmol/l		0.60–1.03 [0.75]	0.8–1.2 (1.0)		♂ 0.83 ± 0.07 ♀ 0.81 ± 0.07	
	(mg/dl)		*[1.46–2.43 [3.00]]*	*[1.94–2.92 (2.43)]*		*[♂ 2.03 ± 0.16* *♀ 1.97 ± 0.16]*	
Iron	µmol/l		17.63–39.48 [28.00]	11.4–21.7 (16.1)			
	(µg/dl)		*[98.49–220.56 [156.42]]*	*[63.7–121.2 (89.9)]*			
Phosphorus	mmol/l		0.47–2.43 [1.07]	0.9–2.2 (1.6)		♂ 1.04 ± 0.21 ♀ 0.91 ± 0.22	0.87–1.65 (1.26)
	(mg/dl)		*[1.46–7.52 [3.31]]*	*2.78–6.81 (4.95)*		*[♂ 3.21 ± 0.64* *♀ 2.81 ± 0.67]*	*[2.7–5.1 (3.9)]*
Uric acid	µmol/l (mg/dl)						5.95–101.12 (23.79) 0.1–1.7 [0.4]

Table 13.7 Lipids and lipoproteins of callitrichids.

Analyte (abbreviation)	Units, SI (conventional)	Common marmoset [16] (*Callithrix jacchus*)	Goeldi's monkey [17] (*Callimico goeldii*)	Cotton-top tamarin [23] (*Saguinus oedipus*)	White-footed tamarin [18] (*Saguinus leucopus*)
Animal number		**48**	**27**	**38**	**20**
Data type		**Range [median]**	**Range (mean)**	**(Mean ± 1 SD)**	**Range (mean)**
High-density lipoprotein cholesterol (HDL Chol)	mmol/l *[mg/dl]*	0.55–2.36 [1.33] *[18.71–80.27 [45.24]]*			
High-density lipoprotein triglycerides (HDL tg)		0.15–0.50 [0.28] *[5.10–17.01 [9.52]]*			
Low-density lipoprotein cholesterol (LDL)		1.34–3.09 [2.20] *[45.58–105.10 [74.83]]*			
Low-density lipoprotein triglycerides (LDL tg)		0.32–1.24 [0.55] *[10.88–42.18 [18.71]]*			
Very-low-density lipoprotein cholesterol (VLDL)		0.02–0.45 [0.11] *[0.68–15.31 [3.74]]*			
Very-low-density lipoprotein triglycerides (VLDL tg)		0.07–1.13 [0.29] *[2.38–38.44 [9.86]]*			
Total cholesterol		2.28–5.09 [3.82] *[77.55–173.13 [129.93]]*	1.2–3.6 (2.3) *[40.82–122.45 [78.23]]*	♂(4.53 ± 1.5) ♀(3.96 ± 0.91) *[♂(153.94 ± 51.04) ♀(134.67 ± 31.04)]*	1.6–3.1 (2.32) *[54.5–103.6 (79)]*
Total triglycerides		0.56–2.63 [1.09] *[19.05–89.46 [37.07]]*	0.2–1.5 (0.6) *[6.8–51.02 [20.41]]*		0.65–2.49 (1.51) *[22–84.8 [51.4]]*

Table 13.8 Serum levels of vitamin D3, metabolites, and parathyroid hormone in select callitrichids and rhesus monkeys.

Analyte (abbreviation)	Units, SI (conventional)	Common marmoset [37] (*Callithrix jacchus*)	Black-tufted marmoset [38] (*Callithrix penicillata*)	Rhesus monkey [37]
Sample size		**17**	**15**	**5**
Data set		**Mean ± SEM**	**Mean ± SD**	**Mean ± SEM**
Calcium	mmol/l *(mg/dl)*	2.15 ± 0.05 *(8.6 ± 0.2)*		2.35 ± 0.08 *(9.4 ± 0.3)*
Ionized calcium	mmol/l *(mg/dl)*		1.0 ± 0.15 *(4.0 ± 0.6)*	
Phosphorus	mmol/l *(mg/dl)*	1.48 ± 0.06 *(4.6 ± 0.2)*		1.39 ± 0.16 *(4.3 ± 0.5)*
25-hydroxyvitamin D	nmol/l *(ng/ml)*	1183.1 ± 239.6 *(474 ± 96)*	154 ± 51.9 *(61.7 ± 20.8)*	124.8 ± 10 *(50 ± 4)*
Calcitriol	pmol/l *(pg/ml)*	1250.6 ± 213.2 *(481 ± 82)*		247 ± 44.2 *(95 ± 17)*
Parathyroid hormone	ng/l *(pg/ml)*	1750 ± 200	275.2 ± 34.1	230 ± 60

Urinalysis

Free catch urine is ideally obtained during a patient voiding or from a clean cage floor. In some laboratory settings, marmosets have been trained to void a urine sample upon command [41]. Urinalysis using the dipstick method including specific gravity determination and microscopic sediment evaluation is recommended [10].

Serology and PCR

Many diseases of callitrichids can result in acute death (Table 13.9). Diagnostic testing is available and relevant for many of these diseases (Table 13.10).

Herpes Viruses

Primates may carry several herpesviruses that cause minimal disease in the natural host, but infection of other New World monkey species causes morbidity and mortality. Saimiriine herpesvirus 1 (HSV-1) (also known as Herpesvirus tamarinus or HVT) is an alphaherpesvirus carried asymptomatically by squirrel monkeys. Infection of marmosets and tamarins results in necrosis of skin, oral mucosa, multiple organs, and is usually fatal. Herpesvirus simplex (HVS), human origin has caused disease similar to HVT in callitrichids with experimental inoculation, but the natural potential for pathogenicity is unknown. At least three herpesviruses have been shown to be oncogenic, often leading to malignant lymphoma in one or more species of callitrichids (*Herpesvirus saimiri, Herpesvirus ateles,* and Epstein–Barr virus) [10]. Serology can be used to screen potential asymptomatic hosts or to confirm diagnosis of affected animals. PCR of whole blood or lesion swabs is available to detect virus in viremic or actively shedding animals.

Measles Virus

Measles (rubeola) infection has resulted in multiple mortalities in a population of *S. oedipus, S. fuscicollis,* and *C. jacchus.* Measle-like disease has occurred in other callitrichid colonies. Clinical signs include swollen eyelids, lethargy, and death ensuing less than a day after first observing illness, rhinorrhea, facial edema, and maculopapular exanthema on the lips and skin. Significant titers to rubeola and evidence of positive seroconversion by selected individuals occurs [42]. Both live and inactivated vaccines were effective in protecting challenged animals [46]. Serology can be used to screen animals for prior exposure to measles virus. Diagnosis in monkeys with clinical signs is confirmed by increasing antibody titers with serology, or by detection of the virus in whole blood, serum, urine, throat swab, or lesion swab by PCR.

Arenavirus

Callitrichid hepatitis (CH) is a highly fatal disease of captive marmosets and tamarins caused by an arenavirus, lymphocytic choriomeningitis virus (LCMV),

Table 13.9 Causes of acute death in callitrichids [3, 11, 28, 42–45].

Etiology	
Viral	Alpha herpes viruses – Herpes Virus Tamarinus (Herpes virus T, Herpesvirus platyrrhinae), herpes virus simplex, lymphocytic choriomeningitis, measles, Encephalomyocarditis virus
Bacterial	*Bordetella bronchiseptica*, Leptospirosis, *Pasteurella multocida, Streptococcus zooepidemicus, Yersinia pseudotuberculosis*
Parasitic	*Toxoplasma gondii, Prosthenorchis elegans, Moniliformis clarki*

Table 13.10 Options for serological and PCR testing of callitrichids.

Company	Address	Further contact information
Charles River Laboratories	RADS, West Coast Laboratory 10788 Roselle Street, San Diego, CA 92121	1.877.274.8371 www.criver.com
VRL Laboratories	P.O. Box 401007540 Louis Pasteur, Suite 200 San Antonio, Texas 78229	www.vrl.net877-615-7275 Fax: 210–615-7771
Zoologix	9811 Owensmouth Ave, Suite 4, Chatsworth CA 91311, USA	www.zoologix.com Phone: 818–717-8880

which is enzootic in house mice worldwide. Clinical signs of LCMV in callitrichids include weakness, anorexia, ataxia, seizures, jaundice, petechiation, and death [43]. Serological testing for LCMV via immunofluorescent assay (IFA) or enzyme-linked immunosorbent assay (ELISA) are available [10].

References

1 Abbott, D.H., Barnett, D.K., Colman, R.J. et al. (2003). Aspects of common marmoset basic biology and life history important for biomedical research. *Comparative Medicine* 53 (4): 339–350.

2 Carroll, J.B., Abbott, D.H., Hindle, J.E., and Martin, R.D. (1990). Urinary endocrine monitoring of the ovarian cycle and pregnancy in Goeldi's monkey (*Callimico goeldii*). *Journals of Reproduction & Fertility* 89: 149–161.

3 Chalmers, D.T., Murgatroyd, L.B., and Wadsworth, P.F. (1983). A survey of the pathology of marmosets (*Callithrix jacchus)* derived from a marmoset breeding unit. *Laboratory Animals* 17: 270–279.

4 Loeb, W.F. (1999). The nonhuman primate. In: *The Clinical Chemistry of Laboratory Animals*, 2nde (ed. W.M. Leob and F. Quimby), 145–162. Ann Arbor: Edward Brothers.

5 Tardif, S.D., Power, M.L., Ross, C.N. et al. (2009). Characterization of obese phenotypes in a small nonhuman primate, the common marmoset (*Callithrix jacchus*). *Obesity* 17: 1499–1505.

6 Porter, L.M. (2007). *The Behavioral Ecology of Callimicos and Tamarins in Northwestern Bolivia*. Upper Saddle River: Prentice Hall.

7 Hodges, J.K. and Eastman, S.A. (1984). Monitoring ovarian function in marmosets and tamarins by the measurement of urinary estrogen metabolites. *American Journal of Primatology* 6: 187–197.

8 Rylands, A.B. (1997). The callirichidae: a biological overview. In: *Marmosets and Tamarins in Biological and Biomedical Research: Proceedings of a Workshop* (ed. C. Pryce, L. Scott and C. Schnell), 1–22. Salisbury: DSSD Imagery.

9 Yamada, N., Sato, J., Wako, Y., and Tsuchitani, M. (2013). Morphological study of progressive glomerulonephropathy in common marmosets (*Callithrix jacchus*). *Toxicologic Pathology* 41 (8): 1106–1115.

10 Richter, C.B. (1984). Biology and diseases of callitrichidae. In: *Laboratory Animal Medicine* (ed. J.G. Fox, B.J. Cohen and F.M. Loew), 353–383. Florida: Academic Press.

11 Ludlage, E. and Mansfield, K. (2003). Clinical care and diseases of the common marmoset (*Callithrix jacchus*). *Comparative Medicine* 53 (4): 369–382.

12 Thomas, J.S. (2004). Introduction to serum chemistries: artifacts in biochemical determinations. In: *Small Animal Clinical Diagnosis by Laboratory Methods* (ed. M.D. Willard and H. Tvedten), 113–116. Saunders.

13 Weiss, D. and Tvedten, H. (2004). The complete blood count and bone marrow examination: general comments and selected techniques. In: *Small Animal Clinical Diagnosis by Laboratory Methods*, 4e (ed. M.D. Willard and H. Tvedten), 14–37. Saunders.

14 Eccleston, E. (1977). Normal haematological values in rats, mice and marmosets. In: *Comparative Clinical Hematology* (ed. R.K. Archer and L.B. Jeffcott), 611–619. Oxford: Blackwell Scientific Publications.

15 Hawkey, C.M., Hart, M.G., and Jones, D.M. (1982). Clinical hematology of the common marmoset *Callthrix jacchus*. *American Journal of Primatology* 3: 179–199.

16 Kuehnel, F., Grohmann, J., Buchwald, U. et al. (2012). Parameters of haematology, clinical chemistry and lipid metabolism in the common marmoset and alterations under stress conditions. *Journal of Medical Primatology* 41 (4): 241–250.

17 Kalaitsidis, F., Lutz, H., and Pryce, C.R. (1999). Hematology and serum chemistry values in captive goeldi's monkeys (*Callimico goeldii*). *Journal of Zoo and Wildlife Medicine* 30 (3): 372–376.

18 Fox, M., Brieva, C., Moreno, C. et al. (2008). Hematologic and serum biochemistry reference values in wild-caught white-footed tamarins (*Saguinus leucopus*) housed in captivity. *Journal of Zoo and Wildlife Medicine* 39 (4): 548–557.

19 Porter, J.A. (1970). Hematologic values of the Panamanian marmoset (*Saguinus geoffroyi*). *American Journal of Veterinary Research* 31 (2): 379–381.

20 Wadsworth, P.F., Hiddleston, W.A., Jones, D.V. et al. (1982). Haematological, coagulation and blood chemistry data in red-bellied tamarins *Saguinus labiatus*. *Laboratory Animals* 16: 327–330.

21 Hawkey, C.M., Knight, J.A., Taffs, L.F. et al. (1983). Red-bellied tamarins (*Saguinus labiatus*): hematologic reference values and hemopathologic responses. *American Journal of Primatology* 4: 33–43.

22 Hawkey, C.M., Hart, M.G., Knight, J.A. et al. (1983). Cotton-top tamarins (*Saguinus oedipus oedipus*): hematologic reference values and hemopathologic responses. *American Journal of Primatology* 5: 231–239.

23 Shukan, E.T., Boe, C.Y., Hasenfus, A.V. et al. (2012). Normal hematologic and serum biochemical values of cotton-top tamarins (*Saguinus oedipus*). *Journal of the American Association for Laboratory Animal Science* 51 (2): 150–154.

24 Bush, M., Custer, R.S., Whitla, J.C., and Smith, E.E. (1982). Hematologic values of captive golden lion tamarins (*Leontopithecus rosalia*): variations with sex, age and heath status. *Laboratory Animal Science* 32 (3): 294–297.

25 Omorphos, S.C., Rice-Evans, C., and Hawkey, C. (1989). Heinz bodies do not modify the membrane characteristics of common marmoset (*Callithrix jacchus*) erythrocytes. *Laboratory Animals* 23: 66–69.

26 Juan-Salles, C., Prats, N., Resendes, A. et al. (2003). Anemia, myopathy, and pansteatitis in vitamin E deficient captive marmosets. *Veterinary Pathology* 40: 540–547.

27 Logan, A.C. and Khan, K.N. (1996). Case report: clinical pathologic changes in two marmosets with wasting syndrome. *Toxicologic Pathology* 24 (6): 707–709.

28 Montali, R.J. and Busch, M. (1999). Diseases of the callitrichidae. In: *Zoo and Wildlife Animal Medicine: Current Therapy 4* (ed. M.E. Fowler and R.E. Miller), 369–375. Philadelphia: WB Saunders Co.

29 Smith, K.M., McAloose, D., Torregrossa, A.M. et al. (2008). Hematologic iron analyte values as an indicator of hepatic hemosiderosis in callitrichidae. *Americal Journal of Primatology* 70: 629–633.

30 da Rocha, R.M. and Harada-Hamel, M.L. Schneider H(1990) ABO Blood Groups in Natural Populations of Callitrichidae (*Platyrrhini,* primates). *Brazilian Journal of Genetics* 13 (3): 531–577.

31 Schulman, F.Y., Montali, R.J., Bush, M. et al. (1993). Dubin-Johnson-like syndrome in golden lion tamarins (*Leotopithicus rosalia rosalia*). *Veterinary Pathology* 30: 491–498.

32 Gatesman, T.J. (1992). Serum amylase values in callitrichids. *Laboratory Animal Science* 42 (1): 46–50.

33 Juan-Salles, C., Marco, A., Ramos-Vara, J.A. et al. (2002). Islet hyperplasia in callitrichids. *Primates* 43 (3): 179–190.

34 Smith, K.M., Calle, P., Raphael, B.L. et al. (2006). Cholelithiasis in four callitrichid species (*Leotopithicus, Callithrix*). *Journal of Zoo and Wildlife Medicine* 37 (1): 44–48.

35 Croll, D., Ausman, L., and Nicolosi, R. (1993). Cholesterol metabolism in new world primates: comparative studies in two tamarin species (*Saguinus oedipus* and *Saguinus fuscicollis*) and the squirrel monkey (*Saimiri sciureus*). *Comparative Biochemical Physiology* 106 (4): 845–853.

36 Wissman, M.A. (1999). Nutrition and husbandry of callitrichids (marmosets and tamarins). In: *Veterinary Clinics of North America Exotic Animal Practice*, vol. 2, 209–240. Elsevier.

37 Yamaguchi, A., Kohno, Y., Yamazaki, T. et al. (1986). Bone in the marmoset: a resemblance to vitamin D-dependent rickets type II. *Calcified Tissue International* 39: 22–27.

38 Teixeira, D.S., Nobrega, Y.K., Valencia, C.E. et al. (2012). Evaluation of 25-hydroxyvitamin D and parathyroid hormone in *Callithrix pencillata* primates living in their natural habitat in Brazil. *Journal of Medical Primatology* 41: 364–371.

39 Ullrey, D.E., Bernard, J.B., Peter, G.K. et al. (1999). Vitamin D intakes by cotton-top tamarins (*Saguinus oedipus*) and associated serum 25-hydroxyvitamin D concentrations. *Zoo Biology* 18: 473–480.

40 Mano, M.T., Potter, B.J., Belling, G.B., and Hetzel, B.S. (1985). Low-iodine diet for the production of severe idodine deficiency in marmosets. *British Journal of Nutrition* 54: 367–372.

41 Kurien, B.T., Everds, N.E., and Schofield, R.H. (2004). Experimental animal urine colletion: A review. *Laboratory Animals* 38: 333–361.

42 Cicmanec, J.L. (1977). Medical problems encountered in a callitrichid colony. In: *The Biology and Conservation of the Callitrichidae* (ed. D.G. Kleiman), 331–336. Washington, D.C.: Smithsonian Inst. Press.

43 Montali, R.J., Connolly, B.M., Armstrong, D.L. et al. (1995). Pathology and immunohistochemistry of callitrichid hepatitis, an emerging disease of captive new world primates caused by lymphocytic choriomeningitis virus. *American Journal of Pathology* 48: 5–15.

44 Montali, R.J., Scanga, C.A., Pernikoff, D. et al. (1993). A common-source outbreak of callitrichid hepatitis in captive tamarins and marmosets. *The Journal of Infectious Disease* 167 (4): 946–950.

45 Weber, M. and Junge, R. (2000). Identification and treatment of *Moniliformes clarki* (Acanthocephala) in cotton-topped tamarins (*Saguinus oedipus*). *Journal of Zoo and Wildlife Medicine* 31 (4): 503–507.

46 Loomis M. (1990). Update of vaccination recommendations for nonhuman primates. *Proceedings of the Association of American Zoological Veterinarians*, (pp. 259–260).

14

Lemurs

Sabrina D. Clark DVM, DACVP (Clinical Pathology)

Department of Pathobiology, College of Veterinary Medicine & Biomedical Sciences, Texas A&M University, College Station, Texas, USA

Introduction

Destruction of Madagascar's forests due to the expansion of the human population continues to bring human and lemur populations closer together [1]. Concerns continue for the loss of lemur species due to the encroachment of the human population, but also for the threat of emerging infectious diseases in humans for which lemurs may serve as reservoirs [1–3]. Understanding of disease through biomedical evaluation is a critical component for recognizing the connection of development of shared infectious diseases between humans and lemurs and for the proper management and care of lemurs, particularly those in captivity, to ensure successful preservation of these species [4]. Establishing baseline values for free-ranging animals allows for the monitoring of various disturbances on these populations and may provide an indication of when aggressive conservation management is needed [2–4]. Only a small amount of clinical data has been collected for lemur species and the number of individuals evaluated within those species has been low. In a few of these species, physiologic data has been gathered from both captive and free-ranging animals to allow comparisons to guide husbandry and environmental and medical management.

Species

Lemurs are strepsirrhine primates that are endemic to the island of Madagascar [5]. While the classification of lemurs continues to evolve on the basis of molecular genetics, five families and 15 genera and from 30 to 101 species and subspecies are currently recognized [5, 6]. Today, only a handful of species are housed in captivity. Ring-tailed lemurs (*Lemur catta*) are the most common of these species found in captivity, so they are the focus of most studies to establish baseline reference values for veterinary care. *Microcebus murinus*, the gray mouse lemur, is a biomedical model for aging research [7, 8]. Common lemur species for which biomedical evaluations has been performed are shown in Table 14.1. Lemurs can be grouped by their primary time of activity as either diurnal (during the day) or nocturnal (at night) [9]. Most lemurs are arboreal, meaning they spend most of their time in trees, but lemurs can be found in habitats ranging from rainforests to desert areas [5, 9]. Lemurs feed primarily on leaves, fruits, and berries, but in nocturnal species or if food is scarce, insects may be incorporated into their diet [9].

Sample Collection

Restraint

In general, anesthesia is needed to obtain blood samples from lemur patients. However, at some facilities, techniques using positive reinforcement training have been utilized to have lemurs station and extend their arms through a port for sample collection to minimize the stress of restraint [9]. Common lemur anesthetic protocols include ketamine combined with diazepam or tiletamine-zolazepam (Telazol®) [3, 10]. Medetomidine or dexmedetomidine and butorphanol combined with ketamine or midazolam can also be used [3, 10]. Lemurs should be fasted adequately prior to any anesthetic induction protocol. Regardless of the anesthetic protocol used, as in domestic species, minimize contact and stimulation with the animal upon initial administration of drugs to allow maximum effect. For small lemurs, face mask or box induction with isoflurane or sevoflurane gas is also effective. Atipamezole and naloxone may be administered intramuscularly to reverse the effects of dexmedetomidine and butorphanol, respectively, once examination and collection is complete.

Exotic Animal Laboratory Diagnosis, First Edition. Edited by J. Jill Heatley and Karen E. Russell.

Table 14.1 Select lemur species.

Common name	Scientific name
Von der Decken's sifaka	*Propithecus verreauxi*
Golden-crowned sifaka	*Propithecus tattersalli*
Gray mouse lemur	*Microcebus murinus*
Red-fronted brown lemur	*Eulemur fulvus*
Red ruffed lemur	*Varecia rubra*
Ring-tailed lemur	*Lemur catta*
White-fronted brown lemur	*Eulemur fulvus*
White ruffed lemur	*Varecia variegate*

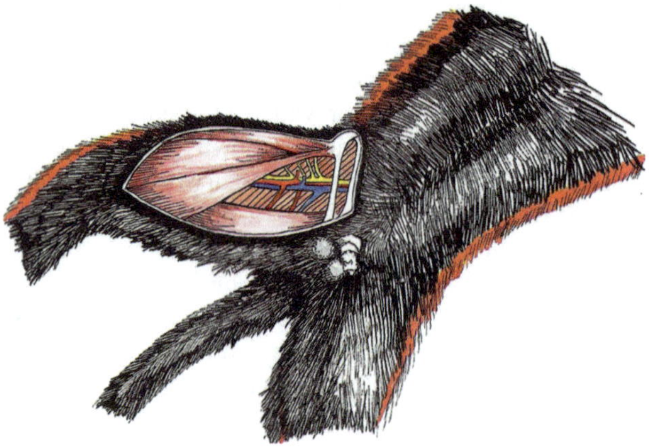

Figure 14.1 Femoral venipuncture of the red ruffed lemur.

More information regarding recommended anesthetic protocols for lemurs is available [11, 12].

Sample Collection

A single blood sample should not exceed 1% of the animal's body weight (10 ml/kg body weight) to avoid hypovolemic shock. To help minimize stress, anesthetic use, and to prevent injury, laboratory-bred blood-sucking bugs can be used collect samples from captive primates [13]. In larger lemurs, once the animal is anesthetized, a venous blood sample can be collected from the jugular, cephalic, or femoral veins (Figure 14.1). Based on the gray mouse lemur's small size, blood is typically drawn from the ear or saphenous veins. Although prosimians are of less zoonotic concern than many other nonhuman primates, appropriate sharps handling procedures for nonhuman primates must be followed.

Sample Handling

For complete blood count and biochemistry panels, blood should be collected into an ethylenediaminetetraacetic (EDTA) anticoagulant tube and a non-anticoagulant tube, respectively, the latter of which should then be allowed to clot (approximately 20–30 min). Once clotted, the non-anticoagulant tube should be centrifuged and the serum separated as soon as possible to minimize erroneous laboratory results due to use of nutrients in the serum by red and white blood cells. Alternately, blood may be collected into lithium heparin tubes for plasma collection, acceptable for many biochemical panels. Blood smears are preferably made immediately after sample collection and prior to contacting anticoagulant but can alternatively be made from the anticoagulant tube as soon as possible to help minimize the distortion of the red and white blood cells for evaluation. Blood smears are routinely stained with a Romanowsky-type stain for evaluation, either manually or through the use of an automatic stainer. A rapid stain, known as Diff-Quik (Dade Behring, Newark, Delaware), is commonly used. Methanol-based stains such as Wright or Wright-Giemsa stains are also available. It is important to recognize that there may be minor variations in the staining quality of the cells depending on the stain chosen. Ideally, blood samples should be processed within 4 h (within 1 h is preferable). Any blood sample that cannot be processed in that time should be refrigerated and then warmed to room temperature prior to evaluation. In most cases, blood can be refrigerated for approximately 12–24 h before storage errors are identified.

Complete Blood Count

Minor differences may occur in hematological values of lemurs depending on species, habitat, free-ranging or captive, sex, or pregnancy [2–4, 14–16]. For ring-tailed lemurs, differences among individuals of different habitats and sexes are not surprising given the small populations analyzed [3]. A recent study assessed age-related changes in hematologic and biochemistry values in wild ring-tailed lemur living at the Bezà Mahafaly special reserve in Madagascar based on three age classes, including young (<5 years), adult (5-9 years), and old (≥10 years) [17]. Values from two studies are listed in Table 14.2. Significant differences identified by Singleton et al. between age and sex are described in the text. The importance of these differences is difficult to interpret until there is a better understanding of the clinical significance associated with the change [3]. Hematologic values in free-ranged ring-tailed lemurs were generally lower compared to those of their captive counterparts [4]. Comparison of pack cell volume (PCV) percentage between captive and free-range lemurs indicates that captive lemurs may be relatively dehydrated (based on higher PCV) despite having continuous access to water [4, 15]. No significant differences in hematologic data were found between male and female brown lemurs [2]. Most lemurs with physical examination

Table 14.2 Hematologic data for lemurs [4, 14, 15, 17, 18].

Analyte (abbreviation)	Units, SI (*conventional*)	Red-fronted brown lemur (*Eulemur fulvus rufus*)	Ring-tailed lemur (*Lemur catta*)	Decken's sifaka (*Propithecus verreauxi deckeni*)	Red ruffed lemur (*Varecia rubra*)	*Gray mouse lemur* (*Microcebus murinus*) [13]
Data format		**Mean ± SD**	**Mean ± SD**	**Mean ± SD**	**Mean ± SD**	**Mean**
Animals sampled		20	20, 44	20	20	86
Pack cell volume (PCV)	%	38.3 ± 5.7	38.7 ± 3.59, 42.3 ± 4.0		45.7 ± 4.38	51.7
Total leukocytes WBC	$10^3/\mu l$	7.76 ± 3.29	4.744 ± 1.129, 7.5 ± 2.4	8.14 ± 3.19	8.55	12 900
Neutrophils	%	40 ± 13.8	49.7 ± 18.3, 36.3 ± 12.7	47.8 ± 20.7	62.8 ± 18.7	30.7
	$10^3/\mu l$		2.33 ± 1.058, 2.6 ± 1.1		5.65	
Band neutrophils	%	0 ± 0	0.694 ± 0.689	0 ± 0	0–10	
	$10^3/\mu l$		0.0368 ± 0.0377		0.159	
Lymphocytes	%	60.2 ± 13.6	41.5 ± 17.9, 51.0 ± 13.6	50.6 ± 19.6	30.5 ± 17.2	59.7
	$10^3/\mu l$		1.987 ± 1.079, 4.0 ± 1.9		2.48 ± 1.10	
Monocytes	%	0.5 ± 0.7	4.9 ± 1.55, 5.9 ± 2.7	0.57 ± 1.0	2.68	4.8
	$10^3/\mu l$		0.236 ± 0.106, 0.42± .19			
Eosinophils	%	0 ± 0	2.38 ± 2.05, 4.8 ± 3.4	0.17 ± 0.8		4.2
	$10^3/\mu l$		0.101 ± 0.0908, .36 ± .29		0.194	
Basophils	%	0.05 ± 0.24	0.333 ± 0.485, 1.8 ± 2.0	0 ± 0		0.6
	$10^3/\mu l$		0.0133 ± 0.0183, .12 ± .13			
Total protein	g/l	69 ± 6	59.7 ± 7.61, 70 ± 5	73 ± 4	65.6 ± 4.03	
	(g/dl)	(6.9 ± 0.6)	(5.97 ± 0.761), (7.0 ± 0.5)	(7.3 ± 0.4)	(6.56 ± 0.403)	

abnormalities had suffered leukocytosis. In a biomedical evaluation of red ruffed lemurs, white blood cell counts were higher in females compared to males [15]. This result may be due to pregnancy; however, the population studied was not subdivided into pregnant versus non-pregnant females [15]. In general, a leukocytosis may be associated with an inflammatory response in these species [3, 19]. In ring-tailed lemurs, age effects were detected in several blood values [17]. Older lemurs had significantly lower numbers of leukocytes, numbers of lymphocytes, lymphocyte percentages, and higher neutrophils percentages and neutrophils:lymphocyte ratio (NLR) compared to young and adult lemurs. These changes were attributed to immunosenescence, which refers to attenuation of immune function associated with aging. Males had significantly higher numbers of leukocytes, neutrophils, and monocytes and a significantly lower percentage of basophils when compared to females at all ages combined. Young females had significantly higher monocyte counts compared to adult and old females and a significantly higher percentage of monocytes when compared to female adults. Old female lemurs had a significantly higher percentage of neutrophils and NLR and a significantly lower number and percentage of lymphocytes compared to young and adult females. Adult and old male lemurs had significantly lower basophil counts than females. Within the old age class, males had significantly higher neutrophils compared to females. Golden-crowned sifaka and ruffed lemurs tend to have neutrophil:lymphocyte ratios >1 [16]. Female lesser mouse lemurs tend to have a lower percentage of lymphocytes compared to males, and the lymphocyte:neutrophil ratio decreases with age [14]. The most common cause of lymphopenia with an equal to higher neutrophil count, resulting in an elevated NLR, is a corticosteroid-induced or "stress" leukogram [15]. External stressors such as transportation, exercise, and restraint have been shown to affect NLR due to glucocorticoid release causing lymphocyte redistribution from blood to other body compartments. In ring-tailed lemurs, the difference in monocyte count between young and adult and older female lemurs is thought to be correlated with decreasing estrogen levels with age, as occurs in women. Eosinophils and basophils participate in a number of processes including hypersensitivity reactions, hemostasis, lipid metabolism, response to parasitic infections, and paraneoplastic conditions. Overall, males had a significantly lower percentage of basophils than female ring-tailed lemurs, but young males had the highest basophil counts. It is postulated that changes in hormones, including thyroid hormone, corticosteroids, sex steroids, and insulin may be attributable to these changes.

The blood smear should be evaluated for erythrocyte and leukocyte morphology, adequacy of platelet numbers, and hemoparasites. Normal leukocyte morphology of lemurs is presented in Figures 14.2–14.8. Because studies have not been performed to determine the significance of morphology changes in lemurs, basic principles derived from domestic species are often applied when evaluating morphologic changes. As in domestic species, anemia can be characterized as morphologic changes of erythrocyte morphology. A manual reticulocyte count is used in most species to determine regeneration, and similarly can be determined to evaluate the degree of regeneration in lemurs. In ring-tailed lemurs, ISIS reports a normal reticulocyte count to be 0.2% [20].

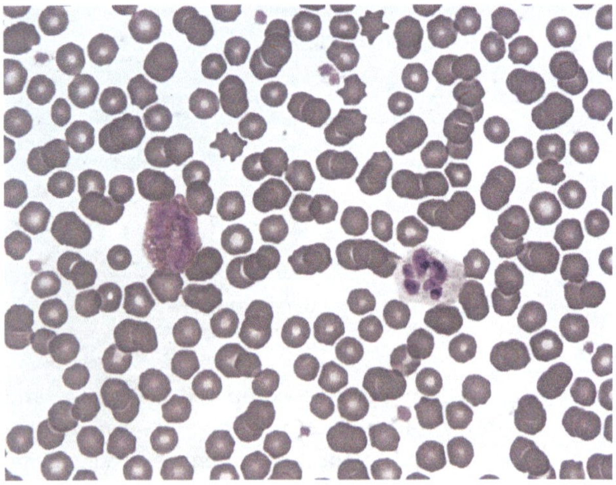

Figure 14.2 Eosinophil (left) and neutrophil (right) of the black-and-white ruffed lemur.

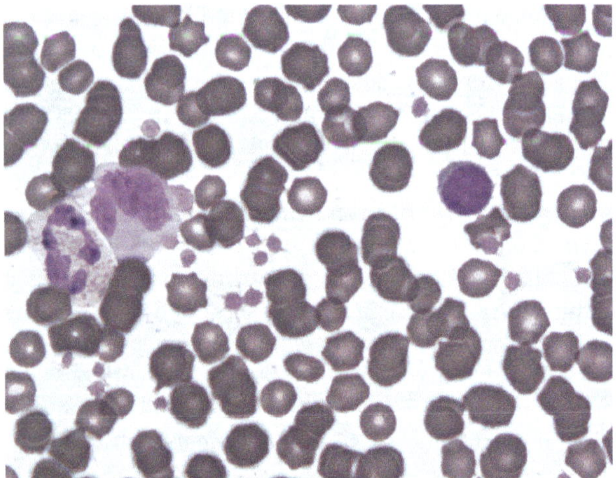

Figure 14.3 From left to right, neutrophil, monocyte, and lymphocyte of the black-and-white ruffed lemur.

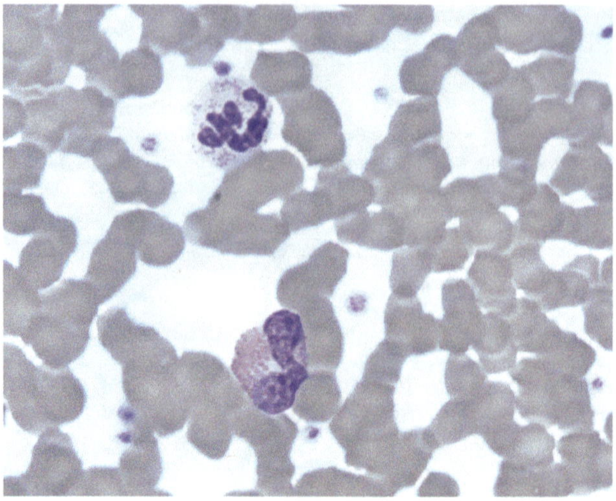

Figure 14.4 Neutrophil (upper) and eosinophil (lower) of the red ruffed lemur.

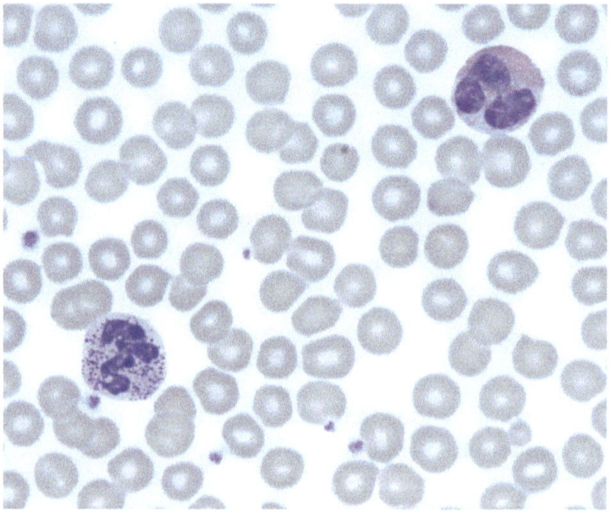

Figure 14.5 Neutrophil (lower left) and eosinophil (upper right) of the crowned lemur.

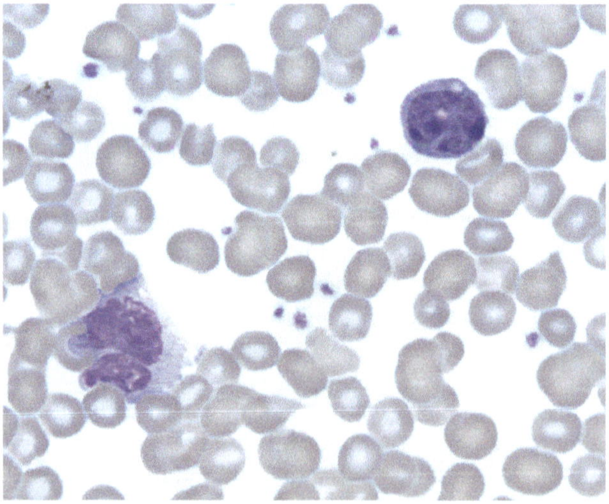

Figure 14.6 Monocyte (lower left) and large lymphocyte (upper right) of the crowned lemur.

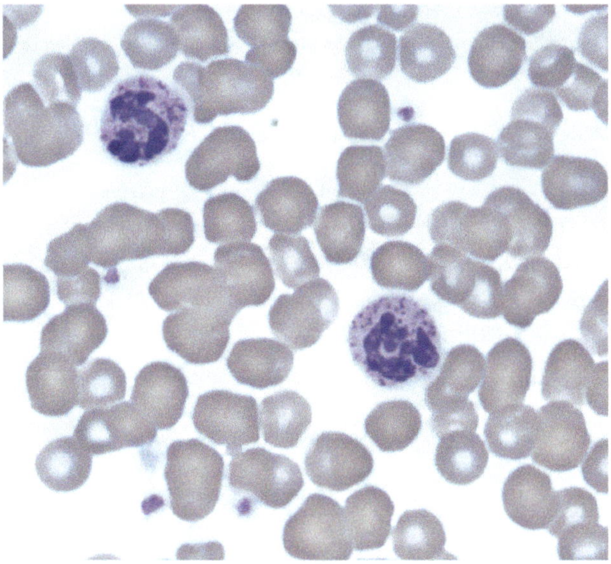

Figure 14.7 Neutrophils of the crowned lemur.

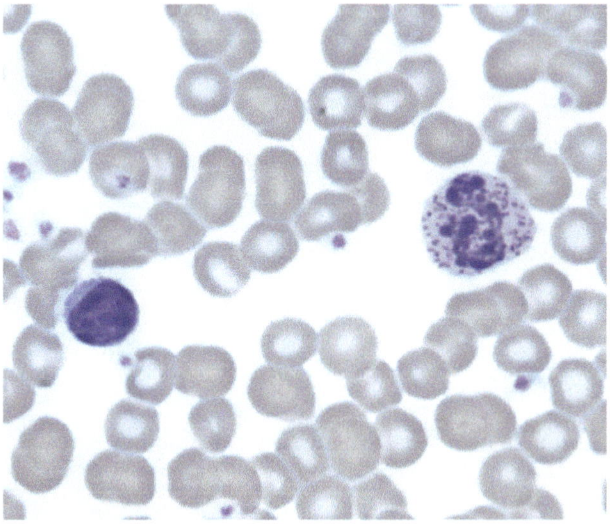

Figure 14.8 Small lymphocyte (lower left) and neutrophil (upper right) of the crowned lemur.

Therefore, the observation of polychromasia on a blood smear is likely minimal. Blood parasites of lemurs include *Plasmodium* (the causative agent of malaria), which was reported in a direct blood smear from a captive black lemur, and microfilariae, which have been reported from direct smears in free-ranging golden-crowned sifaka [16, 21]. Clinical significance in these cases was not determined [16, 21].

Hemostasis (Coagulation Panel) and Blood Types if Known

Data for coagulation times in lemurs has not been published. Some lemurs have B-like antigens on their erythrocytes; therefore, cross-matching prior to transfusion is highly recommended in lemurs [22]. There is one case report of a 16-year-old male ring tailed lemur with iron deficiency anemia who received a blood transfusion from a healthy adult female ring-tailed lemur of the same troop in which a cross-match was not performed. The animal was pre-medicated with diphenhydramine. No adverse reactions following the transfusion were noted. However, four days post-transfusion, the lemur developed edema and intermittent episodes of weakness. There was a concern for a delayed transfusion reaction, so the animal was treated with tapering dosages of prednisone [23].

Biochemical Panel

Minimal data exist for biomedical evaluation in lemurs, and no studies of lemurs have correlated specific chemistry analyte changes with clinical disease (Table 14.3). Most significance of biochemical abnormalities in lemurs is extrapolated from those described in other domestic species.

Liver Enzymes

Hepatic abnormalities in lemurs can be assessed using the enzyme activities of aspartate aminotransferase (AST), alanine aminotransferase (ALT), gamma-glutamyl transpeptidase (GGT), alkaline phosphatase (ALP), and bile acids. While abnormalities in these values may suggest hepatic disease, assays that are liver sensitive or liver specific for lemurs have not yet been established. Differences in liver values among species may be associated with poor or prolonged sample handling if blood is not separated from the serum quickly or kept at elevated temperatures [2, 4]. Although clinically insignificant, this occurred for ALT, ALP, GGT, and total bilirubin from free-range ring-tailed lemurs compared to captive lemurs [4]. AST and ALP activities may also be increased when there is muscle and bone involvement, respectively [3]. ALP elevations have been observed in a family of captive red ruffed lemurs diagnosed with pachydermoperiostosis, a rare form of primary hypertrophic osteoarthropathy (HOA) [24]. Primary HOA was considered owing to the prominent facial abnormalities of each animal and failure to identify a secondary cause [24]. The pathogenesis of this disorder is unclear, although genetics and alterations in fibroblast activity and blood flow likely play a role [24]. ALP was also reported to be increased in a group of captive lemurs that developed bone mineralization abnormalities as a result of secondary hyperparathyroidism due to hypocalcemia induced by hyperphosphatemia [25]. Recurrent multifocal osteomyelitis was reported in a male ruffled lemur, but biochemical abnormalities were not identified [26]. Bile acids and ammonia have not been validated for liver function assessment in lemurs. However, increased concentrations of bile acids

Table 14.3 Biochemical reference ranges for 20 lemurs [4, 15, 17, 18].

Analyte (Abbreviation)	Units, SI (conventional)	Red-fronted brown lemur (*Eulemur fulvus rufus*)	Ring-tailed lemur (*Lemur catta*)	Decken's sifaka (*Propithecus verreauxi deckeni*)	Red ruffed lemur (*Varecia rubra*)
Data format		**Mean ± SD**	**Mean ± SD**	**Mean ± SD**	**Mean ± SD**
Albumin (ALB)	g/l	64 ± 10	43 ± 4	49 ± 4	44.8 ± 4.12
	(g/dl)	6.4 ± 1.0	4.3 ± 0.4	4.9 ± 0.4	4.48 ± 0.412
Alkaline phosphatase (ALP)	U/l	115 ± 145	114.1 ± 42.2	150 ± 68.3	375 ± 137
Amylase	U/l		1034.5 ± 182.6		716
Anion gap (AG)[b]	mM/l		19 ± 2		
Aspartate aminotransferase (AST)	U/l	59.6 ± 31.6	64.6 ± 45.1	78.7 ± 52.7	102
Blood urea nitrogen (BUN)	mmol/l	8.1 ± 5.5	2.6 ± 2.14, 3.21 ± 2.9	18.1 ± 6.5	3.13
	(mg/dl)	22.8 ± 15.3	7.3 ± 6.0, 9 ± 8	50.6 ± 18.1	8.75
Calcium (Ca)	mmol/l	2.4 ± 0.1	1.9 ± 0.1	2.45 ± 0.28	
	(mg/dl)	(9.4 ± 0.4)	(8.1 ± 0.5)	(9.8 ± 1.1)	
Ionized Calcium (iCa)[b]	mM/l		0.92 ± 0.08		
Chloride (Cl)	mEq/l	104.0 ± 4.9	103.4 ± 4.0, 104 ± 4	114.0 ± 6.0	116 ± 12.5
Cholesterol (CHOL)	mmol/l		1.56 ± 0.4		1.26 ± 0.242
	(mg/dl)		60.4 ± 15.3		48.6 ± 9.35
Copper (Cu)	µmol/l	19.4 ± 2.6	12.0 ± 3.30	9.6 ± 1.9	
	(µg/dl)	122.4 ± 16.4	76.5 ± 21	60.7 ± 12.0	
Creatine kinase (CK)	U/l	3446.0 ± 2338.0	4508 ± 2959.9	524.1 ± 390.1	880
Creatinine (CREA)	µmol/l	106 ± 70.7	72 ± 14, 79.6 ± 17.68	53 ± 17.7	87.6
	(mg/dl)	1.2 ± 0.8	0.8 ± 0.2, 0.9 ± 0.2	0.6 ± 0.2	0.99
Gamma-glutamyl transpeptidase (GGT)	U/l	22.9 ± 8.6	13.4 ± 3.7	19.9 ± 6.8	14.5 ± 4.70
Globulin (GLOB)	g/l	5 ± 7	15 ± 4	23 ± 4	18.1 ± 2.86
	(g/dl)	0.5 ± 0.7	1.5 ± 0.4	2.3 ± 0.4	1.81 ± 0.286
Glucose (GLU)	mmol/l	0.08 ± 0.06	10.5 ± 4.4, 9.26 ± 4.5	0.4 ± 0.2	0.555–7.66[a]
	(mg/dl)	1.4 ± 1.0	188.6 ± 80.1, 167 ± 81	7.1 ± 2.7	10.0–138[a]
Lipase	U/l		45.1 ± 31.1		25–31[a]
Magnesium (Mg)	mmol/l		0.896 ± 0.136		1.27 ± 0.219
	(mg/dl)	2.49 ± 0.2	2.18 ± 0.332	2.53 ± 0.4	
Phosphorus (P)	mmol/l	1.7 ± 0.5	1.6 ± 0.3	3.2 ± 0.7	
	(mg/dl)	(5.4 ± 1.5)	(5.0 ± 0.9)	(10 ± 2.3)	
Potassium (K)	mEq/l	5.0 ± 0.8	3.3 ± 0.6, 3.7 ± 0.6	4.1 ± 0.7	5.26 ± 0.848
Sodium (Na)	mEq/l	134.7 ± 5.0	145.0 ± 6.7, 143 ± 3	138 ± 4.4	153 ± 16.9
Na:K			44.4 ± 8.8		28.7 ± 3.18
Total bilirubin	µmol/l	9.7 ± 5.5	6.7 ± 1.6	13.7 ± 5.1	
	(mg/dl)	0.57 ± 0.32	0.4 ± 0.1	0.8 ± 0.3	
Total carbon dioxide (TCO_2)[b]	mmol/L		25 ± 5		
Total protein (TP)	g/l	69 ± 6	58 ± 7, 70 ± 5	73 ± 4	65.6 ± 4.03
	(g/dl)	6.9 ± 0.6	5.8 ± 0.7, 7.0 ± 0.5	7.3 ± 0.4	6.56 ± 4.03
Triglycerides (TRIG)	mmol/l		0.486 ± 0.118		0.136–0.859[a]
	(mg/dl)		(43.0 ± 10.4)		(12.0–76.0)[a]
Zinc (Zn)	µmol/l	21.9–6.9	10.1 ± 3.72	22.2 ± 4.3	19.0
	(µg/dl)	143 ± 43	65.7 ± 24.3	145 ± 28	124

[a] – Min-Max, [b] – Singleton et al., 2018.

can indicate hepatic insufficiency as in other domestic species [27]. Hemosiderosis, a condition of excess iron accumulation in tissues (especially the liver, spleen, duodenum, and bone marrow), is a common disease in captive lemurs. Hemochromatosis occurs when an increase in stored iron causes disease. Hemochromatosis may cause abnormalities in multiple liver analytes including increased concentrations of alkaline phosphatase, bilirubinemia, and bile acids [27]. Hepatic biopsy with Prussian blue stain specific for iron accumulated remains the gold standard for evaluation of liver disease in suspect cases [4].

Muscle Enzymes

Muscle disease may be characterized by elevation in creatine kinase (CK) and AST in lemurs. Muscle damage can occur following administration of anesthetic drugs via intramuscular injection and when animals, particularly those that were free living, were darted and fell from trees, despite measures to minimize trauma [4, 16]. The liver is also a major source of AST, and elevations may be seen with liver disease.

Renal Analytes

Evaluation of renal function is determined by evaluation of blood urea nitrogen (BUN) and creatinine (CREA). Elevations in BUN and CREA, known as azotemia, are associated with decreased glomerular filtration. Azotemia can be classified as prerenal, renal, or postrenal. Renal azotemia is indicated by elevations in BUN and CREA with a concurrent decrease in urine specific gravity indicating a loss of concentrating ability. Free-ranging ring-tailed lemurs have lower BUN and CREA values compared to those of captive lemurs. This likely age-related renal degeneration has been identified in captive lemurs and is a common cause of mortality [4]. BUN may also be influenced by diet, particularly one higher in protein (especially in captivity), GI hemorrhage, and liver function. A study in ring-tailed lemurs showed that males had significantly higher BUN than females. Due to lack of evidence of renal compromise or dehydration, this difference was believed to be attributable to the higher protein consumption in the males, who feed more on leaves compared to pregnant females during the dry season, which was when the study was conducted [17]. In Von der Decken's sifakas, elevations in phosphorus may indicate decreased glomerular filtration, likely owing to a kidney adaption for water conservation [18]. Hyperphosphatemia with concurrent hypocalcemia may develop in chronic renal disease, eventually leading to a secondary hyperparathyroidism. Serum hyperphosphatemia develops as the glomerular filtration rate decreases with kidney disease. This in turn leads to lower serum concentration of ionized calcium. In addition, the synthesis of calcitriol (Vitamin D) is also reduced. Calcitriol acts on the intestine and kidneys to help maintain normal calcium levels. A decrease in both ionized calcium levels and calcitriol concentrations stimulates the parathyroid glands, which then produce increased serum PTH concentrations. Secondary hyperparathyroidism can cause the development of a periosteal reaction of the long bones and has been reported in black lemurs (*Eulemur macaco*) and black-and-white lemurs (*Varecia variegatus variegatus*) [28]. In a case report of black lemurs from two families, several lemurs developed periosteal bone proliferation that was identified on radiographs prior to the detection of renal disease [29]. Renal involvement was confirmed on histopathologic evaluation of the kidneys following euthanasia. The exact etiology of the bone changes associated with renal disease was not identified, but one thought included an immune-mediated cause that resulted in both glomerulonephritis and polyarthritis. Because this syndrome affected two families, an underlying heritable disorder was strongly suspected [29].

Pancreas

Little information is available on interpretation of amylase or lipase in lemurs. Hyperamylasemia was related to decreased glomerular filtration due to dehydration as amylase is filtered by the glomerulus in one study [3]. Concurrent elevations in lipase may also occur as it is also cleared by the kidneys. In domestic species, increased concentrations may indicate pancreatitis, intestinal disease, and hepatic disease; however, increases are not sensitive for these disorders and have not been correlated with disease in lemurs. In free-ranging lemurs, glucose elevations are attributable to stress-induced hyperglycemia as described in other mammals [4]. Diabetes has been reported in lemurs in captivity and linked to obesity [30]. In one study, glucose values of all the samples were low presumably owing to the rapid depletion of serum glucose due to exposure to the blood cells in a warm environment [18]. Therefore, separation of blood cells from serum is crucial to prevent erroneous results. Insulin and glucagon values have not been evaluated in lemurs.

Gastrointestinal and Cardiac Markers

No information is available on gastrointestinal analytes or cardiac troponin or other markers specifically in lemurs. Cardiac troponin I has been used in other nonhuman primates to evaluate for cardiac injury.

Lipids and Lipoproteins

Pathologic levels of lipid or lipoproteins have not been established for lemurs. Similar to other species, elevations in cholesterol and triglycerides are likely associated with metabolic abnormalities and select systemic diseases

[3]. Free-ranging red ruffed lemurs had lower cholesterol levels but higher triglycerides than those in captivity, which was thought to be diet related [15].

Electrolytes

Most differences in electrolyte concentrations are associated with diet, nutrition, and hydration status of lemurs [3, 4, 15, 18]. In free-range animals, electrolyte status is related to water source availability in different habitats [3]. Serum sodium, potassium, chloride, and magnesium concentrations were higher in free-ranging red ruffed lemurs [15]. Sodium, chloride, and osmolality were higher in free-ranging ring-tailed lemurs in marginal habitats where water was less available [3]. Hyperphosphatemia and hypocalcemia can occur in captive lemurs owing to inappropriate dietary Ca:P ratios in the diet [25]. This can also result in captivity due to inadequate exposure to ultraviolet radiation, necessary to synthesize precursors for production of cholecalciferol (Vitamin D), needed for intestinal absorption of calcium [25]. Other causes for elevations in potassium can include sample hemolysis, delayed separation of plasma from erythrocytes, and decreased urinary excretion as described above. Low serum calcium concentrations can cause improper nervous tissue conduction, tetany, convulsions, and/or death. Prolonged delay of separation of blood cells from serum may also result in falsely increased concentrations of magnesium, potassium, and phosphorous [18]. As in other species, hypercalcemia may be observed in younger lemurs due to bone growth. However, in a study of ring-tailed lemurs, young lemurs had significantly lower ionized calcium (iCa) compared to adults [17]. The exact cause for this was not determined, although it was postulated that preanalytical factors during sample collection, which can affect iCa, may have contributed to some of the variation.

Blood Proteins

Blood proteins have a wide variety of specific and important body functions. Total protein (TP) is typically measured as serum protein and includes the components albumin and globulins. When total protein is measured by refractometry on plasma, fibrinogen is also included. In ring-tailed lemurs, plasma TP has been associated with age and sex, with young lemurs having higher TP than adult and older lemurs and females having higher TP than males [17]. Elevations in lemur TP, specifically albumin, may be considered related to dehydration as in other animal species. Additionally, in captive lemurs, higher nutritional planes have been attributed to elevated TP and albumin [1, 31]. Globulin levels reflect an immune system response and increase with infection, inflammation, or neoplasia [18]. Serum protein electrophoresis has not been evaluated in lemur species.

Blood Gases

Compared to other primates, lemurs have a high oxygen carrying capacity which varies depending on the lemur species [32]. Ring-tailed lemurs have blood with a lower affinity for oxygen and a lower concentration of 2,3-diphosphoglycerate compared to black lemurs. Oxygen carrying capacity does not vary with sex in ring-tailed and black lemurs [32]. Hemoglobin structure differs depending on separation via gel electrophoresis.

Vitamins, Minerals and Metals, and Toxins

Hemosiderosis, excessive iron storage in the tissues, is a common problem of captive lemurs [27, 33–35]. Hemochromatosis occurs as iron stores increase to the point of causing disease. Iron is an essential nutrient acquired from the diet that is required for several tissue functions, including hemoglobin synthesis and oxygen transport. However, when uptake of iron exceeds use and loss, iron is stored as hemosiderin in many organs, especially the liver, spleen, and bone marrow. Captive lemur diets are higher in both iron and ascorbic acid (vitamin C), which enhances iron absorption from the intestine. Compared to wild diets, captive diets are also low in tannins which chelate iron, thereby decreasing absorption. While captive diets have been adjusted to minimize hemochromatosis, disease is still common in captive animals. Thus, factors leading to the development of hemochromatosis are likely more complicated than originally believed. For early detection of this disorder, body iron stores should be monitored in captive lemurs [34]. Direct evaluation of tissue biopsy for liver remains the gold standard; however, this diagnostic is impractical for repeated use in the healthy patient. Indirect methods to evaluate total body iron stores include assessing serum iron, total iron binding capacity (TIBC), transferrin saturation, and serum ferritin (Table 14.4) [33]. In many lemur species, serum ferritin correlates with total iron stores although the assay has not been validated in lemurs [3, 33, 34]. However, ferritin is an acute phase protein, and values may increase with inflammation, infection, and hemolysis as well as with liver disease. Therefore, interpret ferritin values in conjunction with the entire patient profile.

Further studies to determine acceptable or necessary vitamin levels for lemurs are needed (Table 14.4). Vitamin levels are influenced by diet and ultraviolet exposure [3, 4, 15]. In free-ranging lemurs, differing vitamin levels between species may also be related to habitat and differing vitamin metabolism [2, 4]. Lemurs have lower carotenoid levels than most other primates [2].

Assessment of blood and hair samples in free-ranging ring-tailed lemurs confirmed lemur exposure to numerous

Table 14.4 Vitamin and mineral data for lemurs [4, 15, 18].

Analyte (abbreviation)	Units, SI (conventional)	Red-fronted brown lemur (*Eulemur fulvus rufus*)	Ring-tailed lemur (*Lemur catta*)	Decken's sifaka (*Propithecus verreauxi deckeni*)	Red ruffed lemur (*Varecia rubra*)
Animals sampled					
25-Hydroxyvitamin D	nmol/l	152.8 ± 43.25	11.3 ± 4.93	27.1 ± 9.73	51.9 ± 15.5
	(ng/ml)	61.1 ± 17.3	4.5 ± 1.97	10.8 ± 3.89	20.8 ± 6.20
Retinol	μmol/l	0.38 ± 0.109	0.659 ± 0.182	1.706 ± 0.372	0.552 ± 0.0871
	(μg/dl)	10.9 ± 3.14	18.9 ± 5.22	48.9 ± 10.67	15.8 ± 2.49
Retinyl palmitate	(μg/dl)	0.8 ± 1.1	0	4.2 ± 2.0	
γ-tocopherol	μmol/l				0.556
	(μg/dl)	13.3 ± 9.56	15.6 ± 5.82	48.0 ± 19.0	23.2
A-tocopherol	μmol/l				4.39
	(μg/dl)	91.3 ± 68.7	195.0 ± 59.8	753.2 ± 368.9	1.89
Lutein + zeaxanthin	(μg/dl)	0	0	1.7 ± 1.59	
β-cryptoxanthin	(μg/dl)	0	0	0	
α-carotene	(μg/dl)	0	0	0	
β-carotene	(μg/dl)	0	0	0	
Lycopene	(μg/dl)	0	0	0	
Iron (Fe)	μmol/l	30.6 ± 14.0	12.8 ± 5.71	32.1 ± 10.1	20.8 ± 8.74
	(μg/dl)	170.8 ± 78	71.4 ± 31.9	179.3 ± 56.6	116 ± 48.8
Total iron binding capacity (TIBC)	μmol/l		43.1 ± 6.69		61.7 ± 9.99
	(μg/dl)	313 ± 69	241 ± 37.4	284.2 ± 82.9	345 ± 55.8
Ferritin	pmol/l		91.9 ± 50.6		135
	(ng/ml)	209.7 ± 148.6	40.9 ± 22.5	149 ± 99.8	59.9

All data given as mean ± SD.

toxins [36]. Exposure was likely owing to chemical environmental contamination, due to human proximity, poor regulation, improper storage and disposal, and agricultural use [36]. The low levels of multiple organochlorine pesticides and toxic metals found were of uncertain biological significance and included aluminum, zinc, boron, phosphorous, silicon, and copper [36].

Hormones

No clinical case of thyroid or adrenal disease has yet been reported in lemur species. However, both primary hyperparathyroidism and secondary hyperparathyroidism due to renal disease and nutrition have been reported in lemurs [24]. In primary hyperparathyroidism, the only chemistry abnormality reported was a continuous elevation in ALP. In these cases, animals developed periosteal proliferations on the long bones, and facial abnormalities, making primary hyperparathyroidism likely [24]. In secondary PTH due to renal disease, azotemia and low calcium levels with increased phosphorous occur. In response to hypocalcemia, parathyroid levels increase while vitamin D concentrations remain low. Secondary bone abnormalities (periosteal reactions) may also occur.

Multiple studies have investigated the reproductive cycles of lemurs, as understanding hormone fluctuations during the estrous cycle is imperative for successful breeding programs in these species with declining population. Both fecal and urinary analysis can provide useful hormonal values [37, 38].

In female lesser mouse lemurs, social conditions also affect the estrous cycle length. Isolated females tend to have shorter cycles than females that can communicate with other females [39]. This increase was related to an extension of the luteal phase of the cycle, which was associated with a decrease in the progesterone concentration during that time period. Females housed with males and other females tend to have individual variations in estrous cycles. Males appear to stimulate the cycle, while being around other females has an inhibitory effect. In females housed with males and other females, the cycle length was inversely related to plasma cortisol concentrations [39]. In the ruffed lemur, estrogen levels are low until the last half of gestation, at which time levels can reach up to 1000 times higher than levels measured at estrus [37]. In Verreaux's sifaka, mating behavior and interest coincided with peak estrogen levels, and estrogen and progesterone levels increase at the end of the conceptive cycle and in late pregnancy [38].

Male hormones have also been evaluated. Red-fronted lemurs have one dominant male and several subordinate males per social group [40]. Androgen levels do not differ between the dominant and subordinate males. Testosterone levels rise with the mating season and correlate with aggression during that time [38]. The highest concentrations of testosterone occur during birthing season, which may relate to aggression associated with infanticide of neonates not sired by the dominant male [40, 41].

Urinalysis

Various techniques for urine collection in both captive and free-ranging lemurs have been described in the literature. Urine can be collected while under anesthesia via manual expression of the bladder, sterile urinary catheterization, or cystocentesis. Additionally, sample collection via opportunistic free-catch or retrieval of urine from the floor has also been performed. Currently, interpretation of the clinical significance of urinalysis findings for lemurs is derived from that known of other nonhuman primate species. In a case of recurrent calcium phosphate urolithiasis in a black-and-white ruffed lemur (*Varecia variegata*), urinalysis demonstrated alkalinity (pH 8) in conjunction with varying degrees of hematuria (minimal to > 100 erythrocytes per high-powered field) [42]. In a red ruffed lemur, urethral obstruction due to a copulatory plug after breeding was detected. Dip stick evaluation of the urine revealed a large amount of protein; however, a sediment exam was not performed [43]. Renal degeneration is a known age-related abnormality and cause of death in older lemurs. [44]. There is one case report of systemic blastomycosis in a 5-year-old male captive red ruffed lemur, diagnosed by fine-needle aspiration and cytologic evaluation of a lung mass originally identified on thoracic radiographs. For confirmation, urine was collected via catheterization for the Blastomyces Quantitative EIA Test, yielding positive results (>14.7 ng/mL) [45]. In a case of a ring-tailed lemur with a renal tumor, mild uremia was reported; however, urinalysis was not done [46]. In six black lemurs with periarticular hyperostosis and renal disease, urinalysis from a mid-stream free catch sample of one of the animals was done, which revealed trace proteinuria with an increased BUN [29].

Serology and Polymerase Chain Reaction (PCR)

A naturally occurring infection of *Ehrlichia chaffeensis* in lemurs has been reported in a lemur colony at the Duke University Primate Center [47]. In a different study, free-ranging lemurs, including ring-tailed lemurs, black lemurs, and black-and-white ruffle lemurs have also been found to test positive for *Anaplasma phagocytophilum* (in addition to *E. chaffeensis*) [48]. Of this same group tested, all lemurs were found to be negative to both *Ehrlichia ewingii* and *Ehrlichia canis* [48]. All these animals appeared clinically normal. One lemur that tested positive for *E. chaffeensis* was found to be slightly hypoproteinemic and had moderate elevations in serum ALT. PCR can be performed on whole blood in EDTA to identify infection.

Captive ring-tail lemurs appear susceptible to toxoplasmosis, and the infection and mortality rates are high [2, 4, 49, 50]. Transmission is due to exposure to free-ranging and captive felids, including feral cats, and zoo staff which may act as fomites [49, 50]. PCR assay may be performed on whole blood in EDTA for *Toxoplasma gondii.*

In a group of 19 ring-tailed lemurs released on St. Catherine's Island, one lemur was positive for infection with *Trypanosoma cruzi* [51]. Free-ranging ring-tailed lemurs have tested serologically positive for antibodies to West Nile virus, simian immunodeficiency virus, but not to herpes simplex virus type 1 [52]. Infection of *Echinococcus multilocularis* was identified by PCR in a four-year-old captive female ring-tailed lemur in Japan and confirmed by gross necropsy [28]. PCR has also been used to screen for *Hemoplasma* spp., *Bartonella* spp., and *Neorickettsia risticii* [3]. In a case of a well-differentiated hepatocellular carcinoma in a ring-tailed lemur, PCR for hepatitis B was negative [53]. A herpesvirus was identified as the cause of encephalitis in a ruffed lemur on the basis of identification of intranuclear inclusions on histopathologic evaluation of neural tissue following necropsy [54]. In a ruffed lemur with osteomyelitis, fungal titers for *Blastomycosis dermatitidis*, *Histoplasma capsulatum*, and *Cryptococcus neoformans* were negative [10].

References

1 Dutton, C.J., Junge, R.E., and Louis, E.E. (2003). Biomedical evaluation of free-ranging ring-tailed lemurs (*Lemur catta*) in Tsimanampetsotsa strict nature reserve, Madagascar. *Journal of Zoo and Wildlife Medicine* 36 (1): 16–24.

2 Rothschild, B.M., Neiffer, D.L., and Marks, S.K. (2011). Pachydermoperiostosis-like disease in captive red ruffed lemurs (*Varecia variegatus rubra*). *Journal of Primatology* 1: 101. doi: 10.4172/jpmt.1000101.

3 Crawford, G.C., Andrews, G.A., Chavey, P.S. et al. (2005). Survey and clinical applications of serum iron, total iron binding capacity, transferring saturation, and serum ferritin in captive black and white ruffled lemurs (*Varecia variegata variegata*). *Journal of Zoo and Wildlife Medicine* 36 (4): 653–660.

4 Kreeger, T.J. and Arnemo, J.M. (2007). *Handbook of Wildlife Chemical Immobilization*, 3e. Terry Kreeger.

5 Junge, R.E. and Louis, E.E. (2005). Preliminary biomedical evaluation of wild ruffed lemurs (*Varecia variegate* and *V.rubra*). *American Journal of Primatology* 66: 85–94.

6 Andrews, G.A., Chavey, P.S., and Crawford, G. (2005). Enzyme-linked immunosorbent assay to quantitate serum ferritin in black and white ruffled lemurs (*Varecia variegate variegata*). *Journal of Zoo and Wildlife Medicine* 36 (4): 648–652.

7 Thomsen, R. and Voigt, C.C. (2006). Non-invasive blood sampling from primates using laboratory-bred blood-sucking bugs (Dipetalogaster maximus; Reduviidae, Heteroptera). *Primates* 47: 397–400.

8 Dhindsa, D.S., Metcalfe, J., and Hoversland, A.S. (1972). Comparative studies of the respiratory functions of mammalian blood IX. Ring-tailed lemur (*Lemur catta*) and black lemur (*Lemur macaco*). *Respiration Physiology* 15: 331–342.

9 Huff, C.G. and Hoogstrall, H. (1963). *Plasmodium lemuris* N. sp from *Lemur collaris*. *Journal of Infectious Diseases* 112 (3): 233–236.

10 Nemeth, N.M., Blas-Machado, U., Cazzini, P. et al. (2012). Well-differentiated hepatocellular carcinoma in a ring-tailed lemur (*Lemur catta*). *Journal of Comparative Pathology* 148 (2–3): 283–287.

11 Goodchild, S. and Schwitzer, C. (2008). The problem of obesity in captive lemurs. *International Zoo News* 55 (6): 353–357.

12 Sondgeroth, K., Blitvich, B., Blair, C. et al. (2007). Assessing flavivirus, lentivirus, and herpesvirus exposure in free-ranging ring-tailed lemurs in southwestern Madagascar. *Journal of Wildlife Diseases* 43 (1): 40–47.

13 Spencer, J.A., Hilton, K.S., Dubey, J.P. et al. (2004). Disseminated toxoplasmosis in a captive ring-tailed lemur (*Lemur catta*). *Journal of Parasitology* 90 (4): 904–906.

14 "Meet the lemurs." lemur.duke.edu. Web. 4 February 2014.

15 West, G., Heard, D., and Caulkett, N. (2007). *Zoo Animal and Wildlife Immobilization and Anesthesia*. Ames, IA: Blackwell Publishing.

16 Der Goukassian, P. (1983). Hematology of the lesser mouse lemur (*Microcebus murinus*). A preliminary study. *Folia Primatologica* 41: 129–136.

17 Singleton, C.L., Sauther, M.A., Cuozzo, F.P., and Youssouf Jacky, I.A. (2018). Age-related changes in hematology and blood biochemistry values in endangered, wild ring-tailed lemurs (*Lemur catta*) at the Bezà Mahafaly special reserve, Madagascar. *Journal of Zoo and Wildlife Medicine* 49 (1): 30–47.

18 Tomson, F.N. and Lotshaw, R.R. (1978). Hyperphosphatemia and Hypocalcemia in lemurs. *Journal of the American Veterinary Medical Association* 173 (9): 1103–1106.

19 Backues, K.A., Hoover, J.P., Bahr, R.J. et al. (2001). Multifocal pyogranulomatous osteomyelitis resembling chronic recurrent multifocal osteomyelitis in a lemur. *JAVMA* 218: 250–253.

20 International Species Inventory System. 2002. Physiologic data reference values [CD-ROM]. Apple Valley, Minn: International Species Inventory System

21 Ankel-Simons, F. (2007). *Primate Anatomy: An Introduction*, 3e, 557. Burlington: Academic Press.

22 Junge, R.E., Dutton, C.J., Knightly, F. et al. (2008). Comparison of biomedical evaluation for white-fronted brown lemurs (*Eulemur fulvus albifrons*) from four sites in Madagascar. *Journal of Zoo and Wildlife Medicine* 39 (4): 567–575.

23 Anderson, K.M. and Wolf, K.N. (2014). Iron deficiency anemia in a ring-tailed lemur (*Lemur catta*) with concurrent chronic renal failure. *Journal of the American Veterinary Medical Association* 244 (4): 471–475.

24 Boraski, E.A. (1981). Renal disease in Prosimians. *Veterinary Pathology* 18: 1–5.

25 Pung, O.J., Spratt, J., Clark, C.G. et al. (1998). *Trypanosoma cruzi* infection of free-ranging lion-tailed macaques (*Macaca silenus*) and ring-tailed lemurs (*Lemur catta*) on St. Catherine's island, Georgia, USA. *Journal of Zoo and Wildlife Medicine* 29 (1): 25–30.

26 Miller, D.S., Sauther, M.L., Hunter-Ishikawa, M. et al. (2007). Biomedical evaluation of free-ranging ring-tailed lemurs (*Lemur catta*) in three habitats at the Beza Mahafaly special reserve, Madagascar. *Journal of Zoo and Wildlife Medicine* 38 (2): 201–216.

27 Muller, S., Oevermann, A., Wenker, C. et al. (2007). A mixed epithelial and stromal tumor of the kidney in a ringtail lemur (*Lemur catta*). *Veterinary Pathology* 44: 243–246.

28 Kondo, H., Wada, Y., Bando, G. et al. (1996). Alveolar hydatidosis in a gorilla and a ring-tailed lemur in Japan. *The Journal of Veterinary Medical Science* 58 (5): 447–449.

29 Sanchez, C.R., Murray, S., and Montali, R.J. (2004). Use of desferoxamine and s-adenosylmethionine to treat hemochromatosis in a red ruffed lemur (*Varecia variegata ruber*). *Comparative Medicine* 54 (1): 100–103.

30 Junge, R.E. and Louis, E.E. (2005). Biomedical evaluation of two sympatric lemur species (*Propithecus verreauxi deckeni* and *Eulemur fulvus rufus*) in Tsiombokibo classified forest, Madagascar. *Journal of Zoo and Wildlife Medicine* 36 (4): 581–589.

31 Donadeo, B.C., Kerr, K.R., Morris, C.L., and Swanson, K.S. (2016). Estimated composition of diets fed to captive black-and-white ruffed lemurs (*Varecia variegata*) at 33 U.S. zoological institutions. *Journal of Zoo and Wildlife Medicine* 47 (1): 150–160.

32 Williams, C.V., Glenn, K.M., Levine, J.F., and Horne, W.A. (2003). Comparison of the efficacy and cardiorespiratory effects of medetomidine-based anesthetic protocols in ring-tailed lemurs (*Lemur catta*). *Journal of Zoo and Wildlife Medicine* 34 (2): 163–170.

33 Barret, M, Junge R. 2012. Lemur disease ecology: linking health, ecosystems viability & conservation in Madagascar. http://media.news.health.ufl.edu/misc/egh/One%20Health%20Newsletter/FDOH%20Newsletters/Vol5Issue4_Fall12.pdf.

34 Fisher, K.E. and Austad, S.N. (2011). The development of small primate models for aging research. *ILAR Journal* 52: 78–88.

35 Dutton, C.J., Junge, R.E., and Louis, E.E. (2008). Biomedical evaluation of free-ranging red ruffed lemurs (*Varecia rubra*) within the Masoala National Park, Madagascar. *Journal of Zoo and Wildlife Medicine* 39 (1): 76–85.

36 Ostner, J., Kappeler, P.M., and Heistermann, M. (2008). Androgen and glucocorticoid levels reflect seasonally occurring social challenges in male redfronted lemurs (*Eulemur fulvus rufus*). *Behavioral Ecology and Sociobiology* 62: 627–638.

37 Williams, C.V., Steenhouse, J.L., Bradley, J.M. et al. (2002). Naturally occurring *Ehrlichia chaffeensis* infection in two prosimian primate species: ring-tailed lemurs (*Lemur catta*) and ruffed lemurs (*Varecia variegata*). *Emerging Infectious Diseases* 8: 1497–1500.

38 Markolf, M., Brameier, M., and Kappeler, P.M. (2011). On species delimitation: yet another lemur species or just genetic variation? *BMC Evolutionary Biology* 11 (216).

39 Perret, M. (1986). Social influences on oestrous cycle length and plasma progesterone concentrations in the female lesser mouse lemur (*Microcebus murinus*). *Journal of Reproduction and Fertility* 77: 303–311.

40 Brockman, D.K., Whitten, P.L., Russel, E. et al. (1995). Application of fecal steroid techniques to the reproductive endocrinology of femal Verreaux's Sifaka (*Propithecus varreauxi*). *American Journal of Primatology* 36: 313–325.

41 Shideler, S.E., Czekala, N.M., Benirschke, K., and Lasley, B.L. (1983). Urinary estrogens during pregnancy of the ruffed lemur (*Lemur variegates*). *Biology of Reproduction* 28: 963–969.

42 Cushing, A.C., Kollias, G., Knafo, E. et al. (2014). Recurrent calcium phosphate urolithiasis in a black-and-white ruffed lemur (*Varecia variegate*). *Journal of Zoo and Wildlife Medicine* 45 (1): 148–152.

43 Chatfield, J.A., Chatfield, J.J., and Chatfield, J.A. (2014). Urethral obstruction with a copulatory plug following natural breeding in a ruffed lemur, *Varecia rubra*. *Journal of Medical Primatology* 43: 115–117.

44 Gould, L. and Scuther, M.L. (2006). *Lemurs: Ecology and Adaption*. New York: Springer.

45 Rosser, M.F., Lindemann, D.M., Barger, A.M. et al. (2016). Systemic blastomycosis in a captive red ruffed lemur (*Varecia rubra*). *Journal of Zoo and Wildlife Medicine* 47 (3): 912–916.

46 Glenn, K.M., Campbell, J.L., Rotstein, D., and Williams, C.V. (2006). Retrospective evaluation of the incidence and severity of hemosiderosis in a large captive lemur population. *American Journal of Primatology* 68: 369–381.

47 Kornegay, R.W., Baldwin, T.J., and Pirie, G. (1993). Herpesvirus encephalitis in a ruffed lemur (*Varecia variegatus*). *Journal of Zoo and Wildlife Medicine* 24: 196–203.

48 Garell, D.M. and Meyers, D.M. (1995). Hematology and serum chemistry values from free-ranging golden crowned sifaka (*Propithecus tattersalli*). *Journal of Zoo and Wildlife Medicine* 26 (3): 382–386.

49 Languille, S., Blanc, S., Blin, O. et al. (2012). The grey mouse lemur: a non-human primate model for ageing studies. *Ageing Research Reviews* 11: 150–162.

50 de Camps, S., Dubey, J.P., and Saville, W.J. (2008). Seroepidemiology of *Toxoplasma gondii* in zoo animals in selected zoos in the Midwestern United States. *Journal of Parasitology* 94 (3): 648–653.

51 Ostner, J., Kappeler, P.M., and Heistermann, M. (2002). Seasonal variation and social correlates of androgen excretion in male redfronted lemurs (*Eulemur fulvus rufus*). *Behavioral Ecology and Sociobiology* 52: 485–495.

52 Yabsley, M.J., Norton, T.M., Powell, M.R., and Davidson, W.R. (2004). Molecular and serologic evidence of tick-borne Ehrlichiae in three species of lemurs from St. Catherines Island, Georgia, USA. *Journal of Zoo and Wildlife Medicine* 35 (4): 503–509.

53 Rainwater, T.R., Sauther, M.L., Rainwater, K.A.E. et al. (2009). Assessment of organochlorine pesticides and metals in ring-tailed lemurs (*Lemur catta*) at Beza Mahafaly special reserve, Madagasgar. *American Journal of Primatology* 71: 998–1010.

54 Junge, R.E., Mehren, K.G., Meehan, T.P. et al. (1994). Periarticular hyperostosis and renal disease in six black lemurs of two family groups. *Journal of the American Veterinary Medical Association* 205 (7): 1024–1029.

15

Other Small New World Monkeys

Megan A. Albertelli DVM, PhD, DACLAM

Department of Comparative Medicine, Stanford University, Stanford, California, USA

Introduction

New World monkeys, also known as neotropical or platyrrhine primates, are a diverse group of animals indigenous to Central and South America. They are generally arboreal, live in a wide range of forest habitats, and may be omnivorous, frugivorous, or insectivorous. Smaller New World monkeys such as members of the families Cebidae (marmosets, tamarins, capuchins, and squirrel monkeys) and Aotidae (owl monkeys) may be found in research settings or zoological exhibits, and most of our clinical pathology knowledge comes from animals in these environments. As with other species, clinical pathology is useful for assessment of general health and nutritional status, disease diagnosis, and subclinical pathogen detection. Because many factors can impact clinical pathology, values such as species, subspecies, diet, housing, wild-caught or captive-bred status, and analyzer and laboratory used, and submitting samples from healthy members of the same colony concurrently with the patient sample can aid in evaluation of the results. Clinical pathology of the callitrichids (marmosets and tamarins) is described in Chapter 13. This chapter will review clinicopathologic parameters useful for the assessment of other small New World monkeys as seen in zoos, private practice, or in research settings: the squirrel monkey, capuchin monkey, and owl monkey.

Species

Squirrel Monkeys

Five species of squirrel monkey make up the genus *Saimiri*, with the common or South American squirrel monkey (*Saimiri sciureus*) and the Bolivian or black-headed squirrel monkey (*Saimiri boliviensis*) found most often in captivity. Squirrel monkeys are generally small, slender primates with agouti body fur, a white mask around the eyes, and a dark snout. *S. saimiri* has an agouti head, while the top of the head is darker than the body in *S. boliviensis*. The body length measures 20–40 cm, and the nonprehensile tail is longer than the body at 35–47 cm [1]. The body weight averages from 500 to 1000 g, with males weighing 25%–30% more than females. Males undergo a seasonal weight gain of approximately 200–300 g prior to breeding, known as the "fatted" condition [2]. Squirrel monkeys have a higher basal metabolic rate than is predicted for their size of approximately 107 kcal/kg per 24 h [3].

Capuchin Monkeys

The genus *Cebus* consists of eight capuchin monkey species. Several of these species may be found in captivity, including the brown or tufted capuchin, also known as the "organ grinder's monkey" (*Cebus apella*), *Cebus capucinus* the white-faced capuchin (*C. capucinus*), and the weeping capuchin (*C. olivaceus*). Capuchins are medium-sized monkeys that average 3–5 kg in body weight and 30–60 cm in body length. The tail also ranges 30–60 cm in length and is functionally prehensile, although it lacks a hairless friction pad at the tip [1, 4]. Males are 25%–35% larger than females and have longer canine teeth. *C. capucinus* and *Cebus olivaceus* have dark brown to black body fur with white chests and faces, while *C. apella* ranges from light brown to black fur with lighter fur on the shoulders and ventrum and has tufts of fur above the ears.

Owl Monkeys

Also known as night monkeys or douroucoulis, these members of the genus *Aotus* were originally grouped as one species (*Aotus trivirgatus*). Recent taxonomic reclassifications list seven to nine species, including *A. trivirgatus*, *Aotus vociferans*, and *Aotus nancymaae*, which may be found in captivity. Owl monkeys are also grouped by

Exotic Animal Laboratory Diagnosis, First Edition. Edited by J. Jill Heatley and Karen E. Russell.

chromosome number and neck fur color, with karyotypes II, III, IV, V, VIII, and IX making up the gray-necked group and I, VI, and VII making up the red-necked group [5]. Owl monkeys are small, nocturnal primates with large eyes, agouti fur on the dorsum, red-brown fur on the ventrum, and black and white markings on the face. Owl monkeys are not sexually dimorphic, with an average body weight of 1 kg and body length of 17–24 cm in length. The nonprehensile tail is longer than the body, ranging from 22–42 cm [1]. The basal metabolic rate in owl monkeys is 18%–24% lower than predicted for a 1 kg mammal [6].

Sample Collection

Restraint

Small New World monkeys can be physically restrained by experienced handlers for sample collection. Personnel should wear heavy leather or welder's-type gloves and clothing with long sleeves in order to avoid bites and scratches from the animal. The monkey is placed dorsally or laterally on a padded surface. The animal's forelimbs at the axillae are held in one hand while the hind limbs are held in the other hand and gently extended caudally (Figure 15.1). A towel or extra glove can be placed near the monkey's head to provide something to grasp and bite during the sampling. Because physical restraint can be stressful, monkeys can be acclimated to the process prior to planned or repeated sampling. In the zoological or private practice setting, it is often prudent to plan for chemical restraint to allow for physical examination as well as sample collection. If an animal cannot be safely controlled with physical restraint, sedation with ketamine (10 mg/kg IM) can be used. Use of ketamine solely or box induction with isoflurane or sevoflurane, as well as combination of ketamine with dexmedetomidine or midazolam should also be considered. However, the fasting status of small primate should always be assessed, as there is risk of regurgitation and aspiration.

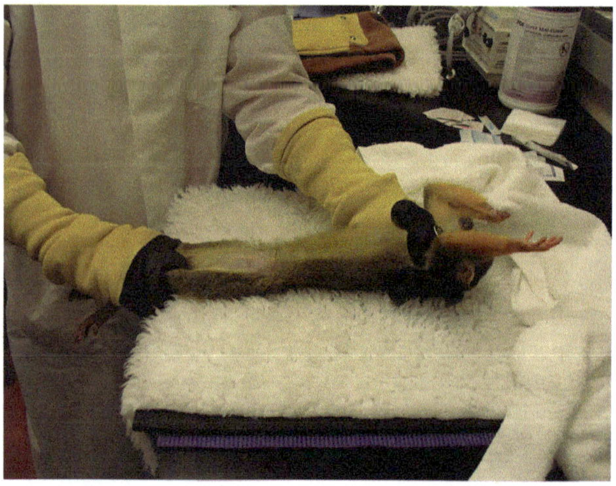

Figure 15.1 Physical restraint of a squirrel monkey.

Venipuncture Sites

The femoral vein and the saphenous vein are the preferred sites for blood collection in small nonhuman primates. The femoral vein is located by finding the femoral pulse on the medial aspect of the thigh and placing a 23–25 gauge (g.) needle just medial to this pulse (Figure 15.2). The saphenous vein is located on the caudal midline of the hind limb and distal to the knee (Figure 15.3). A 25 g. needle is used for sampling; a winged infusion set may facilitate sampling based on the superficial location of the vein [7]. For each site, collection with a 1 or 3 ml syringe is recommended, as vacuum systems will collapse the small vessels. After blood sample collection, application of proper pressure at the venipuncture site is important for hemostasis. This is particularly essential in owl monkeys, as some individuals may hemorrhage from venipuncture sites for prolonged periods of 1 to 5 min [8].

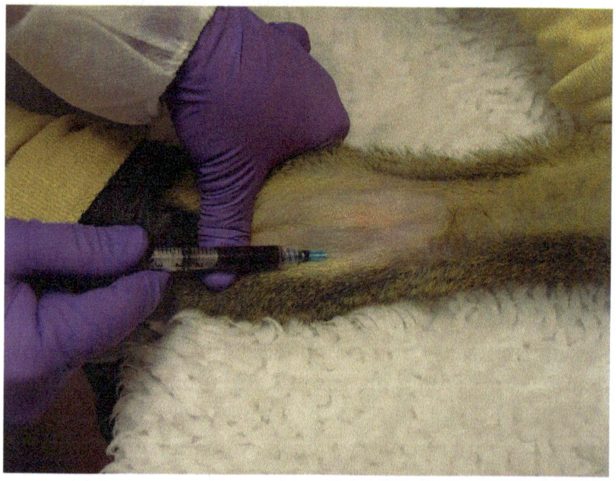

Figure 15.2 Femoral venipuncture site in a squirrel monkey.

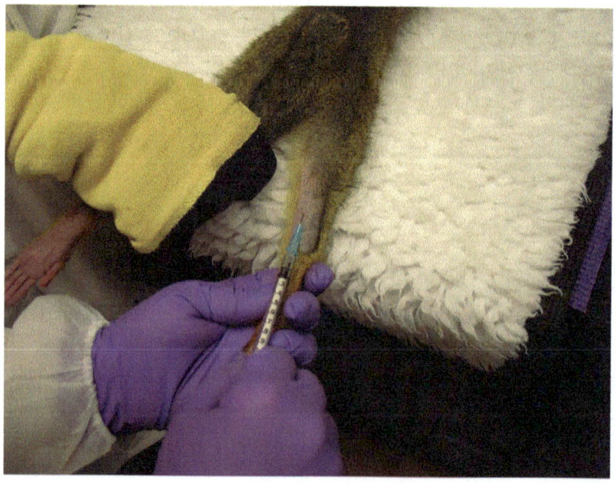

Figure 15.3 Saphenous venipuncture site in a squirrel monkey.

Maximum Safe Volumes for Blood Collection

In small New World monkeys, one must consider maximum safe volumes for blood collection. Although the total blood volume has not been determined in many of these species, the total blood volume in other primates is approximately 6%–7% of the body weight [9]. 7.5%–10% of this total blood volume can be removed safely [10]. Therefore, for a monkey weighing 750 g, 3.4–5.3 ml of blood can be drawn, although only the smallest amount necessary should be collected.

Urine Collection

Free-catch urine collection from the clean floor of a cage is the simplest technique, although this sample may be contaminated with food, water, or feces. If an animal urinates during handling, a cleaner free-catch sample can be obtained [11]. Cystocentesis is difficult due to the small urinary bladder size and location within the pelvic canal, but a 0.5 in., 20 g. needle may be placed 2 cm cranial to the pubis on the midline and directed caudally at a 45° angle and advanced until urine is obtained [11]. Urinary catheterization is extremely difficult and not recommended for routine sample collection in these small primates.

Sample Handling

Small New World primate blood samples are handled similarly to samples from other mammalian species. Ethylenediaminetetraacetic acid (EDTA) is the preferred anticoagulant for complete blood counts; heparin can be used as an alternative anticoagulant, but many result in poorer cell staining of blood smears. The sample should be refrigerated at 4 °C if analysis cannot be performed within 2 to 3 h and should be analyzed within 24 h to avoid artifacts due to RBC swelling. In order to avoid dilution of the sample with excess liquid anticoagulant, BD Microtainer collection tubes (BD, Franklin Lakes, New Jersey) are useful for the collection of small volumes of blood (250–500 μl). Ideally, blood smears should be made immediately after sampling and prior to mixture with an anticoagulant, and can be evaluated with a standard Wright's-type stain. For biochemical panels, blood can be placed in a red top tube for serum collection, or heparinized plasma can also be used. If only a small volume of blood can be obtained, it can be placed in a heparin BD Microtainer for both hematology and biochemical panels.

Complete Blood Count

Ranges for hematologic values of the owl monkey, tufted capuchin monkey, and squirrel monkey are listed in Table 15.1.

Erythrocytes

Squirrel monkey erythrocytes have a relatively small mean corpuscular volume (60 μm^3) which may require adjusting automated hematology analyzers for correct results [15]. Mild-to-moderate anisocytosis is common, and the erythrocytes have central pallor (Figures 15.4–15.11). Annular and target cells are occasionally seen, while spherocytes are rare. In healthy animals, the degree of polychromasia is slight [16], and nucleated red blood cells are rare, although wild-caught animals may show higher levels of nucleated red blood cells compared to captive-bred monkeys [17]. Erythrocyte and hemoglobin levels show diurnal variation in the owl monkey [18]. Female capuchins undergo a 20-day menstrual cycle, which may result in lower levels of erythrocytes, hemoglobin, and hematocrit when compared to males [13]. Parasites may be observed in blood smears, particularly in wild-caught animals. These include microfilariae (multiple species) and *Trypanosoma cruzi* in many neotropical primates, as well as *Plasmodium brasilianum* in squirrel and capuchin monkeys [19]. As with other species, anemia may be due to a number of etiologies. An etiology unique to owl monkeys is vitamin-E-responsive hemolytic anemia. Animals in the gray-necked group may spontaneously develop this condition and present with PCVs of less than 15% [20].

Leukocytes

The total leukocyte number in small New World primates varies widely and may be impacted by a number of factors. Squirrel and owl monkeys bred or maintained in captivity may have increased numbers of total leukocytes compared to wild-caught animals, while captive capuchin monkeys are reported to have lower total leukocyte counts [17, 21, 22]. Animals not acclimated to capture and restraint can exhibit leukocytosis, mature neutrophilia, and lymphopenia associated with stress, while sedation may reverse this response [23]. Owl monkeys in karyotypes II, III, IV, and VI may have elevated levels of eosinophils unrelated to parasitism or other subclinical conditions (idiopathic eosinophilia) [24]. In squirrel monkey blood smears, neutrophils have lobulated nuclei with spherical azurophilic granules (Figure 15.5). Band or other immature cells and toxic changes are rarely seen. Eosinophils have variable nuclear segmentation and small, round orange-red granules (Figure 15.6). Basophils have bilobed nuclei and large purple granules overlying the nucleus (Figure 15.7). Lymphocytes are generally 8–12 μm in diameter with round or oval nuclei and pale blue cytoplasm that may contain granules (Figure 15.8). Larger lymphocytes with pleomorphic nuclei containing coarse strands of chromatin are also seen (Figure 15.9). Reactive lymphocytes with deep blue cytoplasm may be present (Figure 15.10). Monocytes are 15–20 μm in diameter with irregularly shaped, smoothly

Table 15.1 Hematologic reference ranges for New World monkeys.

Cell parameter (abbreviation)	Units, SI (conventional)	*Aotus nancymaae* (owl monkey) ₳ [12]		*Cebus apella* (tufted capuchin) ₳ [13]		*Saimiri boliviensis* (squirrel monkey) ✋ [14]
		Male	**Female**	**Male**	**Female**	**Male**
	Data format	**95% Confidence interval**		**95% Confidence interval**		**95% Confidence interval**
	Animals sampled	**130**	**124**	**12–20**	**13–24**	**38**
Red blood cells	$\times 10^{12}$/l	5.0–7.6	4.4–7.3	4.40–7.05	4.08–6.47	6.46–8.09
Hemoglobin	g/l (g/dl)	131–188 (13.1–18.8)	120–197 (12.0–19.7)	107–167 (10.7–16.7)	100–154 (10–15.4)	128–155 (12.8–15.5)
PCV/HCT	%	41.3–58.0 (PCV)	25.8–57.5 (PCV)	29.0–52.0 (HCT)	28.0–47.1 (HCT)	39.70–50.60 (HCT)
MCV	cubic microns	72.0–87.7	72.3–87	65.0–79.0	65.0–80.0	58.00–65.30
MCH	pg	22.5–29.3	22.6–29.3	20.0–26.0	20.0–26.0	18.2–21.1
MCHC	g/l (g/dl)	305–349 (30.5–34.9)	306–344 (30.6–34.4)	250–380 (25.0–38.0)	290–380 (29.0–38.0)	303–346 (30.3–34.6)
Platelets	10^9/l	207–623	157–690	254.0–527.0	271.0–560.0	277–911
White blood cells	10^9/l	4.7–16.4	4.2–17.6	3.0–15.30	2.8–4.6	4.70–14.60
Neutrophils (absolute)	10^9/l	0.53–9.28	0.15–7.29			
Neutrophils (%)	%	5.3–65.6	3.0–58.8	40.0–87.0	45.0–91.0	13–63
Lymphocytes (absolute)	10^9/l	2.55–12.06	2.28–14.68			
Lymphocytes (%)	%	25.3–87.7	26.9–91.9	11.0–60.0	8.0–53.0	34–76
Monocytes (absolute)	10^9/l	0.00–1.08	0.00–1.19			
Monocytes (%)	%	0.0–10.4	0.0–9.9	0–10.0	0–8.0	1.0–17.0
Eosinophils (absolute)	10^9/l	0.00–2.09	0.00–1.74			
Eosinophils (%)	%	0.0–15.0	0.0–15.9	0–5.0	0–6.0	
Basophils (absolute)	10^9/l	0.00–0.72	0.00–0.65			
Basophils (%)	%	0.0–5.0	0.0–7.2	0–1.0	0–1.0	

Key: Anesthetized with ketamine ₳, Manual restraint ✋.

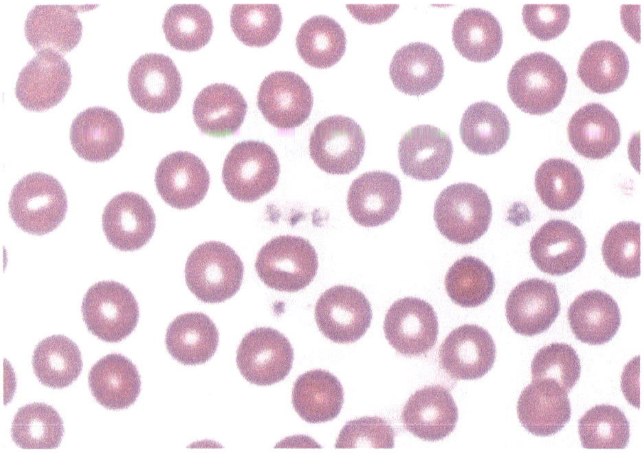

Figure 15.4 Cells in the peripheral blood smear of the squirrel monkey: normal erythrocytes and platelets. (100× objective). *Source:* Photo courtesy of Dr. Jennifer Johns.

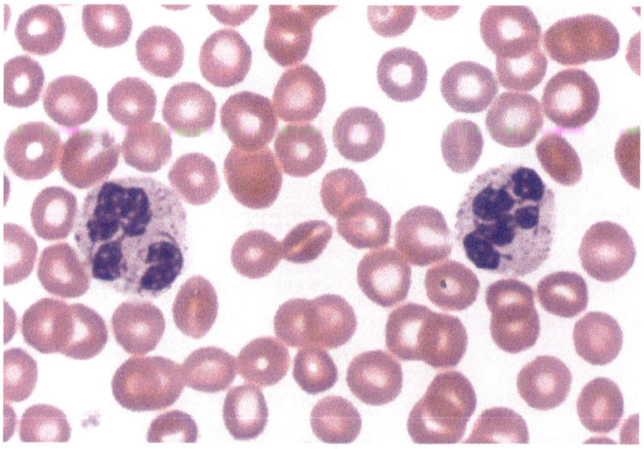

Figure 15.5 Two neutrophils in the peripheral blood smear of a squirrel monkey. (100× objective). *Source:* Photo courtesy of Dr. Jennifer Johns.

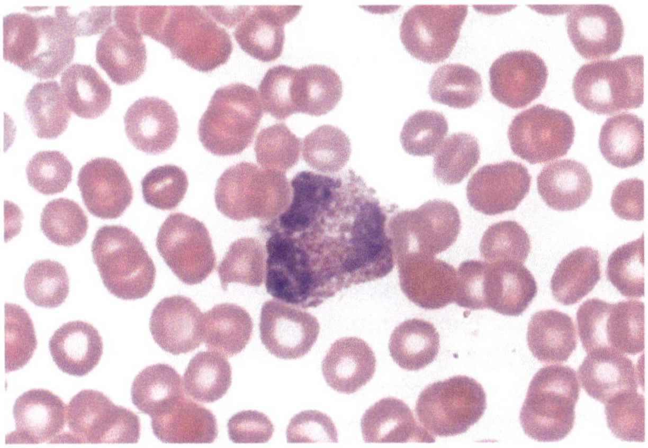

Figure 15.6 An eosinophil in the peripheral blood smear of a squirrel monkey. (100× objective). *Source:* Photo courtesy of Dr. Jennifer Johns.

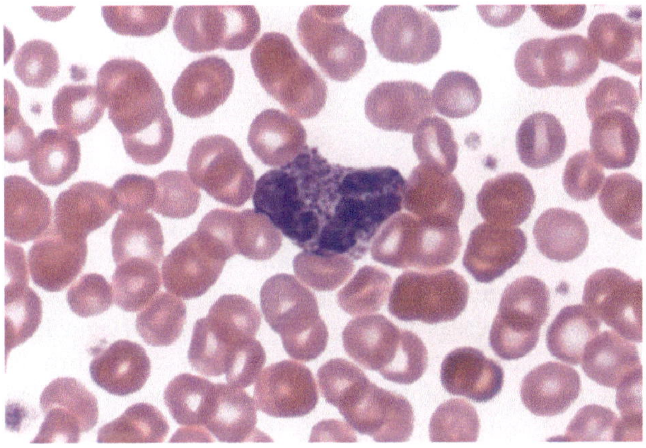

Figure 15.7 A basophil from the peripheral blood smear of a squirrel monkey is present in the center of the image. (100× objective). *Source:* Photo courtesy of Dr. Jennifer Johns.

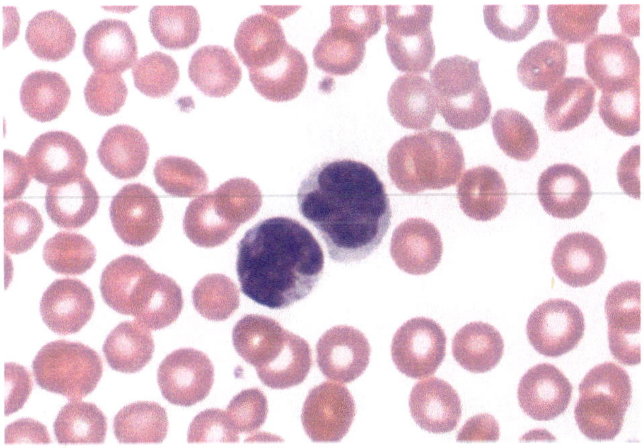

Figure 15.8 Lymphocytes from the peripheral blood smear of a squirrel monkey. The cell on the left contains granular cytoplasm. *Source:* Photo courtesy of Dr. Jennifer Johns.

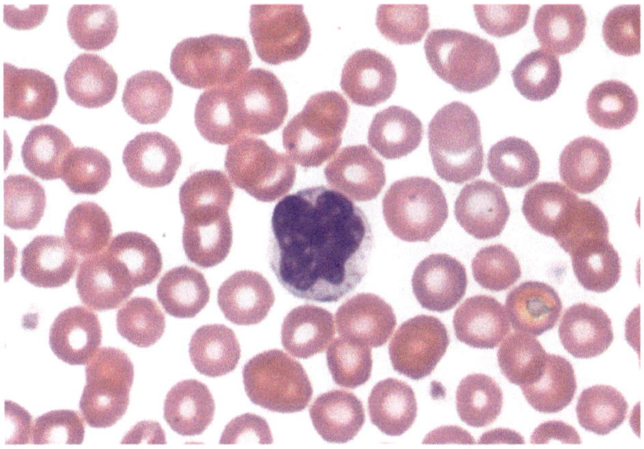

Figure 15.9 A large lymphocyte in the peripheral blood smear of the squirrel monkey. *Source:* Photo courtesy of Dr. Jennifer Johns.

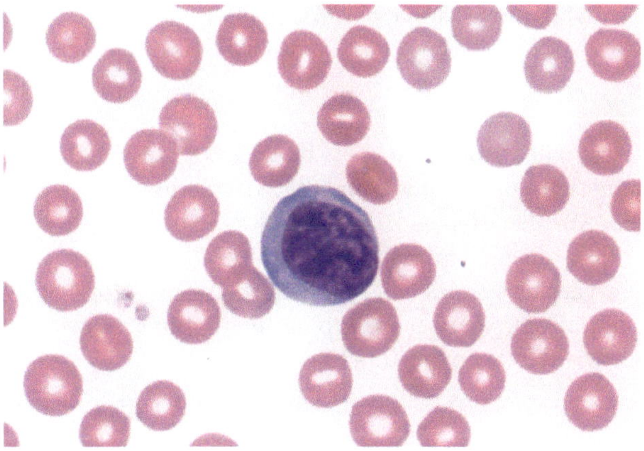

Figure 15.10 A reactive lymphocyte from the peripheral blood smear of a squirrel monkey (100× objective). *Source:* Photo courtesy of Dr. Jennifer Johns.

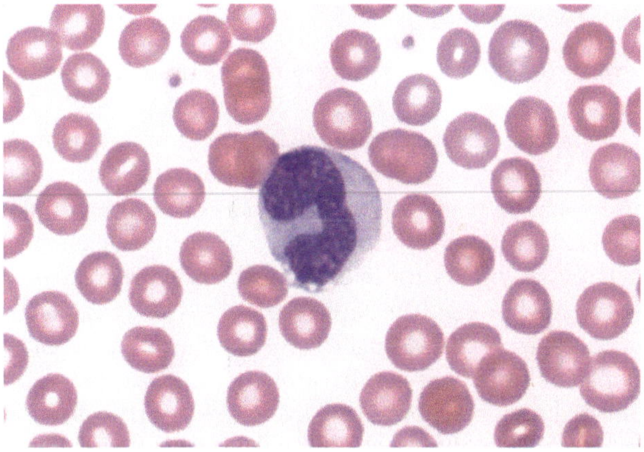

Figure 15.11 A monocyte from the peripheral blood smear of a squirrel monkey. 100× objective. *Source:* Photo courtesy of Dr. Jennifer Johns.

staining nuclei and cloudy blue cytoplasm with very small red granules and occasional vacuoles (Figure 15.11) [16]. Primary hematopoietic disease in New World primates is uncommon, but owl monkeys infected with a variety of herpesviruses may develop lymphocytic leukemia with peripheral atypical and immature lymphocytes [25].

Hemostasis (Coagulation Panel) and Blood Types

Hemostasis

Some owl monkeys may bleed for extended periods of time after venipuncture. This hemorrhage has been associated with long partial and activated partial thromboplastin times and attributed to high levels of antithrombin III [26]. However, other reports have found short activated partial thromboplastin times in the owl monkey (*A. trivirgatus*, 19.6 ± 1.8 s) [8].

Blood Types

All primates express the ABO blood group antigens found in humans. One study found that *S. sciureus* expressed A and AB phenotypes, *Aotus infulatus* expressed only B, while *C. apella* expressed O, A, B, and AB. However, this may vary by species and population. In New World species, salivary and serum typing in the same individual may yield differing results [27].

Biochemical Panel

Biochemical ranges for the owl monkey, tufted capuchin monkey, and squirrel monkey are summarized in Table 15.2.

Liver Enzymes

Similar to other species, serum elevations of alanine transaminase (ALT), aspartate transaminase (AST), serum alkaline phosphatase (SAP), and gamma-glutamyl transpeptidase (GGT) may indicate hepatobiliary disease. Because many of these enzymes occur in multiple tissues, elevations of more than one of these enzymes increase specificity for liver disease. SAP is reported to be extremely variable in squirrel monkeys [30] and is significantly higher in younger monkeys due to an increase in osteoblastic activity in growing animals [31–33]. Elevated total bilirubin may be due to hemolytic disease or hepatobiliary disease. In squirrel monkeys, total bilirubin may vary by species. Bolivian squirrel monkeys develop high bilirubin levels when fasted (34.2 μmol/l [2 mg/dl]) due to increased bilirubin production and decreased UDP-glucuronosyltransferase activity, while levels in other squirrel monkey species remain <8.5 μmol/l (<0.5 mg/dl) when fasted [34].

Muscle Enzymes

Creatine kinase (CK) may be moderately elevated in small New World monkeys due to capture and restraint, intramuscular injection, or trauma. In the owl monkey, CK >160 U/l together with a CK/AST ratio of ≥2 but ≤9 may indicate myocardial infarct [35].

Renal Analytes

As in other species, elevations in blood urea nitrogen (BUN) and serum creatinine are indications of renal disease in nonhuman primates. In glomerulonephropathy (common in squirrel monkeys and owl monkeys), azotemia is accompanied by proteinuria and hypoproteinemia [7, 20].

Pancreas (Endocrine and Exocrine)

Amylase, Lipase, and Pancreatic Lipase-Like Assays

High levels of serum amylase suggest pancreatitis, although this analyte is not specific in some nonhuman primate species. The squirrel monkey produces amylase in the pancreas and liver, but lacks salivary amylase [36]. In a case report of a squirrel monkey with chronic pancreatitis, the animal presented with elevated amylase (447 U/l) and lipase (107 U/l) that increased 3.8- and 2.8-fold respectively over a five-day period [37].

Glucose

Transient hyperglycemia may occur due to capture and restraint stress in unacclimated animals. Hypoglycemia can occur as a primary disorder in squirrel and owl monkeys due to their higher metabolic rates, lower percentage of body adipose tissue, and limited glycogen reserves. Animals present with glucose levels of <2.2 mmol/l (<40 mg/dl) in the squirrel monkey and < 2.8 mmol/l (<50 mg/dl) in the owl monkey. Glucose can be determined with a glucose meter designed for human diabetics, requiring only one to two drops of blood [7, 20].

Electrolytes

Electrolyte levels are similar to other species. Squirrel monkeys maintain normal electrolyte levels despite high circulating cortisol levels through altered cortisol metabolism and excretion [38].

Table 15.2 Biochemical reference ranges for New World monkeys.

Analyte (abbreviation)	Units, SI (conventional)	*Aotus nancymaae* (owl monkey) A [28]		*Cebus apella* (tufted capuchin) A [13]		*Saimiri boliviensis* (Squirrel monkey)[a] [15]
	Gender	Male	Female	Male	Female	Male and female
	Data format	95% Confidence interval		95% Confidence interval		Mean ± SD
	Animals sampled	130	124	12–20	13–24	84–100
Alanine aminotransferase (ALT)	U/l	14.8–89.3	8.1–202.0	22.0–86.0	17.0–111.0	184.2 ± 110.3
Albumin	g/l (g/dl)	35–51 (3.5–5.1)	29–54 (2.9–5.4)	38–54 (3.8–5.4)	38–51 (3.8–5.1)	42 ± 6 (4.2 ± 0.6)
Alkaline phosphatase (ALKP)	U/l	74–2118	98–1557	35–891	31–835	357.9 ± 175.3
Amylase	U/l			37–918	38–771	515.5 ± 188.6
Aspartate aminotransferase (AST)	U/l			27–116	23–125	185.1 ± 95.3
Bilirubin, direct	μmol/l (mg/dl)					3.42 ± 3.42 (0.2 ± 0.2)
Bilirubin, total	μmol/l (mg/dl)	6.8–32.5 (0.4–1.9)	6.8–34.2 (0.4–2.0)	0.51–10.94 (0.03–0.64)	0.17–12.65 (0.01–0.74)	13.7 ± 10.3 (0.8 ± 0.6)
Calcium	mmol/l (mg/dl)	2.10–3.15 (8.4–12.6)	2.15–3.27 (8.6–13.1)	0.50–3.12 (2.0–12.5)	1.2–3.06 (4.8–12.2)	2.4 ± 0.2 (9.6 ± 0.9)
Cholesterol	mmol/l (mg/dl)	2.05–7.77 (79–300)	1.89–6.89 (73–266)	1.92–5.34 (74–206)	1.61–5.78 (62–223)	3.92–1.68 (151.4 ± 64.7)
Creatine kinase (CK)	U/l					562 ± 1379.8
Creatinine	μmol/l (mg/dl)	35.36–129.95 (0.40–1.47)	53.04–146.74 (0.60–1.66)	35.36–129.95 (0.40–1.47)	32.71–115.80 (0.37–1.31)	79.6 ± 17.7 (0.9 ± 0.2)
Gamma-glutamyltransferase (GGT)	U/l	5.3–50.4	3.0–49.6	23.0–94.0	33.0–132.0	56.4 ± 150.4
Glucose	mmol/l (mg/dl)	4.05–11.65 (73–210)	4.22–12.49 (76–225)	2.28–7.33 (41–132)	2.39–10.05 (43–181)	5.69–1.68 (102.6 ± 30.3)
Lactate dehydrogenase (LDH)	U/l			91–795	91–1128	123.2 ± 111.9
Lipase	U/l			52–124	51–164	
Magnesium	mmol/l (mg/dl)			0.62–1.27 (1.52–3.10)	0.41–1.32 (1.0–3.2)	
Phosphorus	mmol/l (mg/dl)	0.45–2.23 (1.4–6.9)	0.65–2.52 (2.0–7.8)	0.47–5.40 (1.5–16.7)	0.51–4.00 (0.2–12.4)	2.23 ± 2.52 (6.9 ± 7.8)
Potassium	mmol/l			2.30–6.60	2.90–5.70	5.7 ± 1.0
Protein, total	g/l (g/dl)	67–96 (6.7–9.6)	65–104 (6.5–10.4)	63–86 (6.3–8.6)	63–88 (6.3–8.8)	69 ± 10 (6.9 ± 1.0)
Protein electrophoresis						
Albumin	%			51.4–69.3	52.6–69.7	
α_1 globulin	%			1.1–2.7	1.2–3.1	
α_2 globulin	%			2.6–15.8	1.5–17.2	
β globulin	%			6.5–19.5	8.2–19.9	
γ globulin	%			9.0–22.5	6.5–20.4	
A/G ratio				1.06–1.95	1.11–1.90	

(*Continued*)

Table 15.2 (Continued)

Analyte (abbreviation)	Units, SI (conventional)	*Aotus nancymaae* (owl monkey) Ⱥ [28]		*Cebus apella* (tufted capuchin) Ⱥ [13]		*Saimiri boliviensis* (Squirrel monkey)[a] [15] ✋
	Gender	Male	Female	Male	Female	Male and female
	Data format	95% Confidence interval		95% Confidence interval		Mean ± SD
	Animals sampled	130	124	12–20	13–24	84–100
Serum iron	mmol/dl (mg/dl)			6.27–35.44 (35–198)	4.12–34.55 (23–193)	
Sodium	mmol/l			130–163	140–158	150.1 ± 7.2
Thyroxine, total (T4)	nmol/l (μg/dl)					M: 38.9 ± 14.2 (3.02 ± 1.1) F: 25.6 ± 10.9 (1.99 ± 0.85)[b] [29]
Triiodothyronine, total (T3)	nmol/l (ng/dl)					M: 0.88 ± 0.34 (57.1 ± 22.2) F: 0.75 ± 0.31 (48.8 ± 20.0)[b] [29]
Triglycerides	mmol/l (mg/dl)			0.15–2.42 (13–214)	0.21–2.23 (19–197)	0.85 ± 0.37 (74.9 ± 32.7)
Urea nitrogen	mmol/l (mg/dl)	2.3–9.6 (6.3–27.0)	1.8–10.0 (5.1–27.9)	2.1–19.6 (6.0–55.0)	2.9–26.1 (8.0–73.0)	13.8 ± 3.6 (38.7 ± 10)

[a] Adults in captivity for ≥5 years [15]. Key: Anesthetized Ⱥ Manual restraint ✋.
[b] n = 9 male and 13 female captive adults [29].

Blood Proteins

As in other species, hyperproteinemia is an indication of dehydration or inflammation, while hypoproteinemia may be due to a number of etiologies including liver, gastrointestinal, and renal diseases as well as hemorrhage. A common cause of hypoproteinemia in New World monkeys is glomerular disease; concurrent findings include proteinuria and azotemia [20]. In the owl monkey, total serum protein levels demonstrate diurnal variation with a fluctuation of about 10%. In one report, the overall serum protein mean was 70.9 g/l, but values were lowest at the beginning of the dark period (67.4 g/L) and highest at the start of the light period (75.2 g/l) [18].

Blood Gases

Arterial blood gas values for squirrel monkeys are included in Table 15.3. Nonsedated animals show a metabolic acidosis (low blood pH and pCO_2) compared to sedated animals, potentially due to increased muscle activity and hyperventilation during capture and restraint [40].

Vitamins, Minerals and Metals, and Toxins

Calcium

Alterations in calcium may occur due to a number of conditions including endocrine disorders, renal disease, nutritional imbalances, and neoplasia. In owl monkeys, hypocalcemia has been reported in chronic renal disease [20], while hypercalcemia has been reported in granulomatous disseminated histoplasmosis [41]. Calcium is usually reported as the total serum calcium concentration, which consists of the physiologically active ionized fraction as well as protein-bound and complexed fractions. In order to correct total calcium levels for variation in albumin or total protein levels in owl monkeys, the following formulas can be used: [42].

$$\text{Adjusted calcium (mg/dl)} = \text{measured calcium}\left(\text{mg/dl}\right) - 0.84[\text{albumin (g/dl)}] + 3.8$$

$$\text{Adjusted calcium (mg/dl)} = \text{measure calcium}\left(\text{mg/dl}\right) - 0.82[\text{total protein (g/dl)}] + 6.5$$

Table 15.3 Arterial blood gas values for squirrel monkeys [39].

Analyte (abbreviation)	Units, SI (conventional)	*Saimiri sciureus* (common squirrel monkey)	*Saimiri boliviensis* (Bolivian squirrel monkey)
pH		7.2 ± 0.02	7.22 ± 0.04
Carbon dioxide partial pressure (PaCO2)	mmHg	23.45 ± 1.59	29.35 ± 2.05
Oxygen partial pressure (PaO2)	mmHg	114.05 ± 2.93	104.80 ± 8.59
Oxygen saturation (SaO2)	%	95.77 ± 0.66	95.88 ± 0.79
Carbon dioxide (CO_2)	mmol/l (or mEq/l)	9.58 ± 0.42	12.70 ± 0.47
Bicarbonate (HCO_3)	mmol/l (or mEq/l)	8.85 ± 0.44	11.78 ± 0.50
Base excess (BE)	mmol/l (or mEq/l)	−17.15 ± 0.53	−14.18 ± 1.56

Data given as mean ± SD, four adult females of each species, manual restraint.

Iron

Serum iron levels show considerable diurnal variation in the owl monkey and can fluctuate by 60% in a bimodal pattern. In one report, daily mean serum iron was 21.2 μmol/l (118 μg/dl), but peaks (mean 27.4 μmol/l [153 μg/dl]) were seen at the beginning of both the dark and light periods, while minimum values (mean 14.9 μmol/l [83 μg/dl]) were observed in the middle of both the dark and light periods [18].

Vitamins

Disease due to deficiency in vitamin A, a fat-soluble vitamin, has been reported in capuchin monkeys (*C. albifrons* and *apella*). Signs included diarrhea, retarded growth, and retinal degeneration when serum levels dropped from normal values of 0.5–0.7 μmol/l (15–20 μg/dl) to <0.2 μmol/l (<5 μg/dl) [43]. Vitamin C (ascorbic acid) is required in the diet of all New World monkeys. In juvenile squirrel monkeys, a common presentation of vitamin C deficiency is acute cephalohematoma, but New World primates may also develop signs of joint pain, gingival hemorrhage, and anemia. Serum ascorbic acid levels can assist in diagnosis of vitamin C deficiency; normal serum levels in the squirrel monkey were 38.0 μmol/l (0.67 mg/dl) in one report but dropped to 7.4 μmol/l (0.13 mg/dl) after three months on a vitamin-C-deficient diet [44]. New World primates not receiving adequate exposure to sunlight require dietary supplementation of vitamin D_3 (cholecalciferol); deficiency results in osteomalacia. The hormonal form of vitamin D found in the serum, 1,25-dihydroxyvitamin D_3, is normally found at approximately 10-fold higher levels in New World monkeys compared to Old World monkeys and apes (2106 ± 309 pmol/l [810 ± 119 pg/ml] compared to 159 ± 13 pmol/l [61 ± 5 pg/ml]) [45]. Vitamin E can be assessed in an animal through measurement of serum or plasma tocopherol levels. Hypovitaminosis E in capuchin monkeys (*C. albifrons* and *apella*) results in a hemolytic, macrocytic, normochromic anemia with reticulocytosis. In one report, anemic monkeys had tocopherol levels of <2.3 μmol/l (<100 μg/dl), while normal animals had levels of >11.6 μmol/l (>500 μg/dl) [46]. Owl monkeys of the gray-necked group are susceptible to a vitamin-E-responsive hemolytic anemia. Plasma α-tocopherol levels in anemia-resistant owl monkeys have been reported at 8.7 ± 4.7 μmol/l (375 ± 203 μg/dl), while anemia-susceptible animals have significantly lower levels (1.0 ± 0.8 μmol/l [45 ± 33 μg/dl]) [47].

Hormones – Thyroid, Adrenal, Reproductive

Thyroid

Generally, New World primates have lower total serum triiodothyronine (T3) and thyroxine (T4) levels than Old World primates, but free T3 and T4 levels are similar between the groups [29, 48]. The owl monkey exhibits diurnal variation; during the day, T4 levels are low, while thyroid-stimulating hormone (TSH) levels are similar to those of other species. However, T3 values rise and TSH values fall when samples are taken at night during the animal's active phase [49]. In male squirrel monkeys, T3 and T4 levels fluctuate throughout the year, ranging from about 0.6 nmol/l (40 ng/dl) (T3) and 28.3 nmol/l (2.2 μg/dl) (T4) during the nonbreeding season to 1.4 nmol/l (92.9 ng/dl) (T3) and 54.1 nmol/l (4.2 μg/dl) (T4) during the breeding season [50].

Cortisol

Some species of New World primates have extremely high levels of total and free serum cortisol without signs of hyperadrenocorticism. Squirrel monkeys in particular have free serum cortisol levels 100-fold higher than humans and Old World primates [51]. Capuchin monkeys may show moderately elevated cortisol, while owl monkeys have cortisol levels similar to those of Old World primates [51, 52]. Squirrel monkeys maintain normal physiologic parameters in the face of high cortisol levels through alterations in cortisol metabolism [38].

Female Reproductive Hormones

Peak steroid hormone levels in New World monkeys are high compared to those in other primates. Squirrel monkeys, as seasonal breeders, have low serum estradiol (<734 pmol/l [<200 pg/ml]) and progesterone (<32 nmol/l [<10 ng/ml]) levels during the nonbreeding season. A 10-fold peak in progesterone indicates the beginning of the breeding season, and during the breeding season cyclic peaks of estradiol >1652 pmol/l (>450 pg/ml) and progesterone >382 nmol/l (>120 ng/ml) occur at 6–12 day intervals [53]. Owl monkeys in captivity are not seasonal breeders and have peaks in estradiol and progesterone every 15–16 days (in one study, estradiol rose from a basal level of 367–734 pmol/l [100–200 pg/ml] to a peak of approximately 2570 pmol/l [700 pg/ml] and progesterone rose from a basal level of about 45 nmol/l [14 ng/ml] to a peak of 795 nmol/l [>250 ng/ml]) [54]. Capuchin monkeys, also not seasonal breeders, have a 18–24 day cycle with estradiol ranging from 257–367 pmol/l (70–100 pg/ml) to a peak of about 1835 pmol/l (500 pg/ml) and progesterone ranging from 10–32 nmol/l (3–10 ng/ml) to a peak of about 223 nmol/l (70 ng/ml) [55].

Male Reproductive Hormones

Squirrel monkeys, as seasonal breeders, have fluctuating testosterone levels throughout the year, ranging from about 173 nmol/l (5000 ng/dl) in the nonbreeding season to about 347 nmol/dl (10 000 ng/dl) during the breeding season [56]. In contrast, testosterone levels in owl and capuchin monkeys do not show seasonality, with a range of about 17–87 nmol/l (500–2500 ng/dl) reported for owl monkeys [57] and 173–382 nmol/l (500–11 000 ng/dl) reported for capuchins [58].

Urinalysis

Urinalysis reference values for the owl monkey and squirrel monkey are listed in Tables 15.4 and 15.5. Because cystocentesis and catheterization are difficult in small primates, urine samples can often only be obtained by free-catch methods. Therefore, urinalysis interpretation

Table 15.4 Urinalysis data for New World monkeys.

Quantitative values [59]	*Aotus nancymaae* (owl monkey)		*Saimiri peruviensis* (squirrel monkey)	
Animals sampled:	62		20	
	Mean ± SD	Range	Mean ± SD	Range
Specific gravity	1.009 ± 0.005	1.002–1.023	1.023 ± 0.006	1.010–1.030
Urine volume (mg/16 h)	81.9 ± 94.7	15–481	23.2 ± 32.0	8–152
Urine creatinine (mg/dl)	34.7 ± 27.6	6.0–135	64.7 ± 30.8	14–159
Urine protein (g/l)	41.2 ± 34.1	4.0–147	21.3 ± 11.0	9–53
Urine protein/creatinine ratio	1.48 ± 1.49	0.26–9.0	0.43 ± 0.49	0.13–2.36
Urine protein loss (mg/kg/day)	45.6 ± 45.4	6.5–256.3	10.5 ± 15.3	2.0–71.2
Endogenous creatinine clearance (ml/min/kg)	2.23 ± 0.67	0.97–4.52	1.65 ± 0.50	0.78–2.47

Table 15.5 Semiquantitative and microscopic urinalysis values for 98 apparently healthy owl monkeys. *(Aotus spp.)* [60].

Semiquantitative values		Microscopic analysis	
Protein	0–3+	Red blood cells	Rare – few (3–5/hpf)
Glucose	0–1+	White blood cells	Rare – occasional
Ketones	0–2+	Epithelial cells	Rare – occasional squamous
Bilirubin	0	Casts	Occasional granular
Urobilinogen	0	Crystals	Few – moderate triple phosphate; rare calcium oxalate
Occult blood	0–4+	Miscellaneous	Occasional renal tubular epithelial cells
pH	6–8.5	Appearance	Light to dark yellow; clear to cloudy

must account for sampling technique and sample quality. If abnormal proteinuria is present, examine the sediment to rule out hemorrhage or inflammation. If these conditions are not present, the urine protein:urine creatinine ratio determines the severity of proteinuria. In the owl monkey, a ratio > 2.5 indicates impaired glomerular function, and the urine protein loss (mg/kg/day) can be calculated as the urine protein:urine creatinine ratio x 29.8 [61]. Proteinuria in New World primates has been reported in glomerulonephropathies in owl and squirrel monkeys, as well as in hypertension due to preeclampsia in many species or subclinical cardiac disease in owl monkeys [7, 20, 35, 62].

Serology and PCR Useful for Small New World Primates

It is highly recommended that you contact the lab regarding sample technique, type, and shipping prior to collecting any samples from New World primates. Based on the increased zoonotic potential of these samples from these species, many standard veterinary diagnostic laboratories may not accept primate samples.

Herpesviruses

Primates may carry several herpesviruses that cause minimal disease in the natural host, but infection of other New World monkey species results in significant morbidity and mortality. Saimiriine herpesvirus 1 (also known as Herpesvirus tamarinus or Herpes T) is an alphaherpesvirus carried asymptomatically by squirrel monkeys. Infection of owl monkeys, marmosets, and tamarins results in severe necrosis of skin, oral mucosa, and multiple organs. Similar disease is seen in owl monkeys when infected with Human herpesvirus 1 or 2 (herpes simplex viruses). Saimiriine herpesvirus 2 (also known as Herpesvirus saimiri type 2 or HVS) is a gammaherpesvirus carried asymptomatically by squirrel monkeys, but rare cases of lymphoma or lymphocytic leukemia have been reported in owl monkeys [63]. Serology can be used to screen potential asymptomatic hosts or to confirm diagnosis of affected animals. PCR of whole blood or lesion swabs is available to detect virus in viremic or actively shedding animals.

Measles Virus

Measles (rubeola) has been documented in many nonhuman primate species, including squirrel and owl monkeys. Animals may be asymptomatic or show clinical signs such fever, diarrhea, pneumonia, and maculopapular rash. Infection or seroconversion can occur after exposure to humans carrying the virus. Serology can be used to screen animals for prior exposure to measles virus. Diagnosis in monkeys with clinical signs is confirmed by increasing antibody titers with serology, or by detection of the virus in whole blood, serum, urine, throat swab, or lesion swab by PCR.

Leptospira

Although naturally acquired leptospirosis is uncommon in nonhuman primates, severe outbreaks have been reported in squirrel monkeys and capuchin monkeys [64, 65]. Signs include fever, icterus, hemorrhage, abortion, and acute death. Serology using the microagglutination test (MAT) can identify *Leptospira* serovars involved in disease outbreaks or be used to screen for potential asymptomatic carriers [66]. PCR of body fluids or tissues can directly detect *Leptospira* and may be particularly useful in the early stages of disease or when poor sample condition decreases the chances of culturing viable bacterial organisms [67].

Encephalitozoon Cuniculi

Infection with *E. cuniculi*, a microsporidian parasite, is usually subclinical in nonhuman primates but can cause seizures and death in young squirrel monkeys; it may also be a factor in decreased reproductive performance in breeding colonies [68]. Serology with indirect immunofluorescence (IFA) and dot enzyme linked immunosorbent assay (dot-ELISA) have been used to screen adult squirrel monkeys for infection [69, 70]. PCR of tissues can be used to confirm the presence of *E. cuniculi* organisms and provide genotype information [71].

References

1 Ankel-Simons, F. (2007). *Primate Anatomy: An Introduction*, 3e. Amsterdam: Academic Press.
2 Hendrickx, A.G. and Dukelow, W.R. (1995). Reproductive biology. In: *Nonhuman Primates in Biomedical Research: Biology and Management* (ed. B.T. Bennett and C.R. Abee), 147–191. San Diego: Academic Press.
3 Malinow, M.R. and Wagner, R. (1966). Oxygen uptake in squirrel monkeys (Saimiri sciurea). *Lab Anim Care* 16 (2): 105–108.
4 Whitney, R.W. (1995). Taxonomy. In: *Nonhuman Primates in Biomedical Research: Biology and Management* (ed. B.T. Bennett, C.R. Abee and R. Henrickson), 33–47. San Diego: Academic Press.

5 Hershkovitz, P. (1983). Two new species of night monkeys, genus Aotus (Cebidae, Platyrrhini): a preliminary report on Aotus taxonomy. *Am. J. Primatol.* 4 (3): 209–243.
6 Le Maho, Y., Goffart, M., Rochas, A. et al. (1981). Thermoregulation in the only nocturnal simian: the night monkey Aotus trivirgatus. *Am. J. Phys.* 240 (3): R156–R165.
7 Abee, C.R. (1985). Medical care and management of the squirrel monkey. In: *Handbook of Squirrel Monkey Research* (ed. L.A. Rosenblum and C.L. Coe). New York: Plenum Press.
8 Mrema, J.E., Johnson, G.S., Kelley, S.T., and Green, T.J. (1984). Activated partial thromboplastin time of owl monkey (Aotus trivirgatus) plasma. *Lab. Anim. Sci.* 34 (3): 295–298.
9 Ageyama, N., Shibata, H., Narita, H. et al. (2001). Specific gravity of whole blood in cynomolgus monkeys (Macaca fascicularis), squirrel monkeys (Saimiri sciureus), and tamarins (Saguinus labiatus) and total blood volume in cynomolgus monkeys. *Contemp. Top. Lab. Anim. Sci.* 40 (3): 33–35.
10 Diehl, K.H., Hull, R., Morton, D. et al. (2001). A good practice guide to the administration of substances and removal of blood, including routes and volumes. *J. Appl. Toxicol.* 21 (1): 15–23.
11 Dysko, R.C. and Hoskins, D.E. (1995). Part B. Collection of biological samples and therapy administration. In: *Nonhuman Primates in Biomedical Research:Biology and Management* (ed. B.T. Bennett and C.R. Abee), 147–191. San Diego: Academic Press.
12 Málaga, C.A., Weller, R.E., Buschbom, R.L., and Ragan, H.A. (1990). Hematology of the wild caught karyotype 1 owl monkey (Aotus nancymai). *Lab. Anim. Sci.* 40 (2): 204–206.
13 Wirz, A., Truppa, V., and Riviello, M.C. (2008). Hematological and plasma biochemical values for captive tufted capuchin monkeys (Cebus apella). *Am. J. Primatol.* 70 (5): 463–472.
14 Kakoma, I., James, M.A., Jackson, W. et al. (1987). Distribution characteristics and relationships between hematologic variables of healthy Bolivian squirrel monkeys. *Lab. Anim. Sci.* 37 (3): 352–353.
15 Bernacky, B.J., Gibson, S.V., Keeling, M.E., and Abee, C.R. (2002). Nonhuman primates. In: *Laboratory Animal Medicine*, 2e (ed. J.G. Fox, L.C. Anderson, F.M. Loew and F.W. Quimby), 675–791. Burlington: Academic Press.
16 Capel-Edwards, K. and Hall, D.E. (1970). Haematological observations on the squirrel monkey. *Folia Primatol.* 12 (2): 142–160.
17 Kakoma, I., James, M., Jackson, W. et al. (1985). Hematologic values of normal Bolivian squirrel monkeys (Saimiri sciureus): a comparison between wild-caught and laboratory-bred male animals. *Folia Primatol.* 44 (2): 102–107.
18 Klein, R., Bleiholder, B., Jung, A., and Erkert, H.G. (1985). Diurnal variation of several blood parameters in the owl monkey, Aotus trivirgatus griseimembra. *Folia Primatol.* 45 (3–4): 195–203.
19 Toft, J.D. II and Eberhard, M.L. (1998). Parasitic diseases. In: *Nonhuman Primates in Biomedical Research* (ed. B.T. Bennett), 111–205. New York: Academic Press.
20 Weller, R.E. (1994). Infectious and noninfectious diseases of owl monkeys. In: *Aotus: The Owl Monkey* (ed. J.F. Baer, R.E. Weller and I. Kakoma), 177–215. San Diego: Academic Press.
21 Porter, J.A. Jr. (1969). Hematology of the night monkey, Aotus trivirgatus. *Lab. Anim. Care* 19 (4): 470–472.
22 Rosner, J.M., Schinini, A., Rovira, T. et al. (1986). Body measurements, hematology, and serum chemistry values of the adult Cebus apella monkey. *J. Med. Primatol.* 15 (4): 295–302.
23 Loomis, M.R., Henrickson, R.V., and Anderson, J.H. (1980). Effects of ketamine hydrochloride on the hemogram of rhesus monkeys (Macaca mulatta). *Lab. Anim. Sci.* 30 (5): 851–853.
24 Beland, M., Bronson, R., Ma, N.S.F. et al. (1981). Karyotypic variation in susceptibility to hemolytic anemia and idiopathic eosinophilia of owl monkeys, Aotus trivirgatus. *Primates* 22 (4): 551–556.
25 Cicmanec, J., Loeb, W., and Valerio, M. (1974). Lymphoma in owl monkeys (Aotus trivirgatus) inoculated with Herpesvirus saimiri: clinical, hematologic and pathologic findings. *J. Med. Primatol.* 3 (1): 8.
26 Loeb, W.F., Cicmanec, J.L., and Wickum, M. (1976). A coagulopathy of the owl monkey (Aotus trivirgatus) associated with high antithrombin III activity. *Lab. Anim. Sci.* 26 (6 Pt 2): 1084–1087.
27 Corvelo, T.C.O., Schneider, H., and Harada, M.L. (2002). ABO blood groups in the primate species of Cebidae from the Amazon region. *J. Med. Primatol.* 31 (3): 136–141.
28 Malaga, C.A., Weller, R.E., Buschbom, R.L., and Ragan, H.A. (1991). Serum chemistry of the wild caught karyotype I night monkey (Aotus nancymai). *Lab. Anim. Sci.* 41 (2): 143–145.
29 Kaack, B., Walker, L., Brizzee, K.R., and Wolf, R.H. (1979). Comparative normal levels of serum triiodothyronine and thyroxine in nonhuman primates. *Lab. Anim. Sci.* 29: 191–194.
30 Hunt, R.D. and Chalifoux, L. (1971). Alkaline phosphatase isoenzymes in the squirrel monkey (Saimiri sciureus). *Am. J. Vet. Res.* 32 (6): 967–974.
31 Beland, M.F., Sehgal, P.K., and Peacock, W.C. (1979). Baseline blood chemistry determinations in the squirrel monkey (Saimiri sciureus). *Lab. Anim. Sci.* 29 (2): 195–199.

32 Riviello, M.C. and Wirz, A. (2001). Haematology and blood chemistry of Cebus apella in relation to sex and age. *J. Med. Primatol.* 30 (6): 308–312.

33 Takeshita, R.S.C., Monteiro, F.O.B., De Miranda Lins e Lins, F.L. et al. (2011). Hematological, hepatic, and renal evaluation in Aotus azarai infulatus. *J. Med. Primatol.* 40 (2): 104–110.

34 Cornelius, C.E. and Freedland, R.A. (1992). Fasting hyperbilirubinemia in normal squirrel monkeys. *Lab. Anim. Sci.* 42 (1): 35–37.

35 Gozalo, A.S., Chavera, A., Montoya, E.J. et al. (2008). Relationship of creatine kinase, aspartate aminotransferase, lactate dehydrogenase, and proteinuria to cardiomyopathy in the owl monkey (Aotus vociferans). *J. Med. Primatol.* 37: 29–38.

36 McGeachin, R.L. and Akin, J.R. (1982). Amylase levels in the tissues and body fluids of several primate species. *Comp. Biochem. Physiol. A Comp. Physiol.* 72 (1): 267–269.

37 Juan-Sallés, C., Prats, N., Ruiz, J.M. et al. (2000). Antioxidant status in a squirrel monkey (Saimiri sciureus) with chronic pancreatitis and degenerative myopathy. *J. Comp. Pathol.* 123 (2-3): 202–206.

38 Scammell, J.G., Westberry, J.M., Sadosky, P.W. et al. (2006). Cortisol metabolism in the Bolivian squirrel monkey (Saimiri boliviensis boliviensis). *Comp. Med.* 56 (2): 128–135.

39 Brizzee, K.R., Ordy, J.M., Dunlap, W.P. et al. (1988). Phenotype and age differences in blood gas characteristics, electrolytes, hemoglobin, plasma glucose and cortisol in female squirrel monkeys. *Lab. Anim. Sci.* 38 (2): 200–202.

40 Manning, P., Lehner, N., Feldner, M., and Bullock, B. (1969). Selected hematologic, serum chemical, and arterial blood gas characteristics of squirrel monkeys (Saimiri sciureus). *Lab. Anim. Care* 19 (6): 831.

41 Weller, R.E., Dagle, G.E., Malaga, C.A., and Baer, J.F. (1990). Hypercalcemia and disseminated histoplasmosis in an owl monkey. *J. Med. Primatol.* 19 (7): 675–680.

42 Weller, R.E., Buschbom, R.L., Ragan, H.A. et al. (1990). Relationship of serum total calcium and albumin and total protein in owl monkeys (Aotus nancymai). *J. Med. Primatol.* 19 (5): 439–446.

43 Hayes, K.C. (1974). Retinal degeneration in monkeys induced by deficiencies of vitamin E or a. *Investig. Ophthalmol.* 13 (7): 499–510.

44 Lehner, N.D.M., Bullock, B.C., and Clarkson, T.B. (1968). Ascorbic acid deficiency in the squirrel monkey. *Proc. Soc. Exp. Biol. Med.* 128 (2): 512–514.

45 Adams, J.S., Gacad, M.A., Baker, A.J. et al. (1985). Serum concentrations of 1, 25-dihydroxyvitamin D3 in Platyrrhini and Catarrhini: a phylogenetic appraisal. *Am. J. Primatol.* 9 (3): 219–224.

46 Ausman, L.M. and Hayes, K.C. (1974). Vitamin E deficiency anemia in old and new world monkeys. *Am. J. Clin. Nutr.* 27 (10): 1141–1151.

47 Meydani, S.N., Nicolosi, R.J., Sehgal, P.K., and Hayes, K.C. (1983). Altered lipoprotein metabolism in spontaneous vitamin E deficiency of owl monkeys. *Am. J. Clin. Nutr.* 38 (6): 888–894.

48 Arbelle, J.E., Gacad, M.A., Spencer, C.A., and Adams, J.S. (1994). Absence of thyroid hormone resistance in vitamin D–resistant new world primates. *Am. J. Primatol.* 32 (3): 215–222.

49 Whittow, G.C., Guernsey, D.L., and Morishige, W.K. (1979). Thyroid activity in a hypometabolic primate, the owl monkey (Aotus trivirgatus). *Arch. Int. Physiol. Biochim.* 87 (5): 963–967.

50 Kaack, B., Walker, M., and Walker, L. (1980). Seasonal changes in the thyroid hormones of the male squirrel monkey. *Arch. Androl.* 4 (2): 133–136.

51 Chrousos, G.P., Renquist, D., Brandon, D. et al. (1982). Glucocorticoid hormone resistance during primate evolution: receptor-mediated mechanisms. *Proc. Natl. Acad. Sci. U.S.A.* 79 (6): 2036–2040.

52 Klosterman, L.L., Murai, J.T., and Siiteri, P.K. (1986). Cortisol levels, binding, and properties of corticosteroid-binding globulin in the serum of primates. *Endocrinology* 118 (1): 424–434.

53 Diamond, E.J., Aksel, S., Hazelton, J.M. et al. (1984). Seasonal changes of serum concentrations of estradiol and progesterone in Bolivian squirrel monkeys (Saimiri sciureus). *Am. J. Primatol.* 6 (2): 103–113.

54 Bonney, R.C., Dixson, A.F., and Fleming, D. (1980). Plasma concentrations of oestradiol-17 beta, oestrone, progesterone and testosterone during the ovarian cycle of the owl monkey (Aotus trivirgatus). *J. Reprod. Fertil.* 60 (1): 101–107.

55 Nagle, C.A., Denari, J.H., Quiroga, S. et al. (1979). The plasma pattern of ovarian steroids during the menstrual cycle in capuchin monkeys (Cebus apella). *Biol. Reprod.* 21 (4): 979–983.

56 Wiebe, R.H., Williams, L.E., Abee, C.R. et al. (1988). Seasonal changes in serum dehydroepiandrosterone, androstenedione, and testosterone levels in the squirrel monkey (Saimiri boliviensis boliviensis). *Am. J. Primatol.* 14 (3): 285–291.

57 Dixson, A.F. and Gardner, J.S. (1981). Diurnal variations in plasma testosterone in a male nocturnal primate, the owl monkey (Aotus trivirgatus). *J. Reprod. Fertil.* 62 (1): 83–86.

58 Nagle, C. and Denari, J. (1982). The reproductive biology of capuchin monkeys. *Int. Zoo Yearb.* 22 (1): 143–150.

59 Weller, R.E., Buschbom, R.L., Málaga, C.A. et al. (1996). Serum and urine biochemical diversity among adult wild-caught Aotus nancymae and Saimiri peruviensis. *J. Med. Primatol.* 25 (1): 46–52.

60 Baer, J.F. (1994). Husbandry and medical management of the owl monkey. In: *Aotus: The Owl Monkey* (ed. J.F. Baer, R.E. Weller and I. Kakoma), 133–164. San Diego: Academic Press.

61 Weller, R.E., Málaga, C.A., Buschbom, R.L. et al. (1991). Protein concentration in urine of normal owl monkeys. *J. Med. Primatol.* 20 (7): 365–369.

62 Ford, E.W., Roberts, J.A., and Southers, J.L. (1998). Urogenital system. In: *Nonhuman Primates in Biomedical Research* (ed. B.T. Bennett, C.R. Abee and R. Henrickson), 311–362. Academic Press.

63 Mansfield, K. and King, J.A. (1998). Viral diseases. In: *Nonhuman Primates in Biomedical Research* (ed. B.T. Bennett, C.R. Abee and R. Henrickson), 311–362. Academic Press.

64 Perolat, P., Poingt, J.P., Vie, J.C. et al. (1992). Occurrence of severe leptospirosis in a breeding colony of squirrel monkeys. *Am. J. Trop. Med. Hyg.* 46 (5): 538–545.

65 Szonyi, B., Agudelo-Flórez, P., Ramírez, M. et al. (2011). An outbreak of severe leptospirosis in capuchin (Cebus) monkeys. *Vet. J.* 188 (2): 237–239.

66 Pinna, M.H., Martins, G., Pinheiro, A.C.O. et al. (2012). Detection of anti-Leptospira antibodies in captive nonhuman primates from Salvador, Brazil. *Am. J. Primatol.* 74 (1): 8–11.

67 Scarcelli, E., Piatti, R.M., Fedullo, J.D.L. et al. (2003). Leptospira spp detection by polymerase chain reaction (PCR) in clinical samples of captive black-capped capuchin monkey (Cebus apella). *Braz. J. Microbiol.* 34 (2): 143–146.

68 Zeman, D.H. and Baskin, G.B. (1985). Encephalitozoonosis in squirrel monkeys (Saimiri sciureus). *Vet. Pathol.* 22 (1): 24–31.

69 Beckwith, C., Peterson, N., Liu, J.J., and Shadduck, J.A. (1988). Dot enzyme-linked immunosorbent assay (dot ELISA) for antibodies to Encephalitozoon cuniculi. *Lab. Anim. Sci.* 38 (5): 573–576.

70 Shadduck, J.A. and Baskin, G. (1989). Serologic evidence of Encephalitozoon cuniculi infection in a colony of squirrel monkeys (Saimiri sciureus). *Lab. Anim. Sci.* 39 (4): 328–330.

71 Asakura, T., Nakamura, S., Ohta, M. et al. (2006). Genetically unique microsporidian Encephalitozoon cuniculi strain type III isolated from squirrel monkeys. *Parasitol. Int.* 55 (2): 159–162.

16

Tortoises and Freshwater Turtles

Charles Innis VMD, DABVP (Reptilian and Amphibian)[1] *and Zdenek Knotek DVM, PhD, DECZM*[2]

[1] *Department of Animal Health, New England Aquarium, Boston, Massachusetts, USA*
[2] *Avian & Exotic Animal Clinic, Faculty of Veterinary Medicine, University of Veterinary & Pharmaceutical Sciences, Brno, Czech Republic*

Introduction

Clinical pathology data can help assess health, diagnosis of disease, and development of prognoses for chelonians. The availability of clinicopathologic data for healthy specimens is increasing, but clinical information regarding the response of clinicopathologic values to specific disease states in these species remains limited. A large body of data has been produced historically in studies of basic chelonian biology and physiology [1, 2]. Many of these studies provide very detailed information about clinicopathologic data for individual species, seasonal effects, sexual differences, and responses to experimental manipulations. Clinicians should seek out this primary literature when interpreting clinicopathologic data for a given species. Clinicopathologic results for turtles may vary with season, age, gender, husbandry, venipuncture site, geographic location, and laboratory methodology [3–18]. Therefore, when such conditions are substantially different from those of published studies, the clinician must use good judgment in making data comparisons and drawing conclusions.

Species

Clinicopathologic data for freshwater turtles and tortoises, to include all non-marine chelonian species, will be reviewed in this chapter. The seven species of sea turtles are discussed only briefly where data are lacking for freshwater turtles and tortoises. The order Chelonia includes two suborders, Cryptodira, or hidden neck turtles, and Pleurodira, or side neck turtles. The majority of species encountered in clinical practice are members of Cryptodira, including species of the families Testudinidae and Emydidae. Well-known species of Testudinidae include Greek, Herman's, and Russian tortoises (*Testudo* spp.), leopard, spur-thigh, red-foot, yellow-foot tortoises (*Geochelone* spp.), and North American tortoises (Gopherus spp.). Well-known members of the Emydidae include box turtles, sliders, and pond turtles (e.g., *Emys, Terrapene, Trachemys, Pseudemys*, and *Chrysemys* spp.). Species for which clinical pathology data are presented are either commonly seen in clinical practice, or members of groups that are underrepresented in clinicopathologic data, for example, side neck turtles (e.g., *Podocnemis, Emydura, Elseya*, and *Phrynops* spp.), soft-shelled turtles (family Trionychidae), snapping turtles (family Chelydridae), family Geoemydidae (e.g., *Hieremys, Ocadia*, and *Mauremys* spp.), and monophyletic groups (e.g., Dermatemydidae). This data set is representative, but not exhaustive, and only includes data from peer-reviewed primary literature. Additional data for Mediterranean tortoises (*Testudo graeca, Testudo hermanni*), Bornean river turtle (*Orlitia borneensis*), Indian flapshell turtle (*Lissemys punctata*), map turtles (*Graptemys* spp.), Asian box turtle (*Cuora amboinensis*), and western pond turtle (*Emys marmorata*) are found in the peer-reviewed literature [15, 19–22]. Other data for species not reported here may be found in review chapters, formularies, and appendices of a number of previously published reptile biology and medicine texts, and in the former International Species Information System (now Species 360: www.species360.org).

Sample Collection

Restraint

Physical restraint is acceptable for blood collection in many chelonian species; however, large or dangerous turtles (e.g., giant tortoises, snapping turtles) may need to be sedated to allow access to venipuncture sites, and to ensure safety of the animals and veterinary staff. Shy species such as some box turtles, may also require chemical restraint for venous access. Detailed discussion

Exotic Animal Laboratory Diagnosis, First Edition. Edited by J. Jill Heatley and Karen E. Russell.

of sedation options for turtles is beyond the scope of this chapter. Injectable agents such as tiletamine-zolazepam, dexmedetomidine, ketamine, alfaxalone, or propofol are often useful [23–28]. Induction of sedation in turtles using gas anesthesia via mask or chamber is generally ineffective.

Blood Volume and Approach to Venipuncture

Blood accounts for 5%–8% body weight in turtles [29, 30]. The total blood volume of the red-eared slider (*Trachemys scripta elegans*) is approximately 80 ml blood per kg body weight [29]. Plasma accounts for 60%–80% of chelonian blood volume and is usually yellowish orange based on plant pigments, or colorless in carnivorous aquatic turtles [31, 32]. Clinically, 10% of the total blood volume can be safely taken from healthy turtles during a single venipuncture [30]. Thus, approximately 5–8 ml of blood can be safely taken from a turtle weighing 1 kg. The volume necessary for common laboratory examination is often much less. Complete blood counts, plasma biochemical analysis, and blood gas analysis can often be completed with less than 1 ml of blood, depending on the methodology. Considerable patience is required for chelonian blood collection. Flow of blood is often intermittent and slow. Gentle negative pressure and fine angular or rotational changes of the syringe position are often required.

Turtle and tortoise blood samples from turtles may be taken from the dorsal coccygeal vein, subcarapacial sinus, dorsal cervical sinus, jugular vein, occipital sinus, ulnar (brachial) venous plexus, femoral venous plexus, and heart [14, 29, 33–39]. Collection of blood by clipping toenails is generally contraindicated based on pain, contamination of the sample with extravascular debris, and risk of infection [36]. For almost all sites, veins are generally not visible externally. In some specimens, the jugular vein may be visible. Syringe volume is selected depending on test requirements. Needle size and length are selected depending on the size of the patient. Needles of 25–20 gauge (g.) and 0.5–5 cm length are useful. Smaller or larger sizes may be needed for juveniles or giant species, respectively. Butterfly catheters are preferred by come clinicians, especially for jugular venipuncture [35]. Disinfection of venipuncture sites with iodine, chlorhexidine, or alcohol is advised.

Dorsal Coccygeal Vein

Dorsal coccygeal (tail vein) venipuncture is practical in medium-sized and larger species, especially for males, which often have a larger tail than females (Figures 16.1 and 16.2). Turtles protect their tail by flexing it under the carapace. To expose the tail, an assistant should hold the turtle's carapace and fix the pelvic limbs in flexion. The phlebotomist grasps and extends the tail firmly so that it cannot flex or rotate. The blood collection site is

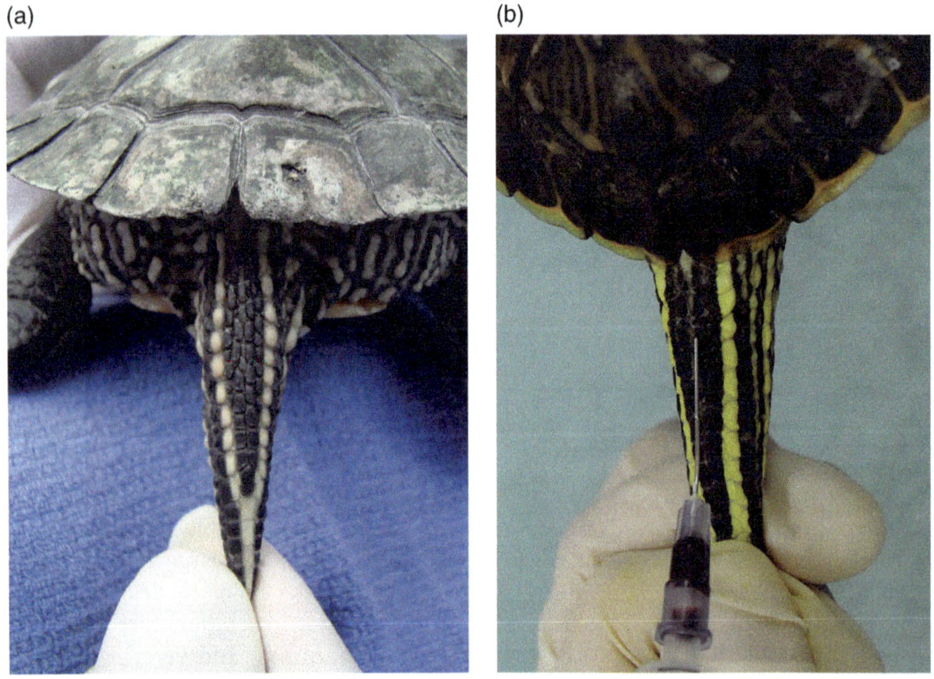

Figure 16.1 (a) Anatomy of the dorsal coccygeal venipuncture site in a male red-eared slider turtle. (b) Dorsal coccygeal venipuncture in a male red-eared slider turtle.

on the dorsal midline of the tail [33, 40, 41]. As the vessel is located relatively superficially, the insertion should be fairly shallow at a 45°–60° angle (no more than 90° from the surface of the tail). After the skin is penetrated, the needle is carefully inserted until it reaches the dorsal surface of the vertebrae while aspirating the plunger of the syringe. Fine changes in angle and depth are then made until the vessel is entered. After the needle is removed, compress the injection site to prevent significant bleeding, which often occurs during this procedure. Aspiration of clear fluid rather than blood may indicate lymph contamination. It is also possible to enter the intrathecal space at this location, leading to collection of cerebrospinal fluid, which may not be the desired sample [42]. Caution is warranted to avoid spinal trauma.

Venipuncture Sites of the Head

The subcarapacial sinus is located on the dorsal midline of the neck just anterior to the eighth cervical vertebra, at the confluence of branches of the jugular veins (Figures 16.3 and 16.4) [34]. It can be approached with the head restrained in extension or retraction. Muscles that turtles use for defensive retraction of the head and neck are very strong, and it is very difficult, or almost impossible, in large animals, to overcome their resistance without sedation. Pulling the head with clamps or forceps is largely ineffective and may lead to injury. If venipuncture is attempted with the head in retraction, there is a risk of movement and biting (especially in aquatic turtles). With the head retracted, gauze pads may be used to apply ventral pressure on the turtle's nose to prevent biting.

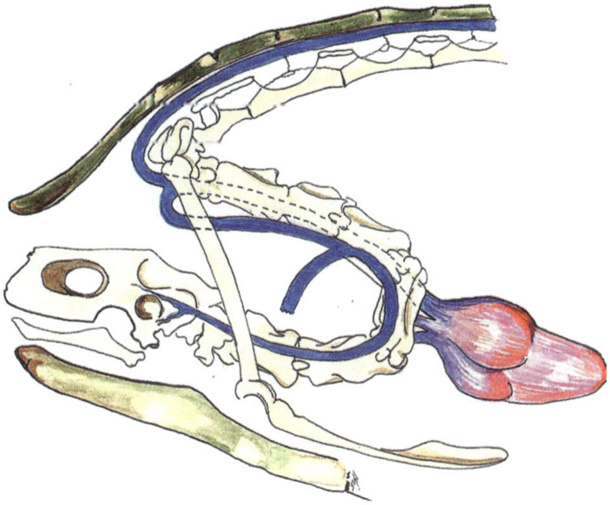

Figure 16.2 Sagittal anatomical diagram of the subcarapacial area for venipuncture of chelonian. Sampling may result in tetraparesis or death if the spinal cord is damaged.

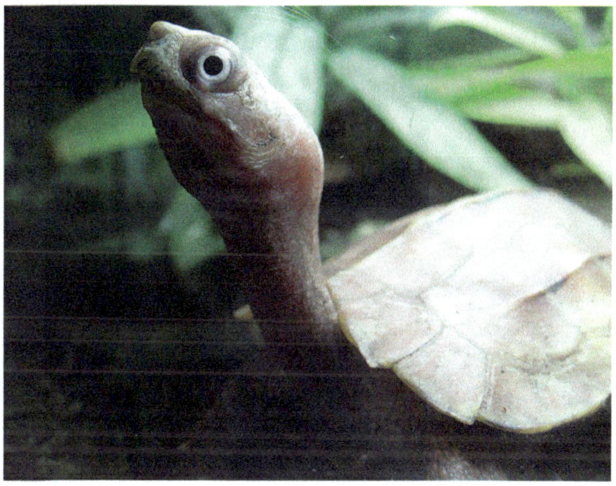

Figure 16.4 Visible jugular vein, as it courses along the left side of the extended neck of a black-breasted leaf turtle, *Geoemyda spengleri*.

(a) (b)

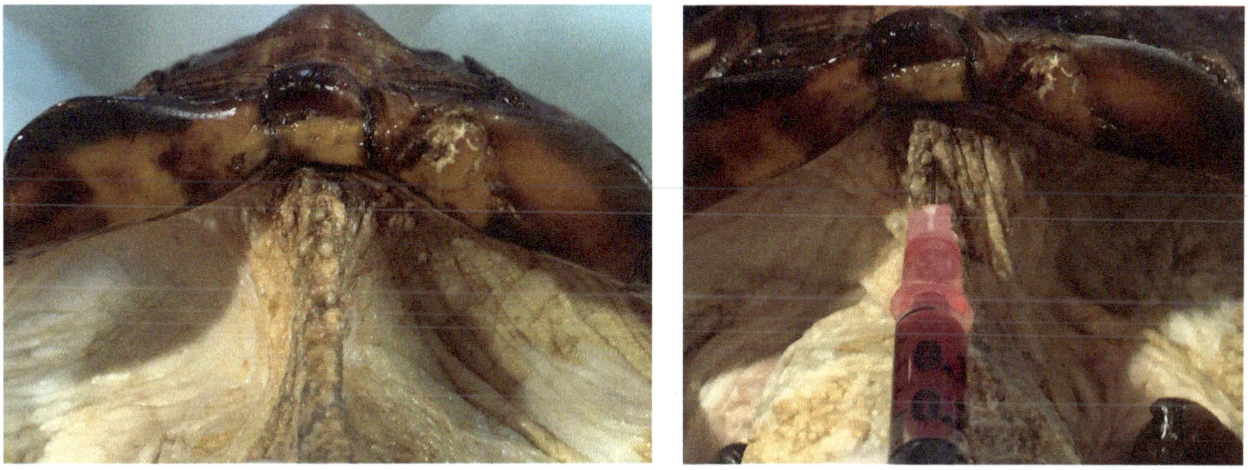

Figure 16.3 (a) Anatomy of the subcarapacial venipuncture site in an Asian pond turtle (*Mauremys mutica*). (b) Subcarapacial venipuncture in an Asian pond turtle (*Mauremys mutica*).

As with the dorsal coccygeal vein, lymph contamination or intrathecal penetration is possible. Several reports of transient or permanent neurologic injury and even death have been described when this site has been used for venipuncture or administration of intravenous anesthetics [43, 44]. Clinicians must use appropriate caution. Venipuncture is accomplished on the dorsal midline under the cranial edge of the carapace, with the needle angled toward the junction of the neck and the carapace until the vertebra is reached. Fine changes in angle and depth are then made until the vessel is entered.

Drawing blood from *dorsal cervical sinus* is similar to collection from the subcarapacial sinus, but the needle does enter under the carapace but rather more anteriorly toward the dorsal surface of the cervical vertebrae at a 45°–60° angle, with the head and neck held in extension. This method does not eliminate the risk of partial contamination of blood with lymph or cerebrospinal fluid (CSF). The *occipital sinus* is located at the base of the skull, lateral to the supraoccipital bone [37, 38]. Venipuncture is accomplished at an angle of 45°–90° from the skin with the head and neck restrained in extension. Lymph contamination is possible.

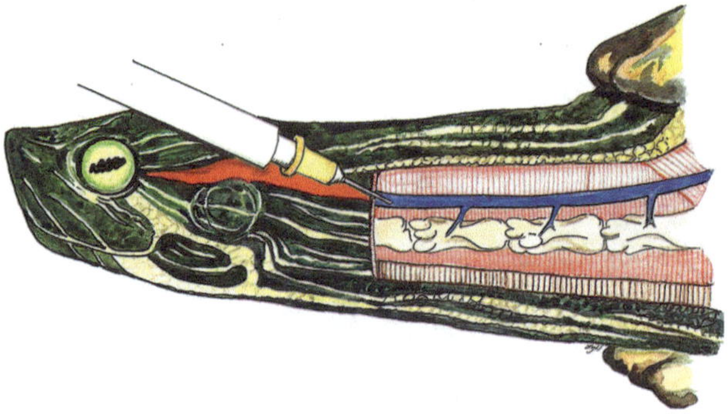

Figure 16.5 Anatomic diagram of jugular venipuncture site in a red-eared slider.

Jugular Veins

In medium-sized and larger turtles, *jugular veins* can often be seen externally, especially with the neck extended (Figure 16.5). If not visible, "blind" venipuncture is often successful. The veins generally run slightly dorsal to the lateral midline of the neck, approximately at the level of the ear (Figures 16.6 and 16.7). Jugular venipuncture may be unsafe for the venipuncturist in large (especially aquatic) turtles that are not sedated. If performed appropriately, this method minimizes the risk of contamination of blood with lymph. The animal

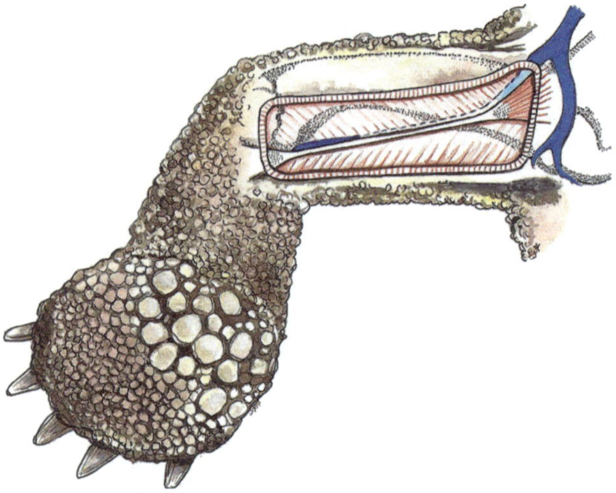

Figure 16.7 Ulnar (brachial) plexus venipuncture in a Burmese star tortoise (*Geochelone platynota*). The right forelimb is extended and abducted cranially, and the needle is inserted dorsal to the biceps toward the elbow.

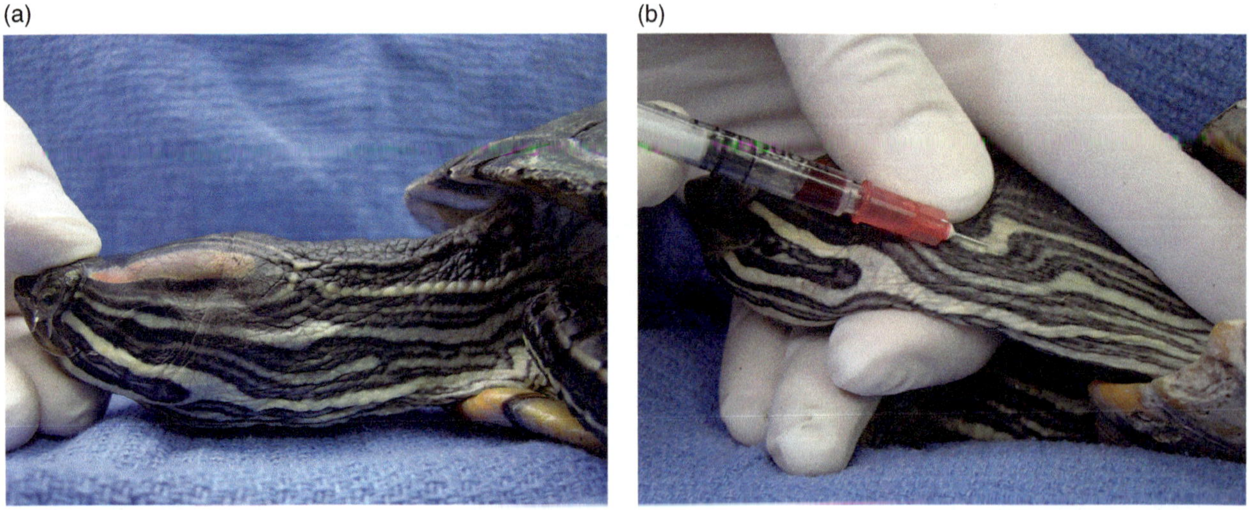

Figure 16.6 (a) Local anatomy and (b) jugular venipuncture in a red-eared slider turtle.

is restrained with the head and neck in extension. The head is slightly rotated and flexed laterally to expose the vein. Compression of the vein at the neck base can help to distinguish the vein from skin folds. Pressure should be applied after completion of venipuncture to prevent hematoma formation.

Venipuncture of the Limbs

Blood may be collected from *ulnar* or *brachial venous plexus* along the posterior aspect of the thoracic limb (Figure 16.8) [14, 45, 46]. For aggressive turtles, the head should be well fixated to prevent biting. This method is less useful in small turtles. The limb should be restrained in an extended position by pulling it slowly and firmly across the head. The needle is inserted at the caudal surface of thoracic limb just anterior to the elbow joint and directed toward the joint. Venipuncture of the femoral venous plexus has been used to collect blood from the diamondback terrapin [39].

Cardiocentesis

Cardiocentesis has been used in turtles for research, but is not the clinician's first choice [29]. A small trephination is made in the plastron at the level of the heart (generally on the midline at the caudal junction of the pectoral scutes). In very young turtles, a needle may directly penetrate the not yet fully mineralized plastron. After blood collection, closure with acrylic or similar materials is recommended. Drawbacks of this technique include the risk of contamination of the sample with pericardial fluid, and risk of damage to the heart.

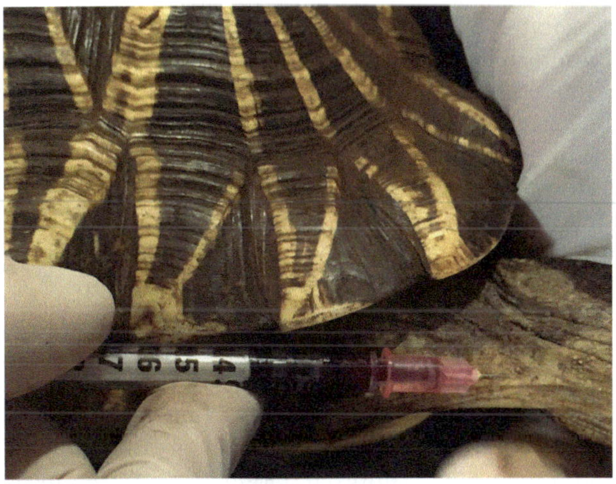

Figure 16.8 Anatomical diagram of the generalized approach for venipuncture of the ulnar vein in chelonian.

Sample Handling

Lymphatic Contamination

Lymphatic contamination will result in many changes to the hematologic sample collected from chelonia, such as decreased packed cell volume, red blood cell (RBC) count, and increased lymphocytes.

Biochemical results can also be influenced by the site from where blood is drawn owing to dilution of blood with lymph or cerebrospinal fluid [8, 10, 14, 47]. Many analytes (glucose, calcium, phosphorus, sodium, urea, and enzymes) have the same concentration in blood plasma, serum, and lymph. However, significantly decreased concentrations of glucose, total protein, potassium, uric acid, aspartate aminotransferase, alanine aminotransferase, lactate dehydrogenase, alkaline phosphatase, calcium, phosphorus, and cholesterol have been seen in lymph-contaminated samples [8, 10, 14]. In iguanas, hemolysis may increase plasma concentrations of potassium, phosphate, total protein, and aspartate aminotransferase (AST) activity; similar changes are presumed for chelonians [48]. Hemolysis results in increased plasma activities of lactate dehydrogenase (LDH) and AST in some reptiles based on high intra-erythrocytic activities of these enzymes [49]; however, it is unclear whether this is true in chelonians.

Anticoagulants

Heparin is generally recommended for anticoagulation of chelonian hematologic and plasma biochemical samples. Commercially available pre-heparinized syringes are ideal, but good results are also obtained using plain syringes that are filled with liquid sodium heparin, which is then forcibly expelled as much as possible [50]. Alternatively, some clinicians prefer to collect the sample with no anticoagulant so that blood smears can be made without the artifactual changes that may be seen with heparin. In this case, blood smears are made immediately, and the remainder of blood is then transferred to commercially available tubes containing lithium heparin. While it is often stated that sodium heparin may affect plasma sodium values, this is generally not true clinically, as long as large volumes of sodium heparin are not used [51]. Additional discussion of heparin effects on biochemical data is provided below. While often used for hematologic analysis in other species, EDTA causes hemolysis in some chelonian species, such as the spiny soft-shelled turtle *(Apalone spinifera)*, Hermann's tortoise *(T. hermanni)*, and Kemp's ridley turtle (*Lepidochelys kempii*) (Innis, personal observation) [16, 47]. For some species [e.g., yellow-blotched map turtle (*Graptemys flavimaculata*), and gopher tortoise (*Gopherus polyphemus*)], EDTA does not cause hemolysis and may actually provide better cellular preservation that heparin [15, 52].

At this time, heparin is recommended, unless specific studies suggest otherwise for a given species. Use of serum for chelonian biochemical analysis is not recommended because of the relatively low volume of serum obtained from a given volume of blood, and the tendency for chelonian serum to sometimes clot even after centrifugation and separation (Innis, personal observation) [30, 31]. AST and (LDH) activities with the reptilian erythrocyte are typically high, although this has not been proved for chelonia [49]. While not specifically investigated in chelonians, hemolysis could result in increased plasma activities of AST and LDH and increased plasma concentrations of potassium, phosphorus, and total protein, as described for other reptiles [48].

Sample Storage

Blood samples should be processed as soon as possible. For the purpose of biochemical examination, centrifuge the blood immediately after collection, separate the plasma, and analyze it immediately, or store it under refrigeration until analysis. If significant delays are expected, the plasma sample may be frozen (ideally at −80 °C) prior to analysis. Despite these general recommendations, a recent study in loggerhead turtles showed no significant changes (except for gamma-glutamyl transferase, GGT) in blood biochemical results when whole blood was stored under refrigeration for 24 h prior to centrifugation and analysis [9]. However, one study showed that delayed separation led to decreased sodium and increased potassium values in two tortoise species [3]. Long-term fasting may affect the biochemical results of turtles [7, 29]; but results of postprandial biochemical analyses are generally not clinically different from results obtained after several days of fasting [53, 54].

Complete Blood Count

Reference intervals for complete blood count vary greatly based on species as well as a number of other factors (Tables 16.1 and 16.2). Chelonian hematologic analysis is conducted manually, with phloxine stain or Natt–Herrick's solution to facilitate cell identification and counting [70, 71]. Estimated leucocyte counts are inherently dependent on blood smear quality and consistency, and may produce discordant results when compared to hemocytometer methods [51]. Different cell counts may be obtained from the same blood sample using different methods [4, 51].

Erythrocytes and Thrombocytes

Chelonian erythrocytes, are the largest of any reptile group and are elliptical and nucleated (Figures 16.9–16.20). Box turtle (Terrapene sp.) erythrocytes live for 600–800 days [72]. Immature erythrocytes are generally more spherical, more basophilic, and have larger nuclei than mature cells. The healthy chelonian blood smear may contain 1–2 immature erythrocytes/100 RBC. Increased numbers of radioiron-labeled erythroblasts were seen within 48 h of blood collection in red-eared sliders, *T.s. elegans* [29]. Reticulocyte percentages of approximately 2%–3% occur in healthy red-eared sliders [30, 73]. Characterization of anemia is on the basis of low hematocrit and subjective assessments of polychromasia, anisocytosis, and numbers of immature erythrocytes. Anemia can occur in turtles with chronic infection, cold-torpor, and exposure to crude oil and organochlorine pesticides [17, 74–76]. Reticulocytosis (7%), anemia (HCT 10%), decreased hemoglobin, and decreased mean corpuscular hemoglobin concentration (MCHC) occurred based on serial bleeding of approximately 20% blood volume over 11 days in red-eared sliders [29]. Increased hematocrit and erythrocyte count can occur in cases of dehydration or prior to hibernation [e.g., box turtle (*Terrapene carolina*) and red-eared slider) [77, 78]. Scant data exist for erythrocyte indices of chelonians (Tables 16.1 and 16.2).

Thrombocytes are also elliptical but generally have a colorless cytoplasm, and are often found in clusters cytologically (Figures 16.1 and 16.2). These characteristics aid in differentiating thrombocytes from lymphocytes, which often have blue cytoplasm, rounder morphology, and are less likely to be clumped. Chelonian thrombocyte morphology, cytochemical staining, and function have been described [79–81]. Thrombocyte counts for reptiles are not routinely determined. Instead, thrombocyte counts are often subjectively estimated as reduced, adequate, or increased. Some studies present thrombocyte data as cells per 100 leucocytes, or include thrombocytes in the differential percentage of leucocytes, while others report more conventional thrombocyte counts (i.e., cells/μl). Reports of clinical thrombocytopenia in turtles appear absent.

Leukocytes

Chelonian leucocytes include heterophils, lymphocytes, eosinophils, basophils, and monocytes (Figures 16.9–16.15, 16.17). Some studies describe azurophils instead of, or in addition to monocytes (Tables 16.1, 16.2). Cytochemical studies of chelonian azurophils demonstrate monocyte-like staining properties [58, 79]. Detailed descriptions of the morphology of chelonian leucocytes, including cell, nuclear, and granule dimensions, histochemical staining, and ultrastructure are available [19, 58, 61, 79, 82–84]. Cell morphology is generally typical of other nonmammalian species. Heterophils and lymphocytes are generally the most numerous cell lines, with relatively lesser numbers of eosinophils, basophils, and monocytes. However, basophils are the most numerous cell line in some North American freshwater species such as the snapping turtle (*Chelydra serpentina*)

Table 16.1 Hematologic data for aquatic turtles.

Analyte	Units, SI (US)	Spiny soft-shelled turtle[a] [47] *Apalone spinifera*	Central American river turtle *Dermatemys mawii*[b,c] [27]	New Guinea snapping turtle[d] [55] *Elseya novaguineae*	Murray River turtle *Emydura macquarii krefftii* [56]	Bog turtle *Glyptemys muhlenbergii*[c,d] [57]	Yellow-headed temple turtle *Hieremys (Heomsemys) annandalii*[d,e,f] [58]	Alligator snapping turtle *Macrochelys temminckii* [59]	Diamond back terrapin *Malaclemys terrapin*[d] [6]	Spanish pond turtle *Mauremys leprosa*[d] [60]	Chinese stripe-necked turtle *Ocadia (Mauremys) sinensis*[b,d] [61]	Geoffroy's side-necked turtle *Phrynops geoffroanus*[d] [62]	Arrau turtle *Podocnemis expansa*[g] [63]	Northern red-bellied cooter *Pseudemys rubriventris*[e] [11]
Sample size & attributes		8–10, Ħ▣	10 Ó-▣ ♂♀ Ħ& ⲁ ☂	58–115 Ħ▣	20–35 ⲁ Ó-▣, healthy	32, Ó-▣, ♂♀, Ħ ⲁ	20♂20♀ ▣ Ħ ⲁ	90–106 ⲁ▣, Ó ♂♀	56–87 ⲁ, Ó-▣, ♂♀	56 ♂ 58♀ ⲁ▣	24♂ 26♀ ⲁ▣ June	36 ⲁ▣	24–28 ♂♀ Ħ, Ó-▣	30 Ħ Ó
Data format		Range	Range	Range	95% CI	Range	Mean ± SD	95% CI	Mean ± SD	95% CI or *[range]*	Central 95th percentile	Mean ± SD	Range	Range of 3 facilities
White blood cell count	×10⁹/l=(×10³/μl)	2.28–18.42	12–30.3	4.2–3.38	14.7–6.27	3–13	11.66 ± 6.59	11.2–13.4	11.3 ± 4.5	3.69–54.7♂ 3.47–5.33♀	4.213–19.627	2.7 ± 0.7♀ 2.8 ± 1.0♂	5.186–6.958	2.750–27.121
Absolute heterophils	x10⁹/l=(×10³/μl)	0.99–6.05[h]		1.4–12.8	6.6–38.9	0.7–3.78	3.43 ± 1.89	4.076–5.355			0–6.934		2.482–3.285	0.514–15.730
Lymphocytes	×10⁹/l=(×10³/μl)	0.38–2.400		0.8–28.4	0.1–15.3	0.98–8.52	1.63 ± 1.06	2.645–3.556			0–3.654		0.73–0.996	0.388–0.9379
Monocytes	×10⁹/l(×10³/μl)	0–0.24		0.6	0.3–0.87	0–0.34					0–0.897			0–0.410
Eosinophils	×10⁹/l=(×10³/μl)	0.99–6.05[h]		0–0.200	0.2-1.9	0–1.54	2.84 ± 1.89	2.276–2.863			1.650–8.930 ♂ 0.450–5.040♀		1.124–1.621	0–1.081
Basophils	×10⁹/l=(×10³/μl)	0.410–14.37		0–3.1	0	0.140–3.8	2.51 ± 1.55	0.813–1.733			0.77–5.150		0.364–0.618	1.127–17.852
Azurophils	×10⁹/l (×10³/μl)			0–5			1.23 ± 0.85	0.56–0.76					0.298–0.458	
Relative heterophils	%	15-57[h]	17–57			11.0-54	29.4 ± 6.88	37–43.3	74.6 ± 13.4	46.9–60.8♂ 52–65.1♀		42.5 ± 6.3♀ 45 ± 7.65♂	44.6–51	
Relative lymphocytes	%	6.0–21	31–63			14–71	14.81 ± 5.88	20.7–25.9	17.7 ± 12.6	4.9–7.7♂ 4.1–7.4♀		13.5 ± 4.86F♀ ♀11 ± 3.34♂	14–16.7	
Relative monocytes	%	0–4	0–7			0–34			2.3 ± 3	2.3–6.5♂ 0–11♀		11 ± 6.44♀ 13.5 ± 5.49♂		
Relative eosinophils	%	15-57[h]	5.0–31			0–22	23.69 ± 5.3	20.2–24.5	1.1 ± 1.9	28.5–42♂ 25.9–39.2♀		16 ± 5.3F ♀15.5 ± 8.11♂	20.6–24.7	
Relative basophils	%	18–78	0–2			2.0–33	21.23 ± 1.9	6.5–10.8	1.6 ± 2.1	*[0–2♂;0–1♀]*		7 ± 2.92♀ 7 ± 4.04♂	6.7–9.0	
Relative azurophils	%						10.73 ± 5.29	5–6.2	3.8 ± 3.5				5.4–7.2	
Hematocrit	l/l (%)	0.125–0.30 (12.5–30)	0.28–0.43 (28–43)	0.26–0.46 (26–46)		0.12–0.33 (12.0–33)	0.14–0.035 (14 ± 3.48)	0.221–0.244 (22.1–24.4)	0.318–0.076 (31.8 ± 7.6)	0.191–0.219♂ 0.172–0.198♀ (19.1–21.9♂ 17.2–19.8♀)	0.18–0.41♂ 0.24–0.45♀ (18–41♂24–45♀)	0.225–0.040♀ 0.24–0.041♂ (22.5 ± 3.99♀ 24 ± 4.1♂)	0.226–0.277 (22.6–27.7)	0.14–0.34 (14–34)
RBC	×10¹²/l(×10⁶/μl)	1.64–2.98	0.44–0.57				0.275 ± 0.094			0.34–0.5♂ 0.27–0.38♀	0.31–0.67	0.59 ± 0.21♀ 0.74 ± 0.27 ♂	0.25–0.3	

(*Continued*)

Table 16.1 (Continued)

Analyte	Units, SI (US)	Spiny soft-shelled turtle[a] [47] *Apalone spinifera*	Central American river turtle *Dermatemys mawii*[b,c] [27]	New Guinea snapping turtle[d] [55] *Elseya novaguineae*	Murray River turtle *Emydura macquarii krefftii* [56]	Bog turtle *Glyptemys muhlenbergii*[c,d] [57]	Yellow-headed temple turtle *Hieremys (Heomsemys) annandalii*[d,e,f] [58]	Alligator snapping turtle *Macrochelys temminckii* [59]	Diamond back terrapin *Malaclemys terrapin*[d] [6]	Spanish pond turtle *Mauremys leprosa*[d] [60]	Chinese stripe-necked turtle *Ocadia (Mauremys) sinensis*[b,d] [61]	Geoffroy's side-necked turtle *Phrynops geoffroanus*[d] [62]	Arrau turtle *Podocnemis expansa*[g] [63]	Northern red-bellied cooter *Pseudemys rubriventris*[e] [11]
Sample size & attributes		**8–10, Ħ₪**	**10 Ó-₪ ♂♀ Ħ& ϡ 🌧**	**58–115 Ħ₪**	**20–35 ϡ Ó-₪, healthy**	**32, Ó-₪, ♂♀, Ħ ϡ**	**20♂20♀ ₪ Ħ ϡ**	**90–106 ϡ₪, Ó ♂♀**	**56–87 ϡ, Ó-₪, ♂♀**	**56 ♂ 58♀ ϡ₪**	**24♂ 26♀ ϡ₪ June**	**36 ϡ₪**	**24–28 ♂♀ Ħ, Ó-₪**	**30 Ħ Ó**
Data format		**Range**	**Range**	**Range**	**95% CI**	**Range**	**Mean ± SD**	**95% CI**	**Mean ± SD**	**95% CI or *[range]***	**Central 95th percentile**	**Mean ± SD**	**Range**	**Range of 3 facilities**
Hb	g/l (g/dl)		18-33[j] (1.8–3.3)				60.8 ± 11.2 (6.08 ± 1.12)		96 ± 11 (9.6 ± 1.1)		35–75 (3.5–7.5)	66.6 ± 21.2♀ 72.2 ± 19.2♂ (6.66 ± 2.12♀ 7.22 ± 1.92♂)	58–72 (5.8–7.2)	
MCV	fl		538.3–811.3				595.3 ± 209.5			*[292.2–2411.8♂ 259.2–2149♀]*	426–921	32.84 ± 7.66 ♀ 32.09 ± 7.42[i]♂	866.7–977.9	
MCH	Pg		33.3–62.3				245.9 ± 91.5				78–151	0.6 ± 0.16♀ 0.49 ± 0.19[i]♂		
MCHC	g/l (g/dl)		500–1036 (50–103.6)[j]				428.5 ± 116.7 (42.8 ± 11.7)				130–210 (13.0–12.0)	312.5 ± 83.2♀ 301.9 ± 80.1♂ (31.25 ± 8.32♀ 30.19 ± 8.01♂)	242–282 (24.4–28.2)	
Thrombocytes	$\times 10^9$/l ($\times 10^3$/μl)				1.1–22.0		10.97 ± 5.4				2.57–14.99		3.34–4.76	

[a] Venipuncture site differences reported.
[b] Seasonal differences reported.
[c] Cell dimension data described.
[d] Sex differences reported.
[e] Geographic differences seen.
[f] Health status differences observed.
[g] See Rossini et al. [64] for female post-nesting data.
[h] Heterophils and eosinophils were reported in aggregate as acidophils.
[i] Data are an order of magnitude lower than most other studies. Suspect error.
[j] Assumed data from manuscript are g/l.
[k] Cytochemical stain data described.
[l] Methodology differences observed.

Table 16.2 Hematologic data for select tortoise species.

Analyte (abbreviation)	Units SI (US)	Chaco tortoise *Chelonoidis chilensis*[a,b] [65]	Aldabra tortoise *Geochelone gigantea*[c] [33]	Radiated tortoise *Geochelone radiata*[a,d,e] [66]	Desert tortoise *Gopherus agassizii*[a,d,f–h] [6]	Gopher tortoise *Gopherus polyphemus*[a,d,i] [52]	Pancake tortoise *Malacochersus tornieri* [67]	Greek tortoise *Testudo graeca*[a] [13]	Hermann's tortoise *Testudo hermanni*[a,j] [13]	Horsfield's tortoise *Testudo horsfieldii*[k,l] [68]	Marginated tortoise *Testudo marginata*[m,o] [14]
Sample Size		150	90	8–10	98	7–17	24–26	12	6	20	7
Attributes		Ó-₪ ♀♂☼	Ó ₪ ♀♂ ⁄	10♂ 8♀ ₪ Ħ☼	₪ ♀♂ ⁄ ☼	7–17 ♀♂ Ħ	♀♂ ⁄	₪ ♀♂ Ħ, June	₪ ♀♂ Ħ, June	₪ ♀♂ Ħ	Ó-₪ ♀♂ Ħ
Data format		Mean ± SD	Mean ± 2SD	Range	95%CI	Mean ± SE	Mean ± SD	Mean ± SD	Mean ± SD	Range	Range
White blood cell (WBC) count	×10^9/l=(×10^3/μl)	11.2 ± 2.5	2.17 ± 1.03 ♂ 2.49 ± 1.07 ♀	5–13♂ 4.3–12♀		15.7 ± 0.908		7.1 ± 1.6	9.8 ± 2.3		2.7–7.8
Heterophils	×10^9/l=(×10^3/μl)		1.51 ± 0.63 ♂ 1.83 ± 0.86 ♀	1.4–6♂ 2.3–5.7♀	0.719–7.159						0.570–3.93
Lymphocytes	×10^9/l=(×10^3/μl)		0.23 ± 0.12 ♂ 0.27 ± 0.15 ♀	2.4–5.2♂ 2.6–5.8♀	0.063–2.746						1.12–5.54
Monocytes	×10^9/l=(×10^3/μl)			0–0.2♂ 0–0.4♀	0–0.324						0–0.310
Eosinophils	×10^9/l=(×10^3/μl)		0.47 ± 0.27 ♂ 0.49 ± 0.39 ♀	0–0.2♂ 0–0.1♀	0–0.95						0–0.86
Basophils	×10^9/l=(×10^3/μl)		0.06♂ 0.05 ± 0.08 ♀	0.4–2.5♂ 0.4–1.5♀	0.062–3.574						
Azurophils	×10^9/l=(×10^3/μl)		0.47♂ 0.61♀		0–0.557						
Thrombocytes	×10^9/l=(×10^3/μl)	6.2 ± 2.5	4 ± 3♂ 5 ± 4♀			12.3 ± 0.11					
Heterophils	%	29 ± 2.3				30.3 ± 3.60[a]				13–45.6	21–77
Lymphocytes	%	25 ± 2.3				56.6 ± 3.68				36.1–75.6	22–71
Monocytes	%	4 ± 2.5				7.4 ± 0.97				0.1–2.1	0–4
Eosinophils	%	32 ± 5				30.3 ± 3.60[a]				2–5.9	0-24
Basophils	%	1 ± 1.3				5.7 ± 0.84				2–7.6	
Azurophils	%	8 ± 2								3.3–12	
Hematocrit	l/l(%)	0.21 ± 0.035 (21.35 ± 3.5)	0.14 ± 0.04♂ 0.18 ± 0.04♀ (14 ± 4♂ 18 ± 4♀)	0.32–0.51♂ 0.23–0.42♀ (32–51♂ 23–42♀)	0.19–0.35♂ 0.18–0.34 ♀(19–34.5 ♂ 18–33.6♀)	0.227 ± 0.012 (22.7 ± 1.18)	0.34 ± 0.38 (34 ± 3.77)	0.28(28)	0.29 ± 0.07 (29 ± 7)		0.21–0.27 (21–27)

(*Continued*)

Table 16.2 (Continued)

Analyte (abbreviation)	Units SI (US)	Chaco tortoise *Chelonoidis chilensis*[a,b] [65]	Aldabra tortoise *Geochelone gigantea*[c] [33]	Radiated tortoise *Geochelone radiata*[a,d,e] [66]	Desert tortoise *Gopherus agassizii*[a,d,f–h] [6]	Gopher tortoise *Gopherus polyphemus*[a,d,i] [52]	Pancake tortoise *Malacochersus tornieri* [67]	Greek tortoise *Testudo graeca*[a] [13]	Hermann's tortoise *Testudo hermanni*[a,j] [13]	Horsfield's tortoise *Testudo horsfieldii*[k,l] [68]	Marginated tortoise *Testudo marginata*[m,o] [14]
Sample Size		150	90	8–10	98	7–17	24–26	12	6	20	7
Attributes		Ó-₪ ♀♂☼	Ó ₪ ♀♂ ⍀	10♂ 8♀ ₪ Ħ☼	₪ ♀♂ ⍀ ☼	7–17 ♀♂ Ħ	♀♂ ⍀	₪ ♀♂ Ħ, June	₪ ♀♂ Ħ, June	₪ ♀♂ Ħ	Ó-₪ ♀♂ Ħ
Data format		Mean ± SD	Mean ± 2SD	Range	95%CI	Mean ± SE	Mean ± SD	Mean ± SD	Mean ± SD	Range	Range
Red blood cell (RBC) count	$\times10^{12}$/l=($\times10^6$/μl)	0.599 ± 0.025	0.28 ± 0.09 ♂ 0.32 ± 0.08 ♀	0.5–1.5♂ 0.5–1.1♀	0.36–1.08♂ 0.39–0.94♀	0.536 ± 0.054		0.67 ± 0.12	0.67 ± 0.15		0.43–0.77
Hemoglobin	g/l (g/dl)	94 ± 13 (9.4 ± 1.3)	35.9 ± 10.6 ♂ 42 ± 10.1 ♀(3.59 ± 1.06♂ 4.21.01 ± ♀)		52–99♂ 41–91♀ (5.2–9.9♂ 4.1–9.1♀)	63.9 ± 3.8 (6.4 ± 0.38)		91 ± 14 (9.1 ± 1.4)	93 ± 13 (9.3 ± 1.3)		52–73 (5.2–7.3)
Mean corpuscular volume (MCV)	fl	356 ± 23	495 ± 65.1 ♂ 544.4 ± 84.3♀		254–638			427 ± 16.3	425.5 ± 12.1		337.7–511.6
Mean corpuscular hemoglobin (MCH)	pg	156 ± 63	132.1 ± 30.2♂ 129.6 ± 19.1 ♀		74–186			137.3 ± 8.1	136.9 ± 6.4		85.7–138.3
Mean corpuscular hemoglobin concentration (MCHC)	g/l (g/dl)	446 ± 57 (44.6 ± 5.7)	268 ± 63 ♂ 242 ± 30 ♀ (26.8 ± 6.3 ♂ 24.2 ± 3.0 ♀)		200–330 (20–30)			322 ± 21 (32.2 ± 2.1)	322 ± 10 (32.2 ± 1.0)		236–286 (23.6–28.6)

[a] Seasonal differences seen.
[b] Suspect unit error for MCV, manuscript cites pg.
[c] Likely lymph or CSF contamination based on description.
[d] Sex differences seen.
[e] Additional data for this species in reference [69].
[f] Methodology differences seen.
[g] Geographic differences seen.
[h] Location data shown for largest sample size; additional data references [5, 6, 10, 46, 68–70].
[i] EDTA, heterophils not differentiated from eosinophils.
[j] Cell dimension data described. Additional data for this species in reference [72].
[k] Cell dimension data described.
[l] Cytochemical stain data described.
[m] Venipuncture site differences seen.
[n] Granulocytes.
[o] Brachial vein.

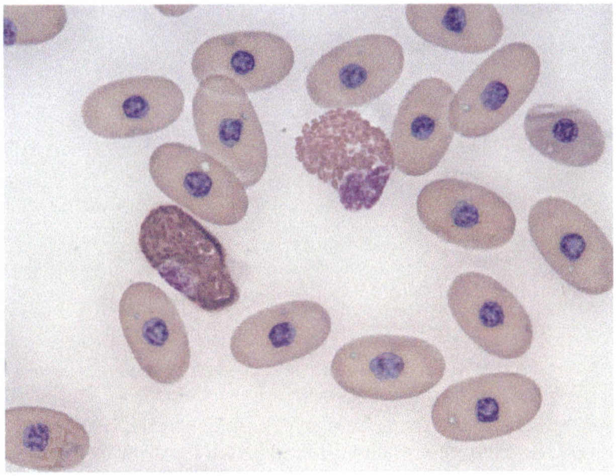

Figure 16.9 Heterophil (left) and eosinophil (right) of the common snapping turtle, *Chelydra serpentina*. Modified Wright's stain.

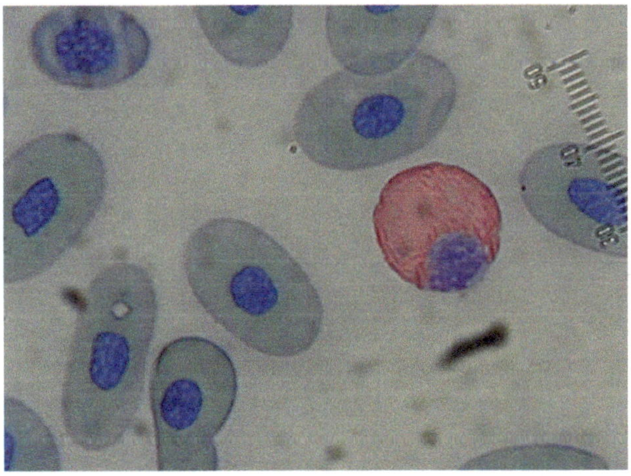

Figure 16.10 Heterophil, northern red-bellied cooter, *Pseudemys rubriventris*. Methanol-based quick stain.

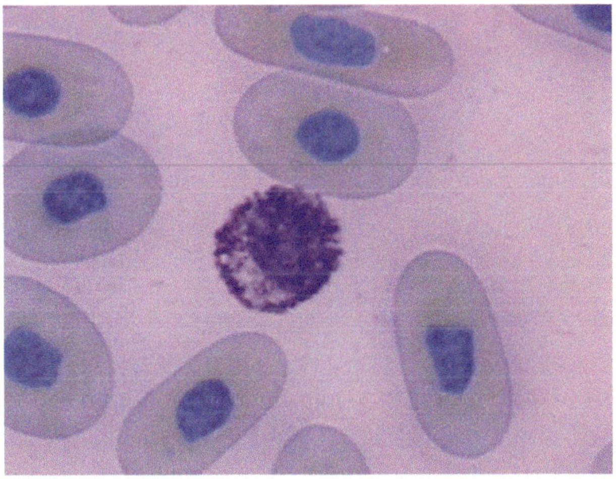

Figure 16.11 Basophil, northern red-bellied cooter, *Pseudemys rubriventris*. Methanol-based quick stain.

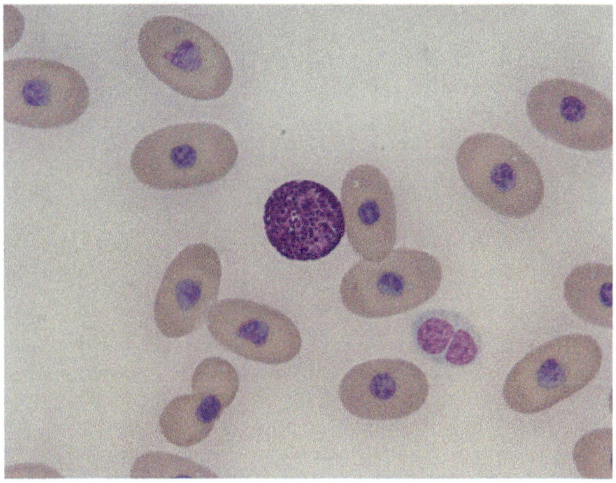

Figure 16.12 Basophil (left) and binucleate lymphocyte (lower right) of the common snapping turtle, *Chelydra serpentina*. Modified Wright's stain.

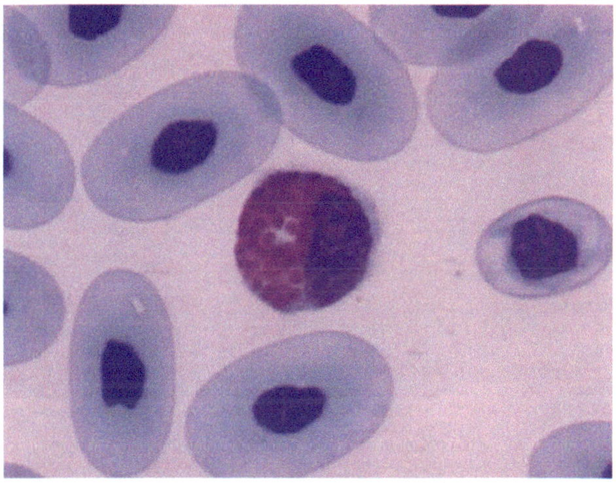

Figure 16.13 Eosinophil, northern red-bellied cooter, *Pseudemys rubriventris*.

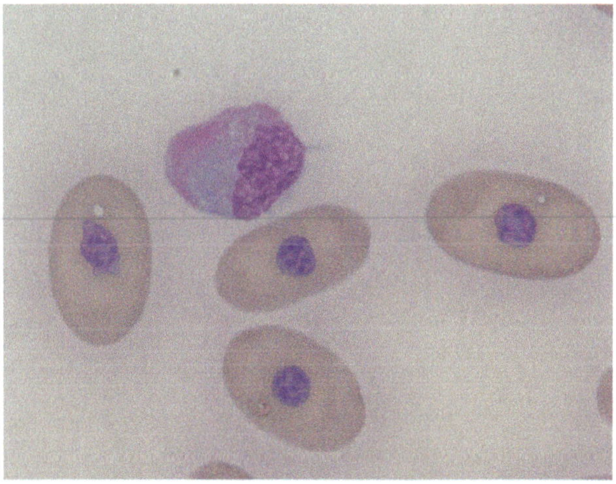

Figure 16.14 Azurophil (Azurophilic monocyte) of the common snapping turtle, *Chelydra serpentina*, modified Wright's stain. Small clear areas, reminiscent of vacuoles, are drying artifacts common to many chelonian species' blood smears.

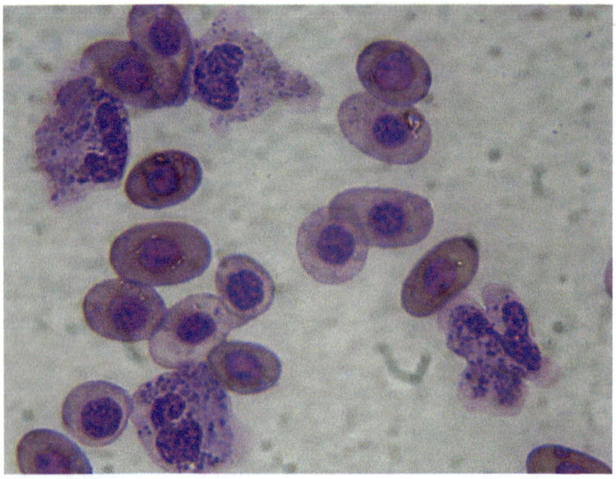

Figure 16.15 Heterophils from a moribund impressed tortoise (*Manouria impressa*) demonstrating toxic degenerative changes. Necropsy revealed severe hepatic infection and necrosis. Methanol-based rapid stain.

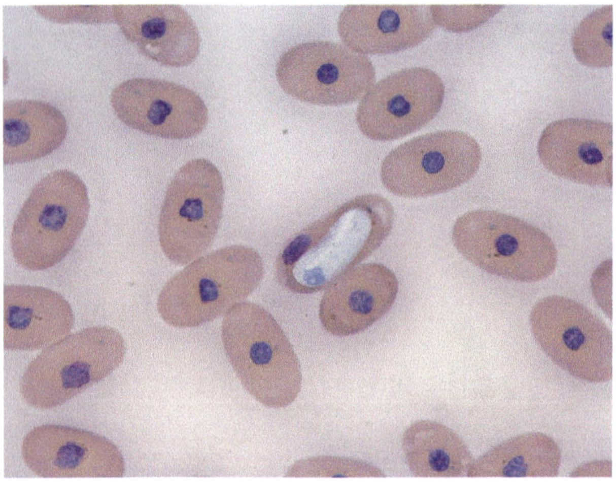

Figure 16.16 Intracytoplasmic hemogregarine in an erythrocyte of the common snapping turtle, *Chelydra serpentina*, modified Wright's stain.

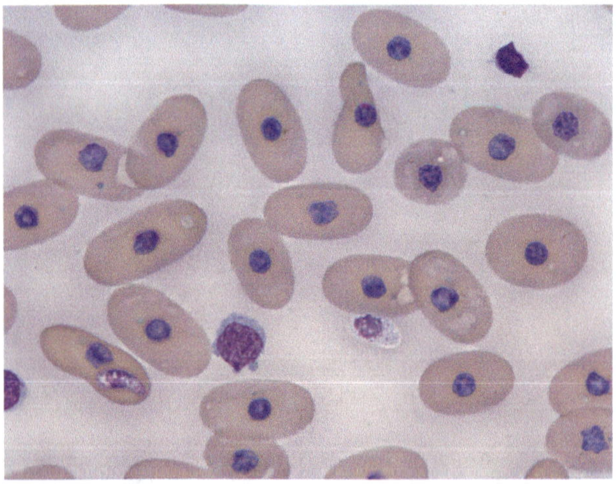

Figure 16.17 Lymphocyte, thrombocyte, intracytoplasmic and extracytoplasmic haemogregarines. Drying artifact manifesting as cytoplasmic clearing is present in multiple erythrocytes of the common snapping turtle, *Chelydra serpentina*, modified Wright's stain.

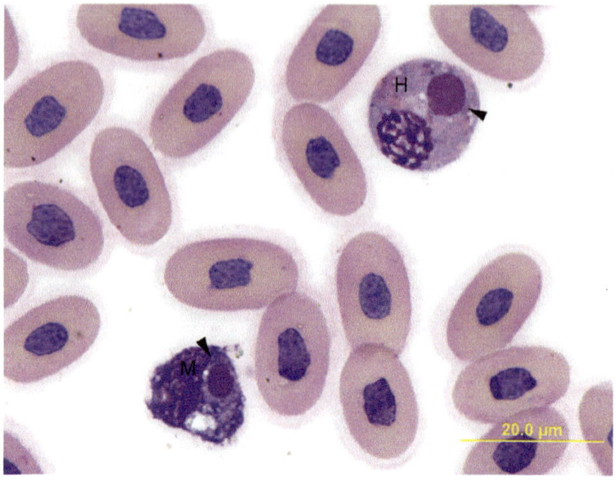

Figure 16.18 Blood smear from an eastern box turtle, *Terrapene carolina carolina*. Pink, granular, round to oval iridoviral inclusions (arrowheads) in a heterophil (H) and monocyte (M). *Source:* Image courtesy of Michael Fry.

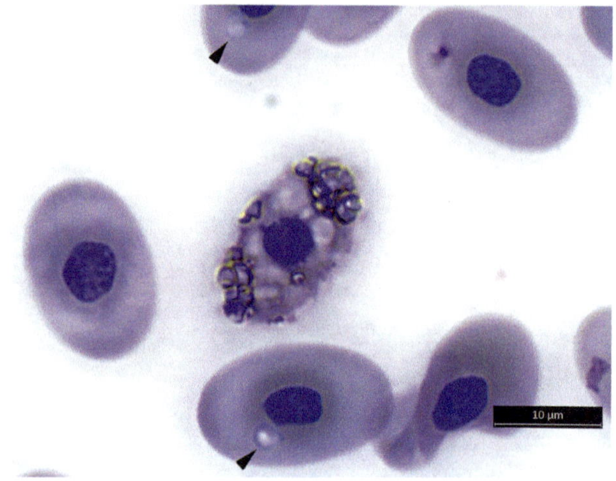

Figure 16.19 Blood smear of a diamondback terrapin, *Malaclemys terrapin* showing an erythrocyte with pleomorphic refractile drying artifact (center) and two erythrocytes with clear inclusions (arrowheads) consistent with degenerate organelles. *Source:* Image courtesy of Nicole Stacy.

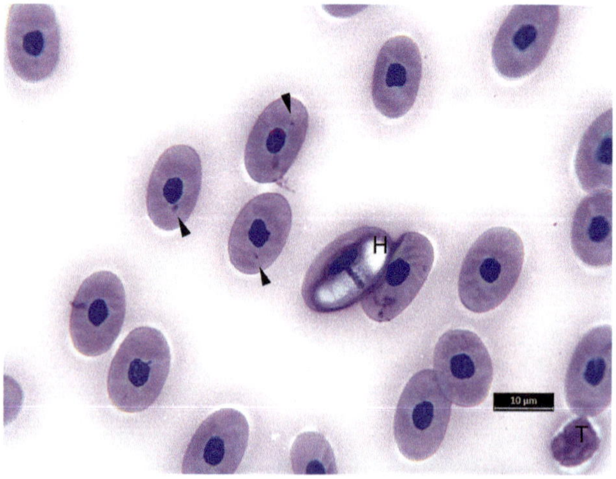

Figure 16.20 Blood smear of a gopher tortoise, *Gopherus polyphemus*, showing an erythrocyte with intracytoplasmic hemogregarine gametocyte (H), other erythrocytes with small distinct basophilic inclusions consistent with degenerate organelles (arrowheads), and a thrombocyte (T). *Source:* Image courtesy of Nicole Stacy.

and red-bellied cooter (*Pseudemys rubriventris*) [11, 85, 86] (Figures 16.11, 16.12). Turtle basophils contain histamine, carry surface immunoglobulins, and have immune capabilities similar to mammalian basophils and mast cells [85, 86].

Abnormal absolute and relative leucocyte counts occur in clinically ill turtles suffering infection, parasitism, cold stunning, crude oil exposure, myeloproliferative neoplasia, mercury exposure, and organochlorine pesticide exposure [5, 21, 56, 75, 76, 87–89]. Winter eosinophilia and lymphopenia occur in the European pond turtle (*Emys orbicularis*) [2]. Lymphopenia was induced by testosterone injection in the Caspian pond turtle (*Mauremys caspica*) [90]. Eosinophilia may or may not be present during parasitism in chelonians [2, 89]. Eosinopenia was induced by experimental cold exposure, while eosinophilia was induced by epinephrine injection in red-eared sliders [91]. Heteropenia was reported during fenbendazole treatment of Hermann's tortoises, although a control group was not used [92]. Degenerative changes of chelonian heterophils including hypersegmentation of nuclei, cytoplasmic vacuolization, and increased cytoplasmic basophilia may occur in the presence of severe infection and tissue necrosis (Figure 16.12).

Hemoparasites

Intracytoplasmic hemogregarine parasites are frequently seen in erythrocytes of free-ranging chelonians, and are generally considered non-pathogenic in moderate numbers (Figure 16.16 and 16.17) [89, 93]. In the presence of concurrent disease, or large numbers, hemogregarines may have an adverse effect [21]. Intracytoplasmic erythrocytic inclusions of unknown etiology were reported in eastern painted turtles (*Chrysemys picta picta*) [94]. Intraerythrocytic inclusions with cytochemical and ultrastructural properties of Heinz bodies were recently identified in loggerhead turtles (*Caretta caretta*) [95]. Intracytoplasmic coccidian merozoites were described in lymphocytes and plasma cells from a radiated tortoise (*Geochelone radiata*) [96]. Single, red, round intracytoplasmic inclusion bodies containing ranavirus were seen in heterophils and mononuclear leucocytes of a moribund eastern box turtle [74]. Inclusions must be differentiated from artifacts of blood smear preparation, drying, fixation, and staining (Figures 16.14 and 16.17).

Hemostasis

Mean coagulation times for eastern box turtles and red-eared sliders were 3.4 min and 14 min for active turtles, respectively, and 4.5 and 10.6 min for hibernating turtles, respectively [97]. Mean and standard deviations (mean ± SD) of prothrombin time, partial thromboplastin time (seconds), and plasma fibrinogen concentration (mg/dL) in healthy radiated tortoises and leopard tortoises (*Geochelone pardalis*) were 26.9 ± 7.3, 88.5 ± 28.2 and 325 ± 372.5; and 24.1 ± 16.1; 30.1 ± 8; and 273.3 ± 30.5 mg/dl, respectively [98]. Times for Quick test and PTT in both terrestrial and aquatic turtles have also been determined [99]. Clinical cases of coagulopathy in turtles appear absent.

Biochemical Panel (Tables 16.3–16.5)

The tissues of origin of commonly measured plasma enzymes have not been determined for freshwater and terrestrial chelonian species. At this time, interpretation is based on extrapolation from limited data available for other reptiles, including one sea turtle species [109–111]. Increased plasma enzyme concentrations in ill turtles are common [77]. Biochemical parameters relevant for assessment of turtles' health state include concentrations of total protein, albumin and globulin, urea, uric acid, calcium, phosphorus, chloride, sodium, potassium, and activity of aspartate aminotransferase (AST), alanine aminotransferase (ALT), alkaline phosphatase (ALP), GGT, creatine kinase (CK), and bile acids. Because creatinine and bilirubin are produced in minimal quantities, they are generally not important to assess for turtles [52, 68, 77, 112, 113].

Liver Biomarkers

In reptiles, biliverdin is a predominant bile pigment. Biliverdin concentrations are not routinely determined by biochemical laboratories, and a commercial assay is unavailable. While not specifically investigated for turtles, yellow-green coloration of plasma could also be caused by increased concentrations of biliverdin as reported in lizards [114]. Hyperbiliverdinemia may result in green discoloration of blood plasma; however, this analyte's utility in determination of liver disease is unknown in chelonia [54]. Bile acids are produced in the liver during metabolism of cholesterol. They emulsify fat in the intestine to produce micelles. The basic structure of primitive reptilian bile acids consists of 3α, 7α-dihydroxy-5ß-cholestan-27-oic acid or trihydroxycoprostanoic acid [115]. All chelonians have another hydroxyl group on the carbon 22 of the side chain, forming sterocholanic acid, and some have a hydroxyl group in the 12 alpha position of the ring. Most bile acids in reptiles are secreted as taurine conjugates [115]. Relatively few studies have evaluated bile acids in turtles (Tables 16.3 and 16.4) [54, 104]. A postprandial increase in bile acids was not seen in red-eared slider turtles [54]. Correlation of bile acids concentrations with histopathologic changes in the liver have not been described for chelonians.

The tissue distribution and utility of many of the analytes commonly used for detection of liver disease in companion mammals have not been determined for freshwater and terrestrial chelonians. In the reptile species that have been evaluated to date, including one

Table 16.3 Biochemical data of select aquatic turtle species.

Analyte	Units SI (US)	Spiny soft-shelled turtle[a] [47] *Apalone spinifera*	Central American river turtle[b,c] [100] *Dermatemys mawii*	New Guinea snapping turtle[d,e] [55] *Elseya novaguineae*	Murray River turtle[f] [56] *Emydura macquarii krefftii*	European pond turtle [101] *Emys orbicularis*	Bog turtle[c,d] [57] *Glyptemys muhlenbergii*
Sample size & attributes		**8–10 ₪Ħ**	**10 Ó-₪ ♂♀ 💧⟩ Ħ**	**58–115 ₪♂♀ Ħ**	**20–35 Ó-₪♂♀ ⟩ healthy**	**10 ₪♂♀ Ħ ⟩**	**32 Ó-₪ ♂♀ ⟩**
Data format		**Range**	**Range**	**95% CI**	**Range**	**Range**	**Range**
Alkaline phosphatase (ALP)	U/l	56–482		28–168	21.6–74.3		
Alanine transaminase (ALT)	U/l	<3–14		0–17		2.9–20.6	
Aspartate transaminase (AST)	U/l	20–122		26–575	69.3–1827.8	82.4–200	28–282
Creatine kinase (CK)	U/l	38–727		53–5644	306.9–93 430		49–1454
Lactate dehydrogenase (LDH)	U/l				773.215 526	575–1880	
Gamma-glutamyl transferase (GGT)	U/l	<5–7				1.0–4.0	
Albumin	g/l (g/dl)	<10–17 (<1–1.7)	8.0–14 (0.8–1.4)	4.0–30 (0.4–3.0)	5.7–19.1 (0.57–1.91)	4.7–11 (0.47–1.1)	3.0–14(0.3–1.4)
Total protein (TP)	g/l (g/dl)	<20–49 (<2–4.9)	20–30 (2.0–3.0)	15–79 (1.5–7.9)	20.4–58.2 (2.04–5.82)	14.7–33.60 (1.47–3.36)	12.0–45(1.2–4.5)
Globulin	g/l (g/dl)				15.3–441.53–4.4	5.2–26.40. 52–2.64	9.0–320.9–3.2
Bilirubin TBIL	μmol/l (mg/dl)		0.171–0.513 (0.01–0.03)	0–0.68 (0–0.4)			
Blood urea nitrogen (BUN)	mmol /l (mg/dl)	1.8–18.6 (5.0–52)	0.7–1.78 (2.0–5)	1.1–28.6 (3.0–80)	0.6–3.9 (1.7–10.9)	7.41–15.96 (20–44.7)	0.7–18.6(2.0–52)
Creatinine	μmol/l (mg/dl)			0–44.2 (0–0.50	10.6–24.3 (0.1–0.270	20.33–86.63 (0.23–0.98)	
Cholesterol	mmol /l (mg/dl)	<1.3–6.2 (<50–238)	2.2–4.4 (86–169)	1.4–10 (55–387)		0.98–1.79 (38–69)	
Glucose	Mmol /l (mg/dl)	1.9–3.2 (34–58)	2.3–5(41–91)	1.27–11.9 (23–215)	0.6–7.2 (11–130)	1.55–4.38 (28–79)	0.3–7.3(5–131)

Yellow-headed temple turtle[d] [58] *Hieremys (Heomsemys) annandalii*	Alligator snapping turtle[g] [59] *Macrochelys temminckii*[g]	Diamond back terrapin[d] [96] *Malaclemys terrapin*	Spanish pond turtle[d] [60] *Mauremys leprosa*	*Chinese stripe-necked turtle*[b,d] [61] *Ocadia (Mauremys) sinensis*	Arrau turtle[h] [63] *Podocnemis expansa*	Northern red-bellied cooter[i] [11] *Pseudemys rubriventris*	Red-eared slider[a] [8, 54] *Trachemys scripta elegans*
20♂ 20♀ ₪♂♀ Ħ ⱻ	**90–106 Ó-₪ ♂♀ ⱻ**	**56–87 Ó-₪ ♂♀ ⱻ**	**56 ♂;58 ♀₪ ⱻ**	**24♂;26♀₪ⱻ June**	**24–28 Ó-₪ ♂♀ Ħ**	**30 Ó Ħ**	**10[j]–36 ₪♀ Ħ**
Mean ± SD	**95% CI**	**Mean ± SD**	**95% CI [range]**	**95% CI**	**Range**	**Range of 3 institutions**	**Range ± SD or [Range][j]**
95 ± 54			31–42 ♂; 39–55 ♀	330–107 ♂ 37–93 ♀			212 ± 131
6 ± 4	20–25.9			0–10 ♂ 0–6 ♀			6–6 ± F
60 ± 39	151.2–184.2	218.1 ± 130.1	[27–531 ♂ 138–184 ♀]	57–153 ♂ 27–138 ♀		51–93	202 ± 217
	213.9–583	4194.1 ± 384	1193–1665 ♂ 1396–2080 ♀			321–1397	1288 ± 195
	5161.5–6272.2		839–1059 ♂ 815–1023 ♀				3625 ± 1236
	7.1–8.0						
4 ± 3 (0.4 ± 0.3)	7–8.1 (0.7–0.81)	13 ± 3 (1.3 ± 0.3)		8.0–28 ♂ 12.0–32 ♀ (0.8–2.8 ♂ 1.2–3.2 ♀)		11.0–19 (1.1–1.9)	[5–16.1♀ (0.5–1.61)]
42 ± 11 (4.2 ± 1.1)	39–44 (3.9–4.4)	41 ± 8 (4.1 ± 0.8)	28–38 ♂31–38 ♀(2.8–3.8 ♂ 3.1–3.8 ♀)	23–70 ♂ 32–70 ♀ (2.3–7 ♂3.2–7 ♀)	30–40 (3.0–4.0)	23–47 (2.3–4.7)	52.6 ± 12.1 (5.26 ± 1.21)
38 ± 10 3.8 ± 1.0		28 ± 6 2.8 ± 0.6		17–401.7-4		10.0–201-2.9	[6.4–20.7♀ 0.64–2.07♀]
5.0 ± 3.6 (14 ± 10)	7.6–10.1 (21.3–28.3)	37.4 ± 19.30 (104.7 ± 54)		1.1–14.63 (3.0–41)	1.1–1.8 (3.0–5.1)	1.4–18.9 (4.0–53)	8.9 ± 6 (53.4 ± 36)
<17.7(<0.2)	23.9–28.3 (0.27–0.32)		20.2–24 ♂ 20–24 ♀ (0.23–0.27 ♂0.23–0.27 ♀)	2.7(0–0.3)			
	1.3–1.7 (50.4–64)		1.9–2.7 ♂ 3.2–4.0 ♀ (73–104 ♂ 124–154 ♀)	0.9–8 ♂ 4–7.8 ♀ (34–310 ♂153–303 ♀)	1.32–1.7 (51–65.1)		2.1–9.8♀ (81–378♀)
2.2 ± 1.1 (40 ± 19)	2.4 ± 2.9 (43.5 ± 52.6)	5.55 ± 3.8 (100 ± 69)	3.1–4.2 ♂ 3.9–5.1 ♀ (56–76 ♂ 70–92 ♀)	3.7–8.3(66–150)	4.7–5.4 (84.9–97.7)	2.5–5.0 (45–91)	3.7 ± 2.6 (66.6 ± 46.8)

(Continued)

Table 16.3 (Continued)

Analyte	Units SI (US)	Spiny soft-shelled turtle[a] [47] *Apalone spinifera*	Central American river turtle[b,c] [100] *Dermatemys mawii*	New Guinea snapping turtle[d,e] [55] *Elseya novaguineae*	Murray River turtle[f] [56] *Emydura macquarii krefftii*	European pond turtle [101] *Emys orbicularis*	Bog turtle[c,d] [57] *Glyptemys muhlenbergii*
Sample size & attributes		8–10 ₪Ħ	10 Ó-₪ ♂♀ 💧⟩ Ħ	58–115 ₪♂♀ Ħ	20–35 Ó-₪♂♀ ⟩ healthy	10 ₪♂♀ Ħ ⟩	32 Ó-₪ ♂♀ ⟩
Data format		Range	Range	95% CI	Range	Range	Range
Calcium	mmol /l (mg/dl)		1.0–2.8 (4.2–11.3)	2.4–5.6 (9.6–22.3)	1.6–3.8 (6.4–15.2)		1.47–7.51 (5.9–30.1)
Ionized calcium (iCa)	Mmol/l	1.04–1.32[k]					
Phosphorous (P)	mmol /l (mg/dl)	0.6–2.3 (2–7.1)		0.03–2.6 (0.1–8.1)	0.6–1.5 (1.9–4.6)	1.13–2.03 (3.5–6.3)	0.48–3.62 (1.5–11.2)
Magnesium (Mg)	mmol /l (mEq/l)				0.8–1.5 (1.6–3.0)		
Total carbon dioxide (TCO2)	mmol /l			7.0–28			
Chloride (Cl)	mmol /l	89–102		74–105	91.5–107.3	89–101	75–110
Potassium (K)	mmol /l	2.6–4.2		1.6–4.4	2.8–6.5	3.1–5.6	2.2–4.4
Sodium (Na)	mmol /l	122–127		110–138	125.9–143.2	118–136	102–148
Uric acid	μmol/l (mg/dl)	<30–131 (<0.5–2.2)	35.7–161 (0.6–2.7)		59.8–280.2 (1–4.7)		18–446(0.3–7.5)
Triglycerides	mmol /l (mg/dl)		0.2–3.7 (18–326)			0.16–0.79 (14–700	
Bile acids	μmol /l (μg/ml)			0–1224 (0–500)[l]			

[a] Venipuncture site differences seen.
[b] Seasonal differences seen.
[c] Wild versus captive differences seen.
[d] Sex differences seen.
[e] Temperature effects seen.
[f] Health status differences seen.
[g] Da4ta for Zn, Cu, As, Se, Hg, Pb, organochlorine also provided.
[h] See also reference [101] for data on post-nesting females.
[i] Institutional differences seen.
[j] Bile acids, ALT, albumin, globulin, cholesterol, uric acid, triglycerides fasting ranges from Knotkova (n = 10 females),found no differences in chemistry data between fasting and postprandial turtles.
[k] iCa not pH corrected.
[l] Range cited as 0–50 mg/dl in manuscript. Suspect unit error, very high value compared to other chelonians when converted to more widely used units (ug/ml or umol/l).

Yellow-headed temple turtle[d] [58] *Hieremys (Heomsemys) annandalii*	Alligator snapping turtle[g] [59] *Macrochelys temminckii*[g]	Diamond back terrapin[d] [96] *Malaclemys terrapin*	Spanish pond turtle[d] [60] *Mauremys leprosa*	*Chinese stripe-necked turtle*[b,d] [61] *Ocadia (Mauremys) sinensis*	Arrau turtle[h] [63] *Podocnemis expansa*	Northern red-bellied cooter[i] [11] *Pseudemys rubriventris*	Red-eared slider[a] [8, 54] *Trachemys scripta elegans*
20♂ 20♀ ₪♂♀ Ħ ⺀	90–106 Ó-₪ ♂♀ ⺀	56–87 Ó-₪ ♂♀ ⺀	56 ♂;58 ♀₪ ⺀	24♂;26♀₪⺀ June	24–28 Ó-₪ ♂♀ Ħ	30 Ó Ħ	10[j]–36 ₪♀ Ħ
Mean ± SD	95% CI	Mean ± SD	95% CI [range]	95% CI	Range	Range of 3 institutions	Range ± SD or [Range][j]
2 ± 0.4 (8 ± 1.8)	2.2–2.4 (8.9–9.7)	3.3 ± 1.3 (13 ± 5)	2.3–2.5 ♂ 3.4–4.7 ♀ (9.2–10 ♂ 13.6–20.4 ♀)			2.2–2.9 (8.8–11.5)	3.6 ± 0.1 (14.4 ± 0.4)
	1.1–1.3 (3.5–3.9)	1.7 ± 0.54 (5.3 ± 1.7)	0.6–0.8 ♂ 0.9–1.2 ♀ (1.9–2.5 ⊥ ♂ 2.78–3.7 ♀)			0.6–2.5 (2–7.8)	1.3 ± 0.1 (4.0 ± 0.3)
							1.3 ± 0.16 (2.57 ± 0.33) [25] *[n = 1]*
	30.4–34.5						
		106.9 ± 9.7					102 ± 4.9
	3.6–3.8	4.9 ± 1	3.2–3.5 ♂ 3.3–3.6 ♀			3.3–5.2	6.3 ± 2.0
	127.2 ± 129.2	148.7 ± 11	131.6–133 ♂ 131.6–134 ♀			132–151	136.8 ± 3.4
89 ± 89 (1.5 ± 1.5)	39–49 (0.65–0.83)	77 ± 54 (1.3 ± 0.9)	73.7–108.3 ♂ 78.1–108.3 ♀ (1.2–1.8 ♂ 1.3–1.8 ♀)	42–113 ♂ 36–77.3 ♀ (0.7–1.9 ♂ 0.6–1.3 ♀)	0.41–0.7 (24.6–40.1)	Dec-77 (0.2–1.3)	1.6–209.4♀ (0–3.5)
	0.4–0.7 (34.8–62.6)			0.4–6.5 ♂ 2.7–10.3 ♀ (34–578 ♂ 235–908 ♀)			0.2–4.4♀ (18–389♀)
						0.9–6.8♀	

Table 16.4 Biochemical data for select tortoise species.

Analyte (abbreviation)	Units SI (US)	Aldabra tortoise *Geochelone gigantea*[a] [40]	Radiated tortoise *Geochelone radiata*[b,c,d] [66]	Desert tortoise *Gopherus agassizii*[b,c,e,f] [6]	Gopher tortoise *Gopherus polyphemus*[b,c] [52]	Pancake tortoise *Malacochersus tornieri*[b] [66]	Greek tortoise *Testudo graeca*[c,g] [12]	Hermann's tortoise *Testudo hermanni*[c] [12]	Horsfield's tortoise *Testudo horsfieldii*[e,h] [68]	Marginated tortoise *Testudo marginata*[i] [14]
Sample size & attributes		**16–44 ♂♀ Ó-₪ ⺀**	**10 M;8F♂♀₪ Ħ☼**	**98♂♀₪⺀ ☼**	**7–17♂♀ Ħ**	**24–26♂♀ ⺀**	**12♂♀₪ Ħ Aug; 9Ħ Mar–Aug[g]**	**6♂♀₪ Ħ, Aug; 9Ħ Mar–Aug[g]**	**20♂♀₪ Ħ**	**7♂♀Ó-₪ Ħ, brachial vein**
Data format		**Mean ± SD**	**Range**	**95%CI**	**Mean ± SE**	**Mean ± SD**	**Mean ± SD; {Min–Max}[g]**	**Mean ± SD {Min–Max}[g]**	**Range**	**Range**
Alkaline phosphatase (ALP)	U/l	217 ± 141		25–114	276 ± 28				105–424	180–295
Alanine transaminase (ALT)	U/l	14.5 ± 5.1	5–17♂;8–15♀	1–5	14.8 ± 4.64				29–71	12.0–24
Aspartate transaminase (AST)	U/l		86–185♂ 65–195♀	24–123♂ 15–78♀	135.8 ± 19.92	157.4 ± 101.69			0.5–1.6	47–98
Creatine kinase (CK)	U/l	192.8 ± 171.1	315–4860♂ 57–377♀		160.3 ± 45.65	492.9 ± 490.09				26–215
Lactate dehydrogenase (LDH)	U/l		3009–6444♂ 515–1595♀							182–882
Gamma-glutamyl transferase (GGT)	U/l		5–9♂;5–6♀							
Albumin	g/l (g/dl)	7.8 ± 4 (0.78 ± 0.4)		10.0–19 (1–1.9)	15.2 ± 1.30 (1.52 ± 0.139)					
Total protein (TP)	g/l (g/dl)	21.4 ± 10.5) (2.14 ± 1.05)		29–53 (2.9–5.3)	31.1 ± 2.3 (3.11 ± 0.23)	31 ± 5.4) (3.1 ± 0.54)	79.9 ± 15.1 (7.99 ± 1.51)	86.6 ± 12.6 (8.66 ± 1.26)	24.3–68.5 (2.43–6.85)	32–39 (3.2–3.9)
Globulin	g/l (g/dl)			17–39 (1.7–3.9)		16 ± 2.9 (1.6 ± 0.29)				
Total bilirubin (TBIL)	μmol/l (mg/dl)		1.71–3.42♂ 1.71–5.13♀ (0.1–0.2♂ 0.1–0.3♀)	0–5.13 (0–0.3)	0.34 ± 0.17 (0.02 ± 0.01)					

Blood urea nitrogen (BUN)	mmol/l (mg/dl)	38.8 ± 23.6 (108.7 ± 66.2)	2.9–12♂ 0.7–3.9♀ (8–34♂ 2–11♀)	0.36–13.2 (1.0–37)	10.8 ± 3.1 (30.1 ± 8.7)		1.4 ± 2 (3.9 ± 0.25)	0.6 ± 0.8 (1.7 ± 2.2)		0.33–1 (0.9–2.8)
Creatinine	μmol/l (mg/dl)	38.89 ± 68.6 (0.51 ± 0.9)	7.6–22.8♂ 7.6–15.2♀ (0.1–0.3♂ 0.1–0.2♀)	15.2–30.4 (0.2–0.4)	21.3 ± 1.6 (0.28 ± 0.021)	15.2 ± 4.6 (0.2 ± 0.06)				0–35.36[j] (0-0.46)
Cholesterol	mmol/l (mg/dl)	1.8 ± 1 (68 ± 40)		0.9–3♂ 1.6–7.3 (33–118♂ 60–281♀)	1.97 ± 0.3 (76.1 ± 11.51)	2.6 ± 1.6 (102.2 ± 62.61)	2.71 ± 0.71 (104 ± 0.02)	3.1 ± 1.3 (120 ± 50)	3–6.5 (116–251)	
Glucose	mmol/l (mg/dl)		1.2–2.8♂ 2.4–3.6♀ (21–52♂ 44–65♀)	3.6–10.3 (65–186)	4.1 ± 0.25 74.5 ± 4.5)	5.3 ± 1.7 (95.1 ± 30.1)	1.46 ± 0.41 (26 ± 7.3)	1.46 ± 0.4 (26 ± 7.2)	8.9–12 (160–216)	0.72–4.66 (13–84)
Calcium (Ca)	mmol/l (mg/dl)	2.3 ± 0.6 (9.3 ± 2.5)	2.7–3♂ 2.3–3.7♀ (10.7–12.3♂ 9–14.9♀)	2.1–3.1♂ 2.8–6♀ (8.6–12.5♂ 11.3–23.9♀)	2.9 ± 0.15 (11.77 ± 0.604)	3.2 ± 0.5 (12.7 ± 2.17)			1.7–2.9 (6.8–11.6)	2.72–5.52 (10.9–22)
Ionized calcium (iCa) (mmol/l)	mmol/l			3.14 ± 0.19 [102], [g]			0.48–1.92 [103], [g]	0.52–2.44 [103], [g]	1.14–2.28 [103], [g]	1.03–2.11 [103], [g]
Phosphorous (P)	mmol/l (mg/dl)	0.7 ± 0.2 (2.2 ± 0.7)	0.9–1.3♂ 1–2.2♀ (2.7–4.1♂ 3.2–6.9♀)	0.36–1.1♂ 0.65–2.1 (1.1–3.3♂ 2.0–6.5♀)	0.67 ± 0.05 (2.07 ± 0.165)	1.0 ± 0.19 (3.1 ± 0.58)			0.7–1.9 (2.2–5.9)	1.32–3.13 (4.1–9.7)
Magnesium (Mg)	mmol/l (mg/dl)			1.4–2.6 (3.5–6.4)	1.7 ± 0.09 (4.09 ± 0.23)					
TCO2	mmol/l		20–28♂ 20–30♀	14–32	25.5 ± 1.65					
Chloride (Cl)	mmol/l			101–138	102.3 ± 4.85	95 ± 6.94				
Potassium (K)	mmol/l		4.3–5.3♂ 4.3–5.2♀	3.7–7.5	5.01 ± 0.325	5.2 ± 0.55			2–4.2	
Sodium (Na)	mmol/l		135–141♂ 129–146♀	127–176	137.7 ± 1.57	122.1 ± 7.3			139–145	124–140
Uric acid	μmol/l (mg/dl)	143 ± 56 (2.4 ± 0.9)	12–36♂ 12.0–60♀ (0.2–0.6♂ 0.2–0.5♀)	155–547 (2.6–9.2)	207 ± 29 (3.48 ± 0.488)	214 ± 105 (3.6 ± 1.77)			37.6–150 (0.6–2.5)	65.43–207.59 (1.1–3.49)

(Continued)

Table 16.4 (Continued)

Analyte (abbreviation)	Units SI (US)	Aldabra tortoise *Geochelone gigantea*[a] [40]	Radiated tortoise *Geochelone radiata*[b,c,d] [66]	Desert tortoise *Gopherus agassizii*[b,c,e,f] [6]	Gopher tortoise *Gopherus polyphemus*[b,c] [52]	Pancake tortoise *Malacochersus tornieri*[b] [66]	Greek tortoise *Testudo graeca*[c,g] [12]	Hermann's tortoise *Testudo hermanni*[c] [12]	Horsfield's tortoise *Testudo horsfieldii*[e,h] [68]	Marginated tortoise *Testudo marginata*[i] [14]
Sample size & attributes		16–44 ♂♀ Ó-₪ ⍀	10 M;8F♂♀₪ Ħ☼	98♂♀₪⍀ ☼	7–17♂♀ Ħ	24–26♂♀ ⍀	12♂♀₪ Ħ Aug; 9Ħ Mar–Aug[g]	6♂♀₪ Ħ, Aug; 9Ħ Mar–Aug[g]	20♂♀₪ Ħ	7♂♀Ó-₪ Ħ, brachial vein
Data format		Mean ± SD	Range	95%CI	Mean ± SE	Mean ± SD	Mean ± SD; {Min–Max}[g]	Mean ± SD {Min–Max}[g]	Range	Range
Triglycerides	mmol/l (mg/dl)		0.3–0.7♂ 1.6–3.4♀ (29–59♂ 146–303♀)	0.07–0.36♂ 0.12–6.8♀ (7–32♂ 11–603♀)	0.36 ± 0.18 (32.1 ± 16.1)					0.8–4.32 (71–382)
Bile acids	µmol/l (µg/ml)		3.3–18♂ 3.1–12.5♀ (1.34–7.35♂ 1.26–5.1)	3.3–18♂ 3.1–12.5♀ (0–0.55)			{15.4–17.9} *[30]* [104]	{17.6–27.3} *[32]* [104]	{20–24.7} *[8]* [104]	

[a] Likely lymph or CSF contamination based on description.
[b] Sex differences seen.
[c] Seasonal differences seen.
[d] Additional data for this species in reference [69].
[e] Geographic differences seen.
[f] Location data shown for largest sample size; ionized calcium data from Rooney [105] n = 8 converted from mEq/l, possible unit error as iCa value much higher than reported in other chelonians; unclear if iCa is pH corrected. For additional data for this species see references [5, 7, 10, 28, 35, 46, 105–107].
[g] Not pH corrected.
[h] Health status differences seen.
[i] Venipuncture site differences seen.
[j] Manuscript lists mmol/l as units for creatinine; suspect error and that it should be µmol/l based on data.

Table 16.5 Protein electrophoresis data for select turtle and tortoise species.

Analyte	Units	Pond slider *Trachemys scripta* [108]	Alligator snapping turtle *Macrochelys temminckii* [59]	Radiated tortoise *Geochelone radiata* [66]	Desert tortoise *Gopherus agassizii* [105]
Data format		**Range**	**Range**	**Range**	**Mean ± SD**
Total protein	g/l	23.8–49.7		44–60 ♂;42–66 ♀	
alpha1	g/l	5.2–15.3 (total alpha)	12 to 15	1–2 ♂;2–5 ♀	5 ± 1
alpha2	g/l		6.9–8.3	11–18 ♂;9–19 ♀	7 ± 2
beta	g /l	8.1–21.7	15–18	7–11 ♂;11–15 ♀	4 ± 2
gamma	g/l	0.4–5.3	0.81–1.0	5–9 ♂;5–8 ♀	9 ± 1
albumin	g/l	6–19.6		14–20 ♂;11–24 ♀	
pre-albumin	g/l			3–6 ♂;2–4 ♀	

species of sea turtle, tissue enzymes such as AST, ALT, ALP, LDH, and CK are widely distributed in many tissues, and cannot be considered specific markers for liver disease. Relatively low plasma activities of ALT and ALP were documented in desert tortoises during hibernation, possibly based on reduced metabolic activity [6]. Relatively high plasma activity of AST was documented in this same study in spring, particularly in males, possibly associated with increased general activity and courtship activity [6]. Gamma-glutamyltransferase concentrations in turtle plasma are often extremely low, and this enzyme has no known diagnostic importance in chelonians [30, 77]. Increased glutamate dehydrogenase (GLDH) activity may indicate hepatocellular necrosis in reptiles; however, most commercial laboratories do not routinely offer this assay [116].

Renal Analytes

Uric acid is the main nitrogenous waste product in many turtle species. Terrestrial turtles are uricotelic, producing mainly uric acid relative to other nitrogenous wastes. Uric acid is formed in the liver and is eliminated through kidneys. The wide range of blood concentrations of uric acid reported in freshwater turtles and tortoises is affected by many factors. Clinically, monitoring of uric acid is important for assessment of kidney function [41, 45]. However, extensive renal damage (two thirds of tissue) may be necessary to cause increases of uric acid [21, 46, 49, 107]. As in other species, uric acid concentrations may increase based on dehydration. To date, postprandial increases in uric acid concentrations have not been noted in chelonians [53].

Urea is the predominant final product of protein metabolism in aquatic turtles. Elimination of urea depends on glomerular filtration. Increased concentrations of urea in reptile plasma can indicate decreased GFR during conditions of poor perfusion or dehydration [12, 41, 52]. Urea values may increase in tortoises during hibernation and dormancy [1, 5–7].

Muscle and Bone Enzymes

CK originates mainly in muscle cells. Increased CK activity may be associated with myopathies, traumas, repeated intramuscular injections, or difficult blood collection [49]. AST plasma activity may also reflect tissue necrosis in generalized health disorders such as endotoxemia and septicemia [49, 117]. ALP activity in plasma of most vertebrates is primarily based on osteoclastic activity and is generally higher in young and rapidly growing animals but may also be released from hepatocytes [49]. Increased ALP activity in adult animals might be expected in cases of bone disease, fracture healing, and hepatopathies [49]. However, specific evidence for these changes is lacking for turtles. LDH is found in reptilian muscle, as well as in liver and erythrocytes [49, 109–111]. The diagnostic value of this enzyme in chelonians is unknown.

Endocrine and Exocrine Pancreas

Glucose is a simple saccharide representing the chief source of energy for cells. Plasma concentrations depend on absorption of glucose in the small intestine, glycogenolysis, and gluconeogenesis. Seasonal differences in glucose concentrations of tortoises associated with ambient temperature occur [12]. Hypoglycemia and hyperglycemia may occur in ill turtles, and causes are presumed similar to those in other species [77, 118]. While several cases of presumptive diabetes mellitus have been reported in turtles, thoroughly documented cases are lacking [107]. Abnormal glucose concentrations may be caused by hepatopathies, anorexia, sepsis, polycythemia, and endocrinopathies [30, 118].

The pancreatic enzymes, lipase, and amylase are rarely measured in chelonians, and the effect of pancreatic disease on their plasma concentrations is not described. Amylase and lipase were specific to the pancreas in loggerhead sea turtles (*Car. caretta*) [109]. Plasma amylase activities were reported as 282–316 U/l for the alligator snapping turtle (*Macrochelys temminckii*); 33–168 (male) and 30–107 (female) U/l for the radiated tortoise; and 258–858 U/l for the European pond turtle [59, 66, 101]. Plasma lipase activities were 7.4–12.6 U/l for *M. temminckii*, and 7–50 (male) and 5–29 (female) U/l for *Ge. radiata* [59, 66].

Beta-hydroxybutyrate (BHB) is a ketone produced during fasting and exercise in mammals to provide an alternate energy source when glucose reserves are insufficient [119]. Increased concentrations of BHB are associated with deranged metabolic conditions such as ketoacidosis [119]. While not widely used clinically, measurement of BHB may provide insight into the metabolic status of turtles. This analyte has been evaluated as a measure of metabolic status in the desert tortoise (*Gopherus agassizii*) and yellow mud turtle (*Kinosternon flavescens*), in which BHB concentrations increase during fasting and drought [7, 120]. Values for BHB of leatherback turtles entangled in fishing gear were an order of magnitude greater than those of healthy, directly captured turtles [112].

Cardiac and Gastrointestinal Biomarkers

Biomarkers to assess gastrointestinal and cardiac health in turtles and tortoises and require further study.

Lipids

Increased concentrations of triglycerides and cholesterol occur in reproductively active female turtles during folliculogenesis [105, 106]. Hyperlipidemia and hypercholesterolemia may also be caused by mobilization of fatty acids from fat deposits during negative energy balance in ill turtles [105]. Decreased triglycerides were documented in leatherback sea turtles entangled in fishing gear [112].

Electrolytes

Sodium is the main extracellular cation and chloride is the main extracellular anion in turtles. Hypernatremia and hyperchloremia are most commonly caused by dehydration or renal failure [30, 49]. Hyponatremia may be associated with diarrhea, renal failure, and ascites (i.e. sequestration of fluids in the "third space" where they cannot be used by the organism) [30, 49]. Hypochloremia may occur in turtles with severe gastric pathology, based on the "chloride trap" effect (Innis personal observation). Potassium is the main intracellular cation which maintains osmolality in cells and assists with acid-base balance. Absorption of potassium takes place mainly in the small intestine, and regulation is performed mainly by the kidneys. Hyperkalemia in turtles can be caused by renal failure, urinary obstruction, acidosis, hemolysis or tissue necrosis [30, 49]. Severe hyperkalemia is associated with a poor prognosis for cold-stunned Kemp's ridley turtles [77, 121]. Assumed causes of hypokalemia include chronic diarrhea, renal failure, ascites, and alkalosis [49].

Blood Proteins

Total protein includes hundreds of proteins that are synthesized mainly in the liver. They maintain appropriate oncotic pressure (especially albumin), which preserves the volume of body fluid; protect the organism from pathogens (e.g., immunoglobulins, complement, and acute phase proteins); support blood coagulation (coagulation factors); and transport of hormones and elements. Causes of hyperproteinemia include hemoconcentration from dehydration, for example, during hibernation [97], and increased globulin concentration from inflammatory processes. Increased albumin concentrations (+30%) were observed in female than in male tortoises in summer, likely from increased production of vitellogenin [12]. Hypoproteinemia and hypoalbuminemia are common in debilitated turtles, and can be caused by impaired liver function (decreased protein synthesis), malabsorption, protein-losing enteropathy, protein-losing nephropathy, plasma or blood loss (burn, hemorrhage), and sepsis [21, 49]. Measurement of albumin by electrophoresis in turtles is more accurate than by the bromcresol green method [122]. Electrophoresis can be used to analyze individual protein fractions (albumin, α-globulins, β-globulins, γ-globulins). Because relatively little data are available for freshwater turtles and tortoises at this time, interpretation of such data in clinical cases is subjective [59, 66, 108, 122].

Blood Gas and Acid–Base Status (Table 16.6 and Table 16.7)

Physiologic studies of the respiratory and metabolic status of freshwater turtles and tortoises, including blood gas, acid–base, and lactate analysis, have been conducted for several decades [123–130]. Most clinical investigations have involved sea turtles [23, 112, 121, 132–134]. Evaluation of blood gas, acid–base, and lactate data is of diagnostic and prognostic importance in these species [121]. While arterial samples are ideal for such analyses, obtaining arterial samples is clinically impractical in most turtles. Most published values for chelonians are for venous samples, yet clearly provide clinically useful information [121].

Body temperature has a significant effect upon interpretation of blood gases and pH in chelonia. As temperature increases, blood pH decreases, and pCO2 and pO2 increase [130, 139]. Most blood analyzers conduct analysis at the normal human body temperature of 37 °C. Should the blood sample be taken from a turtle with body temperature of 25 °C, the analyzer would erroneously report low pH and a high pCO2 and pO2. Ideally,

Table 16.6 Select acid base and blood gas values for turtle and tortoise species.

Species common name	Sample size, type	Analytes	pH	pO2	pCO2	Bicarbonate	Lactate
Scientific name	***Temperature °C***	**Data Type**	**Units**	**mmHg**	**mmHg**	**mmol/l**	**mmol/l**
Common snapping turtle *Chelydra serpentina* [123]	11 mixed ***10***	Mean ± SE	7.876 ± 0.015	53 ± 6.3	15.59 ± 0.6	39.74 ± 0.68	1.89 ± 0.53
Common musk turtle *Sternotherusodoratus* [123]	9 mixed ***10***	Mean ± SE	7.889 ± 0.014	21.4 ± 4.4	10.26 ± 0.6	27.05 ± 1.12	0.85 ± 0.25
Spiny soft-shelled turtle *Apalone spinifera* [123]	16 mixed ***10***	Mean ± SE	7.945 ± ±0.024	35 ± 8	8.11 ± 0.43	24.12 ± 1.2	0.89 ± 0.21
Painted turtle *Chrysemys picta* [123]	15 arterial ***10***	Mean ± SE	7.910 ± 0.012	47.2 ± 7.9	13.35 ± 0.55	36.48 ± 0.93	0.64 ± 0.1
Eastern long-necked turtle *Chelodina longicollis* [124]	11 arterial ***20–22***	Range[a]		40–60			
Fitzroy river turtle *Rheodytes leukops* [125]	30 venous ***25***	Mean ± SD	7.737 ± 0.018	36.5 ± 5.6	8.2–20.3	12.27 ± 0.21	0.4–3.0
Red-bellied short-necked turtle *Emydura subglobosa* [126]	3 arterial ***20***	Mean ± SE	7.76 ± 0.9	58 ± 17	18.6 ± 3.4	33.1 ± 0.2	3.5 ± 1.6
New Guinea snapping turtle *Elseya novaguineae* [126]	5 arterial ***20***	Mean ± SE	7.71 ± 0.02	89 ± 15	19 ± 3	34.9 ± 0.6	0.2 ± 0.1
African helmeted turtle *Pelomedusa subrufa* [126]	6 arterial ***20***	Mean ± SE	7.83 ± 0.03	67 7	19 ± 2	39.8 ± 3	2.7 ± 1.3
Florida soft-shelled turtle *Apalone ferox* [127]	18 arterial ***22–25***	Mean	7.75		14	30	0.5
Pond slider *Trachemys scripta*[b] [25, 127]	28 arterial ***22–25***	Mean	7.8		12	30	2
	12 mixed ***23–25***	Range Ⱥ	7.534–7.834	27.6–109.9	13.6–29.5	21.1–39.3	
Eastern box turtle *Terrapene carolina* [128]	12 mixed ***25***	Mean ± SD	7.68 ± 0.12				
Ornate or western box turtle *Terrapene ornata* [129]	5 arterial ***30***	Mean ± SE	7.56 ± 0.04				3.5 ± 0.48
Desert tortoise *Gopherus agassizii*[c,d] [28, 102]	6 mixed ***25–28.5***[e]	Mean ± SE	7.38 ± 0.05	53.5 ± 16.8	43.8 ± 3.2		
	6Ⱥ, mixed ***25–28.5***[e]		7.57 ± 0.05	112.3 ± 16.8	24 ± 3.2		
	10Ⱥ, mixed ***24a***	Mean ± SE *[range]*	7.38 ± 0.03	*[50–90]*[a]	49.7 ± 3.4	28.8 ± 1.4	
Gopher tortoise *Gopherus polyphemus*[f] [24]	6 arterial ***30–35***	Mean ± SD	7.46 ± 0.04	136.6 ± 8.77	36.42 ± 5.5		
			7.31 ± 0.06 Ⱥ	100.1 ± 23.1 Ⱥ	51.92 ± 10.3 Ⱥ		
Pancake tortoise *Malacochersus tornieri* [130]	4 mixed ***20,35***	Mean	7.64[g] 7.47[h]		15.1[h]	21.4[g] 22.9[h]	

[a] Estimated from graph.
[b] Summary data for anesthetized turtles under ketamine, ketamine/xylazine, or ketamine/midazolam anesthesia; temperature of analysis not reported [25].
[c] Medetomidine anesthesia, atipamezole reversal. Ⱥ 15 min after IV medetomidine, temperature of analysis 37 °C [28].
[d] [131].
[e] Temperature of analysis not reported.
[f] Sevoflurane anesthesia with IPPV 100% O_2, expired sevoflurane 3.75% [24].
[g] 20 °C.
[h] 35 °C.

Table 16.7 Temperature correction formulas for acid base values obtained from chelonians.

Analyte corrected (Abbreviation)	Units	Correction for	Equation	References
pH	pH	Temperature	$pH_{TC} = (0.015 \text{ X } \Delta T) + pH$	[121, 132, 133]
Partial pressure of carbon dioxide (pCO_2)	mmHg	ΔT = 37 °C-patient temperature TC = temperature-corrected	$Pco_{2TC} = Pco_2 \text{ X } 10^{(-0.019 \text{ X } \Delta T)}$	[23, 131, 134, 135]
Partial pressure of oxygen (pO_2)	mmHg		$Po_{2TC} = Po_2 \text{ X } 10^{(-0.0058 \text{ X } \Delta T)}$	[23, 134–136]
Ionized calcium (iCa)	mmol/l	pH cor = corrected	$iCa_{cor} = iCa \text{ X } (1 + [0.53\{pH - pH_{TC}\}])$	[137]
Ionized magnesium (iMg)	mmol/l		$iMg_{cor} = iMg \text{ X } 10^{(-0.2 \text{ X } [pH_{TC} - pH])}$	[138]

blood gas and pH data of ectotherms are generated by an analyzer calibrated to the body temperature of the patient, and the raw data reflect animal values; however, such analyzers are rarely present in clinical settings. Analyzers with automated temperature correction algorithms based on mammalian physiology appear to provide clinically relevant, albeit imprecise, values for pH and pCO2 values, but not pO_2 in chelonia [23, 132]. However, from internal calculations based in human physiology, automated analyzers may not produce accurate hematocrit data for species with nucleated erythrocytes. Thus, any subsequent data (e.g., hemoglobin, SO_2) that are derived from calculations using hematocrit will also be questionable.

Controversy surrounds temperature correction, but the authors recommend that results generated at 37 °C should be mathematically corrected to patient temperature [23, 112, 121, 132, 134, 140]. Additionally, for publication, the raw data, the temperature-corrected data, and the mathematical methods used for temperature correction should be included [134]. The influence of temperature correction becomes greater as temperatures move farther from 37 °C (e.g., a cold-stunned turtle at a body temperature of 6 °C). Preferably, temperature correction for chelonians is conducted using equations specific to ectotherms, derived experimentally for the species of interest. Examples of equations used for Kemp's ridley sea turtles are provided in Table 16.7. Determination of bicarbonate values in turtles are most accurately measured directly using a temperature-calibrated analyzer, which is rarely available clinically [140]. Instead, bicarbonate is often calculated using temperature-corrected pH and pCO2 data and the Henderson Hasselbalch equation, using αCO2- and pK-species-specific constants [23, 112, 121, 132, 134]. These data remain undetermined for many species. Constants determined for select freshwater chelonia include aCO2 = 0.0812, and pK = 6.239 for *Che. serpentina* if pH ≥ 7.99; or pK = 6.305 for decreased pH [141]; and αCO2 and pK of 0.0401 and 6.152, respectively, for the Fitzroy river turtle (*Rheodytes leukops*) [125].

Most chelonians maintain an alkaline blood pH slightly above that of mammals (e.g., pH 7.5–7.9, Table 16.6). Baseline results in the same species vary among different studies [123, 126]. Blood gas values and lactate values are quite variable, and must be interpreted in context. For example, a turtle evaluated after a long voluntary aquatic submergence may have physiologically acceptable derangements that resolve by routine homeostatic mechanisms. Such derangements would be abnormal in the same turtle being maintained out of water in the hospital. A blood pH decrease of approximately 1 unit results in mortality during long-term submergence experiments in several freshwater species [126]. In Kemp's ridley sea turtles, severe respiratory and metabolic acidosis may occur in response to natural hypothermia [121]. Increasing lactate values in these patients are associated with a poor prognosis [121]. Increased lactate concentrations were reported in freshwater turtles injured by vehicles [141].

Measurement of acid–base and blood gas data is useful for anesthetic monitoring of chelonians. [24, 25, 28, 102]. Analytes may vary because of positive pressure ventilation, concentration of inspired oxygen, and type of anesthetic. In desert tortoises, delivery of sevoflurane in 100% oxygen with positive pressure ventilation resulted in a respiratory alkalosis and hyperoxemia [102]. In gopher tortoises, intravenous medetomidine injection resulted in respiratory acidosis and hypoxemia, while in desert tortoises, intramuscular medetomidine injection caused no change in acid–base and blood gas status [24, 28]. Additional clinical study of the blood gas and acid–base status chelonians is encouraged. Documentation and publication of such data for clinical patients (e.g., vehicular trauma, surgical patients) are particularly needed.

Vitamins, Minerals, and Metals and Toxins

Fat-Soluble Vitamins

Vitamins A, D, and E have been measured in the plasma of only a few freshwater turtle and tortoise species (Table 16.8). Preliminary studies suggest that exposure to natural or artificial ultraviolet B light results in increased

Table 16.8 Vitamin data for select chelonian species.

			Analyte	Vitamin A	25OH-Vitamin D	Vitamin E
Species Common name Scientific name	Sample size	Data format	Units SI (US)	μmol /l (μg/dl)	nmol /l (ng /ml)	μmol /l (mg /dl)
Galapagos tortoise [40] *Geochelone gigantea*	14	Mean ± SD		0.24 ± 0.17 (6.9 ± 4.89)		0.7 ± 0.84 (0.03 ± 0.036)
Desert tortoise[a] [106], *Gopherus agassizii*	177	Mean ± 2SD		1.4 ± 0.70 (40 ± 20)		9.98 ± 8.36 ♂ 18.34 ± 11.84♀ (0.43 ± 0.36♂) (0.79 ± 0.51♀)
Pancake tortoise [67] Malacochersus tornieri	17	Mean ± SD		1.57 ± 0.7 (45 ± 20)		α-tocopherol 6.0 ± 3.34 (0.26 ± 0.144) γ-tocopherol 0.74 ± 0.77 (0.032 ± 0.033)
***Testudo* spp.** [142, 143]	19–22	Mean ± SD or [range]			[24.41–32.42 (9.78–13)]	10.44 ± 4.41 ⧗ 6.5 ± 2.8 ⌂ (0.45 ± 0.19 ⧗) (0.28 ± 0.12 ⌂)
Common snapping turtle [144] *Chelydra serpentina*	10	Range				1.16–17.76 (0.05–0.765)
Painted turtle [144] *Chrysemys picta*	49	Range				3.62 29.35 (0.156–1.264)
Alligator snapping turtle [59] *Macrochelys temminckii*	52–60	95%CI		0.48–0.86 (13.8–24.6)	9.95–15.97 (3.99–6.40)	8.36–11.42 (0.36–0.492)
Musk turtle [144] *Sternotherus odoratus*	11	Range				8.87–22.59 (0.382–0.973)
Box turtle [144, 145] *Terrapene carolina*	8	Range				3.34–24.24 (0.144–1.044)
Red-eared slider [146] *Trachemys scripta elegans*	6 + UV ⚡	Mean ± SD			31.4 ± 13.2 71.7 ± 46.9 ⚡ (12.6 ± 5.3) (28.7 ± 18.8⚡)	

[a] Additional data in Jacobson et al. 1991.

25-hydroxyvitamin D values in some chelonian species [146]. However, the minimum plasma 25-hydroxyvitamin D concentration required for maintenance of normal calcium homeostasis is unknown. Vitamin E (plasma α-tocopherol) concentrations were increased in Testudo spp. maintained on an outdoor farm compared to animals from indoor terrariums [142]. Values for Vitamin A in wild desert tortoises and pancake tortoises (*Malacochersus tornieri*) vary depending on season, year, location, and gender [67, 106]. Despite the relatively common clinical diagnosis of vitamin A deficiency in chelonians, plasma concentrations are rarely measured [145].

Minerals

Total plasma calcium and phosphorus data have been determined in most studies of chelonian biochemistry, while total plasma magnesium has been infrequently determined (Tables 16.3 and 16.4). Most freshwater turtles and tortoises have calcium:phosphorus ratios greater than 1.5:1 (Table 16.3). Hypercalcemia and proportional hyperphosphatemia may be seen in female chelonians during folliculogenesis [147]. Estrogen administration causes dose-dependent hypercalcemia and hyperphosphatemia in *Chrysemys picta* and *Tr. scripta elegans* [147]. Parathyroidectomy causes hypocalcemia in *Te. graeca* and Reeve's turtles (*Mauremys reevesii*) [148]. Any disease state that affects parathyroid function may thus affect calcium and phosphorus values. Common disorders include nutritional or renal secondary hyperparathyroidism [149]. Ionized calcium values have been reported for the spiny soft shelled turtle (*A. spinifera*), *Chr. picta*, the desert tortoise (*Go. agassizii*), and *Testudo* sp. (Tables 16.2 and 16.4), and for the marine species *L. kempii*, and leatherback turtles (*Dermochelys coriacea*) [47, 102, 103, 112, 143, 150, 119130]. Hypophosphatemia has been seen in ill free-ranging *Go. agassizii* [5]. Plasma ionized calcium values are loosely correlated with total plasma calcium values in Testudo spp., but total calcium and ionized calcium concentrations are not correlated to plasma albumin values [103]. Ionized magnesium concentrations have been determined for only *L. kempii*, where convalescent values during rehabilitation = 0.44–0.77 mmol/l (10th–90th percentile) [132]. For cold-stunned Kemp's ridley sea turtles, increased ionized calcium and ionized magnesium concentrations upon admission to the hospital correlate with a poor prognosis [121]. This may be related to severe dehydration, reduced renal function, and lactic acidosis. Increased concentrations of total magnesium, total calcium, and ionized calcium occur in experimental hypercapnia in painted turtles and experimental hypoxia in *Che. serpentina* as calcium and magnesium carbonates are mobilized from bone to provide buffering capacity during acidosis [141, 150].

The ionization status of calcium and magnesium is dependent on blood pH [137, 138]; however, no validated correction formulas for reptilian calcium or magnesium have been determined. Reptile values for ionized calcium and ionized magnesium are most valid if sample pH is determined simultaneously. Ionized calcium and ionized magnesium results can be falsely decreased by greater than 14 U heparin per ml of blood [50]. Avoid this issue by using purpose-made lyophilized calcium-balanced heparin syringes [50]. Clinically acceptable results can also be achieved by coating a syringe with liquid sodium or lithium heparin, and then methodically, thoroughly expelling all visible heparin [50].

Iron values of 3.58–18 μmol/l have been noted in healthy wild *G. agassizii*, and 8.96–18.27 μmol/l in captive *E. orbicularis* [6, 101].

Toxins

Data exist for a wide variety of contaminants, including mercury, cadmium, lead, and pesticides in turtles. Lead toxicity associated with blood levels of 3.6 ppm was reported in *Che. serpentina* [151]. Organochlorine pesticides may play a role in the etiology of aural abscesses by inducing vitamin A deficiency, although evidence for this is contradictory [145, 152]. Organochlorine or mercury exposure correlated with abnormal hematologic and plasma biochemical findings in loggerhead sea turtles [75, 87].

Thyroid, Adrenal, and Reproductive Hormones (Table 16.9)

Excellent reviews of clinical reptilian thyroid anatomy and physiology are available [149, 159]. Thyroid hormone concentrations are known in a small number of chelonian species from basic scientific investigation of thyroid physiology. [155, 160–163] Because thyroid function in chelonians is influenced by temperature, sex, age, photoperiod, nutritional state, and season, generalization about "normal" values is complicated [155, 158, 160, 161, 164]. Ideally, thyroid assays are validated prior to diagnostic use in a given species. Such assays are generally not performed by clinical diagnostic laboratories, leaving the clinician in the difficult position of interpreting data of questionable validity. The majority of existing data for chelonians are for total T4, with scant data available for total T3, free T4, or free T3 (Table 16.9). An assay for free T4 was recently validated for Kemp's ridley turtles [165]. Hyperthyroidism has not been diagnosed in chelonians. Relatively elevated free T4 values occur in leatherback turtles entangled in fishing gear, possibly owing to the increased metabolic activity of exertion [166]. Hypothyroidism has been diagnosed clinically in several tortoise species including the African spurred tortoise (*Geochelone sulcata*), Galapagos tortoise (*Geochelone elephantopus*), and Aldabra tortoise (*Geochelone gigantea*). [157, 167, 168] Depressed free T4 values occur in naturally cold-stunned sea turtles, with values increasing during successful rehabilitation [165]. The optimal time for blood collection for thyroid hormone analysis after oral supplementation with thyroxine is unknown in chelonians. Abundant data on adrenal and reproductive endocrinology of chelonians exist [169–171].

Urinalysis

Urine may be collected from chelonians when voided opportunistically, or via prefemoral cystocentesis (blind or ultrasound-guided) or cloacoscopic-assisted bladder catheterization. Physiologic literature regarding chelonian urinary function is available [172], and clinical observations have been reported [173–176]; however, no peer-reviewed chelonian urinalysis data exist. Urine of healthy herbivorous tortoises is generally alkaline. Acidic urine may occur in herbivorous tortoises during hibernation or illness. Recovery of normal urinary pH may be a favorable prognostic sign. Chelonian urine is not concentrated by the kidney, and is generally of low specific gravity. Urinary dipstick and sediment evaluation is useful for documentation of hematuria, proteinuria, ketonuria, pyuria, glucosuria, and so on. Although chelonian urine is not sterile, heavy, pure growth of bacteria or fungi may provide evidence of true infection. Pathogenic renal protozoa such as Hexamita or Entamoeba can be found in turtle urine samples [174].

Table 16.9 Thyroid hormone values for tortoises and freshwater turtles.

Analyte (Abbreviation)	Units SI (US)	Eastern long-necked turtle *Chelodina longicollis*[a] [153]	Painted turtle *Chrysemys picta*[b] [154]	Desert tortoise *Gopherus agassizii*[c] [155]	Sulcata tortoise *Geochelone sulcata* [156]	Galapagos tortoise [157] *Geochelone elephantopus*	Herman's tortoise [158] *Testudo hermanni*	Greek tortoise *Testudo graeca* [158]	Horsfield's tortoise *Testudo horsfieldii* [158]
Sample size, attributes		10, 20–22 °C	44	50 ♂♀	12 ♂♀	5	69	11	11
Data format			Mean ± SE	Mean (±SD) of Min–Max	10–90th percentiles	Mean ± SD			
Thyroxine (T4)	nmol /l	0.69 (0.11)	13 ± 2.3♂ 30.8 ± 7.7♀	0.46 ± 0.12–3.15 ± 0.36 ♂ 0.51 ± 0.1–3.69 ± 0.31 ♀	2.0–9.0	10.39 ± 18.72	12.8 (7)	12.3 (3.9)	9.9 (4.1)
Triiodothyronine (T3)	nmol/l	0.31 (0.03)	(<0.16) not detected	(<0.13) not detected	0–0.8		0.2 (0.1)	0.04 (0.1)	0.1 (0.03)
Free thyroxine (fT4)	pmol/l				3.0–6.0		<0.45	<0.45	<0.45
Free (fT3) triiodothyronine	pmol/l				1.5–4.8		8.1(2.9)	7.2(1.7)	5.6(1.4)

[a] Manuscript provides additional data for 30–32 °C.
[b] See Licht et al. 1985 for male data.
[c] Values seen over a two-year period. Seasonal and sexual differences seen.

Serology and PCR

Serological tests developed for some chelonian species to detect exposure to *Mycoplasma agassizii*, herpesvirus, iridovirus, picornavirus (virus X), and paramyxovirus (ferlavirus) were often developed for specific research and may not be available to the clinician [177–182, 184]. ELISA testing for Mycoplasma is available in the United States. Recently described Western blot assays for *Mycoplasma agassizii* have a relatively high rate of false negative results [177, 181]. PCR testing for Mycoplasma, herpesvirus, iridovirus, adenovirus, and intranuclear coccidiosis of chelonians is available (Table 16.10). Clinicians should consult the

Table 16.10 Laboratories offering serological and PCR assays for chelonian pathogens in the United States and Europe.

Mycoplasma agassizi (ELISA, PCR, culture, sequencing) Dr. Mary Brown University of Florida 1600 SW Archer Rd. BSB Rm B3-30 Gainesville, FL 32610 USA mbbrown@ufl.edu Phone: (352) 294-4029 Lab Phone: (352) 294-4094 or 294-4071 Fax: (352) 846-2781
Herpes, iridovirus, intranuclear coccidia, adenovirus (PCR and sequencing) Dr James Wellehan University of Florida 2015 SW 16th Ave Building 1017 Room V2-238 Gainesville, FL 32608 USA wellehanj@ufl.edu Lab Phone: 352-392-2226 ext 5775 Fax 352-392-5464
Herpes (ELISA) Dr. Francesco C. Origgi Center for Fish and Wildlife Medicine [Zentrum für Fisch- und Wildtiermedizin (FIWI)] Institute of Animal Pathology (Institut für Tierpathologie) College of Veterinary Medicine Vetsuisse Faculty University of Bern Länggassstrasse 122, 3012 Bern-CH francesco.origgi@vetsuisse.unibe.ch Phone: + 41 31 631 2445 Fax: + 41 31 631 2635
Virology Dr. Rachel E. Marschang Institut für Umwelt- und Tierhygiene Universität Hohenheim Garbenstr. 30 70599 Stuttgart Germany rachel.marschang@googlemail.com Phone: +49 (0)711-459-22468 Fax: +49 (0)711-459-22431
Virology and *Mycoplasma agassizii* Dr. Silvia Blahak Veterinaruntersuchungsamt OWL Westerfeldstr. 1 32758 Detmold Germany Silvia.blahak@cvua-owl.de Phone: +49 5231911640 Fax: +495231911503

laboratory prior to sample collection to determine current availability and requirements and to discuss interpretation of results. One should know if the test is validated only for a specific species of turtle or if it can be broadly applied across species. Understanding the significance of positive serological results in chelonians is important. On the basis of the biology of herpesvirus and Mycoplasma, a positive serological result is good evidence of persistent infection. However, a positive serological result for iridovirus may indicate only past exposure without persistent infection, since duration of iridovirus titers is unknown [178].

References

1 Dessauer, H.C. (1970). Blood chemistry of reptiles: physiological and evolutionary aspects. In: *Biology of the Reptilia*, vol. 3 (ed. C. Gans and T.S. Parsons), 1–72. New York: Academic Press. New York.

2 DuGuy, R. (1970). Numbers of blood cells and their variation. In: *Biology of the Reptilia*, vol. 3 (ed. C. Gans and T.S. Parsons), 93–109. New York: Academic Press. New York.

3 Abou-Madi, N. and Jacobson, E. (2003). Effects of blood processing techniques on sodium and potassium values: a comparison between Aldabra tortoises (Geochelone gigantea) and Burmese mountain tortoises (Manouria emys). *Vet. Clin. Pathol.* 32 (2): 61–66.

4 Arnold, J. (1994). White blood cell count discrepancies in Atlantic loggerhead sea turtles: Natt-Herrick vs. Eosinophil Unopette. *Proc. Assoc. Zoo Vet. Tech.* 15–22.

5 Christopher, M.M., Berry, K.H., Henen, B.T., and Nagy, K.A. (2003). Clinical disease and laboratory abnormalities in free-ranging desert tortoises in California (1990–1995). *J. Wildl. Dis.* 39 (1): 35–56.

6 Christopher, M.M., Berry, K.H., Wallis IR Nagy, K.A. et al. (1999). Reference intervals and physiologic alterations in hematologic and biochemical values of free-ranging desert tortoises in the Mojave desert. *J. Wildl. Dis.* 35 (2): 212–238.

7 Christopher, M.M., Brigmon, R., and Jacobson, E.R. (1994). Seasonal alterations in plasma β-hydroxybutyrate and related biochemical parameters in the desert tortoise (Gopherus agassizii). *Comp. Biochem. Physiol. A.* 108: 303–310.

8 Crawshaw, G.J. and Holz, P. (1996). Comparison of plasma biochemical values in blood and blood-lymph mixtures from red-eared sliders, Trachemys scripta elegans. *Bull. Assoc. Rept. Amphib. Vet.* 6 (2): 7–9.

9 Eisenhawer, E., Courtney, C.H., Raskin, R.E., and Jacobson, E.R. (2008). Relationship between separation time of plasma from heparinized whole blood on plasma biochemical analytes of loggerhead sea turtles (Caretta caretta). *J. Zoo Wildl. Med.* 39: 208–215.

10 Gottdenker, N.L. and Jacobson, E.R. (1995). Effect of venipuncture sites on hematologic and clinical biochemical values in desert tortoises (Gopherus agassizii). *Am. J. Vet. Res.* 56: 19–21.

11 Innis, C., Tlusty, M., and Wunn, D. (2007). Hematologic and plasma biochemical analysis of northern red-bellied cooters. *J. Zoo Wildl. Med.* 38 (3): 425–432.

12 Lawrence, K. (1987). Seasonal variation in blood biochemistry of long term captive Mediterranean tortoises (Testudo graeca and T. Hermanni). *Res. Vet. Sci.* 43: 379–383.

13 Lawrence, K. and Hawkey, C. (1986). Seasonal variations in haematological data from Mediterranean tortoises (Testudo graeca and Testudo hermanni) in captivity. *Res. Vet. Sci.* 40: 225–230.

14 López-Olvera, J.R., Montané, J., Marco, I. et al. (2003). Effect of venipuncture site on hematologic and serum biochemical parameters in marginated tortoise (Testudo marginata). *J. Wildl. Dis.* 39: 830–836.

15 Martínez-Jiménez, D., Hernandez-Divers, S.J., Floyd, T.M. et al. (2007). Comparison of the effects of dipotasssium ethylenediaminetetraacetic acid and lithium heparin on hematologic values in yellow-blotched map turtles, Graptemys flavimaculata. *J. Herp. Med. Surg.* 17 (2): 36–41.

16 Muro, J., Ramis, A., Pastor, J. et al. (1998). Effects of lithium heparin and tripotassium EDTA on haematologic values of Hermann's tortoises Testudo hermanni. *J. Zoo Wildl. Med.* 29: 40–44.

17 Mussachia, X.J. and Sievers, M.L. (1956). Effects of induced cold torpor on blood of Chrysemys picta. *Am. J. Phys.* 187: 99–102.

18 Wolf, K.N., Harms, C.A., and Beasley, J.F. (2008). Evaluation of five clinical chemistry analyzers for use in health assessment in sea turtles. *J. Am. Vet. Med. Assoc.* 233: 470–475.

19 De, T.K. and Maiti, B.R. (1981). Differential leucocyte count in both sexes of an Indian soft-shelled turtle (Lissemys punctata punctata). *Z. Mikrosk. Anat. Forsch.* 95: 1065–1069.

20 Keller, K.A., Guzman, D.S.M., Paul-Murphy, J. et al. (2012). Hematologic and plasma biochemical values of free-ranging western pond turtles (Emys marmorata) with comparison to a captive population. *J. Herp. Med. Surg.* 22 (3–4): 99–106.

21 Knotková, Z., Mazanek, S., Hovorka, M. et al. (2005). Haematology and plasma chemistry of Bornean river turtles suffering from shell necrosis and

haemogregarine parasites. *Vet. Med. Czech.* 50 (9): 421–426.

22 Perpiñán, D., Hernandez-Divers, S.M., Latimer, K.S. et al. (2008). Hematology of the Pascagoula map turtle (Graptemys gibbsoni) and the southeast Asian box turtle (Cuora amboinensis). *J. Zoo Wildl. Med.* 39 (3): 460.

23 Chittick, E.J., Stamper, M.A., Beasley, J.F. et al. (2002). Medetomidine, ketamine, and sevoflurane for anesthesia of injured loggerhead sea turtles: 13 cases (1996-2000). *J. Am. Vet. Med. Assoc.* 221: 1019–1025.

24 Dennis, P.M. and Heard, D.J. (2002). Cardiopulmonary effects of a medetomidine-ketamine combination administered intravenously in gopher tortoises. *J. Am. Vet. Med. Assoc.* (10): 1516–1519.

25 Holz, P. and Holz, R.M. (1994). Evaluation of ketamine, ketamine/xylazine, and ketamine/midazolam anesthesia in red-eared sliders (Trachemys scripta elegans). *J. Zoo Wildl. Med.* 25: 531–537.

26 Schumacher, J. and Mans, C. (2014). Anesthesia. In: *Current Therapy in Reptile Medicine and Surgery* (ed. D.R. Mader and S.J. Divers), 134–153. St. Louis: Elsevier Saunders.

27 Schumacher, J. and Yelen, T. (2006). Anesthesia and analgesia. In: *Reptile Medicine and Surgery* (ed. D.R. Mader), 442–452. Philadelphia: WB Saunders Comp.

28 Sleeman, J.M. and Gaynor, J. (2000). Sedative and cardiopulmonary effects of medetomidine and reversal with atipamezole in desert tortoises (Gopherus agassizii). *J. Zoo Wildl. Med.* 31: 28–35.

29 Hirschfeld, W.J. and Gordon, A.S. (1965). The effect of bleeding and starvation on blood volumes and peripheral hemogram of the turtle, Pseudemys scripta elegans. *Anat. Rec.* 153: 317–324.

30 Wilkinson, R. (2004). Clinical pathology. In: *Medicine and Surgery of Tortoises and Turtles* (ed. S. Mac Arthur, R. Wilkinson and J. Myer), 141–187. Oxford: Blackwell.

31 Bolten, A.B. and Bjorndal, K.A. (1992). Blood profiles for wild population of green turtles (Chelonia mydas) in the southern Bahamas. *J. Wildl. Dis.* 28: 407–413.

32 Nakamura, K. (1980). Carotenoids in serum of Pacific green turtle Chelonia mydas. *Bull. Jp. Soc. Sci. Fish.* 46: 909–910.

33 Hart, M.G., Samour, H.J., and Spratt, D.M.J. (1991). An analysis of haematological findings on a feral population of Aldabra giant tortoises (Geochelone gigantea). *Comp. Haematol. Int.* 1 (3): 145–149.

34 Hernandez-Divers, S.M., Hernandez-Divers, S.J., and Wyneken, J. (2002). Angiographic, anatomic, and clinical technique descriptions of a subcarapacial venipuncture site for chelonians. *J. Herp. Med. Surg.* 12 (2): 32–37.

35 Jacobson, E.R., Schumacher, J., and Green, M. (1992). Field and clinical techniques for sampling and handling blood for hematologic and selected biochemical determinations in the desert tortoise (Xerobates agassizii). *Copeia* (1): 237.

36 Johnson, J. (2006). Nail trimming for blood collection from desert tortoises, Gopherus agassizii: panel summary. *J. Herp. Med. Surg.* 16 (2): 61.

37 Martinez-Silvestre, A., Perpinan, D., Marco, I., and Lavin, S. (2002). Venipuncture technique of the occipital venous sinus in freshwater aquatic turtles. *J. Herp. Med. Surg.* 12: 31–32.

38 Owens, D.W. and Ruiz, G.J. (1980). New methods of obtaining blood and cerebrospinal fluid from marine turtles. *Herpetologica* 36: 17–20.

39 Werner, R.E. (2007). Reference hematology and serum chemistry values for the diamondback terrapin Malaclemys terrapin. *Herp. Rev.* 38 (1): 17–22.

40 Ghebremeskel, K., Williams, G., Spratt, D., and Samour, H.J. (1991). Plasma biochemistry of free-living giant tortoises (Geochelone gigantea) on Curieuse Island (Republic of Seychelles). *Comp. Biochem. Physiol.* 99A (1/2): 65–67.

41 Samour, J.H., Hawkey, C.M., Pugsley, S., and Ball, D. (1986). Clinical and pathologic findings related to malnutrition and husbandry in captive giant tortoises (Geochelone spp.). *Vet. Rec.* 118: 299.

42 Rivera, S., Divers, S.J., Knafo, S.E. et al. (2011). Sterilisation of hybrid Galapagos tortoises (Geochelone nigra) for island restoration. Part 2: phallectomy of males under intrathecal anaesthesia with lidocaine. *Vet. Rec.* 168: 78–81.

43 Innis, C., De Voer, M., and Garner, M. (2010). A call for additional study of the safety of subcarapacial venipuncture in chelonians. *Proc. Assoc. Rept. Amphib. Vet.* 8–10.

44 Quesada, R.J., Aiken-Palmer, C., Conley, K., and Heard, D.J. (2010). Accidental submeningeal injection of propofol in gopher tortoises (Gopherus polyphemus). *Vet. Rec.* 167: 494–495.

45 Göbel, T. and Spörle, H. (1992). Blutentnahmetechnik und Serumnormalwerte wichtiger Parameter bei der Griechischen Lanschildkröte (Testudo hermanni hermanni). *Tierarztl. Prax.* 20: 231–234.

46 Rosskopf, W.J. (1982). Normal haemogram and blood chemistry values for California desert tortoises. *Vet. Med. Small Anim. Clin.* 77: 85–87.

47 Perpiñán, D., Armstrong, D.L., and Dórea, F. (2011). Effect of anticoagulant and venipuncture site on hematology and serum chemistries of the spiny softshell turtle (Apalone spinifera). *J. Herp. Med. Surg.* 20 (2–3): 74–78.

48 Benson, K.G., Paul-Murphy, J., and MacWilliams, R. (1999). Effects of hemolysis on plasma electrolyte and chemistry values in the common green iguana (Iguana iguana). *J. Zoo Wildl. Med.* 30 (3): 415–415.

49 Campbell, T.W. (2006). Clinical pathology of reptiles. In: *Reptile Medicine and Surgery* (ed. D.R. Mader), 453–470. Philadelphia: WB Saunders Comp.

50 Shin, C.S., Chang, C.H., and Kim, J.H. (2006). Liquid heparin anticoagulant produces more negative bias in the determination of ionized magnesium than ionized calcium. *Yonsei Med. J.* 47 (2): 191–195.

51 Deem, S.L., Dierenfeld, E.S., Sounguet, G.S. et al. (2006). Blood values in free ranging nesting leatherback sea turtles (Dermochelys coriacea) on the coast of the republic of Gabon. *J. Zoo Wildl. Med.* 37: 464–471.

52 Taylor, R.W. and Jacobson, E.R. (1982). Hematology and serum chemistry of the gopher tortoise, Gopherus polyphemus. *Comp. Biochem. Physiol. A.* 72: 425–428.

53 Anderson, E.T., Minter, L.J., Clarke, E.O. et al. (2011). The effects of feeding on hematological and plasma biochemical profiles in green (Chelonia mydas) and Kemp's ridley (Lepidochelys kempii) sea turtles. *Vet. Med. Internat.* ID 890829. 7 pages, https://doi.org/10.4061/2011/890829.

54 Knotková, Z., Dorrenstein, G.M., Jekl, V. et al. (2008). Fasting and postprandial serum bile acid concentrations in 10 healthy female red-eared terrapins (Trachemys scripta elegans). *Vet. Rec.* 163: 510–514.

55 Anderson, N.L., Wack, R.F., and Hatcher, R. (1997). Hematology and clinical chemistry reference ranges for clinically normal, captive new Guinea snapping turtle (Elseya novaeguineae) and the effects of temperature, sex, and sample type. *J. Zoo Wildl. Med.* 28: 394–403.

56 Flint, M., Limpus, D.J., Limpus, C.J. et al. (2011). Biochemical and hematological reference intervals for Krefft's turtles Emydura macquarii krefftii from the Burnett River catchment, Australia. *Dis. Aquat. Org.* 95 (1): 43–48.

57 Brenner, D., Lewbart, G., Stebbins, M., and Herman, D. (2002). Health survey of wild and captive bog turtles (Clemmys muhlenbergii) in North Carolina and Virginia. *J. Zoo Wildl. Med.* 33: 311–316.

58 Chansue, N., Sailasuta, A., Tangtrongpiros, J. et al. (2011). Hematology and clinical chemistry of adult yellow-headed temple turtles (Hieremys annandalii) in Thailand. *Vet. Clin. Pathol.* 40 (2): 174–184.

59 Chaffin, K., Norton, T.M., Gilardi, K. et al. (2008). Health assessment of free-ranging alligator snapping turtles (Macrochelys temminckii) in Georgia and Florida. *J. Wildl. Dis.* 44 (3): 670–686.

60 Hidalgo-Vila, J., Díaz-Paniagua, C., Pérez-Santigosa, N. et al. (2007). Hematologic and biochemical reference intervals of free-living Mediterranean pond turtles (Mauremys leprosa). *J. Wildl. Dis.* 43 (4): 798–801.

61 Chung, C., Cheng, C., Chin, S. et al. (2009). Morphologic and cytochemical characteristics of Asian yellow pond turtle (Ocadia sinensis) blood cells and their hematologic and plasma biochemical reference values. *J. Zoo Wildl. Med.* 40: 76–85.

62 Zago, C.E.S., Ferrarezi, A.L., Vizotto, L.D. et al. (2010). Hemoglobin polymorphism and hematological profile of Geoffroy's side-necked turtle (Phrynops geoffroanus, Testudines) in the northwestern region of São Paulo state, Brazil. *Genet. Mol. Res.* 9 (2): 721–726.

63 Oliveira-Junior, A.A., Tavares-Dias, M., and Marcon, J.L. (2009). Biochemical and hematological reference ranges for Amazon freshwater turtle, Podocnemis expansa (Reptilia: Pelomedusidae), with morphologic assessment of blood cells. *Res. Vet. Sci.* 86: 146–151.

64 Rossini, M., Blanco, P.A., Marín, E. et al. (2012). Haematological values of post-laying Arrau turtle (Podocnemis expansa) in the Orinoco River. *Venezuela. Res. Vet. Sci.* 92 (1): 128–131.

65 Troiano, J.C. and Silva, M.C. (1998). Valores hematologicos de referencia em Tortuga terrestre Argentina (Chelonoidis chilensis chilensis). *Anacleta Vet.* 18: 47–51.

66 Zaias, J., Norton, T., Fickel, A. et al. (2008). Biochemical and hematologic values for 18 clinically healthy radiated tortoises (Geochelone radiata) on St Catherine's island. *Georgia. Vet. Clin. Pathol.* 35 (3): 321–325.

67 Raphael, B.L., Klemens, M.W., Moehlman, P. et al. (1994). Blood values in free-ranging pancake tortoises (Malacochersus tornieri). *J. Zoo Wildl. Med.* 25 (1): 63–67.

68 Knotková, Z., Doubek, J., Knotek, Z., and Hájkova, P. (2002). Blood cell morphology and plasma biochemistry in Russian tortoises. *Acta Vet. Brno* 71: 191–198.

69 Marks, S.K. and Citino, S.B. (1990). Hematology and serum chemistry of the radiated tortoise (Testudo radiata). *J. Zoo Wildl. Med.* 21: 342–344.

70 Dein, F.J., Wilson, A., Fischer, D., and Langenberg, P. (1994). Avian leucocyte counting using the hemocytometer. *J. Zoo Wildl. Med.* 25: 432–437.

71 Natt, M.P. and Herrick, C.A. (1952). A new blood diluent for counting the erythrocytes and leukocytes of the chicken. *Poult. Sci.* 31: 735–738.

72 Altland, P.D. and Brace, K.C. (1962). Red cell lifespan in the turtle and toad. *Am. J. Phys.* 206 (6): 1188–1190.

73 Sheeler, P. and Barber, A.A. (1964). Comparative hematology of the turtle, rabbit and rat. Comp. Biochem. *Physiol.* 11: 139–145.

74 Allender, M.C., Fry, M.M., Irizarry, A.R. et al. (2006). Intracytoplasmic inclusions in circulating leukocytes from an eastern box turtle (Terrapene carolina carolina) with iridoviral infection. *J. Wildl. Dis.* 42 (3): 677–684.

75 Keller, J.M., Kucklick, J.R., Stamper, M.A. et al. (2004). Associations between organochlorine contaminant concentrations and clinical health parameters in loggerhead sea turtles from North Carolina, USA. *Environ. Health Perspect.* 112: 1074–1079.

76 Lutcavage, M.E., Lutz, P.L., Bossart, G.D., and Hudson, D.M. (1995). Physiologic and clinicopathologic effects of crude oil on loggerhead sea turtles. *Arch. Environ. Contam. Toxicol.* 28: 417–422.

77 Innis, C.J., Ravich, J.B., Tlusty, M.F. et al. (2009). Hematologic and plasma biochemical findings in cold-stunned Kemp's ridley sea turtles (Lepidochelys kempii): 176 cases (2001–2005). *J. Am. Vet. Med. Assoc.* 235: 426–432.

78 Kaplan, H.M. and Rueff, W. (1960). Seasonal blood changes in turtles. *Proc. Anim. Care. Panel.* 10: 63–68.

79 Alleman, A.R., Jacobson, E.R., and Raskin, R.E. (1992). Morphologic and cytochemical characteristics of blood cells from the desert tortoise (Gopherus agassizii). *Am. J. Vet. Res.* 53: 1645–1651.

80 Jacques, F.A. (1963). Blood coagulation and anticoagulant mechanisms in the turtle Pseudemys elegans. *Comp. Biochem. Physiol.* 9 (3): 241–249.

81 Daimon, T., Gotoh, Y., and Uchida, K. (1987). Electron microscopic and cytochemical studies of the thrombocytes of the tortoise (Geoclemys reevesii). *J. Anat.* 153: 185–190.

82 Azevedo, A. and Lunardi, L.O. (2003). Cytochemical characterization of eosinophilic leukocytes circulating in the blood of the turtle (Chrysemys dorbigni). *Acta Histochem.* 105 (1): 99–105.

83 Perpiñán, D. and Sánchez, C. (2009). Morphologic and cytochemical characteristics of blood cells from the European pond turtle (Emys orbicularis) and the Mediterranean pond turtle (Mauremys leprosa). *J. Herp. Med. Surg.* 19 (4): 119–127.

84 Taylor, K. and Kaplan, H.M. (1961). Light microscopy of the blood cells of Pseudemydid turtles. *Herpetologica* 17: 186–192.

85 Mead, K.F., Borysenko, M., and Findlay, S.R. (1983). Naturally abundant basophils in the snapping turtle, Chelydra serpentina, possess cytophilic surface antibody with reaginic function. *J. Immuonl.* 130: 334–340.

86 Sypek, J.P. (1984). Anti-immunoglobulin induced histamine release from naturally abundant basophils in the snapping turtle, Chelydra serpentina. *Dev. Comp. Immunol.* 8: 359–366.

87 Day, R.D., Segars, A.L., Arendt, A.D. et al. (2007). Relationship of blood mercury levels to health parameters in the loggerhead sea turtle (Caretta caretta). *Environ. Health Perspect.* 115: 1421–1428.

88 Frye, F.L. and Carney, J. (1972). Myeloproliferative disease in a turtle. *J. Am. Vet. Med. Assoc.* 161 (6): 595–599.

89 Mihalca, A., Acheălriței, D., and Popescu, P. (2002). Haemoparasites of the genus Haemogregarina in a population of European pond turtles (Emys orbicularis) from Drăgășani, Vâlcea county, Romania. *Sci, Parasitol.* 2: 22–27.

90 Saad, A.H., Torroba, M., Varas, A., and Zapata, A. (1991). Testosterone induces lymphopenia in turtles. *Vet. Immunol. Immunopathol.* 28: 173–180.

91 St. John, R. and Nardone, R.S. (1956). Eosinophil levels of the turtle after exposure to cold and epinephrine. *Am. J. Phys.* 188: 420–422.

92 Neiffer, D.L., Lydick, D., Burks, K., and Doherty, D. (2005). Hematologic and plasma biochemical changes associated with fenbendazole administration in Hermann's tortoises (Testudo hermanni). *J. Zoo Wildl. Med.* 36: 661–672.

93 Davis, A.K. and Sterrett, S.C. (2011). Prevalence of Haemogregarine parasites in three freshwater turtle species in Northeast Georgia. *USAInt. J. Zool. Res.* 7 (2): 156–163.

94 Davis, A.K. and Holcomb, K.L. (2008). Intraerythrocytic inclusion bodies in painted turtles (Chrysemys picta picta) with measurements of affected cells. *Comp. Clin. Pathol.* 17: 51–54.

95 Basile, F., DiSanti, A., Caldora, M. et al. (2011). Inclusion bodies in loggerhead erythrocytes are associated with unstable hemoglobin and resemble human Heinz bodies. *J. Exp. Zool. A Ecol. Genet. Physiol.* 315A: 416–423.

96 Schmidt, V., Dyachenko, V., Aupperle, H. et al. (2008). Case report of systemic coccidiosis in a radiated tortoise (Geochelone radiata). *Parasitol. Res.* 102 (3): 431–436.

97 Hutton, K.E. and Goodnight, C.J. (1957). Variations in the blood chemistry of turtles under active and hibernating conditions. *Physiol. Zool.* 30: 198–207.

98 Seccareccia, V.J., Lloyd, M.I., and Martin, J.C. (1997). Coagulation parameters of clinically normal radiated (Geochelone radiata) and leopard (Geochelone pardalis) tortoises. *Proc. Assoc. Rept. Amphib. Vet.* 89–91.

99 Frommeyer U, Weinzierl F.. Klinisch relevante Blutparameter bei Reptilien. Fortbildungsveranstaltungen der Bayerischen Landestieraerztekammer, Bd. 6 Reptilienmedizin. 2008;80–94.

100 Rangel-Mendoza, J., Weber, M., Zenteno-Ruiz, C.E. et al. (2009). Hematology and serum biochemistry comparison in wild and captive central American river turtles (Dermatemys mawii) in tabasco, Mexico. *Res. Vet. Sci.* 87: 313–318.

101 Metin, K., Türkozan, O., Kargin, F. et al. (2006). Blood cell morphology and plasma biochemistry of the captive European pond turtle Emys orbicularis. *Acta Vet. Brno* 75: 49–55.

102 Rooney, M.B., Levine, G., Gaynor, J. et al. (1999). Sevoflurane anesthesia in desert tortoises. *J. Zoo Wildl. Med.* 30: 64–69.

103 Eatwell, K. (2009). Comparison of total calcium, ionized calcium and albumin concentrations in the plasma of captive tortoises (testudo species). *Vet. Rec.* 165: 466–468.

104 Montesinos A, Martinez R, Jimenez A. Proc. 27th WSAVA/FECAVA/AVEPA Congress. Plasma bile acids concentration in tortoises: reference values and histopathologic findings of importance for interpretation. 2002;2:125.

105 Jacobson, E.R., Gaskin, J.M., Brown, M.B. et al. (1991). Chronic upper respiratory tract disease of free-ranging desert tortoises (Xerobates agassizii). *J. Wildl. Dis.* 27: 296–316.

106 Dickinson, V.M., Jarchow, J., and Trueblood, M.H. (2002). Hematology and plasma biochemistry reference range values for free-ranging desert tortoises in Arizona. *J. Wildl. Dis.* 38 (1): 143–153.

107 Frye, F.L. (1991). *Biomedical and Surgical Aspects of Captive Reptile Husbandry*, 2e, vol. 1. Melbourne: Krieger Publishing.

108 Gimenez, M., Saco, Y., Pato, R. et al. (2010). Plasma protein electrophoresis of Trachemys scripta and Iguana iguana. *Vet. Clin. Pathol.* 39 (2): 227–235.

109 Anderson, E.T., Socha, V.L., Gardner, J. et al. (2013). Tissue enzyme activities in the loggerhead sea turtle (Caretta caretta). *J. Zoo Wildl. Med.* 44 (1): 62–69.

110 Ramsay, E.C. and Dotson, T.K. (1995). Tissue and serum enzyme activities in the yellow rat snake (Elaphe obsoleta quadrivittata). *Am. J. Vet. Res.* 56: 423–428.

111 Wagner, R.A. and Wetzel, R. (1999). Tissue and plasma enzyme activities in the juvenile green iguanas. *J. Am. Vet. Med. Assoc.* 60 (2): 201–203.

112 Innis, C., Merigo, C., Dodge, K. et al. (2010). Health evaluation of leatherback turtles (Dermochelys coriacea) in the northwestern Atlantic during direct capture and fisheries gear disentanglement. *Chel. Cons. Biol.* 9 (2): 205–222.

113 Knotková, Z., Knotek, Z., and Hájková, P. (2000). Plasma biochemistry of chelonians of the Geochelone group. *Proc. Eur. Assoc. Zoo Wildl. Vet.* 281–285.

114 Austin, C.C. and Jessing, K.W. (1994). Green-blood pigmentation in lizards. *Comp. Biochem. Physiol.* 109A: 619–626.

115 Schaffner, F. The liver. In: *Biology of the Reptilia*, Morphology G: Visceral Organs, vol. 19 (ed. C. Gans and A.S. Gaunt), 485–531. Ithaca, NY: Society for the Study of Amphibians and Reptiles.

116 Lomas, A. and Waters, M. (2000). The potential use of plasma glutamate dehydrogenase activity for the evaluation of hepatocellular damage in reptiles. *Proc. Brit. Vet. Zool Soc.* 32.

117 Hernandez-Divers, S.J. and Cooper, J.E. (2006). Hepatic lipidosis. In: *Reptile Medicine and Surgery* (ed. D.R. Mader), 806–813. St Louis: Saunders Elsevier.

118 Stahl, S. (2006). Hyperglycemia in reptiles. In: *Reptile Medicine and Surgery*, 2e (ed. D. Mader), 822–830. St. Louis: Elsevier.

119 Laffel, L. (1999). Ketone bodies: a review of physiology, pathophysiology and application of monitoring to diabetes. *Diabetes Metab. Res. Rev.* 15: 412–426.

120 Chilian WM. Master's Thesis. Texas Tech University. Lubbock, TX. Physiological strategies of dormancy of *Kinosternon flavescens*. 1976;1–53.

121 Keller, K., Innis, C., Tlusty, M.F. et al. (2012). Metabolic and respiratory derangements associated with death in cold-stunned Kemp's ridley turtles (Lepidochelys kempii): 32 cases (2005-2009). *J. Am. Vet. Med. Assoc.* 240 (3): 317–323.

122 Müller, K. and Brunnberg, L. (2010). Determination of plasma albumin concentration in healthy and diseased turtles: a comparison of protein electrophoresis and the bromcresol green dye-binding method. *Vet. Clin. Pathol.* 39 (1): 79–82.

123 Ultsch, G.R., Herbert, C.V., and Jackson, D.C. (1984). The comparative physiology of diving in north American freshwater turtles. I. Submergence tolerance, gas exchange, and acid-base balance. *Physiol. Zool.* 57 (6): 620–631.

124 Burggren, W., Smits, A., and Evans, B. (1989). Arterial O_2 homeostasis during diving in the turtle Chelodina longicollis. *Physiol. Zool.* 62 (3): 668–686.

125 Gordos, M.A., Franklin, C.E., Limpus, C.J., and Wilson, G. (2004). Blood-respiratory and acid–base changes during extended diving in the bimodally respiring freshwater turtle Rheodytes leukops. *J. Comp. Physiol. B.* 174 (4): 347–354.

126 Crocker, C.E., Ultsch, G.R., and Jackson, D.C. (1999). The physiology of diving in a north-temperate and three tropical turtle species. *J. Comp. Physiol. B.* 169 (4–5): 249–255.

127 Bagatto, B. and Henry, R.P. (1999). Exercise and forced submergence in the pond slider (Trachemys scripta) and softshell turtle (Apalone ferox): influence on bimodal gas exchange, diving behaviour and blood acid–base status. *J. Exp. Biol.* 202: 267–278.

128 Gaumer, A.E.H. and Goodnight, C.J. (1957). Some aspects of the hematology of turtles as related to their activity. *Am. Midl. Nat.* 58: 332–340.

129 Gatten, R.E. Jr. (1975). Effects of activity on blood oxygen saturation, lactate, and pH in the turtles Pseudemys scripta and Terrapene ornata. *Physiol. Zool.* 48 (1): 24–35.

130 Wood, S.C., Lykkeboe, G., Johansen, K. et al. (1978). Temperature acclimation in the pancake tortoise, Malacochersus tornieri: metabolic rate, blood pH, oxygen affinity and red cell organic phosphates. *Comp. Biochem. Physiol. A.* 59 (2): 155–160.

131 Nunn, J.F., Bergman, N.A., Bunatyan, A., and Coleman, A.J. (1965). Temperature coefficients for pCO2 and PO2 of blood in vitro. *J. Appl. Physiol.* 20 (1): 23–26.

132 Innis, C., Tlusty, M., Merigo, C., and Weber, E.S. (2007). Metabolic and respiratory status of cold-stunned Kemp's ridley sea turtles (Lepidochelys kempii). *J. Comp. Physiol. B.* 177: 623–630.
133 Moon, D.Y., Mackenzie, D.S., and Owens, D.W. (1997). Simulated hibernation of sea turtles in the laboratory: I. Feeding, breathing frequency, blood pH, and blood gases. *J. Exp. Zool.* 278: 372–380.
134 Harms, C.A., Mallo, K.M., Ross, P.M., and Segars, A. (2003). Venous blood gases and lactates of wild loggerhead sea turtles (Caretta caretta) following two capture techniques. *J. Wildl. Dis.* 39: 366–374.
135 Ashwood, E.R., Kost, G., and Kenny, M. (1983). Temperature correction of blood-gas and pH measurements. *Clin. Chem.* 29: 1877–1885.
136 Roughton, F.J.W. and Severinghaus, J.W. (1973). Accurate determination of O2 dissociation curve of human blood above 98.7% saturation with data on O2 solubility in unmodified human blood from 0° to 37°C. *J. Appl. Physiol.* 35: 861–869.
137 Fogh-Anderson, N. (1981). Ionized calcium analyzer with built in pH correction. *Clin. Chem.* 27: 1264–1267.
138 Ising, H., Bertschat, F., Günther, T. et al. (1995). Measurement of free magnesium in blood, serum and plasma with an ion sensitive electrode. *Eur. J. Clin. Chem. Biochem.* 33: 365–371.
139 Reeves, R.B. (1977). The interaction of body temperature and acid-base balance in ectothermic vertebrates. *Annu. Rev. Physiol.* 39: 559–586.
140 Nicol, S.C., Glass, M.L., and Heisler, N. (1983). Comparison of directly determined and calculated plasma bicarbonate concentration in the turtle Chrysemys picta bellii at different temperatures. *J. Exp. Biol.* 107: 521–525.
141 Reese, S.A., Jackson, D.C., and Ultsch, G.R. (2002). The physiology of overwintering in a turtle that occupies multiple habitats, the common snapping turtle (Chelydra serpentina). *Physiol. Biochem. Zool.* 75 (5): 432–438.
142 Köelle, P., Wiedemann, A., and Kienzle, E. (2011). Vitamin E in plasma of reptiles. *Proc. Assoc. Rept. Amphib. Vet.* 182.
143 Eatwell, K. (2008). Plasma concentrations of 25-cholecalciferol in 22 captive tortoises (testudo sp.). *Vet. Rec.* 162: 342–345.
144 Dierenfeld, E.S. (1989). Vitamin E deficiency in zoo reptiles, birds, and ungulates. *J. Zoo Wildl. Med.* 29: 3–11.
145 Holladay, S.D., Wolf, J.C., Smith, S.A. et al. (2001). Aural abscesses in wild-caught box turtles (Terrapene carolina):possible role of organochlorine-induced hypovitaminosis A. *Ecotox. Environ Saf.* 48: 99–106.
146 Acierno, M.J., Mitchell, M.A., Roundtree, M.K., and Zachariah, T. (2006). Effects of ultraviolet radiation on 25-hydroxyvitamin D3 synthesis in red-eared slider turtles (Trachemys scripta elegans). *Am. J. Vet. Res.* 67: 2046–2049.
147 Clark, N.B. (1967). Influence of estrogens upon serum calcium, phosphate and protein concentrations of fresh-water turtles. *Comp. Biochem. Physiol.* 20: 823–834.
148 Oguro, C., Tomisawa, A., and Matuoka, N. (1974). Effect of parathyroidectomy on the serum calcium and phosphorus in the tortoise. *Testudo graeca. Zoo. Mag.* 83: 201–202.
149 Rivera, S. and Lock, B. (2008). The reptilian thyroid and parathyroid glands. *Vet. Clin. North Am. Exotic. Anim. Pract.* 11: 163–175.
150 Silver, R.B. and Jackson, D.C. (1986). Ionic compensation with no renal response to chronic hypercapnia in Chrysemys picta belli. *Am. J. Phys. Regul. Integr. Comp. Phys.* 251: 1228–1234.
151 Borkowski, R. (1997). Lead poisoning and intestinal perforations in a snapping turtle (Chelydra serpentina) because of fishing gear ingestion. *J. Zoo Wildl. Med.* 28 (1): 109–113.
152 Sleeman, J.M., Brown, J., Steffen, D. et al. (2008). Relationships among aural abscesses, organochlorine compounds, and vitamin a in free-ranging eastern box turtles (Terrapene carolina carolina). *J. Wildl. Dis.* 44 (4): 922–929.
153 Hulbert, A.J. and Williams, C.A. (1988). Thyroid function in a lizard, a tortoise and a crocodile, compared with mammals. *Comp. Biochem. Physiol.* 90A (1): 41–48.
154 Sawin, C.T., Bacharach, P., and Lance, V. (1981). Thyrotropin-releasing hormone and thyrotropin in the control of thyroid function in the turtle, Chrysemys picta. *Gen. Comp. Endocrinol.* 45: 7–11.
155 Franco, K.H., Famini, D.J., Hoover, J.P., and Payton, M.E. (2009). Serum thyroid values for African spurred tortoises (Centrochelys [formerly Geochelone] sulcata). *J. Herpetol Med. Surg.* 19 (2): 47–49.
156 Kohel, K.A., MacKenzie, D.S., Rostal, D.C. et al. (2001). Seasonality in plasma thyroxine in the desert tortoise, Gopherus agassizii. *Gen. Comp. Endocrinol.* 121: 214–222.
157 DiGesualdo, C.L., West, G., Brown, T.R., and Hoover, J.P. (2004). Determining normal thyroid hormone status in Galapagos tortoises (Geochelone elphantopus), then comparing normal levels to thyroid levels of Galapagos tortoises suspected of hypothyroidism. *Proc. Am. Assoc. Zoo Vet.* 546–547.
158 Buehler, I. (2006). Veterinary doctorate dissertation, veterinary faculty, Ludwig-Maximilians-university,

Munich, Germany. *Thyroid parameters in common veterinary practice presented in tortoise species.* 1–139.

159 Boyer, T. and Steffes, Z.J. (2011). Reptilian thyroid anatomy, physiology and disease. *Proc .Assoc. Rept. Amphib. Vet.* 18–35.

160 Licht, P., Breitenbach, G.L., and Congdon, J.D. (1985). Seasonal cycles in testicular activity, gonadotropin, and thyroxine in the painted turtle, Chrysemys picta, under natural conditions. *Gen. Comp. Endocrinol.* 59: 130–139.

161 Licht, P., Denver, R.J., and Pavgi, S. (1989). Temperature dependence of in vitro pituitary, testis, and thyroid secretion in a turtle, Pseudemys scripta. *Gen. Comp. Endocrinol.* 76: 274–285.

162 Sarkar, S., Sengupta, A., Chaudhuri-Sengupta, S., and Maiti, B. (2007). Thyroid responses to altered photoperiod in the soft-shelled turtle Lissemys punctata punctata. *Acta Biol. Hung.* 58 (1): 11–19.

163 Semple, R.E. (1975). Seasonal changes in thyroid activity in turtles native to Ontario, Canada. *J. Physiol.* 245 (2): 115–117.

164 Sengupta, A., Ray, P.P., Chaudhuri Sengupta, S., and Maiti, B.R. (2003). Thyroidal modulation following hypo- and hyperthermia in the soft-shelled turtle Lissemys punctata Bonnoterre. *Eur. J. Morphol.* 41 (5): 149–154.

165 Hunt, K.E., Innis, C., and Rolland, R.M. (2012). Corticosterone and thyroxine in cold-stunned Kemp's ridley sea turtles (Lepidochelys kempii). *J. Zoo Wildl. Med.* 43: 479–493.

166 Hunt, K.E., Innis, C.J., Merigo, C., and Rolland, R.M. (2016). Endocrine responses to diverse stressors of capture, entanglement and stranding in leatherback turtles (Dermochelys coriacea). *Conservation Physiology* 4 (1): https://doi.org/10.1093/conphys/cow022.

167 Frye, F.L. and Dutra, F.R. (1974). Hypothyroidism in turtles and tortoises. *Vet. Med. Small Anim. Clin.* 69: 990–993.

168 Norton, T.M., Jacobson, E.R., Caligiuri, R., and Kollias, G.V. (1989). Medical management of a Galapagos tortoise (Geochelone elephantopus) with hypothyroidism. *J. Zoo Wildl. Med.* 20 (2): 212–216.

169 Cash, W.B., Holberton, R.L., and Knight, S.S. (1997). Corticosterone secretion in response to capture and handling in free-living red-eared slider turtles. *Gen. Comp. Endocrinol.* 108 (3): 427–433.

170 Kuchling, G. (1999). The reproductive biology of the chelonia. *Zoophysiology* 38: 1–223.

171 Rostal, D.C., Lance, V.A., Grumbles, J.S., and Alberts, A.C. (1994). Seasonal cycle of the desert tortoise (Gopherus agassizii) in the eastern Mojave Desert. *Herpetol. Monogr.* 8: 72–82.

172 Dantzler, W.H. and Schmidt-Nielsen, B. (1966). Excretion in the fresh-water turtle (Pseudemys scripta) and desert tortoise (Gopherus agassizii). *Am. J. Phys.* 210: 198–210.

173 Gibbons, P.M., Horton, S.J., and Brandl, S.R.W. (2000). Urinalysis in box turtles, Terrapene species. *Proc. Assoc. Rept. Amphib. Vet.* 161–168.

174 Divers, S.J. and Innis, C.J. (2006). Renal disease in reptiles: diagnosis and clinical management. In: *Reptile Medicine and Surgery*, 2nde (ed. D.R. Mader), 878–892. St. Louis: Elsevier.

175 Innis, C.J. (1997). Observations on urinalyses of clinically normal captive tortoises. *Proc. Assoc. Rept. Amphib. Vet.* 109–112.

176 Köelle, P. (2000). Urinalysis in tortoises. *Proc. Assoc. Rept. Amphib. Vet.* 111–114.

177 Hunter, K.W., Dupre, S.A., Sharp, T. et al. (2008). Western blot can distinguish natural and acquired antibodies to mycoplasma agassizii in the desert tortoise (Gopherus agassizii). *J. Microbiol. Methods* 75: 464–471.

178 Johnson, A.J., Wendland, L., Norton, T.M. et al. (2010). Development and use of an indirect enzyme-linked immunosorbent assay for detection of iridovirus exposure in gopher tortoises (Gopherus polyphemus) and eastern box turtles (Terrapene carolina carolina). *Vet. Microbiol.* 160–167.

179 Marschang, R.E., Rösler, R., Degan, M.A., and Papp, T. (2011). Detection of antibodies against paramyxoviruses in tortoises. *Proc. Assoc. Rept. Amphib. Vet.* 114.

180 Marschang, R.E. and Schneider, R.M. (2007). Antibodies to viruses in wild-caught spur-thighed tortoises (Testudo graeca) in Turkey. *Vet. Rec.* 161: 102–103.

181 Wendland, L.D., Klein, P.A., Jacobson, E.R., and Brown, M.B. (2010). Mycoplasma agassizii strain variation and distinct host antibody responses explain differences between enzyme-linked immunosorbent assays and western blot assays. *Clin. Vaccine Immunol.* 17 (11): 1739–1745.

182 Johnson, A.J., Morafka, D.J., and Jacobson, E.R. (2006). Seroprevalence of mycoplasma agassizii and tortoise herpesvirus in captive desert tortoises(Gopherus agassizii) from the greater Barstow Area,Mojave Desert, California. *J. Arid Environ.* 67: 192–201.

183 Heatley, J.J., Wohl, J., and Mitchell, M. (2006). Determination of electrolyte, acid-base, and venous blood gas parameters in critically injured Emydid turtles. *Proc. Assoc. Rept. Amphib. Vet.* 87–88.

184 Origgi, F.C., Romero, C.H., Bloom, D.C. et al. (2004). Experimental transmission of a herpesvirus in Greek tortoises (Testudo graeca). *Vet. Pathol.* 41: 50–61.

17

Snakes

Jen Brown DVM, DACVP (Clinical Pathology)[1], Tim Tristan DVM, DABVP (Reptilian and Amphibian)[2] and J. Jill Heatley DVM, MS, DABVP (Avian, Reptilian, Amphibian), DACZM[3]

[1] Rochester, New York, USA
[2] Texas Sealife Center, Corpus Christi, Texas, USA
[3] Department of Small Animal Clinical Sciences, College of Veterinary Medicine & Biomedical Sciences, Texas A&M University, College Station, Texas, USA

Introduction

The hematology and clinical chemistry of snakes continue to develop as more research and information are obtained. Reference intervals published for snake species vary widely. Diversity results from individual patient factors (intrinsic and extrinsic), blood collection techniques, laboratory methodology, and environmental parameters. Patient variables include factors such as age, sex, reproductive status, temperature, geographical location, season, nutrition, captivity status, brumation/hibernation status, and stress. Blood collection variables include location, sample handling, and contamination. Laboratory variables include methodology, individual laboratory quality control and quality assurance, staff experience and staff training, and lack of standardized leukocyte identification techniques and reference ranges for individual snake species. These many variables may affect results and make the establishment and interpretation of reference intervals for snakes challenging. Further complicating the interpretation, most reference intervals do not record the many factors which affect biochemical or hematologic analytes. Therefore, published reference intervals should be interpreted with caution and used only as an estimate or guide. Decision levels allow application of published values to those obtained from a specific laboratory or hospital, to facilitate a response above or below a certain value of an analyte. However, decision levels have not been established for most snakes. Ideally, a set of hematologic and clinical chemistry values should be obtained from healthy snakes maintained with specified, optimal environmental and nutritional parameters to provide best comparison to health when these patients become ill.

Species

Snakes are characterized by their lack of limbs and eyelids, their tubular elongate body, and their carnivorous diet. Body morphology reduces the number of options for hematologic sampling. As widely radiated, highly evolved squamates, snake species have a variety of lifestyles and a plethora of attendant physiologic adaptations. While the reader may note that much information is drawn from studies of captive and free-living venomous snakes, the authors do recommend or advocate these creatures as patients in private practice. "Hot" snakes are somewhat overrepresented in the scientific literature likely owing to the human need for production of antivenoms. However, species commonly seen as exotic pets by the veterinarian are largely limited to the non-venomous species of the genera Colubridae and Boidae.

Sample Collection

Restraint

Blood samples can often be collected from snakes using manual restraint. However, in the case of venomous, large, or aggressive species, general anesthesia or chemical restraint may be required. Appropriate handling, restraint, and treatment of venomous species requires specialized handling skills, techniques, and equipment for the safety of both humans and snakes. The reader may consult excellent texts review sedation or anesthetic regimens appropriate for snakes including injections of tiletamine/zolazepam, propofol, or isoflurane or sevoflurane administered via induction chamber [1].

Exotic Animal Laboratory Diagnosis, First Edition. Edited by J. Jill Heatley and Karen E. Russell.

Sample Volume

The blood volume of reptiles varies among species, but is approximately 5%–8% of the body weight [2–4]. Marine snakes tend to have higher blood volume. Sea snakes of the genus *Hydrophis* and the file snake, *Acrochordus gramdatus*, have blood volumes of greater than 9% of their bodyweight [4]. Blood volume may also substantially decrease in some species of snake owing to activity [3]. Resting blood volumes (mean ± SE) of the western rat snake *Elaphe (Pantherophis) obsoleta* and prairie rattlesnake *Crotalus viridis* were 6.07 ± 0.40% and 6.41 ± 0.06% of the body mass, respectively [5]. Snake species may tolerate withdrawal of up to 10% of their blood volume for a single sample when healthy, but only approximately 0.2–1 ml of whole blood is needed for most routine hematologic studies [6]. In the research setting, larger volume percentages of blood may be repeatedly removed over an extended time period with apparent detrimental effect; limits for serial blood sampling have yet to be clearly defined for these species [4, 7].

Sample Collection Sites of the Snake

Common collection sites include the ventral coccygeal or tail vein, the ventricles of the heart, and less commonly, the palatine or vertebral veins.

Tail or Ventral Coccygeal Vein

One of the most common venipuncture sites used in snakes is the ventral coccygeal vein, or tail vein. This vessel is accessed in the portion of the tail located 25%–50% distal to the cloaca. Needle gauges of 25–22 gauge (g.) and lengths of 5/8–1½ in., with an attached syringe of 1–5 ml, are common choices depending on the patient size. The needle is inserted at a 45°–90° angle at the midline, under a ventral midline scale. Advance the needle in a craniodorsal direction, while maintaining slight negative pressure. Should the needle make contact with a vertebral body, withdraw it a small amount until blood flows into the syringe. Directing the needle tip slightly further cranial or caudal may also facilitate blood flow. Avoid attempting ventral coccygeal venipuncture close to the vent, to avoid damage to the hemipenes of males or musk glands of females (Figures 17.1–17.3).

Cardiac

Cardiocentesis is the preferred method of snake venipuncture for nonvenomous species >300 g [8]. However, cardiocentesis requires adequate patient immobilization, venipuncture skill, and patience. Cardiocentesis has been used for serial sampling of snakes (>120 blood samples obtained over 120 days) without apparent ill effect in the laboratory setting [7].

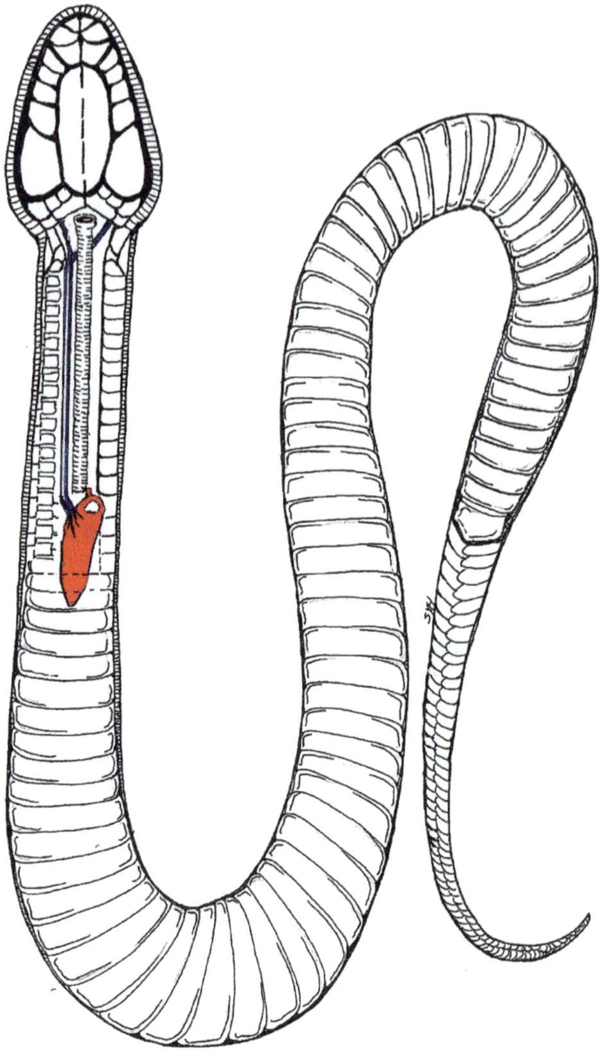

Figure 17.1 Generalized cardiac position of the snake. The ventricle is routinely used for venipuncture. Snake heart position is mobile and also varies based on genera [10–13].

However, as a general rule for the snake patient, only three attempts at cardiocentesis should be made in a single sampling episode [9]. Euhydration and the preferred optimum body temperature should be established for the patient prior to reattempting cardiocentesis.

Because the heart is a mobile organ to allow food passage, it must be located and stabilized prior to cardiocentesis. The location of the heart in snakes varies depending on physiologic and anatomic adaptations. In terrestrial and arboreal species, the heart is located from 15% to 20% of the snake's total length from the head. In totally aquatic species, the heart is located from 25% to 45% of the snake's total length from the head (Figure 17.4) [10, 11]. Similarly, in boids, the heart tends to be more caudally located in relational total patient body length than in colubrids [12, 13]. Cardiac location may be determined by a number of methods. In all methods, the snake must first be restrained and stabilized, often in

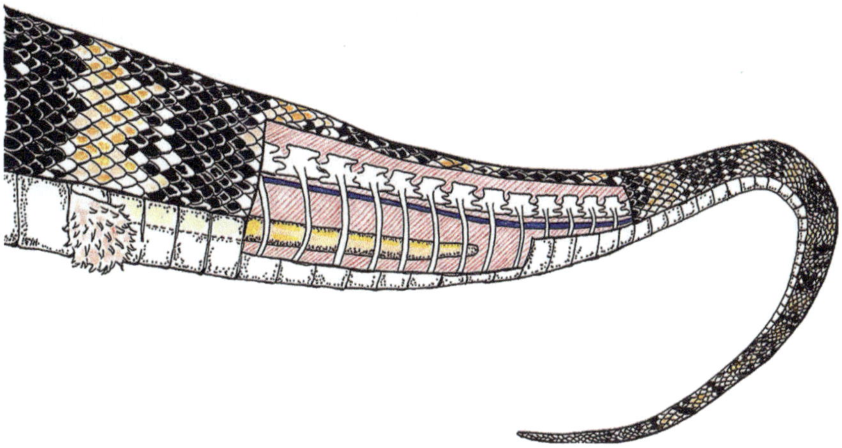

Figure 17.2 Local anatomy for approach to the ventral coccygeal vein of the male snake. The spiny hemipene is exteriorized at the cloaca as the hemipene pouch is shown as it extends caudally 12 scales. The ventral coccygeal vein is depicted in blue as it courses below the coccygeal vertebrae.

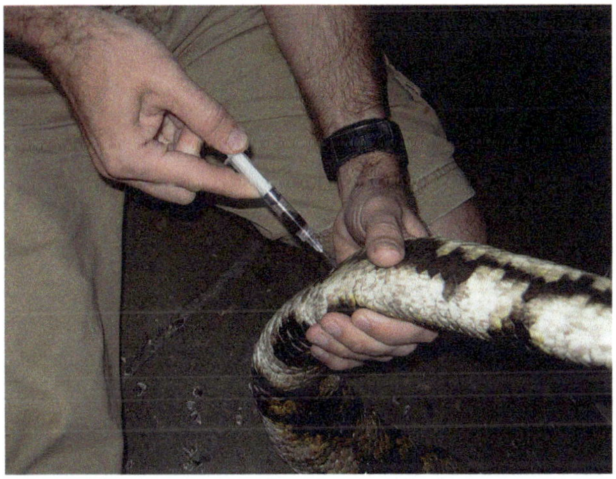

Figure 17.3 Approach for venipuncture of the tail veins of a large snake.

dorsal recumbency. Hold the patient parallel to the clinicians' sightline, and observe heart contractions as rhythmic pulsations of the ventral scutes. Heart localization may also be determined by "heart-slip" as the thumb is gently moved down the ventral aspect of the snake for palpation, and the heart is felt to slip past the thumb. Direct palpation may also be used. Translucency and lack of skin pigment of some species may allow direct visualization of the heart or transillumination via cool fiber-optic light or ophthalmoscope. Ultrasound or Doppler may also be used to locate the heart.

Stabilization of the heart within the coelomic cavity is necessary to avoid iatrogenic trauma to the heart or local structures. Hemoptysis as a complication of cardiocentesis has been observed in a patient which was not properly restrained for this procedure. More than one method may be used for cardiac stabilization depending on patient size and temperament. In very large, muscular snakes, cardiac stabilization may not be possible with physical restraint alone. Place the thumb and index finger cranial and caudal to the heart, to gently stabilize the organ in smaller species. In larger species, stabilization may only be possible caudal thumb placement. A 22–25 g. 1–1½ in. needle attached to a 1–6 ml syringe is then inserted at a 45° angle under the scute and directed craniodorsally into the ventricle [14]. Blood should enter the syringe slowly with each heartbeat and is withdrawn with gentle aspiration. Preheparinization of the syringe, or a hurried approach to cardiocentesis, is not generally necessary because of the protracted clotting time expected in reptiles. Avoid excess negative pressure upon the syringe plunger to allow the heart to refill. If the patient cannot be physically restrained or moves unexpectedly during blood collection, remove the needle immediately to prevent cardiac laceration or damage to surrounding internal vessels and structures.

Palatine Vein

The palatine-pterygoid veins in the ventral aspect of the dorsal palate of the oral cavity have been used for blood collection in large snakes (Figure 17.5). However, blood collection from this site is uncommon because of difficulties with physical restraint, contamination of the sample, and difficulty in providing hemostasis, resulting in hematoma formation. Sample collection is straightforward; however, small needle size and a steady hand are recommended. Placement of gel foam or other biologically friendly clotting agents or simple application of pressure to the venipuncture site may reduce blood loss or hematoma formation. This venipuncture site is not recommended for use in patients with stomatitis ("mouth rot").

Sample Handling

Lithium heparin is the most commonly used anticoagulant in snakes, likely because it allows assessment of CBC and plasma biochemistries from the same sample. While EDTA may cause cell lysis in some snake species, it has been suitable for use in some including the yellow rat

Table 17.1 Hematologic reference data for snakes.

Analyte (abbreviation)	Units, SI (US)	Boa constrictor [128] *Boa constrictor*	Reticulated [128] python (*Python reticulatus*), Ball python (*Python regius*), Burmese python (Python *molurus*)	Ball python [25] *P. regius*	Gopher snake [20] *Pituophis melanoleucas catenifer*
Sample Size and attributes		**90**	**38**	**20**	**22**
Data format		**Range**	**Range**	**Range**	**Range**
Lymphocytes	$\times 10^9$/l ($\times 10^3$/μl)			82–13268	
Monocytes	$\times 10^9$/l ($\times 10^3$/μl)			0–428	
Eosinophil	$\times 10^9$/l ($\times 10^3$/μl)				
Basophil	$\times 10^9$/l ($\times 10^3$/μl)			0–588	
Neutrophil	%	0–15	0–20		
Lymphocytes	%	10–60	10–60	1–49	
Monocytes	%	0–3	0–3	0–2	
Eosinophil	%	0–3	0–3		
Basophil	%	0–20	0–10	0–4	
Packed cell volume (PCV)	l/l (%)	24–40	25–40	10.5–28	15–38
Hemoglobin	g/l g/dl×10			3.41–8.79	
RBC	$\times 10^{12}$/l ($\times 10^6$/μl)	1.0–2.5($\times 10^4$ mm^3)	1.0–2.5($\times 10^4$ mm^3)		

snake, the brown tree snake, *Boiga irregularis*, and the king cobra, *Ophiophagus hannah* [10, 15, 16]. Other options for anticoagulation of snake blood samples include sodium heparin and ammonium heparin [17]. Heparinized samples should be processed soon after sample collection, as heparin imparts a blue tinge to blood smears and causes leukocyte and thrombocyte clumping, resulting inaccurate cell counts. Blood smears are best made during the blood collection process, using fresh blood without the addition of anticoagulant. Staining is recommended as soon as the smear is dry, to allow the most accurate interpretation.

The effects of time or storage type upon analytes of blood samples from snake species have been only minimally assessed. Samples from Burmese pythons collected into heparin-coated syringes and transferred to containers with the anticoagulants lithium heparin, K3-EDTA, or sodium citrate and/ or bovine serum albumin were evaluated for biochemical and cellular changes on the basis of time and anticoagulant [18]. Addition of bovine serum albumin failed to show advantage owing to cell preservation, and sodium-citrated samples stored at 4 °C had notable hemolysis at 12 h post sample storage [18]. In contrast, python blood samples placed into lithium heparin, or K3-EDTA, and refrigerated at 4 °C for up to 24 h had similar hematologic results to those immediately processed [18]. Heparinized blood samples of pythons had potassium concentrations that increased and glucose concentrations that decreased over time. In blood samples obtained from free-living anacondas, *Eunectes murinus*, those processed within 12 h of collection exhibit increased concentrations of glucose, total CO2, total bilirubin, and iron and decreased lactate concentrations and lactate dehydrogenase activities than samples processed after cold storage for one to two days prior to processing [19]. Thus, snake blood samples are best evaluated within 24 h of collection (or less) and may be refrigerated at 4 °C for best results.

Plasma is the preferred sample for biochemical assessment because of the increased sample volume obtained compared with serum. Additionally, low thromboplastin activity and strong natural circulating antithrombin tend to cause unpredictable and prolonged clot formation [20]. Typically, plasma is colorless, although some snakes (e.g., pythons) have a yellow-green colored plasma owing

Table 17.2 Biochemical reference data for snakes.

Analyte (abbreviation)	Units, SI (US)	Red-tailed boa constrictor [128] *Boa constrictor*	Common boa constrictor [129] *Constrictor constrictor imperator*	Reticulated [128] python (*Python reticulatus*), Ball python (*P. regius*), Burmese python (*P. molurus*)	Ball python [25] *Python regius*	Gopher snake [20] *Pituophis melanoleucas cenifer*
Sample number, type		**90, Serum**	**5, Serum**	**38, Serum**	**20, Plasma**	**22, Plasma**
Data format		**Range**	**Range**	**Range**	**Range**	**Range**
Albumin: Globulin			0.7–1.1			
Albumin	g/l (g/dl)		25–39 (2.5–3.9)			16–21 (1.6–2.1)
Alkaline phosphatase (ALP)	U/l = (units/l)		242–652		63–145	8.8–133
Alanine aminotransferase (ALT)	U/l = (units/l)		0–20		3–22	10.9–65
Aspartate (AST) aminotransferase	U/l = (units/l)	5–35	1–30	5–30	15–77	16.2–127
Calcium	mmol/l (mg/dl)	2.5–5.5 (10–22)	3.5–5.9 (14.0–23.7)	2.5–5.5 (10–22)	2.8–3.8 (11.3–15.3)	3–3.9 (13–15.7)
Chloride	mmol/l =(mEq/l)		104–124			109–148
Cholesterol	mmol/l (mg/dl)		1.37–3.57 (53–138)			
Creatinine	µmol/l (mg/dl)	8.84–26.5 (<0.1–0.3)	6.19 (0–0.07)	8.84–26.5 (<0.1–0.3)		8.84–53 (0.1–0.6)
Globulin	g/l (g/dl)		29–44 (2.9–4.4)			
Glucose	mmol/l (mg/dl)	0.55–3.33 (10–60)	1.0–3.4 (18–61)	0.55–3.33 (10–60)	1.4–1.8 (25–32)	1.32–7.1 (24–129)
Lactate dehydrogenase	U/l = (units/l)	30–300	52–287	40–300		
Phosphorus	mmol/l (mg/dl)		0.84–1.6 (2.6–4.9)		0.74–1.7 (2.3–5.3)	0.81–1.8 (2.5–5.7)
Potassium	mmol/l =(mEq/l)	3.0–5.7	3.6–7.1	3.0–5.7		3.6–10
Sodium	mmol/l = (mEq/l)	130–152	152–166	130–152		161–180
Total bilirubin[a]	µmol/l (mg/dl)		3.42–6.84 (0.2–0.4)			
Total protein	g/l (g/dl)	46–80 (4.6–8)	58–83 (5.8–8.3)	50–80 (5–8)	43–59 (4.3–5.9)	28–73 (2.8–7.3)
Triglyceride[a]	mmol/l (mg/dl)		0–0.09 (0–8)			
Urea[a]	mmol/l (mg/dl)	<0.35–3.6 (<1–10)	0–1.79 (0–5)	0.35–3.6 (<1–10)		0.6–1.79 (1–5)
Uric acid	Umol/l (mg/dl)	71.4–345 (1.2–5.8)	166.5–368.8 (2.8–6.2)	71.4–333.1 (1.2–5.6)	107.1–297.4 (1.8–5)	

[a] Analytes provided for information but seldom clinically used for diagnosis of snakes.

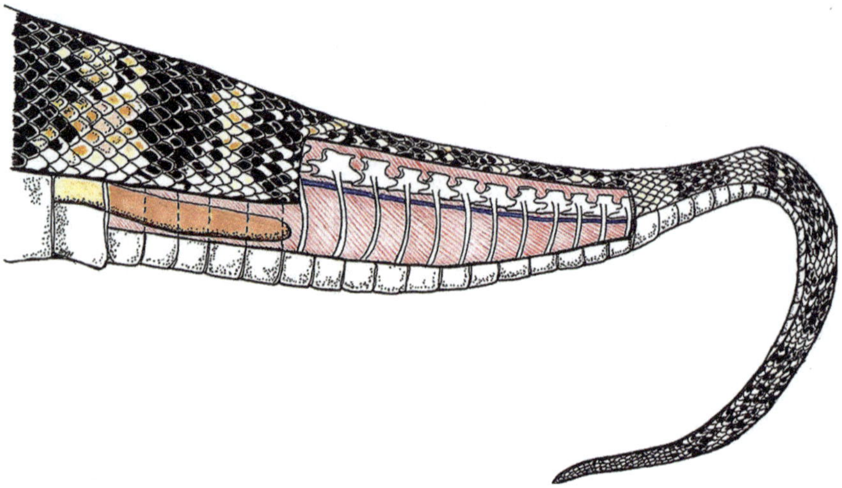

Figure 17.4 Local anatomy for approach to the ventral coccygeal vein of the female snake. The vein is depicted in blue as it courses below the coccygeal vertebrae, above the vestigial pouch which extends only 5 scales caudal to the vent in the female.

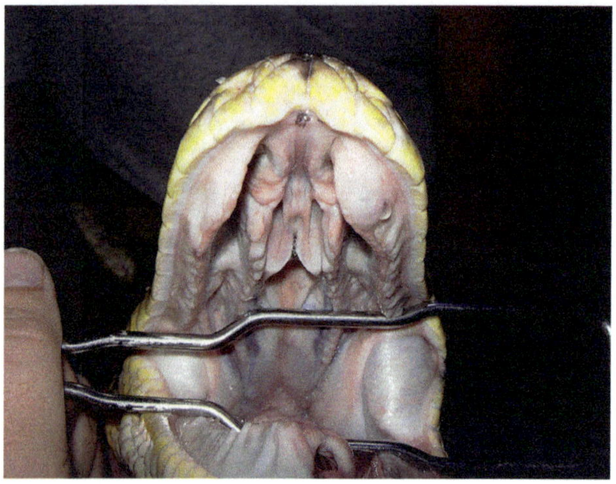

Figure 17.5 Approach for venipuncture of the palatine veins of a large snake.

to carotenoid and riboflavin pigments [17]. Chemistry analyzers that use dry reagents and reflectance photometry can be used for biochemical analysis of reptile plasma or serum, and most of these require only a small sample size (~0.5 ml).

Lymphatic contamination is a frequent complication in reptile venipuncture because of the close association of the lymphatic vessels and sinuses and the veins. Lymph dilution may be identified during blood collection by clear fluid entering the syringe before the blood or blood that appears thin and anemic when withdrawn. In these cases, blood may be redrawn. Venipuncture of the caudal tail vein of snakes may result in some degree of lymphodilution, while cardiocentesis decreases the possibility of lymph dilution. However, should clear fluid be withdrawn during cardiocentesis, one must endeavor to differentiate this fluid from that of pericardial fluid [17]. For hemograms, lymphatic dilution may occur from samples acquired from snakes, and lower packed cell volume (PCV), TP, azurophils, and total white cell count are expected in these samples [21]. In sea snakes, observable lymphatic dilution of sample collected from the tail veins resulted in multiple biochemical changes including decreased concentrations of albumin, alkaline phosphatase (ALP), calcium, cholesterol, globulin, total protein (via multiple methods of measurement), and increased sodium [21]. Clinically, lymphatic dilution is of most concern in causing the erroneous diagnosis of monocytosis, azurophilia or anemia, and hypoproteinemia in snake species. Nonetheless, the authors highly recommend using, rather than discarding, this sample for determination of appropriate biochemical values and serological or other appropriate diagnostic purposes.

Complete Blood Count

Erythrocyte, leukocyte, and thrombocyte counts of snakes are most often determined by hemocytometer techniques as most automated cell counters cannot differentiate between the nucleated thrombocytes, erythrocytes, and leukocytes of reptiles. The stain type and counting methods used may significantly affect cell counts reported in snakes. The clinician should be aware of the methods used to determine cell counts for their patients.

Erythrocytes

Methods

The total erythrocyte count and thrombocyte count in snakes can be determined by manual or automated methods [14]. The manual methods involve diluting whole blood with solutions to dilute, lyse, and stain cells (Eosin or Natt and Herrick's) and then loading the mixture into a hemocytometer for counting. Automated methods require electric cell counter adjustment to accommodate reptile erythrocytes and are not commonly available for clinical use. Ophidian PCV can be determined by microhematocrit centrifugation. Snake hemoglobin molecules are diverse; nevertheless, hemoglobin concentration of snake erythrocytes can be measured by automated methods, such as the hemoglobinometer (Coulter Electronics, Hialeah, Florida) or cyanmethemoglobin reagent–blood mixture method [14, 20, 22].

Morphology and Normal Physiology

Hematopoiesis occurs in the bone marrow of the spine and ribs of the *Boa constrictor*; the corn snake, *Elaphe guttata*; and the African house snake, *Lamprophis fulaginosus*; and in the spleen and bone marrow of *Bothrops jararaca* [23]. Mature erythrocytes of snakes are larger than those of birds and mammals, yet smaller than amphibian erythrocytes [24]. Among the reptiles, snake erythrocyte size is deceded only by lizard erythrocytes [25, 26]. As an example, Indian Rock Python MCV ranges from 290 to 333 fl [27]. Snake erythrocytes are round to elliptical in shape with homogeneous, orange-pink cytoplasm (Figure 17.6). The snake erythrocyte nucleus is central, has dense chromatin, and is round to oval to scalloped. Small, round to irregularly shaped basophilic intracytoplasmic inclusions commonly observed in snake erythrocytes are likely degenerate organelles on the basis of electron microscopy, but have sometimes been erroneously attributed to Pirhemocyton infection [9, 24, 27]. Vacuoles, refractile clear areas, and intracellular hemoglobin crystallization are addition artifacts that may be noted in erythrocyte cytoplasm of snakes [27].

Erythroplastids (anucleate erythrocytes) are rarely observed in the peripheral blood of snakes; <5% of the RBC count is considered an incidental finding [27]. Immature RBC, polychromatic erythroblasts, often with cytoplasmic vacuolation, may also occasionally be found (up to 1%) in the peripheral circulation of healthy snakes [27, 28]. In healthy snakes, slight anisocytosis and mild polychromasia can be present, and rare mitotic erythrocytes may also be seen [28]. Polychromasia is recognized by more basophilic cytoplasm and a less dense nuclear chromatin pattern. Finding low numbers (<1% RBC count) of polychromatic red blood cells (polychromatophils) is expected in snakes which are young or undergoing ecdysis; no clinical significance is generally attributed to this finding [9]. Reticulocytes can be enumerated with use of a vital stain such as new methylene blue. In snakes, cells counted as true reticulocytes have a ring of aggregated reticulum surrounding the nucleus, and these cells are polychromatophilic in the peripheral blood film. The reticulocyte count in healthy adult snakes is typically less than 1% of circulating erythrocytes. Increased numbers may be observed in neonates and in snakes undergoing ecdysis [29]. Because reptilian chromatophils are generally smaller than mature RBCs, a decreased MCV results [17].

Erythrocyte concentrations of snakes tend to be lower than those of lizards but higher than those of chelonians [20]. Total erythrocyte count, hemoglobin concentration, and PCV are influenced by physiologic and environmental factors. The hematocrit of sea snakes tends to be higher than that of most other snakes, and seasonal variation also occurs [30]. No consistent differences in red blood cell count or hematocrit were found when freshwater and terrestrial snakes were compared [31]. Typically, erythrocyte concentration is higher before and during brumation, and lower afterward. In a captive South American rattlesnake, *Crotalus durissus terrificus*, erythrocyte concentration, hematocrit, and hemoglobin concentration were 17%–30% higher in winter [32]. In the grass snake, *Natrix natrix natrix*, erythrocyte concentration, hemoglobin concentration, and hematocrit were higher during hibernation than prior to hibernation [32]. However, in some captive temperate viper species, hibernation did not affect erythrocytic values [33].

Age, sex, reproductive status, body size, captivity, and other factors may also affect RBC parameters of snakes. Erythrocyte numbers were higher in younger Indian grass snakes, *Natrix stolata* [34]. Erythrocyte size and PCV also increased with increasing body weights in this species [34]. Erythrocyte concentration tends to be higher in males than in females of some species such as the eastern massasauga rattlesnake, *Sistrurus catenatus catenatus*, and the grass snake, *N. natrix natrix* [35, 36].

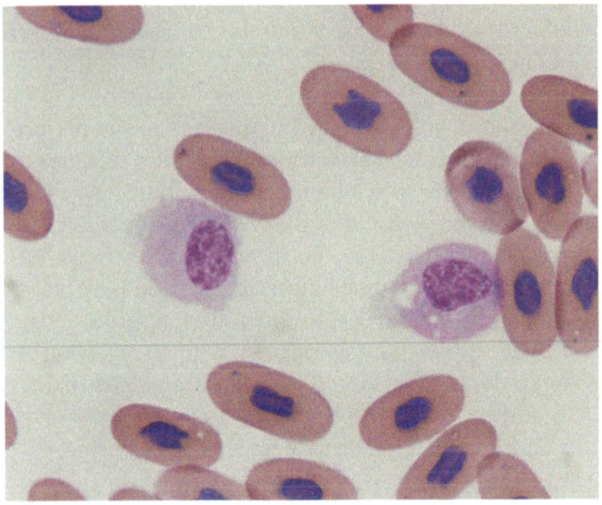

Figure 17.6 Monocytes and red blood cells of a ball python *(Python regius)* Modified Wright Giemsa stain. Note the commonly observed vacuolation of the monocytes and the degenerate organelles seen as eccentrically located small dark purple dots in the RBC. Also shown are small clear areas in the RBC, a common preparation artifact in snake blood smears.

In the grass snake and asp viper, *Vipera aspis*, erythrocyte concentration, hematocrit, and hemoglobin concentration decrease during the mating period, increase after the mating period, and remain increased until late autumn [36]. Male grass snakes have higher hemoglobin and PCV than females [36]. In king cobras, higher RBC was found in captive-bred than in wild-caught animals [37]. Starvation results in decreased RBC, PCV, and hemoglobin concentrations in the checkered keelback, *Xenochrophis piscator*, which rebound upon treatment with erythropoietin and L-thyroxine [38].

Erythrocyte Abnormalities

Anemia of snakes is typically diagnosed when the PCV is less than 20%. However, the ball python, *Python regius*, has a lower PCV (16%–21%) in health and depending on seasonal variation [25, 39]. A common cause of anemia in snakes is chronic disease resulting in decreased erythrocyte production. Differentials for decreased red blood cell production in snakes are similar to those for other companion mammals and include chronic renal or hepatic failure, infection, gastrointestinal disease, neoplasia, improper diet and environment, and from toxin exposure [9, 39]. Anemia in snakes may also occur secondary to hemorrhage caused by trauma, parasitism, ulcers, or coagulopathies [40]. Lastly, anemia can occur secondary to hemolysis because of septicemia, parasitemia, viremia, or toxemia (e.g., zinc toxicity) [41]. In free-ranging anacondas, *Eu. murinus*, in Venezuela, female anacondas were more likely to have been injured than males and had lower PCVs [19]. Anemia can be regenerative or nonregenerative as in mammals; however, the regenerative response in reptiles is slow and prolonged [42]. Moderate to marked anisocytosis, poikilocytosis, basophilic stippling, increased numbers of reticulocytes and possibly earlier erythrocytes (e.g. rubricytes), binucleated erythrocytes, abnormal nuclear shapes, and/or mitoses may be observed in the peripheral blood smear of snakes with regenerative anemias or those suffering severe inflammation, malnutrition, starvation, or undergoing emergence from brumation [30]. The regenerative response in snakes is very slow as reptilian erythrocytes have a longer life span (600–800 days) and slower turnover [43]. To the best of our knowledge, basophilic stippling is associated with a regenerative response, secondary to iron deficiency and lead toxicosis; and hypochromasia observed with iron deficiency or chronic inflammatory disease have not yet been documented in snakes.

Thrombocytes

Snake thrombocytes are oval to fusiform cells with clear to pale basophilic cytoplasm that occasionally contains few small, round, dark pink azurophilic granules [44]. Nuclei are central, round to oval, and have dense, dark chromatin [44]. In snakes suffering severe inflammatory disease, thrombocyte nuclear shape may become more irregular, pleomorphic, or slightly lobulated [27]. Snakes thrombocytes are cytochemically periodic acid-Schiff (PAS) positive [16, 44]. Activated thrombocytes become rounded in shape, and the cytoplasm commonly contains vacuoles [45]. Activated thrombocytes aggregate and likely play an important physiologic role in clot formation. In snakes, thrombocyte aggregation and clumping may be more likely to occur with the anticoagulant heparin than with potassium EDTA [18, 46]. Thrombocyte counting via staining and hemocytometer methods are seldom clinically pursued. Rather, a thrombocyte estimate is provided on the basis of observation of a blood smear. On the peripheral blood smear, normal thrombocyte numbers in reptiles range from 25 to 350 per 100 leukocytes [47].

Thrombocyte numbers may be influenced by external factors such as season. Thrombocyte concentrations are 15%–20% higher in summer in the South American rattlesnake, *C. durissus terrificus* [32]. In snakes, clinical reports of thrombocytopenia or thrombocytosis remain anecdotal, likely because of the current methodological challenges in quantitation of these cells. Presumed causes of thrombocytopenia and thrombocytosis in snakes would likely be similar to those described in mammals such as increased peripheral use of thrombocytes or decreased thrombocyte production of bone marrow disorder. The presence of immature thrombocytes in the peripheral blood of affected snakes is consistent with a regenerative response to thrombocytopenia [17].

Leukocytes

Total WBC

The total leukocyte count is obtained by semidirect or direct methods (Table 17.1). In the semidirect method, acidophilic granulocytes (heterophils and eosinophils) are stained with phloxine B solution and counted in a hemocytometer. This method may underestimate the white blood cell count because most snakes primarily have lymphocytes. Additionally, a differential cell count is performed on a blood film stained with Romanowsky-type stains (e.g., Wright Giemsa). This method requires an accurate leukocyte differential from the blood smear, and when a heteropenia exists, the total leukocyte count may be falsely elevated. The direct method uses Natt and Herrick's stain for leukocytes, which are counted in a hemocytometer to calculate the total leukocyte count. This method may be more appropriate in snakes, as the semidirect method relies on the predominance of acidophilic granulocytes, and in most snakes, lymphocytes are the predominant circulating leukocyte [16, 20, 32, 35, 39,

48]. Limitations of the direct method include a falsely increased total leukocyte count if small lymphocytes are not differentiated from thrombocytes. A rough estimate of the total number of leukocytes per microliter can be obtained by multiplying the average number of leukocytes per 40× objective field (a minimum of 10 fields should be counted) by 1500. However, if leukocytes are not evenly distributed on the smear (e.g., leukocyte clumps present), this estimate is inaccurate [49].

Evaluation of leukocyte morphology on a stained blood smear is key because of the limitations of current methods of leukocyte enumeration. The leukocytes of snakes consist of granulocytes (heterophils, eosinophils, and basophils) and mononuclear cells (lymphocytes, monocytes, and azurophils). Leukocytosis in snakes is typically associated with inflammatory disease, especially that of infectious etiology and occasionally neoplastic diseases [50]. Chronic disease, especially coupled with poor husbandry and suboptimal temperatures, may result in leukopenia. Environmental temperature and season can affect leukocyte numbers. As in other ectotherms, snakes with inadequate environmental heat sources or poor husbandry may become immunocompromised and fail to mount an appropriate inflammatory response, despite severe infection. In some snake species, such as the South American rattlesnake, *C. durissus terrificus*, total leukocyte concentrations are 15%–20% higher in the summer months [32, 51–56]. Blood samples collected from free-living anacondas, *Eu. murinus*, within a day of capture had increased azurophils and decreased lymphocyte counts and chloride concentrations than samples collected 2–10 days after capture, which is suggestive of a stress response in this species [57].

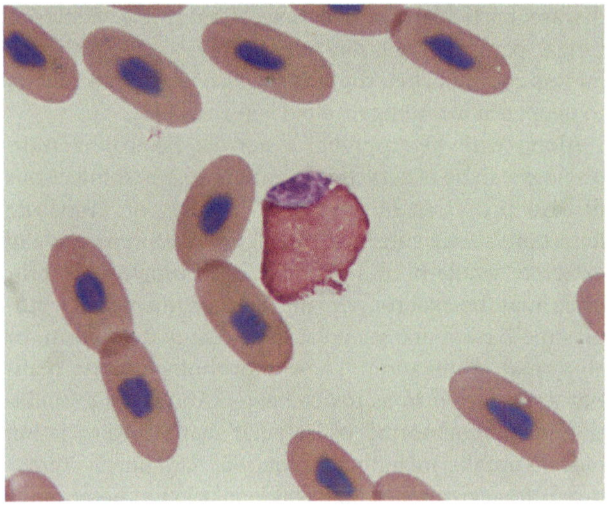

Figure 17.7 Heterophil of a ball python *(Python regius)*. Modified Wright Giemsa stain.

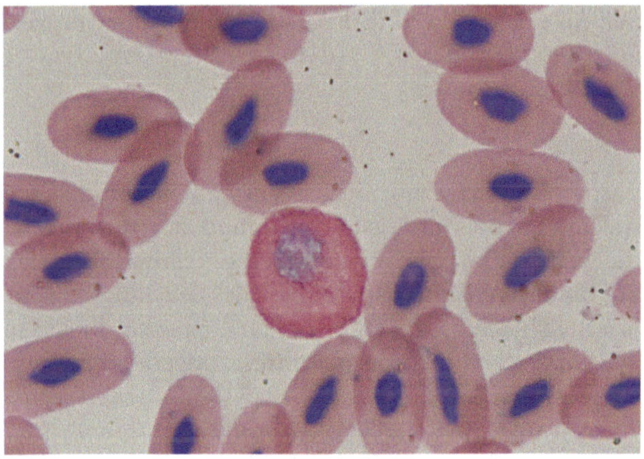

Figure 17.8 Ball python heterophil with the focus adjusted to highlight the oblong pink granules. Modified Wright Giemsa stain, 1000x magnification.

Heterophils

Heterophils vary in diameter between snake species from approximately 12 to 20 µm [16, 27, 36, 48]. Heterophils have clear, abundant cytoplasm containing bright orange-red to orange-brown fusiform-shaped granules in most snakes (Figures 17.7 and 17.8) [24, 58]. However, some species have darker blue purple granules, resembling those of the iguana heterophil [27]. In snakes, heterophil granules may be so small, pleomorphic, poorly formed, and numerous that their shape is difficult to distinguish [17]. Two morphologically distinct forms of snake heterophils have been described as having either irregularly oval or elongate granules [16, 17, 44, 48, 59]. These forms may represent different stages of cell maturation each with differing staining intensity [60]. Heterophil nuclei of snakes are typically eccentric, round to oval, and have densely clumped chromatin [24].

Snake heterophils so far studied are ALP negative, similar to the mammalian neutrophil. However, unlike neutrophils, heterophil granules are mostly peroxidase negative except for a few snake species such as *Bothrops jararaca* [60]. King cobra, *O. hannah*, heterophil granules stained positive for Sudan black B (SBB), alpha-naphthyl acetate esterase (ANAE), and beta-glucuronidase (B-Glu) [47, 48, 61].

Heterophil concentration is influenced by many environmental factors. Heterophil concentrations are highest in *V. aspis* during the summer months and lowest during hibernation or brumation in the winter months [60]. In king cobras, lower heterophils occurred in captive-bred than in wild-caught animals [62]. The primary function of heterophils in snakes is thought to be phagocytosis, particularly of microbes [58]. In free-ranging anacondas, *Eu. murinus*, females had higher heterophil counts and were more likely to have been injured than males [19]. As in other species, heterophilia in snakes can often be related to stress (glucocorticoid-induced); inflammatory disease, particularly of infectious etiology (e.g., bacterial, fungal, parasitic); or is due to tissue injury [24]. Although far less common, heterophilia can also be seen secondary to neoplasia including myeloid leukemia [43].

Along with heterophilia, abnormal heterophil morphology can be observed in inflammatory and infectious disease processes in snakes [27]. Toxic or immature heterophils may enter peripheral circulation in cases of extreme, whole-body inflammation. Immature heterophils may be macrocytic and contain increased cytoplasmic basophilia, vacuolated or foamy cytoplasm, or abnormal granulation. These morphologic abnormalities are referred to as toxic change. Abnormal granulation includes abnormal or irregular shapes and variation in stain uptake, including presence of dark purple immature primary granules [27]. Degranulation of heterophils may occur with toxic change; however, other signs of toxicity must also be present, as degranulation is a common artifact of preparation in squamates [27, 63]. Lobulation and hypersegmentation of heterophil nuclei may also be observed with severe inflammatory disease in snakes [27].

Eosinophils

Eosinophils, have not been identified in some snake species, such as the eastern diamondback rattlesnake; the ball python, *P. regius*; and the yellow rat snake, *Elaphe obsoleta quadrivittata* [15, 25, 59], but do occur in others such as the king cobra, *O. hannah*; Burmese python, *Python molurus bivittatus*; reticulated python, *Python reticulatus*; African rock python, *Python sebae*; a green tree python, *Chondropython viridis*; and *Boa constrictor, Boa constrictor* [16, 24, 58, 64]. Eosinophils may represent a second heterophil type in snakes [15, 33, 59, 61].

King cobras have eosinophils with light basophilic purple, round spherical, bulging granules similar to those of iguanas, which may obscure the nucleus [16]. Other snake eosinophils are typically described as having spherical to slightly oval cytoplasmic granules that are reddish, orange, or magenta in color, and nuclei that are eccentric and round to oval [24, 65]. When present, snake eosinophils are relatively larger than those of other reptilian species [26, 46]. Eosinophil numbers of snakes vary with season and are lowest in the summer months and highest during brumation [48, 66]. Eosinophilia has been associated with parasitic infestation, such as trematodiasis in boa constrictors [67]. In a recent study of *Rhabdias* spp. parasitism in the South American rattlesnake or cascabel, *C. durissus terrificus*, increased granulocytes occurred in parasitized animals when compared to nonparasitized animals [62]. The significance of eosinopenia in snakes, if any, remains unknown [17].

Basophils

Basophils are smaller cells containing large numbers of dark purple, metachromatic granules that commonly obscure the nucleus (Figure 17.9). These granules may be both round and spiculate and are best visualized using alcohol fixation and Romanowsky-type stains, as water-based stains may cause partial dissolution or expulsion of the granules [27]. Free basophil granules in the blood smear may require differentiation from parasites, bacteria, or RBC remnants [27]. In king cobras, *O. hannah*, basophil granules stain positive for PAS, SBB, ANAE, and B-Glu, while in the eastern diamondback rattlesnake, *Crotalus adamanteus*, basophils stained only PAS positive [16, 59]. Snake basophil nuclei are central to paracentral, round, and have dense chromatin. Electron microscopy further reveals a dense oval nucleolus [43]. Snake basophils do appear to have surface immunoglobulins and release histamine during degranulation, according to cytochemical and ultrastructural studies [47, 68, 69].

Basophil numbers vary depending on species. Some snakes such as the common brown water snake, *Lycodonomorphus rufulus*; the rhombic night adder, *Causus rhombeatus*; the red-lipped or herald snake, *Crotaphopeltis hotamboeia*; the stripe bellied sand snake, *Psammophis subtaeniatus subtaeniatus*; the black-necked spitting cobra, *Naja nigricollis*; the glossy-bellied racer, *Coluber ventrimaculatus*; and Brazilian pit vipers, *Bot. jararaca*, tend to have higher numbers of basophils than other snake species [70, 71]. Basophilia attributable to hemoparasitic or viral infections has not been specifically documented in snakes.

Lymphocytes

Both small and large lymphocytes circulate in healthy snakes and are the most numerous blood leukocyte in many snake species, such as the eastern massasauga

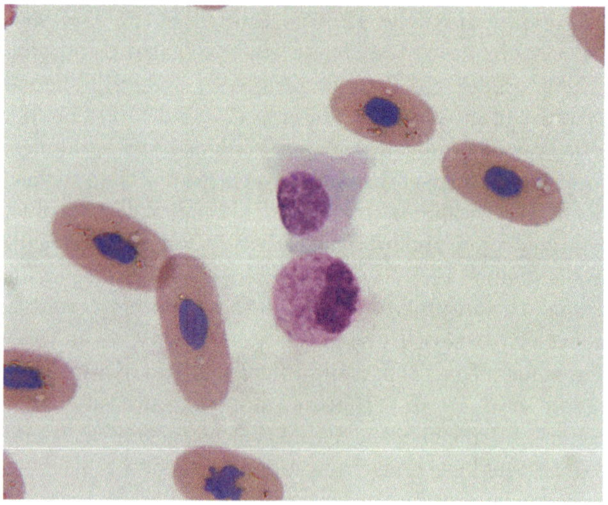

Figure 17.9 Monocyte (uppermost white blood cell) and a basophil (lower) from a ball python *(Python regius)*.

rattlesnake, *S. catenatus catenatus*; South American rattlesnake, *C. durissus terrificus*; sidewinder, *Crotalus cerastes*; several *Bothrops* species; king cobras, *O. hannah*; brown tree snakes, *Boi. irregularis*; eastern diamondback rattlesnakes, *C. adamanteus*; and puff-faced water snakes, *Homalopsis buccata* [16, 32, 35, 39, 48, 65, 72]. Snakes have both T- and B-like lymphocytes. In the diadem snake, *Spalerosophis diadema*, and the Japanese striped snake, *Elaphe quadrivirgata*, T lymphocytes predominate in the thymus, spleen, and peripheral blood [43]. During the winter and summer months, in the Schokari sand racer, *Psammophis schokari*, T-lymphocyte-specific antigen was not detected in the thymus, spleen, or peripheral blood [60]. The small lymphocytes of snakes resemble those of mammals and birds, having high nuclear to cytoplasmic ratios, scant amounts of light blue cytoplasm, and a central to eccentric, round to oval to slightly cleaved nucleus with dense, clumped chromatin (Figure 17.10). In contrast, large lymphocytes have more cytoplasm that may contain azurophilic granules [65]. Additionally, the nucleus stains lighter than small lymphocyte nuclei. In the king cobra, *O. hannah*, lymphocytes are cytochemically positive for PAS, ANAE, acid phosphatase (AcP), and B-Glu [48]. Snake lymphocytes may be less deformable than those of birds [27]. Snake plasma cells are rarely seen in peripheral blood [20]. They have moderate amounts of deep blue cytoplasm with a perinuclear clear zone (Golgi zone), and an eccentric round nucleus with dense chromatin. Snake plasma cells are similar ultrastructurally to those of other species, having rough and smooth endoplasmic reticulum, and a prominent Golgi apparatus [43]. Plasma cell appearance in the peripheral blood of snakes is presumed to extend from immune stimulation as occurs in other species.

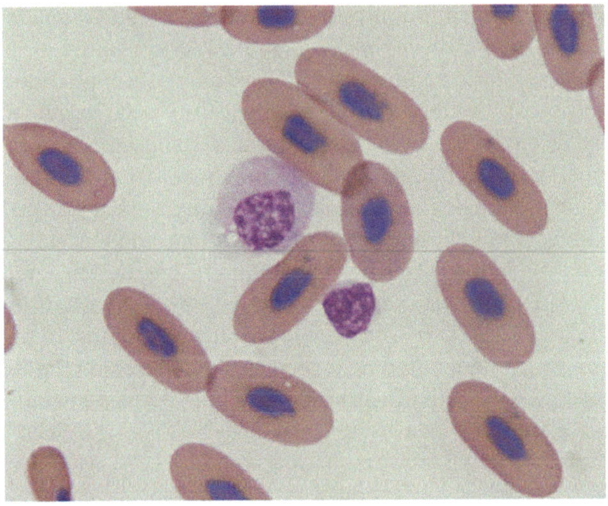

Figure 17.10 A monocyte (larger, uppermost white blood cell) and lymphocyte from a ball python *(Python regius)*. Modified Wright Giemsa stain.

Snake lymphocyte concentrations can be influenced by several external factors. Lymphocyte numbers may vary with season, tending to be highest in summer and lowest in winter, at least partially, because hibernation, which occurs in winter, causes decreased lymphocyte concentrations [33, 66]. In some species, including *Vipera berus* and *V. aspis*, sex is also a significant factor, with higher lymphocyte concentrations in females [37, 47, 73, 74]. In contrast, the free-ranging female anacondas, *Eu. Murinus*, had lower lymphocyte concentrations than males, but were also more likely to have been injured in this study [19]. Lymphocytes are affected by temperature. As expected in all ectotherms, snakes housed in environments that are too cold may have a markedly suppressed or absent immune response. In king cobras, increased lymphocytes concentrations occurred in captive-bred compared to wild-caught animals [16].

Lymphocytosis is observed with inflammation, wound healing, ecdysis, viral infection, and parasitic infestations, while lymphopenia occurs secondary to stress, immunosuppression (from disease or cold temperatures), or malnutrition [70]. Blood samples collected from free-living anacondas, *Eu. murinus*, within a day of capture had decreased lymphocyte counts and other changes in samples collected 2–10 days after capture suggestive of a stress response in this species [19]. Extreme leukocytosis (>100 000 cells/μl), attributable primarily to lymphocytosis, has been in early stages on inclusion body disease of boid snakes [6]. Relative lymphopenia has been reported in a controlled study of Cascabel infected with *Rhabdias* spp. [62]

Hematopoietic malignancies, specifically lymphoid, are among the most common neoplasms in snakes, yet they have been only rarely and sporadically reported. Among these, lymphoproliferative disorders are most common, and are most frequently reported in vipers (particularly cobras and urutus) [75]. Lymphosarcoma has been diagnosed in an eastern kingsnake, *Lampropeltis getulus getulus*; a rhinoceros viper, *Bitis nasicornis*; a California kingsnake, *L. g. californiae*; and a red-tail boa (*boa constrictor constrictor*) [42, 64, 76]. Most reported leukemias are lymphoid in origin, although myeloproliferative disease has occurred in an Aruba island rattlesnake, *Crotalus unicolor*, and a carpet python, *Morelia spilota cheynei* [77]. Chronic lymphocytic leukemia diagnosed in an Asian cobra, *Naja naja kaouthia*, and a diamond python, *Morelia spilota spilota*, were each determined to be of T cell origin [78].

Monocytes

Monocytes occur in snakes and are large round to ameboid cells with lower nuclear to cytoplasmic ratios than lymphocytes. They have moderate to large amounts of blue-gray cytoplasm that may contain clear, round vacuoles (Figures 17.6, 17.9, and 17.10). Nuclei are pleomorphic, ranging from round to oval to reniform, and have lighter, less condensed chromatin compared to lymphocytes [27, 36].

Azurophils are large mononuclear cells commonly found in snakes which are controversial among clinical pathologists and researchers. Some consider azurophils a variation of monocytes (azurophilic monocytes), while others suggest that azurophils are a separate, distinct cell type. Azurophils appear similar to monocytes apart from the presence of few to many fine, dust-like eosinophilic to azurophilic cytoplasmic granules (Figure 17.11). Snake azurophils may be a distinct cell type with function similar to the mammalian neutrophil on the basis of morphological and cytochemical properties [29]. Thus, some clinical pathologists advocate that azurophils be tallied separately from standard monocytes in snake differential cell counts [9, 16, 48]. In some snake species, azurophils are the second most common leukocyte and may normally account for up to 35% of the circulating white blood cells. The eastern massasauga rattlesnake, *S. catenatus catenatus*; king cobra; and the puff-faced water snake, *H. buccata*, have higher azurophil than heterophil concentrations, and the azurophil is the predominant leukocyte in some species of *Boa constrictors* and rat snakes [16, 32, 39, 48, 59, 79].

Azurophilia, with or without a left shift, is associated with inflammatory and infectious diseases in snakes, especially in acute phases of disease [27, 42]. Cells resembling mammalian monocytes may be reactive azurophils [15, 17]. Azurophilia has been reported in association with severe, spreading necrosis of the tail, multiple abscesses, cellulitis, and muscle necrosis. Increased cytoplasmic vacuolation, scalloping of the cell membrane, and excessive lobation of the nucleus have been reported as cellular changes in azurophils associated with severe inflammation in snakes [27].

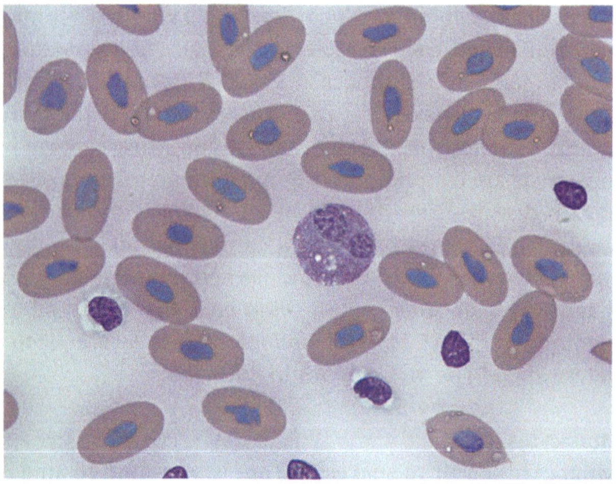

Figure 17.11 Blood smear from an adult reticulated python, Modified Wrights stain, shown at 1000× magnification. The azurophil is the large purple leukocyte with small granules.

In snakes, circulating monocytes or macrophages may contain melanin (melanomacrophage), lipid vacuoles, nucleoproteinaceous debris, phagocytized erythrocytes (erythrocytophagocytic macrophages), hemosiderin from erythrocytes (siderophagocytes) or intracellular bacterial organisms. Such cells have occurred for greater than two months post surgically but have also been associated with infectious disease (particularly sepsis), neoplastic disease, or delayed sample processing. [9, 80] *Chlamydia* spp. inclusions were identified, via microscopy and PCR, in peripheral monocytes of captive emerald tree boas with pneumonia [77].

Monocytes and azurophils appear minimally affected by season in most species, but increase in the Brazilian *Boa constrictor, Boa constrictor amarali*, in winter [54]. Monocytes are affected by sex [54]. Female eastern massasauga rattlesnakes, *S. catenatus catenatus*, have lower absolute azurophil counts than males [35]. Monocytosis in snakes occurs with inflammatory disease, especially bacterial and parasitic diseases that cause granuloma formation (e.g., mycobacteriosis) [58]. In king cobras, fewer circulating azurophils occurred in captive-bred than in wild-caught animals [16]. Blood samples collected from free-living anacondas, *Eu. murinus*, within a day of capture had increased azurophils and other changes in samples collected 2–10 days after capture, suggestive of a stress response in this species [19].

Hemoparasites and Other Hemic Infectious Agents

A variety of hemoparasites can be identified on the peripheral blood smear of snakes, the most common of which are hemogregarine protists [27]. The genus *Hepatozoon* commonly infects terrestrial and aquatic snakes, and *Karyolysus* spp. infects tree snakes [81]. These genera cannot be differentiated through light microscopy, as they appear cytologically similar and thus are often referred to as a group as hemogregarines. In most snakes, hemogregarine infections do not cause clinical disease. However, immunocompromised snakes with severe infections may suffer anemia, and a correlation of hemogregarine presence in circulation and *Hepatozoon* liver granulomas has been reported in snakes [82, 83]. Further, hemogregarine infection in an unnatural, unadapted host species would be expected to cause clinical inflammatory disease [82]. In the neotropical rattlesnake, *Crotalus durissus collilineatus*, wild-caught snakes had an infection rate of 38.3%, while no *Hepatozoon* sp. infection was detected in the captive-bred animals. Uninfected snakes' had increased weight, length, and weight:length ratios and fewer immature RBC than those of the infected animals [84].

Hemogregarines have a sausage-shaped gametocyte (gamont) with a central, eccentric, or saddle nucleus. The organism may surround or displace the erythrocyte nucleus or create a bulge in the cytoplasm, deforming the cell [58, 85]. Erythrocytes usually contain only a single gametocyte, but may rarely contain two. Even more rarely gamonts may be found extracellularly, or in other cells such as the azurophil [48, 81]. Meronts of hemogregarines may also occur in the cytoplasm of red or less commonly white blood cells [81].

Snakes may occasionally be infected with *Plasmodium* blood parasites, often of the *Hemoproteus* genera. Infection has been associated with hemolytic anemia but many snakes are not clinically affected. *Hemoproteus* can undergo merogony and gametogony in reptilian erythrocytes. Thus, gametocytes, meronts, and trophozoites may occur in erythrocyte cytoplasm and extracellularly. Trophozoites are small, round, signet-ring structures. The gametocytes can be differentiated from those of hemogregarines by the presence of hemozoin, intracytoplasmic refractile pigment granules. *Plasmodium* spp. gametocytes typically greatly distort the erythrocyte, enlarging the cell and markedly displacing the nucleus to the periphery. For more detailed information, the reader is referred to additional texts on this subject [81]. *Serpentoplasma* is a genus of protozoan parasite which rarely infects snake erythrocytes. Piroplasms of this organism are recognized by 1–2 μm diameter, round to pleomorphic signet-ring-shaped intracytoplasmic basophilic inclusions, usually in small aggregates, surrounded by a clear vacuole [81].

Trypanosomes are extracellular flagellate protozoa of which infection, although commonly lifelong, does not usually cause clinical illness. Trypomastigotes can be identified by their blade-like shape with an undulating membrane and single flagellum [81]. A related nonpathogenic protozoan that only rarely infects snakes is *Sauroleishmania*. Amastigotes are found in the cytoplasm of thrombocytes, lymphocytes, monocytes, or azurophils [81]. They are approximately 1.5–5 μm in diameter, round to oval organisms with basophilic cytoplasm containing an oval deeply eosinophilic to red nucleus and bar-shaped kinetoplast [81]. *Microfilaria* are common extracellular hemoparasites that are typically incidental findings, as most affected snakes are clinically healthy [81]. These organisms have only rarely been documented to cause illness, as the case of *Macdonaldius oschei* infection of captive Asiatic pythons, as they reside in the mesenteric arteries [86]. Blood smear examination can support the diagnosis of bacterial and viral diseases in snakes. The bacteria *Chlamydophila* spp. inclusions were identified, via microscopy and PCR, in peripheral monocytes of captive emerald tree boas with pneumonia [77].

Iridovirus (genus *Ranavirus*), snake erythrocyte virus, can cause severe anemia in snakes [41]. This viral inclusion was formerly described as the hemoparasite *Pirhemocyton* spp., but was reclassified on the basis of transmission electron microscopy, which revealed viral particles [87]. Viral inclusions may be observed in erythrocytes of affected snakes. Two types of inclusion are described. One type of iridoviral erythrocyte inclusion is granular and pink to dark purple and of viral origin. The other SEV inclusion is oval, rectangular, or hexagonal and flat in shape, and pale, translucent orange-pink in color, flat, crystalline, and composed of lipids and proteins from cellular and viral origin [72, 88]. These inclusions are reported in several snake species, such as the peninsula ribbon snake, *Thamnophis sauritus sackeni*; fer-de-lance, *Bothrops moojeni*; and the northern water snake, *Nerodia sipedon sipedon*, which were anemic and/or had hypochromic erythrocytes [41, 71, 87]. Infection progression has been linked to increasing crystalline inclusion size; occasionally, two inclusions in a single RBC are noted [39].

Inclusion body disease is an infectious disease affecting captive boas and pythons worldwide, causing high morbidity and mortality. *Boa constrictors*, *Boa constrictor constrictor*, and Burmese pythons, *Python molurus bivittatus*, appear highly susceptible and frequently affected by this disease [89]. The etiologic agent is now thought to be an arenavirus on the basis of PCR [90]. Antemortem diagnosis of this disease can be difficult; however, intracytoplasmic inclusion bodies may be observed most commonly in lymphocytes, or less commonly in heterophils, erythrocytes, basophils, and thrombocytes in peripheral blood smears [9, 17]. Buffy coat preparations may increase the likelihood of identifying inclusions, particularly in lymphocytes. The inclusions are variably sized, round to oval, and homogeneous. Romanowsky-type staining reveals inclusions of a pale basophilic nature, while hematoxylin and eosin staining creates pale moderately eosinophilic inclusions [9]. Inclusions may completely fill the cytoplasm and push the nucleus of leukocytes aside, creating a half-moon appearance [9]. Identification of inclusions on the blood film is considered diagnostic [9]; lack of the presence of inclusions does not rule out inclusion body disease (IBD) infection or disease. Additional discussion of IBD diagnosis is found in the subsection "Arena Virus and Inclusion Body Disease" under the section "PCR and Serology Useful in Snakes."

Hemostasis, Blood Types, Transfusions, and Cross-Matching

Despite extensive study of the effect of snake venom on human hemostasis, little study of snake hemostasis or blood types appear extant. The findings of a single study of *Elaphe obsoleta* suggest that erythrocytes and leukocytes both produce eicosanoids, to facilitate snake hemostasis [91].

Biochemical Panel

Plasma and serum biochemical analytes for select snake species are provided in Table 17.2. Lymphatic dilution may cause the following abnormalities of biochemistry parameters in snakes: decreased ALP albumin (calcium cholesterol globulin, total protein, sodium, and protein), and increased sodium increased [21]. The best-documented guide for enzyme use pertinent to snakes remains a single study of tissue enzyme activities performed in rat snakes as summarized in Table 17.3. Further research in other species, especially those boids common in the pet trade, is warranted to facilitate assessment of snake organ health. Multiple serum chemistry parameters may be affected by the hibernation cycle in some species, but apparently do not affect plasma chemistries in others [33, 92].

Liver Enzymes and Biomarkers

Lactate dehydrogenase (LDH) and aspartate aminotransferase (AST) occur in high concentrations in the liver of snakes, similar to birds and mammals. Because AST is not liver specific, increased activity may occur secondary to hepatocellular injury, muscle damage, or from generalized disease (e.g., toxemia, septicemia). Lack of liver specificity for LDH suggests this enzyme may increase with hepatocellular damage, skeletal or cardiac muscle injury, or hemolysis. Both alanine aminotransferase (ALT) and ALP occur in many tissues, and do not occur in high concentrations in the liver of snakes [46]. Thus, increased activities of ALP and or ALT do not indicate hepatocellular damage in snakes. In snakes, the primary end product of hemoglobin breakdown is biliverdin. Liver insufficiency or failure may increase biliverdin concentrations in peripheral blood, which may impart a green color to plasma. However, no assay for biliverdin is currently commercially available.

Hepatic lipidosis is a relatively common disease in captive, sedentary, overfed snakes, nonbreeding female snakes and those with low metabolic rates, such as black-headed pythons, *Aspidites melanocephalus*, and womas (Ramsay's python, *Aspidites ramsayi*) [50]. Female snakes typically accumulate lipid in hepatocytes and coelomic fat bodies for follicle development and yolk formation and deposition. If the stored fat goes unused, hepatic lipidosis may occur [50]. Affected snakes may have increased AST, LDH, ALT, gamma-glutamyltransferase (GGT), and ALP activities [50]. In wild-caught yellow rat snakes, *Elaphe obsoleta quadrivittata*, the major enzyme activities found in the liver were LDH and AST, but the kidney also exhibited moderate activities of LDH, AST, alanine transaminase, and creatine kinase (CK). No GGT activity was found in serum or tissues analyzed [46].

In evaluation of serum chemistry parameters of the Egyptian cobra, *Naja haje haje*, in correlation with the hibernation cycle, markedly decreased activities of LDH, GPT, GOT, and AP activities in response to hibernation may have contributed to functional impairment [92].

Muscle Enzymes

CK activity is specific to muscle and present in high concentration in myocytes of snakes, particularly in skeletal muscle [46]. Thus, increased plasma CK activity would be expected to occur with myocyte damage, exertion, or increased catabolism, which can occur with struggling during restraint, trauma, seizures, intramuscular injections, chronic cachexia, or systemic infections affecting skeletal and/or cardiac muscle. Anecdotally, activities of CK may also increase in snakes with gastrointestinal disease, causing damage to intestinal smooth muscle [61]. Snake myocyte damage could also result in increased AST and LDH activity of plasma, mimicking hepatic disease. In wild-caught yellow rat snakes, *Elaphe obsoleta quadrivittata*, skeletal muscle, and heart exhibited high CK activity. Serum CK activity was increased in rat snakes compared to other reptiles studied [46]. With hibernation, CK levels have been noted to be markedly decreased, as with the Egyptian cobra *Naja haje haje* [92].

Kidney Biomarkers

Snake kidneys cannot concentrate urine because they lack the loop of Henle. Secretion of soluble nitrogenous wastes such as urea that require water for excretion would be maladaptive for terrestrial snakes, especially desert species. The primary nitrogenous wastes excreted by snakes are uric acid and urate salts, which are eliminated as semi-solids [159]. The diagnosis of renal insufficiency in snakes can be challenging, as serum or plasma urea nitrogen and creatinine are not markers of renal disease. Plasma or serum urea nitrogen (blood urea nitrogen, BUN) are commonly low in snake plasma, do not reliably increase with renal disease, but may increase because of dehydration and dietary protein intake. Creatinine concentrations are low in snake plasma and increase only when renal failure is severe [46]. Assays for creatinine are not readily available. In a study of free-ranging anacondas, *Eu. murinus*, male anacondas had higher ALP, creatinine, and amylase values, for which no cause was attributed by the author, but may have been due to dehydration [19].

In wild-caught yellow rat snakes, *Elaphe obsoleta quadrivittata*, the kidney had moderate activities of LDH, AST, alanine transaminase, and CK, while snake renal tubules contain AST, creatinine phosphokinase (CPK), LDH, ALP, and GGT [46]. Renal enzyme activity increases with renal disease, but concomitant increases are not typically seen in peripheral blood as these enzymes are removed by the kidneys [46]. As in rats and mice, assay of urinary enzymes may be more valid for diagnosis of snake renal disease, but investigation is lacking. Increased plasma activity of AST observed may be attributed to the wide tissue distribution of this enzyme; increased AST is not a reliable indicator of renal disease in snakes [46]. Increased GGT activity could serve as a urinary marker of renal disease in some snakes, but further research and validation is needed [46].

Plasma uric acid concentration can be a useful analyte to evaluate the snake kidney, within limits. Hyperuricemia is commonly associated with renal insufficiency, as diseased kidneys cannot properly excrete uric acid. However, increased plasma uric acid concentrations are rare unless renal function is severely compromised. Diseases resulting in such dysfunction include bacterial infection, nephrotoxicity (e.g., aminoglycosides), and nephrocalcinosis [46]. However, uric acid concentrations of snakes may also increase with gout or after a high-protein meal. Therefore, uric acid concentrations are neither a sensitive nor specific analyte for renal disease [46]. However, renal disease and gout typically result in a more marked increase in uric acid concentration (greater than twofold) which can result in secondary visceral and articular gout [46]. Advanced diagnostics such as nuclear scintigraphy, CT, MRI, and renal clearance of radioactive contrast material or iohexol have been investigated as renal function tests, but are not routinely clinically used in snakes [46]. Nuclear medicine may be used to evaluate the kidneys of snakes; in the corn snake, *Elaphe gutatta gutatta,* imaging via injection of the radiopharmaceutical 99mTc-MAG3 shows promise for evaluation of renal function [93]. Among free-ranging anacondas, *Eu. murinus,* injured anacondas had significantly lower uric acid levels than did uninjured ones [19].

Glucose

In snakes, glucose levels are regulated by insulin and glucagon released from the mixed pattern of pancreatic beta and alpha cells, respectively, found within the snake pancreatic islets [94]. Intraperitoneal administration of insulin in grass snakes causes hypoglycemia, with the degree of decrease in glucose concentration proportional to the dose administered [95]. Snakes appear highly sensitive to insulin, and snake insulin has high affinity for mammalian insulin receptors [96]. However, glucose concentration of snakes is also affected by a variety of physiologic and environmental factors. Glucose concentrations vary depending on snake species and gender [97]. In the eastern massasauga rattlesnake, *S. catenatus catenatus,* lower blood glucose concentrations occurred in females, possibly because of increased glucose use for folliculogenesis, and to replace energy lost to parturition [79]. Insulin and glucagon activity, and therefore glucose concentration, are also affected by temperature [96]. Thus, serial plasma glucose measurements are recommended, and recording snake and or ambient temperature at sampling are recommended. As in mammals, obtaining only a single glucose measurement may not provide a complete assessment of the patient's glucose concentrations.

Plasma glucose can be measured with automated chemistry analyzers or glucometers; glucometer values underestimate the true glucose concentration by approximately 20%, and become less accurate as glucose concentrations decrease [96]. Hyperglycemia in snakes occurs most commonly owing to iatrogenic glucose administration or stress hyperglycemia due to epinephrine or corticosteroid release [96, 97]. Stress hyperglycemia is exemplified by the grass snake, *N. natrix natrix.* In this species, repeated blood sampling and cardiac puncture resulted in hyperglycemia [97]. Clinical snake pancreatitis or diabetes mellitus diagnosed via biochemical means was not found in a literature search. Hypoglycemia in snakes may occur because of starvation or malnutrition, septicemia, or severe hepatobiliary disease. Blood glucose decreased in the Egyptian cobra in response to hibernation [92]. Free-ranging male anacondas had significantly higher amylase values [19]; the utility of this analyte is snakes remains unproved. In this same study, reduced glucose concentrations in samples with delayed processing occurred [19].

Electrolytes

Electrolyte values for apparently healthy snakes are provided in Table 17.3. In snakes, the most common cause of hypernatremia (<160 mEq/l) is likely dehydration. Hyponatremia may occur with sodium loss through gastrointestinal disease (e.g., diarrhea) or renal failure, from salt gland excretion in marine species, or from iatrogenic causes such as excessive administration of sodium poor fluids. Hyperchloremia (>130 mEq/l) is presumed likely to occur in snakes suffering dehydration, renal insufficiency, or salt gland pathology [98]. Hypochloremia (<100 mEq/l) is rare in snakes, but can occur with chloride loss due to gastrointestinal disease or overhydration with chloride-poor fluids. Blood samples collected from free-living anacondas, *Eu. murinus,* within a day of capture

Table 17.3 Relative enzyme activities of select organs of wild-caught yellow rat snakes [46].

ORGAN	Enzyme activity, units/ gram of tissue	
	>200	>50, <150
Liver	LDH	AST, ALT
Kidney	LDH, ALT, CK, AST	ALP
Muscle	CK	LDH
Heart	CK	LDH, AST

Table 17.4 Select trace elements from whole blood of free-living water snakes [19, 109, 130, 131].

Element	Northern water snake *Nerodia sipedon*			Banded water snake *Nerodia fasciata*	Brown water snake *Nerodia taxispilota*	Cottonmouth *Agkistrodon piscivorus*	Anaconda *Eunectes murinus*
Data	Mean ± SE n = 18, NJ PPB wet weight	Mean ± SE n = 36, TN PPB wet weight	Mean ± SE n = 34, SC PPB wet weight	Mean ± SE n = 34 ppm, dry weight	Mean ± SE N = 9 ppm, dry weight	Mean ± SE N = 5 ppm, dry weight	Mean ± SD [Range] N = 12 ppm
Arsenic	20 ± 8	15 ± 2	246 ± 35	0.3 ± 0.03	0.4 ± 0.08	0.3 ± 0.10	–
Copper				0.6 ± 0.04	0.3 ± 0.04	0.6 ± 0.10	1.1 ± 0.5[0.4–1.7]
Iron				236 ± 12	220 ± 228	190 ± 39	1.4 ± 0.8[0.7–3.4]
Lead	108 ± 18	49 ± 6	56 ± 13	0.1 ± 0.01	0.04 ± 0.01	0.04 ± 0.02	–
Mercury	126 ± 26	417 ± 42	400 ± 47	0.4 ± 0.05	0.7 ± 0.15	0.1 ± 0.04	–
Selenium	560 ± 108	1090 ± 58	378 ± 30	0.4 ± 0.03	1 ± 0.09	0.6 ± 0.2	–
Zinc				11 ± 0.5	13 ± 1	8 ± 1	13.8 ± 2.5[10–18.4]

had decreased chloride concentrations compared to samples collected 2–10 days after capture, which may have reflected euhydration in snakes sampled on the day of capture [19]. In this same study, sodium concentrations varied depending on the snake capture site [19]. Artifactual increases in potassium and phosphate concentrations due to hemolysis in blood samples, caused by potassium release from blood cells has not been documented for snake species. Etiologies of hyperkalemia (>6 mEq/l) in snakes are presumed similar to those of other species and include renal failure due to decreased excretion by the diseased kidneys, iatrogenic oversupplementation or dietary excess, or due to potassium leaving cells and entering plasma as occurs in severe metabolic acidosis. Hyperkalemia has been reported in a western hognose snake, *Heterodon nasicus,* with metastatic ductal adenocarcinoma [63]. As in other species, snake hypokalemia (<2 meq/l) is presumed to occur owing to multiple mechanisms including increased loss through the gastrointestinal tract secondary to intestinal disease, dietary potassium deficiency, such as occurs in refeeding syndrome and because of severe metabolic alkalosis, due to movement of potassium into the cell. Few of these causes of electrolyte abnormalities have been definitively diagnosed or documented in snakes; however, the author (JJH) has experience one case of refeeding syndrome in a constrictor species in which plasma potassium values were reported as 0 mg/dl.

Plasma/Serum Protein

Gender, reproductive status, and season can affect total protein concentrations of snakes. Estrogen secretion during folliculogenesis in female snakes results in a transient hyperproteinemia based on hyperglobulinemia, as globulins needed for yolk production (vitellogenins) are produced [99]. In king cobras, *O. hannah,* higher protein concentrations occurred in winter compared to spring, and plasma protein concentrations were increased in wild-caught snakes compared to captive snakes [16]. Similarly in the Egyptian cobra, decreased serum protein concentrations occur during hibernation, and an increase in total non-protein nitrogen (NPN) and serum uric acid, and a fall in urea, creatinine, ammonia, and free amino acids levels indicate increased protein catabolism in hibernating animals [92].

Plasma proteins are most accurately measured by protein electrophoresis followed by the biuret method and, finally, refractometry. However, expense, laboratory methodologies, and technical difficulty progress in a similar manner. Thus, while refractometry is most often used owing to its simple and inexpensive technique, the information provided for snakes may be unreliable [17, 56]. Hyperproteinemia in snakes occurs with dehydration or chronic inflammatory disease. Infectious disease can cause significant elevations in alpha, beta, and gamma globulins [79]. Plasma proteins were increased in Cascabel infected with *Rhabdias* spp. compared to those that were not [62].

Hypoproteinemia is most commonly the result of chronic malnutrition, but can also occur with maldigestive or malabsorptive disease, protein-losing enteropathies (e.g., intestinal parasitism), severe blood loss, and chronic hepatic or renal disease [79]. In experimentally *Hepatozoon*-infected king cobras, *O. hannah,* and hematozoa-infected puff-faced water snakes, *H. buccata,* plasma protein fibrinogen decreased in parasitized compared to unaffected snakes [16, 48]. Heat precipitation may provide an estimate of fibrinogen concentrations, as an indication of acute inflammation, but has received little investigation in snakes [17]. In the Egyptian cobra, *Naja haje haje*, total lipids decreased, while total cholesterol and triglycerides concentrations did not change significantly during winter hibernation [92].

Blood Gases, Acid/Base

Snake blood pH is typically 7.5–7.7 at 23–25 °C, although in some snakes pH may be more acidic (<7.4) [88, 100]. High environmental temperature or excitement decreases pH, while low temperatures and anesthesia may increase pH [88]. The bicarbonate/carbonic acid system is considered the primary buffering system in snakes [100]. Decreased TCO2 due to evaporation from plasma in samples which were delayed in processing has been reported in a study of the anaconda, *Eu. murinus* [19]. In experimentally staged agonistic encounters of male copperheads, *Agkistrodon contortrix*, plasma lactate concentrations were not correlated with body mass, length, behavior duration, or season. However, 1 h post encounter, lactate concentrations (given as mM ± SEM) of winners [6.47 ± 0.89] and controls [6.38 ± 0.63] were lower those of losers [10.37 ± 0.89] [101].

Vitamins, Minerals, Metals, and Toxins

Calcium, Phosphorus, and Vitamin D

In snakes, calcium homeostasis is maintained by regulation via parathyroid hormone, calcitonin, and activated vitamin D3 (1,25 dihydroxycholecalciferol). Exogenous administration of Vitamin D3 to the smooth water snake, *Enhydris enhydris*, and the freshwater snake, *Natrix piscator*, increases serum calcium and inorganic phosphorus levels [102, 103]. Environment and reproductive status also greatly influence calcium metabolism. Vitamin D3 stimulates absorption of calcium and phosphorus by the intestine and becomes "active" with exposure to UV radiation (290–320 nm wavelength) in many reptiles, but this has yet to be demonstrated in snakes [29]. Photochemical activation is especially important for diurnal basking reptiles. During follicular development prior to ovulation, estrogen and reproductive activity cause an increased total calcium due to increased protein-bound calcium [104]. In the freshwater snake, *N. piscator*, exogenous prolactin administration induces progressive increases in serum calcium [103]. In the eastern massasauga rattlesnake, *S. catenatus catenatus*, females had higher calcium and phosphorus concentrations than males [105]. Although not routinely measured in snakes, ionized calcium concentrations (physiologically active calcium) likely provide the most accurate assessment of true calcium status.

Hypercalcemia is typically diagnosed when plasma total calcium is greater than 20 mg/dl. However, in free-living indigo snakes (*Drymarchon* spp.), a physiologic hypercalcemia has been documented (average calcium concentration of 159 mg/dl); concentrations of this magnitude appear rare in captive indigo snakes [106]. Hypercalcemia in snakes is most frequently caused by over-supplementation of calcium and/or vitamin D3, while less likely differentials to consider include primary hyperparathyroidism, pseudohyperparathyroidism, and osteolytic bone disease.

Hypocalcemia occurs with dietary deficiencies in calcium and/or vitamin D3, excessive dietary phosphorus, metabolic alkalosis, hypoalbuminemia, or far less likely, hyperparathyroidism. Hypocalcemia can also develop in snakes with severe chronic renal insufficiency as a result of renal secondary hyperparathyroidism [29]. Nutritional calcium or vitamin D3 deficiencies and/or the lack of proper UVB light may result in metabolic bone disease (nutritional secondary hyperparathyroidism), but this disease tends to occur less commonly in snakes because of their whole prey diet. Nevertheless, captive snakes fed all-meat diets can develop bone disease from dietary calcium and phosphorus imbalance (NSHP) [20, 93]. Diamond pythons, *Morelia spilota spilota*, indigo snakes, *Drymarchon corais*, some aquatic species, the insectivorous rough and smooth green snakes, *Opheodrys aestivus* and *O. vernalis*, and other arboreal, diurnal snakes may be at increased disease risk for NSHP, although further research is needed [93, 107].

Phosphorus concentrations are increased in healthy indigo snakes, *Drymarchon* spp., in comparison to other species, with an average phosphorus concentration of 35 mg/dl [106]. In other snake species, hyperphosphatemia occurs most commonly with excessive dietary phosphorus, hypervitaminosis D, and renal insufficiency. In the freshwater snake, *N. piscator*, exogenous prolactin administration induces progressive increases in serum phosphorous [103]. An artifactual hyperphosphatemia is presumed to occur in snakes if serum or plasma is not immediately separated from the clot, owing to phosphorus release from erythrocytes in the clot. However, phosphorus concentrations within snake blood cells, or in samples which have and have not clotted, have not been specifically determined. Rarely, anecdotal differentials for causes of phosphorous concentration abnormalities in snakes include severe tissue trauma and osteolytic bone disease as causes of increased phosphorous and starvation or dietary phosphorus deficiency as causative of decreased phosphorus [17, 29, 107].

Vitamins

In captive corn snakes, *El. guttata*, plasma concentration of 25-hydroxyvitamin D3 of snakes provided supplemental lighting (196 ± 16.73 nmol/l) were greater than those of control snakes (57.17 ± 15.28 nmol/l) [108]. However, plasma vitamin D3 concentrations necessary or recommended for snake health have yet to be determined. Plasma values for the E vitamins alpha tocopherol and gamma tocopherol, and the vitamin A retinol obtained from 12 free-living anacondas, *Eu. murinus,* were (mean ± SD, range expressed as μg/ml) 12.5 ± 6.5, 5.9–23.7; 0.4 ± 0.2, 0.2–0.9; and 0.08 ± 0.06, 0.03–0.24; respectively.

Lead/Zinc

Heavy metal toxicity in captive snakes appears rare, likely owing to dietary and environmental control, as well as a lack of baseline plasma metal values for most species. Studies of trace element accumulation in free-living water snakes suggest that tissues samples have greater sensitivity for assessment of bioaccumulation than whole blood [109]. In free-ranging anacondas, *Eu. murinus,* captured in Venezuela, zinc levels were elevated (13.8 ± 2.5 ppm) as compared with normal values for mammals and birds, and copper concentration were increased in males compared to females [19]. In free-living snakes, toxicity from exposure to coal combustion wastes and accumulation of the trace elements arsenic, cadmium, and selenium manifested at an increased metabolic rate, but no plasma or blood concentrations of these elements were determined [110]. Although water snakes appear to be good bioaccumulators and reasonable environmental sentinels, species and tissue accumulation variability may obscure scientific or clinical assessment [109]. Some blood trace element measurements from select snake species are provided in Table 17.4.

Acetylcholinesterase Inhibitors and Other Environmental Toxins

Cases of organophosphate toxicity in captive snakes occur, but have not been reported in the literature. Certainly these pesticides as well as synthetic pyrethrins, delivered by a variety of methods, are toxic and have caused death in snakes in investigation of control methods for invasive or venomous species [111]. However, plasma concentrations of acetylcholinesterase or other pesticides consistent with either health or intoxication have not been determined for any snake species to our knowledge [112]. The diamondback water snake, *Nerodia rhombifer,* blotched water snake, *N. erythrogaster,* and the cottonmouth, *Agkistrodon piscivorus,* were collected from Texas sites with toxification from intensive agricultural or industrial activities for over the last 50 years [113]. Dichlorodiphenyldichloroethylene (DDE) concentrations were 3.0 ppm in whole blood of a diamondback water snake at one site, similar to plasma concentrations of peregrine falcons, *Falco peregrinus,* in 1978–1979. Despite these findings, a gravid, apparently health female was captured at this site, suggesting snakes may be less sensitive to these environmental toxins. In free-living anacondas, plasma assay for chlorinated pesticide residues and polychlorinated biphenyls (PcBs) failed to identify these compounds [19].

Hormones

Endocrine and reproductive hormones are not commonly evaluated clinically in snakes. Endocrine function appears to parallel mammals, apart from the environmental influence over these systems in ectotherms [114]. For example, the thyroid function of snakes is typically

Table 17.5 Select laboratories offering PCR and serology diagnostics of use in snake species.

Test Available	Organisms	Laboratory
PCR & Sequencing, Serology Culture	Adenoviruses, Arenaviruses Astroviruses, Chlamydiales, Cryptosporidium, Ferlaviruses, Herpesviruses, Iridoviruses, Microsporidians, Mycobacteria, Mycoplasmas, Orthoreoviruses, Papillomaviruses, Paramyxoviruses, Pentastomids, Ranaviruses	Zoo Medicine Infectious Disease Testing Laboratory, University of Florida, College Of Veterinary Medicine, UF Veterinary Diagnostic Labs2015 SW 16TH AV, RM VS-50GAINESVILLE, FL 32608-1166 352-294-4420 http:// labs.vetmed.ufl.edu/sample-requirements/ zoo-med-infections/
0PCR	*Cryptosporidium* Genus *Cryptosporidium saurophilum, Cryptosporidium serpentis, Entamoeba invadens,* Arenavirus (inclusion body disease) Ferlavirus (OPMV) Sunshine Virus, West Nile Virus	Research Associates Laboratory 14556 Midway Road, Dallas, TX 75244. Phone: (972)960-2221 Fax: (972)960-1997 www.vetdna.com
PCR	Paramyxovirus I *Cryptosporidium* spp.	Veterinary Molecular Diagnostics 5989 Meijer Dr., Suite 5 Milford, OH 45150 Tel: 513.576.1808 Fax: 513.576.0031 www.vmdlabs.com
RT-PCR, in situ hybridization	Ophidian Paramyxovirus	INFECTIOUS DISEASES LABORATORY 110 Riverbend Rd, Riverbend North, Room 150 University of Georgia, Athens, GA 30602 Email: idllab@uga.edu Office: 706.542.8092 Fax: 706.583.0843 Lab: 706.542.5812

slower at lower temperatures [114]. However, the resting metabolic rate of a cool-temperature species, the adder, *V. berus*, was higher than that an age- and weight-matched desert species, the horned viper, *Cerastes cerastes gasperetti*, likely owing to cold adaptation [115]. Higher resting metabolic rates occur in younger snakes than adults, supporting age-related effects in thyroid function. Snakes possess both thyroid and parathyroid glands.

Thyroid

The thyroid gland governs metabolic rate, endocrine function, growth, ecdysis, and reproduction [114]. Thyroid hormone levels in snakes appear to be lower than in mammals; though diagnostic tests measuring mammalian thyroid hormones are not sensitive enough for use in snakes. [Rivera]. A high-sensitivity radioimmunoassay can measure total T4 in snakes, and has been used in corn snakes, *El. guttata*; ball pythons, *P. regius*; red-tailed boas, *Boa constrictor*; and milk snakes, *Lampropeltis triangulum* [116]. Hyperthyroidism has been diagnosed in snakes undergoing frequent ecdysis. Thyroid neoplasia also occurs in snakes [114].

Parathyroid

The parathyroid glands maintain calcium homeostasis. Secondary hyperparathyroidism can occur in snakes with chronic renal failure or dietary calcium deficiency [114]. Clinical diagnosis is based on exam, imaging, and calcium (bound and or ionized), phosphorous, and vitamin D concentrations, rather than on parathyroid hormone levels, which are not routinely measured in snakes.

Adrenal, Corticosteroids

Hyperadrenocorticism or hypoadrenocorticism have not been reported as clinical syndromes in snake species. However, corticosterone, the main adrenal hormone of snakes, has been evaluated in some snake species as indication of health or stress, via radioimmunoassay. In experimentally staged agonistic encounters of 58 male copperheads, *Agkistrodon contortrix*, plasma corticosterone concentrations [mean ± SD ng/ml] were highest in losers [63.49 ± 15.00] and significantly less in winners [29.67 ± 13.70] and controls [21.59 ± 10.10] [117].

In laboratory-housed western diamondback rattlesnake males, *Crotalus atrox*, plasma corticosterone concentrations [mean ng/ml] of snakes handled for 5 min [50 ± 25] were higher than those only handled at 15 min for blood collection [30 ± 15]. Similarly, sample collection delay from 15 to 30 min post handling also resulted in increased plasma corticosterone concentrations [145 ± 20] in this study [118]. In free-living brown tree snakes, *Boi. irregularis*, trapping and handling were associated with twofold to fourfold increases in corticosterone when compared to free-ranging snakes. In free-ranging snakes, corticosterone concentrations [mean ± SE ng/ml] of females [8.71 ± 1.82] were about twice as high as those of males [4.41 ± 0.77] [119]. Plasma corticosterone concentrations increase dramatically in late gestation of some snake species and return to baseline after parturition in reproductive females [120]. In summary, the clinician should be aware that snakes secrete corticosterone secondary to trap, capture, and handling; conspecific agonistic behaviors; and in late gestation. Further, corticosteroid-related changes in hematology or biochemistry should be considered when reviewing assay results in free-living, late-gestation, or stressed captive snakes.

Reproductive Hormones

Reproductive hormones are not routinely measured for clinical assessment of reproduction in snakes; imaging and palpation are more common clinical procedures to facilitate reproductive diagnosis. However, reproductive hormones have been measured for research purposes in both captive and free-living snake species. Clinical use of reproductive hormones is further hampered by overrepresentation of temperate and viperid nonpet species in the scientific literature and by the variety of reproductive strategies of snakes. Because a paucity of hormone concentrations have been determine for snake species commonly maintained as exotic pets, no specific hormonal values are provided here. However, the reader is encouraged to consult an extensive recent review by Taylor et al. for further information. Below is a limited summary of reproductive hormones as they clinically relate to snake reproduction [120].

In females, increased plasma concentrations of plasma 17β-estradiol coincide with vitellogenesis, reflecting its role in the production of vitellogenin by the liver. Similarly, plasma progesterone is often elevated during gestation (ovulation-oviposition) in viviparous and some oviparous species, owing to its role of pregnancy maintenance. A slightly increase of testosterone may occur at the beginning of mating activities in some species, as this steroid is a precursor to 17β-estradiol. In the Chinese cobra, *Naja naja*, and some species of marine snakes, increased T has also been associated with vitellogenesis [121]. Corticosterone increases substantially during late gestation in *Crotalus atrox*, but returns to baseline along with progesterone after parturition.

In males, increased plasma testosterone concentrations are associated with spermatogenesis, spermatogenic activity, hypertrophy of the sexual segment of the kidney, and mating/breeding behavior. It should be noted that in some temperate species, these activities do not occur simultaneously; mating may occur in a time period distinct from spermatogenesis; thus, two separate peaks may occur. Similarly, year-round spermiogenesis, mating, and the absence of seasonal trends in have been observed in some tropical snake species. In staged experimental agonistic encounters of male copperheads,

Agkistrodon contortrix, only correlated with late summer, a time of testicular recrudescence in this species, but not body length, mass, duration of agonistic behaviors, winning, losing, or loafing [117]. Plasma steroid hormone concentrations of viperids appear relatively increased compared to most other snakes and vertebrates [120]. Gonadotropins have received little scientific attention in snakes of clinical relevance; in the species most studied (*N. naja*), the relationship between gonadotropin concentrations, steroid hormone secretion, and the reproductive cycle is not straightforward [121]. Thyroid hormones may also be involved in snake reproduction owing to the linkage between temperature and reproductive activity; however, much more study is needed in this and many other areas of snake reproductive endocrinology.

Urinalysis

Likely because of the infrequency of urination and the routine admixture of urine and feces of snakes, urinalysis remains infrequently performed in these species. As snakes lack urinary bladders, and have ureters which empty into the cloacal urodeum, voided urine is not sterile, and contamination with materials released from the genital or gastrointestinal tracts is presumed. Reference values for urinalysis, or an assessment of the utility or validity of this technique, or lack thereof, for use in diagnosis in snakes are currently unavailable.

PCR and Serology Useful for Snakes

Table 17.5 provides an overview of select PCR and Serologic test available which may be useful in snakes.

Cryptosporidium

Cryptosporidium serpentis is an apicomplexan parasite that commonly infects the gastrointestinal tract of snakes. This organism is intermittently shed in feces, and thus gastric lavage is preferred to detect organisms. PCR is the most commonly used and readily available test for diagnosis. However, cryptosporidia are acid-fast positive organisms, and this test may be performed in-house [122]. The most sensitive diagnostic method is the immunofluorescent antibody (IFA) stain (Merifluor, Meridian Diagnostic, Cincinnati, Ohio) [122]. Six weeks after fecooral infection with *C. serpentis*, serum antibodies may be detected via ELISA, which detects exposure or active infection [122]. Many species of cryptosporidium exist and infect snakes (e.g., *Cryptosporidium saurophilum*), and PCR, IFA, and serology may not detect all species of cryptosporidium [123].

Entamebiasis

Entameoba invadens may subclinically infect turtles or tortoises but result in debilitation and death in snakes. Diagnosis may be accomplished via PCR of gastrointestinal tract excretions, or direct fecal or regurgitant wet mount exam for protozoa may be attempted [31].

Paramyxoviruses

Ophidian Paramyxoviruses or Ferlaviruses (OPMV), including the recently discovered, distantly related OPMV Sunshine virus, are important viral pathogens of snakes [122, 124, 125]. All viperid species are likely susceptible to infection, which may also occur in colubrid, boid, and elapid snakes. These viruses affect the snake neurorespiratory system and commonly also cause nonspecific clinical signs such as lethargy and inappetence. Diagnosis of OPMV infection may be accomplished with histology, immunohistochemistry, electron microscopy, virus isolation, and in situ hybridization [122, 124]. However, in recent years, RT-PCR testing has been able to identify OPMVs from organ or swab samples. The most sensitive RT-PCR involves detection of OPMV by targeting a segment of the L-gene which encodes the RNA dependent RNA polymerase [122, 124]. In the live snake in which OPMV infection is suspected, respiratory secretions would constitute a reasonable sample.

Paramyxoviral exposure may be determined by commercially available hemagglutination inhibition which may be performed on snake plasma or serum; a positive titer only indicates exposure to OPMV. One cannot infer viral presence or shedding status from a single serology result. A rising titer over a two- to four-week interval

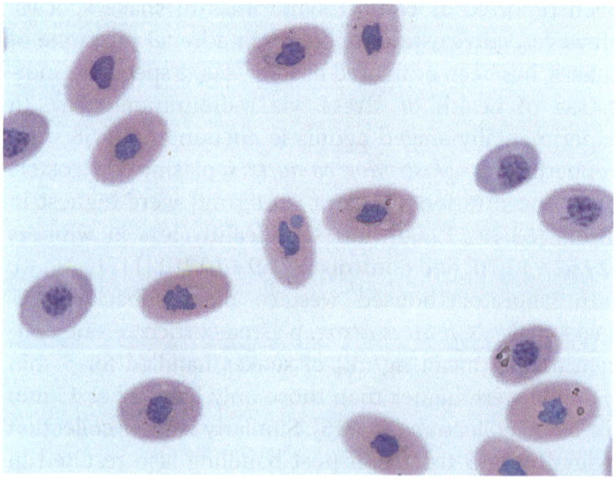

Figure 17.12 Blood smear from a red-tailed *Boa constrictor, Boa constrictor,* which upon necropsy had eosinophilic inclusions typical of inclusion body disease (IBD) in multiple organs. Buffy coat submitted for PCR testing was positive for reptarena virus, common boa strain. The inclusion body in the red blood cell is a light blue when subjected to modified Wrights stain, shown at 1000× magnification.

provides supportive evidence for recent OPMV infection. However, viral shedding or disease is not known to be reliably predicted via serology.

Arenavirus and Inclusion Body Disease (IBD)

Arenavirus has recently been proposed as causative of IBD of snakes [90]. IBD disease causes multisystem illness, predominantly neurological, in affected snakes, which are commonly boids and pythons. Intracytoplasmic inclusions may be observed in peripheral blood cells and visceral epithelial cells (Figure 17.12) [126]. PCR for arenavirus is commercially available; to the best of our knowledge, virus isolation is not commercially available for clinical diagnosis. Western blot can be used to detect IBD protein in peripheral blood or tissue biopsy of the liver, but it is also not commercially available [126].

West Nile Virus

On the basis of limited experimental data, it appears that snakes may be infected with West Nile virus, become viremic, shed virus, and develop neutralizing antibodies [127]. Commercially available PCR assays should detect viral shedding of WNV, and or other encephalitis viruses in snakes.

References

1 Wojtaszek, J.S. (1991). Haematology of the grass snake Natrix natrix natrix. *Comparative Biochemistry and Physiology Part A: Physiology* 100A (4): 805–812.
2 Jacobson, E.R. (1993). Blood collection techniques in reptiles: laboratory investigations. In: *Zoo and Wild Animal Medicine Current Therapy*, 3e (ed. M. Fowler) 144–152. WB Saunders Company.
3 Lillywhite, H.B. and Smits, A.N. (1984). Lability of blood volume in snakes and its relation to activity and hypertension. *The Journal of Experimental Biology* 110: 267.
4 Lillywhite, H.B., Smits, A.W., and Feder, M.E. (1988). Body fluid volumes in the aquatic snake, Acrochordus granulatus. *Journal of Herpetology* 22 (4): 434–438.
5 Lillywhite, H.B. (1987). Circulatory adaptations of snakes to gravity. *American Zoologist* 27: 81–95.
6 Jacobson, E.R. (2007). *In Infectious Diseases and Pathology of Reptiles CRC*. Boca Raton: Press Taylor and Francis Group.
7 Isaza, R., Andrews, G.A., Coke, R.L., and Hunter, R.P. (2004). Assessment of multiple cardiocentesis in ball pythons (Python regius). *Journal of the American Association for Laboratory Animal Science* 43 (6): 35–38.
8 Murray MJ. 2000. Ch 20. Reptilian Laboratory Medicine: 185–189
9 Stahl, S.J. (2003). Diseases of the reptile pancreas. *The Veterinary Clinics of North America. Exotic Animal Practice* 6: 191–212.
10 Lamirande, E.W., Bratthauer, A.D., Fisher, D.C., and Nichols, D.K. (1999). Reference hematologic and plasma chemistry values of brown tree snakes (Boiga irregularis). *Journal of Zoo and Wildlife Medicine* 30: 516–520.
11 Sherif, M. and El Ridi, R. (1992). Natural cytotoxic cell activity in the snake Psammophis sibilans. *Immunobiology* 184 (4–5): 348–358.
12 Gartner, G.E., Hicks, J.W., Manzani, P.R. et al. (2010). Phylogeny, ecology, and heart position in snakes. *Physiological and Biochemical Zoology* 83 (1): 43–54.
13 HE, M.C. (1999). Organ location in snakes for diagnostic and surgical evaluation. In: *Zoo & Wildlife Medicine Current Therapy 4* (ed. M.E. Fowler and R.E. Miller), 243–248. Philadelphia: WB Saunders.
14 Brown, C. (2010). Cardiac blood sample collection from snakes. *Laboratory Animals* 39 (7): 208–209.
15 Dotson, T.K., Ramsey, E.C., and Bounous, D.I. (1995). A color atlas of blood cells of the yellow rat snake. *Compendium on Continuing Education for the Practicing Veterinarian* 17: 1013–1026.
16 Salakij, C., Salakij, J., Apibal, S. et al. (2002). Hematology, morphology, Cytochemical staining, and ultrastructural characteristics of blood cells in king cobras (Ophiophagus hannah). *Veterinary Clinical Pathology* 31 (3): 116–126.
17 Skoczylas, R. and Sidorkiewicz, E. (1974). Studies on the blood sugar level in the grass snake (Natrix natrix L.). *Comparative Biochemistry and Physiology, Part A: Molecular & Integrative Physiology* 48 (3): 439–456.
18 Harr, K.E., Raskin, R.E., and Heard, D.J. (2005). Temporal effects of 3 commonly used anticoagulants on hematologic and biochemical variables in blood samples from macaws and Burmese pythons. *Veterinary Clinical Pathology* 34 (4): 383–388.
19 Calle, P.P., Rivas, J., Munoz, M. et al. (1994). Health assessment of free-ranging anacondas (*Eunectes murinus*) in Venezuela. *Journal of Zoo and Wildlife Medicine* 25 (1): 53–62.
20 Mader, D.R., Horvath, C.C., and Paul-Murphy, J. (1985). The hematocrit and serum profile of the gopher snake (Pituophis melanoleucas catenifer). *Journal of Zoo Animal Medicine* 139–140.
21 Gillett, A.K., Flint, M., Hulse, L. et al. (2015 Jun 30). Haematological and biochemical reference intervals for three species of hydrophiine sea snakes (Hydrophis curtus, H. Elegans and H. Peronii) in Australia. *The Veterinary Journal* 204 (3): 275–281.
22 Persson, B., Zaidi, Z.H., and Jörnvall, H. (1990). Sea snake (Microcephalophis gracilis) hemoglobin: primary structure and relationships to other forms. *Journal of Protein Chemistry* 9 (5): 533–541.

23 Dabrowski, Z., Sano Martins, I.S., Tabarowski, Z. et al. (2007). Haematopoiesis in snakes (Ophidia) in early postnatal development. *Cell and Tissue Research* 328: 291–299.

24 Reagan, W.J., Rovira, A.R.I., and DeNicola, D.B. (2013). *Veterinary Hematology: Atlas of Common Domestic and Non-domestic Species*. Wiley.

25 Johnson, J.H. and Benson, P.A. (1996). Laboratory reference values for a group of captive ball pythons (Python regius). *American Journal of Veterinary Research* 57 (9): 1304–1307.

26 Saint Girons, M.C. (1970). Morphology of the circulating blood cell. In: *Biology of Reptilia*, vol. 3 (ed. C. Gans and T. Parsons). New York: Academic Press.

27 Hawkey, C.M. and Dennett, T.B. (1989). *A Colour Atlas of Comparative Veterinary Haematology*. Wolfe Publishing Ltd.

28 Stacy, N.I., Alleman, A.R., and Sayler, K.A. (2011). Diagnostic hematology of reptiles. *Clinics in Laboratory Medicine* 31 (1): 87–108.

29 Sykes, J.M., Schumacher, J., Avenell, J. et al. (2006). Preliminary evaluation of 99mTechnetium diethylenetriamine pentaacetic acid, 99mTechnetium dimercaptosuccinic acid, and 99mTechnetium mercaptoacetyltriglycine for renal scintigraphy in corn snakes (Elaphe guttata guttata). *Veterinary Radiology & Ultrasound* 47 (2): 222–227.

30 Heatwole, H. and Dunson, W.A. (1987). Hematological parameters of some marine snakes. *Journal of Experimental Marine Biology and Ecology* 113 (3): 289–300.

31 Baeyens, D.A., Patterson, M.W., and McAllister, C.T. (1979). Hematology as related to diving characteristics of *Elaphe obsolete, Nerodia erythrogaster, Nerodia fasciata* and *Nerodia* rhombifera. *Arkansas Academy of Science Proceedings* 33: 17–18.

32 Tucunduva, M., Borelli, P., and Silva, J.R. (2001). Experimental study of induced inflammation in the Brazilian boa (boa constrictor constrictor). *Journal of Comparative Pathology* 125: 174–181.

33 Dutton, C.J. and Taylor, P. (2003). A comparison between pre- and posthibernation in morphometry, hematology and blood chemistry in viperid snakes. *Journal of Zoo and Wildlife Medicine* 34 (1): 53–58.

34 Chouhey, B.J. and Singh, N.K. (1977). Some aspects of hematology of an Indian grass snake Natrix stolata in relation to sex and size. *Folia Haematologica* 104 (1): 75–84.

35 Allender, M.C., Mitchell, M.A., Phillips, C.A. et al. (2006). Hematology, plasma biochemistry, and antibodies to select viruses in wild-caught eastern massasauga rattlesnakes *(Sistrurus catenatus catenatus)* from Illinois. *Journal of Wildlife Diseases* 42 (1): 107–114.

36 Wojtaszek, J.S. (1992). Seasonal changes of circulating blood parameters in the grass snake Natrix natrix natrix L. *Comparative Biochemistry and Physiology Part A Physiology* 103 (3A): 461–471.

37 Saad, A.H. and Shoukey, N. (1988). Sexual dimorphism on the immune responses of the snake Psammophis sibilans. *Immunobiology* 177: 404–419.

38 Ohlendorf, H.M., Hothem, R.L., and Aldrich, T.W. (1988). Bioaccumulation of selenium by snakes and frogs in the San Joaquin Valley, California. *Copeia* 1998 (3): 704–710.

39 Troiano, J.C., Vidal, J.C., Gould, J. et al. (1997). Haematological reference intervals of the south American rattlesnake (Crotalus durissus terrificus) in captivity. *Comparative Haematology International* 7 (2): 109–112.

40 Heath, K.B. (1983). Fatal parasitic anemia in a green vine snake. *Veterinary Medicine, Small Animal Clinician* 78 (7): 1095–1096.

41 West, G., Heard, D., and Caulkett, N. (eds.) (2008). *Zoo Animal and Wildlife Immobilization and Anesthesia*. Wiley Antonio FB: Chapter 20. Venomous Reptile Restraint and Handling, 337–350. Bertelson MF,Chapter 21. Squamates (Snakes and Lizards) 351–365.

42 Jacobson, E.R., Seely, J.C., and Novilla, M.N. (1980). Lymphosarcoma associated with viral-like intranuclear inclusions in a California kingsnake (Colubridae: Lampropeltis). *Journal of the National Cancer Institute* 65 (3): 577–583.

43 Frye, F.L. (1991). Hematology as applied to clinical reptile medicine. In: *Biomedical and Surgical Aspects of Captive Reptile Husbandry*, 2e, vol. 1 (ed. F. Fl), 209–277. Melbourne FL: Kreiger.

44 Bounous, D.I., Dotson, T.K., Brooks, R.L., and Ramsay, E.C. (1996). Cytochemical staining and ultrastructural characteristics of peripheral blood leucocytes from the yellow rat snake (Elaphe obsoleta quadrivitatta). *Comparative Haematology International* 6 (2): 86–91.

45 Sano-Martins, I.S., Jared, C., and Brunner, A. (1994 Dec 1). Ultrastructural alterations in thrombocytes of the snake Waglerophis merremii after activation by ADP. *Comparative Haematology International* 4 (4): 226–231.

46 Ramsay, E.C. and Dotson, T.K. (1995). Tissue and serum enzyme activities in the yellow rat snake (Elaphe obsoleta quadrivitatta). *American Journal of Veterinary Research* 56 (4): 423–428.

47 Taylor EN, Denardo DF. 2010. Hormones and reproductive cycles in snakes. Hormones and reproduction of vertebrates, 3:355.

48 Salakij, C., Salakij, J., Suthunmapinunta, P., and Chanhome, L. (2002). Hematology, morphology and ultrastructure of blood cells and blood parasites from puff-faced watersnakes (Homalopsis buccata). *Kasetsart Journal (Natural Science)* 36: 35–43.

49 Wang, T., Fernandes, W., and Abe, A.S. (1993). Blood pH and O2 homeostasis upon CO2 anesthesia in the rattlesnake (Crotalus durissus). *Snake* 25: 21–26.

50 Skovgaard, N., Møller, K., Gesser, H., and Wang, T. (2009). Histamine induces postprandial tachycardia through a direct effect on cardiac H2-receptors in pythons. *American Journal of Physiology. Regulatory, Integrative and Comparative Physiology* 296 (3): R774–R785.

51 El Ridi, R., Badir, N., and El Rouby, S. (1981). Effect of seasonal variation on the immune system of the snake, Psammophis schokari. *Journal of Experimental Zoology* 216: 357–365.

52 Farag, M.A. and El Ridi, R. (1985). Mixed leukocyte reaction (MLR) in the snake *Psammophis siblans. Immunology* 55: 173–181.

53 Klenk, K. and Komar, N. (2003). Poor replication of West Nile virus (New York 1999 strain) in three reptilian and one amphibian species. *The American Journal of Tropical Medicine and Hygiene* 69 (3): 260–262.

54 Machado, C.C., Silva, L.F.N., Ramos, P.R.R., and Takahira, R.K. (2006). Seasonal influence on hematologic values and hemoglobin electrophoresis in Brazilian boa constrictor amarali. *Journal of Zoo and Wildlife Medicine* 37 (4): 487–491.

55 Sidorkiewicz, E. and Skoczylas, R. (1974). Effect of insulin on the blood sugar level in the grass snake (Natrix natrix L.). *Comparative Biochemistry and Physiology Part A: Physiology* 48 (3): 457–464.

56 Simpson, M. (2006). Hepatic lipidosis in a black-headed python (Aspidites melanocephalus). *The Veterinary Clinics of North America. Exotic Animal Practice* 9 (3): 589–598.

57 Campbell, K.R., Campbell, T.S., and Burger, J. (2005). Heavy metal concentrations in northern water snakes (Nerodia sipedon) from east fork Poplar Creek and the Little River, East Tennessee, USA. *Archives of Environmental Contamination and Toxicology* 49 (2): 239–248.

58 Montali, R.J. (1988). Comparative pathology of inflammation in the higher vertebrates (reptiles, birds and mammals). *Journal of Comparative Pathology* 99: 1–26.

59 Alleman, A.R., Jacobson, E.R., and Raskin, R.E. (1999). Morphologic, cytochemical staining, and ultrastructural characteristics of blood cells from eastern diamondback rattlesnakes (Crotalus adamanteus). *American Journal of Veterinary Research* 60 (4): 507–514.

60 Egami, M.I. and Sasso, W.S. (1988). Cytochemical observations of blood cells of *Bothrops jaracaca. Revista Brasileira de Biologia* 48: 155–159.

61 Mitchell, M.A. and Diaz-Figueroa, O. (2005). Clinical reptile gastroenterology. *The Veterinary Clinics of North America. Exotic Animal Practice* 8: 277–298.

62 Santos, K.R., Takahira, R.K., Rall, V.L. et al. (2008). Pulmonary, microbiological and hematological changes in Crotalus durissus terrificus (Serpentes, Viperidae) parasitized by nematodes of the genus Rhabdias (Nematoda, Rhabdiasidae). *Arquivo Brasileiro de Medicina Veterinaria e Zootecnia* 60 (3): 667–674.

63 Strik, N.L., Alleman, A.R., and Harr, K.E. (2007). Circulating inflammatory cells. In: *Infectious Diseases and Pathology of Reptiles* (ed. E.R. Jacobsen), 167–218. Boca Raton FL: CRC Press.

64 Schilliger, L., Selleri, P., and Frye, F.L. (2011). Lymphoblastic lymphoma and leukemic blood profile in a red-tail boa (boa constrictor constrictor) with concurrent inclusion body disease. *Journal of Veterinary Diagnostic Investigation* 23: 159–162.

65 MacMahon, J.A. and Hamer, A.H. (1975). Hematology of the sidewinder (Crotalus cerastes). *Comparative Biochemistry and Physiology Part A: Physiology* 51 (1): 53IN755–53IN5458.

66 Wozniak, E.J. and Telford, S.R. (1991). The fate of Hepatozoon species naturally infecting Florida black racers and watersnakes in potential mosquito and soft tick vectors and histological evidence of pathogenicity in unnatural host species. *International Journal for Parasitology* 21: 511–516.

67 Myers, T.S. (1971). Renal trematodiasis in a boa constrictor (constrictor constrictor). *Laboratory Animal Science* 21 (3): 423–425.

68 Lipps, B.V. and Khan, A.A. (2001). The presence of pharmacological substances myoglobin and histamine in venoms. *Journal of Venomous Animals and Toxins* 7: 1. accessed 25 Mar 2015.

69 Spadacci-Morena, D.D., Jared, C., Antoniazzi, M.M. et al. (1998). Comparative cytomorphology of maturing Amphisbaenian (Amphisbaena alba) and snake (Waglerophis merremii) erythroid cells with regard to haemoglobin biosynthesis. *Comparative Haematology International* 8 (1): 7–15.

70 Irizarry, A.R. (2010). *Hematology of Reptiles in Schalm's Veterinary Hematology*, 6e, 1004–1012. Ames: Blackwell Publishing Ltd.

71 Johnsrude, J.D., Raskin RE Hoage, A.Y. et al. (1997). Intraerythrocytic inclusions associated with iridoviral infection in fer de lance (Bothrops moojeni) snake. *Veterinary Pathology* 34: 235–238.

72 Troiano, J.C., Vidal, J.C., Gould, E.F. et al. (2000). Hematological values of some Bothrops species (Ophidia-Crotalidae) in captivity. *Journal of Venomous Animals and Toxins Including Tropical Diseases* 6 (2): 194–204.

73 Duguy, R. (1970). Numbers of blood cells and their variations. In: *Biology of Reptilia*, vol. 3 (ed. C. Gans and T. Parsons). New York: Academic Press.

74 Saad, A.H. (1989). Sex associated differences in the mitogenic responsiveness of snake blood lymphocytes. *Developmental and Comparative Immunology* 13 (3): 225–229.

75 Frye, F.L. and Kass, L. (1990). Characterization of neoplastic cell type in subacute baso-eosinophilic myelogenous leukemia in a snake. *Herpetopathologica* 2 (1): 63–71.

76 Jacobson, E.R., Calderwood, M.B., French, T.W. et al. (1981). Lymphosarcoma in an eastern Kingsnake and a rhinoceros viper. *Journal of the American Veterinary Medical Association* 179 (11): 1231–1235.

77 Lock, B., Heard, D., Dumore, D. et al. (2001). Lymphosarcoma with lymphoid leukemia in an Aruba island rattlesnake, Crotalus unicolor. *Journal of Herpetological Medicine and Surgery* 11: 19–23.

78 Raiti, P., Garner, M.M., and Wojcieszyn, J. (2002). Lymphocytic leukemia and multicentric T-cell lymphoma in a diamond python, Morelia spilota spilota. *Journal of Herpetological Medicine and Surgery* 12: 26–29.

79 Allender, M.C., Junge, R.E., Baker-Wylie, S. et al. (2015). Plasma electrophoretic profiles in the eastern Massasauga (Sistrurus catenatus) and influences of age, sex, year, loaction and snake fungal disease. *Journal of Zoo and Wildlife Medicine* 46 (4): 767–773.

80 George, G.W., Holmberg, T.A., Riggs, S.M. et al. (2008). Circulating siderophagocytes and erythrophagocytes in a corn snake (Elaphe guattata) after ceolomic surgery. *Veterinary Clinical Pathology* 37 (3): 308–311.

81 Tosunoğlu, M., Gül, Ç., Yilmaz, N., and Topyildiz, H. (2011). Hematological reference intervals of some snake species in Turkey. *Turkish Journal of Zoology* 35 (2): 237–243.

82 Wright, A. and Jones, I.C. (1957). The adrenal gland in lizards and snakes. *Journal of Endocrinology* 15 (1): 83–99.

83 Zwart, P. (2006). Renal pathology in reptiles. *Veterinary Clinics Exotic Animal Practice* 9: 129–159.

84 Motta, R.O., Cunha, L.M., Leite, R.C. et al. (2011). Hepatozoon ssp.(Apicomplexa: Hepatozoidae) infection and selected hematological values of the Neotropical rattlesnake, Crotalus durissus collilineatus (Linnaeus, 1758)(Serpentes: Viperidae), from Brazil. *Journal of Zoo and Wildlife Medicine* 42 (3): 399–407.

85 Ball, G.H. (1958). A haemogregarine from a water snake, Natrix piscator taken in the vicinity of Bombay, India. *The Journal of Protozoology.* 5 (4): 274–281.

86 Reichenbach-Klinke, H. and Elkan, E. (2013). *The Principal Diseases of Lower Vertebrates*. Elsevier.

87 Daly, J.J., Mayhue, M., Menna, J.H. et al. (1980). Virus like particles associated with Pirhemocyton inclusion bodies in the erythrocytes of a water snake, Nerodia erythrogaster flavigaster. *The Journal of Parasitology* 66: 82–87.

88 Wellehan, J.F.X., Strik, N.I., Stacy, B.A. et al. (2008). Characterization of an eryrthocytic virus in the family iridoviridae from a peninsula ribbon snake (Thamnophis sauritus sackenii). *Veterinary Microbiology* 131: 115–122.

89 Chang, L. and Jacobsen, E.R. (2010). Inclusion body disease. *A worldwide infectious disease of Boid Snakes: a review Journal of Exotic Pet Medicine* 19 (3): 216–225.

90 Stern, W.A., Velguth, K.E., and D'Agostino, J. (2010). Metastatic ductal adenocarcinoma in a western hognose snake (Heterodon nasicus). *Journal of Zoo and Wildlife Medicine* 41 (2): 320–324.

91 Herman, C.A., Wang, X., and Gronert, K. (1997). Biosynthesis of thromboxane by snake (Elaphe obsoleta) erythrocytes and the requirement of eicosanoid production for blood clotting. *Biochimica et Biophysica Acta (BBA) - General Subjects* 1334 (1): 23–27.

92 Al-Badry, K.S., El-Deib, S., and Nuzhy, S. (1992 Mar 1). Changes in serum chemistry parameters of the Egyptian cobra (Naja haje haje) in correlation with the hibernation cycle. *Journal of Thermal Biology* 17 (2): 111–4.35.

93 Sykes, K.L. and Klukowski, M. (2009). Effects of acute temperature change, confinement and housing on plasma corticosterone in water snakes, Nerodia sipedon (Colubridae: Natricinae). *Journal of Experimental Zoology Part A: Ecological Genetics and Physiology* 311 (3): 172–181.

94 Moscona, A.A. (1990). Anatomy of the pancreas and Langerhans islets in snakes and lizards. *The Anatomical Record* 227: 232–244.

95 Silva, L.F.N., Riana-Costa, C.C.M., Ramos, P.R.R., and Takahira, R.K. (2011). Seasonal influence on biochemical profile and serum protein electrophoresis for boa constrictor amarali in captivity. *Brazialian Journal of Biology* 71 (2): 517–520.

96 Steinman, A., Banet-Noach, C., Simanov, L. et al. (2006). Experimental infection of common garter snakes (Thamnophis sirtalis) with West Nile virus. *Vector Borne and Zoonotic Diseases* 6 (4): 361–368.

97 Srivastav, A.K. and Rani, L. (1989). Serum calcium and inorganic phosphorus levels of the freshwater snake Sinonatrix piscator (formerly Natrix piscator) in response to calcitonin treatment. *Canadian Journal of Zoology* 67 (5): 1335–1337.

98 Chabaud, A.G. and Frank, W. (1960). Description of the microfilaria of Macdonaldius oschei. *Annales de Parasitologie Humaine et Comparée* 36: 133.

99 Dessauer, H.C., Fox, W., and Gilbert, N.L. (1956). Plasma calcium, magnesium and protein of viviparous colubrid snakes during estrous cycle. *Experimental Biology and Medicine* 92 (2): 299–301.

100 Sykes, J.M. and Klaphake, E. (2008). Reptile hematology. *Veterinary Clinics Exotic Animal Practice* 11: 481–500.

101 Schuett, G.W. and Grober, M.S. (2000). Post-fight levels of plasma lactate and corticosterone in male copperheads, Agkistrodon contortrix (Serpentes,

Viperidae): differences between winners and losers. *Physiology & Behavior* 71 (3): 335–341.

102 Kagwade, M.V. and Padgaonkar, A.S. (1994 Oct 1). Effects of vitamin-d (3) administration on the levels of serum-calcium and inorganic phosphorus in the smooth water snake, enhydris-enhydris (schneider). *Zoological Studies* 33 (4): 319–321.

103 Srivastav, A.K., Srivastav, S.K., Singh, S., and Norman, A.W. (1995 Oct). Effect of various vitamin D metabolites on serum calcium and inorganic phosphate in the freshwater snake Natrix piscator. *General and Comparative Endocrinology* 100 (1): 49–52.

104 Alcobendas, M., Castanet, J., Martelly, E., and Milet, C. (1992). Phosphate and calcium level variations in the plasma of the snake Vipera aspis during the annual cycle and the reproductive period. *Herpetological Journal* 2 (2): 42–47.

105 Lance, V.A., Cort, T., Masuoka, J. et al. (1995). Unusually high zinc concentrations in snake plasma, with observations on plasma zinc concentrations in lizards, turtles and alligators. *Journal of Zoology (London)* 235: 577–585.

106 Drew, M.L. (1994). Hypercalcemia and hyperphosphatemia in indigo snakes (Drymarchon corais) and serum biochemical reference values. *Journal of Zoo and Wildlife Medicine: Reptile and Amphibian March* 25 (1): 48–52.

107 Stinner, H.N. (1982 Mar 1). Ventilation, gas exchange and blood gases in the snake, Pituophis melanoleucus. *Respiration Physiology* 47 (3): 279–298.

108 Acierno, M.J., Mitchell, M.A., Zachariah, T.T. et al. (2008). Effects of ultraviolet radiation on plasma 25-hydroxyvitamin D3 concentrations in corn snakes *(Elaphe guttata). American Journal of Veterinary Research* 69 (2): 294–29762.

109 Burger, J., Murray, S., Gaines, K.F. et al. (2006). Element levels in snakes in South Carolina: differences between a control site and exposed site on the Savannah River site. *Environmental Monitoring and Assessment* 112 (1–3): 35–52.

110 Hopkins, W.A., Rowe, C.L., and Congdon, J.D. (1999). Elevated trace element concentrations and standard metabolic rate in banded water snakes (Nerodia fasciata) exposed to coal combustion wastes. *Environmental Toxicology and Chemistry* 18 (6): 1258–1263.

111 Savarie, P.J., Bruggers, L. 1999. Candidate repellents, oral and dermal toxicants, and fumigants for brown tree snake control. In Problem Snake Management: The Habu and the Brown Treesnake, eds. G. H. Rodda, Y. Sawai, D. Chiszar, and H. Tanaka, 417–422. Ithaca: Cornell University Press.

112 Schmidt SR. 2003. *R*eptile Cholinesterase Characterization and Use in Monitoring Anti-Cholinesterases.

113 Clark, D.R., Bickham, J.W., Baker, D.L., and Cowman, D.F. (2000). Environmental contaminants in Texas, USA, wetland reptiles: evaluation using blood samples. *Environmental Toxicology and Chemistry* 19 (9): 2259–2265.

114 Rivera, S. and Lock, B. (2008 Jan 31). The reptilian thyroid and parathyroid glands. *The Veterinary Clinics of North America. Exotic Animal Practice* 11 (1): 163–175.

115 Al-Sadoon, M.K. (1991). Metabolic rate-temperature curves of the horned viper, Cerastes cerastes gasperetti, the moila snake, Malpolon moilensis, and the adder, Virera berus. *Comparative Biochemistry and Physiology Part A: Physiology* 99 (1–2): 119–122. **Metabolic rate-temperature curves of the horned viper, *Cerastes cerastes gasperetti*, the moila snake, *Malpolon moilensis*, and the adder, *Virera berus*.**

116 Greenacre, C.B., Young, D.W., Behrend, E.N. et al. (2001). Validation of a novel high sensitivity radioimmunoassay procedure for measurement of total thyroxine concentration in psittacine birds and snakes. *American Journal of Veterinary Research* 62 (11): 1750–1754.

117 Schuett, G.W., Harlow, H.J., Rose, J.D. et al. (1996). Levels of plasma corticosterone and testosterone in male copperheads (Agkistrodon contortrix) following staged fights. *Hormones and Behavior* 30 (1): 60–68.

118 Schuett, G.W., Taylor, E.N., van Kirk, E.A., and Murdoch, W.J. (2004). Handling stress and plasma corticosterone levels in captive male western diamond-backed rattlesnakes (Crotalus atrox). *Herpetological Review* 35 (3): 229–232.

119 Mathies, T., Felix, T.A., and Lance, V.A. (2001). Effects of trapping and subsequent short-term confinement stress on plasma corticosterone in the brown treesnake (Boiga irregularis) on Guam. *General and Comparative Endocrinology* 124 (1): 106–114.

120 Telford, S.R. (2008 Oct 7). *Appendix: The Identification of Reptilian Hemoparasites. Hemoparasites of the Reptilia. Color Atlas and Text*, 357–368. CRC Press.

121 Bona-Gallo, A., Licht, P., MacKenzie, D.S., and Lofts, B. (1980). Annual cycles in levels of pituitary and plasma gonadotropin, gonadal steroids, and thyroid activity in the Chinese cobra (Naja naja). *General and Comparative Endocrinology* 42 (4): 477–493.

122 Paiva, P.R., Grego, K.F., Lima, V.M. et al. (2013 Nov 15). Clinical, serological, and parasitological analysis of snakes naturally infected with Cryptosporidium serpentis. *Veterinary Parasitology* 198 (1): 54–61.

123 Richter, B., Kübber-Heiss, A., Weissenböck, H., and Schmidt, P. (2008). Detection of cryptosporidium spp., Entamoeba spp. and Monocercomonas spp. in the gastrointestinal tract of snakes by in-situ hybridization. *Journal of Comparative Pathology* 138 (2): 63–71.

124 Abbas, M.D., Marschang, R.E., Schmidt, V. et al. (2011). A unique novel reptilian paramyxovirus, four atadenovirus types and a reovirus identified in a concurrent infection of a corn snake (Pantherophis guttatus) collection in Germany. *Veterinary Microbiology* 150 (1): 70–79.

125 Hyndman, T.H., Shilton, C.M., Doneley, R.J., and Nicholls, P.K. (2012). Sunshine virus in Australian pythons. *Veterinary Microbiology* 161 (1): 77–87.

126 Banajee, K.H., Chang, L.W., Jacobson, E.R. et al. (2012). What is your diagnosis? Blood film from a boa constrictor. *Veterinary Clinical Pathology* 41 (1): 158.

127 Stenglein, M.D., Sanders, C., Kistler, A.L. et al. (2012). Identification, characterization, and in vitro culture of highly divergent arenaviruses from boa constrictors and annulated tree boas: candidate etiological agents for snake inclusion body disease. *MBio* 3 (4): e00180–e00112.

128 Rosskopf, W.J., Woerpel, R.W., and Yan off, S.R. (1982). Normal hemogram and blood chemistry values for boa constrictors and pythons. *Veterinary Medicine, Small Animal Clinician* 77: 822–823.

129 Choidini, R.J. and Sundberg, J.P. (1982). Blood chemical values of the common boa constrictor. *American Journal or Veterinary Research.* 43: 1701–1702.

130 Burger, J., Campbell, K.R., Campbell, T.S. et al. (2005). Use of skin and blood as nonlethal indicators of heavy metal contamination in northern water snakes (*Nerodia sipedon*). *Archives of Environmental Contamination and Toxicology* 49: 232–238.

131 Burger, J., Campbell, K.R., Murray, S. et al. (2007). Metal levels in blood, muscle and liver of water snakes (Nerodia spp.) from New Jersey, Tennessee and South Carolina. *Science of the Total Environment* 373 (2): 556–563.

132 Arikan, H., Göçmen, B., Atatür, M.K. et al. (2009). Morphology of peripheral blood cells from various Turkish snakes. *North-Western Journal of Zoology* 5 (1): 61–73.

133 Bryant, G.L., Fleming, P.A., Twomey, L., and Warren, K.A. (2012). Factors affecting hematology and plasma biochemistry in the southwest carpet python (Morelia spilota imbricata). *Journal of Wildlife Diseases* 48 (2): 282–294.

134 Campbell, T.W. and Ellis, C.K. (2013). *Avian and Exotic Animal Hematology and Cytology*, 2005–2007. Wiley.

135 Fudge, A.M. (ed.) (2000). *Laboratory Medicine: Avian and Exotic Pets*, 376–399. Philadelphia: Saunders.

136 Garner, M.M., Hernandez-Divers, S.M., and Raymond, J.T. (2004). Reptile neoplasia: a retrospective study of case submissions to a specialty diagnostic service. *Veterinary Clinics Exotic Animal Practice* 7: 653–671.

137 Gillilan, L.A. and Conklin, R.E. (1938). Removal of foreign substances by the lymphatics of the snake lung. *The American Journal of Physiology* 123 (3): 598–607.

138 Jacobsen, E.R., Adams, H.P., Geisbert, T.W. et al. (1997). Pulmonary lesions in experimental ophidian paramyxovirus pneumonia of Aruba island rattlesnakes, Crotalus unicolor. *Veterinary Pathology* 34: 450–459.

139 Jaensch, S.M. and Raidal, S.R. (2006). Peripheral erythrophagocytosis in two reptiles. *Comparative Clinical Pathology* 15 (2): 113–116.

140 Jones, D.E. and Holladay, S.D. (2006). Excretion of three heavy metals in the shed skin of exposed corn snakes (Elaphe guttata). *Ecotoxicology and Environmental Safety* 64 (2): 221–225.

141 Lance, V. (1975). Studies on the annual reproductive cycle of the female cobra Naja naja – I. Seasonal variation in plasma cholesterol. *Comparative Biochemistry and Physiology* 52A: 519–52555.

142 Lance, V. (1976). Studies on the annual reproductive cycle of the female cobra, Naja naja. Seasonal variation in plasma inorganic ions. *Comparative Biochemistry and Physiology Part A: Physiology* 53 (3): 285–289.

143 Mansour, M.H., El Ridi, R., and Badir, N. (1980 Aug). Surface markers of lymphocytes in the snake, Spalerosophis Diadema. I. Investigation of lymphocyte surface markers. *Immunology* 40 (4): 605.

144 Marquardt, W.C. and Yaeger, R.G. (1967). The structure and taxonomic status of Toddia from the cotton-mouth snake Agkistrodon piscivorous leucostoma. *The Journal of Protozoology* 14: 726–731.

145 McDaniel, R.C., Grunow, W.A., Daly, J.L., and Plummer, M.V. (1984). Serum chemistry of the diamond-backed water snake (Nerodia rhombifera rhombifera) in Arkansas. *JWD* 20: 44–46.

146 Mills, G.L. and Taylaur, C.E. (1971). The distribution and composition of serum lipoproteins in eighteen animals. *Comparative Biochemistry and Physiology Part B: Comparative Biochemistry* 40 (2): 489–501.

147 Moço, T.C., O'Dwyer, L.H., Vilela, F.C. et al. (2002). Morphologic and morphometric analysis of Hepatozoon spp.(Apicomplexa, Hepatozoidae) of snakes. *Memórias do Instituto Oswaldo Cruz* 97 (8): 1169–1176.

148 Moore, I.T., Lemaster, M.P., and Mason, R.T. (2000). Behavioural and hormonal responses to capture stress in the male red-sided garter snake, Thamnophis sirtalis parietalis. *Animal Behaviour* 59 (3): 529–534.

149 Moore, I.T., Lerner, J.P., Lerner, D.T., and Mason, R.T. (2000). Relationships between annual cycles of testosterone, corticosterone, and body condition in male red-spotted garter snakes, Thamnophis sirtalis concinnus. *Physiological and Biochemical Zoology* 73 (3): 307–312.

150 Papp, T., Pees, M., Schidt, V., and Marschang, R.E. (2010). RT-PCR diagnosis followed by sequence characterization of paramyxoviruses in clinical samples from snakes reveals concurrent infections within populations and/or individuals. *Veterinary Microbiology* 144: 466–472.

151 Pati, A.K. and Thapliyal, J.P. (1984). Erythropoietin, testosterone, and thyroxine in the erythropoietic response of the snake, Xenochrophis piscator. *General and Comparative Endocrinology* 53 (3): 370–374.

152 Ridi, R.E., Badir, N., and Rouby, S.E. (1981). Effect of seasonal variations on the immune system of the snake, Psammophis schokari. *Journal of Experimental Zoology* 216 (3): 357–365.

153 (a) Schumacher, J., Jacobson, E.R., Homer, B.L., and Gaskin, J.M. (1994). Inclusion body disease in boid snakes. *Journal of Zoo and Wildlife Medicine* 25 (4): 511–524. (b) Selleri P, Hernandez-Divers SJ. 2006. Renal Diseases of Reptiles.:16d1–174.

154 Seymour, R.S. (1987). Scaling cardiovascular physiology in snakes. *American Zoologist* 27: 97–109.

155 Srivastav, A.K. and Rani, L. (1990 Dec 1). Prolactin-induced hypercalcemia and hyperphosphatemia in the freshwater snake Natrix piscator. *Canadian Journal of Zoology* 68 (12): 2702–2704.

156 Sypik, J. and Borysenko, M. (1988). Reptiles. In: *Vertebrate Blood Cells Cambridge* (ed. A.F. Rawley and N.A. Ratcliff). Cambridge University: Press.

157 Wozniak, E.J., Telford, S.R., and McLaughlin, G.L. (1994). Employment of PCR in the molecular differentiation of reptilian hemogregarines and its application to preventative zoological medicine. *Journal of Zoo and Wildlife Medicine* 25: 538–549.

18

Lizards

Stephen J. Divers DECZM (Zoo Health Management, Herpetology) DACZM, FRCVS[1] and Melinda S. Camus DVM, DACVP[2]

[1] *Department of Small Animal Medicine and Surgery, College of Veterinary Medicine, University of Georgia, Athens, Georgia, USA*
[2] *Department of Veterinary Pathology, College of Veterinary Medicine, University of Georgia, Athens, Georgia, USA*

Introduction

The accumulation of species specific reference ranges continues to be slow for lizards. Most publications fall short of the standardized requirements necessary to establish true reference ranges, and some fail to take into account the significant effects of gender, age, season, reproductive status, diet, and feeding schedule [1]. Zoological practitioners should strive to adhere to established procedures in domestic animal clinical pathology, with respect to consistent collection, handling, and laboratory practices.

Despite the recent interest and reviews in reptile clinical pathology, much detailed data can still only be found outside of the veterinary literature, and often in scientific units which are less familiar to most US clinicians. Given the frequency with which the clinician may be forced to evaluate a clinical pathology report without an appropriate reference range, referring to older chapters can still be rewarding and complementary to this summary chapter [2–8]. This chapter was submitted in January 2012 and has not been updated. Readers are encouraged to review the literature after this date for any important updates or changes.

Species

Lizards, are of the Order Squamata (with snakes), Suborder Lacertilia (Sauria), a widespread and diverse group of vertebrates with nearly 6000 extant species, found on all continents except Antarctica, and ranging from a few centimeters to 3m in total length. Bearded dragons (Agamidae), chameleons (Chamaeleonidae), iguanas (Iguanidae), geckos (Eublepharidae, Gekkonidae), and monitors (Varanidae) are commonly presented for veterinary diagnosis.

Anatomy and Physiology

Most lizards are quadruped with pentadactyl limb anatomy, and all possess a three-chambered heart, although oxygenated and deoxygenated blood are functionally separated. Most lizards have an obvious tail, a common site for venipuncture. Lizards possess similar visceral organs as found in mammals, often differing in size and position. Lizards lack a distinct diaphragm; most species possess a single coelomic cavity.

The gastrointestinal organ system consists of the buccal cavity, esophagus, stomach, small and large intestines and cloaca, and the accessory digestive organs the liver and pancreas [9]. While the gross appearance of many digestive organs is similar to those of mammals, histological differences exist, often as an adaptation to diet [10]. The generic lizard pancreas is composed of three limbs, one each associated with the bile duct, duodenum, and the spleen. The pancreas possesses endocrine and exocrine roles, just as in mammals; however, the structure varies [9]. Variable pancreatic secretions of amylase, chymotrypsin, trypsin, carboxypeptidase, elastase, lipase, and chitinase have been reported [9].

Investigation of liver and kidney disease and dysfunction is a common diagnostic concern, and therefore these are described in more detail. The macroscopic appearance, gall bladder location, and blood supply of the liver of reptiles differs little from those of other vertebrates. Liver shape varies depending on animal morphology; liver weight comprises 3%–4% of the body weight in most squamates. Shape and mass can fluctuate depending on the time of year and nutritional and/or reproductive status [11]. The liver mainly originates from the endodermal gut, usually consists of two lobes, and varies in color from pale tan to black. The saurian

Exotic Animal Laboratory Diagnosis, First Edition. Edited by J. Jill Heatley and Karen E. Russell.

liver has less well-defined lobules than the mammalian liver, despite similar portal architecture. In many lizard species, the lobule structure is replaced by cords of hepatocytes and melanin pigmentation. The saurian liver metabolizes fat, protein (including globulin), and glycogen and produces nitrogenous waste products and clotting factors. These functions may vary as the animal progresses from embryo to adult, and be affected by seasonal changes, especially hibernation and estivation [11].

In the green iguana, the paired, lobulated kidneys are dark brown, elongate, taper cranially and cadually and lie dorsally in the pelvic canal. They are separated cranially and conjoined caudally. The ureters are visible from the caudal quarter of the ventral kidney surface as they course cranially, running medial to the renal portal vessels and entering the urodeum at the urinary papillae of the urodeum. The urethral opening is located in the ventral midline of the urodeum and connects to the bladder via a short wide urethra. The bladder has a large capacity for the storage of fluid and urates prior to elimination. The kidneys are supplied by arterial blood from the renal arteries and with venous blood from the renal portal veins [12]. The lobular structure of the kidney is well developed in the iguana. The intralobular artery is accompanied by the intralobular (efferent) vein and surrounded by an extensive network of peritubular portal arterioles. The numerous glomeruli are well vascularized. The renal portal system is a continuation of the caudal vein in the iguana, but in other lizards may include venous drainage from the caudal viscera or hind limbs [13, 14].

The saurian kidney is metanephric, has only a few thousand nephrons, and lacks an ansa nephroni. Thus, concentration of urine by the kidney to higher than plasma osmolality is not thought to occur in lizards. In the iguana, the glomeruli are well developed, although those nearer the surface are simpler, consisting of fewer capillary loops [12]. A typical nephron consists of the glomerulus connected by a thin, ciliated neck segment to the proximal tubule. A narrow, ciliated intermediate segment connects the relatively long proximal tubule to the shorter distal tubule, which leads to the collecting duct.

Precise control of glomerular filtration rate (GFR) and tubular function is not well understood in lizards. On the basis of a number of studies, lizard GFR may be affected by hydration status, arginine vasotocin or oxytocin administration, temperature, and the number of functional glomeruli [15–21]. In some species that possess an alternate method for salt excretion (e.g., nasal salt glands of the sand monitor *Varanus gouldii*), dramatic elevations of plasma osmolarity may not cause the expected decrease in GFR, because mechanisms for postrenal reabsorption of water from the cloaca, colon, or bladder are well developed [22]. Most, but not all lizards, possess a bladder.

Tubular function includes the regulation of water, sodium, potassium, hydrogen ion, calcium, phosphorus, and nitrogenous compounds [16]. Urea and creatinine are considered useless for renal evaluation of lizards owing to the small or variable quantities produced [23]. Ammonia appears to be a significant nitrogenous waste product in the tuatara (*Sphenodon* sp.) [24]. The most important nitrogenous waste product of most lizards is urate (or uric acid), which is freely filtered by the glomerulus [25]. In species thus far examined, tubular secretion of urate occurs in the proximal tubule [16]. Urate secretion requires the active transport of urate against a diffusion gradient from the blood into the proximal tubular cell and passive diffusion into the lumen of the proximal tubule [16]. In tubules with greatly reduced GFR and tubular flow, the passive diffusion of urate into the lumen ceases as urate concentrations equalize across the luminal membrane [16]. The proximal tubular secretion of urate is dependent upon and directly associated with the glomerular filtration rate. Urate complexed with various ions, potassium, and urinary proteins forms a colloidal suspension that passes from the nephron into the collecting duct. In the cloaca, colon, or bladder, the acidification of urine through hydrogen ion secretion or bicarbonate absorption, combined with water reabsorption, leads to the precipitation of uric acid [16]. Failure to adequately excrete urate leads to hyperuricemia, gout, and death [26].

Electrolytes, including sodium and potassium, are freely filtered by the glomerulus. Most of the ultrafiltrate sodium (and water) is reabsorbed from the nephron, collecting duct, colon, cloaca, or bladder. In hydrated geckos (*Hemidactylus* sp.) and iguanids (*Phrynosoma* sp. and *Tropidurus* sp.), 15%–46% of glomerular filtered sodium is excreted in urine [16]. Isosmotic sodium reabsorption occurs in the proximal tubule. However, as the osmolarity of ureteral urine is generally lower than plasma, fluid reabsorbed from the distal tubule must vary from isosmotic to hyperosmotic [16]. In many species, colon, cloaca, or bladder are more important sites for the regulation of sodium excretion and water reabsorption than the kidneys. Control of sodium and potassium regulation has been poorly studied in reptiles, but AVT, aldosterone, and temperature have been shown to exert significant effects [16]. Finally, the theoretical ineffectiveness of furosemide in these species, owing to the lack of the loop of Henle, has not been confirmed experimentally. In lizards, furosemide exerts significant diuretic effects by increasing sodium, chloride, potassium, and water losses from the kidney, colon, cloaca, and bladder [27–29].

Sample Collection

The blood volume of reptiles varies between 4% and 8% of the body weight, and in general, 10% of the total blood volume (i.e., 0.4–0.8 ml/kg) can be safely collected from healthy reptiles [30]. Sample size should be lessened in the ill or injured patient. Patient safety should always be considered prior to obtaining samples. Lymphatic or cerebrospinal fuid (CSF) contamination is common during reptile venipuncture, but appears less likely to occur in lizards compared to other reptiles, especially chelonians.

Handling and Restraint

Lizards vary in size, strength, and temperament, and therefore a variety of handling techniques are required to cover most practical situations and permit physical examination [31]. Tegus and monitors have powerful bites, while the green iguana can use their claws and tail for defense. Large lizards are best restrained with the forelimbs held laterally against their body and the hind limbs held laterally against the tail base. Lizards can be wrapped in a towel to aid restraint. Smaller lizards can be restrained around the pectoral girdle holding the forelimbs against the coelom, although care is required not to impair respiratory movements. Never grasp a lizard by the tail as many species can perform autotomy and drop their tails in an attempt to evade predation. Restricting the vision of these animals is often the simplest way to facilitate handling, and a towel placed over the head will often induce calm. Chemical restraint is not usually necessary for saurian venipuncture; however, excellent references exist for saurian chemical immobilization and anesthesia, and tiletamine/zolazepam, propofol, sevoflurane, and alphaxone are commonly used drugs in these species [32].

Blood Collection Sites

The most clinically useful vessel is the *caudal vein*, often referred to as the tail vein (Figures 18.1 and 18.2). The needle is positioned in the ventral midline between 20% and 80% down the tail and advanced at 45–60° in a craniodorsal direction, while maintaining slight negative pressure (Figures 18.3–18.5). If a coccygeal vertebra is encountered, the needle is withdrawn slightly and redirected either

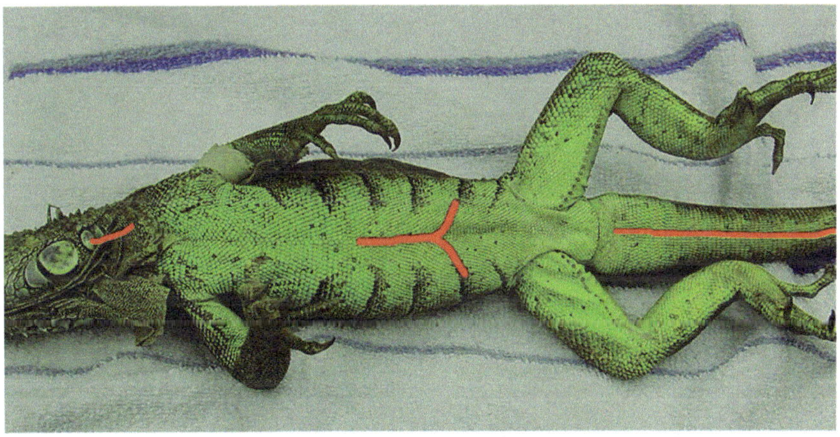

Figure 18.1 Ventral view of a green iguana, depicting from left to right the positions of the right jugular, anastomosing pelvic veins forming the large ventral abdominal vein, and the caudal (tail) vein. *Source:* Courtesy of Stephen J. Divers and Melinda Camus.

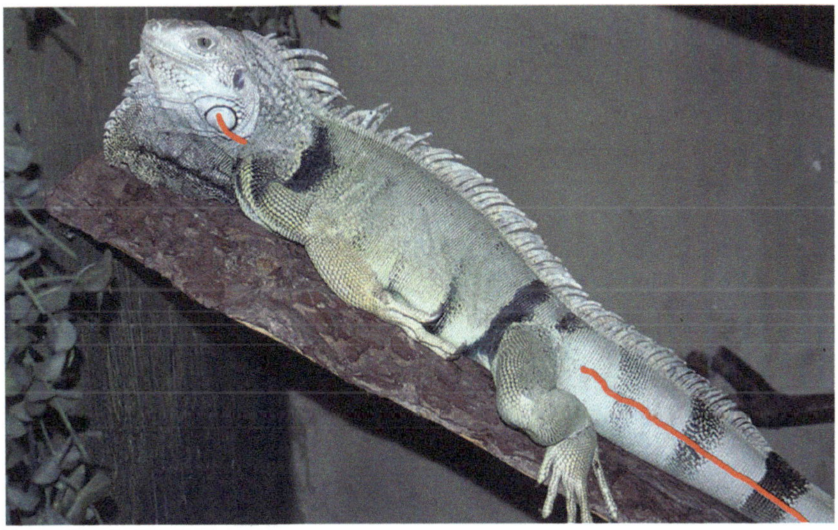

Figure 18.2 Lateral view of a green iguana, depicting from left to right the positions of the right jugular and caudal (tail) veins. *Source:* Courtesy of Stephen J. Divers and Melinda Camus.

further craniad or caudad. Care should be taken to avoid the hemipenes in male lizards. An alternative approach, more useful for large or ventrodorsally compressed species, is to insert the needle from the lateral midline (Figure 18.6). The needle is advanced at 45–60° in a craniomedial direction, aiming just ventral to the lateral processes of the coccygeal vertebrae. Lymphatic or CSF contamination may be more likely with the lateral approach.

Lizards possess a large *ventral abdominal vein* (formed by the joining of the pelvic veins) that courses within a suspensory ligament just below the linea alba. This vessel is most easily entered in the mid-caudal coelomic region. The needle is positioned in the ventral midline and advanced in a craniodorsal direction. Apart from the risks of puncturing the gastrointestinal tract or bladder, it is difficult to apply pressure to this vessel, which makes post-venipuncture hemorrhage a potential complication.

Jugular vein venipuncture is also practical, especially in the larger iguanids and monitor lizards. The jugular veins lie lateral and deep, and are seldom visible even when caudally occluded by digital pressure. For most species, the tympanum is a useful anatomical landmark. The lizard is restrained in lateral recumbency, and the needle inserted behind the tympanum (Figure 18.7). In

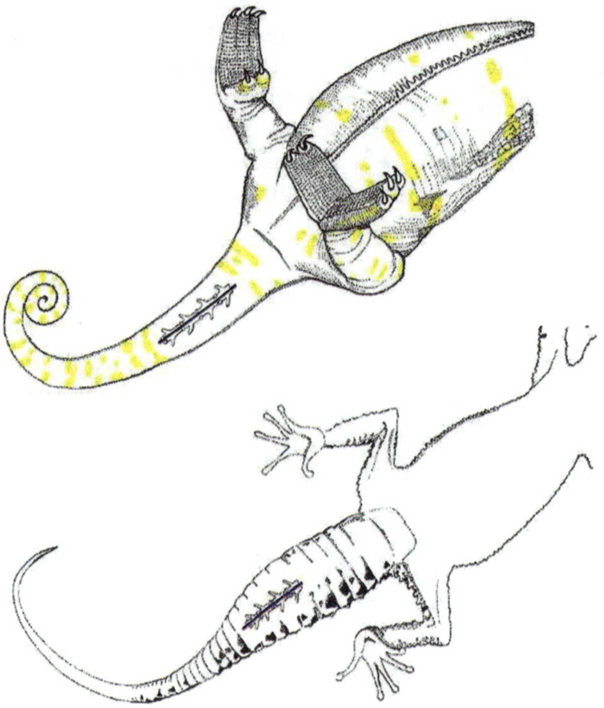

Figure 18.3 Diagrammatic view of the caudal (tail) vein in a chameleon and a gecko.

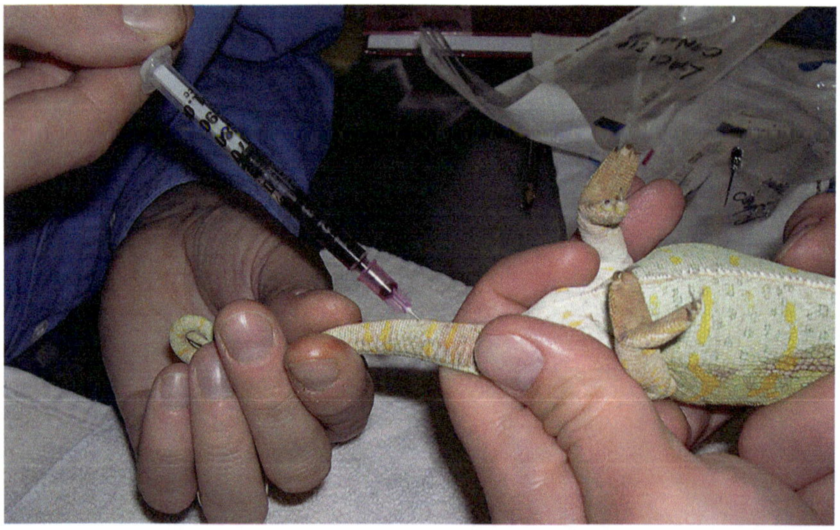

Figure 18.4 Caudal (tail) vein venipuncture in a chameleon utilizing the ventral approach. *Source:* Courtesy of Stephen J. Divers and Melinda Camus.

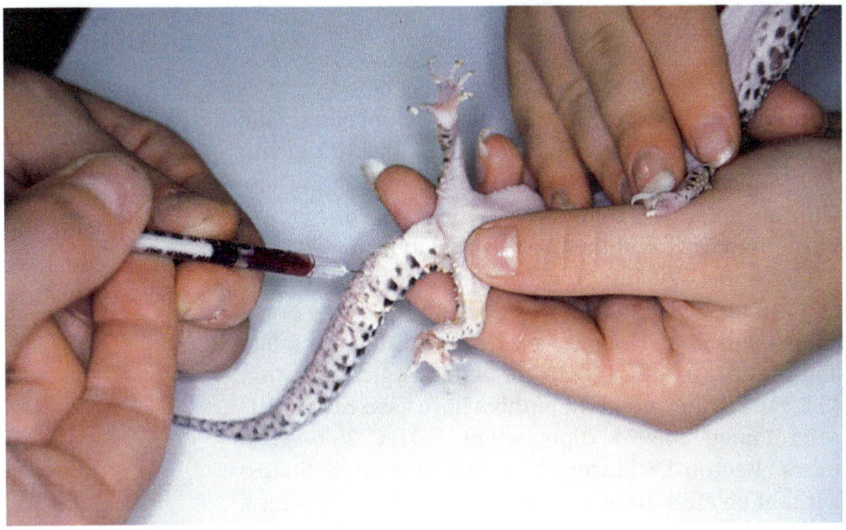

Figure 18.5 Caudal (tail) venipuncture in a leopard gecko utilizing the ventral approach. Geckos are especially prone to autotomy and may shed their tails during conscious venipuncture. Therefore, venipuncture of sensitive species is better performed under light anesthesia or sedation. *Source:* Courtesy of Stephen J. Divers and Melinda Camus.

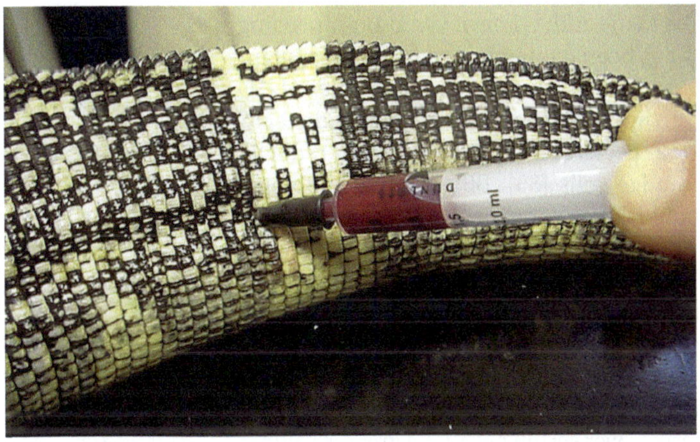

Figure 18.6 Caudal (tail) venipuncture in a monitor lizard utilizing the lateral approach between the dorsal and ventral coccygeal muscle groups. *Source:* Courtesy of Stephen J. Divers and Melinda Camus.

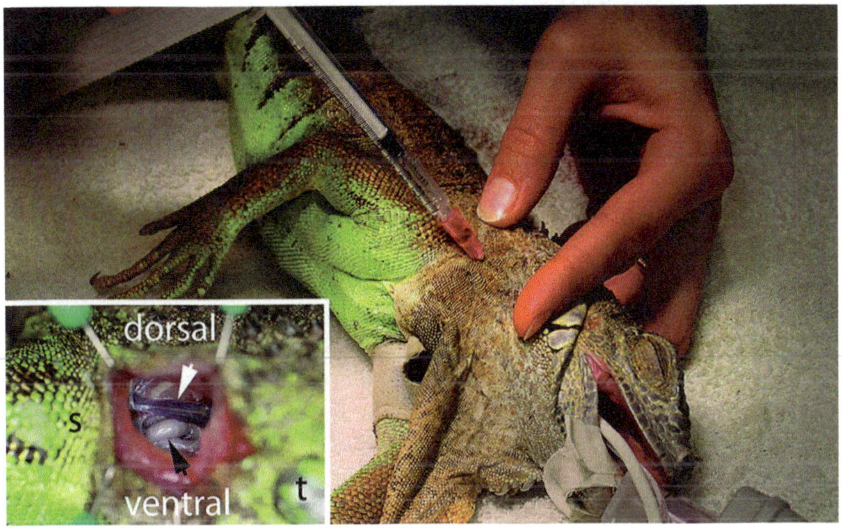

Figure 18.7 Jugular venipuncture in a green iguana. Insert – dissected view of the lateral cervical area demonstrating the point of the shoulder (s) and tympanic membrane (t) landmarks, and the jugular vein (white arrow) and carotid artery (black arrow). *Source:* Courtesy of Stephen J. Divers and Melinda Camus.

chameleons, an extension of the jugular vein may be accessed behind the casque as it courses vertically along the inside of this bony structure. This vein has been called the casque vein.

Cardiocentesis in lizards is not considered safe because the heart cannot be stabilized. Similarly, use of the axillary plexus, orbital sinus, and toenail clip is generally clinically unwarranted, and ethically less acceptable.

Sample Handling

Common materials used for collection of blood samples from lizards include 27–23 gauge (g.) needles, and 0.3–3 cm^3 syringes dependent upon the size of the animal. Superficial disinfection of the venipuncture site with an antiseptic solution is recommended, but will most often not facilitate vessel visualization.

The anticoagulant of choice for use in lizards is heparin for biochemistry; however, studies in the green iguana and water dragon have demonstrated the safety and superiority of CaEDTA for hematologic evaluation [33, 34]. Furthermore, the authors have used EDTA (BD Microtainer 365974 dipotassium EDTA 250–500 µl tubes, Becton-Dickinson, New Jersey, United States) without deleterious effects in a variety of lizard species, and is unaware of any adverse effects when this anticoagulant is used for lizard hematology. A fresh blood smear should be made at the time of venipuncture using blood that has not been contaminated by anticoagulant (i.e., the last drop in the syringe). In some studies of lizard blood, coverslip-to-slide and bevel-edge slide technique created a preferred monolayer with reduced numbers of smudge cells [35]. Blood for hematologic evaluation should ideally be processed within 1 h. Delays can be accommodated by refrigerating the EDTA tube, but deterioration will occur. Do not refrigerate blood smears, as water condensation may damage cell morphology. Freezing blood will result in cell lysis [36].

For biochemical analyte determinations, heparinized plasma is preferred over serum because a greater volume of plasma is harvested per unit of blood, sample analysis can occur without waiting for clot formation, and to prevent formation of fibrin clots, which interfere with analysis. Differences between serum and plasma in green iguanas were [36] higher total protein, albumin, and globulin concentrations and higher AST concentrations in plasma; while plasma ALT was lower than serum ALT. Nonetheless, plasma provided reasonable approximations for serum biochemical values. Small blood tubes containing lithium heparin with plasma separators are useful in reptile practice as they come in a variety of sizes, as small as 400 µl (BD Microtainer 365985 lithium heparin with PST gel separator 400–600 µl blood tubes, Becton-Dickinson). Moderate hemolysis in the green iguana increases phosphorus levels, while marked hemolysis significantly increases phosphorus, potassium, total protein, and AST [36]. Samples are best processed immediately. However, for a delay of 1–48 h, separate plasma immediately from the cellular fraction, and keep refrigerated or, in field conditions, keep on ice. If delays exceed two days, freezing at −80 °C will preserve most chemical constituents. Frozen–thawed plasma should be thoroughly mixed prior to processing.

Complete Blood Count

Erythron

Like all reptiles, lizards possess nucleated erythrocytes. The complete blood count includes packed cell volume (PCV), total red blood cell count (TRBC), hemoglobin content (Hg), total white blood cell count (TWBC), and a differential leukocyte count and qualitative blood smear evaluation (Figures 18.8–18.12). Less commonly, mean corpuscular hemoglobin (MCH), mean corpuscular volume (MCV) and mean corpuscular hemoglobin concentration (MCHC) are also determined. Published hematology results for clinically healthy lizards are summarized in Tables 18.1–18.4. Few of these observed ranges are true reference ranges, on the basis of criteria

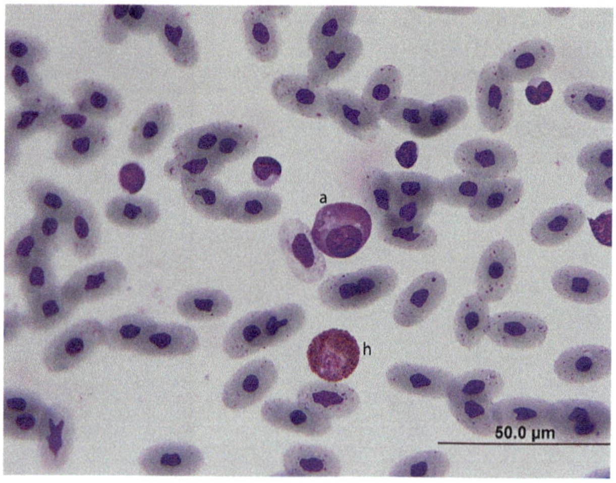

Figure 18.8 Azurophil (a) and heterophil (h), bearded dragon (*Pogona vitticeps*), modified Wright's stain. *Source:* Courtesy of Stephen J. Divers and Melinda Camus.

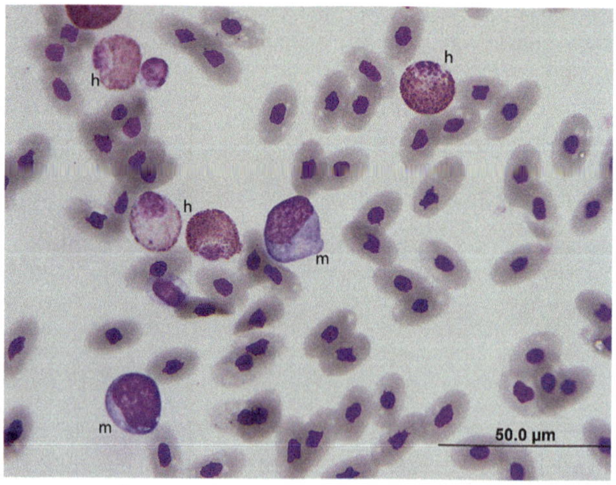

Figure 18.9 Heterophils (h) and monocytes (m), bearded dragon (*Pogona vitticeps*), modified Wright's stain. *Source:* Courtesy of Stephen J. Divers and Melinda Camus.

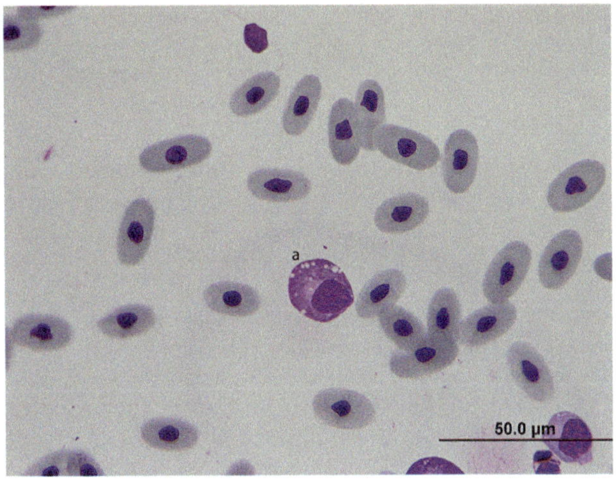

Figure 18.10 Azurophil (a), bearded dragon (*Pogona vitticeps*), modified Wright's stain. *Source:* Courtesy of Stephen J. Divers and Melinda Camus.

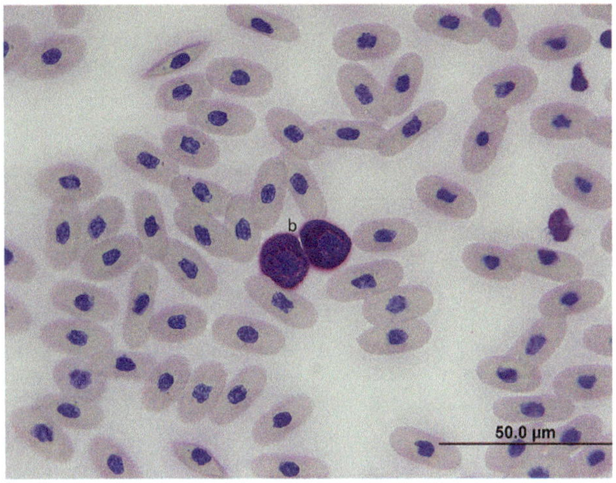

Figure 18.12 Basophils (b), bearded dragon (*Pogona vitticeps*), modified Wright's stain. *Source:* Courtesy of Stephen J. Divers and Melinda Camus.

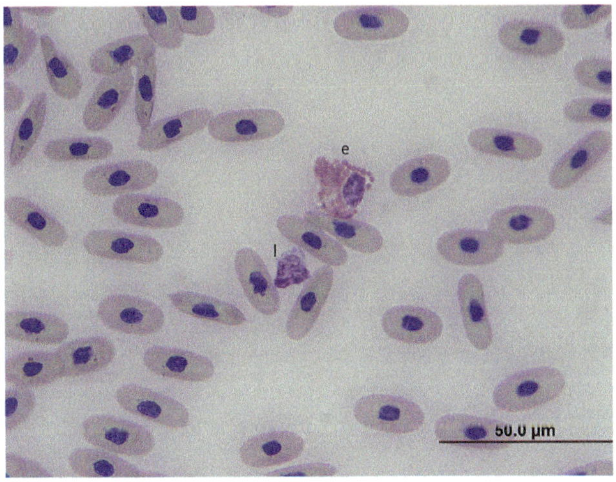

Figure 18.11 Eosinophil (e) and lymphocyte (l), bearded dragon (*Pogona vitticeps*), modified Wright's stain. *Source:* Courtesy of Stephen J. Divers and Melinda Camus.

for reference range determination as stipulated by the American Society for Veterinary Clinical Pathology [1]. The TRBC of lizards tends to be lower than those of mammals and birds, and there tends to be an inverse relationship between erythrocyte number and erythrocyte size. The PCV of lizards is commonly between 20% and 40%, although some publications have indicated values up to 60% in clinically healthy animals [51]. Reptiles are often more tolerant of hemoconcentration than mammals, and desert-adapted species will naturally permit hemoconcentration to levels that would be fatal to many mammals. Anemia is not uncommon in reptiles, and is often observed as a consequence of chronic disease. Lizards tend to have the smallest red blood cell (RBC) size and the highest RBC count when compared to other reptilian orders.

Leukon

The leukocyte cell types are divided into granulocytes (heterophils, eosinophils, and basophils) and agranulocytes (lymphocytes and monocytes). Azurophils were considered a distinct cell type, but are now widely thought to belong to the monocyte cell lineage. The lizard TWBC is performed manually because nucleated erythrocytes and thrombocytes confuse most automated hematology counters. The two methods commonly used are the direct method using Natt and Herrick and the indirect method using phloxine B [3]. Considerable variation exists in total and differential leukocyte counts between taxa, and within the same species, with respect to sex, age, and season [8, 43, 46, 52]. Few hematologic reference ranges exist that have identified and separated out these major factors (Table 18.1). Use caution when evaluating the complete blood count of an individual on the basis of a published range for which age, sex, reproductive status, and season are not stated. Collection of baseline hematology data from captive individuals on a regular basis to create an individual's own observed range is recommended. Leukocyte morphology for the granulocytes varies widely between lizard species, with some lizards exhibiting blue rather than pink granules in their eosinophils, as is true in the iguana and some members of the family Teiidae. In the case of the sick lizard, reference to a published range may be unavoidable; however, a lack of documented leukocyte responses to specific insults and diseases exists. Most leukocyte functions of lizards are extrapolated from knowledge of mammalian hematology and clinical observations rather than experimentation [3]. Nevertheless, leukocytosis (often heterophilia and azurophilia) is associated with inflammatory and infectious conditions, while lymphocytosis can occur in cases of lymphatic neoplasia [48, 53, 54].

Table 18.1 Hematologic values for the Iguanidae [33, 37–39].

		Green iguanas (*Iguana iguana*) Ħ			Allen Cays rock iguana (*Cyclura cychlura inornata*) [39]
Cell parameter (abbreviation)	**Units, SI (US)**	**Indoor [37]**	**Outdoor [38]**	**Indoors [33]**	**Free-ranging**
Anticoagulant		**Heparin**	**Heparin**	**EDTA**	**Lithium heparin**
Animals sampled		**10, 32 [33, 37]**	**48**	**32**	**18**
Data given as		**Min-max [37] min-max range; mean ± standard deviation [33]**	**Min-max range; mean ± standard deviation**	**Min-max range; mean ± standard deviation**	**Min-max range, mean ± standard deviation**
Packed cell volume (PCV)	%	25–38 [37] 40.1–42.4 [33] 41.3 ± 3.2	29–47	40.9–43.2; 42.1 ± 3.2	23–42; 29 ± 4
Packed cell volume (PCV)	%		29–38; 34 ± 4♂ 33–44; 38 ± 4♀		
Red blood cell (RBC) count	×10^6^/µl ×10^12^/l	1.0–1.9 [37]	1.0–1.8		
Hemoglobin (Hg)	g/l (g/dl)	60–100 [37] (6.0–10.0)	67–122 (6.7–12.2) 67–102; 86 ± 2 ♂ (6.7–10.2; 8.6 ± 0.2)♂ 91–122; 10.6 ± 1.2♀ (9.1–12.2; 10.6 ± 1.2)♀		
Mean corpuscular volume (MCV)	fl µm^3^	165–305 [37]	228–331		
Mean corpuscular hemoglobin (MCH)	Pg	48–78 [37]			
Mean corpuscular hemoglobin concentration (MCHC)	g/l (g/dl)	200–380 [37] (20–38)	227–280; 251 ± 23♂ (22.7–28.0; 25.1 ± 2.3)♂ 249–310; 279 ± 27♀ (24.9–31.0; 27.9 ± 2.7)♀		
Fibrinogen	µmol/l (mg/dl)		2.94–8.82 (100–300)		
Total white blood cell (WBC) count	×10^3^/µl ×10^9^/l	3–10 [37] 8.50–11.96; 10.20 ± 4.70 [33]	8.0–25.2	12.45–15.91; 14.2 ± 5.50	2.75–12.50; 6.91 ± 2.57
Lymphocytes	×10^3^/µl ×10^9^/l	0.5–5.5 [37] 4.91–7.98; 6.44 ± 4.00	5.0–17.2	6.99–10.05; 8.52 ± 4.39	0.34–2.54; 1.28 ± 0.68
Monocytes	×10^3^/µl ×10^9^/l	0.0–0.1 [37] 0.41–0.63; 0.61 ± 0.36	0.2–2.7	0.70–1.08; 1.06 ± 0.69	0.00–0.77; 0.24 ± 0.19
Azurophils	×10^3^/µl ×10^9^/l	0.0–1.7 [37] Included with monocytes	Included with monocytes	Included with monocytes	0.00–0.16; 0.04 ± 0.06
Heterophils	×10^3^/µl ×10^9^/l	0.35–5.2 [37] 2.34–3.77; 3.06 ± 1.60	0.6–6.4	3.67–5.10; 4.38 ± 2.03	1.19–7.12; 4.25 ± 1.84
Eosinophils	×10^3^/µl ×10^9^/l	0.0–0.3 [37] 0.02–0.11; 0.06 ± 0.09	0.0–0.4	0.03–0.13; 0.09 ± 0.18	0.00–0.56; 0.12 ± 0.17
Basophils	×10^3^/µl ×10^9^/l	0.0–0.5 [37] 0.01–0.09; 0.05 ± 0.08	0.1–1.2	0.05–0.13; 0.10 ± 0.13	0.00–1.12; 0.52 ± 0.30
Thrombocytes		22 slides [38] adequate 10 slides clumping		32 slides adequate 0 slides clumping	

Free-living ⅄ Captive Ħ All analyses performed manually. Diluents were ammonium oxalate [37], Phloxine B [33] and Natt & Herrick [39]. Stains were May-Grünwald/Giemsa [37], Wright Giemsa [38], modified Wright's stain [33], and Quick Dip [39].

Table 18.2 Hematological values for Corytophanidae, Crotaphytidae, and Helodermatidae [40–43].

Cell parameter (abbreviation)	Units, SI (US)	Green or plumed basilisk (*Basiliscus plumifrons*) [41] ⅄	Collared lizards ⅄ (*Crotaphytus collaris*) [43]	Mexican beaded lizard ⅄ (*Heloderma horridum*) [42]	Gila monster Ħ [40] (*Heloderma suspectum*)
Anticoagulant		**Heparin**	**Heparin**	**Heparin**	**EDTA**
Data format		**Min-max; mean ± SD**	**Min-max; mean ± SE**	**Min-max; mean ± SD**	**Min-max; mean ± SD**
Animals sampled		**20**	**126**	**16**	**16**
Packed cell volume (PCV)	%	20–52; 31 ± 8		28–41; 36 ± 4	22–50; 37 ± 8
Red blood cell (RBC) count	$\times 10^6/\mu l$ $\times 10^{12}/l$		0.68–1.54; 0.96 ± 0.03	0.70–1.09; 0.86 ± 0.10	0.22–0.67; 0.5 ± 0.13
Hemoglobin (Hg)	g/l (g/dl)		53–129; 88.6 ± 2.4 (5.3–12.9; 8.86 ± 0.24) 63–129; 95.9 ± 4.2♂ (6.3–12.9; 9.59 ± 0.42) 53–120; 85.1 ± 2.6♀ (5.3–12.0; 8.51 ± 0.26)	70–109; 89 ± 10 (7.0–10.9; 8.8 ± 1.0)	60–95; 74 ± 9 (6.0–9.5; 7.4 ± 0.9)
Mean corpuscular volume (MCV)	fl μm^3		218–493; 328 ± 9	360.8–511.4; 432.8 ± 45.2	415–1773; 812 ± 370
Mean corpuscular hemoglobin (MCH)	Pg		51–151; 94 ± 3	81.4–122.9; 108.7 ± 11.4	
Mean corpuscular hemoglobin concentration (MCHC)	g/l (g/dl)		180–370; 290 ± 510 (18–37; 29 ± 51) 231–336; 291 ± 6♂ (23.1–33.6; 29.1 ± 0.6) ♂ 185–368; 287 ± 7♀ (18.5–36.8; 28.7 ± 0.7) ♀	225.7–287.6; 246.5 ± 17.5 (22.6–28.8; 24.6 ± 1.8)	140–360; 209 ± 53 (14.0–36.0; 20.9 ± 5.3)
White blood cell (WBC) count	$\times 10^3/\mu l$ $\times 10^9/l$	3.9–35.5; 18.7 ± 8.4		2.86–7.30; 4.61 ± 1.65	3.30–6.40; 4.72 ± 0.84
Lymphocytes		0.8–7.4; 3.6 ± 2.2		0.3–1.2; 0.72 ± 0.27	0.58–3.39; 1.54 ± 0.80
Monocytes		0.1–4.2; 1.4 ± 1.2		0.03–0.15; 0.03 ± 0.04	0.00–0.19; 0.07 ± 0.08
Azurophils		Included with monocytes		0.17–2.29; 0.93 ± 0.67	0.00–1.14; 0.38 ± 0.27
Heterophils		3.1–24.1; 13.2 ± 5.9		1.38–4.44; 2.61 ± 0.99	1.35–3.31; 2.17 ± 0.61
Eosinophils		0.0–0.0; 0.0 ± 0.0		0.06–0.57; 0.29 ± 1.18	0.00–0.00; 0.00 ± 0.00
Basophils		0.19–0.39; 0.28 ± 0.0		0.03–0.16; 0.04 ± 0.05	0.21–1.05; 0.57 ± 0.23

Wright Giemsa stain [40–42], Phloxine B diluent [41, 42], Natt and Herrick [40], analyses performed manually [40, 42], blood collected from orbital sinus. Significant differences existed depending on sex and season [43]. Free-living ⅄, Captive Ħ.

Hemostasis and Blood Types

It is often thought that reptile blood clots slower than mammals [4, 55]. The slow clotting is believed to be due to the low thromboplastin activity of reptile blood and the high circulating antithrombin activity to compensate for sluggish blood flow [55]. However, studies investigating clotting times and pathways in reptiles have been limited. A preliminary investigation in green iguanas has demonstrated that clotting times may not be too dissimilar to mammalian clotting times [56]. Plasma fibrinogen is present in all species studied and forms a fibrin clot in the presence of thrombin [4]. Blood

Table 18.3 Hematologic values for the Agamidae and Teiidae [34, 44–47].

Cell parameter (abbreviation)	Units, SI (US)	Chinese water dragon Ħ (*Physignathus cocincinus*) [34]	Spiny-tailed lizard ⟩ (*Uromastyx* spp.) [44]	Blanford's rock agama Ħ (*Psammophilus blanfordanus*) [45]	Argentine black & white tegu Ħ (*Tupinambis merianae*) [46, 47]	Red tegu Ħ (*Tupinambis rufescens*) [46]
Data format		Multiple [34]	Min-max; mean ± SE	Min-max	Mean ± SD	Mean ± SD
Animals sampled		12	76	100	100	100
Packed cell volume (PCV)	%	32–40; 35	14.9–44.5; 29.7 ± 0.7		26 ± 2	24 ± 4
Red blood cell (RBC) count	$\times 10^6/\mu l$ $\times 10^{12}/l$		0.33–4.1; 0.78 ± 0.05	0.53–1.02	0.96 ± 0.13	0.93 ± 0.13
Hemoglobin (Hg)	g/l (g/dl)		33–174; 99.3 ± 2.6 (3.3–17.4; 9.93 ± 0.26)	45–52 (4.5–5.2)	118 ± 24 (11.8 ± 2.4)	100 ± 25 (10.0 ± 2.5)
Mean corpuscular volume (MCV)	fl μm^3		119.5–614; 415.5 ± 9.3		276 ± 24	230 ± 32
Mean corpuscular hemoglobin (MCH)	pg		1.2–203.5; 133.6 ± 3.5		117 ± 13	104 ± 13
Mean corpuscular hemoglobin concentration (MCHC)	g/l (g/dl)		222–413; 326 ± 4 (22.2–41.3; 32.6 ± 0.4)		420 ± 60 (42 ± 6)	450 ± 40 (45 ± 4)
Fibrinogen	μmol/l (g/l)		0.0–17.6; 5.29 ± 0.29 (0.0–6.0; 1.8 ± 0.1)			
Total white blood cell (WBC) count	$\times 10^3/\mu l$ $\times 10^9/l$	11.7–18.2; 13.5 ± 5.1	1.0–8.1; 3.10 ± 0.17	12.6–21.1	16.6 ± 2.5	18.2 ± 2.4
Lymphocytes		5.6–9.5; 7.2 ± 3.0	0.27–4.05; 0.99 ± 0.08	3.65–9.92	7.56 ± 0.50	8.22 ± 0.78
Monocytes		0.4–1.9; 1.1	0.0–0.5; 0.04 ± 0.01	0.13–2.53	0.86 ± 0.07	1.29 ± 0.23
Azurophils		0.0–0.6; 0.0	Included with monocytes	Included with monocytes	1.75 ± 0.17	1.81 ± 0.13
Heterophils		3.9–6.9; 5.1 ± 2.4	0.59–5.36; 2.00 ± 0.12	2.77–8.02	2.02 ± 0.22	2.09 ± 0.24
Eosinophils		0.1–0.3; 0.2 ± 02	0.00–0.20; 0.04 ± 0.01	1.01–3.08	4.03 ± 0.04	4.42 ± 0.06
Basophils		0.2–0.8; 0.5 ± 0.5	0.00–0.33; 0.03 ± 0.01	0.13–1.90	0.34 ± 0.01	0.36 ± 0.01
Thrombocytes			2.9–22.9; 9.58 ± 0.94		7.6 ± 4.7	9.3 ± 2.3

All analyses performed manually, anticoagulants were heparin and diluent was Natt-Herrick's diluent excepting [34, 44]. Stains were Wright [34], Wright Giemsa [44], Giemsa [45], and May-Grünwald and Giemsa [46, 47]. EDTA anticoagulant, Phloxine B diluent, 95% confidence intervals or min-max ranges, medians or means, and standard deviations variably reported [34].

Used EDTA anticoagulant and either phloxine B or Natt and Herrick's diluent.

No significant differences between genders, age, or season [47].

Table 18.4 Hematological values for the Scincidae, Varanidae, Lacertidae, and Chamaeleonidae [48–51].

Cell parameter (abbreviation)	Units, SI (US)	Prehensile-tailed skink (*Corucia zebrata*)[a] [51] Ħ	Crocodile monitor (*Varanus salvadorii*)[a] [49]	El Hierro giant lizard (*Gallotia simonyi*)[b] [50]	Common chameleon ♂♀ (*Chamaeleo chamaeleon*)[c] [48]
Animal number		20	5	9	8
Packed cell volume (PCV)	%	24–60; 35 ± 9	28–49; 38 ± 3	31 ± 4	10–33; 24 ± 4
Red blood cell (RBC) count	$\times 10^6/\mu l$ ($\times 10^{12}/l$)	0.84–1.43; 1.45 ± 0.29		1.08 ± 0.26	0.4–1.7; 0.8 ± 0.4
Hemoglobin (Hg)	g/l (g/dl)	74–116; 95.8 ± 13.3 (7.4–11.6; 9.6 ± 1.3)		73.2 ± 12.1 (7.3 ± 1.2)	<50–104 (<5.0–10.4)
Mean corpuscular volume (MCV)	fl μm^3	152–600; 263 ± 116		290 ± 41	
Mean corpuscular hemoglobin (MCH)	pg	42–111; 69 ± 17		70.4 ± 8.8	
Mean corpuscular hemoglobin concentration (MCHC)	g/l (g/dl)	170–560; 280 ± 80 (17–56; 28 ± 8)		239 ± 20 (23.9 ± 2.0)	
Total white blood cell (WBC) count	$\times 10^3/\mu l$ ($\times 10^9/l^1$)	3.93–22.4; 12.36 ± 4.39	8.79–17.0; 12.49 ± 3.02	6.00 ± 2.29	12.5–56.2; 31.2 ± 15.0
Lymphocytes		0.3–4.7; 2.67 ± 1.73	1.37–2.57; 1.87 ± 0.45	0.82 ± 0.47	
Monocytes		0.0–1.0; 0.07 ± 0.22	0.14–0. 36; 0.24 ± 0.09	0.10 ± 0.08	
Azurophils		0.4–4.8; 2.76 ± 1.52	3.43–5.82; 4.45 ± 0.89	1.27 ± 0.74	
Heterophils		1.02–6.40; 4.39 ± 1.60	3.53–9.32; 5.94 ± 2.11	2.34 ± 1.02	
Eosinophils		0.0–3.0; 0.56 ± 0.86	0.00–0.00; 0.00 ± 0.00	0.22 ± 0.24	
Basophils		0.1–4.3; 1.92 ± 1.33	0.12–0.41; 0.22 ± 0.11	1.23 ± 1.25	
Thrombocytes				19.4 ± 4.9	

Data presented as min-max; mean ± SD, analyses performed manually with heparin as anticoagulant.
Natt and Herrick's diluent, and May-Grünwald stain.
[a] Phloxine B and Wright Giemsa stain [49, 51].
[b] Natt and Herrick's diluent and Wright's stain [50].
[c] *Gallotia intermedia* (*n* = 4) and *Gallotia bravoana* (*n* = 6) also reported in the paper but excluded from table due to low numbers of animals [48].

transfusions are uncommon in reptile practice as most severe anemias are chronic in nature. Blood typing is seldom performed; however, red cell isoantigens have been described in lizards. The physiologic determinants of blood types exist in lizards [57]. Transfusions should be intraspecific, following a simple slide agglutination test.

Biochemical Panel

Published biochemical data are summarized for Iguanidae (Table 18.5), Agamidae, and Teiidae (Table 18.6), Scincidae, Chamaeleonidae and Lacertidae (Table 18.7), and Varanidae and Helodermatidae (Table 18.8) [23, 34, 37–42, 44, 48–51, 58–66]. Interpret references values with caution as within the same species, sex, season, nutrition, and management can affect biochemical values. Given these variations, biochemical profiles collected from a healthy individual may prove the most useful reference for that individual.

Liver Analytes

A standard group of biochemical tests useful for the diagnosis of liver disease has not been established [11]. In juvenile green iguanas, moderate activities of lactate dehydrogenase (LDH) and AST were found in many tissues, making diagnostic differentiation impossible [67]. ALT and ALKP activities were also low but found in a variety of tissues. ALT, ALKP, AST, and LDH seem of limited use in identifying hepatocellular damage. The diagnostic value of gamma glutamyl transferase (GGT) and GLDH are largely unknown. Recent research at the university of Georgia evaluated liver enzyme changes in the green iguana following a carbon tetrachloride toxic insult [56]. Results indicated that AST, LDH and SDH increased dramatically, ALT increased less, and GGT and ALKP showed no change.

Table 18.5 Biochemical data from Iguanidae [23, 37–39, 58–64].

Analyte (abbreviation)	Units, SI (US)	Green iguana[a,b,c,d,e,f,g] [23, 37, 38, 59–61, 64] *(Iguana iguana)*	Desert iguana Ħ *(Dipsosaurus dorsalis)*[h] [62]	Allen Cays rock iguana ⅁ *(Cyclura cychlura inornata)*[i] [39]	Ricord's iguana ⅁ *(Cyclura ricordii)*[i] [63]	Green or plumed basilisk ⅁ *(Basiliscus plumifrons)*[e] [58]
Animals sampled		10^b [37] 7^f [61] 51 [38] 21^d [59] 23^a [23] 11^g [64] 47^g [60]	34	37	23	19
Data format		Min-max; mean ± SD^{c,f} [38, 61] 95% CI; mean ± SD^{a,g} [23, 64] Min-max; mean or median ± SD^e [60] min-max^b [37]	Min-max; mean	Min-max; Mean ± SD	Min-max; Median ± SD	Min-max; Mean ± SD
Albumin	g/l (g/dl)	21–28 (2.1–2.8)₪⌂^{b,f} [37, 61] 13–30 (1.3–3.0) Ӽ^c [38] 13–30;20 ± 5 (1.3–3.0; 2.0 ± 0.5)♂^{c} Ӽ^c [38] 15–30; 24 ± 4) (1.5–3.0; 2.4 ± 0.4)♀Ӽ^c [38] 0.2–0.5 ∞♀Ӽ^c [38] 18–23; 21.2 ± 1.6 (1.8–2.3; 2.12 ± 0.16)ÓӼ^d [59] 18–33; 30.8 ± 7.7 (1.8–3.3; 3.08 ± 0.77)₪Ӽ^d [59] 9.1–30.1;20.1 ± 4.6(0.91–3.01; 2.02 ± 0.46)⌂₥^{e} [60] 9.6–27.6 (0.96–2.76) ♂⌂₥^{e} [60] 22–26; 25 ± 2 (2.2–2.6) ⌂♂^{a,g} [23, 64] 13.5–30.3 (1.35–3.03)♀⌂₥^{e} [60]	16–30; 23 (1.6–3.0; 2.3)	14–33; 20 ± 4 (1.4–3.3; 2.0 ± 0.4)	16–27; 22 ± 3 (1.6–2.7; 2.2 ± 0.3)	13–26; 18 ± 0.3 (1.3–2.6; 1.8 ± 0.3)
Albumin:globulin		0.3–1.0 Ӽ^c [38]males, non-reproductive females, and juveniles	1.0–2.3; 1.7			
Anion gap	mmol/l mEq/l	12.1–41.0 Ӽ^c [38]				
Alkaline phosphatase (ALP)	IU/l U/l	50–290 ₪⌂^{b,f} [37, 61] 14–90 Ӽ^c [38]	4–30; 14			
Aspartate (AST, SGOT) aminotransferase	IU/l IU/l	5–52 ₪⌂^{b,f} [37, 61] 7–102 Ӽ^c [38] 35.3–122.7; 57.0 ± 30.6 ÓӼ^d [59] 11.2–53.2; 27.0 ± 11.3 ₪Ӽ^d [59] 11–41; 20⌂₥^{e} [60] 5–9⌂♂^{g}[23, 64] 11–41; 18♂⌂₥^{e} [60] 16–40; 21♀⌂₥^{e} [60]	34–400; 179	11–85; 29 ± 16 12–50; 23 ± 10 ♂ 11–85; 37 ± 20 ♀	16–143; 42 ± 29	19–115; 48 ± 26

Alanine transferase (ALT)	IU/l IU/l	5–68 ₪⌂^{b,f} [37, 61] 4–96 X^{c} [38]				
Bile acids Unknown feeding schedule	μmol/l (μg/dl)	0.47–18.16; 3.97 (20–710; 160) ⌂₥^{e} [60]		0.9–38.3; 10.6 ± 20.2 (37–1565; 433 ± 825)	0–27; 7.0 ± 7.0 (0–1103; 286 ± 286)	
Preprandial		2.6–30.3; 7.5 ± 7.8 (1.06–12.38; 3.06 ± 3.19) ⌂♂^{a,g} [23, 64]				
Postprandial 3 h		5.2–71.5; 33.3 ± 22.0 (2.12–29.21; 13.60 ± 8.99) ⌂♂^{a,g} [23, 64]				
Postprandial 7.5 h		15.2–44.1; 32.5 ± 8.4 (6.21–18.01; 13.28 ± 3.43) ⌂♂^{a,g} [23, 64]				
Blood urea nitrogen (BUN)	mmol/l (mg/dl)		0.36–1.78; 0.86 (1.0–5.0; 2.4)		0.0–0.5; 0.18 ± 0.12 (0.0–1.4; 0.5 ± 0.35)	
Total calcium	mmol/l (mg/dl)	2.2–3.5(3.8–14.0) ₪⌂^{b,f} [37, 61] 2.15–3.52; 2.83 ± 0.30 (8.6–14.1;11.3 ± 1.2) X ♂^{c} [38] 2.70–3.50; 3.13 ± 0.25 (10.8–14.0; 12.5 ± 1.0)XΦ♀^{c} [38] 5.53–11.88; 8.13 ± 3.3 (22.5–47.5; 32.5 ± 13.2) ∞♀^{c} [38] 2.73–3.60; 3.20 ± 0.23 (10.9–14.4; 12.8 ± 0.93) X^{d} [59] 2.30–6.42; 3.40 ± 1.07 (9.20–25.68; 13.61 ± 4.27) ⌂₥^{e} [60] 2.44–3.58; 3.01 ± 0.28 (9.75–14.35; 12.05 ± 1.15)♂⌂₥^{e} [60] 2.18–3.84; 3.01 ± 0.42 (7.03–13.71; 12.04 ± 1.16) Φ♀⌂₥^{e} [60] 2.47–6.41; 3.11 (9.90–25.68; 12.45)∞♀⌂₥^{e} [60] 2.47–6.41; 3.11 (9.90–25.68; 12.45)∞♀⌂₥^{e} [60]	1.9–7.4; 2.65 (7.6–29.6; 10.6)	1.85–11.75; 3.25 ± 2.30) (7.40–47.0; 13.03 ± 9.20) 2.02–2.90; 2.51 ± 0.24) ♂ (8.10–11.60; 10.06 ± 0.95) ♂ (1.85–11.75; 4.18 ± 3.26) 11–85; 37 ± 20 ♀ (7.4–47.0; 16.7 ± 13.0) 11–85; 37 ± 20 ♀	2.2–5.6; 3.1 ± 0.5 (8.80–22.40; 12.40 ± 2.00)	2.08–3.10; 2.65 ± 0.33 (8.3–12.4; 10.6 ± 1.3)

(*Continued*)

Table 18.5 (Continued)

Analyte (abbreviation)	Units, SI (US)	Green iguana[a,b,c,d,e,f,g] [23, 37, 38, 59–61, 64] (*Iguana iguana*)	Desert iguana Ħ (*Dipsosaurus dorsalis*)[h] [62]	Allen Cays rock iguana ⦣ (*Cyclura cychlura inornata*)[i] [39]	Ricord's iguana ⦣ (*Cyclura ricordii*)[i] [63]	Green or plumed basilisk ⦣ (*Basiliscus plumifrons*)[e] [58]
Ionized calcium	mmol/l (mg/dl)	1.22–1.62; 1.47 ± 0.11 (4.88–6.48; 5.88 ± 0.44) Χ[d] [59] 1.34–1.42; 1.38 ± 0.10 (5.36–5.68; 5.52 ± 0.40) ⌂♂[a,g] [23, 64]				
Carbon dioxide (CO_2)	mmol/l mEq/l	15.1–24.7 Χ[c] [38]	2.0–17.0; 8.6			
Cholesterol	mmol/l (mg/dl)	2.7–8.6 (104–332) ₪⌂[b,f] [37, 61] 2.12–5.54; 4.17 ± 0.91 (82–214; 161 ± 35) Χ ♂[c] [38] 5.28–8.99; 6.60 ± 1.06 (204–347; 255 ± 41)ΧΦ♀[c] [38] 6.55–11.27; 8.78 ± 2.36 (253–435; 339 ± 91)Χ∞♀[c] [38] 3.78–7.40 (142–286) ⌂♂[a,g] [23, 64]	2.59–10.33; 6.29 (100–399; 243)	0.98–4.90; 2.51 ± 0.87 (38–189; 97 ± 34)	0.4–5.2; 1.5 ± 1.0 (15–201; 58 ± 39)	
Chloride	mmol/l mEq/l	113–129 Χ[c] [38]	112–155; 120	108–141; 118 ± 7	76–121; 103 ± 11	
Creatinine	mmol/l mg/dl		17.7–159.1; 44.2 (0.2–1.8; 0.5)			
Creatinine phosphokinase (CPK)	IU/l IU/l	74–4912; 495⌂ₘ[e] [60] 30–1045⌂♂[a,g] [23, 64]	700–14 240; 4507	256–13 053; 2342 ± 2573	145–12 363; 3275 ± 3274	2497–8893; 6323 ± 2074
Fibrinogen	μmol/l (mg/dl)	2.94–8.82 (100–300)Χ[c] [38]				
Globulin	g/l (g/dl)	25–43(2.5–4.3)₪⌂[b,f] [37, 61] 25–52 (2.5–5.2)Χ[c] [38] 49–67; 55 ± 1 (4.9–6.7; 5.5 ± 1.0)Χ ∞♀[c] [38] 29.9–60.8;42.1 ± 7.4(2.99–6.08;4.21 ± 0.74)⌂ₘ[e] [60] 35–39; 37 ± 6 (3.5–3.9; 3.7 ± 0.6) ⌂♂[a,g] [23, 64]	8–24; 15 (0.8–2.4; 1.5)	17.0–47.0; 28.6 ± 5.9 (1.7–4.7; 2.9 ± 0.6)	35–64; 51 ± 9 (3.5–6.4; 5.1 ± 0.9)	16–47; 26 ± 7 (1.6–4.7; 2.6 ± 0.7)
Gamma glutamyl transferase (GGT)	IU/l IU/l	0–3₪⌂[b,f] [37, 61]				

Glucose (adults)	mmol/l (mg/dl)	9.4–16.0₪⌂^{b,f} [37, 61] (169–288) ₪⌂^{b,f} [37, 61] 3.9–145.3 (70–258)₪⚔^{c} [38] 7.3–19.6;15.2 ± 3.9 (131–335; 273 ± 71)Ó⚔^{c} [38] 6.4–13.5;9.5 ± 2.7(115–244; 171 ± 49) ₪⚔^{d} [59] 11.5–18.6;15.0 ± 3.7(207– 335;271 ± 66)Ó⚔^{d} [59] 4.8–14.8; 9.2 ± 2.1 (87–270; 165 ± 38)⌂₥^{e} [60]	14.2–31.9; 19.7 (255–575; 355)	7.49–15.00; 10.5 ± 2.18 (135–270; 189 ± 39)	9.4–18.0; 12.2 ± 2.8 (169–324; 220 ± 50)	2.8–15.4; 10.7 ± 2.7 (108–279; 193 ± 48)
Lactate dehydrogenase (LDH)	IU/l IU/l	49–226⌂♂^{a,g} [23, 64]	145–2915; 788			
Phosphorus	mmol/l (mg/dl)	1.5–3.0₪⌂^{b,f} [37, 61] (4.6–9.3) ₪⌂^{b,f} [37, 61] 0.9–3.0 (2.8–9.3)⚔^{c} [38] 2.7–5.7; 3.9 ± 1.6 (8.4–17.5; 12.0 ± 5.0)♀⚔ ∞^{c} [38] 0.9–2.5; 1.6 ± 0.5 (2.8–7.8; 4.8 ± 1.4) ₪⚔^{d} [59] 2.4–2.9; 2.5 ± 0.5 (7.3–9.0; 7.6 ± 1.4)Ó⚔^{d} [59] 0.88–2.27; 1.51 ± 0.34 (2.73–7.03; 4.69 ± 1.08)⌂₥^{e} [60] 1.21–1.44; 1.32 ± 0.28 (3.8–4.5; 4.1 ± 0.9) ⌂♂^{a,g} [23, 64]	0.9–3.2; 1.8 (2.8–10.0; 5.5)	0.78–4.20; 1.72 ± 0.74 (2.40–13.00; 5.31 ± 2.30)	1.0–2.6; 1.8 ± 0.4 (3.10–8.05; 5.57 ± 1.24)	1.32–3.00; 1.81 ± 0.52 (4.1–9.3; 5.6 ± 1.6)
Potassium	mmol/l mEq/l	2.0–6.1 ⚔^{c} [38] 3.74–7.34; 5.42 ± 0.78⌂₥^{e} [60] 2.5–2.8; 2.6 ± 0.4⌂♂^{a,g} [23, 64]	0.4–7.0; 2.6	1.80–5.90; 3.66 ± 1.06	0.8–6.0; 3.6 ± 1.3	2.3–7.9; 5.4 ± 1.7
Sodium	mmol/l mEq/l	152–172 ⚔^{c} [38] 144–175; 157 ± 7⌂₥^{e} [60] 147–149; 148 ± 3⌂♂^{a,g} [23, 64]	137–245; 164		124–193; 163 ± 15	142–167; 154 ± 7
Total thyroxine (T_4)	nmol/l (ng/ml)	2.98–4.65 (0.17–0.27) ₪⌂^{f} [61]				

(*Continued*)

Table 18.5 (Continued)

Analyte (abbreviation)	Units, SI (US)	Green iguana[a,b,c,d,e,f,g] [23, 37, 38, 59–61, 64] (*Iguana iguana*)	Desert iguana Ħ (*Dipsosaurus dorsalis*)[h] [62]	Allen Cays rock iguana ⅓ (*Cyclura cychlura inornata*)[i] [39]	Ricord's iguana ⅓ (*Cyclura ricordii*)[i] [63]	Green or plumed basilisk ⅓ (*Basiliscus plumifrons*)[e] [58]
Triglycerides	mmol/l (mg/dl)	0.6–7.8₪⌂[b,f] [37, 61] (53–690) ₪⌂[b,f] [37, 61]			0.16–3.4; 0.77 ± 0.78 (14–300; 68 ± 69)	
Total bilirubin	µmol/l (mg/dl)	1.7–53.0 (0.1–3.1) ⴳ[c] [38]	1.71–8.55; 3.42 (0.1–0.5; 0.2)			
Total protein	g/l (g/dl)	50–78(5.0–7.8) ₪⌂[b,f] [37, 61] 42–76) (4.2–7.6) ⴳ[c] [38] 70–82; 75 ± 6(7.0–8.2; 7.5 ± 0.6) ⴳ ∞♀[c] [38] 42–52; 48 ± 4 (4.2–5.2; 4.8 ± 0.4) Óⴳ[d] [59] 52–76; 49 ± 17 (5.2–7.6; 4.9 ± 1.7) ₪ⴳ[d] [59] 46.6–87.9;62.2 ± 9.4(4.66–8.79;6.22 ± 0.94)⌂₥[e] [60] 51–65 (5.1–6.5) ⌂♂[a,g] [23, 64]	24–54; 38 (2.4–5.4; 3.8)	31–80; 48 ± 9) (3.1–8.0; 4.8 ± 0.9)	52–91; 72 ± 10 (5.2–9.1; 7.2 ± 1.0)	31–66; 44 ± 16 (3.1–6.6; 4.4 ± 1.6)
Uric acid	µmol/l (mg/dl)	70–140 (1.2–2.4) ₪⌂[b,f] [37, 61] 42–399(0.7–6.7) ⴳ ∞♀[c] [38] 30–320; 150 ± 170(0.6–5.48; 2.54 ± 1.14)⌂₥[e] [60] 181–263; 222 ± 100 (3.0–4.4; 3.7 ± 1.7)⌂♂[a,g] [23, 64]	142.8–791.1; 333.1 (2.4–13.3; 5.6)	0.0–475.8; 105.3 ± 119.0 (0.00–8.00; 1.77 ± 2.00)	46.8–514.6; 172 ± 129 (0.79–8.65; 2.89 ± 2.17)	35.7–172.5; 101.1 ± 47.6 (0.6–2.9; 1.7 ± 0.8)

[a] Analyses performed using whole blood with a Heska I-Stat EG7+ and heparinized plasma with an Hitachi 912 chemistry analyzer [23];
[b] Analyses performed using plasma and a Technicon RA1000 chemistry analyzer [37];
[c] Analyses performed using plasma and a Ciba Corning 550 Express chemistry analyzer [38];
[d] Analyses performed using plasma and Heska I-Stat EG7+ or Ciba Corning 550 Express chemistry analyzer [59];
[e] Analyses performed using heparinized whole blood and an Abaxis VetScan chemistry analyzer; 382 year olds [58, 60];
[f] Analyses performed using plasma and fluorescence polarization immunoassay and an Abbot TDX analyzer [61];
[g] Analyses performed using plasma and an Hitachi 912 chemistry analyzer [64];
[h] Analyses performed using serum and a Technicon SMAC chemistry analyzer, $n = 34$; min-max ranges, means and standard deviations reported [62];
[i] Analyses performed using plasma and a Hitachi 747-200 chemistry analyzer [39, 63].

Table 18.6 Biochemical values for the Agamidae and Teiidae [34, 44, 58, 65].

Analyte (abbreviation)	Units, SI (US)	Chinese water dragon (*Physignathus cocincinus*)[a] [34] ⌂ Ħ	Spiny-tailed lizards (*Uromastyx* spp.)[b] [44] ⺀	Bearded dragons (*Pogona vitticeps*)[a] [58] Ħ⌂♂	Bearded dragons (*Pogona vitticeps*)[c] [65] Ħ ⌂
Animal number		**12–26**	**76**	**11**	**100**
Data format		**Min-max; median ± SD**	**Min-max; mean ± SE**	**Min-max; median ± SD**	**25th–75th Quartiles**
Albumin	g/l (g/dl)	16–30; 22 ± 3; 21–23 (1.6–3.0; 2.2 ± 0.3; 2.1–2.3)	12–31; 20 ± 10 (1.2–3.1; 2.0 ± 0.1)	21–41; 31 ± 6 (2.1–4.1; 3.1 ± 0.6)	18–30 (1.8–3.0)
Alkaline phosphatase (ALP)	IU/l U/l		5.9–139.3; 30.8 ± 3.2		200–734
Alanine transferase (ALT)	IU/l U/l				1–8
Aspartate (AST, SGOT) aminotransferase	IU/l U/l	8–52; 16.5		21–85; 40 ± 20 (21–85; 40 ± 20)	4–15♂ 6–21♀
Blood urea nitrogen (BUN)	mmol/l (mg/dl)	0.71–1.07; 0.71 ± 0.11 (2.0–3.0; 2.0 ± 0.3)	0.0–1.07; 0.20 ± 0.03 (0.0–3.0; 0.56 ± 0.08)		
Total calcium	mmol/l (mg/dl)	2.4–4.0 (3.1 ± 0.53; 2.9–3.33) 9.4–16.0 (12.4 ± 2.1; 11.6–13.3)	1.80–3.30; 2.47 ± 0.04 (7.2–13.2 (9.88 ± 0.18))	2.55–3.40; 2.91 ± 0.25 (10.2–13.6; 11.65 ± 1.01)	2.98–3.23 (11.9–12.9) ♂ 3.08–4.13 (12.3–16.5) ♀
Chloride	mmol/l mEq/l				102–116
Cholesterol	mmol/l (mg/dl)		1.66–7.64; 4.17 ± 0.18 (64–295; 161 ± 7)		4.01–6.11 (155–236) ♂ 5.34–7.72 (206–298) ♀❄ 5.88–9.66 (227–373) ♀✿
Creatinine	mmol/l (mg/dl)		7.63–228.75; 30.5 ± 3.05 (0.1–3.0; 0.40 ± 0.04)		
Creatinine phosphokinase (CPK)	IU/l U/l	19 6630; 1747 ± 214	141–10 016; 1778 ± 235	236–4404; 1622 ± 1219	4.38–67.37 (262–4034)
Gamma glutamyl transferase (GGT)	IU/l U/l		0.0–5.0 (0.79 ± 0.12)		
Glucose	mmol/l (mg/dl)	6.22–23.8; 8.71 ± 3.44 (112–428; 157 ± 62)	3.76–19.74; 11.12 ± 0.33 (67.7–355.6; 200.4 ± 6.0)	8.54–13.99; 11.09 ± 1.65 (154–252; 200 ± 30)	10.88–19.76 (196–356)
Glutamic oxaloacetic transaminase (GOT)	IU/l U/l		28.5–172.0; 73.1 ± 4.6		
Glutamic pyruvic transaminase (GPT)	IU/l U/l		2.4–34.8; 11.0 ± 0.78		
Globulin	g/l (g/dl)	34–72; 47 ± 9; 45–53 (3.4–7.2; 4.7 ± 0.9; 4.5–5.3)		20–32; 27 ± 3 (2.0–3.2; 2.7 ± 0.3)	22–34 (2.2–3.4) ♂ 28–40 (2.8–4.0) ♀
Lactate dehydrogenase (LDH)	IU/l U/l		22.0–899.0; 209.6 ± 24.9		56–516
Magnesium	mmol/l (mg/dl)		0.86–4.19; 1.44 ± 0.04 (2.1–10.2; 3.5 ± 0.1)		
Phosphorus	mmol/l (mg/dl)	1.10–2.65; 1.84 ± 0.42; 1.61–2.10 (3.4–8.2; 5.7 ± 1.3; 5.0–6.5)		0.97–2.13; 1.58 ± 0.31 (3.0–6.6; 4.9 ± 0.9)	1.16–1.81 (3.6–5.6)

(Continued)

Analyte (abbreviation)	Units, SI (US)	Chinese water dragon (*Physignathus cocincinus*)[a] [34] ⌂ Ħ	Spiny-tailed lizards (*Uromastyx* spp.)[b] [44] 🦎	Bearded dragons (*Pogona vitticeps*)[a] [58] Ħ⌂♂	Bearded dragons (*Pogona vitticeps*)[c] [65] Ħ⌂
Animal number		12–26	76	11	100
Data format		Min-max; median ± SD	Min-max; mean ± SE	Min-max; median ± SD	25th–75th Quartiles
Plasma osmolality (measured)	mOsm/kg			295.4 ± 9.35	
Potassium	mmol/l mEq/l	1.7–5.7; 4.2 ± 0.8; 3.8–4.5 (1.7–5.7; 4.2 ± 0.8; 3.8–4.5)		4.4–5.1; 4.8 ± 0.3	3.4–4.6
Sodium	mmol/l mEq/l	138–163; 150 ± 7; 147–153 (138–163; 150 ± 7; 147–153)		150–165; 156 ± 5	148–158
Triglycerides	mmol/l (mg/dl)				0.92–3.67 (81–325)
Total protein	g/l (g/dl)		26–74; 40 ± 10 (2.6–7.4; 4.0 ± 0.1)	46–73; 57 ± 7 (4.6–7.3; 5.7 ± 0.7)	45–64 (4.5–6.4) ☼ 41–62 (4.1–6.2) ❄♂ 48–69 (4.8–6.9) ❄♀
Uric acid	µmol/l (mg/dl)	83–208; 137 ± 42; 113–161 (1.4–3.5; 2.3 ± 0.7; 1.9–2.7)	18–434; 173 ± 12 (0.3–7.3; 2.9 ± 0.2)c	130–460; 290 ± 100 (2.2–7.7; 4.9 ± 1.7)	274–714 (4.6–12.0) 190–399 (3.2–5.7) ☼

[a] Analyses performed using plasma and an Abaxis VetScan [34, 58].
[b] Analyses performed using serum and UDICHEM-RASTA chemistry analyzer [44].
[c] Analyses performed using plasma and a Fuji Dri-chem 7000v analyzer [65].

Table 18.7 Biochemical values for Scincidae, Chamaeleonidae, and Lacertidae [48, 50, 51].

Analyte (abbreviation)	Units, SI (US)	Prehensile-tailed skink (*Corucia zebrata*)[a] [51] Ħ	Common chameleon (*Chamaeleo* 🦎♀ *chamaeleon*)[b] [48]	El Hierro giant lizard (*Gallotia simonyi*)[c] [50] Ħ
Animal number		20	8	15
Data format		Min-max; mean ± SD	Min-max; mean ± SD	Mean ± SD
Albumin	g/l (g/dl)			24.9 ± 4.1 (2.49 ± 0.41)
Alkaline phosphatase (ALP)	IU/l U/l			39.7 ± 22.9
Alanine transferase (ALT)	IU/l U/l			18.0 ± 9.3
Aspartate (AST, SGOT) aminotransferase	IU/l U/l	<4–76; 19 ± 22	122–271; 218 ± 52	39.7 ± 26.4
Bile acids unknown feeding schedule	µmol/l (µg/dl)			42.0 ± 48.7 (17.2 ± 19.89)
Blood urea nitrogen (BUN)	mmol/l (mg/dl)			0.97 ± 0.41 2.72 ± 1.15

(*Continued*)

Table 18.7 (Continued)

Analyte (abbreviation)	Units, SI (US)	Prehensile-tailed skink (*Corucia zebrata*)[a] [51] Ħ	Common chameleon (*Chamaeleo* ♂♀ *chamaeleon*)[b] [48]	El Hierro giant lizard (*Gallotia simonyi*)[c] [50] Ħ
Animal number		**20**	**8**	**15**
Data format		**Min-max; mean ± SD**	**Min-max; mean ± SD**	**Mean ± SD**
Total calcium	mmol/l (mg/dl)	2.75–5.30; 3.30 ± 0.54 (11.0–21.2; 13.2 ± 2.17)		2.80 ± 0.23 (11.2 ± 0.92)
Chloride	mmol/l (meq/l)	123–129; 124 ± 6		150.4 ± 13.6
Cholesterol	mmol/l (mg/dl)	0.28–6.53; 3.73 ± 1.55 (11–252; 144 ± 60)		6.29 ± 1.65 (243 ± 64)
Creatinine phosphokinase (CPK)	IU/l U/l	27–940; 210 ± 260	331-1000+; 482 ± 106	4048 ± 3904
Fibrinogen	(mg/dl)	0.0–14.7; 2.21 ± 4.35 (0–500; 75 ± 148)		
Glucose	mmol/l (mg/dl)	3.89–6.77; 5.54 ± 0.75 (70–122; 100 ± 14)	11.21–31.58; 20.09 ± 5.83 (202–569; 362 ± 105)	6.67 ± 2.04 (120 ± 37)
Globulin	g/l (g/dl)			α1 4.93 ± 1.1 (α1 0.49 ± 0.11) α2 3.48 ± 1.3 (α2 0.35 ± 0.13) β 11.1 ± 3.1 (β 1.11 ± 0.31) γ 6.03 ± 0.8 (γ 0.60 ± 0.08)
Lactate dehydrogenase (LDH)	IU/l U/l			720 ± 242
Phosphorus	mmol/l (mg/dl)	0.90–2.16; 1.20 ± 0.39 (2.8–6.7; 3.7 ± 1.2)		1.68 ± 0.45 (5.20 ± 1.39)
Potassium	mmol/l mEq/l	1.4–5.0; 3.6 ± 0.8		1.01 ± 0.27
Sodium	mmol/l mEq/l	145–167; 158 ± 5		182.9 ± 8.8
Triglycerides	mmol/l (mg/dl)			0.49 ± 0.47 (43.6 ± 41.6)
Total protein	g/l (g/dl)	50–80; 65 ± 8 (5.0–8.0; 6.5 ± 0.8)	36–57; 47 ± 7 (3.6 5.7; 4.7 ± 0.7)	58.4 ± 77.2 (5.8 ± 7.7)
Uric acid	μmol/l (mg/dl)	<18–184; 95 ± 62 (<0.3–3.1; 1.6 ± 1.05)	<12–416; 232 ± 143 (<0.2–7.0; 3.9 ± 2.4)	117.8 ± 50.6 (1.98 ± 0.85)

Gallotia intermedia (n = 4) and *Gallotia bravoana* (n = 6) also reported in the paper but excluded from table due to low numbers of animals.
[a] Analyses performed using plasma and a Kodak Ektachem DT60 chemistry analyzer [51].
[b] Analyses performed using heparinized plasma and a Reflotron analyzer [48].
[c] Analyses performed using heparinized plasma and a Clima chemistry analyzer [50]

The bile acids of reptiles have been extensively studied as evolutionary biomarkers [11]. The 3α,7α,12α,24R-tetrahydroxy-5β-cholestan-27-oic acid of lizards is an intermediate in the formation of cholic acid in snakes and mammals. In healthy green iguanas, fasted 3α hydroxyl-bile acid levels were reported as 7.5 ± 7.8 μmol/l, with feeding producing a significant increase between 3 and 7.5 h. Unfortunately, many published ranges that include bile acids fail to indicate the fasting period prior to sampling. Lizards should be fasted for 48 h prior to obtaining a baseline. The lizard should then be gavage fed approximately 10 ml/kg (10 kcal/kg) of an enteral feeding formula, followed by a second blood sample 7 to 8 h later. Postprandial concentrations above 50 μmol/l may indicate compromised liver function. Little information is available regarding the bile pigments and their

Table 18.8 Biochemical values for captive Varanidae and Helodermatidae [37, 42, 49, 66].

Analyte (abbreviation)	Units, SI (US)	Crocodile monitor ♂ (*Varanus salvadorii*)[a] [49]	Dumeril's monitor (*Varanus dumerili*)[b] [66] ♂	Mexican beaded lizards ♀ (*Heloderma horridum*)[c] [42]	Gila monster ♂ & ♀ (*Heloderma suspectum*)[d] [40]
Data format		min-max range; mean ± SD	mean ± SD	Min-max; mean ± SD	Min-max; mean ± SD
Animal number		5	8	16	16
Albumin	g/l (g/dl)	34.80–38.10; 36.70 ± 1.60(3.48–3.81; 3.67 ± 0.16)	27.0 ± 3.3 (2.7 ± 0.33)	9–14; 12 ± 2 (0.9–1.4; 1.2 ± 0.2)	
Albumin: globulin				0.0–0.3; 0.2 ± 0.1	
Anion gap	mmol/l mEq/l	28.36–38.00; 31.3 ± 3.86			
Alkaline phosphatase (ALP)	IU/l (U/l)	31.17–43.08; 36.95 ± 5.56		7.0–47.0; 20.0–10.3	
Alanine transferase (ALT)	IU/l (U/l)	27.45–114.75; 71.63 ± 42.81		10.0–25.0; 16.9 ± 5.0	
Amylase	IU/l (U/l)		1997 ± 447	1234–3673; 2384 ± 783	
Aspartate (AST, SGOT) aminotransferase	IU/l U/l	25.2–47.8; 33.8 ± 8.67	48.7 ± 22.9	13–50; 32 ± 11	20–66; 42 ± 13
Bile acids (unknown feeding schedule)	µmol/l (µg/dl)				0.06–1.35; 0.40 ± 0.33 (2.6–55.1; 16.2 ± 13.3)
Blood urea nitrogen (BUN)	mmol/l (mg/dl)	1.07–1.25; 1.12 ± 0.071 (3.00–3.50; 3.15 ± 0.20)		0.0–0.71; 0.26 ± 0.25 (0–2; 0.73 ± 0.7)	2.1–10.7; 5.4 ± 2.1 (6–30; 15 ± 6)
Total calcium	mmol/l (mg/dl)	3.53–22.87; 8.53 ± 8.35 (14.2–91.7; 34.2 ± 33.5)	4.05 ± 0.48 (16.2 ± 1.92)	2.35–4.55; 3.16 ± 0.71 (9.4–18.2; 12.7 ± 2.9)	2.55–3.35; 3.05 ± 0.20 (10.2–13.4; 12.2 ± 0.8)
Ionized calcium	mmol/l (mg/dl)				1.09–1.50; 1.26 ± 0.10 (4.36–6.00; 5.04 ± 0.40)
Carbon dioxide (CO_2)	mmol/l (meq/l)	10.0–17.25; 15.40 ± 3.03			
Chloride	mmol/l (meq/l)	121–129; 124 ± 3	111 ± 7	116–125; 121 ± 3	
Cholesterol	mmol/l (mg/dl)	1.21–21.28; 1.55 ± 0.40 (46.75–82.27; 59.75 ± 15.61)	4.62 ± 1.53 (178 ± 59)		
Creatinine	µmol/l (µg/dl)			17.7–44.2; 33.6 ± 8.0 (0.2–0.5; 0.38 ± 0.09)	
Creatine (CPK) (phospho)kinase	IU/l U/l	443–1468; 969 ± 468		43–107; 180 ± 120	144–1812; 600 ± 457
Gamma glutamyl transferase (GGT)	IU/l U/l			0.0–16.0; 1.9 ± 3.7	
Glucose	mmol/l (mg/dl)	7.02–9.52; 8.27 ± 1.02 (126–171; 149 ± 18)	4.55 ± 1.39 (82 ± 25)	2.77–6.49; 4.64 ± 0.97 (50–117; 84 ± 18)	0.22–6.05; 2.68 ± 1.34 (4.0–109; 48.3 ± 24.2)
Globulin	g/l (g/dl)	41.9–71.3; 55.2 ± 11.5 (4.2–7.1; 5.5.2 ± 1.2)	43.5 ± 9.0 (4.35 ± 0.9)		

(*Continued*)

Table 18.8 (Continued)

Analyte (abbreviation)	Units, SI (US)	Crocodile monitor ♁ (*Varanus salvadorii*)[a] [49]	Dumeril's monitor (*Varanus dumerili*)[b] [66] ♁	Mexican beaded lizards ♀ (*Heloderma horridum*)[c] [42]	Gila monster ♁ & ♀ (*Heloderma suspectum*)[d] [40]
Lactate dehydrogenase (LDH)	IU/l U/l	166–353; 279 ± 71		92–585; 266 ± 166	
Lipase	IU/l U/l			0.0–13.0;4.5 ± 3.6	
Magnesium	mmol/l (mg/dl)			1.27–1.44; 1.13 ± 0.15 (3.1–3.5; 2.8 ± 0.4)	
Osmolarity	Osm/l (mOsm/l)			0.29–0.31; 0.30 ± 0.01 (291–315; 3.4 ± 7.7)	
pH					7.48–7.79; 7.66 ± 0.09
Phosphorus	mmol/l (mg/dl)	1.82–4.37; 2.65 ± 1.04 (5.63–13.55; 8.2 ± 3.32)	1.57 ± 0.42 (4.86 ± 1.30)	0.77–1.58; 1.08 ± 0.27 (2.4–4.9; 3.4 ± 0.9)	0.36–2.78; 1.10 ± 0.58 (1.1–8.6; 3.4 ± 1.8)
Potassium	mmol/l mEq/l	4.48–5.16; 4.76 ± 0.31	6.84 ± 0.72	5.26–7.35; 5.84 ± 0.70	2.8–4.6; 3.9 ± 0.5
Sodium	mmol/l mEq/l	168–176; 171 ± 3	163 ± 7	145–159; 155 ± 5	140–151; 144 ± 3
Direct bilirubin	μmol/l (mg/dl)			0.0–6.8; 4.3 ± 4.6 (0.0–0.4; 0.25 ± 0.27)	
Total bilirubin	μmol/l (mg/dl)			0.0–65.0; 20 ± 24 (0.0–3.8; 1.2 ± 1.4)	
Total protein	g/l (g/dl)	79.0–110.2; 92.2 ± 11.7 (7.90–11.02; 9.22 ± 1.17)	70.5 ± 10.4 (7.05 ± 1.04)	32–75; 61 ± 12 (3.2–7.5; 6.1 ± 1.2)	5.4–6.9; 6.3 ± 0.5 (54–69; 63 ± 5)
Uric acid	μmol/l (mg/dl)	116.6–244.5; 170.1 ± 63.6 (1.96–4.11; 2.86 ± 1.07)	210.6 ± 87.9 (3.54 ± 1.48)	60–440; 150 ± 100 (1.1–7.4; 2.49 ± 1.60)	583–1469; 999 ± 250 (9.8–24.7; 16.8 ± 4.2)

[a] Analyses performed using plasma and Hitachi 747–200 clinical chemistry analyzer [49].
[b] Samples collected after a six-day fast; analyses performed using plasma, Hitachi 911 chemistry analyzer [66].
[c] Analyses performed using serum and Beckman Synchron CX7 dry chemistry analyzer [42].
[d] Analyses performed using plasma and Cobas Roche chemistry analyzer [40].

metabolism in lizards. Some skink species (*Prasinohaema* spp.) have high levels of biliverdin [68]. Concentrations of biliverdin in the plasma of *P. flavipes*, *P. prehensicauda*, and *P. virens* are 714 ± 79 μmol/l, 1020 ± 624 μmol/l, and 819 ± 89 μmol/l, respectively.

Muscle Enzymes

CK activity is high in skeletal and cardiac muscle, and low in other iguanid tissues, and increased plasma concentrations may indicate muscle damage [67]. AST and LDH occur many tissues and are less muscle-specific; however, isoenzymes of LDH exist in squamate reptiles, and further work could demonstrate their diagnostic value [69].

Renal Analytes

Increased plasma concentrations of nitrogenous metabolites are poor indicators of renal function because they can be affected by hydration status and because pathologic changes tend to occur late in the course of disease. Over 90% of nitrogenous excretion in lizards is in the form of uric acid or urates, with hyperuricemia or uremia seldom evident before terminal renal failure [16, 70]. In clinical practice, urea and creatinine are poor indicators of renal disease in most species because of their low production and variable excretion [16, 23, 26, 70]. Of the lizards, only the tuatara excretes urea as a consistent fraction of urinary nitrogen, although bladder urea levels have been reported in some lizards, including *Anolis carolinensis* and *Lacerta viridis* [71]. Low or undetectable levels of urea occur in the green iguana [37]. Creatinine and creatine values have been described in a limited number of healthy and renal-diseased iguanas. Creatinine production and excretion appear too variable for useful clinical interpretation, and creatine, like uric acid, only rises late in the course of renal disease [72]. In green iguanas, calcium:phosphorus ratios may become inverted in many, but not all, cases of renal failure [23, 73].

The ranges for sodium and potassium determined in previous studies may assist in the evaluation of electrolyte changes during disease. However, significant regulation of sodium and potassium is possible at extrarenal sites (e.g., nasal salt glands). Hyponatremia and hyperkalemia may be expected from dysfunction of the distal tubules, cloaca, colon, bladder, or distal extrarenal salt glands, but a more detailed evaluation is necessary in healthy animals and those with renal disease [70].

Activities of other enzymes, including AST, CK, and LDH, may increase during renal disease, but their wide tissue distribution makes them poorly specific markers of renal damage [67, 70, 74]. Tubular disease may result in increased urinary loss of the brush border enzyme, GGT; however, further studies are necessary to confirm this theory. Severe glomerular disease may increase urinary loss of albumin and lead to hypoalbuminemia. Acute renal inflammation is uncommon, but may result in leukocytosis and elevated fibrinogen. Chronic disease may lead to secondary renal hyperparathyroidism due to inadequate hydroxylation of vitamin D_3 by the kidneys or phosphate retention resulting in hypocalcemia and increased parathyroid hormone secretion [70, 75, 76].

Iohexol clearance studies have proved useful for determination of GFR in iguanas [23]. Iohexol excretion assays are commercially available and do not require bladder or ureteral catheterization or expensive equipment or radioisotopes to perform. This technique for renal function evaluation in reptiles can be performed in private practice. Iohexol is excreted solely by glomerular filtration with negligible extrarenal elimination. The plasma clearance of iohexol (PCI) can be determined with analysis of plasma iohexol concentration over time after a single intravenous injection [23]. The rate of clearance of iohexol from plasma is used to estimate GFR by dividing the iohexol dose by the area under the curve (AUC) because elimination is solely by glomerular filtration. In the healthy green iguanas, GFR was 14.78–18.34 ml/kg/hr (95% confidence interval) [23]. Iguanas with renal disease had reductions in GFR even in the absence of other clinical or biochemical signs. A suggested protocol for measurement of GFR in iguanas (and potentially other reptiles) is shown in Table 18.9 GFR has been calculated for several species using clearance methods (Table 18.10) [23, 71].

Table 18.9 Glomerular filtration rates of lizards [23, 71].

Species	GFR ml/kg h	Animal condition
Puerto Rican gecko	10.4 ± 0.77	
House gecko (*Hemidactylus* sp.)	3.33 ± 0.37	Dehydrated
	24.3	Water-loaded
Green iguana (*Iguana iguana*)	16.56 ± 3.90	Healthy males, iohexol excretion

Table 18.10 Protocol to measure glomerular filtration rate of lizards.

Contact the Diagnostic Center for Population and Animal Health (Michigan State University, East Lansing, MI 48824, (517) 353–1683, www.ahdl.msu.edu) to check for any changes to the blood collection and submission requirements for iohexol assay and GFR calculation
Ensure the reptile is hydrated and fasted for 24 h.
Weigh accurately, and inject 75 mg/kg iohexol intravenously (intravenous catheterization reduces the risks of perivascular injection that invalidates the results) at time 0.
Collect three 0.5 ml blood samples at 4, 8, and 24 h after injection. Separate and store plasma on ice.
Record the exact times of blood collection.
Send these details with the three separated plasma samples on ice to the Diagnostic Center for Population and Animal Health for iohexol assays and GFR calculation.

Pancreas

An extensive review of the structure of the reptilian pancreas has been published [77]. Amylase is almost exclusively restricted to the pancreas in iguanas, and should therefore prove useful for the evaluation of pancreatic disease [67]. Unfortunately, only amylase values for Dumeril's monitors and beaded lizards have been published (Table 18.8) [42, 66].

Care must be taken when identifying a hyperglycemic reptile as diabetic. The stress of handling for blood collection and environmental temperature can cause a physiological hyperglycemia [78]. Therefore, the diagnosis of diabetes mellitus should rely on demonstrating a persistent hyperglycemia, preferably using a hands-free glucose monitoring system (Guardian Real-Time Continuous Glucose Monitoring System, Medtronic, California, United States), and confirmed by pancreatic biopsy.

Gastrointestinal and Cardiac

Apart from the wide distribution of enzymes such as LDH, enzyme activities in intestinal tissues appear low and of poor diagnostic value [67]. Low blood albumin and total protein may indicate protein-losing enteropathies or the long-term starvation associated with chronic intestinal disease. Increased CK activities have been documented in the heart of iguanas, but no cardiac specific markers have been established for lizards [67].

Lipids and Lipoproteins

Lipids provide for vitellogenesis and act as an energy store during hibernation/estivation and fasting. Hepatic lipid reserves of species studied are highest in females just before hibernation and lowest in males in late hibernation [79]. Fats are transported from the intestinal tract and the fat bodies to the liver in the form of unesterified fatty acids [11]. All fat transportation away from the liver is in an esterified form, being protein-bound as lipoproteins. These very-low-density lipoproteins are recycled as low-density lipoprotein fragments. The formulation of phospholipids and cholesterol is also under hepatic regulation, again from lipid precursors. Cholesterol and triglycerides undergo a natural and physiological elevation during vitellogenesis and prehibernation; increased lipoprotein concentrations occur in cases of gross obesity and hepatic lipidosis [80].

Electrolytes

The water balance varies between species and is affected by diet and environmental conditions [24]. Plasma electrolyte concentrations for lizards are shown in Tables 18.5–18.8. Wide ranges indicate the importance of known populations of single species for reference range determination. Causes of electrolyte disturbances in lizards should include the usual mammalian differentials such as intestinal and renal disease, iatrogenic, excessive fluid therapy, and dehydration, but disorders of the salt gland should also be considered [2].

Blood Proteins

Total protein levels for lizards may vary between 24 and 110 g/l, depending on species, age, sex, reproductive status, and season. Females exhibit the highest protein levels during estrogen-induced vitellogenesis, often associated with increased concentrations of albumin and globulins. The Biuret method is more accurate for total protein determination than the refractometer. Hyperproteinemia can be associated with dehydration or hyperglobulinemia associated with chronic inflammatory conditions. Unpublished data from the University of Georgia for male green iguanas are summarized in Table 18.11, along with a recent publication for female iguanas [81]. The six standard protein fractions were identified, and albumin did not differ in serum or plasma. However, plasma samples yielded higher total globulins based on higher beta$_2$, and gamma globulins. The α, β, and γ globulins are expected to increase with infectious diseases. Recent research at the University of Georgia indicates that in the bearded dragon, bromocresol green (BCG) determinations for albumin are inaccurate compared to protein electrophoresis. Therefore, albumin values determined using BCG should be considered inaccurate from bearded dragons, and probably most reptiles.

Blood Gases

Arterial and venous blood gases determined for the green iguana demonstrate a circadian rhythm (Table 18.12) [82]. Blood pH in the iguana varies between 7.18 and 7.40 at 37 °C (or 7.17–7.47 when corrected to 30 °C). However, pH decreases with increasing temperature and increases during anesthesia likely owing to reduced ventilation and increased CO_2 [2].

Table 18.11 Plasma protein electrophoresis values of healthy green iguanas (*Iguana iguana*) [81].[a]

Analyte	Units (US)	Captive subadult males[a]	Captive adult females[b] [81]
Animals sampled		20	14
Total protein	g/l (g/dl)	56.0–69.5; 62.6 ± 4.9 (5.6–6.95; 6.26 ± 0.49)	40.9–74.1; 56.7 ± 12.0
Albumin	g/l (g/dl)	17.2–24.6; 20.9 ± 2.1 (1.72–2.46; 2.09 ± 0.21)	13.9–30.6; 19.3 ± 4.6
Total globulin	g/l (g/dl)	34.9–49.0; 41.7 ± 4.7 (3.49–4.90; 4.17 ± 0.47)	
α_1-globulins	g/l (g/dl)	1.5–7.6; 2.5 ± 1.3 (0.15–0.76; 0.25 ± 0.13)	4.2–12.3; 8.8 ± 2.6
α_2-globulins	g/l (g/dl)	5.0–9.5; 6.5 ± 1.6 (0.50–0.95; 0.65 ± 0.16)	
β_1-globulins	g/l (g/dl)	12.1–20.9; 15.3 ± 3.6 (1.21–2.09; 1.53 ± 0.36)	15.9–37.5; 25.3 ± 8.0
β_2-globulins	g/l (g/dl)	5.1–16.3; 8.3 ± 4.2 (0.51–1.63; 0.83 ± 0.42)	
γ-globulins	g/l (g/dl)	2.6–13.9; 5.1 ± 3.4 (0.26–1.39; 0.51 ± 0.34)	1.2–7.4; 4.0 ± 2.9
Albumin:globulin		0.37–0.64; 0.51 ± 0.08	0.41–0.78; 0.57 ± 0.14

Analyses performed using heparinized plasma, agarose gel plates.

[a] Unpublished data determined in clinical pathology laboratory, University of Georgia.

[b] Analyses performed using heparinized plasma, cellulose acetate plates, and quantified by densitometry [81].

Table 18.12 Arterial and venous blood gas values for 37 °C in 15 conscious green iguanas (*Iguana iguana*) breathing room air [82].

Analyte	Units	Arterial	Venous
pH		7.29 ± 0.11 (7.38 ± 0.12)	7.31* (7.36 ± 0.13)
Pco_2	mm Hg	42 ± 9 (32 ± 7)	49* (36 ± 7)
Po_2	mm Hg	81 ± 19† (54 ± 15) [94 ± 21† (64 ± 16)]	46 ± 23(30 ± 15)
Lactate	mmol/l	2.7 ± 1.1	2.3*
Bicarbonate	mmol/l	20 ± 4	22 ± 5
Total CO_2	mmol/l	22 ± 4	24 ± 5
Base excess	mmol/l	−6.3 ± 5.5	−5 ± 6
Sao_2	%	92 ± 6 [95 ± 3]	84* [49*]
SPo_2	%	86 ± 6	
RR	breaths/min	28 ± 6	27 ± 6

Data presented as mean ± SD unless indicated otherwise: *Values are reported as medians. Values in parentheses are corrected for a body temperature of 30 °C. SPo_2 = Oxygen saturation measured by pulse oximetry. When afternoon values were significantly different, they are listed (in brackets).

Minerals, Metals, and Toxins

Calcium and phosphorus represent a pivotal dynamic within lizards, and disruption is the cause of common disease (e.g., secondary nutritional hyperparathyroidism). Total calcium values can vary dramatically with species, age, gender, and reproductive status; however, physiologically active ionized calcium is more tightly regulated (Table 18.13) [38, 59]. Common causes of hypocalcemia include dietary deficiencies of calcium and vitamin D_3, phosphorus excess, alkalosis, hypoalbuminemia, or hypoparathyroidism [2, 3]. Physiologic hypercalcemia can occur in reproductively active females, or in any animal overly supplemented with vitamin D_3 and calcium. Rare differentials include primary hyperparathyroidism, pseudohyperparathyroidism, and osteolytic bone diseases. Hypophosphatemia is often associated with starvation or nutritional deficiency. Hyperphosphatemia is most commonly associated with dietary excess, hypervitaminosis D, or renal disease. 25-Hydroxyvitamin D_3 levels have been determined for several species of free-ranging lizards (Table 18.13) [83, 85]. Several trace minerals and heavy metals have also been reported for *Iguana iguana* and *Varanus komodoensis* [83, 84].

Hormones

Total thyroxine (T4), free T4, and T3 levels have been determined in some lizard species. Peaks of T4 and T3 are often related to pre- and posthibernation, and ecdysis [86]. Total thyroxine of seven green iguanas ranged from 2.98 to 4.65 nmol/l (0.17 to 0.27 μg/ml) [61]. Ranges of free T4 and T3 (triiodothyronine) levels in male Indian garden lizards (*Calotes versicolor*) were 0.02–0.60 pmol/l (0.16–4.63 ng/ml) and 0.0–2.7 nmol/l (0.0–1.76 ng/ml), respectively, during the course of the year.

Urinalysis

Urinalysis is less helpful in lizards than in mammals. As the reptilian kidney cannot concentrate urine, urine specific gravity is of limited use in the assessment of renal function. Because urine passes through the urodeum of the cloaca before entering the bladder (when a bladder is present), urine is often nonsterile. Further, electrolyte and water changes can occur across the bladder or cloacocolonic membrane [28]. Nevertheless, lizard urine samples are useful for assessments of inflammation and infection and for identification of renal casts.

Urine may be collected from the enclosure floor or examination table, by free-catch, or cystocentesis. A more representative and less contaminated sample is usually obtained by cystocentesis. However, the potential danger of post-sampling leakage of unsterile urine into the coelom does exist. Urine collected with cystocentesis may not be representative of renal urine with respect to electrolyte composition and osmolarity. Such samples are often unsterile, although a heavy pure microbiologic growth should alert the clinician to potential infection. A more detailed review of urine collection and urinalysis can be found elsewhere [70]. A complete urinalysis examination includes gross evaluation of the urine, microscopic evaluation of the sediment, and chemical analysis (often using standard urine chemistry dipsticks). Most reptile urinalysis data comes from chelonians and should be consulted, as lizard specifics are currently lacking.

Table 18.13 Vitamin, trace mineral, and heavy metal levels in select lizard species [83–85].

Analyte	Units, SI (US)	Komodo dragon ♂ & ♀ (*Varanus komodoensis*)[a] [83]	Green iguana ♀ (*Iguana iguana*)[b] [84]	Rhinoceros iguana (*Cyclura cornuta*)[b] [85]	Ricord's iguana (*Cyclura ricordii*)[b] [85]
Data format		**Min-max range, mean ± SD or median**	**Min-max range; mean ± SD**	**Min-max range; mean ± SD**	**Min-max range; mean ± SD**
Animal number		**77**	**20**	**20**	**20**
Vitamin A	μmol/l (μg/ml)	0.10–0.85; 0.25 (2.87–24.36; 7.16)			
Vitamin E	μmol/l	2–23; 6 (0.09–0.99; 0.26)			
25- hydroxyvitamin D_3	nmol/l(ng/ml)	117–324; 183 ♂ (47–130; 73) ♂ 4–97; 29 ♀ (2–39; 12) ♀		260–369; 332 ♂ (104–148; 133) ♂	250–1118; 554 ♂ (100–448; 222) ♂
Selenium	μmol/l (μg/l)	0.7–3.3; 1.9 (55–260; 150)			
Molybdenum	μmol/l	<0.4			
Magnesium	mmol/l (mEq/l)	0.84–1.86; 1.34 (1.68–3.72; 2.68)			
Iron	μmol/l (μg/dl)	11–22; 15 (61–123; 84)			
Boron	μmol/l	≤20			
Chromium	nmol/l (μg/l)	<0.2 (<0.01)			
Cobalt	μmol/l (μg/l)	<0.3 (<18)			
Copper	μmol/l (μg/dl)	10.0–24.4; 15.2 (64–155; 97)			
Lead (whole blood)	μmol/l (μg/dl)		0.00–0.82; 0.29 ± 0.14 (0–17; 6 ± 3)		
Zinc (plasma)	μmol/l (μg/dl)	41.2–163.7; 49.1 ♀ (269–1070; 321) ♀ 31.8–74.4; 50.9 ♂ (208–486; 333) ♂	20.4–71.9; 41.0 ± 12.7 (133–470; 268 ± 83)		

[a] Analyses performed using heparinized plasma or serum at various commercial laboratories [83].
[b] Analyses performed with EDTA whole blood (lead) and heparinized plasma (zinc) using a PerkinElmer 5100 atomic absorption spectrometer [84, 85].

Serology and PCR

A hemagglutination inhibition assay against paramyxovirus antibodies was developed and used to screen caiman lizards (*Dracaena guianensis*), spiny-tailed iguanas (*Ctenosaura bakeri, C. similis*), green iguanas (*I. iguana rhinolopha*), and Mexican lizards (*Xenosaurus* and *Abronia*) [87]. Many bacterial, viral, and fungal PCR tests are commercially available. As these depend upon the identification of pathogen DNA but not the host's immune system; they can be employed using lizard samples.

References

1 Friedrichs, K.R., Harr, K.E., Freeman, K.P. et al. (2012). ASVCP reference interval guidelines: determination of de novo reference intervals in veterinary species and other related topics. *Vet Clin Pathol* 41: 441–453. https://doi.org/10.1111/vcp.12006.

2 Heatley, J.J. and Russell, K. (2019). Hematology. In: *Maders Reptile and Amphibian Medicine and Surgery*, 3e (ed. S. Divers and S. Stahl), 301–318. Elsevier.

3 Heatley, J.J. and Russell, K. (2019). Clinical chemistry. In: *Maders Reptile and Amphibian Medicine and*

Surgery, 3e (ed. S. Divers and S. Stahl), 319–332. Elsevier.

4 Dessauer, H.C. (1970). Blood chemistry of reptiles: physiological and evolutionary aspects. In: *Biology of the Reptilia, Volume 3, Morphology C* (ed. C. Gans and T.S. Parsons). London: Academic Press.

5 Duguy, R. (1970). Numbers of blood cells and their variation. In: *Biology of the Reptilia, Volume 3, Morphology C* (ed. C. Gans and T.S. Parsons). London: Academic Press.

6 Fudge, A.M. (2000). Section two: reptilian laboratory medicine. In: *Laboratory Medicine: Avian and Exotic Pets* (ed. A.M. Fudge). Philadelphia, PA: WB Saunders Co.

7 Girons, M.C. (1970). Morphology of the circulating blood cells. In: *Biology of the Reptilia, Volume 3, Morphology C* (ed. C. Gans and T.S. Parsons). London: Academic Press.

8 Strik, N., Alleman, A.R., and Harr, K.E. (2007). Circulating inflammatory cells. In: *Infectious Diseases Pathology of Reptiles – Color Atlas and Text* (ed. E.R. Jacobson). London: Taylor & Francis.

9 Skoczylas, R. (1978). Physiology of the digestive tract. In: *Biology of the Reptilia*, vol. 8 (ed. C. Gans and K.A. Gans). London: Academic Press.

10 Jacobson, E.R. (2007). Overview of Reptile Biology, Anatomy and Histology. In: *Infectious Diseases and Pathology of Reptiles* (ed. E.R. Jacobson), 1–130. Taylor and Francis.

11 Schaffner, F. (1998). The liver. In: *Biology of the Reptilia, Volume 19, Morphology G, Visceral Organs* (ed. C. Gans and A.S. Gaunt), 485–531. Society for the Study of Amphibians and Reptiles.

12 Guo, M., Ditrich, H., and Splechtna, H. (1996). Renal vasculature and uriniferous tubules in the common iguana. *Journal of Morphology* 229: 97–104.

13 Benson, K.G. and Forrest, L. (1999). Characterization of the renal portal system of the common green iguana (*Iguana iguana*) by digital subtraction imaging. *Journal of Zoo and Wildlife Medicine* 30: 235–241.

14 Holz, P.H. (1999). The reptilian renal portal system – a review. *Bulletin of the Association of Reptilian and Amphibian Veterinarians* 9: 4–9.

15 Bradshaw, S.D. and Bradshaw, F.J. (2002). Arginine vasotocin: site and mode of action in the reptilian kidney. *General and Comparative Endocrinology* 126: 7–13.

16 Dantzler, W.H. (1976). Renal function (with special emphasis on nitrogen excretion). In: *Biology of the Reptilia, Physiology A* (ed. C. Gans and W.R. Dawson). London: Academic Press.

17 Dantzler, W.H. and Schmidt-Nielson, B. (1966). Excretion in fresh-water (*Pseudemys scripts*) and the desert tortoise (*Gopherus agassizii*). *The American Journal of Physiology* 210: 198–210.

18 Ranges, H.A., Chasis, H., Goldring, W., and Smith, H.W. (1939). The functional measurement of a number of active glomeruli and tubules in kidneys of normal and hypertensive subjects. *The American Journal of Physiology* 126: 103.

19 Schmidt-Nielson, B. and Davies, L.E. (1968). Fluid transport and tubular intercellular spaces in reptilian kidneys. *Science (New York, N.Y.)* 159: 1105–1108.

20 Shoemaker, V.H., Licht, P., and Dawson, W.R. (1966). Effects of temperature on kidney function in the lizard *Tiliqua rugosa*. *Physiological Zoology* 39: 244–252.

21 Templeton, J.R. (1964). Cardiovascular response to temperature in the lizard *Sauromalus obesus*. *Physiological Zoology* 37: 300–306.

22 Green, B. (1972). Aspects of renal function in the lizard, *Varanus gouldii*. *Comparative Biochemistry and Physiology* 42: 747–756.

23 Hernandez-Divers, S.J., Stahl, S.J., Stedman, N.L. et al. (2005). Renal evaluation in the healthy green iguana (Iguana iguana): assessment of plasma biochemistry, glomerular filtration rate, and endoscopic biopsy. *Journal of Zoo and Wildlife Medicine* 36: 155–168.

24 Minnich, J.E. (1982). The use of water. In: *Biology of the Reptilia, Volume 12, Physiology C* (ed. C. Gans and F.H. Pough). London: Academic Press.

25 Bordley, J. and Richards, A.N. (1933). Quantitative studies of the composition of glomerular urine. VII. The concentration of uric acid in glomerular urine of snakes and frogs, determined by an ultramicroadaption of Folin's method. *The Journal of Biological Chemistry* 101: 193–221.

26 Hernandez-Divers, S.J. (2003). Green iguana nephrology: a review of diagnostic techniques. *The Veterinary Clinics of North America* 6: 233–250.

27 Badia, P., Gomez, T., Diaz, M., and Lorenzo, A. (1987). Mechanisms of transport of Na+ and Cl– in the lizard colon. *Comparative Biochemistry and Physiolology Part A* 87: 883–887.

28 Ehrenspeck, G. and Voner, C. (1985). Effect of furosemide on ion transport in the turtle bladder: evidence for direct inhibition of active acid-base transport. *Biochimica et Biophysica Acta* 817: 318–326.

29 Stephens, G.A. and Robertson, F.M. (1985). Renal responses to diuretics in the turtle. *Journal of Comparative Physiology* 155: 387–393.

30 White, F.N. (1976). Circulation. In: *Biology of the Reptilia, Volume 5, Physiology A* (ed. C. Gans and W.R. Dawson). London: Academic Press.

31 Divers, S.J. (1999). Clinical evaluation of reptiles. *The Veterinary Clinics of North America* 2: 291–331.

32 West, G., Heard, D., and Caulkett, N. (2007). *Zoo and Wild Animal Immobilization and Anesthesia*, 656. Wiley-Blackwell.

33 Hanley, C.S., Hernandez-Divers, S.J., Bush, S., and Latimer, K.S. (2004). Comparison of dipotassium EDTA and lithium heparin on hematologic values in the green iguana (*Iguana iguana*). *Journal of Zoo and Wildlife Medicine* 35 (3): 328–332.

34 Mayer, J., Knoll, J., Innis, C., and Mitchell, M.A. (2005). Characterizing the hematologic and plasma chemistry profiles of captive Chinese water dragons, *Physignathus cocincinus*. *Journal of Herpetological Medicine and Surgery* 15: 45–52.
35 Perpinan, D., Hernandez-Divers, S.M., and Hernandez-Divers, S.J. (2006). Comparison of three different techniques to produce blood smears from green iguanas, *Iguana iguana*. *Journal of Herpetological Medicine and Surgery* 16: 99–101.
36 Finkelstein, A.D., DiGesualdo, C.L., and Hoover, J.P. (2003). Comparison of biochemical profile values from paired plasma and serum samples of green iguanas, *Iguana iguana*, and red-tailed boa constrictors, *Boa constrictor*. *Journal of Herpetological Medicine and Surgery* 13: 5–9.
37 Divers, S.J., Redmayne, G., and Aves, E.K. (1996). Haematological and biochemical values of 10 green iguanas (*Iguana iguana*). *The Veterinary Record* 138: 203–205.
38 Harr, K.E., Alleman, A.R., Dennis, P.M. et al. (2001). Morphologic and cytochemical characteristics of blood cells and hematologic and plasma biochemical reference ranges in green iguanas. *JAVMA* 218: 915–921.
39 James, S.B., Iverson, J., Greco, V., and Raphael, B.L. (2006). Health assessment of Allen cays rock iguana, *Cyclura cychlura inornata*. *Journal of Herpetological Medicine and Surgery* 16: 93–97.
40 Cooper-Bailey, K., Smith, S.A., Zimmerman, K. et al. (2011). Hematology, leukocyte cytochemical analysis, plasma biochemistry, and plasma electrophoresis of wild-caught and captive-bred Gila monsters (*Heloderma suspectum*). *Veterinary Clinical Pathology* 40: 316–323.
41 Dallwig, R.K., Paul-Murphy, J., Thomas, C. et al. (2011). Hematology and clinical chemistry values of free-ranging basilisk lizards (*Basiliscus plumifrons*) in Costa Rica. *Journal of Zoo and Wildlife Medicine* 42: 205–213.
42 Espinosa-Aviles, D., Salomon-Soto, V.M., and Morales-Martinez, S. (2008). Hematology, blood chemistry, and bacteriology of the free-ranging Mexican beaded lizard (*Heloderma horridum*). *Journal of Zoo and Wildlife Medicine* 39: 21–27.
43 Olmeda, R. (1985). Hematological variations in the collared lizard, Crotaphytus collaris (Saura: Iguanidae). *Copeia* 3: 782–784.
44 Naldo, J.L., Libanan, N.L., and Samour, J.H. (2009). Health assessment of a spiny-tailed lizard (*Uromastyx* spp.) population in Abu Dhabi, United Arab Emirates. *Journal of Zoo and Wildlife Medicine* 40: 445–452.
45 Parida, S.P., Dutta, S.K., and Pal, A. (July 2011). Hematological and plasma biochemistry in Psammophilus blanfordanus (Sauria: Agamidae). *Comparative Clinical Pathology* 28: 1–8.
46 Troiano, J.C. and Gould, E.G. (2011). Interspecific differences in the hematological reference intervals in Tupinambis from Argentina (Sauria-Teiidae). *Comparative Clinical Pathology* 20: 309–312.
47 Troiano, J.C., Gould, E.G., and Gould, I. (2008). Hematological reference intervals in argentine lizard Tupinambis merianae (Sauria - Teiidae). *Comparative Clinical Pathology* 17: 93–97.
48 Cuadrado, M., Diaz-Paniagua, C., Quevedo, M.A. et al. (2002). Hematology and clinical chemistry in dystocic and healthy post-reproductive female chameleons. *Journal of Wildlife Diseases* 38: 395–401.
49 Fontenot, D.K., Lamberski, N., and Pfaff, S. (2004). Physical, hematologic, and plasma biochemistry values of five crocodile lizards, *Varanus salvadorii*. *Journal of Herpetological Medicine and Surgery* 14: 5–9.
50 Martinez Silvestre, A., Rodriguez Dominguez, M.A., Mateo, J.A. et al. (2004). Comparative haematology and blood chemistry of endangered lizards (Gallotia species) in the Canary Islands. *The Veterinary Record* 155: 266–269.
51 Wright, K.M. and Skeba, S. (1992). Hematology and plasma chemistries of captive prehensile-tailed skinks (*Corucia zebrata*). *Journal of Zoo and Wildlife Medicine* 23: 429–432.
52 Acuna, M.L. (1974). The hematology of the tropical lizard, Iguana iguana - seasonal variations. *Herpetologica* 30: 299–303.
53 Folland, D.W., Johnston, M.S., Thamm, D.H., and Reavill, D. (2011). Diagnosis and management of lymphoma in a green iguana (*Iguana iguana*). *Journal of the American Veterinary Medical Association* 239: 985–991.
54 Schultze, A.E., Mason, G.L., and Clyde, V.L. (1999). Lymphosarcoma with leukemic blood profile in a savannah monitor lizard (*Varanus exanthematicus*). *Journal of Zoo and Wildlife Medicine* 30: 158–164.
55 Hackett, E. and Hann, C. (1967). Slow clotting of reptile bloods. *Journal of Comparative Pathology* 77 (2): 175–180.
56 Divers, S.J. (2019). Hepatology. In: *Maders Reptile and Amphibian Medicine and Surgery*, 3e (ed. S.J. Divers and S.J. Stahl), 649–668. Elsevier.
57 Hildemann, W.H. (1962). Immunogenetic studies of amphibians and reptiles. *Annals of the New York Academy of Science* 97: 139–152.
58 Dallwig, R.K., Mitchell, M.A., and Acierno, M.J. (2010). Determination of plasma osmolality and agreement between measured and calculated values in healthy adult bearded dragons (*Pogona vitticeps*). *Journal of Herpetological Medicine and Surgery* 20: 69–73.
59 Dennis, P.M., Bennett, R.A., Harr, K.E., and Lock, B.A. (2001). Plasma concentration of ionized calcium in healthy iguanas. *JAVMA* 219: 326–328.
60 Grant, K.R., Thode, H.P., Connor, S., and Johnston, M.S. (2009). Establishment of plasma biochemical reference values for captive green iguanas, Iguana iguana, using a point-of-care biochemistry analyzer. *Journal of Herpetological Medicine and Surgery* 19: 23–28.
61 Hernandez-Divers, S.J., Knott, C.D., and MacDonald, J. (2001). Diagnosis and surgical treatment of thyroid

adenoma-induced hyperthyroidism in a green iguana (*Iguana iguana*). *Journal of Zoo and Wildlife Medicine* 32: 465–475.
62 Kopplin, R.P., Tarr, R.S., and Iverson, C.N.M. (1983). Serum profile of the iguanid lizard (*Dipsosaurus dorsalis*). *Journal of Zoo and Wildlife Medicine* 14: 30–32.
63 Maria, R., Ramer, J., Reichard, T. et al. (2007). Biochemical reference intervals and intestinal microflora of free-ranging Ricord's iguanas (*Cyclura ricordii*). *Journal of Zoo and Wildlife Medicine* 38: 414–419.
64 McBride, M., Hernandez-Divers, S.J., Koch, T. et al. (2006). Preliminary evaluation of pre- and post-prandial 3α-hydroxy bile acids in the green iguana (*Iguana iguana*). *Journal of Herpetological Medicine and Surgery* 16: 129–134.
65 Tamukai, K., Takami, Y., Akabane, Y. et al. (2011). Plasma biochemical reference values in clinically healthy captive bearded dragons (*Pogona vitticeps*) and the effects of sex and season. *Veterinary Clinical Pathology* 40: 368–373.
66 Bertelsen, M.F., Kjelgaard-Hansen, M., Howell, J.R., and Crawshaw, G.J. (2007). Short-term biological variation of clinical chemical values in Dumeril's monitors (*Varanus dumerili*). *Journal of Zoo and Wildlife Medicine* 38: 217–221.
67 Wagner, R.A. and Wetzel, R. (1999). Tissue and plasma enzyme activities in juvenile green iguanas. *American Journal of Veterinary Research* 60: 201–203.
68 Austin, C.C. and Jessing, K.W. (1994). Green-blood pigmentation in lizards. *Comparative Biochemistry and Physiology Part A: Physiology* 109: 619–626.
69 Aleksiuk, M. (1971). An isoenzymic basis for instantaneous cold compensation in reptiles: lactate dehydrogenase kinetics in *Thamnophis sirtalis*. *Comparative Biochemistry and Physiology Part B: Comparative Biochemistry* 40: 671–681.
70 Divers, S.J. and Innis, C. (2019). Urology. In: *Maders Reptile and Amphibian Medicine and Surgery*, 3rde (ed. S. Divers and S. Stahl), 624–648. Elsevier.
71 Roberts, J.S. and Schmidt-Nielson, K. (1969). Renal ultrastructure and excretion of salt and water by three terrestrial lizards. *The American Journal of Physiology* 211: 476–486.
72 Boyer TH, Getzy D, Vap L, Innis C. Clinicopathologic findings of twelve cases of renal failure in Iguana iguana. Proceedings of the Proc ARAV, Tampa, 1996, p. 113.
73 Innis, C., Hawes, M., Stone, M., and Seymour, R. (1999). What's your diagnosis? – case 2. *Bulletin of the Association of Reptilian and Amphibian Veterinarians* 9: 50–52.
74 Suedmeyer, K. (1995). Hypocalcaemia and hyperphosphataemia in a green iguana, Iguana iguana, with concurrent elevation of serum glutamic oxalic transaminase. *Bulletin of the Association of Reptilian and Amphibian Veterinarians* 5: 5–6.
75 Elder, G. (2002). Pathophysiology and recent advances in the management of renal osteodystrophy. *Journal of Bone and Mineral Research* 17: 2094–2105.
76 Malluche, H.H. and Monier-Faugere, M.C. (1999). Understanding and managing hyperphosphatemia in patients with chronic renal disease. *Clinical Nephrology* 52: 267–277.
77 Miller, M.R. and Lagios, M.D. (1970). The pancreas. In: *Biology of the Reptilia, Volume 3, Morphology C* (ed. C. Gans and T.S. Parsons). London: Academic Press.
78 Callard, G.V., Chan, S.W.C., and Callard, I.P. (1975). Temperature effects on ACTH-stimulated adrenocortical secretion and carbohydrate metabolism in the lizard. *Journal of Comparative Physiology B: Biochemical, Systemic, and Environmental Physiology* 99: 271–277.
79 Ji, X. and Wang, P.C. (1990). Annual cycle of lipid contents and caloric values of carcass and some organs of the gecko (*Gekko japonicus*). *Comparative Biochemistry and Physiology* 96A: 267–271.
80 Divers, S.J. (2019). Hepatic lipidosis. In: *Maders Reptile and Amphibian Medicine and Surgery* (eds Divers SJ and Stahl SJ). 3rd edition, Elsevier. Pp 1312–1313.
81 Gimenez, M., Saco, Y., Pato, R. et al. (2010). Plasma protein electrophoresis of *Trachemys scripta* and *Iguana iguana*. *Veterinary Clinical Pathology* 39: 227–235.
82 Hernandez, S.M., Schumacher, J., Lewis, S.J. et al. (2011). Selected cardiopulmonary values and baroreceptor reflex in conscious green iguanas (*Iguana iguana*). *American Journal of Veterinary Research* 72: 1519–1526.
83 Gillespie, D., Frye, F.L., Stockham, S.L., and Fredeking, T. (2000). Blood values in wild and captive Komodo dragons (*Varanus komodoensis*). *Zoo Biology* 19: 495–509.
84 Burns, R.P. and Paul-Murphy, J. (2009). Determination of lead and zinc concentrations in the blood and liver of the captive common green iguana (*Iguana iguana*). *Journal of Zoo and Wildlife Medicine* 40: 495–500.
85 Ramer, J.C., Maria, R., Reichard, T. et al. (2005). Vitamin D status of wild Ricord's iguanas (*Cyclura ricordii*) and captive and wild rhinoceros iguanas (*Cyclura cornuta cornuta*) in the Dominican Republic. *Journal of Zoo and Wildlife Medicine* 36: 188–191.
86 Kar, A. and Chandola-Saklani, A. (1985). Circulating thyroid hormone concentrations in relation to seasonal events in the male Indian garden lizard, Calotes versicolor. *General and Comparative Endocrinology* 60: 14–19.
87 Jacobson, E.F. and Origgi, C. (2007). Serodiagnostics. In: *Infectious Diseases and Pathology of Reptiles* (ed. E. Jacobson). Boca Raton, FL: CRC Press.

19

Amphibians*

María J. Forzán PhD, DACVP[1] and Barbara S. Horney DVM, PhD, DACVP (Clinical Pathology)[2]

[1] College of Veterinary Medicine, University of Long Island, Brookvale, New York, USA
[2] Department of Pathology and Microbiology, University of Prince Edward Island, Charlottetown, Canada

Introduction

Clinical pathology as a tool for health evaluation can be as useful in amphibians as in higher vertebrates. The stoic nature of the amphibian patient and the great variety of species in the class make it difficult to interpret external health clues easily. Unfortunately, diagnostically relevant information for hematology and clinical chemistries of amphibians is scarce. Most reports concerning native North American species are compiled with a biologic or ecologic perspective [1–5]. Reports on laboratory frogs (*Xenopus* sp.) are more clinically oriented, but in both instances the number of subjects studied is frequently small [6, 7]. Published information is restricted to two orders: Anura (frogs and toads) and Caudata (salamanders and newts). Clinical pathology information is completely lacking for Caecilians, members of Apoda which resemble earthworms. The study of amphibian hematology and clinical chemistry is further complicated by numerous and varied species, differences present within a species depending on its life stage, and the great influence that environmental factors have on amphibian physiology. Amphibian medicine would benefit from studies conducted under established guidelines, such as those by the American Society for Veterinary Clinical Pathology (ASVCP). The paucity of laboratory-specific or even published reference intervals often necessitates the use of conspecifics for comparative assessment of normal parameters. Conspecifics used as reference individuals must not only be of the same species but also of a similar age (tadpole, juvenile, or adult), fed and housed in the same way, and sampled at the same time of day and under equal conditions of temperature and humidity as the individual in question.

Inclusion criteria for species presented here are that the data has been derived from at least 10 subjects, determined through known and acceptable methodologies, and contain diagnostically relevant analytes. Information has been standardized following the recommendations of the ASVCP and is presented as mean (reference interval = mean ± 2 standard deviations, or 95%CI) or median (reference interval = 2.5th–97.5th percentile) for normally and non-normally distributed data, respectively. When distribution of the data was not known, normality was assumed. Data based on one to nine individuals can be found in the International Species Information System (ISIS, 2002 edition, www.isis.org) for the American toad as well as for cane toads (*Bufo* [Anaxyrus] *americanus* and *Bu. marinus*, respectively). Intervals provided are for guidance only: interpretation of results must include consideration for the amphibian's clinical presentation, results from conspecifics, and the variability of differing analyzer and laboratory methodologies. Furthermore, one should be cautious about relying on reference values for a different species, even one closely related to the patient's, as this may result in misleading diagnostic information [8].

Species

Modern amphibians comprise over 4000 species and can be divided into three orders, each with a distinct external morphology: Anura (frogs and toads, the stereotypical amphibians), Caudata (salamanders and their aquatic counterparts, the newts, both of lacertilian shape), and Apoda (caecilians, worm-like and often blind) [8].

*A slightly edited and revised version has previously been published as an Invited Review article in *Veterinary Clinical Pathology*, 2017 46(1): 11–33, under the title "Amphibian Clinical Pathology: A Review."

Exotic Animal Laboratory Diagnosis, First Edition. Edited by J. Jill Heatley and Karen E. Russell.

Amphibians are becoming more common as pets, are used as models for numerous infectious and non-infectious diseases in the laboratory, and have declining free-living populations. Free-living amphibian species are often studied as indicators of ecological health. Caudata and Anura, the salamander and frog groups, primarily those few native, exotic, or laboratory species, are most likely to be encountered by the clinician (Table 19.1).

Table 19.1 Amphibian species commonly kept as pets or laboratory subjects.

Family	Common name	Scientific name	IUCN status
Ambystomatidae	Eastern Tiger Salamander	*Ambystoma tigrinum*	LC
	Mexican axolotl	*Ambystoma mexicanum*[a]	CE
	Marbled salamander	*Ambystoma opacum*	LC
	Spotted salamander	*Ambystoma maculatum*	LC
Bombinatoridae	Oriental fire-bellied toad	*Bombina orientalis*	LC
Bufonidae	African toad	*Amietophrynus regularis*	LC
	Cane toad	*Rhinella marina*	LC
	Cururu (Rococo) toad	*Rhinella schneideri*	LC
	Gulf Coast toad	*Incilius nebulifer*	LC
Calyptocephalellidae	Helmeted water toad	*Calyptocephalella gayi*	VU
Ceratophryidae	Argentine horned (Pac-man) frog	*Ceratophrys ornata*	NT
	Brazilian horned frog	*Ceratophrys aurita*	LC
	Cranwell's horned frog	*Ceratophrys cranwelli*	LC
	Pacific horned frog	*Ceratophrys stolzmanni*	VU
Dendrobatidae	Black-legged dart frog	*Phyllobates bicolor*	NT
	Dyeing poison frog	*Dendrobates azureus*	LC
	Golden poison frog	*Phyllobates terribilis*	EN
	Golfodulcean poison dart frog	*Phyllobates vittatus*	EN
	Green& black poison dart frog	*Dendrobates auratus*	LC
	Kõkoé poison dart frog	*Phyllobates aurotaenia*	NT
	Lovely poison frog	*Phyllobates lugubris*	LC
	Strawberry poison dart frog	*Oophaga pumilio*	LC
Eleutherodactylidae	Puerto Rican coquí	*Eleutherodactylus coqui*	LC
Hemiphractidae	Andean marsupial tree frog	*Gastrotheca riobambae*	EN
	Peru marsupial frog	*Gastrotheca peruana*	LC
Hylidae	Black-eyed (Morelet's) tree frog	*Agalychnis moreletii*	CR
	Bleating tree frog	*Phyllobates bicolor*	LC
	Blue Mountains tree frog	*Litoria citropa*	LC
	Broad-palmed frog	*Litoria latopalmata*	LC
	Brown tree frog	*Litoria ewingii*	LC
	Cuban tree frog	*Osteopilus septentrionalis*	LC
	Dainty green tree frog	*Litoria gracilenta*	LC
	Eastern dwarf tree frog	*Litoria fallax*	LC
	Green and golden bell frog	*Litoria aurea*	VU
	Green (White's) tree frog	*Litoria caerulea*	LC
	Growling (southern bell) grass frog	*Litoria raniformis*	EN
	Leaf green tree frog	*Litoria phyllochroa*	LC

Table 19.1 (Continued)

Family	Common name	Scientific name	IUCN status
	Littlejohn's tree frog	*Litoria littlejohni*	LC
	Mimic poison frog	*Ranitomeya [Dendrobates] imitator*	LC
	Splendid tree frog	*Litoria splendid*	LC
	Mountain stream tree frog	*Litoria barringtonensis*	DD
	Peron's tree frog	*Litoria peronii*	LC
	Phantasmal poison frog	*Epipedobates tricolor*	LC
	Red-eyed tree frog (Australia)	*Litoria chloris*	LC
	Red-eyed tree frog (Central America)	*Agalychnis callidryas*	LC
	Striped rocket frog	*Litoria nasuta*	LC
	Tyler's tree frog	*Litoria tyleri*	LC
	Waxy monkey leaf frog	*Phyllomedusa sauvagii*	LC
	Whistling tree frog	*Litoria verreauxii*	LC
	White-lipped tree frog	*Litoria infrafrenata*	LC
Hyperoliidae	Argus reed frog	*Hyperolius argus*	LC
Mantellidae	Black-eared mantella	*Mantella milotympanum*	CE
	Golden mantilla	*Mantella aurantiaca*	CE
Microhylidae	False tomato frog	*Dyscophus guineti*	LC
	Tomato frog	*Dyscophus antongilii*	NT
<u>Myobatrachidae</u>	Corroboree frog	*Pseudophryne corroboree*	CR
	Great barred frog	*Mixophyes fasciolatus*	LC
	Ornate burrowing frog	*Limnodynastes ornatus*	LC
	Spotted grass frog	*Limnodynastes tasmaniensis*	LC
	Striped marsh frog	*Limnodynastes peronii*	LC
	Sudell's frog	*Neobatrachus sudelli*	LC
Pipidae	African clawed frog	*Xenopus laevis*	LC
	African (tropical) clawed frog	*Xenopus tropicalis*	LC
	African (Zaire) dwarf frog	*Hymenochirus boettgeri*	LC
Pyxicephalidae	African bullfrog (pixie frog)	*Pyxicephalus adspersus*	LC
Ranidae	American bullfrog	*Rana [Lithobates] catesbeiana*	LC
	Northern leopard frog	*Rana [Lithobates] pipiens*	LC
	Wood frog	*Rana sylvatica [Lithobates sylvaticus]*	LC
Rhacophoridae	Mossy frog	*Theloderma corticale*	DD
Rhinodermatidae	Darwin's frog	*Rhinoderma darwinii*	VU
Salamandridae	California newt	*Taricha torosa*[a]	LC
	Eastern newt	*Notophthalmus viridescens*	LC
	Lorestan newt	*Neurergus kaiseri*[a]	CR
	Oriental fire-bellied newt	*Cynops orientalis*	LC
	Taricha newts	*Taricha* sp.[a]	LC

Nomenclature includes suggested changes [43] but follows traditional phylogeny (www.amphibiaweb.org). Families known to produce toxic secretions are <u>underlined</u>. International Union for Conservation of Nature (IUCN) status [44]: least concern (LC), vulnerable (VU), near threatened (NT), endangered (EN), critically endangered (CE), data deficient (DD). Tail autotomy [9]: does not occur ([a]).

Amphibian Physiology and Anatomy

Amphibians tolerate wide fluctuations in the osmolality and composition of their plasma. This adaptation is essential to conserve water since amphibian kidneys are incapable of concentrating urine above the osmolality of plasma. In general, larvae and aquatic adults, such as those in the genus *Xenopus*, excrete ammonia (ammonotelia) through the kidneys, skin, and gills, while terrestrial species convert ammonia in the liver into urea (ureotelia) [8, 9]. Adults of some species of tree frogs, such as the waxy monkey tree frog (*Phyllomedusa sauvagii*), more concerned about water conservation, excrete uric acid (uricotelia) as the end product of protein metabolism even if their larvae, which are developing in a more aquatic environment, are ureotelic [8, 9]. Endocrine organs in amphibians vary morphologically but have similar functions to those in other vertebrates. Adrenal glands (also called interrenal glands, given their location) produce three types of steroids in amphibians: aldosterone, corticosterone, and cortisol [8, 9].

Particularly important to frogs and salamanders inhabiting the northern hemisphere are adaptations for winter survival (overwintering or hibernation). Overwintering frogs and salamanders have increased fibrinogen, shock proteins, and glucose-transport proteins, and produce ice-nucleating proteins in the blood to guide ice formation. They also accumulate low-molecular-weight carbohydrates (glycerol or glucose) in tissues and blood and increase plasma osmolality through dehydration. These changes lower the freezing point of tissues and ensure that ice forms in extracellular compartments, sparing cells from shearing damage [10, 11].

Metamorphosis occurs exclusively but not invariably in amphibians and is a complicated process that transforms an aquatic limbless larva into a tetrapod adult. During metamorphosis glucocorticoid and thyroxine levels rise, and shifts in lymphocyte populations are required to develop tolerance to a barrage of new adult antigens and a new definition of self [8, 9]. Changes in plasma biochemistry occur in metamorphosing amphibians. Serum proteins, particularly albumin, increase drastically as metamorphosis progresses in order to increase the osmotic pressure of blood and thus its water-retaining capacity [9].

Amphibian hearts have two atria and one ventricle. The interatrial septum is fenestrated in most salamanders and complete in frogs. Blood from the caudal end of the body will pass through the kidney before entering the postcaval vein, which may affect drugs administered to the caudal aspect of the body [10]. A lack of lymph nodes is balanced by a well-developed lymphatic vasculature which often courses parallel to large blood vessels. As in other vertebrates, lymph drains into the bloodstream [12]. Because of the mixing of arterial and venous blood in the single ventricle, most blood samples from amphibians, even those obtained from the heart, are considered mixed venous samples.

The site of hematopoiesis varies depending on the species. Frogs produce lymphoid, myeloid, and thrombocytic cells in their bone marrow; erythrocytes are only produced in the spleen of adults, while erythropoiesis occurs primarily in the liver of froglets and in the kidneys of tadpoles. Salamanders produce lymphoid and myeloid cells in their bone marrow, and erythroid cells in the spleen. In newts, hematopoiesis occurs exclusively in the liver, kidney, thymus, and spleen [9].

Individuals in captivity have relatively long life spans. Native species like the American toad (*Bu.* [*Anaxyrus*] *americanus*) that would live for 5–10 years in the wild can reach 35 years of age in captivity [13]. Exotic species that are often kept as pets, such as the bumblebee poison dart frog (*Dendrobates leucomelas*) or the fire-bellied toad (*Bombina bombina*), can live for 12 years or more.

Sample Collection and Handling

Plastic or nitrile gloves (without talcum powder), rinsed with dechlorinated water, are best for handling frogs or salamanders [10]. Gloves protect the delicate skin of the patient, and reduce handler exposure to zoonotic pathogens or toxins. Amphibians can carry zoonotic pathogens such as *Salmonella* spp. [14] and *Mycobacterium marinum* [15], and some species produce toxic secretions [16]. Poison frogs, found in South America (some dendrobatidis and bufonids), Madagascar (mantellids), and Australia (myobatrachids), have striking colorations that both mark them as undesirable prey and make them appealing pets (Table 19.1). Poison frogs have specialized skin glands that secrete toxic alkaloids. As poisonous compounds in frogs come from dietary sources, individuals maintained in captivity and fed non-poisonous arthropods will not be able to synthesize the alkaloids [16]. The exception is the corroboree frog (*Pseudophryne corroboree*), which synthesizes toxic alkaloids regardless of the food source [17].

Minimize handling to avoid removing the protective mucus layer that maintains skin moisture, and to decrease temperature exchange between the handler and the amphibian patient. Amphibians are poikilotherms (ectotherms) and rely on a combination of environmental temperature, heat or cold-seeking behavior, peripheral vascular control, and color changes to maintain their body temperature. An amphibian's temperature is dependent on the immediate environment and has significant influence on hematologic and biochemical parameters. Thus, increasing the patient's body temperature may alter test results in the sample collected [8]. Collect samples from animals kept at their optimum

Table 19.2 Ambient temperature gradients recommended for amphibians based on the type of species and habitat [8].

		Temperature (°C)	
Type of species	Habitat type	Min	Max
Terrestrial amphibians	Tropical lowland	24	30
	Tropical montane	18	24
	Subtropical	21	27
	Temperate (winter hibernation)	18 (10)	24 (16)
Aquatic amphibians (includes larvae of terrestrial species)	Tropical lowland	24	30
	Tropical montane	18	24
	Subtropical	21	27
	Temperate, stream	16	21
	Temperate, pond (Winter hibernation)	18 (9)	24 (15)

temperature range, which depends on the species, season, and life stage (Table 19.2).

Clinical examination and observation of the patient before sample collection should include assessing posture, blink reflex (touch the eyes gently), righting reflex (place patient on its back and watch it right itself), and withdrawal reflex (extend the limbs and watch their retraction) [8]. Loss of any of these reflexes or abnormal posture may indicate serious illness and influence your decision to take a blood sample and the volume that should be collected [18]. Always calculate the volume of blood that can be safely drawn from of a frog or salamander to avoid causing metabolic disturbances, morbidity, or mortality. Minimal total blood volumes (TBVs) are 7%–10% of the body weight in terrestrial amphibians and 13%–25% in aquatic ones [18] (Figure 19.1). No more than 5%–10% of the TBV should be drawn: usually only 5% from sick individuals and up to 10% from healthy ones (safe volume to draw, SVD).

Choice of equipment and technique of blood collection from frogs, salamanders, or tadpoles depends on the size of the animal and its anatomical characteristics. Specifics for size and vein approach are given below in each section. Generally, one chooses 0.3–3 ml syringes and 27–23 gauge (g.) needles. Superficial topical anesthetics such as lidocaine or benzocaine creams or gels (EMLA™ cream or Orajel™) may be used. Lithium or ammonium heparin is the preferred anticoagulant for amphibians, unless the blood is intended for bacterial culture. One may flush the needle and syringe with the liquid solution or use heparinized capillary tubes, such as Fisherbrand® Microhematocrit (Fisher Scientific Cat. no. 22-362-566) 75-mm-long size capillary tubes, (*not to be confused with* other shorter microhematocrit tubes) or green-cap Microtainer® collection tubes (BD Cat. no. 365965, coated with dry lithium heparin).

Cardiocentesis

Cardiac puncture can be used in any species, but this invasive procedure has potential life-threatening complications such as cardiac standstill, atrial fibrillation, and pericardial tamponade. Anesthesia is necessary and may be achieved by submerging the amphibian in a buffered solution of 0.02%–0.1% (0.2–1 g/l) tricaine methanesulfonate (MS222), or a solution of benzocaine (Orajel™, or similar gels) at 0.005%–0.01% for larvae and 0.02%–0.03% for adults. Rinsing the patient with clean dechlorinated water after the procedure is finished will allow excretion of the MS222 and is necessary for patient recovery if benzocaine is used. Place the anesthetized tadpole, frog, or salamander on its back on a moist paper towel; the cardiac pulse is either observed or detected using a Doppler probe placed near the manubrium. A small 25 or 27 g. needle is inserted into the ventricle, at a 45°–60° angle to the skin, and blood is drawn either by placing a capillary tube in the hub of the needle or by gently aspirating with a 0.3, 1, or 3 ml syringe [8, 18]. When successfully employed, cardiocentesis is the collection method most likely to yield the largest volume of blood, but it is not without its disadvantages. The amphibian heart is easily displaced within the coelomic cavity, making it a moving target. Furthermore, the bi-lobulated liver wraps tightly around the heart and may be punctured during cardiocentesis. Although the use of MS222 has been suggested to interfere with bacterial culture from samples taken under anesthesia [19], this is a misconception based on a laboratory study [20] that is irrelevant to routine bacterial cultures from animal samples.

Facial Vein

The facial and musculocutaneous veins can be sampled in ranid frogs and those with similar cranial anatomy, such as tree frogs and toads. The facial vein courses parallel to the upper jaw toward the commissure of the mouth, becoming the musculocutaneous vein as it passes the tympanum. Holding the frog in one hand to expose only the head, quickly insert and withdraw a small-caliber needle through the skin between the upper jawline and the rostral side of the tympanum, in the slightly sunken triangle formed by the back of the eye, the front of the tympanum, and the maxillary bone (Figure 19.2). Insertion follows a 30° angle to the skin, in a rostrocaudal direction to access the facial vein, or in the opposite direction to access the musculocutaneous vein. This external collection method punctures the vein and releases blood onto the skin surface for collection with a capillary tube [21]. Needles should be 30 g. for frogs weighing under 25 g, and 25–27 g. for larger frogs. After collection, gentle pressure over the area achieves hemostasis. The area may be disinfected using the antiseptic spray Bactine® before or after blood collection. Depending on sampling

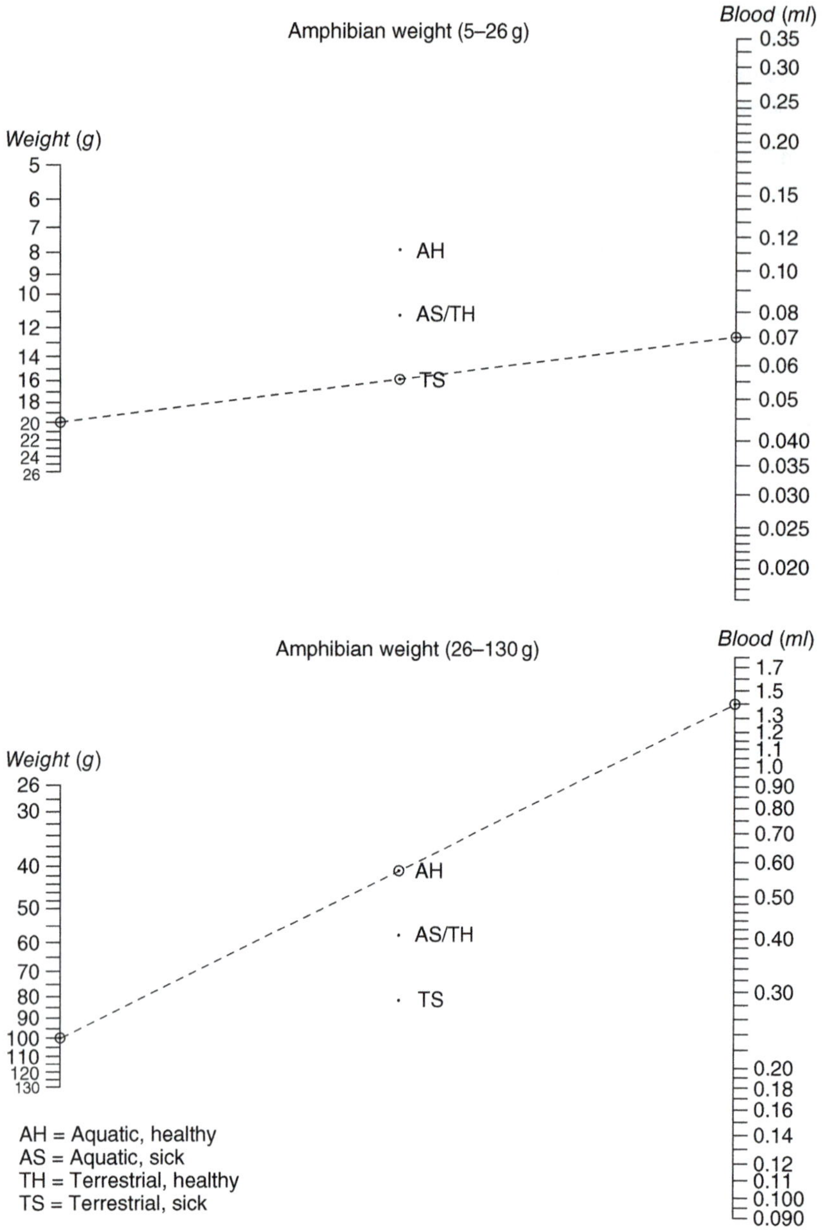

Figure 19.1 Normograph to calculate blood volume that can be drawn from an amphibian. Draw a line from the left column (body weight) through the type of species and health status (AH = aquatic healthy, AS = aquatic sick, TH = terrestrial healthy, TS = terrestrial sick): the right column indicates the volume that can be drawn safely. Conservatively, the graph is based on total blood volumes (TBVs) of 14% and 7% of body weight for aquatic and terrestrial species, respectively; safe volumes to draw are 5% and 10% from sick and healthy animals, respectively.

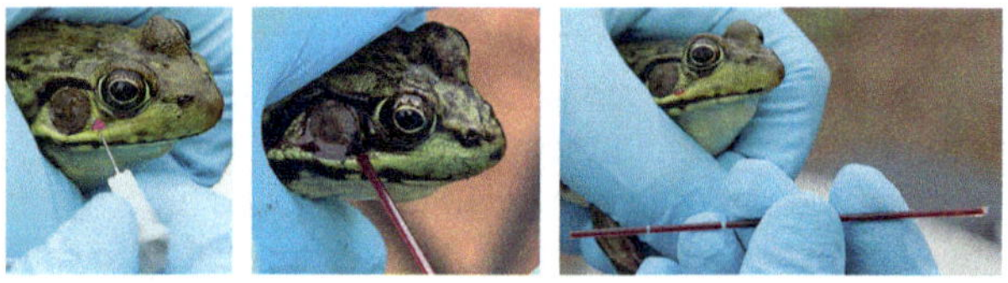

Figure 19.2 Facial vein venipuncture. Area where 27–30 g. needle should be quickly inserted and withdrawn is marked in pink (left). Collection with a heparinized capillary tube is aided by tilting the capillary toward the ground (center). Hemostasis is quickly achieved after a few seconds of gentle pressure in the area (right).

conditions, 0.02–0.07 ml of blood (the latter loosely corresponding to the volume collected in one ammonium heparin capillary tube, Fisherbrand) can be collected from small frogs; in large frogs, the puncture will yield larger volumes. Tilting the capillary tube earthward uses gravity to facilitate blood flow and increases the speed of collection and the blood volume obtained. Warmer environmental temperatures facilitate blood flow. This technique does not require anesthesia and may be applied repeatedly, barring excessive sampling volumes.

Femoral and Abdominal Veins

Venipuncture of the femoral and ventral abdominal veins can be performed on relatively large amphibians. The veins should be visible through the skin unless the individual is darkly pigmented, in which case transillumination can facilitate visualization. Needles should be 27–30 g., depending on the size of the animal. While syringes can range from 0.3 to 3 ml, avoid aggressive aspiration and vessel collapse. The technique cannot be used in small individuals. As the ventral abdominal vein runs parallel to lymphatic vessels, lymph contamination may lead to a false interpretation of anemia, lymphocytosis, or hypercalcemia [8].

Lingual Venous Plexus

The lingual venous plexus may be accessed in most frogs over 25 g, but cannot be used in species with unsuitable tongue anatomy such as the pipid frogs, for example, African clawed frogs, *Xenopus* spp. Carefully open the mouth with a rigid but smooth instrument, such as a rubber spatula. Draw the tongue forward to expose the lingual venous plexus (Figure 19.3). Puncture the plexus with a 25- or 27 g. needle, and collect the blood oozing out with a capillary tube [8]. Releasing the tongue and allowing the frog to close its mouth usually suffices to stop the bleeding. The contamination of the sample with saliva, a major disadvantage of this technique, can be reduced by gently rubbing the lingual surface with a cotton swab prior to sampling. This method, however, is cumbersome for the practitioner and uncomfortable for the frog.

Ventral Caudal Vein

Venipuncture of the ventral caudal tail vein, which courses immediately beneath the vertebrae, is practical for use in salamanders and newts. For salamanders weighing less than 80 g, a 27 g. needle is needed; in salamanders over 80 g, 25 g. needles may be used [8]. Blood is slowly drawn into a 0.3–1 ml syringe. At least two thirds of the Plethodontidae family, which includes most wild salamanders from northeastern North America, are capable of autotomy. Autotomy is the ability to willfully detach the tail at predetermined zones of breakage (cleavage points), so that if a salamander is caught by it, or if it feels threatened or injured, it may shed its tail to facilitate escape and therefore predation [9]. The tail may fully or completely regenerate, but the coloration and internal structure may differ from the original. Therefore, one must take care when using the technique on wild-caught North American salamanders as they may lose their tail during sampling. The Mexican axolotl (*Ambystoma mexicanum*), a common pet species, does not undergo tail autotomy [9].

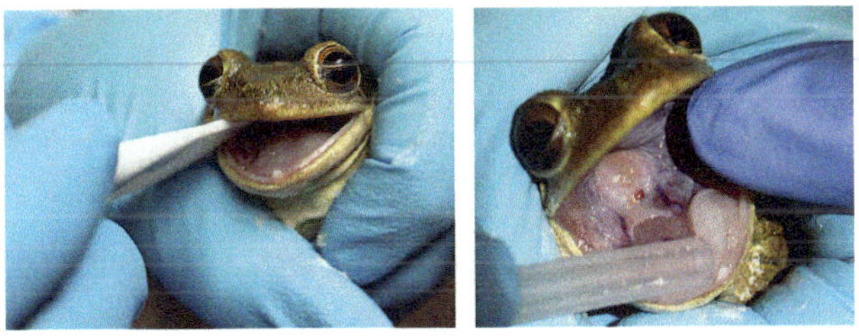

Figure 19.3 Lingual plexus venipuncture. Gently open the mouth of the frog with a soft instrument, such as a rubber spatula (left). Bringing the tongue forward, the venus plexi behind and beneath the tongue are exposed (right) and may be punctured with a 27 g. needle to collect blood with a capillary tube.

Appendage Amputation

Tail clipping is used in salamanders and tadpoles; toe clipping is used in frogs. These techniques are more commonly used in field studies than in a clinical setting and are the least advisable options for blood collection. The procedures are painful, so the use of local anesthetic, such as 2% lidocaine, is recommended. Application of an antiseptic, such as Bactine, may prevent secondary bacterial infections. If toe clipping is performed, amputation should occur at the interphalangeal joint, no more than one digit should be removed per limb, and the digit chosen must not be involved in normal behavior of the species (burrowing, climbing, amplexus, nest excavation, or propulsion) to avoid endangering the viability of wild populations [8]. Tail and toe clipping will result in short- or long-term disfiguration. Furthermore, and perhaps more importantly, toe clipping provides either a small volume of blood or, often, none at all.

Urine Collection

Collection of urine from amphibians is dependent on chance. Although most species have a small urinary bladder, catheterization or cystocentesis are not usually performed [8]. Some individuals will urinate when they are captured or initially handled, but most will not, particularly if they have spent time in a transport container before being handled. Standard urinalysis tests (specific gravity/density, urea, ammonia, uric acid, etc.) can be run in amphibian samples to varying relevance. For instance, specific gravity will not indicate renal function but will reflect plasma density (see urinalysis section) [8, 9]. Urinalysis should be performed within a few hours of collection for best results.

Sample Handling

Given the small size of most amphibians, unless blood collection is terminal, only small sample volumes may be obtained. However, small amounts will suffice to obtain

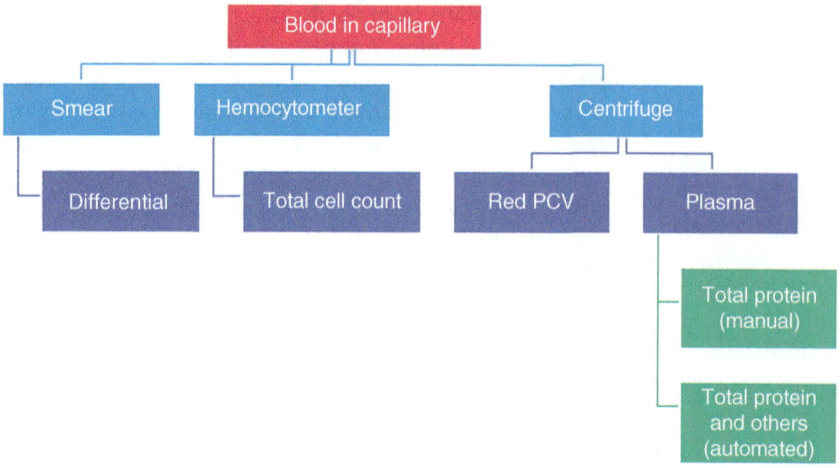

Figure 19.4 Stepwise algorithm to maximize diagnostic information obtained from amphibian blood samples.

a complete blood cell count (CBC), make a blood smear for a differential count, evaluate morphology and detect hemoparasites, determine the red packed-cell volume (PCV), and measure total protein and other select chemical analytes. Prioritization of the sample depends on the analysis desired, but the best use of a small blood sample (0.07 ml or less) is to prepare a blood smear, determine the CBC count, PCV, and total protein. More voluminous samples allow for plasma biochemistry analysis. Blood can be collected directly into a capillary tube or into a syringe and then transferred to heparinized capillary tube(s) or Microtainer(s) depending upon the volume.

One should prioritize analyses to derive the most diagnostic data, particularly from small samples (Figure 19.4). First, use a small drop from the heparinized capillary tube (Fisherbrand) or syringe immediately after collection to make a blood smear. Actively air-dry the blood smear and fix or stain (Wright-Giemsa or Diff-Quik) within 24–48 h for best results. Then, transfer the exact amount of blood necessary for a CBC count (generally 10–25 µl) into a purpose-specific micropipette, such as the discontinued Unopette® or the currently available Bryopette®, to be mixed with pre-measured dye, such as a Natt-Herrick solution (Figure 19.5). Finally, plug the capillary tube and centrifuge it to measure erythrocyte PCV, and separate plasma to measure total solids (protein) with a refractometer. If more than one capillary tube is collected, pool the plasma together, skip the refractometer, and use an automated benchtop analyzer for expanded biochemical analysis. Alternatively, plasma can be shipped to a diagnostic laboratory, where a more accurate total protein measurement can be obtained, and additional analytes, such as urea, albumin, globulins, cholesterol, triglycerides, and plasma enzymes, can be measured. Diagnostic laboratories have equipment capable of processing minute amounts of plasma but need to be contacted prior to shipping to ensure that the amount submitted is sufficient.

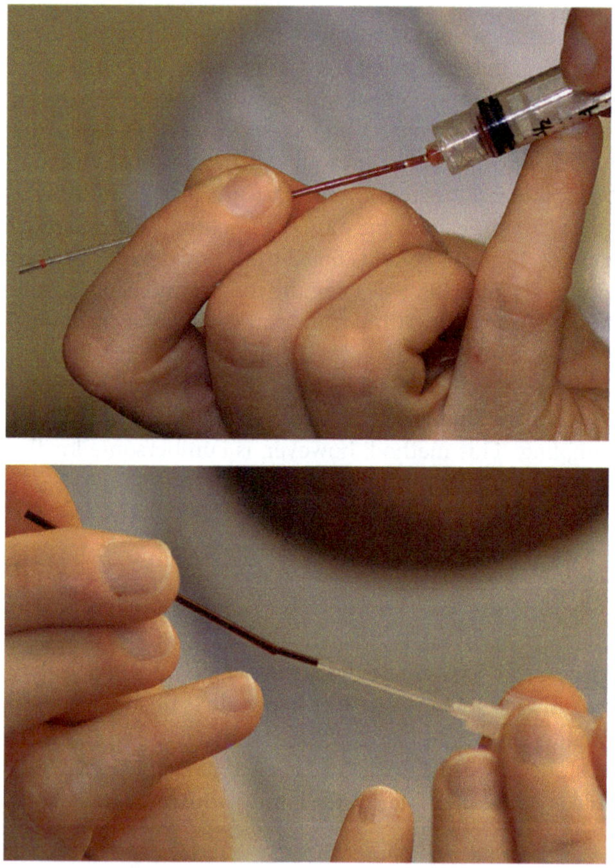

Figure 19.5 Capillary action allows for transfer of blood from syringe to heparinized capillary tube (top) and from capillary tube to Unopette® (bottom) or to any other pipette capable of measuring exactly a 20µl volume to be used for the blood cell count.

Complete Blood Cell Count (CBC) (Tables 19.3 and 19.4)

Cell Counting

Hemocytometry remains the most accurate method available for the amphibian complete blood count (including white blood cell, red blood cell, and thrombocyte

Table 19.3 Hematologic reference intervals for select anuran species.

Analyte (abbreviation)	Units, SI Conventional	American bullfrog (*Rana catesbeiana*) [2] Ħ	Northern leopard frog (*R. pipiens*) [4] ›	Wood frog (*R. sylvatica*) [23]	African clawed frog (*Xenopus laevis*) [6] Ħ	African (tropical) clawed frog (*Xenopus tropicalis*) [24] Ħ	Sapito de jardín (*Bufo* [*Rhinella*] *fernandezae*) [45] ›	Green (White's) tree frog (*Litoria caerulea*) [25] ›	White-lipped tree frog (*L. infrafrenata*) [25] ›
Data type				Mean (reference interval)^a				Median (reference Interval)^b	
Sample size		302	12–56	26–40	10	33–41	17	80	66
WBC	$\times10^9$/l $\times10^3$/μl	20.5 (11.3–29.7)	5.5 (0.7–10.3)	7.65 (2.2–13.1)	4.59 (2.92–9.16)	20.7 (11.5–36.0)^b	4.5 (1.18–7.82)	15.9 (6.7–34.9)	21 (6.5–47.9)
Absolute neutrophils	$\times10^9$/l $\times10^3$/μl			0.46 (0–0.9)		11.8 (5.7–26.7)^b	0.79 (0.43–1.15)	3.3 (0.9–7.7)	4.2 (0.6–17.1)
Relative neutrophils	%	60.9 (36.1–85.7)	26.5 (3.7–49.3)	6.83 (0.4–13.3)	26.5 (7.5–45.5)	54.7 (26.7–82.7)	19 (0–45.8)	21.5 (7–42)	20 (5–50.3)
Absolute eosinophils	$\times10^9$/l $\times10^3$/μl			0.09 (0–0.25)^b		0.2 (0–1.0)^b	0.19 (0.11–0.27)	0.4 (0–3.1)	0 (0–2)
Relative eosinophils	%	5.8 (2.6–9)	7.3 (3.1–11.5)	1.55 (0–4.5)^b	1.2 (0–5)	1.2(0–4.0)^b	5 (0–13.6)	2 (0–11)	0 (0–10.6)
Absolute basophils	$\times10^9$/l $\times10^3$/μl			0.8 (0.1–1.5)		0.4 (0–1.1)^b	1.34 (0.78–1.9)	0 (0–1.1)	0 (0–4)
Relative basophils	%	3.5 (1.1–5.9)	4.4 (0–10.6)	10.65 (5.9–14.8)^b	40.5 (16.5–64.5)	2.2 (0–7.0)^b	32 (0–76.5)	0 (0–7)	0 (0–31)
Absolute lymphocytes	$\times10^9$/l $\times10^3$/μl			5.76 (1.3–10.2)		7.2 (2.6–11.7)	1.71 (1.15–2.27)	10.7 (3.9–27.1)	12.2 (3.2–34.7)
Relative lymphocytes	%	26.8 (17–36.6)	53.4 (23.8–83)	76.85 (63.7–90.0)	30.1 (6.3–53.9)	37.2 (11.8–60.7)	41 (0–82.68)	67.5 (40.2–88)	70 (33.4–85)
Absolute monocytes	$\times10^9$/l $\times10^3$/μl			0.13 (0–0.35)^b		1.0 (0.2–2.5)^b	0.01 (0–0.03)	1.3 (0.3–4.7)	1.1 (0.1–6.9)
Relative monocytes	%	2.9 (0.7–5.1)	11 (1.4–20.6)	1.64 (0–3.4)	1.6 (0–4)	4.7 (1.0–10.0)^b	1 (0–2.52)	7 (2–18)	6 (1–21.3)
RBC	$\times10^{12}$/l $\times10^6$/μl	0.42 (* 1.82)	0.32 (0.16–0.48)	0.41 (0.25–0.57)	0.75 (0.53–1.09)	1.5 (1.0–2.0)	0.505 (0.24–0.76)	0.74 (0.42–1.02)	0.72 (0.4–1.12)
Red packed-cell volume (PCV)	%	30.1 (19.3–40.9)		29.5 (18.6–40.5)		40 8 (27.3–54.4)		38 (23–48)	30 (19.4–48.6)
Hemoglobin	g/l g/dl	68 (38.4–97.6) 6.8 (3.84–9.76)	67.5 (27.5–107.5) 6.75 (2.75–10.75)				91.8 (35.8–147.8) 9.18 (3.58–14.78)	93 (41–126) 9.3 (4.1–12.6)	70 (33–117) 7 (3.3–11.7)
Hematocrit (Ht)	%		24.65 (5.51–43.79)				27.37 (12.01–42.73)		
Thrombocytes	$\times10^9$ /l $\times10^3$ /μl		7.3 (1.1–13.5)	8.3 (1.3–15.2)	18.52 (12–24.88)	14.6 (6.8–22.5)	4.81 (0–15.1)	27.3 (13.3–49.1)	31.9 (20–62.5)
Blood pH			7.36 (7.06–7.66)						

Key: Free-living › Captive Ħ.
Reference interval = 95%CI^a or 2.5th–97.5th percentile^b distribution of original data: normal (Rc, Xt), non-normal (Rf, Lc, Li, Xt^b), unknown (Rp, Xl). Values below zero or incompatible with life are reported as 0 and *, respectively.

Table 19.4 Hematologic reference intervals for select Caudata species.

Analyte (abbreviation)	Units, SI Conventional	Japanese newt (*Cynops pyrrhogaster*) [46] ⅄	Eastern hellbender (*Cryptobranchus alleganiensis alleganiensis*) [3] ⅄	Ozark hellbender (*C. a. bishopi*) [3] ⅄
Sample size		23	37–38	42
WBC	$\times 10^9$ /l $\times 10^3$ /μl		3.9 (2.7–5.1)	4.6 (3.7–5.5)
Relative neutrophils[h]	%	28 (3.06–52.94)	30.3 (21.3–39.2)	35.1 (29.2–41.1)
Relative eosinophils	%	4 (0–10.72)	4.1 (1–7.3)	10.9 (8.8–13)
Relative basophils	%	57 (26.3–87.7)	6.9 (4.3–9.4)	4.3 (2.7–6)
Relative lymphocytes	%	3 (0–6.84)	54.6 (43.7–65.6)	49.3 (41.8–56.8)
Relative monocytes	%	6 (0–15.58)	1.1 (0–2.3)	0.6 (0–1.3)
RBC	$\times 10^{12}$ /l $\times 10^6$ /μl	2.28 (0–5.1)		
Hematocrit (Ht)	%	40 (21.78–58.22)	36.1 (31.7–40.6)	44.3 (41.3–47.4)
Thrombocytes	$\times 10^9$ /l $\times 10^3$ /μl	Not identified or counted	Clumped, not counted	Clumped, not counted

All data reported as mean (reference interval = 95%CI) and calculated from a single population (Cp) or various populations weighted by sample size (Caa, Cab). Distribution of original data: normal (Caa, Cab), unknown (Cp). Values below zero are reported as 0.
Key: Free-living ⅄, Captive Ħ.

determinations), as automated analyzers cannot differentiate between amphibian erythrocytes, leukocytes, and thrombocytes. However, this method is time consuming (20–30 min to complete counts of the three blood cell types) and requires experience and skill, so it is avoided by all but the most resolute clinicians and researchers. Hemocytometry provides a better estimate than indirect methods from back-calculations on blood smears and is the appropriate way to establish reference intervals for a species. Natt-Herrick's solution can be stored in refrigeration for up to 2 years. The solution can be purchased from a laboratory or university, or from a commercial provider in pre-measured pipetters.

Distinguishing between erythrocytes, leukocytes, and thrombocytes of the amphibian patient can be challenging. Scanning the stained blood smear of the amphibian in question is helpful to gauge the shape and size of the species' blood cells before beginning the hemocytometer count. Although cell counting is best performed soon after collection, Natt-Herrick's solution contains formalin, so it maintains cellular integrity for several days, even months [24]. Distinguishing cell types, however, becomes difficult in older samples as color differences are lost and leukocytes tend to aggregate and may thus be confused with thrombocytes. Aggregation or clumping of leukocytes will also make white blood cell counts less accurate.

Published CBCs in amphibians are rare; most rely on indirect determinations from smears rather than on hemocytometer counts and follow different sampling and analyzing techniques, so that their value to diagnostic investigation is minimal. Intentional or unwitting inclusion of thrombocytes when reporting white blood cells (WBC) counts further limits validity of some reports. The clinician should be wary of reports that do not mention thrombocytes specifically, as these cells could have been mistakenly counted as lymphocytes. Lacking specific information regarding a particular amphibian species, interpretation of abnormalities usually follows generalities established for related species or, more frequently, other vertebrates. This extrapolation makes assumptions that are unproved in amphibians. The CBC count and differential count from a conspecific of similar age and maintained at equal environmental conditions will be helpful in the interpretation of results from a particular individual.

Red Blood Cells (RBCs)

Amphibian erythrocytes (red blood cells, RBC) vary in size depending on the species but are ovoid and generally larger than those found in most other vertebrates [8, 22]. Amphibian erythrocytes are nucleated, both in larvae and adults, except in a few species of salamanders, such as the slender salamanders of the genus *Batrachoseps*, where large proportions are anucleated [8]. Erythrocytes become smaller and reduce their endoplasmic reticulum throughout metamorphosis. When using a Natt-Herrick solution, erythrocytes are commonly the largest cells, ovoid, with a pale staining cytoplasm and slightly darker nucleus; immature erythrocytes have a slightly darker cytoplasm, are smaller and may be bit rounder, but they usually retain their ovoid shape and are larger than leukocytes or thrombocytes (Figure 19.6).

RBCs are counted via hemocytometry or estimated via PCV. Cell morphology and proportional abnormalities in the RBCs, such as conspicuously immature erythrocytes (slightly smaller than other RBCs and with bluer cytoplasm) (Figure 19.8), and circulating intra- or extracellular pathogens can be identified through the microscopic examination of the blood smear.

RBC counts vary among amphibian species, mainly because of differences in erythrocyte size, so values for one species are of little use as a reference for another. Because of this difference in size, the PCV of two different species may be similar, while their RBC counts are different. For instance, RBCs in wood frogs (*Rana sylvatica* or *Lithobates sylvaticus*) are roughly twice as large as those from African (tropical) clawed frogs (*Xenopus tropicalis*) so that even if their PCV is similar (30% (19–41) vs. 41% (27–54), respectively) their actual RBC numbers are quite different (0.4 (0.3–0.6) and 1.5 (1–2) $\times 10^{12}\,l^{-1}$, respectively) [23, 24]. A drop in the PCV, probably along with a reduced RBC count and an increase in the percentage of immature erythrocytes, has been found in intense infections with intraerythrocytic parasites, such as *Hepatozoon* spp., in wild green frogs, *Rana* [*Lithobates*] *clamitans* (Fielding et al., manuscript in preparation) and with unidentified hemogregarines in Australian tree frogs, *Litoria caerulea* and *Litoria infrafrenata* [25]. In American bullfrogs (*Rana* [*Lithobates*] *catesbeiana*) PCV tends to increase as the environmental temperature decreases in the winter [26].

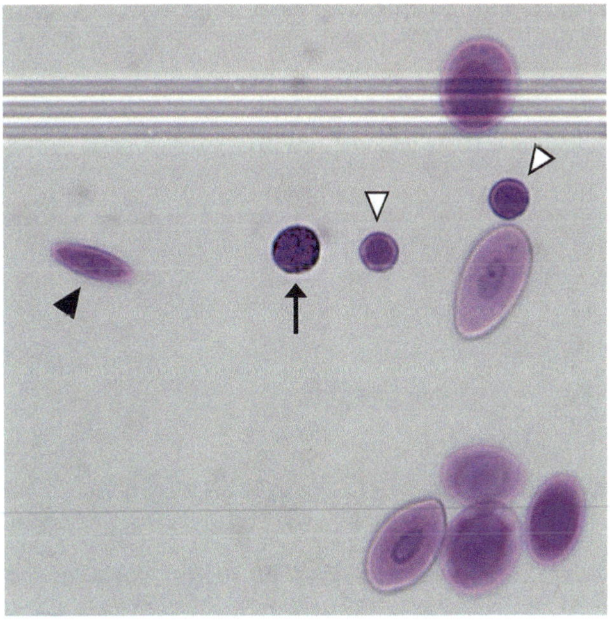

Figure 19.6 Blood cells in hemocytometer (Neubauer) chamber stained with Natt-Herrick's solution. Erythrocytes (largest, unmarked cells), leukocyte with dark granules (arrow), ovoid thrombocyte (black arrowhead), and challenging cells (white arrowheads) that require fine adjustments of the microscope focus plane to identify: dark blue cytoplasm indicates a leukocyte, pale cytoplasm indicates a thrombocyte. Lines across the field mark the border of the chamber, 40×.

Thrombocytes

Amphibian thrombocytes are often ovoid, occasionally round, and have a dark nucleus. Unlike lymphocytes, however, chromatin in thrombocytes is not randomly clumped but condensed at the center of the nucleus, and their cytoplasmic edges are seldom smooth (Figure 19.7). With Natt and Herrick's stain, thrombocytes are ovoid or round, smaller than the erythrocytes, and with a pale blue cytoplasm lighter than that of the leukocytes (Figure 19.6). Amphibian thrombocytes are analogous to mammalian platelets. Thrombocytes are calculated via hemocytometer counting; estimation using only direct examination of the blood smear is usually impeded by clumping and uneven distribution.

White Blood Cells (WBCs)

Leukocytes (WBCs) in amphibians include lymphocytes, monocytes, eosinophils, basophils, and neutrophils or heterophils (Figure 19.7) [22]. As neither heterophils nor neutrophils contain visible cytoplasmic granules in images recorded for amphibian species, this chapter will use the term neutrophil. Leukocytes are round, with less cytoplasm than erythrocytes or thrombocytes, that stains dark blue to black and sometimes include dark granules when stained with Natt and Herrick's solution (Figure 19.6). WBC numbers are calculated via hemocytometry. A stained smear is used to examine and differentiate each type of blood cell, determine the proportion of each type and, by relating that proportion to the WBC count obtained with the hemocytometer, establish the absolute numbers of each type of leukocyte. Morphology and proportional abnormalities in the blood cells, such as toxic change or the presence of atypical lymphocytes

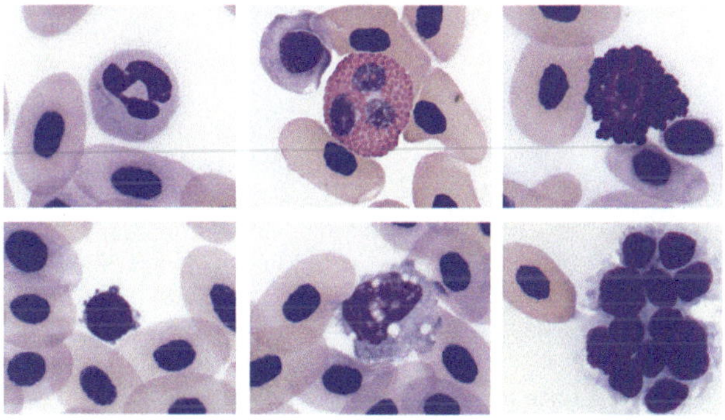

Figure 19.7 Leukocytes and thrombocytes of the green frog (*Rana* [*Lithobates*] *clamitans*). Clockwise from top left: neutrophils, eosinophil, basophil, thrombocytes (clumped), monocyte, and lymphocyte. Wright-Giemsa stain, 100×.

and circulating intra- or extracellular pathogens, can be identified through examination of the blood smear. Atypical cells, often difficult to categorize, are not uncommon in amphibian smears (Figures 19.8 and 19.9). Leukocytes in amphibians are thought to have similar inflammatory and immune functions as those in other vertebrates, but published information on WBC counts is scattered and fragmented [8, 9].

Attribution of specific significance to parameters outside reference intervals is challenging. Metamorphosis alters amphibian metabolism, and the elevated levels of glucocorticoids required may result in neutrophilia and lymphocytopenia [8, 9]. However, the precise effects of metamorphosis on the numbers or proportions of circulating leukocytes are poorly described and understood, due to varying research methodologies among researchers and small numbers of animals per study. Similarly, an increase in the N:L (neutrophil:lymphocyte) ratio can be associated with increased plasma cortisol, and thus is considered an indicator of stress [27]. The N:L ratio is, however, nonspecific and needs to be compared to an N:L ratio from conspecifics of the same age, sex, and environmental conditions. A small study in American bullfrog tadpoles suffering from chytridiomycosis-associated depigmentation of oral tissues suggests that severely affected animals may have a higher proportion of neutrophils than those with mild lesions [28]. In reptiles, blue-gray intracytoplasmic viral inclusions have been reported in circulating leukocytes infected with ranavirus [29], while immunohistochemical staining has detected virus in circulating lymphocytes of European common frogs, *Rana temporaria* [30]. In wood frogs experimentally infected with Frog virus 3 (*Ranavirus* sp.), bright pink-red intracytoplasmic inclusions developed in circulating leukocytes [23].

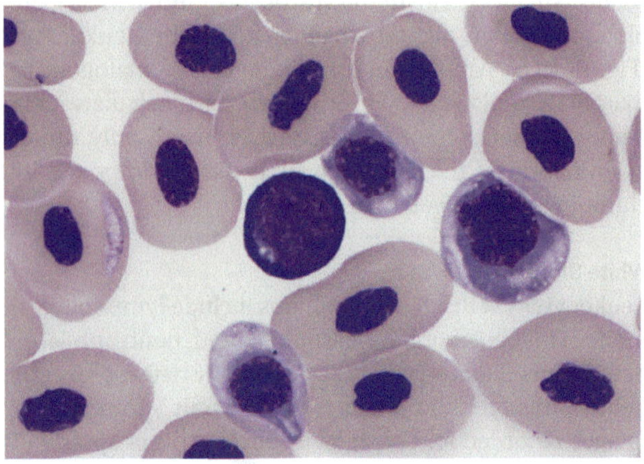

Figure 19.8 Blood smear from a green frog (*Rana [Lithobates] clamitans*). Among the three immature erythrocytes (blue-staining cytoplasm), there is an atypical cell with a generous round nucleus and little deep blue cytoplasm which may be an activate lymphocyte or an erythrocyte in an early stage in development. Wright-Giemsa stain, 100×.

Hemoparasites

Hemoparasites are detected via direct examination of the dried stained blood smear or via PCR. Hemoparasites found on examination of amphibian blood smears include, but are not restricted to, intraerythrocytic merozoites of *Hepatozoon* sp., and various stages of *Trypanosoma* spp. in the plasma (Figure 19.10). These parasites can be found in wild-caught individuals or captive-bred colonies with outdoor access. Frogs acquire

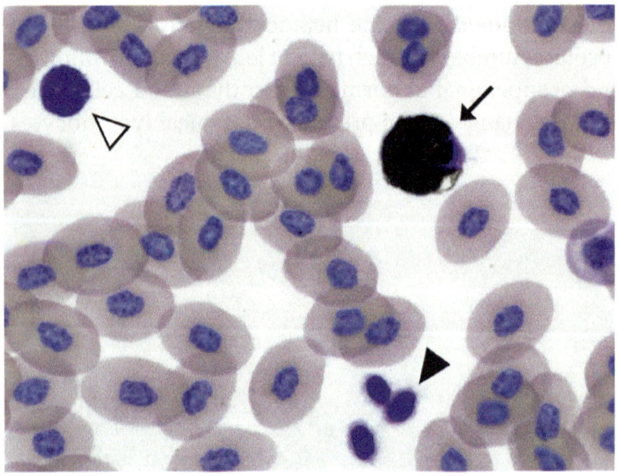

Figure 19.9 Cuban tree frog (*Osteopilus septentrionalis*), blood cell with a cytoplasm full of fine black (melanin) granules (arrow). Thrombocytes are small and ovoid, with raggedy cytoplasmic edges and often cluster together (black arrowhead); lymphocytes are round, slightly larger, with deep blue cytoplasm and clumped nuclear chromatin. Wright-Giemsa stain, 100×.

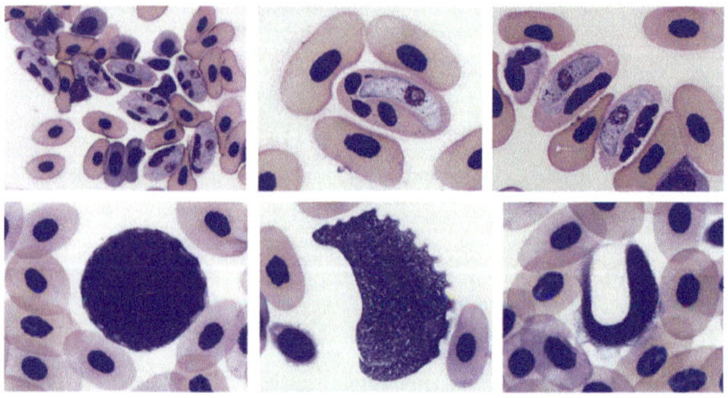

Figure 19.10 Hemoparasites of green frogs (*Rana [Lithobates] clamitans*). Gamonts of *Hepatozoon* sp. in the cytoplasm of erythrocytes: intense infection accompanied by numerous immature erythrocytes with blue cytoplasm (top left); nuclear fragmentation (top middle and right) associated with *H. clamatae* infection; concurrent infection with *H. clamatae* and *H. catesbianae*. The latter does not fragment the nucleus (top right). *Trypanosoma* sp. stages in infected frogs: spherical form (bottom left) and trypomastigote stages with a visible undulating membrane (middle and right bottom). Wright-Giemsa stain, 40× (top left) and 100×.

Hepatozoon spp. infections solely by feeding on infected *Culex* spp. mosquitoes, while the mosquitoes must bite infected individuals to become vectors [31]. Interestingly, some frog trypanosomes remain in the renal vasculature during the night and circulate systemically only during the daytime: to detect infection, it is best to sample at mid-day [32]. Infection with *Trypanosoma* spp. has not been linked to clinical disease.

Biochemical Panel

Most biochemical tests, including those for all analytes mentioned in this section, may be run on plasma as well as serum, so blood collected for hematology with a heparinized syringe or capillary tube may also be used for biochemistry panels. The normal color of amphibian plasma ranges from clear to yellow or even blue, as in the case of the Japanese giant salamander, *Andrias japonicus*, and the white-lipped tree frog, *L. infrafrenata* [8, 25]. Plasma should be separated immediately after centrifugation and then kept refrigerated or frozen until processed or shipped to a diagnostic laboratory. Ideally, reference intervals should be determined from conspecifics not only of similar age and environment, but also sampled and tested by the same method, as lack of consistency in methodology diminishes the validity of reference intervals. Biochemical panels have been determined for only few amphibian species (Tables 19.5 and 19.6). Patchy information is available on alterations in other species or groups. Almost nothing is known of the diagnostic significance of hepatic, pancreatic, muscular, or cardiac enzymes in amphibian blood.

Freeze-tolerant overwintering amphibians such as wood frogs (*Rana sylvatica* [*L. sylvaticus*]), spring peepers (*Pseudacris* [*Hyla*] *crucifer*) and western chorus frogs (*Pseudacris triseriata*), accumulate low-molecular-weight carbohydrates (glucose or, less frequently, glycerol) in tissues and blood [11], and thus have a physiologic glucosuria if sampled soon after thawing or during frozen hibernation. In wood frogs that have recently thawed (1 h) after hibernation, blood glucose levels can be >400 mmol/l (>7000 mg/dl), while glucose in individuals that have not undergone freezing is only around 1.5 mmol/l (27 mg/dl). In another freeze-tolerant species, the gray tree frog (*Hyla versicolor*), response is dependent on age: glucose levels of adults remain unchanged during freezing, while glycerol concentrations increase from 6.8 to 423 mmol/l; immature gray tree frogs have a mild increase in both glycerol (0.1–16.3 mmol/l) and glucose (1.46–25.9 mmol/l) [11].

Captive Cuban tree frogs (*Osteopilus septentrionalis*) are prone to obesity and corneal lipidosis, which are associated with marked increases in serum cholesterol and triglycerides. Cuban tree frogs affected with corneal lipidosis have cholesterol levels averaging 27.5 mmol/l or 1062 mg/dl, while cholesterol in wild-caught, non-affected frogs averages 3.86 (0–8.26, 95%CI) mmol/l or 149 (0–319, 95%CI) mg/dl [33]. Australian green tree frogs, also known as White's tree frogs (*L. caerulea*), are also prone to obesity and corneal lipidosis [8], but no information regarding the cholesterol levels of affected or non-affected individuals is available.

Renal function and/or hydration status can be evaluated through measurement of nitrogen waste products in plasma. One must measure the appropriate form of nitrogen, remembering that the type of waste product in amphibians depends on species-specific adaptations to native environments: ammonia for aquatic adults and larvae (ammonotelic), urea for adult terrestrial amphibians (ureotelic), and uric acid for some tree frogs (uricotelic) [8, 9].

Electrolytes, Osmolality, and Blood Gases

Osmolality, the concentration of active particles in an aqueous solution, in this case serum or plasma, is usually closely associated with the hydration state and the concentration of the most diagnostically important electrolytes: sodium and potassium. Various methods of measuring osmolality and electrolytes exist; most require relatively large amounts of serum or plasma, so their determination may not be feasible except for amphibians of significant size.

Amphibians are tolerant of wide fluctuations in the osmolality and composition of their plasma. This adaptation results in great variability in clinical chemistry parameters that depends on environmental and physiological conditions and complicates interpretation of results. Overwintering frogs and salamanders intentionally undergo dehydration; thus, healthy animals close to or in hibernation should have increased plasma osmolality [9, 10]. In green (White's) tree frogs (*L. caerulea*), reduced plasma osmolality, sodium, potassium, magnesium, and chloride concentrations were found in six cases of severe *Batrachochytrium dendrobatidis*-infection (chytridiomycosis) [34]. Wild-caught mountain yellow-legged frogs, *Rana muscosa*, infected with *Ba. dendrobatidis* develop hyponatremia and hypokalemia, while acid–base balance and blood gases remain unaffected [35].

Proteins

Blood proteins (albumin, globulins, total protein, fibrinogen, and others) may be measured by refractometry, biochemical means (bromcresol green or Biuret method),

Table 19.5 Biochemical reference intervals for blood of select Anuran species.

Analyte (abbreviation)	Units, SI (Conventional)	American bullfrog (*Rana catesbeiana*) Ħ [2]	Cuban tree frog (*Osteopilus septentrionalis*) [33] ⋋	African clawed frog (*Xenopus laevis*) [7] Ħ	African (tropical) clawed frog (*Xenopus tropicalis*) [24] Ħ	Green (White's) tree frog (*Litoria caerulea*) [25] ⋋	White-lipped tree frog (*Litoria infrafrenata*) [25] ⋋
Sample size		**302**	**29**	**166**	**24**	**80**	**66**
Data format				**Mean (reference interval)[a]**		**Median (reference interval)[b]**	
Albumin/globulin		0.54 (0.3–0.78)		0.7 (0–3.28)			
Albumin	g/l g/dl	15.8 (9.2–22.4) 1.58 (0.92–2.24)		10 (0–35.8) 1 (0–3.58)			
Alkaline phosphatase (ALP)	U/l	157 (155.1–158.9)		148 (19–277)			
Alanine aminotransferase (ALT)	U/l	12.4 (10.52–14.28)		21 (0–46.8)			
Amylase	U/l			270 (0–682)			
Aspartate aminotransferase (AST)	U/l			453 (0–1587)		91 (30–362)	67 (26–370)
Bilirubin, total	μmol/l mg/dl			1.2 (0–6.35) 0.07 (0–0.33)			
Bilirubin, indirect	μmol/l mg/dl			0.8(0–5.9) 0.05 (0–0.3)			
Bilirubin, direct	μmol/l mg/dl			0.3 (0–5.45) 0.02 (0–0.28)			
Ca	mmol/l mg/dl	2.08 (1.38–2.78) 8.31 (6.89–9.73)		2.2 (0.9–3.49) 8.9 (3.7–14.0)		2.94 (2–4.4)	2.45 (1.8–4.7)
Cl	mmol/l mEq/l	108.6 (96–121.2) 108.6 (96–121.2)		82.5 (67–98) 82.5 (67–98)			
Cholesterol	mmol/l mg/dl	1.6 (0.88–2.32) 61.8 (34.0–89.6)	3.86 (0–8.26) 149 (0–319)	6.01 (0–14) 232 (0–541.2)			
Creatine phosphokinase (CPK)	U/l	432 (262–602)		1658 (0–6502)		470 (75–2555)*	399 (73–3420)
Creatinine	μmol/l mg/dl	42.7 (21.14–64.26) 0.48 (0.24–0.73)		35.4 (0–262.2) 0.4 (0–2.98)			
Fe	μmol/l μg/dl	25.43 (14.8–36.0) 142.1 (82.7–201.1)					
Fibrinogen	g/l mg/dl	7.9 (5.7–10.1) 0.268–0.7 (193.1–343.54)					
Globulin	g/l g/l			23 (0–48.77) 2.3 (0–4.88)			

Glucose	mmol/l mg/dl	2.77 (1.43–4.11) 49.9 (25.8–74.0)		2.9 (0.07–5.73) 53 (1.46–104.54)		3.6 (1.9–6) 64.9 (34.2–108.1)	3.3 (2–6.8) 59.4 (36–122.5)
Gamma glutamyl transferase (GGT)	U/l			4 (0–29.8)			
Lactate dehydrogenase (LDH)	U/l	117 (73–161)		1809 (0–4592)			
Lipase	U/l			98 (0–201)			
P	mmol/l mg/dl	2.85 (1.69–4.01) 8.82 (5.23–12.41)		2.39 (0.84–3.94) 7.4 (2.25–12.55)		1.33 (0.72–2.64)	1.3 (0.6–2.7)
K	mmol/l mEq/l	3.62 (2.2–5.04) 3.62 (2.2–5.04)		4 (1.42–6.58)		5.9 (3.2–9.5)	3.7 (1.9–3.1)
Na	mmol/l mEq/l	118.6 (96.2–141) 118.6 (96.2–141)		123 (97.2–148-0.8)		110 (101–123)	106 (99–114)
Total protein	g/l g/dl	43.4 (30.2–56.6) 4.34 (3.02–5.66)		33 (7.23–58.77) 3.3 (0.72–5.88)	39.1 (24.2–54.0)	62 (39–85.9)	35 (18–56.3)
Triglycerides	mmol/l mg/dl	0.48 (0.26–0.7) 42.5 (23–61.9)	0.4 (0–1.12) 35.4 (0–99.1)	1.3 (0–3.36) 117 (0–297.38)			
Urea Urea nitrogen (BUN)	mmol/l mg/dl	3 (1.76–4.24) 8.4 (4.93–11.9)		1.8 (0–11.1) 5 (0–30.8)			
Uric acid	μmol/l mg/dl	79.7 (0–422.1) 1.34 (0–7.1)		11.89 (0–165.2) 0.2 (0–2.78)		25 (4–86)	12 (0–27)**

Reference Interval = 95%CI[a] or 2.5th–97.5th percentile[b]. Data distribution: normal (Rc, Xt), non-normal (Lc, Li), unknown (Os, Xl). Values below zero or incompatible with life are reported as 0 and *, respectively. *n = 78, **n = 65.

Key: Free-living ♀, Captive Ħ.

Table 19.6 Biochemical reference intervals for blood of select Caudata species.

Analyte (abbreviation)	Units, SI (Conventional)	Eastern hellbender (*Cryptobranchus alleganiensis alleganiensis*) [1] ϡ		Eastern hellbender (*C. a. alleganiensis*) [3] ϡ	Ozark hellbender (*C.a. bishopi*) [3] ϡ
Sample size		**Variable ♂**	**Variable ♀**	**37–38**	**42**
Albumin	g/l	12.2 (10.6–13.8)	11.9 (9.5–14.3)	9.8 (7.9–11.7)	11.3 (9.3–13.2)
	g/dl	1.2 (1.1–1.4)	1.2 (0.9–1.4)	1 (0.8–1.2)	1.1 (0.9–1.3)
Aspartate aminotransferase (AST)	U/l	74.52 (0–150.72)	76.48 (0–170.72)	128.1 (84.8–171.5)	147.2 (117.1–177.4)
Ca	mmol/l	2.0 (1.72–2.28)	2.7 (1.66–3.74)	2.3 (1.9–2.7)	3 (2.7–3.3)
	mg/dl	8.0 (6.7–9.0)	10.9 (6.7–15.1)	9.3 (7.7–10.8)	12.1 (11–13.3)
Cl	mmol/l			84.3 (81.7–86.9)	80.8 (79.0–82.7)
	mEq/l				
Creatine phosphokinase (CPK)	U/l	661.7 (0–2239.1)	488.52 (0–1088.7)	3703 (641–6765)	972 (0–3100)
Globulin	g/l	26 (0–65.8)	20.3 (8.5–32.1)	21.7 (19.8–23.6)	22.3 (20.3–24.2)
	g/dl	2.6 (0–6.6)	2.0 (0.8–3.2)	2.2 (2.0–2.4)	2.2 (2.0–2.4)
Glucose	mmol/l	1.29 (0.59–1.99)	1.2 (0.6–1.8)	1.5 (0.9–2.1)	1.6 (1.1–2)
	mg/dl	23.2 (10.6–35.8)	21.6 (10.8–32.4)	26.7 (31–5.6)	29.3 (21.6–37.1)
P	mmol/l	1.66 (0.8–2.52)	1.65 (0.77–2.53)	1.6 (1.2–2)	2.2 (2–2.4)
	mg/dl	5.14 (2.48–7.8)	5.1 (2.38–7.83)	4.9 (0–9.9)	6.9 (6.3–7.5)
K	mmol/l	5.07 (2.23–7.91)	4.38 (2.02–6.74)	4.2 (3.4–5.0)	5.1 (4.5–5.6)
	mEq/l	5.07 (2.23–7.91)	4.38 (2.02–6.74)	4.2 (3.4–5.0)	5.1 (4.5–5.6)
Na	mmol/l	110.83 (109.33–112.33)	111 (108.6–113.4)	106.5 (104.3–108.8)	106.3 (104.7–107.9)
	mEq/l	110.83 (109.33–112.33)	111 (108.6–113.4)	106.5 (104.3–108.8)	106.3 (104.7–107.9)
Total protein	g/l	31.5 (19.1–43.9)	31.9 (20.7–43.1)	31.8 (29–34.6)	32.5 (30.6–34.5)
	g/dl	3.15 (1.91–4.39)	3.19 (2.07–4.31)	3.2 (2.9–3.5)	3.3 (3.1–3.4)
Urea	mmol/l			0.8 (0.2–1.4)	1 (0.6–1.5)
	mg/dl			2.5 (0.7–4.2)	3 (1.8–4.2)
Uric acid	µmol/l			21.3 (13.5–29.2)	23.8 (17.3–30.3)
	mg/dl			0.4 (0.2–0.5)	0.4 (0.3–0.5)

All data reported as mean (reference interval = 95%CI); calculated from various populations weighted by sample size (Caa, Cab [18]). Distribution of original data: normal (Caa, Cab), unknown (Cp). Values below zero are reported as 0.
Key: Free-living ϡ, Captive Ħ.

or protein electrophoresis. Total protein in blood includes albumin and globulins and is commonly estimated from the refractive index measured with a refractometer or calculated via spectrophotometric methods (Biuret reaction) used in reference laboratories. Refractometry is a quick, dependable, and inexpensive way of measuring total protein in serum or plasma. Total protein results obtained with the refractometer may, however, be artificially inflated and unreliable when other solid analytes occur in high concentrations in the plasma or serum. A refractometer reading above the reference interval, or significantly higher than the reading from a conspecific, should be confirmed through chemical protein measurement, as high concentrations of bilirubin, cholesterol, and triglycerides increase the refractive index of plasma [22]. The Biuret reaction (used by most reference laboratories) is the most reliable method of measuring *total protein*, and it is recommended over refractometry if a concentration of other solid analytes such as cholesterol and triglycerides is suspected. Although changes in osmolarity may influence the total protein measured by refractometry, the effect is seldom clinically significant.

The test used by most in-house automated analyzers to measure albumin is based on the chemical binding of albumin to bromcresol green dye. Since binding varies depending on the animal species, it may not be valid in all amphibians. Also, it is the least reliable method in two species of Australian tree frogs [25]. If plasma is red tinged, suggesting hemolysis, neither Biuret nor bromcresol reactions will yield valid protein or albumin measurements.

Plasma electrophoresis (EPH) calculates the relative concentrations of the various protein classes and determines the concentrations of albumin and globulins when run alongside an accurate measurement of total protein concentration. This is the most accurate, most time-consuming, and most expensive method for measuring proteins. It requires only very small amounts of plasma or serum (~5 µl) and may be the most appropriate when measuring albumin and globulin in at least some species of amphibians [25]. If the test is run on plasma, heparin and fibrinogen bands or spikes may be present. The validity of clinical parameters such as acute phase proteins or monoclonal gammopathies as determined by EPH in amphibians is unknown.

Metamorphosis requires an increase in protein concentrations from a relatively low level in tadpoles to a concentration equal to, or slightly higher than, the baseline of adults [9]. Total protein in plasma of American bullfrog tadpoles (*Rana* [*Lithobates*] *catesbeiana*) increases incrementally during metamorphosis from 14.6 g/l in the early larval stages to 51.6 g/l in froglets [36], values that are close to the upper end of the adult intervals (43 [30–56] g/l) [2]. Albumin levels also increase during metamorphosis of bullfrogs: from 0.6 g/l in early tadpole stages to 8.9 g/l in froglets [36], a concentration close to that of adult frogs (16 [9–22] g/l) [2]. Hibernating (overwintering) amphibians have increased fibrinogen, shock proteins, and glucose-transport proteins [10]. Differential diagnoses for non-physiologic increases in total protein include active inflammation (globulin fraction) or dehydration (albumin portion). Decreased total protein may reflect a poor diet or suggest liver, gastrointestinal, or renal disease [8].

Vitamins, Minerals, Metals, and Toxins

Calcium metabolism in some amphibian species changes with the season and life stage: In adults, it increases in spring and summer, decreasing in winter, while in tadpoles calcium increases as they approach metamorphosis [37]. In free-ranging eastern hellbenders (*Cryptobranchus alleganiensis*) (Table 19.6) [1] and wild-caught African clawed frogs (*Xenopus laevis*) [7], calcium levels are slightly higher in females than males. A similar trend is suggested for American bullfrogs (*Rana* [*Lithobates*] *catesbeiana*) [38]. Although metabolic bone disease in frogs has been reported, information on calcium concentration in amphibian plasma or on the Ca:P ratio are largely unavailable. If metabolic bone disease is suspected, whole-body radiographic examination is indicated to detect folding fractures, cortical thinning, or decreased bone density [39]. Metabolic bone disease in large amphibians may also be associated with a diet that includes rats or mice, as the high levels of vitamin A contained in the rodents are thought to interfere with the absorption and use of vitamin D [8].

Heavy metals (Hg, Pb, Cd, Cr, and Co) in whole blood of free-ranging adult Ozark and eastern hellbenders (*Cryptobranchus alleganiensis alleganiensis* and *C. a. bishopi*, respectively) have been reported [3]. Eastern hellbenders may have higher levels of Hg and Pb, while Co may be higher in the Ozark subspecies. However, since none of the sites sampled included individuals from both subspecies, difference in levels between Ozark and eastern hellbenders are difficult to distinguish from the effect of location. Ranges incorporating all animals sampled (µg/g of whole blood) are Hg (0.08–0.65), Pb (0.013–0.180), Co (0.07–1.41), Cr (0.13–6.87), and Cd (<0.002–0.11). Mercury levels in general increase proportionally to body mass and length.

Although hypovitaminosis A is a commonly mentioned clinical concern in captive amphibians and has been associated with squamous metaplasia of the lingual and oral mucosas [40], little validation or assay comparison of whole blood or plasma vitamin A has been performed in amphibian species. Similarly, little or no information is available on plasma or blood levels of vitamin D.

Hormones

Although amphibians have been the laboratory species of choice when studying endocrinology, and reviews on amphibian endocrinology exist [41], most of the available information has little or no clinical application. Free-ranging female whistling frogs (*Litoria ewingii*) exhibit a marked increase in plasma corticosterone (from <1.8 to 13.8 ng/ml) after an episode of acute stress (24 h of captivity) [27], suggesting that some responses may resemble those of other vertebrates.

Urinalysis

Amphibian kidneys cannot concentrate urine above the osmolality of plasma. Therefore, in amphibians, urine specific gravity/density is not an indicator of renal function but a reflection of plasma density. A more relevant analyte to measure may be ammonia, as its excretion increases during metabolic acidosis, particularly following episodes of exhaustive exercise when ammonia concentration in urine may rise to over 200% the reference level [8]. Crystals may be seen in urine from tadpoles fed on oxalate-rich vegetables, such as spinach or kale. Development of oxalate crystals occurs in their mesonephri and usually results in death a few days after metamorphosis [42]. Urinalysis reference intervals are provided for the American bullfrog (*Rana* [*Lithobates*] *catesbeiana*) [2] (Table 19.7). Renal disease is one differential for the edematous amphibian (Figure 19.12).

Table 19.7 Urinalysis reference intervals for American bullfrog (*Rana* [*Lithobates*] *catesbeiana*).

Analyte (abbreviation)	American bullfrog [2] Ħ
Sample size	302
Data format	Mean (95% confidence interval)
Specific gravity	1.0075 (1.0007–1.0143)
pH	6.68 (5.26–8.1)

Serology and PCR Useful in Amphibians

PCR tests for the diagnosis of chytridiomycosis, caused by the fungus *Ba. dendrobatidis* (Bd), and ranavirus infection require a skin swab (Bd) or a tissue sample (ranavirus). Unfortunately, the most reliable sample to diagnose ranavirus infection is a lethal sample of liver: tail clips can be diagnostic in septicemic salamanders

Table 19.9 Water quality parameters for amphibians [8].

Parameter	Measure
Temperature	16–20 °C, salamanders 16–24 °C, temperate frogs 22–28 °C, tropical lowland frogs 18–23 °C, tropical highland frogs
pH	6.5–8.5
Salinity	0–5 ppt
Hardness	75–150 mg/l
Alkalinity	15–50 mg/l
Dissolved oxygen	>80% saturation
Carbon dioxide	<5 mg/l
Un-ionized ammonia	<0.02 mg/l
Nitrite	<1 mg/l
Nitrate	<50 mg/l
Chlorine	undetectable

Table 19.8 Diagnostic laboratories for PCR testing of amphibian samples.

Laboratory	Contact person	PCR tests
Pisces Molecular, 1600 Range Street, Suite 201, Boulder CO 80301, USA. Ph: (303) 546–9300, www.pisces-molecular.com	John Wood, jwood@pisces-molecular.com	Ranavirus, *Batrachochytrium dendrobatidis* (chytrid fungus)
CSIRO Livestock Industries, Australian Animal Health Laboratory, Private Bag 24 (Ryrie Street), Geelong, Victoria 3220, Australia. Ph: 61–3 5227 0000, www.csiro.au	Alex Hyatt, alex.hyatt@csiro.au	

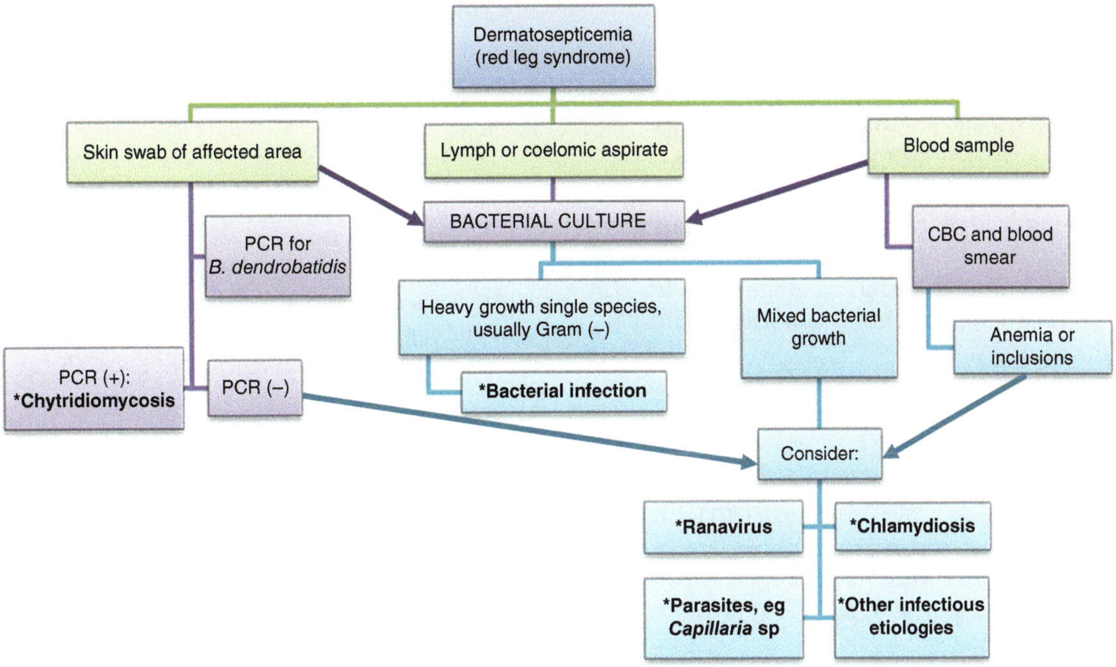

Figure 19.11 Diagnostic diagram for dermatosepticemia in amphibians.

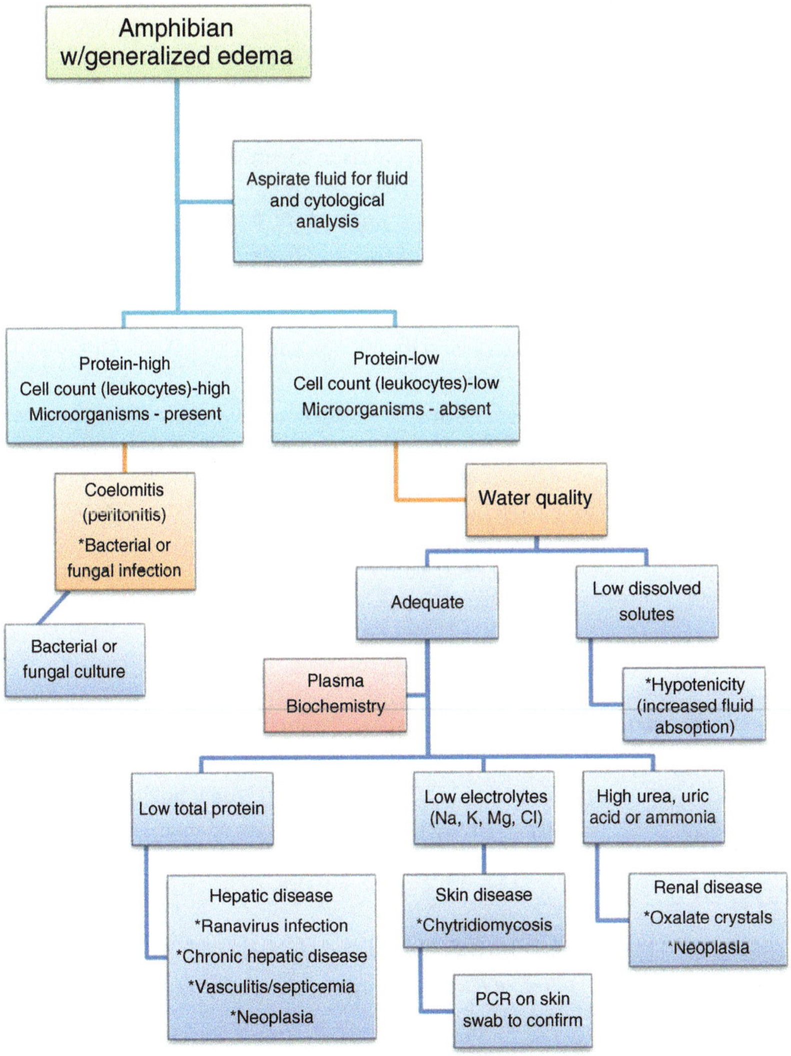

Figure 19.12 Diagnostic diagram for edematous amphibian.

and tadpoles, but are not advisable in subclinical individuals; toe clips are usually non-diagnostic in juvenile or adult frogs. Samples are placed in 70% ethanol (prepared with PCR-quality distilled water) or kept dry, depending on the instructions from the diagnostic laboratory of analysis (Table 19.8). Serological testing for exposure to various infectious agents in amphibians is sometimes performed for research but is not routinely performed in the clinical setting.

Water Quality Parameters for Amphibians

Water quality of amphibian enclosures or surrounding environment can be measured with commercial aquarium kits (Table 19.9). Water quality should be assessed on a regular basis for the pet or laboratory-maintained amphibian and for amphibians suffering edema, dermatosepticemia, or other illness (Figures 19.11 and 19.12).

References

1 Burgmeier, N.G., Unger, S.D., Meyer, J.L. et al. (2011). Health and habitat quality assessment for the eastern hellbender (*Cryptobranchus alleganiensis alleganiensis*) in Indiana, USA. *Journal of Wildlife Disease* 47 (4): 836–848.

2 Coppo, J.A., Mussart, N.B., and Fioranelli, S.A. (2005). Blood and urine physiological values in farm-cultured *Rana catesbeiana* (Anura:Ranidae) in Argentina. *Revista de Biologia Tropical* 53 (3–4): 545–559.

3 Huang, C.C., Xu, Y., Briggler, J.T. et al. (2010). Heavy metals, hematology, plasma chemistry, and parasites in adult hellbenders (*Cryptobranchus alleganiensis*). *Environmental Toxicology and Chemistry* 29 (5): 1132–1137.

4 Rouf, M.A. (1969). Hematology of the leopard frog, *Rana pipiens*. *Copeia* 1969 (4): 682–687.

5 Solis, M.E., Bandeff, J.M., and Huang, Y. (2007). Hematology and serum chemistry of Ozark and eastern hellbenders (*Cryptobranchus alleganiensis*). *Herpetologica* 63 (3): 285–292.

6 Hadji- Azimi, I., Coosemans, V., and Canicatti, C. (1987). Atlas of adult *Xenopus laevis* hematology. *Developmental and Comparative Immunology* 11: 807–874.

7 Wilson, S., Felt, S., Torreilles, S. et al. (2011). Serum clinical biochemical and hematologic reference ranges of laboratory-reared and wild-caught *Xenopus laevis*. *Journal of the American Association for Laboratory Animal Science* 50 (5): 635–640.

8 Wright, K.M. and Whitaker, B.R. (2001). *Amphibian Medicine and Captive Husbandry*, 1e. Krieger Publishing Co.

9 Duellman, W.E. and Trueb, L. (1994). *Biology of Amphibians*. The Johns Hopkins University Press.

10 O'Malley, B. (2005). *Clinical Anatomy and Physiology of Exotic Species*, 1e. Elsevier Saunders.

11 Storey, K.B. and Storey, J.M. (1986). Freeze tolerance and intolerance s strategies of winter survival in terrestrially-hibernating amphibians. *Comparative Biochemistry and Physiology* 83A (4): 613–617.

12 Ecker, A. (1889). *The Anatomy of the Frog (Translated by George Haslam)*, 449. Oxford, England: Clarendon Press.

13 Tyning, T.F. (1990). *Guide to Amphibians and Reptiles*, 1e. Little Brown and Company.

14 CDC (2010). Multistate outbreak of human *Salmonella typhimurium* infections associated with aquatic frogs, United States, 2007–2008. *Morbidity and Mortality Weekly Report* 58 (51&52): 1433–1436.

15 Marthinho, F. and Heatley, J.J. (2012). Amphibian mycobacteriosis. *Veterinary Clinics of North America: Exotic Animal Practice* 15: 113–119.

16 Saporito, R.A., Norton, R.A., Andriamaharavo, N.R. et al. (2011). Alkaloids in the mite *Scheloribates laevigatus*: further alkaloids common to oribatid mites and poison frogs. *Journal of Chemical Ecology* 37: 231–218.

17 Richards N. 2007. Western Sydney Institute of TAFE, Richmond, Captive Animal Management 1068, Lecturers Graeme Phipps and Jacki Salkeld. Online. January 25, 2012.

18 Heatley, J.J. and Johnson, M. (2009). Clinical technique: amphibian hematology: a practitioner's guide. *Journal of Exotic Pet Medicine* 18 (1): 14–19.

19 Cecala, K.K., Price, S.J., and Dorcas, M.E. (2007). A comparison of the effectiveness of recommended doses of MS-222 (tricaine methanesulfonate) and Orajel® (benzocaine) for amphibian anesthesia. *Herpetological Review* 38 (1): 63–66.

20 Fedewa, L.A. and Lindell, A. (2005). Inhibition of growth for select gram-negative bacteria by tricaine methane sulfonate (MS-222). *Journal of Herpetological Medicine and Surgery.* 15 (1): 13–17.

21 Forzán, M.J., Vanderstichel, R.V., Ogbuah, C.T. et al. (2012). Blood collection from the facial (maxillary)/ musculo-cutaneous vein in true frogs (family Ranidae). *Journal of Wildlife Diseases* 48 (1): 176–180.

22 Thrall, M.A. (2006). *Veterinary Hematology and Clinical Chemistry*, 1e. Blackwell Publishing.

23 Forzán, M.J., Smith, T.G., Vanderstichel, R.V. et al. (2016). Hematological reference intervals for *Rana sylvatica* (*Lithobates sylvaticus*) and effect of infection with frog virus 3 (*Ranavirus* sp, Iridoviridae). *Veterinary Clinical Pathology* 45 (3): 430–443.

24 Maxham, L.A., Forzán, M.J., Hogan, N.S. et al. (2016). Hematological reference intervals for *Xenopus tropicalis* with partial use of automatic counting methods and reliability of long-term stored samples. *Veterinary Clinical Pathology* 45 (2): 291–299.

25 Young, S., Warner, J., Speare, R. et al. (2012). Hematologic and plasma biochemical reference intervals for health monitoring of wild Australian tree frogs. *Veterinary Clinical Pathology* 41 (4): 478–492.

26 Weathers, W. (1975). Circulatory responses of *Rana catesbeiana* to temperature, season, and previous thermal history. *Comparative Biochemistry and Physiology, Part A* 51: 43–52.

27 Coddington, E.J. and Cree, A. (2005). Effect of acute captivity stress on plasma concentrations of corticosterone and sex steroids in female whistling frogs, *Litoria ewingi*[sic]. *General and Comparative Endocrinology* 100: 33–38.

28 Davis, A.K., Keel, M.K., Fereira, A., and Maerz, J.C. (2010). Effects of chytridiomycosis on circulating white blood cells distributions of bullfrog larvae (*Rana catesbeiana*). *Comparative Clinical Pathology* 19: 49–55.

29 Allender, M.C., Fry, M.M., Irizarry, A.R. et al. (2006). Intracytoplasmic inclusions in circulating leukocytes from an eastern box turtle (*Terrapene carolina carolina*) with iridoviral infection. *Journal of Wildlife Diseases* 43 (2): 677–684.

30 Cunningham, A.A., Tems, C.A., and Russell, P.H. (2008). Immunohistochemical demonstration of ranavirus antigen in the tissues of infected frogs (*Rana temporaria*) with systemic haemorrhagic or cutaneous ulcerative disease. *Journal of Comparative Pathology* 318: 3–11.

31 Boulianne, B., Evans, R.C., and Smith, T.G. (2007). Phylogenetic analysis of *Hepatozoon* species (Apicomplexa:Adeleorina) infecting frogs of Nova Scotia, Canada, determined by ITS-1 sequences. *Journal of Parasitology* 93 (6): 1435–1441.

32 Southworth, G.C., Mason, G., and Seed, J.R. (1968). Studies on frog Trypanosomiasis. I. A 24-hour cycle in the parasitemia level of *Trypanosoma rotatorium* in *Rana clamitans* from Louisiana. *Journal of Parasitology* 54 (2): 255–258.

33 Shilton, C.M., Smith, D.A., Crawshaw, G.J. et al. (2001). Corneal lipid deposition in Cuban tree frogs (*Osteopilus septentrionalis*) and its relationship to serum lipids: an experimental study. *Journal of Zoo and Wildlife Medicine* 32 (3): 305–319.

34 Voyles, J., Berger, L., Young, S. et al. (2007). Electrolyte depletion and osmotic imbalance in amphibians with chytridiomycosis. *Diseases of Aquatic Organisms* 77: 113–118.

35 Voyles, J., Vredenburg, V.T., Tunstall, T.S. et al. (2012). Patophysiology in mountain yellow-legged frogs (*Rana muscosa*) during a chytridiomycosis outbreak. *PLoS One* 7 (4): e35374.

36 Feldhoff, R.C. (1971). Quantitative changes in plasma albumin during bullfrog metamorphosis. *Comparative Biochemistry and Physiology* 40B: 733–739.

37 Stiffler, D.F. (1993). Amphibian calcium metabolism. *Journal of Experimental Biology* 184: 47–61.

38 Cathers, T., Lewbart, G.A., Correa, M., and Stevens, J.B. (1997). Serum chemistry and hematology values for anesthetized American bullfrogs (*Rana catesbeiana*). *Journal of Zoo and Wildlife Medicine* 28 (2): 171–174.

39 King, J.D., Muhlbauer, M.C., and James, A. (2011). Radiographic diagnosis of metabolic bone disease in captive bred mountain chicken frogs (*Leptodactylus fallax*). *Zoo Biology* 30: 254–259.

40 Rodriguez, C.E. and Pessier, A.P. (2014). Pathologic changes associated with suspected hypovitaminosis A in amphibians under managed care. *Zoo Biology* 33: 508–515.

41 Denver, R.J., Glennemeier, K.A., and Gc, B. (2002). Endocrinology of complex life cycles: amphibians. In: *Hormones, Brain and Behavior*, vol. 2 (ed. D. Pfaff, A. Arnold and A. Etgen), 469–513. San Diego: Academic Press.

42 Forzán, M.J., Ferguson, L.V., and Smith, T.G. (2015). Calcium oxalate nephrolithiasis and tubular necrosis in recent metamorphs of *Rana sylvatica* (*Lithobates sylvaticus*) fed spinach during the premetamorphic (tadpole) stage. *Veterinary Pathology* 52 (2): 384–387.

43 Frost, D.R., Grant, T., Faivovich, J.N. et al. (2006). The amphibian tree of life. *Bulletin of The American Museum of Natural History* 297: 370.

44 IUCN 2012. The IUCN Red List of Threatened Species. Version 2012.2. Online. 17 October 2012.

45 Cabagna-Zenklusen, M.C., Lajmanovich, R.C., Attademo, A.M. et al. (2011). Hematology and blood cell cytochemistry of *Rhinella fernandezae* (Amphibia: Anura) from Espinal and Delta-Islands of Paraná River, Argentina. *Revista de Biologia Tropical* 59 (1): 17–28.

46 Pfeiffer, C.J., Pyle, H., and Asashima, M. (1990). Blood cell morphology and counts in the Japanese newt (*Cynops pyrrhogaster*). *Journal of Zoo and Wildlife Medicine* 21 (1): 56–64.

Webliographies

amphibiaweb.org — Information on amphibian biology and conservation, listing of worldwide species, with photos and life history details.amphibians.org — IUCN Amphibian Specialist Group, information on conservation and other wild and captive population topics

www.amphibianark.org — Information on captive husbandry.www.asvcp.org – Information on establishing reference intervals for animal species.

www.carcnet.ca — Canadian Herpetological Society (formerly Canadian Amphibian and Reptile Conservation Network and Canadian Association of Herpetologists), information on Canadian native species of amphibians.

www.naturewatch.ca — Information on native North American frog and toad species.

20

Fish

Stephen A. Smith MS, DVM, PhD

Department of Biomedical Sciences and Pathobiology, VA/MD College of Veterinary Medicine, Blacksburg, Virginia, USA

Introduction

Fish have been kept as ornamental species for over 2000 years, with contemporary aquarists keeping fish in home aquaria and backyard ponds for almost 200 years. Of greater than 30 000 species of freshwater, marine, and brackish water fish described, only a small fraction has successfully entered the commercial aquarium and ornamental pond markets. With their increasing popularity as companion animals, clients are increasingly requesting veterinary care and services for their fish. Thus, clinical pathology becomes essential to providing proper diagnostic and therapeutic recommendations for the prevention and control of diseases for these animals. Unfortunately, even though the techniques used to obtain and process diagnostic samples for clinical pathology are similar to those of other animals, interpretation of results can be difficult based on the lack of reference values for individual species of fish and the potential inaccuracy inherent in extrapolating values from similar or closely related species of fish. In addition, factors such as environmental conditions, seasonality, stress, age, gender, reproductive status, husbandry, and diet may significantly affect the values obtained.

Species

Over 800 varieties of freshwater tropical fish and close to 200 species of marine fish are currently available commercially, each having their own unique diversity in morphology, biology, physiology, habitat requirements, behavior, and dietary needs. Common freshwater aquarium species include guppies and mollies, swordtails and platies, freshwater angelfish, cichlids, tetras, barbs, danios, rainbow fish, loaches, killifish, betas, and various types of catfish, while common marine species include marine angelfish, butterfly fish, anthias, gobies, tangs, blennies, wrasses, damsels, and clownfish (Tables 20.1 and 20.2). Backyard ornamental pond species include carp (including ornamental carp, i.e., koi), goldfish, grass carp, orfe, and the channel catfish (Table 20.3). Species commonly maintained for laboratory research include the zebra fish, medaka, fathead minnows, tilapia, trout, and channel catfish (Table 20.4).

General Fluid Balance and Osmoregulation in Fish

Living and surviving in an aqueous environment requires specialized physiologic and anatomic adaptations for fish to maintain internal fluid and ion homeostasis. The external environment of fish is either hyposmotic (e.g., freshwater fish) or hyperosmotic (e.g., marine fish). The gills, a semipermeable thin layer of epithelial cells, are the primary site of osmoregulation in teleost fish [1–3]. Other organs such as the skin, kidney, and gastrointestinal tract also contribute to the regulation of fluid and ion balance.

In freshwater fish, external forces present a constant influx of water (favoring a hypervolemic state), up to 50% of their body water volume per hour. Internally, forces favor ion depletion (the efflux of ions). To counteract these forces, freshwater fish drink little to no water and produce copious amounts of dilute urine (polyuria). The kidneys of freshwater fish are generally larger compared to those of marine fish, based mainly on the high volume of water excreted. The glomerular filtration rate (GFR) of freshwater fish is high when compared to that of marine fish [2]. Freshwater fish also reabsorb almost all Na^+ and Cl^- ions via the gills and kidneys. Clinically, this becomes important when managing or reducing stress in fish patients, and in cutaneous wound management.

Marine teleosts are presented with the opposite situation as freshwater fish. Their environmental conditions

Exotic Animal Laboratory Diagnosis, First Edition. Edited by J. Jill Heatley and Karen E. Russell.

Table 20.1 Common freshwater tropical fish species kept as pets in home aquariums.

Common name	Scientific name
Freshwater angelfish	*Pterophyllum* spp.
Guppies and mollies	*Poecilia* spp.
Swordtails and platies	*Xiphophorus* spp.
Cichlids	*Melanochromis* spp., multiple genera
Tetras	*Hyphessobrycon* spp., multiple genera
Barbs	*Puntius* spp.
Danios	*Devario* spp.
Rainbow fish	*Glossolepis* spp., multiple genera
Loaches	*Chromobotia* spp., multiple genera
Killifish	*Nothobranchius* spp., multiple genera
Gourami	*Trichopodus* spp., multiple genera
Siamese fighting fish (Beta)	*Betta splendens*
Catfish	*Corydoras* spp., *Clarias* spp., *Hypostomus* spp., *Synodontis* spp.

Table 20.2 Common marine fish species kept as pets in home aquariums.

Common name	Scientific name
Marine angelfish	*Pomacanthus* spp., multiple genera
Butterfly fish	*Chaetodon* spp., multiple genera
Anthias	*Pseudanthias* spp.
Gobies	Multiple genera
Tangs	*Acanthurus* spp., multiple genera
Blennies	Multiple genera
Wrasses	*Thalassoma* spp., multiple genera
Damsels	Multiple genera
Clownfish	*Amphiprion* spp., multiple genera.

Table 20.3 Common ornamental fish species kept in backyard ponds.

Common name	Scientific name
Carp, koi	*Cyprinus carpio carpio*
Goldfish	*Carassius auratus*
Grass carp	*Ctenopharyngodon idella*
Orfe	*Leuciscus idus*
Channel catfish	*Ictalurus punctatus*

Table 20.4 Common fish species maintained for laboratory research.

Common name	Scientific name
Zebra fish	*Danio rerio*
Medaka	*Oryzias latipes*
Fathead minnow	*Pimephales promelas*
Goldfish	*Carassius auratus*
Tilapia	*Tilapia spp., Oreochromis* spp., *Sarotherodon* spp., *Steatocranus* spp.
Trout and salmonid	*Oncorhynchus* spp., *Salmo* spp., *Salvelinus* spp.
Channel catfish	*Ictalurus punctatus*

favor loss of body fluids (leaning toward dehydration) and an increased body salt content. Saltwater fishes' strategy includes polydipsia, up to 10%–20% of their body weight daily; active reabsorption of water in the urinary bladder; and active excretion of ions (Na^+, Cl^-, and K^+) by mitochondrial-rich branchial chloride cells, which are more numerous in saltwater fish compared to freshwater fish [4]. Divalent ions, such as Mg^{2+} and SO_4^{2-}, are excreted in feces (80%) and in the urine via the kidneys [2]. Urine production in saltwater fish is relatively small, about 1%–2% of their body weight daily. The GFR increases occur in euryhaline (capable of adapting to a wide range of salinities) species when moving from a high-salinity environment to freshwater to counter the changing osmotic conditions [2].

Elasmobranchs (e.g., sharks, rays, and skates) counter the marine environmental pressure of dehydration and excess ion influx via the active secretion of salt by the rectal glands and by actively raising the blood osmolality with high levels of serum urea concentrations [1–3, 5]. Interestingly, the plasma of most shark species, even euryhaline species such as the bull shark (*Carcharhinus leucas*), have blood that is isosmotic to seawater.

Clinical Importance of Osmoregulatory Disruption

The fishes' osmoregulatory ability can be decreased during times of stress (e.g., poor water quality, handling and transport, and infectious disease). Stress causes the release of many chemical mediators into the bloodstream, including epinephrine. Epinephrine causes reduced permeability of gill epithelia, resulting in a net increase of water in the body and blood ion loss in freshwater fish, and a net loss of water and an increased ion influx in saltwater fish. In addition, marine species may also stop drinking as a result of elevated catecholamine levels in the bloodstream, compounding the problem [6]. Elevated catecholamine levels in freshwater fish cause an acute rise in water influx based on gill epithelial permeability changes. An increase in diuresis occurs to compensate for the increased fluid volume, resulting in an electrolyte imbalance due to ion depletion.

The addition of salt (NaCl) to the water, 1–6 ppt depending on the species, can reduce the osmotic gradient and subsequently help to decrease the energy required for osmoregulation in freshwater fish [2, 6]. This strategy can be used for treatment and in transport situations to reduce stress of freshwater fish. External parasite control, primarily for protozoans, is an added benefit of increasing water salinity (usually >0.3%) for freshwater fish.

Marine species may experience a reduction in osmoregulatory energy expenditure and some external parasite control from a gradual, temporary reduction in salinity [2]. Dehydration in sick or stressed saltwater fish can be treated with oral or intracoelomic fluid therapy at a rate of 1%–3% of the body weight [2]. Fluid choices include hypotonic saline (0.45%), normal saline (0.9%), and other balanced electrolyte solutions [2]. The administration of short-acting corticosteroids, such as dexamethasone, can increase excretion of sodium and increase water uptake by the intestine and urinary bladder. A bath of 10 mg/ml dexamethasone may be useful in reducing the deleterious effects of stress, improving appetite, and reducing inflammation in marine fish [2].

In either saltwater or freshwater fish, physical damage to the gills, skin, or kidneys can result in mild to severe, sometimes fatal, alterations in osmoregulation. Because of this, wounds such as cutaneous ulcers should be treated aggressively to minimize their impact on osmoregulation. Sedation may also be used to reduce stress in fish during handling, transport, hospitalization, and other stress-inducing situations [6].

Water Quality Parameters of Clinical Importance

Water quality is one of the most important considerations when clinically evaluating the health of fish. The most common water quality parameters typically evaluated include temperature, pH, ammonia, nitrites, and nitrates, but depending on the species of fish being presented, may also include evaluating salinity (e.g., marine and brackish water species), dissolved oxygen, hardness, and alkalinity [7, 8]. Chlorine and chloramines may also need to be evaluated if new or replacement water has been recently added to the aquarium or pond. Most species of fish have an optimal temperature range, and deviation outside this range, either above or below, can have a detrimental effect on the health of fish [9]. There are cold-water species of fish (7–18 °C, i.e., trout), cool water species of fish (16–23 °C, i.e., Koi and goldfish), and warm water species of fish (21–32 °C, i.e., tropical fish, catfish, and tilapia); thus, the temperature requirement of each species should be noted when evaluating water quality parameters. The pH of the water should also be within an acceptable range for the species, generally between 6.8 and 7.2 for freshwater fishes and 8.0–8.5 for marine fishes. Some species of fish have specific pH requirements, while others are tolerant of a wide variation in the pH. Again, deviation outside the acceptable range of pH can have a detrimental effect on the health of the fish. Nitrogenous compounds (i.e., ammonia, nitrites, and nitrates) from metabolic waste products, feces, and uneaten feed all contribute to the overall level of ammonia in an aquarium or pond. The pH of the water will determine how much of the ammonia is unionized (NH_3), which is more toxic to fish than the ionized form (NH_4+). Various bacteria are able to convert the ammonia to nitrites and then to relatively less toxic nitrates. As a general rule, levels of ammonia, nitrite, and nitrate should be as close to 0 mg/l as possible. Overt clinical signs of suboptimal or poor water quality in fish can include anorexia, lethargy, increased opercular rate, dyspnea, gasping or piping at the surface, clamped fins, changes in coloration, and acute or chronic mortality (Table 20.5).

Sample Collection

Restraint

All sampling techniques described below can be performed on unanesthetized fish, but light sedation facilitates physical management of the fish, reduces the stress of the procedures on the fish and clinician, reduces the risk of injury to the fish, and makes the technique less complicated to perform. Use of gloves cleaned in dechlorinated water and having adequate available water treated and assessed for fish well-being available is recommended. The most common anesthetic used to sedate fish is tricaine methanesulfonate (MS-222). This compound is the only FDA-approved anesthetic for food fish and has a 21-day withdrawal period. The MS-222 is added to the fish's water, and the depth and time of sedation or anesthesia can be controlled by varying the concentration and length of time the fish is exposed to the anesthetic water [11–13]. The typical anesthetic dosage of MS-222 ranges from 50 to 150 mg/l water depending on the species of fish involved, the health of the patient, and the properties of the water used to anesthetize the fish. Induction dosages for short procedures are often higher (75–125 mg/l) than those used for maintenance in longer procedures (50–75 mg/l). The anesthetic mixture

Table 20.5 Water quality parameters and clinical signs associated with water quality abnormalities, adapted [10].

Water quality parameter ***(acceptable level)***	**Clinical signs of toxicity**	**Treatment**	**Comments**
Ammonia *0 ppm*	• Lethargy • Anorexia • Increased opercular rate • Convulsions/coma • Gill hyperplasia • Death	• Frequent water changes • Reduce or stop feeding • Reduce stocking density (overpopulation) • Add ammonia binding compounds • Monitor by frequent testing	• Ammonia more toxic at higher pH and water temperatures • Ammonia levels in new systems must be monitored • New tank syndrome • Chemicals and drugs that adversely affect biofiltration bacteria can lead to increased ammonia concentrations
Nitrite *0 ppm*	• Gasping/piping • Opercular flaring • Increased respiratory rate • Lethargy • Dyspnea • Pale gills • Death	• Frequent water changes • Add 0.01%–0.02% sodium chloride to freshwater system • Monitor by frequent testing	• Newly established systems • Nitrite binds hemoglobin (Hb) forming methoxyhemoglobin, or "Brown blood" disease. • Chloride competitively inhibits nitrite uptake across the gills
Nitrate *<50 ppm*	• Chronic stress • Growth suppression • Blindness • Immune suppression? • Buoyancy disorders?	• Water changes • Addition of vegetation	• Algal blooms may occur with increased nitrate levels
pH *6.8–7.2 for freshwater fish* *8.0–8.5 for marine fish*	Low pH • Tremors, hyperactivity • Increased mucus production • Stress • Sudden deaths High pH • Skin and gill cloudiness • Acute and chronic stress	Low pH • Water changes • Add buffering agents • Measure ammonia before changing pH acutely! High pH • Water changes • Add buffering agents • Remove excess vegetation – photosynthesis consumes CO_2 & increases pH	• Acceptable pH varies with species of fish • Small pH changes are less stressful than large, rapid changes • Most fish can adapt to a stable pH
Dissolved oxygen (DO) *6–10 ppm*	• Dyspnea • Increased opercular rate • Gasping, piping • Lethargy • Mortalities	• Add aeration or pure oxygen • Decrease feeding, stocking density • Reduce temperature • 3% hydrogen peroxide (0.5 ml/l) carefully added to water in emergency situations	• Lowest DO occurs at dawn (before plant photosynthesis) • Large fish succumb first (higher oxygen requirement) • Medication such as formalin can reduce DO • Biofilter requires adequate oxygen to function – monitor ammonia after DO returns to normal
Alkalinity *100–180 ppm*		• Water changes • Baking soda can raise alkalinity in a low pH crisis ("pH crash")	• Alkalinity levels decrease prior to pH decrease
Chlorine *0 ppm*	• Signs of hypoxia/dyspnea • Gill necrosis • Hemolytic anemia • Acute mortalities	• Immediate water change with dechlorinated water • Lower water temperature to reduce oxygen demand • Add oxygenated water or bubble oxygen into water	• Dechlorinate all water with water changes • Use dechlorinators containing sodium thiosulfate (3.5–10 mg/l) or vigorous aeration for 24 h

should be buffered with bicarbonate as MS-222 tends to acidify the water, and water should always be aerated to prevent hypoxia. For recovery, the fish is placed back into water without the anesthetic. Benzocaine hydrochloride, eugenol, propofol, and ethanol have also been used for restraint of fish.

Fin Clip, Skin Scrape, and Gill Clip

One of the most important and useful diagnostic tools used in clinical medicine of fish are the non-lethal biopsies that include skin scrapes, fin snips, and gill snips [14–16]. These techniques are inexpensive, simple to perform, and provide immediate diagnostic information. They are used primarily to diagnose external parasitic, bacterial, and fungal infections, but can also be used in the diagnosis of specific viral infections (e.g., lymphocystis) in fish and the occurrence of suboptimal water qualities (Figure 20.1a–c).

The skin scrape is a superficial sampling of the external mucous layer of the skin. This is obtained by using a coverslip to gently scrape a small area of the skin of the fish in an anterior-to-posterior (cranial to caudal) direction or at the edge of a skin lesion to collect a sample of the mucous at the edge of the coverslip (Figure 20.2a) [16]. The sample is then placed face down in a drop of water from the aquarium or pond on a microscope slide and the wet mount observed under the microscope for potential external pathogens. Avoid using too much pressure to obtain the sample as this could remove scales from the fish and traumatize the skin. The fin snip (or fin clip) is used less commonly than the skin scrape and is the removal of a small piece of the distal tip of one of the fins for examination in a wet mount. This technique usually provides similar information as the skin scrape but is more traumatic. Fin snipping should never be used on display or show fish as the sampled fin may not heal with a normal appearance after sampling. The gill biopsy (or gill clip) is the removal of the distal tips of a few gill filaments from the gill and examination of the tissue in a wet mount under the microscope (Figure 20.2b) [16]. This traumatic technique will cause the cut edges of the gill

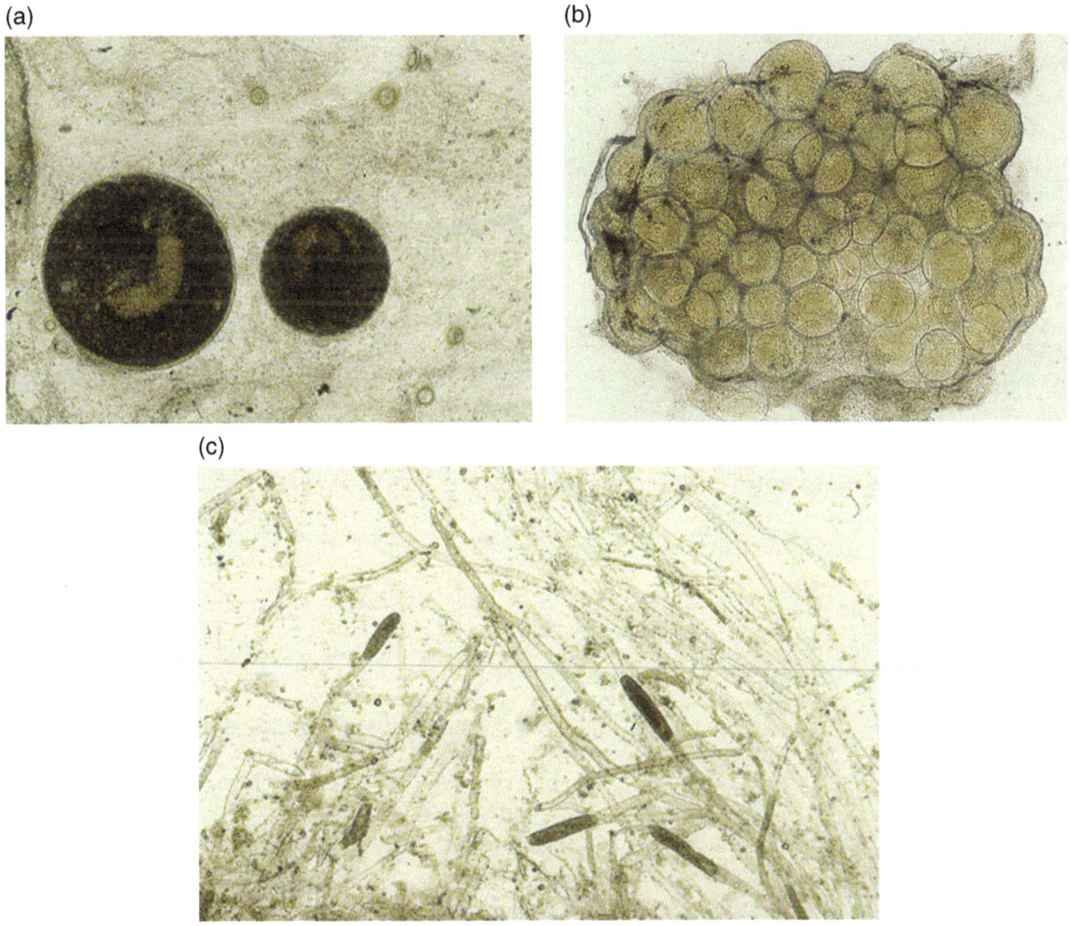

Figure 20.1 Examples of diagnoses from wet mounts using non-lethal samples. (a) Two large *Ichthypphthirius multifiliis* parasites and several small *Trichodina* sp. parasites in a gill clip from an Oscar, *Astronotus ocellatus*. (b) A clump of lymphocystis virus infected cells in a skin scrape of a glass fish, *Parambassis ranga*. (c) *Saprolegnia* sp. in a skin scrape of a yellow perch, *Perca flavescens*.

(a) (b)

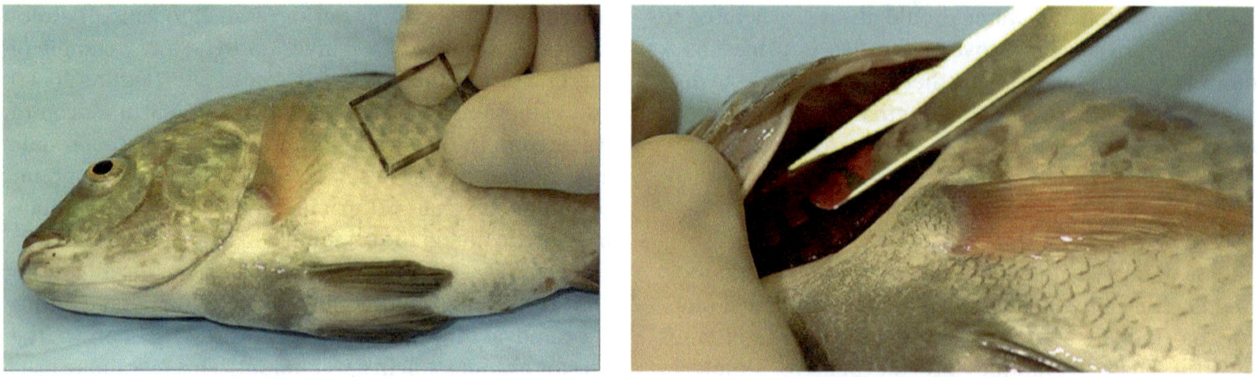

Figure 20.2 Non-lethal biopsies obtained from fish, *Oreochromis* sp. (a) A skin scrape can be obtained by using a coverslip (outlined in blank) to gently scrape a small amount of mucus from the skin surface. (b) A gill biopsy (or gill snip) may be obtained by carefully removing only the distal tips of a few filaments from the gill.

filament to bleed for a short time, but the gill filament is usually completely replaced with normal tissue within three to four weeks.

Wet mounts are evaluated for the presence of living protozoan parasites and some larger helminthes, such as monogeneans and crustacean parasites [17, 18]. Protozoan parasites can range in size from the size of a red blood cell (10–12 μm) as in the case of *Ichthyobodo necatrix* to as large as 1 mm with *Ichthyophthirius multifiliis* of freshwater fish and *Cryptocaryon irritans* of saltwater fish. Low numbers of bacteria may commonly be observed in the mucous of the skin and gills of normal fish; however, increased numbers of bacteria associated with a lesion is suggestive of a potential bacterial pathogen. Identification of particular species of bacteria can be made by observing certain characteristics of the bacteria, such as the flexing movement or column formation of *Flexibacterium* spp. or the acid-fast staining characteristic of *Mycobacterium* sp. Fungal infections, for example, *Saprolegnia* spp. and *Aphanomyces* spp., are diagnosed by observing hyphal elements in the mucous sample of the skin or in the mucous or tissue of gill samples. An indirect assessment of the water quality from which the fish was maintained can also be made by the observation of excessive mucous present on the gills and the presence of epithelial hyperplasia as manifested by clubbing of individual gill filaments or the fusion of adjacent gill filaments [19].

(a) (b)

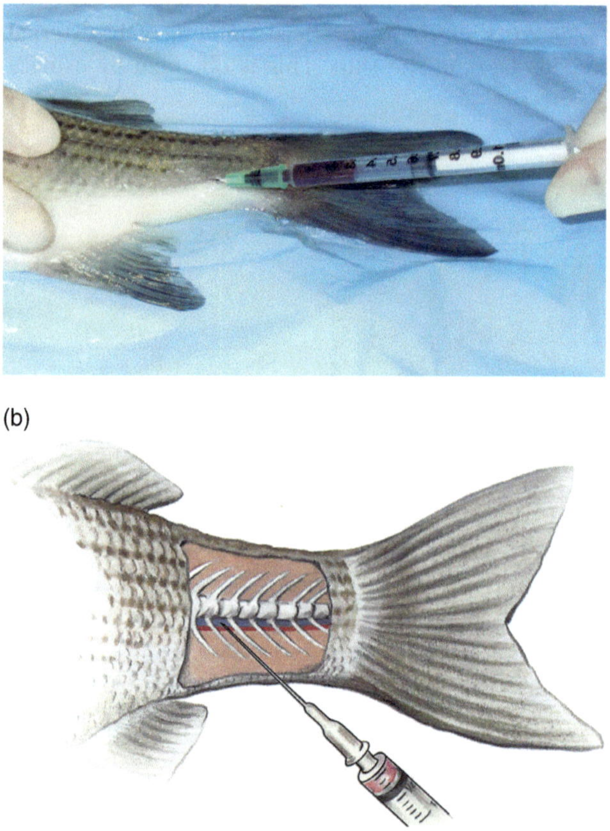

Figure 20.3 Lateral approach for sampling blood from the caudal vessels of a sedated striped bass (*Morone saxatilis*) using a 3.0 ml syringe with a 1.5 in. 23 g. needle. (a) Photo, (b) illustration. *Source:* Drawing courtesy T. Lawrence.

Venipuncture

A clinically acceptable blood sample can be readily obtained from most fish species. The caudal vessels are the most common blood-sampling site and yield a mixed arterial and venous sample (Figure 20.3). A ventral or lateral approach is most often used [20]. Cardiac puncture has an increased risk of patient mortality and is not recommended for use in companion species. For most biochemical analytes, plasma is preferred over serum [21]. Lithium heparin is the preferred anticoagulant for use in most tests and with most fish species [21, 22]. As fish blood clots quickly, the needle and syringe may need to be heparinized prior to blood collection. Because some serological tests may require unheparinized whole blood, attention to test sample requirements in advance is recommended. A blood volume collection of 0.5%–1.0% of the body weight can be safely taken from most fish. In most cases, 1.0 ml can be taken from 100 g fish and up to 3.0 ml in larger fish, such as koi [22]. Most venipuncture in fish can be accomplished using with a 1.5 in. 21–23 gauge (g.) needle on a 1.0 or 3.0 ml syringe. A 0.5 in. 25 g. needle on a tuberculin (1 ml) syringe can be used for small fish. Blood should be transferred immediately to a blood tube containing an anticoagulant to minimize clotting. Clumped, clotted, or hemolyzed blood samples should be discarded.

Hematology

Biochemical tests and complete blood counts (CBCs) are valuable diagnostic tools in determining the cause of disease in many species. However, reference intervals, normal hematologic parameters, and interpretation of those values are not available for most pet fish species. Published hematologic data exists for important food fish species (e.g., trout, channel catfish, tilapia, striped bass, winter flounder, sturgeon, pangasius and yellow perch), but these values are not always applicable to pet and ornamental fish [23–30]. Selected hematology and biochemical reference values of a few common pet species, that is, koi, goldfish, pacu, and zebra fish are provided (Tables 20.6 and 20.7) [22, 33–36]. Environmental conditions such as water quality (i.e., temperature, pH, ammonia, nitrite, nitrate, etc.) can affect many analytes [22, 31, 37, 38]. Capture and handling stressors, sampling technique, age, gender, reproductive status, photoperiod, diet, activity level, and test methodology are other factors that affect the results of a CBC and serum or plasma biochemistry analytes [21, 28, 37].

Interpretation of Blood Results

Interpretation of results in fish is challenging when compared to more common terrestrial species. Nucleated red blood cells and platelets prohibit the use of most automated analyzers used for mammalian blood counts. Manual evaluation using the hemocytometer chamber method is the most common technique [22]. Few clinical studies have been published, but more are expected in future as the expansion of pet fish medical care continues. Recently, two studies evaluated the use of in-house blood analyzers for fish [39, 40]. The discussion on interpretation below highlights some published studies to guide the fish clinician.

Blood Cell Morphology

Most fish blood cell types appear to have a morphology and function similar to mammalian blood cell (Figure 20.4). Erythrocytes are the most numerous blood cell type and are nucleated. Reticulocytes, frequently present in significant numbers in blood smears, are easily recognized by their smaller size and slightly basophilic cytoplasm. Thrombocytes vary in shape depending on their activation state, changing from spiked or oval to round cells as they activate, and may have a segmented or oval nucleus. Lymphocytes can be divided into small or large lymphocytes, though functional differences have not been documented. Neutrophils are one of the largest fish blood cells (Figures 20.5 and 20.6). The cytoplasm of the neutrophils may have a grainy appearance and a less

Table 20.6 Mean hematology reference values for common pet and ornamental species.

Hematology	Koi/carp, *C. carpio* [31, 32]	Goldfish, *Carassius auratus* [31]	Pacu, *Colossoma brachypomus* [33]	Zebra fish, *Danio rerio* [28]
Red blood cells (10E6/μl)	1.67, 1.81	1.61	1.68	3.02
White blood cells (10E3/μl)	37.8, 24.0	52.3	33.5	NR
Lymphocytes (%)	88–93, 79.1	51.4 ± 1.32	84.0	82.95 ± 5.47
Monocytes (%)	0.5–2.0, 2.9	0.4 ± 0.19	4.0	9.68 ± 2.44
Neutrophils (%)	3.0–10.0, 10.9	5.0 ± 1.32	NR	7.10 ± 4.75
Eosinophils (%)	0.5–1.0, NR	0.3 ± 1.13	0.3	0.15 ± 0.53
Basophils (%)	0.5–1.5, 4.5	0.2 ± 0.29	NR	0.13 ± 0.40
Thrombocytes (%)	NR, NR	39.7 ± 3.04	NR	NR
Heterophil (%)	NR, NR	NR	5.2	NR
Monocyte (%)	NR, NR	NR	4.0	NR
Granular-lymphocytoid (%)	NR, NR	NR	4.7	NR

NR = not reported.

Table 20.7 Mean biochemistry reference values for common pet and ornamental species.

Biochemistry analyte (SI units)	Koi/carp, *C. carpio* [31]	Goldfish, *Carassius auratus* [31]	Pacu, *Piaractus brachypomus* [13]	Zebra fish, *Danio rerio* [28]
Sodium (mmol/l)	130.3 ± 1.4	131–136	150.4	NR
Chloride (mmol/l)	125.2 ± 1.8	112–113	138.7	NR
Potassium (mmol/l)	2.93 ± 0.11	2.6–3.2	3.93	6.8 ± 1.0
Calcium (mmol/l)	2.125 ± 0.1[a]	2.1–2.4[a]	2.7[a]	3.675 ± 0.575[a]
Phosphorus (mmol/l)	2.23 ± 0.1[a]	NR	2.35[a]	7.20 ± 0.5[a]
Magnesium (mmol/l)	1.23 ± 0.16[a]	0.70–0.78[a]	NR	NR
Total protein (g/l)	25–35[a]	6–32[a]	NR	52 ± 5[a]
Osmolarity (mOsm/l)	274 ± 3	294.6 ± 2.06	NR	NR
Albumin (g/l)	7.6–8.5[a]	NR	8.6[a]	30 ± 2[a]
Glucose (mmol/l)	1.67–2.61[a]	1.58 ± 0.53[a]	NR	82.2 ± 12.0 g/dl
Cholesterol (mmol/l)	3.83 ± 0.60[a]	NR	NR	NR
Creatinine (μmol/l)	7.07 ± 0.88[a]	NR	27.4[a]	61.8 ± 17.7[a]
BUN (mmol/l)	0.89 ± 0.2[a]	NR	NR	1.14 ± 0.1[a]
ALP (U/l)	NR	NR	NR	2.0 ± 4.5
ALT (U/l)	NR	NR	NR	367.0 ± 25.3
AST (U/l)	NR	NR	49.1	NR
LDH (U/l)	NR	NR	237.8	NR

NR = not reported.
[a] Original published values converted to SI units, except for glucose for zebra fish.

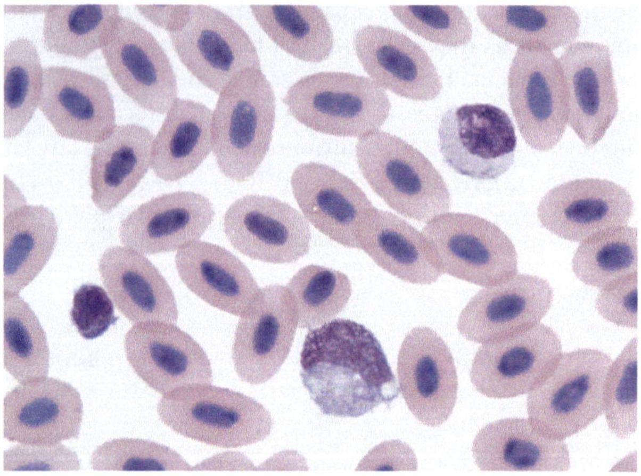

Figure 20.4 Blood smear from a koi, *Cyprinus carpio*, 1000× magnification, modified Wright's stain. Among the nucleated red blood cells, a monocyte is present centrally, and a small lymphocyte in the upper left.

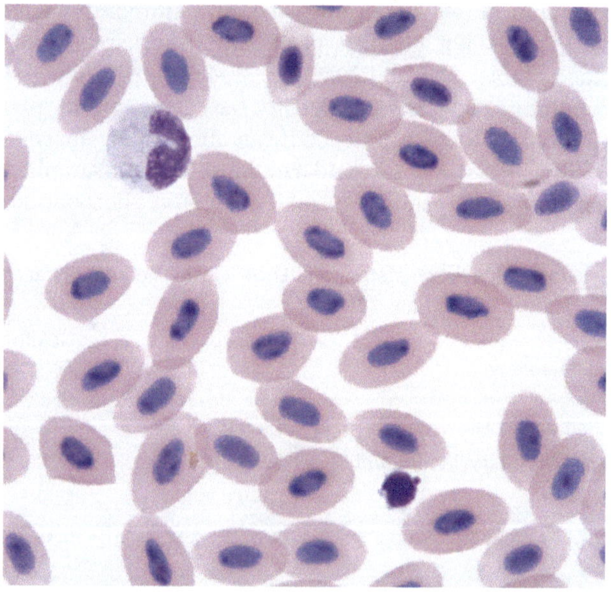

Figure 20.5 Blood smear from a koi, *Cyprinus carpio*, 1000× magnification, modified Wright's stain. A neutrophil is shown in the upper left and a small lymphocyte in the lower right.

dense, euchromatic nucleus and is usually oval to kidney bean shaped. Heterophils are similar to neutrophils but with pale eosinophilic to lavender granules in the cytoplasm. Fish species usually have either neutrophils or heterophils, although some species may have both. Functional differences between fish neutrophils and heterophils have also not been documented. Monocytes are round cells with a deep blue cytoplasm and a round to horseshoe-shaped nucleus. Eosinophils are infrequently observed in fish blood, but are the same size or slightly smaller than neutrophils with distinct eosinophilic granules in the cytoplasm. Basophils are rarely observed in

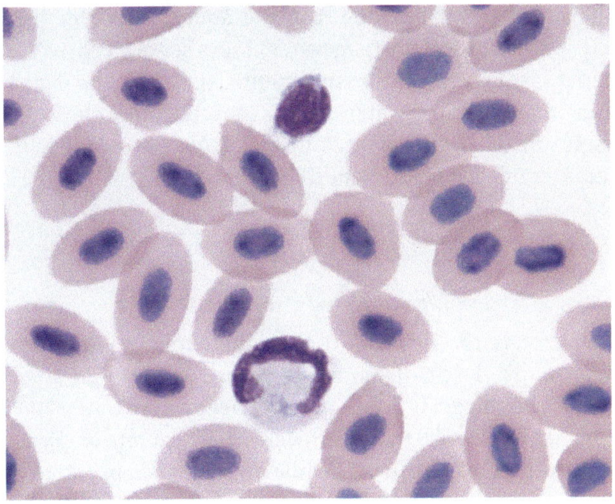

Figure 20.6 Blood smear from a koi, *Cyprinus carpio*, 1000x magnification, modified Wright's stain. A neutrophil appears near the bottom, while a small lymphocyte appears above.

fish and are similar to mammalian basophils in morphology. A more in-depth review of morphology and function of fish blood cells is available [41].

CBC Abnormalities

Packed cell volume (PCV) results can vary within and between species depending on age, gender, activity level, diet, stocking density, and water quality [37]. Active species such as tuna have higher normal PCV levels, while young fish, elasmobranchs, and bottom dwellers have lower PCVs [37]. Male fish tend to have higher PCVs when compared to female fish of the same age and sex [22]. Obligate air breathers also have higher PCVs [42]. Anemia is typically associated with a PCV less than 20, except in some shark species, where a PCV of 20 or less is normal [37]. Anemia in fish has been associated with elevated ammonia and nitrite levels, hypoxia, heavy metal toxicities, poor acclimation to captivity, nutritional disorders including starvation, increased stocking density, the use of chlorinated water, stress response, bacterial and viral diseases, inflammatory disease, and parasitism [37, 42–44]. A temporary reduction in hemoglobin levels, red blood cell counts, and PCV has been observed 24 h after oral administration of praziquantel in common carp, *Cyprinus carpio*, at a therapeutic dosage level [45]. These changes were reversed when measured again at 96 h post treatment. An increased PCV (>45) is associated with dehydration (marine fish), hypoxia (marine and freshwater fish), stress, and anesthesia (MS-222 and benzocaine) [37, 46]. The response to hypoxia can be rapid, and in some cases can occur in less than 1 h [15]. Increased water temperature can cause an elevated PCV in both goldfish and koi [22, 43].

White blood cell changes occur with many diseases and adverse environmental conditions. A stress leukogram in fish reveals a leukopenia with a lymphopenia and granulocytosis [37]. Elevated white blood cell counts can be found in freshwater fish held at higher water temperatures and those with sepsis [22, 43]. A decreased total white count can be found during starvation [43]. Increased lymphocyte counts can be found in normal juvenile fish, husbandry-related disorders, and any disease that stimulates the immune system [37]. Lymphopenia is associated with disorders that cause immune suppression such as stress and bacterial sepsis, and has also been found in ciliated protozoan infections [37, 43, 44]. Inflammation from several causes, including external parasitism, is often accompanied by granulocytosis. Granulocytosis is also seen in sharks with bacterial septicemia, and neutrophilia can occur in other fish species with septicemia [37]. Increases in the eosinophil count can sometimes occur with disorders causing inflammation, including parasitism, but is not consistently observed.

Hemostasis and Coagulation

Hemostasis and coagulation mechanisms in fish are similar to those found in mammals [29]. The primary cell involved in hemostasis in the fish is the thrombocyte, which is the equivalent of the platelet in mammals. Both the intrinsic and extrinsic coagulation pathways have been identified in fish, as well as many of the same coagulation factors found in mammals. Many factors can influence the coagulation process in fish including stress, nutritional status, exposure to chemicals, liver damage, vitamin K-deficiencies, vascular abnormalities, thrombocyte disorders, and coagulation factor deficiencies [29]. Normal thrombocyte number, clotting time, prothrombin time, activated partial thromboplastin time, and fibrinogen levels have been reported in the literature for only a few species, making these assays difficult to use and interpret diagnostically for fish [29, 47–49].

Biochemical Abnormalities

Liver and Muscle Enzymes

Muscle damage secondary to capture, anesthesia, and excess tissue trauma during sampling can increase creatine kinase (CK) levels, similar to other species. Alanine aminotransferase (ALT) appears to be the most liver-specific enzyme in koi for a common in-house blood analyzer [10]. A significant increased plasma enzyme activity of ALT was measured 96 h after a single oral dose of praziquantel in common carp, *C. carpio* [45].

Glucose

Lowered blood glucose levels are seen as a response to hepatic disease or injury and sepsis [50]. This is likely owing to impairment of the liver's ability to maintain normal glucose levels [45]. Blood glucose can be elevated during stress, anesthesia, hypoxia, and as an initial response in bacterial septicemia [43, 46, 51].

Vitamins, Minerals, Metals, and Toxins

Serum calcium levels have been observed to be elevated in gravid females, although additional reference interval studies are needed to substantiate this observation [40].

Blood Proteins

Total protein levels are found to be decreased in males and fish with bacterial septicemia, starvation, chronic stress, renal, and hepatic diseases, during spawning, and failure to acclimate to captivity [22, 43, 44]. Starvation is also accompanied by a decrease in blood urea nitrogen (BUN) [42]. Serum protein levels can be increased in female cyprinids (koi and goldfish) and cyprinids held at higher water temperatures [22]. In one study, rockfish with poor body condition had reduced total protein, albumin, glucose, cholesterol, and phosphorus values [36].

Renal, Gill, and Electrolytes

Elevated BUN, serum sodium, and chloride levels in marine fish can be indicative of gill disease [39, 44]. Elevated BUN, and decreased sodium and chloride levels can be observed in freshwater fish with gill disease [22]. Renal disease in marine fish can be accompanied by elevations in magnesium and sulfate levels and an elevation in creatinine [44]. Marine cold-water fish, for example, rockfish (*Sebastes* sp.) with exophthalmia, had decreased total protein, albumin, sodium, calcium, and chloride concentrations when compared to values taken from clinically normal fish [39]. These findings may have resulted from chronic, low-level malnutrition secondary to the cause of exophthalmia (Figure 20.6).

Hormones

There are currently very few clinical applications for hormone measurements in fish, although numerous research publications exist describing hormone levels and their alteration under varying circumstances. In addition to measuring serum or plasma cortisol levels, several assays have been developed to measure cortisol and a few other hormones in the aquarium water [52, 53]. The results of cortisol water assays seem to correlate with plasma cortisol measurement. Therefore, the use of non-invasive tank water assays may become clinically useful in the future as this method offers the ability to reduce collection and handling stress on the fish.

Urinalysis

Fish excrete the majority of their metabolic waste products in the form of ammonia primarily through their gills. The biggest difference between freshwater and marine species is that freshwater fish excrete copious amounts of dilute urine, while marine fish produce a small amount of concentrated urine. Interestingly, trimethylamine oxide, a stabilizer of proteins like urea, is present in the urine of marine teleosts but does not appear to be present in the urine of freshwater fishes [54]. Urinalysis is currently not a diagnostic test used in clinical medicine of fish. Urine is difficult to collect from a fish without catheter placement, and there is very little data available on the value of any results acquired [55].

Serology

The use of serology for the detection of disease agents in pet or ornamental fish is in its infancy. A number of ELISA and PCR assays are used in the research setting for the diagnosis and/or confirmation of disease in production (i.e., food) fish, while a few serological assays are available in the research setting for a small number of viral diseases of ornamental pond fish (e.g., koi, carp, and goldfish). These include an antibody and PCR assay for CyHV-3 (Koi Herpes Virus) in Koi and a PCR assay for CyHV-2 (Cyprinid Herpesvirus-2) in goldfish [56–58]. The antibody assay for KHV has also been used as a prepurchase screening test to determine previous exposure to KHV and identify latent carriers. In addition, there are a few research laboratories that have developed serological assays for betanodavirus, iridoviruses, and ranaviruses in fish [32, 59, 60]. Unfortunately, few serological assays have met the standards needed for validation as standard diagnostic methods; however, further development of serological methodology will hopefully advance the use of serology for routine diagnostic purposes.

References

1 Evans, D.H., Piermarini, P.M., and Choe, K.P. (2005). The multifunctional fish gill: dominant site of gas exchange, osmoregulation, acid-base regulation, and excretion of nitrogenous waste. *Physiological Review* 85: 97–177.

2 Greenwell, M.G., Sherrill, J., and Clayton, L.A. (2003). Osmoregulation in fish: mechanism and clinical implications. *Veterinary Clinics of North America: Exotic Animal Practice* 6: 169–189.

3 Raidal, S.R. and Raidal, S.L. (2006). Comparative renal physiology of exotic species. *Veterinary Clinics of North America: Exotic Animal Practice* 9 (3): 13–31.

4 Fontenot, D.K. and Neiffer, D.L. (2004). Wound management in teleost fish: biology of the healing process, evaluation, and treatment. *Veterinary Clinics of North America: Exotic Animal Practice* 7 (1): 57–86.

5 Weber, E.S. (2005). Gastroenterology for the piscine patient. *Veterinary Clinics of North America: Exotic Animal Practice* 8 (2): 247–276.

6 Harmon, T.S. (2009). Methods for reducing stressors and maintaining water quality associated with live fish transport in tanks: a review of the basics. *Reviews in Aquaculture* 1: 58–66.

7 Fisher, J.P. (2000). Facilities and husbandry (large fish models). In: *The Laboratory Fish* (ed. G.K. Ostrander), 23–24. Baltimore: Academic Press and 33–34.

8 Shelton, J.L. (2009). Water quality. In: *Fundamentals of Ornamental Fish Health* (ed. H.E. Roberts), 39–45. Hoboken, NJ: Wiley-Blackwell.

9 Johansen, R., Needhan, J.R., Colquhoun, D.J. et al. (2006). Guidelines for health and welfare monitoring of fish used in research. *Laboratory Animal* 40: 323–340.

10 Roberts, H.E. (2010). Freshwater ornamental fish. In: *BSAVA (British Small Animal Veterinary Medical Association) Manual of Exotic Pets*, 5e (ed. A. Meredith and C. Johnson-Delaney). Wiley.

11 Harms, C.A. (1999). Anesthesia in fish. In: *Zoo and Wild Animal Medicine, Current Therapy*, 4e (ed. M.E. Fowler and R.E. Miller), 158–163. Philadelphia: WB Saunders.

12 Harms, C.A. and Bakal, R.S. (1995). Techniques in fish anesthesia. *Journal of Small Exotic Animal Medicine* 3: 19–25.

13 Neiffer, D.L. and Stamper, M.A. (2009). Fish sedation, anesthesia, analgesia, and euthanasia: considerations, methods, and types of drugs. *ILAR Journal* 50: 343–360.

14 Reavill, D. and Roberts, H.E. (2007). Diagnostic cytology of fish. *Veterinary Clinics of North America: Exotic Animal Practice* 10: 207–234.

15 Roberts, H.E., Weber, E.S., and Smith, S.A. (2009). Chapter 17: Nonlethal diagnostic techniques. In: *Fundamentals of Ornamental Fish Health* (ed. H.E. Roberts), 172–184. Hoboken, NJ: Wiley-Blackwell.

16 Smith, S.A. (2002). Non-lethal clinical techniques used in the diagnosis of fish diseases. *Journal of the American Veterinary Medicine Association* 220: 1203–1206.

17 Gratzek, J.B. (1988). Tropical fish medicine. Parasites associated with ornamental fish. *Veterinary Clinics of North America: Small Animal Practice* 18 (2): 375–399.

18 Smith, S.A. and Roberts, H.E. (2009). Chapter 8: parasites of fishes. In: *Fundamentals of Ornamental Fish Health* (ed. H.E. Roberts), 102–112. Hoboken, NJ: Wiley-Blackwell.

19 Roberts, H.E. and Smith, S.A. (2011). Disorders of the respiratory system in pet and ornamental fish. *Veterinary Clinics of North America: Exotic Animal Practice* 14: 179–206.

20 Southgate, P.J. (2001). Laboratory techniques. In: *BSAVA Manual of Ornamental Fish*, 2e (ed. W.H. Wildgoose), 91–101. Gloucester: British Small Animal Veterinary Association.

21 Hrubec, T.C. and Smith, S.A. (1999). Differences between plasma and serum samples for evaluation of blood chemistry values in rainbow trout, channel catfish, hybrid tilapias and hybrid striped bass. *Journal of Aquatic Animal Health* 11: 116–122.

22 Groff, J.M. and Zinkl, J.G. (1999). Hematology and clinical chemistry of cyprinid fish. *Veterinary Clinics of North America: Exotic Animal Practice* 2 (5): 741–776.

23 Dye, V.A., Hrubec, T.C., Dunn, J.L., and Smith, S.A. (2001). Hematology and serum chemistry values for winter flounder (*Pleuronectes americanus*). *International Journal of Recirculation Aquaculture* 2: 37–50.

24 Hrubec, T.C., Smith, S.A., Robertson, J.L. et al. (1996a). Comparison of hematological reference intervals between culture system and type of hybrid striped bass. *American Journal of Veterinary Research* 57: 618–623.

25 Hrubec, T.C., Smith, S.A., Robertson, J.L. et al. (1996b). Blood biochemical reference intervals for sunshine bass (*Morone chrysops* × *Morone saxatilis*) in three culture systems. *American Journal of Veterinary Research* 57: 624–627.

26 Hrubec, T.C., Cardinale, J., and Smith, S.A. (2000). Hematology and plasma chemistry reference intervals for cultured tilapia (*Oreochromis* hybrid). *Veterinary Clinical Hematology* 29: 7–12.

27 Hrubec, T.C. and Smith, S.A. (2004). Hematology and blood chemistry reference intervals for yellow perch (*Perca flavescens*) raised in recirculation systems. *International Journal of Recirculating Aquaculture* 5: 29–42.

28 Knowles, S., Hrubec, T.C., Smith, S.A., and Bakal, R.S. (2006). Hematology and plasma chemistry reference intervals for cultured shortnose sturgeon (*Acipenser brevirostrum*). *Veterinary Clinical Pathology* 35 (4): 434–440.

29 Tavares-Dias, M. and Oliveira, S.R. (2009). A review of the blood coagulation system of fish. *Revista Brasileira de Biociências* 7: 205–224.

30 Tavares-Dias, M. and Ruas de Moraes, F. (2007). Leukocyte and thrombocyte reference values for

channel catfish (*Ictalurus punctatus*), with an assessment of morphologic, cytochemical, and ultrastructural features. *Veterinary Clinical Pathology* 36: 49–54.

31 Hrubec, T.C., Robertson, J.L., and Smith, S.A. (1997a). Effects of temperature on haematologic and biochemical profiles of sunshine bass (*Morone chrysops* × *Morone saxatilis*). *American Journal of Veterinary Research* 58: 126–130.

32 Munday, B.L., Kwang, J., and Moody, N. (2002). Betanodavirus infections of teleost fish: a review. *Journal of Fish Diseases* 25: 127–142.

33 Sakamoto, K., Lewbart, G.A., and Smith, T.M. (2001). Blood chemistry values of juvenile red pacu (*Piaractus brachypomus*). *Veterinary Clinical Pathology* 30 (2): 50–52.

34 Murtha, J.M., Qi, W., and Keller, E.T. (2003). Hematologic and serum biochemical values for zebrafish (*Danio rerio*). *Comparative Medicine* 5: 37–41.

35 Tocidlowski, M.E., Lewbart, G.A., and Stoskopf, M.K. (1997). Hematologic study of red pacu (*Colossoma brachypomum*). *Veterinary Clinical Pathology* 26 (3): 119–125.

36 Tripathi, N.K., Latimer, K.S., and Burnley, V.V. (2004). Hematologic reference intervals for koi (*Cyprinus carpio*), including blood cell morphology, cytochemistry, and ultrastructure. *Veterinary Clinical Pathology* 33 (2): 74–83.

37 Clauss, T.M., Dove, A.D.M., and Arnold, J.E. (2008). Hematologic disorders of fish. *Veterinary Clinics of North America: Exotic Animal Practice* 11: 445–462.

38 Hrubec, T.C., Robertson, J.L., and Smith, S.A. (1997b). Effects of ammonia and nitrate concentration on hematologic and serum biochemical profiles of hybrid striped bass (*Morone chrysops* × *Morone saxatilis*). *American Journal of Veterinary Research* 58: 131–134.

39 Harrenstien, L.A., Tornquist, S.J., Miller-Morgan, T.J. et al. (2005). Evaluation of a point-of-care blood analyzer and determination of reference ranges for blood parameters in rockfish. *Journal of the American Veterinary Medical Association* 226 (2): 255–265.

40 Palmeiro, B.S., Rosenthal, K.L., Lewbart, G.A., and Shofer, F.S. (2007). Plasma biochemical reference intervals for koi. *Journal of the American Veterinary Association* 230 (5): 708–712.

41 Hrubec, T.C. and Smith, S.A. (2010). Chapter 126. Hematology of fish. In: *Schalm's Veterinary Hematology*, 6e (ed. D.J. Weiss and K.J. Wardrop), 995–1004. Ames: Wiley-Blackwell.

42 Stoskopf, M. (1993b). Clinical pathology of freshwater tropical fishes. In: *Fish Medicine* (ed. M. Stoskopf), 543–545. Philadelphia: WB Saunders.

43 Stoskopf, M. (1993c). Clinical pathology of carp, goldfish, and koi. In: *Fish Medicine* (ed. M. Stoskopf), 450–453. Philadelphia: WB Saunders.

44 Stoskopf, M. (1993d). Clinical pathology of marine tropical fishes. In: *Fish Medicine* (ed. M. Stoskopf), 614–617. Philadelphia: WB Saunders.

45 Sudova, E., Piackova, V., Kroupova, H. et al. (2009). The effect of praziquantel applied *per os* on selected haematological and biochemical indices in common carp (*Cyprinus carpio* L.). *Fish Physiology and Biochemistry* 35: 599–605.

46 Ross, L.G. and Ross, B. (2008). *Anaesthetic and Sedative Techniques for Aquatic Animals*, 3e, 222. Oxford: Blackwell Publishing.

47 Fujikata, A. and Ikeda, Y. (1985). Blood coagulation and clotting test in carp. *Bulletin of the Japanese Society of Scientific Fisheries* 51: 933–939.

48 Pavlidis, M., Berry, M., Kokkari, C., and Kentouri, M. (1999). Prothrombin time, activated partial thromboplastin time and fibrinogen values in Mediterranean marine teleosts. *Fish Physiology and Biochemistry* 21: 335–343.

49 Smit, G.L. and Schoonbee, H.J. (1988). Blood coagulation factors in the freshwater fish *Oreochromis mossambicus*. *Journal of Fish Biology* 32: 673–677.

50 Juopperi T. 2003. Fish Clinical Pathology. Presented at Fish Health Management Continuing Education, Course, NC State College of Veterinary Medicine.

51 Velisek, J., Svobodova, Z., and Piackova, V. (2005). Effects of clove oil anaesthesia on common carp (*Cyprinus carpio* L.). *Veterinarni Medicina* 50 (6): 269–275.

52 Ellis, T., James, J.D., Stewart, C., and Scott, A.P. A non-invasive stress assay based upon measurement of free cortisol released into the water by rainbow trout. *Journal of Fish Biology* 65: 1233–1252.

53 Scott, A.P. and Ellis, T. (2007). Measurement of fish steroids in water – a review. *General and Comparative Endocrinology* 153: 392–400.

54 Grafflin, A.L. and Gould, R.G. (1936). Renal function in marine teleosts: II. The nitrogenous constituents of the urine of sculpin and flounder, with particular reference to trimethylamine oxide. *Biological Bulletin* 70: 16–27.

55 Stoskopf, M. (1993a). Clinical examination and procedures. In: *Fish Medicine* (ed. M. Stoskopf), 62–78. Philadelphia: WB Saunders.

56 Gilad, O., Yun, S., Andree, K.B. et al. (2002). Initial characteristics of koi herpesvirus and development of a polymerase chain reaction assay to detect the virus in koi, *Cyprinus carpio koi*. *Diseases of Aquatic Organisms* 48: 101–108.

57 Gilad, O., Yun, S., Zagmutt-Vergara, F. et al. (2004). Concentrations of a herpes-like virus (KHV) in tissues of experimentally infected *Cyprinus carpio koi* as

assessed by real-time TaqMan PCR. *Diseases of Aquatic Organisms* 60: 179–187.

58 Goodwin, A.E., Merry, G.E., and Sadler, J. (2006). Detection of the herpesviral haematopoietic necrosis disease agent cyprinid herpesvirus 2 in moribund and healthy goldfish: validation of a quantitative PCR diagnostic method. *Diseases of Aquatic Organisms* 69: 137–143.

59 Weber, E.S., Waltzek, T.B., Young, D.A. et al. (2009). Systemic iridovirus infection in the Banggai cardinalfish (*Pterapogon kauderni* Koumans 1933). *Journal of Veterinary Diagnostic Investigations* 21: 306–320.

60 Whittington, R.J., Becker, J.A., and Dennis, M.M. (2010). Iridovirus infections in finfish - critical review with emphasis on ranaviruses. *Journal of Fish Diseases* 33 (2): 95–122.

21

Aquatic Invertebrates

Nadia Stegeman DVM, MPH[1], Matthew Allender DVM, MS, PhD, DACZM[2], Jill Arnold MS, MT (ASCP)[3] and Christopher J. Bonar VMD, DACZM[4]

[1] *Animal Health Associates, Eugene, Oregon, USA*
[2] *Wildlife Epidemiology Laboratory, College of Veterinary Medicine University of Illinois, Urbana, Illinois, USA*
[3] *National Aquarium Baltimore, Baltimore, Maryland, USA*
[4] *Dallas Zoo, Dallas, Texas, USA*

Introduction

Invertebrates are defined by their lack of spine and include nine phyla, including Arthropoda, Echinodermata, and Mollusca. The species vary markedly in physiology. This chapter is an overview of clinical information for common species in the aquarium trade. Much information was extracted from data of case-control studies rather than from studies to establish normal values. The resulting biases, including small sample size, should be accounted for when using these values. Furthermore, techniques and protocols used to monitor health parameters in vertebrates have rarely been evaluated or validated for invertebrates. However, many of these techniques are useful in assessment of alterations in homeostasis of aquatic invertebrates.

General diagnostic testing useful for many aquatic invertebrates include assessment of hemolymph color and clotting, hemocyte counts, and species-specific determination of hemolymph biochemical analytes, enzymes, and gases. This chapter focuses on interpretation of the characteristics of hemolymph in display animals (Tables 21.1–21.5). Additionally, information from species in aquaculture, those outside of the aquarium trade, wild populations, and those used for physiologic research are also incorporated herein. We will summarize the limited research published on other diagnostic samples, ranging from crustacean urine to gastropod perivitelline fluid.

Environmental factors commonly affecting physiology include dissolved oxygen levels, temperature, pH, salinity, total alkalinity, hardness, and levels of ammonia, nitrite, nitrate, and chloride. Mild elevations in ammonia and nitrite have been reported to affect the immune response of shrimp, prawns, and abalone [1–5]. Values described in this chapter should be evaluated in light of the study of environmental parameters. However, several useful values and trends among invertebrates are similar to those of vertebrates, and can be adapted for clinical use. Assessment of clinicopathologic parameters of aquatic invertebrates should coincide with assessment of environmental parameters, such as water quality, to render these values most useful. For this reason, in order to evaluate population health, baseline values for a specific population living under defined conditions should be established. An approach to the clinicopathologic assessment of aquatic invertebrates is delineated in Box 21.1

Overview of Aquatic Invertebrate Species

Invertebrates are not only increasingly popular display animals, but also are also used in research and are a popular human food source. Common captive species of aquatic invertebrates include the Arthropoda, which include Chelicerata (horseshoe crabs) and the crustaceans (crab, shrimp/prawn, lobster, and mantis shrimp; Table 21.1); the echinoderms (urchins, sea stars, and sea cucumbers – Table 21.2); and the molluscs (bivalves: oysters, mussels, and scallops – Table 21.3), cephalopods (cuttlefish, octopus, and squid – Table 21.4), and gastropods (slugs and snails – Table 21.5).

Exotic Animal Laboratory Diagnosis, First Edition. Edited by J. Jill Heatley and Karen E. Russell.

Table 21.1 Arthropods: Horseshoe crabs and decapod crustaceans.

Horseshoe crab	**Family limulidae**
American horseshoe crab	*Limulus polyphemus*
Crabs	**Infraorders Brachyura and Anomura**
Anemone hermit crab	*Dardanus* spp.
Arrow crab, yellowline arrow crab	*Stenorhynchus seticornis*
Blue leg hermit crab	*Phimochirus* spp.
Cone shell hermit crab	*Trizopagurus/Ciliopagurus* spp.
Decorator crab, Camposcia crab	*Camposcia retusa*
Decorator crab, spider decorator crab, coral crab, Conical spider crab	*Xenocarcinus* spp.
Dwarf zebra hermit crab	*Coenobita* spp.
Emerald crab, green clinging crab	*Mithraculus sculptus*
Hermit crabs, various	*Calcinus, Clibanarius* spp.
Mini crab, fiddler crab, calling crab	*Uca* spp.
Porcelain crab, Anemone crab	*Neopetrolisthes ohshimai*
Red claw crab	*Sesarma bidens*
Red reef or scarlet hermit crab	*Paguristes* spp.
Sally lightfoot crab, nimble spray crab, short crab, Urchin crab	*Percnon gibbesi*
Stone, king crab	*Lithodes* spp.
Trapezia Pocillopora/Acropora crab	*Trapezia* spp.
Lobster and crayfish	**Infraorders Achelata and Astacidea**
American lobster	*Homarus americanus*
Blue crayfish	*Procambarus* spp.
Purple and orange lobster, red lobster, Debelius's reef lobster	*Enoplometopus debelius*
Red lobster, Hawaiian reed lobster, hairy reef lobster	*Enoplometopus* spp.
Slipper lobster, sculptured slipper lobster	*Parribacus antarcticus*
Spiny blue lobster, painted rock lobster	*Panulirus versicolor*
Shrimp	**Suborder Natantia**
Bumblebee shrimp, striped bumblebee shrimp	*Gnathophyllum americanum*
Camel shrimp, dancing shrimp, hinge-beak shrimp, candy shrimp	*Rhynchocinetes durbanensis*
Coral banded shrimp	*Stenopus hispidus*
Fire, peppermint, cleaner shrimp	*Lysmata* spp.
Ghost shrimp, glass shrimp, grass shrimp	*Palaemonetes* spp.
Glass anemone shrimp, Pacific Clown Anemone shrimp	*Periclimenes brevicarpalis*
Harlequin shrimp, Blue Clown shrimp	*Hymenocera elegans* or *elegans*
Pistol shrimp, snapping shrimp	*Alpheus* spp., *Synalpheus* spp.
Red Cherry shrimp, Yellow shrimp	*Neocaridina davidi*
Saron shrimp	*Saron* spp.
Sexy anemone shrimp	*Thor amboinensis*
Singapore flower, bamboo shrimp, wood shrimp, Asian filter shrimp, fan shrimp	*Atyopsis moluccensis*
Snowball shrimp, blue pearl shrimp, amber-orange pearl shrimp	*Neocaridina* cf. *zhangjiajiensis*
Tiger shrimp, Amano algae-eating, crystal shrimp, green shrimp, orange sunkist shrimp, bee shrimp, blue bee shrimp, crystal red shrimp, golden bee shrimp, orange bee shrimp, white bee shrimp, orange tiger shrimp, black tiger shrimp, blue tiger shrimp, red tiger shrimp	*Caridina* spp.
Viper shrimp, African filter shrimp, Gabon shrimp	*Atya gabonensis*
Mantis shrimp	**Stomatopod**
Mantis shrimp	*Squilla mantis*

Table 21.2 Echinoderms: Urchins, sea cucumbers and sea stars.

Common names Echinoderms	Scientific names Echinodermata
Black sea urchin	*Tetrapygus niger*
Chilean sea urchin	*Loxechinus albus*
Common sea star	*Asterias rubens*
Green sea urchin	*Strongylocentrotus droebachiensis*
Red sea urchin	*Strongylocentrotus franciscanus*
Rock-boring urchin, rock urchin, short-spined urchin	*Echinometra lacunter*
Shore sea urchin, green sea urchin	*Psammechinus miliaris*
Variegated sea urchin, green sea urchin	*Lytechinus variegatus*
Sea cucumber	*Holothuria glaberrima*

Table 21.3 Common molluscs – bivalves: Clams, mussels, oysters, and scallops.

Common name	Scientific name
Clams	**Bivalvia**
Blue/green lipped mussel	*Perna canaliculus*
Clam	*Hippopus* spp.
Common bay scallop	*Argopecten irradians*
Common oyster	*Crassostrea virginica*
Common quahog clam	*Mercenaria campechiensis*
Coquina	*Donax variabilis*
Flame scallop	*Lima* spp.
Freshwater clam	*Corbicula* spp.
Freshwater mussel	*Elliptio* spp.
Giant clam	*Tridacna* spp.
Giant heart cockle	*Dinocardium robustum*
Mussel	*Modiolus americanus*
Pen shell	*Atrina rigida*, or *A. serrate*
Sculptured venus clam	*Chione cancellata*
Southern shipworm	*Bankia gouldi*; *Teredo navalis*
Spiny and rock oysters	*Spondylus* spp.
Sun ray venus clam	*Macrocallista nimbosa*
Surf clam	*Spisula solidissima*

Restraint of and Hemolymph Collection from Aquatic Invertebrates

Restraint required for sampling aquatic invertebrates varies by species. For hemolymph sampling, many studies report use of physical restraint alone. Some species require sedation for sampling for safety of both the handler and patient. Knowledge of an individual species' defense mechanisms is crucial in determining the optimal restraint technique. For example, octopods have sharp beaks and species like the blue-ringed octopus (*Hapalochlaena* spp.) have powerful neurotoxins in their saliva. Additionally, octopod hemolymph sampling sites are often at the level of the mantle, in close proximity to major organs. There is a paucity of information on chemical or physical restraint in other aquatic invertebrates, and their effects on the hematology of the species, which is a fertile area for clinical research.

Table 21.4 Molluscs – cephalopods: Cuttlefish, octopus, squid, and nautilus.

Common name	Scientific name
Cephalopods	**Coleoidea and nautiloidea**
Common cuttlefish, European cuttlefish	*Sepia officinalis*
Common octopus	*Octopus vulgaris*
Giant Pacific octopus, North Pacific giant octopus	*Enteroctopus dofleini*; *Octopus dofleini*
Lesser octopus, curled octopus	*Eledone cirrhosa*
Long-finned inshore squid, long-finned squid	*Loligo pealei*
Nautilus	*Nautilus pompilius*

Invertebrate blood is composed of hemolymph, which is involved in nonspecific innate immunity and has no capacity for adaptive immunity. In general, an open circulatory system is present in some molluscs and arthropods in which a fluid is contained in the dominant body cavity or hemocoel. The fluid, usually called hemolymph, bathes the organs directly without distinction between blood and interstitial fluid. In this case, the hemolymph fluid acts as both blood and interstitial fluid. The closed circulatory system of cephalopods, some molluscs, and echinoderms is characterized by the presence of blood vessels [5]. Differing circulatory systems are not taxon specific. These physiologic differences direct clinician determination of hemolymph access points. The process of sample collection in each body design is described below. Safe sample size or sample volumes which have been associated with morbidity, as well as sample volumes expected depending on the hemolymph collection site, are detailed under each invertebrate class below (when known). Known contraindications, if any, for that collection site are also noted. Additionally, appropriate sample handing is also detailed under each taxon of aquatic invertebrate. Non-powder gloves are advised for use in all aquatic invertebrates as is cleaning the sampling site prior to collection with 70%–80% ethanol.

Table 21.5 Molluscs – gastropods.

Common name	Scientific name
Snails and slugs	**Gastropods**
Abalone racer/fuzzy tiger, Taiwan abalone, green abalone	*Haliotis asinina, H. diversicolor supertexta, H. fulgens*
Apple snail, golden apple snail	*Pomacea canaliculata, P. bridgesi, P. depressa, P. lineata*
Assassin snail, killer snail, bumble bee snail	*Clea helena, Anentome helena*
Black Japanese trap door snail, Chinese mystery snail, Asian apple snail, Chinese apple snail, Japanese trapdoor snail, mud snail, Oriental mystery snail, tanisha, rice snail	*Viviparus malleatus*
Bumble bee snail	*Pusiostoma mendicaria*
Conehead algae eater, Star Snail, Turbo Snail, Turbo Grazer Snail, Turban Snail, Top Shell Snail, and Astraea Star Snail	*Astraea* spp., *Astraea tecta*
Dark Cerith, Florida Cerith; Stocky Cerith, True Cerith	*Cerithium atratum, C. litertatum*
Giant ramshorn snail	*Marisa cornuarietis, Planorbarius corneus*
Lettuce Nudibranch	*Tridachia crispata*
Madagascar Nucleus Cowrie, Panther Cowrie, Money Cowrie, Arabian Cowrie, Tiger Cowrie	*Cypraea nucleus, C. patherina, C. moneta, C arabica, C. tigris*
Malaysian trumpet snail, red-rimmed melania, Malayan burrowing snail	*Melanoides tuberculata*
Margarita snail, Pink Margarita Snail, Stomatella Limpet Snail, Little Margarite Snail, Pearly Topped Snail	*Margarites pupillus*
Mexican turbo, Top Shell Snail, Turban Snail	*Turbo fluctuosa*
Nerite snail	*Nerita* spp.
Queen Conch	*Strombus gigas*
Ramshorn snail	*Helisoma trivolvis (Planorbella trivolvis), Biomphalaria alexandrina*
Red foot algae snail, Norris Top Snail, Red Foot Moon Snail, and Smooth Brown Turban	*Norrisia norrisi*
Sea hare	*Aplysia spp.*
Super Tongan Nassarius Snail, Super Sand Snail	*Nassarius distortus*
Trochus banded snail	*Trochus spp.*
Turban snail, Tectus snail	*Tectus fenestratus*
Velvet sea slug	*Chelidonura varians*

Arthropods: Chelicerates: Horseshoe Crabs

Hemolymph is most often collected from the pericardial sinus through the arthrodial membrane (Figure 21.1). Wiping the arthrodial membrane with alcohol or chlorhexidine may therefore reduce the potential for clotting due to contamination at the entrance of the needle into the exoskeleton. Flexing the opisthosoma ventrally to expose the arthrodial membrane facilitates sampling with a 21–23 gauge (g.) needle with a 1 or 3 ml syringe. Larger volumes can be collected with a 14 g. needle [6, 111]. Smaller hemolymph samples can also be taken from any of the soft exoskeleton joints on any of the legs, but these are often more contaminated and yield small volumes (<0.5 ml) [6]. The total volume of hemolymph in adult horseshoe crab has been estimated with a mean of 25% body weight, that is, linearly associated with body weight and non-linearly correlated with prosomal width and inter-ocular width [6]. Total hemolymph volume that can be safely harvested has not been established, but has been reported to be between 50 and 150 ml for an adult [7, 111].

Arthropods: Crustaceans

Hemolymph can be obtained from the sinus beneath the arthrodial membrane in the American lobster, *Homarus americanus*, by inserting a needle into the ventrum at about a 45° angle to the body surface (Figure 21.12) and again in the blue crab by inserting the needle between two segments of the flexed chela. Using a 22 g. needle and a 1–3 ml syringe, hemolymph is obtained by puncturing the dorsal carapace, anteriolateral to the heart, with the needle used to aspirate hemolymph from the pericardial sinus [8, 9]. In the red rock crab, *Cancer productus*, this site yielded 0.2–0.4 ml in crabs weighing approximately

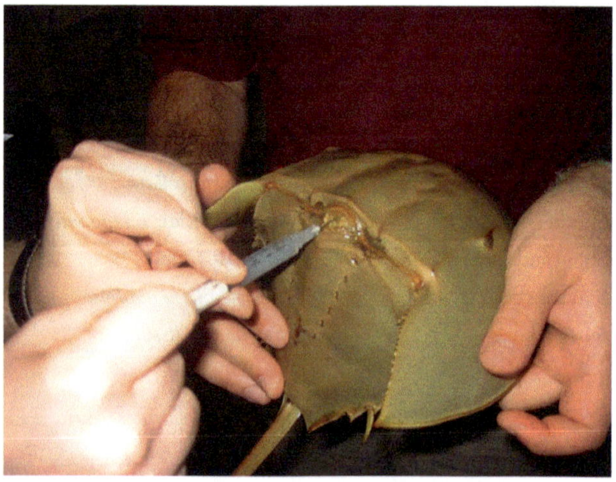

Figure 21.1 Hemolymph collection from the pericardial sinus of a horseshoe crab (*Limulus polyphemus*) via the arthrodial membrane. *Source:* Photo courtesy of Matt Allender.

21 g [10]. This technique is used in many physiologic studies; however, follow-up studies of morbidity following the iatrogenic carapacial puncture were lacking. A similar method has also been used in crayfish weighing as little as 6 g; one study obtained 0.1 ml hemolymph samples dorsally from the pericardial sinus between the carapace and first abdominal segment using a 0.5-ml syringe fitted with a 27 g. needle. A collection method utilizing direct cardiocentesis, often after drilling a hole in the carapace for accuracy, has also been described [11]. Use of a 22 g. needle directed into the ventral sinus to terminally collect 30 ml of hemolymph from a 400 to 500 g lobster has also been reported [12].

Prebranchial – In crustaceans, both venous and arterial sites are accessible. For a venous sample, a commonly used prebranchial phlebotomy site is through the arthrodial membrane at the base of the fifth leg using a 22–23 g. needle on a 1–3 ml syringe [13]. In a crab with a carapacial length of 5–7 cm, 1–2 ml of hemolymph were obtained from this site [8].

Chelae – Another arthrodial membrane between the prosoma and opisthosoma can be used to target the cardiac sinus (Figure 21.2) [8]. Hemolymph also can be collected from crayfish via pipet after breaking off a periopod or cheliped [14]. In display animals, this open method is best relegated to a last resort.

Echinoderms

Hemolymph from sea urchins can be collected from the perivisceral coelom with a 1–3 ml syringe with a 21–26 g., 0.5–0.75 in. needle attached, and inserted adjacent to the oral disc [15–18]. The needle should be directed in between the spines adjacent to oral disc on the ventral surface of the animal (Figure 21.3). Hemolymph should be collected with the patient in water to avoid a respiratory or metabolic acidosis induced by air exposure [16].

Mollusks: Bivalves

Bivalve sampling sites include the adductor muscle sinus, pericardial sinus and ventricle, and the venous sinus just beyond the mantle (this will yield extrapallial fluid). In smaller bivalves such as the mussel, *Elliptio complanata*, one can use a 25 g. 5/8 in. needle to penetrate between valves (valves may be held agape with a knife and tissue forceps) into the sinus in the white anterior adductor muscle (Figure 21.4). The needle should be directed parallel to the anterior edge of the valves [20]. In a 50 g animal, this sampling site yielded 0.5 ml. Other attempts for collection from the pericardial sinus, or cardiac ventricles, through a drilled hole or gaping valves lacked accuracy and resulted in 100% mortality (Figure 21.5). Needle insertion through the mantle to obtain extrapallial fluid yielded a maximum of 0.2 ml. Although magnesium, phosphorous, ammonia, protein,

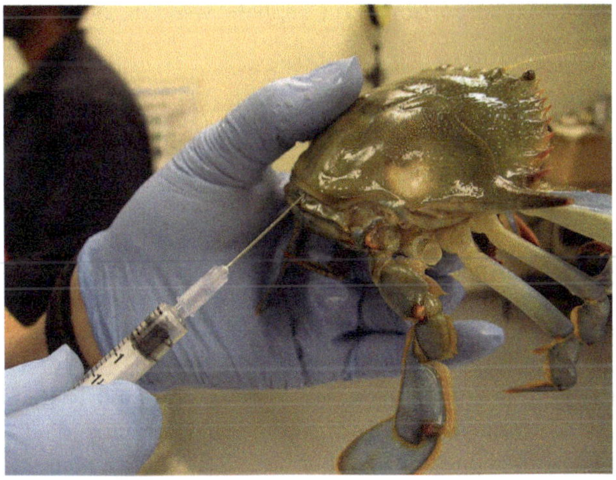

Figure 21.2 Hemolymph collection from a blue crab *(Callinectes sapidus)* between prosoma and opisthosoma. Note that hemolymph is often initially clear but turns blue upon exposure to air.

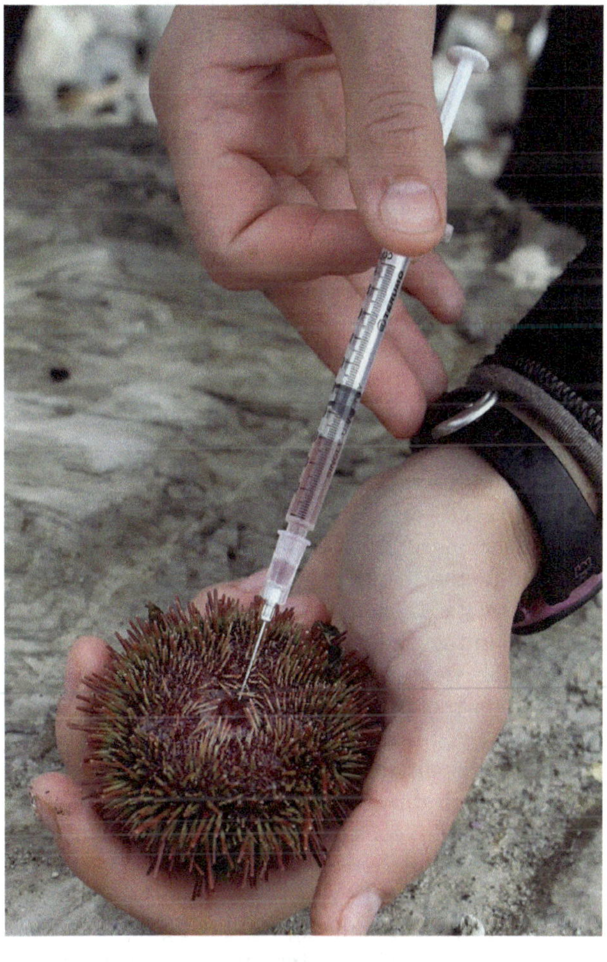

Figure 21.3 Hemolymph collection from a sea urchin by a needle inserted into the perivisceral coelom by a needle inserted adjacent to the oral disc.

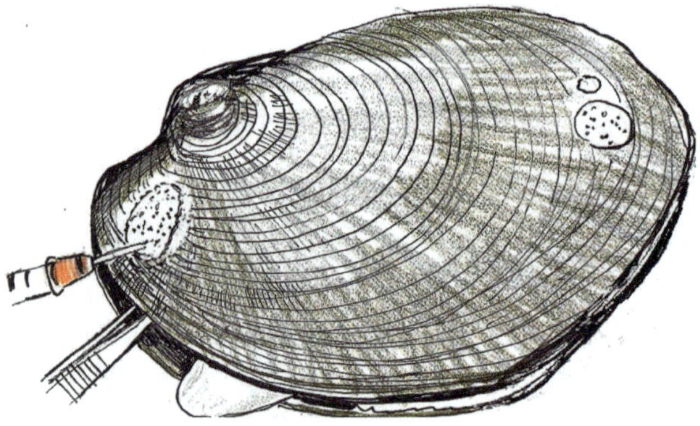

Figure 21.4 Non-lethal approach to hemolymph collection from the adductor muscle of a freshwater bivalve (*Elliptio complanata*). *Source:* Redrawn from Ref. [20].

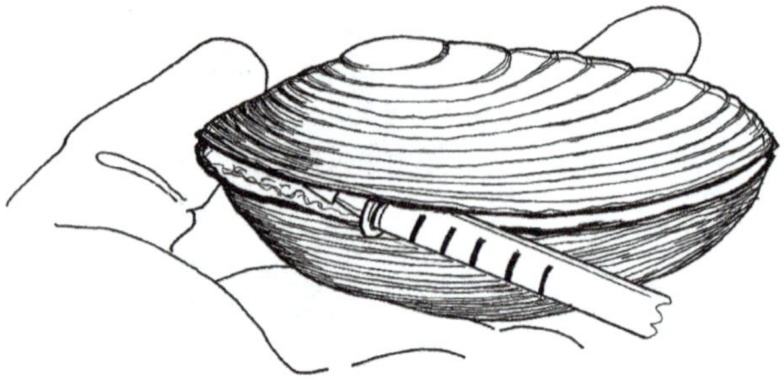

Figure 21.5 Lethal approach through the shell to hemolymph collection from the adductor muscle, pericardial sinus, or cardiac ventricles of a freshwater bivalve (*Elliptio complanata*). *Source:* Adapted from Ref. [20].

sodium, potassium, and chloride showed no significant difference between ventricular chamber and adductor sinus sampling sites, calcium levels were significantly different between the two sites [20]. In larger bivalves such as clams, sampling can be accomplished with a 19 g., 38 mm needle inserted midway between the inlet and outlet siphons with the needle angled into the body of the clam [21] (Figure 21.5). The sample is obtained from the venous sinus located in the mantle tissue, between the edge of the mantle and the inside of the shell. A trend in total extractable blood volume has been demonstrated in the giant clam: for every 8 cm shell length, hemolymph yield is about 10 ml [22]. Other sampling methods for molluscs include accessing the pericardial sac in oysters through a hole drilled in the ligament holding the shells together, or in clams by inserting a needle through this ligament. After sampling, the hole may be filled with epoxy (Figure 21.6). Removal of 500–800 µl of hemolymph in bivalves weighing an average of 8.24 g has been reported. Extraction of 0.5–1 ml hemolymph from bivalves ranging 9.6–129.2 g in weight has also been performed [20]. Ten milliliter of hemolymph for every 8 cm of mantle has been extracted safely in the giant clam (*Tridacna crocea*) [22].

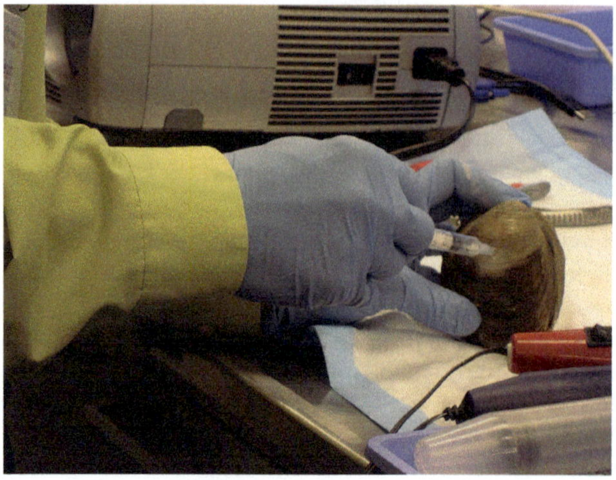

Figure 21.6 Lethal bivalve sampling: After drilling a hole, penetrate adductor muscle and pericardial sinus.

Mollusks: Cephalopods

In octopod cephalopods weighing more than 250 g, hemolymph can be collected from the branchial blood vessel using a 21–27 g. needle with a 1–3 ml syringe [23]. Using a dorsal approach through the mantle in octopods, the aorta may be sampled using ultrasound or endoscopy to identify the vessel lying adjacent to the crop [24]. Total hemolymph volume for the giant (Figure 21.5) Pacific octopus (*Enteroctopus dofleini*) is approximately 5.8% of the body weight [25], but the safe sampling volume is not established. One study demonstrated success with a sample volume of 0.3 ml/100 g BW [26]. The hemolymph vascular system of the coleoid squid (*Illex illecebrosus*) has been described and may prove useful when selecting alternative hemolymph sampling sites [27]. Collection of hemolymph has been accomplished in cuttlefish (*Sepia* sp.) from the cephalic peribuccal blood sinus and from the muscular portion of the cephalic vein [28, 29].

Mollusks: Gastropods

Gastropod hemolymph collection can be divided into methods that do and do not involve puncturing the shell. Certain collection sites outside the heart may yield a mix of fluids, such as pallial fluid, which is thought to be a mixture of hemolymph and urine [30]. For gastropods with hemal pores, such as snails of *Lymnaea* spp., persistent stimulation of either the foot or operculum results in expulsion of extracellular fluid (ECF). The fluid enters the pulmonate cavity via the hemal pore and is then ejected through the pneumostome, which can be identified by the appearance of bubbles. This fluid can be collected via a pipette [31]. Alternatively, in snails less than 50 g, a needle inserted 5 mm below the pneumostome with a 25 g. needle may allow hemolymph aspiration. In snails weighing between 50 and 200 g, this point is

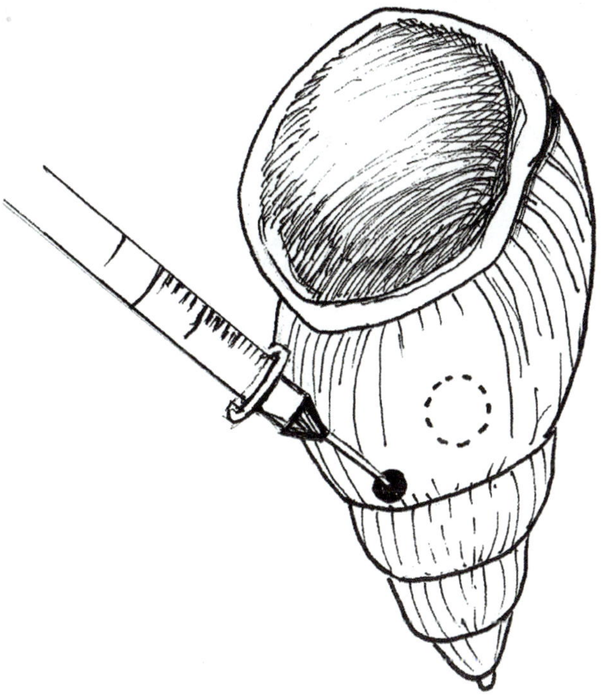

Figure 21.7 Method for sampling hemolymph from a Lymnaeid snail. The dotted lines depict the albumin gland. *Source:* Redrawn from Ref. [19].

approximately 20 mm below the pneumostome [32]. As a complete full-body withdrawal can expel up to 60% of the hemolymph volume in a lymnaeid snail [30], repeated sampling with this technique could cause patient morbidity or mortality. Other snail studies involve irritation (needle or scalpel) of the foot followed by hemolymph collection with a capillary tube or pipette [33, 34]. In abalone, hemolymph can also be collected from the branchial vein with a 5 ml syringe and a 1 in., 20 g. needle [35], or the pallial sinus using a 1 ml syringe with a 25 g. needle [2]. Finally, in the sea slug (*Aplysia* spp.), 0.5 ml of hemolymph can be extracted at the level between the rhinophores and parapodia near the foot using a 16 g. needle and a 1 ml syringe [36]. Alternatively, one may file a notch in each valve to create an opening and then insert the needle into the adductor sinus through the adductor muscle [37]. Methods involving pre-drilling a hole are as follows [19]. Hold the snail spire down, and use a dissecting needle to make an access hole over the sinus. Insert a 27 g. needle attached to a 1–3 ml syringe into the sinus area adjoining the suture of the whorl and apical to the yellowish albumin gland (Figure 21.7). This site yielded 0.1 ml of hemolymph from snails with a minimum shell length of 25 mm. Similar methods include pre-drilling a hole penetrating the posterior mantle cavity for collection from the perivisceral sinus in pulmonate and prosobranch snails [38], or from the efferent branchial vein in prosobranch snails [39].

Sample Handling

Analytical Procedures

Methods for total and differential hemocyte counts (THC and DHC, respectively) have been reported for a number of species. One study determined that automated cell counts yielded variable results compared to manual counts using a Neubauer hemocytometer, especially noting the poor correlation for samples from nonintermoult American lobsters [12].

Arthropods: Chelicerae: Horseshoe Crabs

There is no ideal anticoagulant for use with horseshoe crab hemolymph. Horseshoe crabs have a unique component of their hemolymph, *Limulus* amoebocyte lysate (LAL), which induces clotting in the presence of Gram-negative endotoxin [40]. Due to the LAL, bacterial contamination of the tubes or surfaces of the tubes will lead to white precipitates in any tube, regardless of anticoagulant contained therein. Therefore, sterile procedures are often the most successful. EDTA has been shown to prevent aggregation of the amoebocytes when diluted 1:20 [41]. Lithium heparin tubes have also been used successfully to perform hemocyte evaluation [42]. Temperature may also play a role in aggregation of amoebocytes, as amoebocytes in saline at lower temperatures are slower to clot than at higher temperatures [41]. Storage parameters are unknown and likely depend on the analyte; therefore, for most biochemical analytes, storage at −80 °C is recommended as a precaution against analyte degradation.

Arthropods: Crustaceans

Crustacean hemolymph clots quickly, and thus sampling requires the use of an anticoagulant. Options include EDTA, citrate, L-cysteine, glutaraldehyde, and formalin [43]. A formula for the blue crab (*Callinectes sapidus*) has been reported that included two calcium chelating compounds (EDTA and citrate) [44]. Another formula has been reported for the American lobster (*H. americanus*) using an artificial seawater solution that also contained formaldehyde to preserve the cells [12]. Hemolymph (0.5 ml) was drawn into a syringe containing 4.5 ml of cold anticoagulant. Alternatively, lobster hemolymph was collected and 200 μl immediately transferred into 800 μl cold 10% neutral buffered formalin, without using an anticoagulant [45]. Collection with cooled (5 °C) plastic and glass syringes followed by sample placement in sterile sealed vials on ice after collection is common [10, 46]. Some blood gas studies used ice cold 8% perchloric acid to deproteinize the sample prior to analysis [9, 47]. However, this and other established crustacean anticoagulants may not be readily available to clinicians [45, 48]. Some blood gas studies report that samples may be maintained without anticoagulant on ice for 1 h without affecting values [13, 49]. To deter hemocyte movement for cellular analysis in crayfish, ice cold 4% formaldehyde was added to the sample in equal volumes of sample to diluent [50].

Echinoderms

Variegated sea urchin (*Lytechinus variegatus*) hemolymph destined for cell counts can be preserved by placement in EDTA and storage at 4 °C until analysis [17, 51]. Black sea urchin (*Diadema antillarum*) hemolymph was stored in lithium heparin Microtainers (Microtainer: Becton-Dickenson, 1 Becton Dr., Franklin Lakes, NJ 07417 U.S.A.) and stored on wet ice to make smears [16]. Appropriate safe hemolymph sample volumes have not been described for echinoderms; however, a 1.0 ml sample was safely removed from 70 to 100 g green sea urchins from Maine [17]. Hemolymph should be placed in sterile serum tubes to assess color, clotting characteristics, and sample consistency [17]. Fresh hemolymph smears should be made on glass slides and air-dried to allow for coelomocyte expansion up to 10-fold [17, 51].

Mollusks: Bivalves

No anticoagulant is recommended in these species as untreated hemocytes at ambient temperature maintain a high level of viability (80%–93%) for up to 24 h [52]. Hemocytes need only be exposed to L-cysteine (25 mg/ml, pH 8.0) just prior to slide preparations for morphological analysis [52]. While specific invertebrate anticoagulants do exist, they are not common in veterinary practice. Studies have used no anticoagulant for cytology, or for centrifugation of samples, kept samples on ice for chemical analysis. After centrifugation, plasma samples have been stored at −80 °C for later measurements [53]. Immediate use of a hemocytometer to obtain a total blood count after sampling has been reported [20]. The remaining hemolymph was centrifuged and the supernatant extracted and frozen for chemical analysis. Invertebrate hemocytes tend to display high mobility, even after collection, making cytological analysis challenging. To address this, hemolymph may be combined with a solution of 1% formalin in TBS (0.05 M Tris–buffered saline, pH 8.4) as a fixative [54]. For examination of the cellular morphology of bivalve hemolymph, a dry slide cytologic technique may also be used. In this technique, 100 µl of fresh hemolymph were placed on a slide and maintained at 20 °C for 5 min to allow hemocytes to settle prior to fixation for 5 min in seawater containing 2.5% glutaraldehyde. Slides were rinsed for 2 min in distilled water, dehydrated in 96% ethanol for one minute, and air-dried prior to staining [54]. Other than the effects of clotting on cell count, interferences are rarely reported. In one study, samples were held on ice in polyethylene tubes prior to analysis to inhibit aggregation and were stored in a −20 °C freezer overnight prior to measuring clinical chemistries [20].

Mollusks: Cephalopods

There is no ideal anticoagulant for cephalopod hemolymph. One protocol describes adding 100 ml sample to 900 ml of marine anticoagulant (pH 7.00) (NaCl, 2.63 g : 100 ml; glucose, 1.8 g : 100 ml; tri-sodium citrate, 0.088 g/ml; citric acid, 0.055 g : 100 ml) containing ethylene glycol-bis (b-aminoethylether) N,N,N′,N′-tetraacetic acid (0.029 g : 100 ml) [26].

Mollusks: Gastropods

Anticoagulants used in physiology studies, such as phosphate buffered saline, are unlikely to be readily found in a veterinary setting. Like many crustacean hemolymph studies, gastropod studies tend to employ immediate use of a hemocytometer to determine the hemogram with samples kept in an ice-bath or frozen without anticoagulant after sampling [55–57]. In gastropods, as with other invertebrates with open circulatory systems, sampling location affects analyte levels. For example, in lymnaeid snails, the ionic content of pallial fluid and hemolymph is different [30]. Clinicians utilizing blind sampling methods should consider sampling site when interpreting hemolymph chemistries.

Hemolymph Assessment

Hemolymph Appearance

Assessment of gross appearance of hemolymph is the first step in hemolymph evaluation. Hemolymph from healthy crabs is described as clear or bluish while, bacteremic blood appears milky, and blood with ciliates is increased in turbidity [58]. Unlike most vertebrates, the most common invertebrate oxygen-carrying pigment, hemocyanin, is free in the hemolymph rather than confined to a cell. For this reason, when most invertebrate blood is exposed to air, it generally takes on a bluish tint. However, low levels of hemocyanin can cause a very pale blue coloration.

Cellular Assessment

In most invertebrates, the numbers, types, and function of hemocytes are still under debate. Discrepancies can be attributed to variation of staining techniques, sampling techniques, and choice of anticoagulants as well as interpretation in combination with stage of cell maturity [57, 59, 110]. Most invertebrates have a main phagocytic immune cell, which, regardless of name, is similar in structure and morphology to the vertebrate macrophage [59]. For the purposes of this chapter, we will refer to the two cell types as hyalinocytes (agranulocytes) and granulocytes while acknowledging that these may be different life stages of the same cell type in some species. As many parasites, bacteria, viruses, and fungus can be seen with light microscopy, assessment of a hemolymph smear may provide critical information for a diagnosis. When other animals are available, collecting hemolymph from healthy animals for comparison, housed in the same environment if possible, is recommended (Table 21.6).

Total Hemocyte Count

Methods for THCs vary, and most are performed manually using a counting chamber. Blue crab hemolymph can be directly loaded into a Neubauer hemocytometer if diluted in equal volumes of anticoagulant [44]. Neubauer hemocytometer can be used to count 1:10 diluted lobster hemolymph in cold anticoagulant [12]. One published account used a KOVA Glasstic slide 10 with quantitative grids for lobster hemolymph diluted 1:5 in. 10% formalin [12].

Differential Hemocyte Counts (DHCs)

The hemocyte morphology may be sufficiently distinct in the hemocytometer to perform a differential count [44]. Preparing the hemolymph using a cytocentrifuge

Table 21.6 Biochemical reference ranges for Horseshoe crab, *Limulus polyphemus* [7, 60].

Analyte	Units, SI (US)	Sample size (N)	Mean, *median* (95% CI, *10–90 Percentile*)
Osmolality	mOsm	50	950
Total protein	g/l (g/dl)	50	0.85 (8.15)
Glucose	mmol/l (mg/dl)	50	3.25 (58.5)
Creatinine	umol/l (mg/dl)	50	53.4 (0.7)
Cholesterol	mmol/l (mg/dl)	50	0.021 (0.8)
Sodium	mmol/l (mEq/l)	50	389.5
Potassium	mmol/l (mEq/l)	50	12.5
Chloride	mmol/l (mEq/l)	50	445.1
Calcium	mmol/l (mg/dl)	50	39
Magnesium	mmol/l (mg/dl)	50	 96.1
Phosphorus	mmol/l (mg/dl)	50	1.1 (3.4)
Triglycerides	mmol/l (mg/dl)	50	5.3 (0.06)
Amylase	Units/l = U/l	50	9.3
Lipase	U/l	50	32.7
Alkaline phosphatase	U/l	50	12.1
Aspartate aminotransferase	U/l	50	5.4
Gamma-glutamyltransferase	U/l	50	0.92
pH		10	*7.12* (7.04–7.17)
pCO_2	mm Hg	10	*7.1* (6.26–8.07)
pO_2	mm Hg	10	90.5 (60.73–102.7)
HCO_3-	mm Hg	10	2.1 (1.8–2.7)

has also been reported to successfully produce slide preparations that can be stained with commercially available Romanowsky stains [12]. Others have used hematoxylin and eosin or toluidine blue [61].

Arthropodas: Chelicerates

The hemolymph of the American horseshoe crab has only one cell, the amoebocyte (Figure 21.8) [63, 111]. Causes of changes in amoebocyte numbers (relative or absolute) in hemolymph have not been established, as baseline reference ranges for the horseshoe crab do not exist. However, it may be expected that relative increases should be documented and may indicate infection, injury, or nonspecific inflammation.

Arthropodas: Crustaceans

The presence of endotoxin stimulates the crustacean coagulation system and leads to hemocyte lysis; all sampling material must be free of this ubiquitous contaminant [43]. In crustaceans, clotting time may be prolonged by viremia, bacteremia, and protozoal hemolymph infection. The corresponding pathogens including reo-like viruses, vibrios, aeromonads, aerococci ("gaffkemia"), histophagous ciliates ("bumper car disease"), and amoebae ("gray crab disease") may also be visible on hemolymph smear [43].

A minimum of two major cell types, hyalinocytes and granulocytes, have been documented in crustaceans. The smaller of the two cells, the hyalinocytes, are associated with coagulation and, in some species, phagocytic activity. Hyalinocytes tend to decrease during molting and may be associated with post-molt tanning of the cuticle [43]. The larger cell type, the granulocyte, is phagocytic in some species and often associated with encapsulating larger pathogens such as fungal hyphae [8]. A third type called the semi-granulocyte, possibly an intermediate stage, was described in the blue crab (Figure 21.9) [61]. Granulocytes may also be involved in coagulation [43]. In crustaceans, the THC has been reported to increase with high tide, during emersion, after wounding and bleeding, and after exposure to a low concentration of sewage [43]. THC decreases in high temperatures, low temperatures, preceding molt, during starvation, with zymosan or bacteria (live and dead) exposure, after polychlorinated biphenyl (PCB) or cadmium exposure, and after exposure to a high concentration of sewage (Table 21.7).

Echinoderms

Coelomocytes of the echinoderms vary by species, size, immune status, and physiologic factors [17, 66–70]. Four sea urchin coelomocyte types that have been described include phagocytic amoebocytes (60%–70%), vibratile cells (15%–20%), red spherule cells (5%–10%), and colorless spherule cells (5%–10%) [17]. Phagocytic coelomocytes are the key cell in innate immunity which eliminates microorganisms through phagocytosis [17, 67]. Coelomocyte counts in green sea urchins (*Strongylocentrotus droebachiensis*) increased independently of pathogens with temperatures to 10 °C, but declined at both lower and higher temperatures [17]. Red spherule coelomocytes increase with stress and polluted seawater and can characterize captive husbandry issues [15, 17]. Four different coelomocytes have been identified in the sea cucumber (*Holothuria*

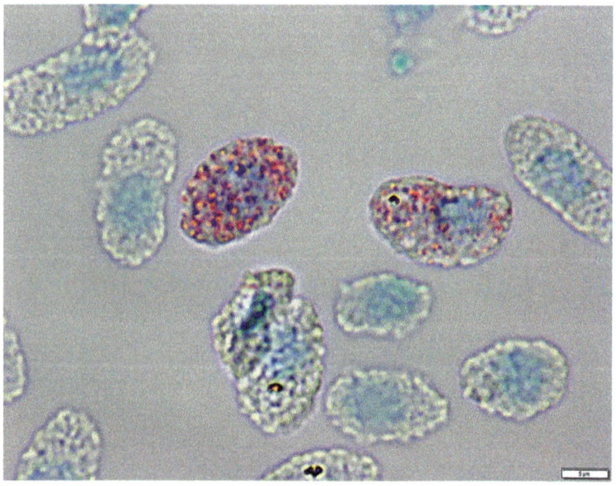

Figure 21.8 Horseshoe crab, *Limulus polyphemus*, hemocytes collected in cold anticoagulant [44] 1:4 dilution, followed immediately by a 50 µl aliquot diluted into 200 µl 10% neutral buffered formalin. A 100 µl aliquot was spun in a cytocentrifuge, and the slide was stained with Hema-3 (Protocol, Fisher Scientific, Kalamazoo, Michigan) modified by diluting Solution II (1 ml stain +100 ml RO water). Nearly all the hemocyte granules stained clear, and some cells contained azurophilic granules.

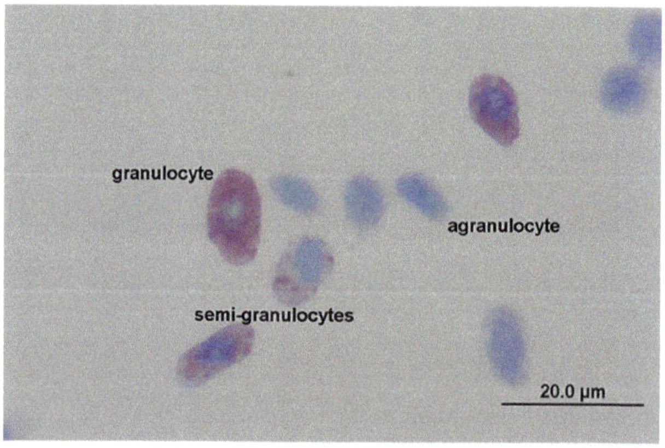

Figure 21.9 Blue crab, *Callinectes sapidus*, hemocytes collected in cold anticoagulant [44] 1:4 dilution, followed immediately by a 50 µl aliquot diluted into 200 µl 10% neutral buffered formalin. A 100 µl aliquot was spun in a cytocentrifuge, and the slide was stained with Hema-3 (Protocol, Fisher Scientific, Kalamazoo, Michigan) modified by diluting Solution II (1 ml stain +100 ml RO water).

Table 21.7 Reference ranges for crustaceans.

Analyte (abbreviation)	Units (SI)	Sample size (N)	*Procambarus clarki* [64]	*Uca pugilator* [58, 65]	*Uca pugnax* and *Uca pugilator* [58, 65]	*Homarus americanus* [45, 55]
Attributes						
Cells (no distinction RBC vs. WBC)	$\times 10^6/\mu l$ vs. $\times 10^3/\mu l$	26				4.4 vs. 2.07
Total lipids		14		115.5 ± 30.7		
TP	g/l (g/dl)	170 260 (17; 26)	85 ± 27 (8.5 ± 2.7)			17–83 (1.7–8.3)
ALT	U/l	30				14–33
GLDH	U/l	30				11–13
Ammonia	μmol/l	22				66.0–223.3
SDH	U/l	30				0–8
AST	U/l	30				11–14
BUN	mM/l	28			20 ± 1.28	
TG	mmol/l	21				0.08–0.35
Lipase	U/l	30				9–15
Cholesterol	mmol/l	24				0.008–0.07
Glucose	mmol/l (mg/dl)	0.389; 1.33 (7; 24)		0.505–0.128 (9.1 ± 2.3)		
Osmolarity	mOsm/kg (mmol/l)	28 (28)			0.497 ± 0.12	
Sodium (Na)	mmol/l	5	166.4 ± 5.9*		328 ± 4.40	346 ± 529
Chloride (Cl)	mmol/l	5	196.5 ± 4.3*		537 ± 7.75	
Potassium (K)	mmol/l	5	4.19 ± 0.15*		11 ± 0.32	4.7–25.3
Magnesium (Mg)	mmol/l	5	2.69 ± 0.15*		46 ± 2.55	7.7–12.7
Calcium (Ca)	meq/l	5	9.15 ± 0.54*		16 ± 1.35	15.9–26.2
HCO_3	mM	5	9.94 ± 0.56*			15.4–64
pH		5	7.930 ± 0.22*			7.76–8.23
Lactate	mmol/l	24				0.0–0.1
pCO_2	torr	5	3.64 ± 0.18*			
Copper		12		1.37 ± 0.25		
Sulfate		28			42 ± 1.26	

All data presented as mean ± SD unless presented as *Median* and/or (95% confidence interval). *Arterial sample for Procambarus.

glaberrima), which we have listed in descending order of prevalence: lymphocytes, phagocytes, spherulocytes, and giant cells [71]. Four cell types have also been observed in the common sea star: phagocytes (95%), amoebocytes, vibratile cells, and hemocytes [72]. The three starfish amoebocyte groups are classified on the basis of size [66]. The cell concentrations of the two largest and more numerous of these groups (G2 and G3) were modulated by immune stimulation, while the group of smallest, less numerous cells (Gl) was unaffected [66]. Moderate relative increases in total coelomocyte counts in the sea star were seen within 6 h of amputation [72]. Experimental exposure of sea cucumbers to certain pathogens increased total coelomocytes, particularly lymphocytes and phagocytes [71].

Mollusks: Bivalves

Like other invertebrates, bivalves lack an acquired immunity equivalent to that of vertebrates. They rely solely on innate mechanisms, including phagocytic, cytotoxic, and inflammatory responses by hemocytes in addition to lysosomal enzymes and lytic/cytotoxic molecules in the serum for defense [73]. Bivalve hemocytes also assist in wound and shell repair, nutrient digestion, transport, and excretion [74]. The THC of bivalves is affected by seasonal changes, temperature, size, gender, maturity, food availability, and molt status [54, 75–77]. Body condition index, protein content, and hemocyte size may also be greatly affected by seasonal variation, while only hemolymph protein was documented to differ by location where the animal was found. The interaction of location and season affects the mobility and particle binding ability of hemocytes in oysters, demonstrating the need to establish locale baseline before interpreting analytes for abnormalities [78]. A decrease in both THC and granulocytes in parasitized mussels has been documented, suggesting a tendency for invertebrate hemocytes to degranulate in response to parasitism [54]. Disease process affects both the THC and the differential cell count of bivalves. In bivalves, bacteremia may contribute to a rapid fall in circulating hemocytes. However, bacteria are also found in the hemolymph of clinically normal cold marine bivalves [78]. The total cell count may also remain unchanged, but changes in the differential count may indicate disease processes. During parasitism, *Mytilus galloprovincialis* showed a decrease in granular and an increase in agranular hemocytes [54]. Circulating hemocytes in the gill vein of an oyster are illustrated in Figure 21.10. In a comparison of four freshwater mussel species of two different genera, cell differentials were genus specific at baseline and for the first month in captivity, although THCs between genera differed significantly at two weeks and again in November. Both genera showed predominantly eosinophilic granulocytes throughout the study. These findings demonstrate pronounced taxonomic and seasonal differences, as well as an effect of captivity on hemocytes [52].

Mollusks: Cephalopods

In cephalopods, mature hemocytes are also called secondary leukoblasts or leukocytes [79]. Hemocytes are believed to play a role in ingestion of food particles, phagocytosis and killing, and tissue repair [80]. Hemocytes increase in response to inflammatory or pathogen stimulation histologically, but little information exists about the peripheral response [23, 26, 79, 81]. Cephalopods also increased hemocytes in response to increased temperature [26]. Circulating hemocytes from an octopus are illustrated in Figure 21.11.

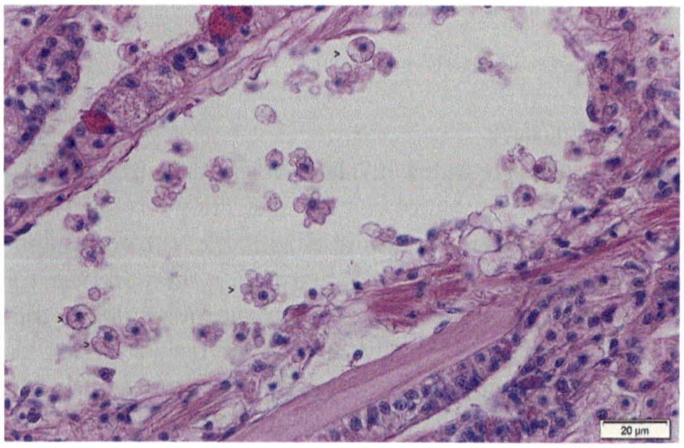

Figure 21.10 Hemocytes (granulocytes) from a Chesapeake oyster, *Crassostrea virginica* (arrowheads), H&E stain, magnification 40×. *Source:* Photo courtesy of Chris Dugan, Maryland Department of Natural Resources Cooperative Oxford Laboratory, Oxford, Maryland.

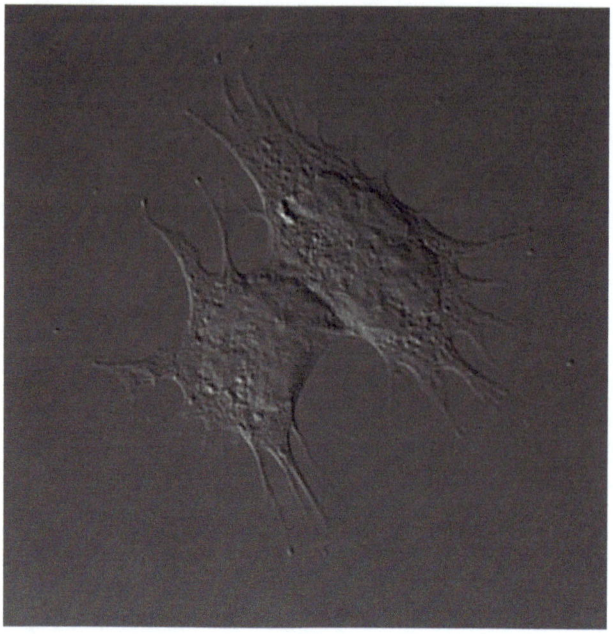

Figure 21.11 Hemocytes from an adult *Euprymna scolopes* (Hawaiian bobtail squid): differential interference contrast (DIC) microscopy of a paraformaldehyde fixed specimen; magnification 40×. *Source:* Photo courtesy of Bethany Rader, PhD, Southern Illinois University.

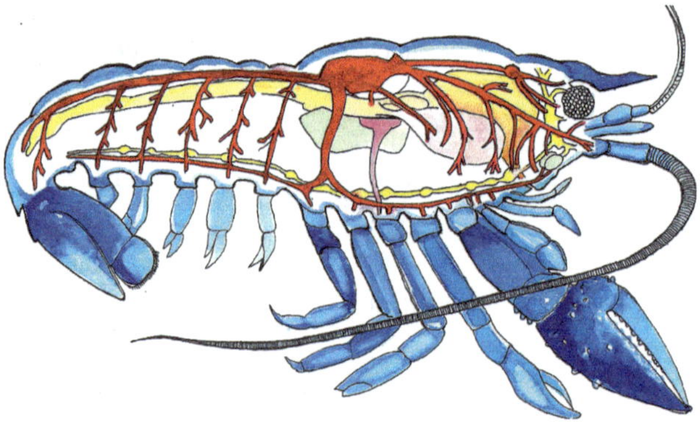

Figure 21.12 Diagram of generalized circulation of the lobster.

Mollusks: Gastropods

Abalone with severe shell pathology had a low proportion of circulating stem cells and an increased number of hyalinocytes [35, 62].

Hemostasis

Clotting time can help assess the disease state of aquatic invertebrates, as slow clotting, in comparison to that of healthy animals, is abnormal [22]. In lobsters, alanine aminotransferase (ALT) and aspartate aminotransferase (AST) decrease in "warmer months," coincident with absent hemolymph clotting [82]. Poor clotting may also be due to hemocytopenia [83]. In bivalves, agglutination titers were unaffected by parasitism but strongly affected by the stage of the reproductive cycle [54].

Enzymes

Some analytes indicate similar processes across groups of animals. However, the ability to extrapolate other analytes in function and location from vertebrates to invertebrates is not universal. Readily available blood chemistry analyzers may also not be validated for the species in question. Enzyme activity will be affected by reaction conditions such as substrate, temperature, and pH. For these reasons, reference intervals for enzyme activity must be considered laboratory and automated analyzer specific [45]. These restrictions should be kept in mind while interpreting blood chemistries.

Enzymology studies for the crustaceans are scarce, but may be helpful in pinpointing diseased organs. In the American lobster, AST, ALT, sorbitol dehydrogenase (SDH), glutamate dehydrogenase (GD), amylase (AMY), and lipase (LIP) were analyzed in plasma, serum, heart, antennal gland, proximal intestine, hepatopancreas, abdominal muscle, and hemocyte lysate. The hepatopancreas was generally the only source of AMY. AST and ALT were found in all tissues, with the heart containing the most activity. The highest GD activity was found in the heart, although other tissues had low levels. LIP activity was low and primarily found in proximal intestine tissue. Activity of SDH was low and widely distributed. While tissue injury of some organs can lead to elevated enzyme levels in the blood, damage to the antenna gland and proximal intestine do not lead to elevated blood enzyme levels [55]. Although knowing the location of certain enzymes in organs is helpful, hemolymph enzyme levels do not always reflect organ levels. For example, in the crab *Scylla serrata*, exposure to naphthalene caused decreased acid phosphatase, ALKP, AST, ALT, and lactate dehydrogenase (LDH) in the hepatopancreas and ovary, although these levels increased in the hemolymph [84].

In a comparison of enzyme levels following transportation with possible hypoxia, The American lobster (*H. americanus)* experienced increased ALT and AST up to 10-fold in samples taken two days after, versus samples taken six days after, a stressful event. A similar pattern, though less dramatic, occurs with lipase. In contrast, enzyme levels in *H. americanus* experimentally infected with gaffkemia did not significantly change. Gaffkemia was confirmed in both the antenna gland and hepatopancreas [45]. These findings suggest that enzymology may not be a sensitive or specific marker for bacteremia, but may increase during physiologically stressful events [45].

Bacteremic lobsters experience an initial increase in THC for the first three days, followed by a decrease to 2× from baseline by day 5. THC levels continued to drop to a decrease by 10%–15% of initial values [45]. A drop in THC occurred in white shrimp, *Litopenaeus vannamei*, infected with white spot syndrome [85]. Parasitism correlates with an altered biochemical profile of crustaceans. In the sand crabs infected with *Hematodinium australis*, animals showed elevated urea, elevated creatinine, hyperglycemia, and an ALT 2.5 times the upper limit of normal. Activities of AST were unchanged [86]. In lobsters, ALT and AST decrease in "warmer months," coincident with absent hemolymph clotting [82]. Poor clotting may also be due to hemocytopenia [83]. Altered ALT and AST values may indicate decreased total and differential hemocyte counts rather than, or in addition to, release of these enzymes from tissues [45]. Interpretation of both hemogram and hemolymph chemistries together may help a clinician decipher causes of abnormalities. Serum values of AST, ALT, and GD were higher than those in plasma, likely due to release of enzymes from hemocytes during coagulation, and serum is therefore preferred for analysis over plasma in crustaceans [55]. Decreased ALT, AST, and GD occur when comparing serum analyzed at 5 and 22 h post phlebotomy when stored at 4 °C [55]. While same-day analysis is recommended, it is not always possible. Stable enzyme activity using samples refrigerated (2–4 °C) for up to four days or frozen at −20 °C for six weeks has been reported for lobsters [55].

Mollusks: Bivalves, Cephalopods, and Gastropods

One study of Manila clams found different effects on alanine aminotransferase activity depending on the type of heavy metal exposure [87]; as with other molluscs, in gastropods bacteremia can lead to a rapid fall in circulating hemocytes [88]. However, in some pathologies, the opposite may occur. Shell length has been correlated with hemolymph glucose, AST, and ALT levels in wild *Elliptio complanata*. The smallest bivalves had the highest values of these analytes. In contrast, calcium and bicarbonate were positively correlated with length [89]. In a comparison of four freshwater mussel species differences, ALT, AST, and ALP were found between genera [3]. These findings demonstrate pronounced taxonomic and seasonal differences, as well as an effect of captivity on electrolytes [52]. THC is used as a general health parameter in gastropod medicine. In abalone with severe shell pathology, THC was elevated [35]. Shell disease of abalone led to hyperglycemia and low urea. While still within the reference range, diseased animals had higher total protein, LDH, AST, calcium, iron, sodium, and potassium [35].

Glucose

Crustaceans

In crustaceans, glucose has been reported to increase during the winter season, during low tide, salinity shock, after molt, during periods of hypoxia, emersion or hypercarbia, during handling, after injections, after dichlorophenol exposure, and after formalin exposure [43]. In some species, hemocytes have significant stores of glycogen, which may contribute to the hyperglycemia during stress [43]. Glucose decreases before molt, during fasting, with gaffkemia (*Aerococcus viridans* bacteremia), with amoebae in the hemolymph [43].

Parasitism correlates with an altered chemical profile in crustaceans. In sand crabs infected with *H. australis*, animals showed hyperglycemia [86].

Echinoderms

Perivisceral coelomic fluid in sea urchins is similar to seawater, but also contains low quantities of sugars [51, 67].

Mollusks: Bivalves, Cephalopods, and Gastropods

Shell length has been inversely correlated with hemolymph glucose levels in wild eastern elliptio freshwater mussel (*E. complanata).* The smallest bivalves had the highest values of these analytes. In contrast, calcium and bicarbonate were positively correlated with length [20]. Intermediary metabolism in bivalves has some parallels to their vertebrate counterparts. For example, while mussels lack pancreatic tissue and do not make insulin, the gut epithelium produces an insulin-like substance which is modulated by glucose levels in the hemolymph. Glucose metabolism is regulated by the production of these substances by gut epithelium [90]. Insulin-like substance secretion is, in turn, modulated by hemolymph glucose concentrations. In the giant clam, glucose concentration is cyclical, with maximum day time levels being up to 3.2 fold higher than nighttime minimums [21]. Shell disease of abalone led to hyperglycemia [35]. Knowledge of the underlying physiology, feedback systems, and analyte origin will greatly assist the clinician with blood chemistry trend interpretation, even in the absence of an established reference range (Table 21.8).

Blood Protein and Lipids

Unlike vertebrates, the major lipoprotein in invertebrates is high-density lipoprotein (HDL) [42].

Arthropods – Crustaceans

In crustaceans, hemocyanin accounts for up to 70% of the total hemolymph protein. Hemocyanin levels increase with low salinity or moderate hypoxia and decrease with low temperatures, during and after molt, during starvation, with severe hypoxia, after hemolymph loss (serial bleeding), and after ammonia exposure [43]. Depending on the species, hemocyanin levels may increase or decrease when exposed to dilute media [43]. In crustaceans, protein decreases during winter, low temperature, high temperature, during and after molt, during fasting, during starvation, with inadequate nutrition, after hemolymph loss (serial bleeding), and with ammonia exposure [4, 43]. Protein may also increase with low salinity and atrazine exposure [43].

Echinoderms

Perivisceral coelomic fluid in sea urchins is similar to seawater, but higher in potassium, and contains low quantities of lipids, proteins, sugars, and coelomocytes [51, 67].

Mollusks: Bivalves, Cephalopods, and Gastropods

Analytes of bivalves are highly prone to influence by external factors. Protein levels of bivalves were unaffected by parasitism but strongly affected by the stage of the reproductive cycle [54]. A positive correlation between gravidity and hemolymph protein was seen in the freshwater mussel, *E. complanata* [20]. Repeated sampling decreases hemolymph copper but not protein [20, 26]. In contrast to an elevated protein in abalone, *Helisoma* snails challenged with bacteria showed a progressive hypoalbuminemia but no evidence of hyperglobulinemia [91]. Shell disease of abalone led to hyperglycemia and low urea. While still within the reference range, diseased animals also had higher total protein [35].

Blood Gases, Electrolytes, Acid–Base Balance, and Respiration

As in other poikilotherms, many physiological factors, including immune response, acid–base balance, and electrolyte balance are affected by the environment. In terms of osmoregulation, aquatic invertebrates may be either osmoconformers or osmoregulators. Similarly, in regard to ionic regulation, aquatic invertebrates may be either ionoconformers or ionoregulators. Most marine invertebrates are osmoconformers, equilibrating their ECF osmolarity with the surrounding water. While osmoconformers may be termed ionoconformers due to the total ionic concentration matching that of the

Table 21.3 Reference values for echinoderms.

Analyte (abbreviation)	Species	Units, SI (US)	Mean/*median*	95% CI/10–90%ile	Min/max	Sample number	Sample information	Reference
Sample size, attributes								
Coelomocyte count	*Strongylocentrotus droebachiensis*	$\times 10^6$ cells/l ($\times 10^3$ cells/μl)	4.756	4.7184–4.7896		275	Highest cell counts seen at temperature of 10 °C	[17]
Phagocytic coelomocyte	*S. droebachiensis*	$\times 10^6$ cells/l ($\times 10^3$ cells/μl	2.1527	2.1357–2.1697		275	Lowest cell counts seen at temperature of 13 °C	[17]
Red spherule cell	*S. droebachiensis*	$\times 10^6$ cells/l ($\times 10^3$ cells/μl)	3.326	3.3036–3.3484		275	Highest cell counts seen at temperature of 10 °C	[17]
Colorless spherule cell	*S. droebachiensis*	$\times 10^6$ cells/l ($\times 10^3$ cells/μl)	1.2916	1.2732–1.310		275	Lowest cell counts seen at temperature of 13 °C	[17]
Coelomocyte count	*S. droebachiensis*	$\times 10^6$ cells/l ($\times 10^3$ cells/μl)	0.9743	0.9587–0.9899		275	Highest cell counts seen at temperature of 10 °C	[17]
Phagocytic coelomocyte	*S. droebachiensis*	$\times 10^6$ cells/l ($\times 10^3$ cells/μl)	1.2711	0.1139–0.1403		275	Lowest cell counts seen at temperature of 13 °C	[17]
Red spherule cell	*S. droebachiensis*	$\times 10^6$ cells/l ($\times 10^3$ cells/μl)	1.665	1.6512–1.6788		275	Highest cell counts seen at temperature of 10 °C	[17]
Colorless spherule cell	*S. droebachiensis*	$\times 10^6$ cells/l ($\times 10^3$ cells/μl)	0.0663	0.0505–0.0821		275	Lowest cell counts seen at temperature of 13 °C	[17]
Phagocytic coelomocyte	*Echinometra lacunter*	$\times 10^6$ cells/l ($\times 10^3$ cells/μl)	5.144	4.348–5.940	1.800–9.750	NR		[68]
Red spherule cell	*E. lacunter*	$\times 10^6$ cells/l ($\times 10^3$ cells/μl)	1.288	0.784–1.792	0.400–3.500	NR		[68]
Colorless spherule Cell	*E. lacunter*	$\times 10^6$ cells/l ($\times 10^3$ cells/μl)	0.207	0.125–0.289	0–0.200	NR		[68]
Vibratile cells	*E. lacunter*	$\times 10^6$ cells/l ($\times 10^3$ cells/μl)	0.038	0.020–0.056	0–0.700	NR		[68]
Coelomocyte count	*Lytechinus variegatus*	$\times 10^5$ cells/l ($\times 10^3$ cells/μl)	2.752.7	0.5275–4.9779		80	Mouth down position drawn from oral region	[51]
Phagocytic coelomocyte	*L. variegatus*	$\times 10^5$ cells/l ($\times 10^3$ cells/μl)	2.016	0.3932–3.6388		80	Mouth down position drawn from oral region	[51]
pH	*Psammechinus miliaris*		7.53	7.31–7.75		20		[18]
PCV	*Tetrapygus niger*	l/l (%)	0.00917 (0.917)	0.00514–0.0113 (0.514–1.13)		26	Spring	[16]
TS	*T. niger*	g/l (mg/dl)	34 (3.4)	32.7–36.6 (3.27–3.66)		26	Spring	[16]

(Continued)

Table 21.8 (Continued)

Analyte (abbreviation)	Species	Units, SI (US)	Mean/*median*	95% CI/10–90%ile	Min/max	Sample number	Sample information	Reference
Sample size, attributes								
pH	*T. niger*		7.07	7.04–7.12		43	Spring	[16]
pCO_2	*T. niger*	mm Hg	8.07	7.83–8.32		43	Spring	[16]
pO_2	*T. niger*	mm Hg	122.3	116.34–128.27		50	Spring	[16]
HCO_3	*T. niger*	mmol/l	2.2	1.7–3.9		43	Spring	[16]
PCV	*Loxechinus albus*	l/l (%)	0.01 (1)	0.00–0.031 (0–3.1)	0.00–0.04 (0–4)	18	Spring	[16]
TS	*L. albus*	mg/dl	3.4	3.39–3.73	3.3–4	18	Spring	[16]
pH	*L. albus*		7.23	7.16–7.29		16		[12]
pCO_2	*L. albus*	mm Hg	8.88	8.62–9.14		16		[12]
PO_2	*L. albus*	mm Hg	115.18	105.91–124.44		17		[12]
HCO_3	*L. albus*	mOsm/kg (mmol/l)	3.82	3.32–4.32		16		[12]

environment, they are usually ionoregulators to some degree, using transport mechanisms to excrete some ions and maintain other ions in their ECF at optimal concentrations. Some animals like the brine shrimp, *Artemia*, can either osmoconform or osmoregulate depending on environmental conditions. Freshwater invertebrates are osmoregulators and ionoregulators, expending energy to be hyperosmotic and maintain an ECF ionic composition different from the surrounding environment. In crustaceans, sodium and chloride have been reported to increase during high temperature and decrease with low salinity, during molt, and after nitrite exposure [43]. Among invertebrates, metabolic responses to hypercapnia vary between taxonomic groups [53].

Arthropods: Chelicerates

The American horseshoe crab's unique anatomic and physiologic adaptations to changing environmental conditions, in particular, those of oxygen depletion, make hemolymph gas analysis at various environmental conditions of practical importance [92]. Furthermore, changes in acid–base balance and ventilatory status have been linked to alterations in immune responses in other invertebrates. Decreases in pH are seen with short-term hypoxia and due to metabolic acidosis or with long-term hypoxia due to respiratory acidosis [60].

Arthropods: Crustaceans

As other invertebrates, crustaceans can adapt their osmoregulatory approach to their environment. In the hermit crab *Clibanarius vittatus*, hemolymph is regulated to be hyperosmotic in low salinities (5%–50%). However, the maintenance of osmolality changes to maintenance of an osmotic concentration at salinities greater than 20%. Hemolymph chloride ion concentration is regulated hyperionic to the external medium in lower salinities (<15‰) and is hypoionic at medium to high salinities. These changes occur without a change in percentage body water, indicating the crab is an effective volume regulator when in its shell [93]. Osmoregulation is affected by salinity, pH, dissolved oxygen, turbidity, size, nutrition, age, and molt stage [43]. Thus, interpretation of analytes should occur while also observing water parameters and the life stage (Table 21.9).

Blood gas analysis approaches change with lifestyle. Supralittoral zone crustaceans breathe air using lung-like specializations of the linings of the branchial chamber. Littoral species, like the green crab (*Carcinus maenas*), retain some contact with the water via branchial water stores while exposed to air, compensating internally for an initial acidosis. Sublittoral species have not developed these adaptations [94]. Similar to many vertebrate poikilotherms, the ventilator drive in the green crab, *C. maenas*, is set by oxygen requirements rather

Table 21.9 Reference data for bivalve molluscs [20–22].

Analyte (abbreviation)	Units SI (USA)	*Tridacna gigas*	*Tridacna crocea*	*Elliptio complanata*	Sample size
Sample size, attributes		**Mean (*median*) ± SD**	**Mean (*median*) ± SD**	**Mean (median) ± SD, [95% CI]**	
Cells (no distinction)	Million cells/ml		0.3–2.6	[0.25–2.3]	6
Eosinophilic hemocyte	%		48.2 ± 7.6		6
Agranular hemocyte	%		49.4 ± 8.8		6
Morula hemocyte	%		6.9 ± 3.0		6
Total protein/total solids	μg/ml (mg/dl)	259 ± 35		[19.5–142.8] (mg/dl)	6
Ammonia	μmol/l			[<10–138]	380
AST	/μl			[<4–38]	374
Glucose	mg/dl			[<2–4]	372
Sodium (Na)	M	0.51 ± 0.02			6
Chloride (Cl)	M	0.57 ± 0.01			6
Potassium (K)	mM	10.1 ± 3.6			6
Magnesium (mg)	mM	53 ± 2		[1.6–3.8](mg/dl)	6
Calcium (Ca)	mM (mg/dl)	9.5 + 3		[13.1–23.7] (mg/dl)	6
Phosphorus (P)	mg/dl			[<0.3–0.9]	374
HCO_3	mmol/l			[<5–12]	375

than by hemolymph CO_2 levels. When exposed to a hypoxic medium, hyperventilation and CO_2 excretion lead to respiratory alkalosis, which is compensated by metabolic acidosis (a decline in bicarbonate) within 16 h [49]. Another study in green crabs revealed that both hyperoxia and low water alkalinity led to hypercapnic acidosis. Water parameters should be assessed along with the acid–base interpretation of any crustacean water breather [95]. Parasitism correlates with an altered biochemical profile of crustaceans. In sand crabs (*Portunus pelagicus*) infected with *H. australis*, animals showed pronounced hyperkalemia and hyperphosphatemia, but infection produced no effect on sodium, chloride, and calcium [86].

In contrast to this, the sublittoral lobster *Homarus gammarus*, when exposed to air for 12–14 h, mitigated hypoxemia via conserved oxygen bound to hemocyanin. An accompanying increase in $PaCO_2$ (1.13 kPa) and lactic acid (9.0 mmol/l), though the animals were not acidotic (pHa 7.71), was also noted due to an elevation in buffer base (HCO_3a 21.7 mmol/l). Once resubmerged, PaO_2 and $PaCO_2$ normalized within 1 h, and HCO_3a and lactate normalized by 24 h. Late premolt lobsters, and those severely hypoxic and acidotic, were unable adjust, and experienced a 75% mortality rate upon resubmersion [94].

Hemolymph pH in crustaceans is inversely related to temperature and salinity [43]. Acidosis, while generally not seen in crustaceans secondary to hypoxia, is seen during exercise. In the blue crab, *C. sapidus*, lactic acidosis and elevated PCO_2 occurred after 1 h of swimming. While lactate levels climbed steadily over the hour, hemolymph pH hit its nadir at 15 min. This disparity is may be due to the branchial ion exchange process and a sixfold increase in ammonia excretion. While pH compensated fairly quickly, lactate levels took longer to normalize [96].

Echinoderms

Perivisceral coelomic fluid in sea urchins is similar to seawater, but higher in potassium [51, 67]. Hemolymph gas analysis has been performed for two species of sympatric sea urchins in Peru [16]. Inherent differences in baseline values for each species highlight the importance of establishing reference ranges for each species and various environmental conditions. When comparing the hemolymph gas values of black sea urchin sampled in and out of water, the pH and pO_2 were significantly lower and the pCO_2 significantly higher in those submerged [16]. Similarly, experimental exposure to acidified seawater in the shore sea urchin (*Psammechinus miliaris*) results in acidosis and hypercapnia [18]. These findings reinforce the need to standardize methods for sample collection, as well as provide exceptional husbandry for these species. Severe acidosis in sea urchins causes mortalities [18], and may also decrease components of the innate immune system as in other invertebrate classes.

Mollusks: Bivalves, Cephalopods, and Gastropods

In smaller bivalves such as the mussel, *E. complanata*, the sample site can affect values. While magnesium, phosphorous, ammonia, protein, sodium, potassium, and chloride showed no significant difference between the ventricular chamber and adductor sinus sampling sites, calcium levels were significantly different (Table 21.10).

Osmoregulation in bivalves is, in general, similar to teleosts in the same environment. Most marine invertebrates are isosmotic and osmoconformers, but ionic regulators. As opposed to species in areas of high salinity that experience a continual loss of water and net gain of ions [100], freshwater species continually gain water and lose ions. However, the approach to osmoregulation may change in freshwater species dependent on environmental salinity, among other factors. For example, the unionid clam (*Lampsilis teres*) is a hyperosmotic and hyperionic regulator when the ambient osmolality is less than 50 mOsm and an osmotic and ionic conformer when the environmental osmolality is above 50 mOsm. Tissue hydration in *L. teres* does not change in animals acclimated to higher salinities, suggesting that the animals are good volume regulators [56]. Unionid clams and other freshwater bivalves excrete ammonium and hydrogen ions, while chloride is exchanged for bicarbonate and hydroxide [100]. However, osmotic concentrations of unionid clams are only 25%–50% of other freshwater bivalves [100]. While gills uptake sodium and chloride in inionid clams, the kidneys are the main route of water excretion with an accompanying net ionic loss to the environment [100].

Ionic regulation can be species specific, even in similar environments. In the marine oyster *Crassostrea gigas*, immersion in acidic hypercapnic seawater (pH 7.68, kPa PCO2 0.15) caused marked extracellular acidosis, a 20% decrease in PO_2 levels, and a small increase in bicarbonate levels. With these blood gas changes, calcium, and sodium levels dropped, while potassium levels increased [53]. This is in contrast to the Mediterranean mussel, *M. galloprovincialis*, which responded to acidic hypercapnic seawater (pH 7.3, 0.6 kPa PCO2) with an extracellular drop in pH, and an increase in bicarbonate and calcium [101]. In the case of *Mytilus*, the elevated bicarbonate and calcium levels arise from shell dissolution to compensate for the extracellular acidosis [92]. Most bivalves can switch to anaerobic metabolism in response to hypoxic conditions to circumvent the need for high levels of oxygen [19].

Table 21.10 Reference values for cephalopod molluscs.

Analyte	Species	Units (SI)	Mean/*median*	95% CI/10–90%	Min/max	Reference
Hemocytes	*Eledone cirrhosa*	$\times 10^9$ cells/l ($\times 10^3$ cells/μl)	0.011			[26]
Progesterone	*Octopus vulgaris*	nmol/l (ng/ml)	2.67 (0.84)			[97]
Testosterone	*O. vulgaris*	nmol/l (ng/ml)	0.017 (0.5)			[97]
17B-estradiol	*O. vulgaris*	nmol/l (ng/ml)	0.294 (0.08)			[97]
Hemolymph pH	*Loligo pealei*		7.64	7.6–7.68		[98]
Hemolymph pH	*L. pealei*			7.42–7.45		[98]
Fecal estrogen	*Enteroctopus dofleini*	nmol/l (ng/g)		3.67–99.39		[99]
Fecal progesterone	*E. dofleini*	nmol/l (ng/g)		44.35–231.71		[99]
Fecal testosterone	*E. dofleini*	nmol/l (ng/g)		9.3–18.18		[99]
Fecal corticosterone	*E. dofleini*	nmol/l (ng/g)		6.32–30.38		[99]
Protein	*E. cirrhosa*	g /l (g/dl)	116			[26]

Within the bivalves are those that remain immersed and those that vacillate between immersion and emersion. Many intertidal and estuarine bivalves have evolved respiratory compensations for short times of emersion, while shallow freshwater bivalves must be able to withstand longer, less predictable periods of emersion. Examples include valve gaping and aerial gas exchange and the use of shell $CaCO_3$ for buffering acidosis and hypoxia. These lead to a spike in both calcium and bicarbonate during a period of hypercapnia. These abilities may be decreased in species only recently invasive to the freshwater habitat. Understanding the ecology of the species of interest will provide insight into expected analyte trends. In a comparison of four freshwater mussel species in two genera, significant differences in sodium, potassium, chloride, and magnesium occur depending on genera [52]. Both genera, however, showed declines in sodium and chloride in the first month in captivity and exhibited marked increases in all electrolyte values in November, five months after transport to captivity. These findings demonstrate pronounced taxonomic and seasonal differences, as well as an effect of captivity on electrolytes [52].

Gastropod molluscs may be subcategorized as Prosobranchs, Opisthobranchs, and Pulmonates based on respiratory physiology. Those with rudimentary lungs also known as pulmonary sacs are the pulmonates, and while prosobranchs and opisthobranchs lack these pulmonary sacs. Air enters the sac via the pneumostome, a landmark for venipuncture of pulmonates. In addition to dermal CO_2 exchange employed by other gastropods, pulmonates use ventilation for gas exchange [102]. Like their air-breathing crustacean counterparts, in comparison to water-breathing animals, ventilation is reduced and internal PCO_2 increases, with the resulting extracellular acidosis compensated for by increases in hemolymph bicarbonate [102]. Pulmonates maintain bicarbonate levels up to fivefold higher than gill-breathing prosobranch snails, allowing greater ability to buffer respiratory acidosis secondary to hypoxemia [38].

Like other molluscs, osmoregulatory approaches of the snail are environmentally responsive. To accommodate increases in ambient osmolality, freshwater molluscs increase the circulating amino acid pool, though some species have a larger capacity to do so. In the snail *Pomacea bridgesii*, hemolymph is hyperosmotic and hyperionic when in osmolalities below 100 mOsm (Table 21.11).

Oxygen binding of hemocyanin increases relatively in both Antarctic and temperate cephalopods with increasing temperature and pH, which can be monitored by measuring serial hemolymph gases during disease [105]. Abalone suffering shell disease had increased sodium and potassium [35].

Vitamins, Minerals, Metals, and Toxins

Echinoderms

Concentrations of heavy metals in the sea urchin are only available for tissues [17]. Elevated levels of several metals, but most notably zinc cause toxic effects on sea urchin embryos [106]. Effects worsen when zinc is accompanied by manganese, lead, iron, and copper [106].

Mollusks: Bivalves, Cephalopods, and Gastropods

One study of Manila clams found different effects on alanine aminotransferase activity depending on type of heavy metal exposure [87]. Repeated sampling decreases hemolymph copper [26]. Calcium was positively correlated with shell length in wild eastern elliptio (*E. complanata*) [20]. In unionid clams, exposure to acidic water (pH 4.0–4.5) caused mild hypercalcemia [107]. In a comparison of four freshwater mussel species, significant differences in magnesium were found between genera [52]. Shell disease of abalone led to higher calcium and iron in diseased animals, although values were still within the reference range [35].

Hormones

Mollusks: Bivalves, Cephalopods, and Gastropods

At this time, hormones are rarely evaluated for clinical purpose in vertebrates, and endocrinopathy remains clinically undemonstrated. Fecal sex hormone analysis of captive giant Pacific octopuses found that one female demonstrated a spike in fecal estrogen on the day of observed breeding [99].

Urinalysis and Assessment of Nitrogen Metabolism

Urinalysis may be of questionable use in aquatic invertebrates as some lack a closed urinary system or urinary bladder. However, evaluation of nitrogen

Table 21.11 Reference ranges for gastropod molluscs.

Analyte (abbreviation)	Units SI (US)	*Biomphalaria alexandrina* [103]	*Haliotis diversicolor supertexta* [2]	*Haliotis iris* [104]	*Planorbis corneus* [34]	*Pomacea bridgesi* [38, 39]	*Pomacea canaliculata* [42]	*Pomacea depressa* [39]	*Pomacea lineata* [39]
Sample size, attributes									
Number (N)		50	10	70	10	6–8	5–10	6	6–7
Cells (no distinction RBC vs. WBC) [range]	$\times 10^6$/l ($\times 10^3$/μl)		2.102 ± 0.146	*10.2* ± 0.8 [8.8–11.6]					
Type 1 hemocyte	%			*22* ± 1 [19–25]					
Type 2 hemocyte	%			*46* ±2 [42–51]					
Type 3 hemocyte	%			*31* ± 3 [26–36]					
Total protein (TP)	mg/ml (g/l)			*19.9* ± 0.7 [18.6–21.2]	12.16 ± 13	3.46 ± 0.17			
Alanine aminotransferase (ALT)		25.6 ± 4.1 (mg/ml)		*2.78* ±0.43 [1.95–3.96]					
Alkaline phosphatase (ALP)	U/l	0.25 ± 0.34 (mg/ml)				63.2 ± 31.80			
Lactate dehydrogenase (LDH)	U/l			*8.51* ± 0.6 [6.93–10.44]					
Aspartate aminotransferase (AST)		18.45 ± 2.3 (mg/ml)		*5.47* ± 0.55 [4.38–6.56]					
Blood urea nitrogen (BUN)	mM/l			*0.3* ± 0.04 [0.29–0.45]					0.07 ± 0.03
Uric Acid (UA)	mmol/l							0.04 ± 0.04 (mgN/dl)	0.09 ± 0.03 (mgN/dl)
Amylase				0.*247* ± 0.042 [0.158–0.389]		3.78 ± 1.74			
Cholesterol	mmol/l								
Glucose	mg/dl			*0.0018* ± 0.0001		5.02 ± 1.70			
Total lipids	μg/ml						[127–210]		
Osmolality (H_2O)					99 ± 1				
Sodium (Na)	mmol/l			*461* ± 6 [450–474]				55.7 ± 1.8	49.8 ± 1.3
Chloride (Cl)	mmol/l							52.0 ± 2.0	41.3 ± 1.8
Potassium (K)	mmol/l			*10.9* ± 0.2 [10–11.6]				3.0 ± 0.2	2.4 ± 0.1
Calcium (Ca)	meq/l			*11.89* ± 0.13 [11.64–12.15]					
HCO_3	mm								
pH									

Box 21.1 Approach to Clinicopathologic Assessment of an Aquatic Invertebrate

1) Handle species appropriately, record temperature and water quality parameters.
2) Plan for appropriate sample storage:
   a) Ice
   b) Immediate centrifugation
   c) Anticoagulant preparation.
3) Sample, observe hemolymph color.
4) Prepare hemolymph smears.
5) Fix aliquot for hemolymph cell count in formalin.
6) Point of care analysis for blood gases or other analytes.
7) Observe hemolymph clotting time.
8) Freeze prior to biochemical or enzyme analysis.

metabolism pathways can prove worthwhile in some species. Knowledge of expected excretion products is essential for accurate interpretation of results. Gastropods have different nitrogen metabolism approaches across taxa. For example among snails, prosobranchs are uricotelic, while all pulmonates make urea via the ornithine cycle. However, only non-helicid pulmonates accumulate urea [108]. Ammonia, urea, and uric acid were measured in the ramshorn snail (*Biomphalaria glabrata*) before and after starvation. While uric acid was not detectable during either sampling, both ammonia and urea increased after five days of starvation [109]. Taxon-specific metabolism data may therefore guide clinical interpretation of analyte abnormalities.

References

1 Cheng, W., Liu, C.H., and Chen, J.C. (2002). Effect of nitrite on interaction between the giant freshwater prawn *Macrobrachium rosenbergii* and its pathogen *Lactococcus garvieae*. *Diseases of Aquatic Organisms* 50: 189–197.
2 Cheng, W.T., Hsiao, I.S., and Chen, J.C. (2004). Effect of nitrite on immune response of Taiwan abalone *Haliotis diversicolor supertexta* and its susceptibility to *Vibrio parahaemolyticus*. *Diseases of Aquatic Organisms* 60: 157–164.
3 Le Moullac, G. and Haffner, P. (2000). Environmental factors affecting immune responses in Crustacea. *Aquaculture* 191: 121–131.
4 Liu, C.H. and Chen, J.C. (2004). Effect of ammonia on the immune response of white shrimp *Litopenaeus vannamei* and its susceptibility to *Vibrio alginolyticus*. *Fish & Shellfish Immunology* 16: 321–334.
5 Berzins, I. (2011). Diagnostic techniques and sample handling. In: *Invertebrate Medicine* (ed. G. Lewbart), 263–274. Wiley-Blackwell.
6 Hurton, L., Berkson, J., and Smith, S. (2005). Estimation of total hemolymph volume in the horseshoe crab *Limulus polyphemus*. *Marine and Freshwater Behaviour and Physiology* 38: 139–147.
7 Smith, S.A., Berkson, J.M., and Barratt, R.A. (2002). Horseshoe crab (*Limulus polyphemus*) hemolymph, biochemical and immunological parameters. *Proceedings of the International Association for Aquatic Animal Medicine* 33: 101–102.
8 Noga, E.J. (2011). Crustaceans. In: *Invertebrate Medicine* (ed. G. Lewbart), 179–193. Wiley-Blackwell.
9 Van Wettere, A. and Lewbart, G.A. (2007 Jan 1). Cytologic diagnosis of diseases of invertebrates. *Veterinary Clinics: Exotic Animal Practice.* 10 (1): 235–254.
10 Defur, P.L., Mcmahon, B.R., and Booth, C.E. (1983). Analysis of Hemolymph oxygen levels and acid-base status during emersion Insitu in the red rock crab, *Cancer productus*. *Biological Bulletin* 165: 582–590.
11 Vermeer, G.K. (1987). Effects of air exposure on desiccation rate, hemolymph chemistry, and escape behavior of the spiny lobster, *Panulirus argus*. *Fishery Bulletin* 85: 45–51.
12 Battison, A., Cawthorn, R., and Horney, B. (2003). Classification of *Homarus americanus* hemocytes and the use of differential hemocyte counts in lobsters infected with *Aerococcus viridans* var. homari (Gaffkemia). *Journal of Invertebrate Pathology* 84 (3): 177–197.
13 Tylerjones, R. and Taylor, E.W. (1988). Analysis of hemolymph and muscle acid-base status during aerial exposure in the crayfish *Austropotamobius pallipes*. *Journal of Experimental Biology* 134: 409–422.
14 Gutzmer, M.P. and Tomasso, J.R. (1985). Nitrite toxicity to the crayfish *Procambarus-clarkii*. *Bulletin of Environmental Contamination and Toxicology* 34: 369–376.
15 Matranga, V., Toia, G., Bonaventura, R., and Muller, W.E.G. (2000). Cellular and biochemical responses to environmental and experimentally induced stress in sea urchin coelomocytes. *Cell Stress & Chaperones* 5: 113–120.
16 Jankowski G., Allender M., Adkesson M., Cardeña M., Garcia F., Guerrero P., Majluf P. 2011. Hemolymph gas analysis in the black sea urchin (*Tetrapygus niger*) and the red sea urchin (*Loxechinus albus*) using an iSTAT point of care analyzer. Presented at International Association of Aquatic Animal Medicine Annual Conference, Las Vegas
17 Haskell, S. (2008). *Pathogenic Impacts on the Green Sea Urchin (Strongylocentrotus droebachiensis) in the Gulf of Maine*, 216. Davis: University of California-Davis.

18 Miles, H., Widdicombe, S., Spicer, J.I., and Hall-Spencer, J. (2007). Effects of anthropogenic seawater acidification on acid-base balance in the sea urchin *Psammechinus miliaris*. *Marine Pollution Bulletin* 54: 89–96.
19 Friedl, F.E. (1961). Studies on larval *Fascioloides magna*. 4. Chromatographic analyses of free amino acids in the hemolymph of a host snail. *Journal of Parasitology* 47: 773–776.
20 Gustafson, L.L., Stoskopf, M.K., Bogan, A.E. et al. (2005). Evaluation of a nonlethal technique for hemolymph collection in *Elliptio complanata*, a freshwater bivalve (Mollusca: Unionidae). *Diseases of Aquatic Organisms* 65: 159–165.
21 Rees, T.A.V., Fitt, W.K., Baillie, B., and Yellowlees, D. (1993). A method for temporal measurement of hemolymph composition in the Giant clam symbiosis and its application to glucose and glycerol levels during a Diel cycle. *Limnology and Oceanography* 38: 213–217.
22 Nakayama, K., Nomoto, A.M., Nishijima, M., and Maruyama, T. (1997). Morphological and functional characterization of hemocytes in the giant clam *Tridacna crocea*. *Journal of Invertebrate Pathology* 69: 105–111.
23 Malham, S.K., Lacoste, A., Gelebart, F. et al. (2002). A first insight into stress-induced neuroendocrine and immune changes in the octopus *Eledone cirrhosa*. *Aquatic Living Resources* 15: 187–192.
24 Stoskopf, M.K. and Oppenheim, B.S. (1996). Anatomic features of *Octopus bimaculoides* and *Octopus digueti*. *Journal of Zoo and Wildlife Medicine* 27: 1–18.
25 Martin, A.W., Harrison, F.M., Huston, M.J., and Stewart, D.M. (1958). The blood volumes of some representative molluscs. *Journal of Experimental Biology* 35: 260–279.
26 Malham, S.K., Coulson, C.L., and Runham, N.W. (1998). Effects of repeated sampling on the haemocytes and haemolymph of *Eledone cirrhosa* (Lam.). *Comparative Biochemistry and Physiology A-Molecular and Integrative Physiology* 121: 431–440.
27 Bradbury, H.E. (1971). Technique for demonstrating blood vascular system of squid. *Canadian Journal of Zoology* 49: 505–506.
28 Beuerlein, K., Ruth, P., Westermann, B. et al. (2002). Hemocyanin and the branchial heart complex of *Sepia officinalis*: are the hemocytes involved in hemocyanin metabolism of coleoid cephalopods? *Cell and Tissue Research* 310: 373–381.
29 Gore, S.R., Harms, C.A., Kukanich, B. et al. (2005). Enrofloxacin pharmacokinetics in the European cuttlefish, *Sepia officinalis*, after a single i.v. injection and bath administration. *Journal of Veterinary Pharmacology and Therapeutics* 28: 433–439.
30 Schlichter, L.C. (1981). Ion relations of hemolymph, pallial fluid, and mucus of *Lymnaea stagnalis*. *Canadian Journal of Zoology-Revue Canadienne De Zoologie* 59: 605–613.
31 Wood, E.J., Corfield, G.C., and Siggens, K.W. (1981). Biosynthesis of hemocyanin in *Lymnaea stagnalis* L (Gastropoda). *Comparative Biochemistry and Physiology B-Biochemistry & Molecular Biology* 69: 877–880.
32 Cooper, J.E. (1994). Bleeding of pulmonate snails. *Laboratory Animals* 28: 277–278.
33 Michelson, E. (1966). Specificity of hemolymph antigens in taxonomic discrimination of medically important snails. *Journal of Parasitology* 52: 466–468.
34 Ottaviani, E. (1984). Composition of the serum hemolymph of *Planorbis porneus* (Gastropoda, Pulmonata). *Comparative Biochemistry and Physiology B-Biochemistry & Molecular Biology* 78: 585–589.
35 Nollens H.H., Keogh J.A., Probert P.K. 2003. Effect of shell lesions on survival, growth, condition, reproductive capacity and hematology of the New Zealand blackfoot abalone, *Haliotis iris*. Presented at 34th Annual Conference of the International Association of Aquatic Animal Medicine.
36 Levenson, J., Byrne, J.H., and Eskin, A. (1999). Levels of serotonin in the hemolymph of *Aplysia* are modulated by light/dark cycles and sensitization training. *Journal of Neuroscience* 19: 8094–8103.
37 Williams, D.L. (1999). Sample taking in invertebrate veterinary medicine. *Veterinary Clinics of North America* 2 (3): 777–801.
38 Scholnick, D.A., Snyder, G.K., and Spell, A.R. (1994). Acid-base status of a pulmonate land snail (*Helix aspersa*) and a prosobranch amphibious snail (*Pomacea bridgesi*) during dormancy. *Journal of Experimental Zoology* 268: 293–298.
39 Little, C. (1968). Aestivation and ionic regulation in 2 species of *Pomacea* (Gastropoda Prosobranchia). *Journal of Experimental Biology* 48: 569–585.
40 Levin, J. and Bang, F.B. (1968). Clottable protein in *Limulus* – its localization and kinetics of its coagulation by endotoxin. *Thrombosis Et Diathesis Haemorrhagica* 19: 186–197.
41 Kenney, D.M., Belamarich, F.A., and Shepro, D. (1972). Aggregation of horseshoe crab (*Limulus polyphemus*) amebocytes and reversible inhibition of aggregation by Edta. *Biological Bulletin* 143: 548–567.
42 Heras, H. and Pollero, R.J. (2002). Lipoproteins from plasma and perivitelline fluid of the apple snail *Pomacea canaliculata*. *Biocell* 26: 111–118.
43 Noga, E.J. (2000). Hemolymph markers in crustacean health. In: *Recent Advances in Marine Biotechnology* (ed. M. Fingerman and R. Nagabhushanam), 124–163. Science Publishers.

44 Wenli C., Shields J. 2007. Characterization and primary culture of hemocytes from the blue crab, *Callinectes sapidus*. In: Transactions of the Chinese Crustacean Society. In: Cai SL (ed) 5th World Chinese Symposium for Crustacean Aquaculture. Vol 5: 25–35.

45 Basti, D., Bricknell, I., Chang, E.S., and Bouchard, D. (2010). Biochemical reference intervals for the resting state in the adult lobster, *Homarus americanus*. *Journal of Shellfish Research* 29 (4): 1013–1101.

46 Ellis, B.A. and Morris, S. (1995). Effects of extreme pH on the physiology of the Australian Yabby *Cherax destructor* – acute and chronic changes in Hemolymph carbon-dioxide, acid-base and ionic status. *Journal of Experimental Biology* 198: 395–407.

47 Walker R.L. 1993. Using crustaceans to illustrate the principles of osmoregulation, acid-base balance, and respiratory physiology. Presented at Proceedings of the 7th and 8th Workshop/Conferences of the Association for Biology Laboratory Education (ABLE).

48 Soderhall, K. and Smith, V.J. (1983). Separation of the hemocyte populations of *Carcinus maenas* and other marine decapods, and prophenoloxidase distribution. *Developmental and Comparative Immunology* 7: 229–239.

49 Burnett, L.E. and Bridges, C.R. (1981). The physiological-properties and function of Ventilatory pauses in the crab *Cancer pagurus*. *Journal of Comparative Physiology* 145: 81–88.

50 Taylor, S., Landman, M.J., and Ling, N. (2009). Flow cytometric characterization of freshwater crayfish hemocytes for the examination of physiological status in wild and captive animals. *Journal of Aquatic Animal Health* 21: 195–203.

51 Borges, J.C.S., Jensch, B.E., Garrido, P.A.G. et al. (2005). Phagocytic amoebocyte sub populations in the perivisceral coelom of the sea urchin *Lytechinus variegatus* (Lamarck, 1816). *Journal of Experimental Zoology Part A-Comparative Experimental Biology* 303A: 241–248.

52 Valentine, H.K. (2011). *Methods in Health Assessment of Freshwater Mussels, Amblema plicata and Quadrula spp*. Columbus: Ohio State University.

53 Lannig, G., Eilers, S., Portner, H.O. et al. (2010). Impact of ocean acidification on energy metabolism of oyster, *Crassostrea gigas*-changes in metabolic pathways and thermal response. *Marine Drugs* 8: 2318–2339.

54 Santarem, M.M., Robledo, J.A.F., and Figueras, A. (1994). Seasonal changes in hemocytes and serum defense factors in the blue mussel *Mytilus palloprovincialis*. *Diseases of Aquatic Organisms* 18: 217–222.

55 Battison, A. (2006). Tissue distribution and hemolymph activity of six enzymes in the American lobster (*Homarus americanus*): potential markers of tissue injury. *Journal of Shellfish Research* 25: 553–560.

56 Jordan, P.J. and Deaton, L.E. (1999). Osmotic regulation and salinity tolerance in the freshwater snail *Pomacea bridgesi* and the freshwater clam *Lampsilis teres*. *Comparative Biochemistry and Physiology A-Molecular and Integrative Physiology* 122: 199–205.

57 Yoshino, T.P. and Davis, C.D. (1983). Surface-antigens of *Biomphalaria- glabrata* (Gastropoda) hemocytes – evidence for linkage-independence of some hemolymph-like surface-antigens and con-A receptor-bearing macromolecules. *Journal of Invertebrate Pathology* 42: 8–16.

58 Spindlerbarth, M. (1976). Bacterial-infection in common shore crab *Carcinus maenas* and fiddler crab *Uca pugilator*. *Marine Biology* 36: 1–4.

59 Ottaviani, E. (2011). Immunocyte: the invertebrate counterpart of the vertebrate macrophage. *Isj-Invertebrate Survival Journal* 8: 1–4.

60 Allender, M.C., Schumacher, J., George, R. et al. (2010). The effects of short- and long-term hypoxia on Hemolymph gas values in the American horseshoe crab (*Limulus polyphemus*) using a point-of-care analyzer. *Journal of Zoo and Wildlife Medicine* 41: 193–200.

61 Clare, A.S. and Lumb, G. (1994). Identification of haemocytes and their role in clotting in the blue crab, *Callinectes sapidus*. *Marine Biology* 118: 601–610.

62 Shields, J.D., Perkins, F.O., and Friedman, C.S. (1996). Hematological pathology of wasting syndrome in black abalone. *Journal of Shellfish Research* 15: 498.

63 Murer, E.H., Levin, J., and Holme, R. (1975). Isolation and studies of granules of Amebocytes of *Limulus polyphemus*, horseshoe crab. *Journal of Cellular Physiology* 86: 533–542.

64 Morgan, D.O. and McMahon, B.R. (1982). Acid tolerance and effects of sublethal acid exposure on iono-regulation and acid-base status in two crayfish *Procambarus clarki* and *Oroconectes rusticus*. *Journal of Experimental Biology* 97: 241–252.

65 Green, J.W., Harsch, M., Barr, L., and Prosser, C.L. (1959). The regulation of water and salt by the fiddler crabs, *Uca Pugnax and Uca pugilator*. *Biological Bulletin* 116 (1): 76–87.

66 Coteur, G., Corriere, N., and Dubois, P. (2004). Environmental factors influencing the immune responses of the common European starfish (*Asterias rubens*). *Fish & Shellfish Immunology* 16: 51–63.

67 Chia, F.S. and Xing, J. (1996). Echinoderm coelomocytes. *Zoological Studies* 35: 231–254.

68 de Faria, M.T. and da JRMC, S. (2008). Innate immune response in the sea urchin *Echinometra lucunter* (Echinodermata). *Journal of Invertebrate Pathology* 98: 58–62.

69 Edds, K.T. (1993). Morphological and cytoskeletal transformation in sea urchin coelomocytes. In: *Blood Cells of Marine Invertebrates: Experimental Systems in*

Cell Biology and Comparative Physiology (ed. W.D. Cohen), 53–74. New York: A.R. Liss Publisher.

70 Gross, P.S., Clow, L.A., and Smith, L.C. (2000). SpC3, the complement homologue from the purple sea urchin, *Strongylocentrotus purpuratus*, is expressed in two subpopulations of the phagocytic coelomocytes. *Immunogenetics* 51: 1034–1044.

71 Ramirez-Gomez, F., Aponte-Rivera, F., Mendez-Castaner, L., and Garcia-Arraras, J.E. (2010). Changes in holothurian coelomocyte populations following immune stimulation with different molecular patterns. *Fish & Shellfish Immunology* 29: 175–185.

72 Pinsino, A., Thorndyke, M.C., and Matranga, V. (2007). Coelomocytes and post-traumatic response in the common sea star *Asterias rubens*. *Cell Stress & Chaperones* 12: 331–341.

73 Roch, P. (1999). Defense mechanisms and disease prevention in farmed marine invertebrates. *Aquaculture* 172: 125–145.

74 Cheng, T.C. (1981). Bivalves. In: *Invertebrate Blood Cells: General Aspects, Animals without True Circulatory Systems to Cephalopods* (ed. N.A. Ratcliffe and A.F. Rowley), 233–300. New York: Academic Press.

75 Oliver, L.M. and Fisher, W.S. (1995). Comparative form and function of oyster *Crassostrea virginica* Hemocytes from Chesapeake Bay (Virginia) and Apalachicola Bay (Florida). *Diseases of Aquatic Organisms* 22: 217–225.

76 Soudant, P., Paillard, C., Choquet, G. et al. (2004). Impact of season and rearing site on the physiological and immunological parameters of the manila clam *Venerupis (=Tapes, =Ruditapes) philippinarum*. *Aquaculture* 229: 401–418.

77 Mosca, F., Narcisi, V., Cargini, D. et al. (2011). Age related properties of the Adriatic clam *Chamelea gallina* (L. 1758) hemocytes. *Fish & Shellfish Immunology* 31: 1106–1112.

78 Olafsen, J.A., Mikkelsen, H.V., Glaever, H.M., and Hansen, G.H. (1993). Indigenous bacteria in hemolymph and tissues of marine bivalves at low-temperatures. *Applied and Environmental Microbiology* 59: 1848–1854.

79 Cowden, R.R. and Curtis, S.K. (1973). Observations on living cells dissociated from leukopoietic organ of *Octopus briareus*. *Experimental and Molecular Pathology* 19: 178–185.

80 Jenkin, C.R. (1976). Factors involved in the recognition of foreign material by phagocytic cells from invertebrates. In: *Comparative Immunology* (ed. J.J. Machalonis), 80–97. New York: Wiley.

81 Bullock, A.M., Polglase, J.L., and Phillips, S.E. (1987). The wound-healing and Hemocyte response in the skin of the lesser octopus *Eledone cirrhosa* (Mollusca, Cephalopoda) in the presence of *Vibrio tubiashii*. *Journal of Zoology* 211: 373–385.

82 Dove, A.D.M., Sokolowski, M.S., Bartlett, S.L., and Bowser, P.R. (2005). Spatio-temporal variation in serum chemistry of the lobster, *Homarus americanus* Milne-Edwards. *Journal of Fish Diseases* 28: 663–675.

83 Martin, G.G. and Hose, J.E. (1995). Circulation, the blood, and disease. In: *Biology of the Lobster Homarus americanus* (ed. J.R. Factor), 465–495. San Diego, CA: Academic Press.

84 Vijayavel, K. and Balasubramanian, M.P. (2006). Fluctuations of biochemical constituents and marker enzymes as a consequence of naphthalene toxicity in the edible estuarine crab *Scylla serrata*. *Ecotoxicology and Environmental Safety* 63: 141–147.

85 Yeh, S.P., Chen, Y.N., Hsieh, S.L. et al. (2009). Immune response of white shrimp, *Litopenaeus vannamei*, after a concurrent infection with white spot syndrome virus and infectious hypodermal and hematopoietic necrosis virus. *Fish & Shellfish Immunology* 26: 582–588.

86 Hudson, D.A. (1995). Biochemical parameters of the serum of the sand crab, *Portunus pelagicus*, with reference to the parasitic dinoflagellate, *Hematodinium australis*. *Bulletin of the European Association of Fish Pathology* 15: 201–205.

87 Blasco, J. and Puppo, J. (1999). Effect of heavy metals (Cu, Cd and Pb) on aspartate and alanine aminotransferase in *Ruditapes philippinarum* (Mollusca: Bivalvia). *Comparative Biochemistry and Physiology C-Pharmacology Toxicology & Endocrinology* 122: 253–263.

88 Ottaviani, E. (1989). Selected decrease of hemocytes of the fresh-water snail *Planorbariuscorneus* (L) (Gastropoda, Pulmonata) after bacteria injection. *Experientia* 45: 368–369.

89 Gustafson, L.L., Stoskopf, M.K., Showers, W. et al. (2005). Reference ranges for hemolymph chemistries from *Elliptio complanata* of North Carolina. *Diseases of Aquatic Organisms* 65: 167–176.

90 Fisher, W.S., Oliver, L.M., and Edwards, P. (1996). Hematologic and serologic variability of eastern oysters from Apalachicola Bay, Florida. *Journal of Shellfish Research* 15: 555–564.

91 Cheng, T.C. (1969). An electrophoretic analysis of hemolymph proteins of snail *Helisoma duryi normale* experimentally challenged with bacteria. *Journal of Invertebrate Pathology* 14: 60–81.

92 Towle, D.W. and Henry, R.P. (2003). Coping with environmental changes: physiological challenges. In: *The American Horseshoe Crab* (ed. C.N. Schuster, R.B. Barlow and H.J. Brockman), 224–244. Cambridge, MA: Harvard University Press.

93 Sharp, M.S. and Neff, J.M. (1980). Steady-state hemolymph osmotic and chloride-ion regulation and percent body-water in *Clibanarius vittatus* (Decapoda, Anomura) from the Texas Gulf-coast. *Comparative Biochemistry and Physiology A-Physiology* 66: 455–460.

94 Whiteley, N.M. and Taylor, E.W. (1992). Oxygen and acid-base disturbances in the hemolymph of the lobster *Homarusc gammarus* during commercial transport and storage. *Journal of Crustacean Biology* 12: 19–30.
95 Truchot, J.P. (1984). Water carbonate alkalinity as a determinant of hemolymph acid-base-balance in the shore crab, *Carcinus maenas* – a study at 2 different ambient PCO_2 and PO_2 levels. *Journal of Comparative Physiology* 154: 601–606.
96 Booth, C.E., Mcmahon, B.R., Defur, P.L., and Wilkes, P.R.H. (1984). Acid-base regulation during exercise and recovery in the blue-crab, *Callinectes sapidus*. *Respiration Physiology* 58: 359–376.
97 D'Aniello, A., Di Cosomo, A., Di Cristo, C. et al. (1996). Occurrence of sex steroid hormones and their binging proteins in *Octopus vulgaris* Lam. *Biochemical and Biophysical Research Communications* 227: 782–788.
98 Howell, B.J. and Gilbert, D.L. (1976). pH-temperature dependence of hemolymph of squid, *Loligo pealei*. *Comparative Biochemistry and Physiology A-Physiology* 55: 287–289.
99 Larson, S.E. and Anderson, R.C. (2010). Fecal hormones measured within giant Pacific octopuses *Enteroctopus dofleini*. *Journal of Aquatic Animal Health* 22: 152–157.
100 McMahon, R.F. (1991). Mollusca: Bivalvia. In: *Ecology and Classification of North American Freshwater Invertebrates* (ed. J.H. Thorp and A.P. Covich), 315–399. San Diego: Academic Press.
101 Carballal, M.J., Villalba, A., and Lopez, C. (1998). Seasonal variation and effects of age, food availability, size, gonadal development, and parasitism on the hemogram *of Mytilus galloprovincialis*. *Journal of Invertebrate Pathology* 72: 304–312.
102 Barnhart, M.C. (1992). Acid–base regulation in pulmonate mollusks. *Journal of Experimental Zoology* 263: 120–126.
103 Mohamed, R. (2011). Impact of profenophos (pesticide) on infectivity of *Biomphalaria alexandrina* snails with *Schistosoma mansoni* miracidia and on their physiological parameters. *Open Journal of Ecology* 1 (2): 41–47.
104 Nollens, H.H., Keogh, J.A., and Probert, P.K. (2004). Haematological pathology of shell lesions in the New Zealand abalone, *Haliotis iris* (Mollusca: Gastropoda). *Comparative Clinical Pathology* 12: 211–216.
105 Zielinski, S., Sartoris, F.J., and Portner, H.O. (2001). Temperature effects on hemocyanin oxygen binding in an Antarctic cephalopod. *Biological Bulletin* 200: 67–76.
106 Kobayashi, N. and Okamura, H. (2005). Effects of heavy metals on sea urchin embryo development. Part 2. Interactive toxic effects of heavy metals in synthetic mine effluents. *Chemosphere* 61: 1198–1203.
107 Pynnonen, K. (1995). Changes in acid-base status, gases and electrolytes in the hemolymph of freshwater Unionids during continuous and intermittent exposure to acid water. *Annales Zoologici Fennici* 32: 355–363.
108 Horne, F.R. and Barnes, G. (1970). Reevaluation of urea biosynthesis in Prosobranch and Pulmonate snails. *Zeitschrift Fur Vergleichende Physiologie* 69: 452–457.
109 Becker, W. and Schmale, H. (1975). Nitrogenous products of degradation – ammonia, urea and uric-acid – in Hemolymph of snail *Biomphalaria glabrata*. *Comparative Biochemistry and Physiology A-Physiology* 51: 407–411.
110 Dyrynda, E.A., Law, R.J., Dyrynda, P.E.J. et al. (1997). Modulations in cell-mediated immunity of *Mytilus edulis* following the 'Sea Empress' oil spill. *Journal of the Marine Biological Association of the United Kingdom* 77: 281–284.
111 Smith, S.A. (2011). Horseshoe crabs. In: *Invertebrate Medicine* (ed. G. Lewbart), 133–142. Wiley-Blackwell.

22

Terrestrial Invertebrates

Trevor T. Zachariah DVM, MS, DACZM

Brevard Zoo, Sea Turtle Healing Center, Melbourne, Florida, USA

Introduction

The traditional role of invertebrates in veterinary medicine has been as parasites or disease vectors of vertebrate animals, with a subsequent paucity of information regarding medical care of invertebrates. However, there is a growing interest in the field, as evidenced by the recent publication of the second edition of Lewbart's *Invertebrate Medicine* and an increasing number of journal articles and various book chapters. The interest is growing partly in response to a need for such information. Many large and small captive invertebrate collections are maintained for research, display, commercial sales, and hobbies. Many species are crucially involved in agriculture, especially the honeybee (*Apis mellifera*). This has become more apparent in the last decade with the recognition in the United States of colony collapse disorder and its various potential etiologies [1, 2]. The role of invertebrates in biodiversity loss and conservation has also recently been gaining more recognition [3, 4].

Like much of invertebrate medicine, the use of clinical pathology to determine health and disease in these animals is in its infancy. Much work remains to be done to establish basic reference intervals for hematologic and biochemical components of hemolymph for most species, as well as to evaluate those components for changes in response to disease conditions. This chapter will introduce the reader to evaluation of the body fluids of terrestrial invertebrates for health assessment. However, given the breadth of the topic and the numerous species it could involve, the reader is encouraged to seek out more detailed information in the primary scientific literature as needed.

Species

A partial list of the terrestrial invertebrate species included in this chapter or commonly found in captivity can be found in Table 22.1.

Arachnids are likely the most common types of invertebrates used for both public and private display. This is primarily due to the fear and awe that they invoke in many people, but also due to their relatively simple husbandry requirements and long life spans (e.g., some female tarantulas can reach over 30 years in age) [5]. Tarantulas all belong to the family Theraphosidae, which consists of 120 genera and more than 930 species [6]. Scorpions belong to the order Scorpiones, which consists of approximately 700 species [7].

Tarantula external anatomy consists of two body segments, the prosoma (cephalothorax) and opisthosoma (abdomen), connected by a narrow region called the pedicel. A dorsal carapace and a ventral sternum connected circumferentially by a flexible membrane make up the prosoma. Attached to it are six pairs of appendages: the chelicerae bearing the fangs, a pair of pedipalps used for mating and prey handling, and four pairs of walking legs. At the caudal end of the opisthosoma is a pair of spinneret appendages for manipulating silk.

Internally, the prosoma houses the paired venom glands, ganglia comprising the primitive centralized nervous system, stomach, cartilaginous rudimentary endoskeleton, and a large amount of musculature. The endoskeleton and muscles within the prosoma allow the carapace and sternum to be moved in relation to one another, thus changing the pressure of the hemolymph throughout the body cavity and into the appendages. This is important for extension of the appendages. Tarantulas have striated muscles, similar to that of vertebrates, but only for contraction.

The opisthosoma contains the majority of the internal organs. The midgut is extensive with many diverticula, some of which may extend into the prosoma. Excretory organs called Malpighian tubules are also present, and both empty into the stercoral pocket located just cranial to the anus. The reproductive organs and silk glands also are found in the opisthosoma.

Exotic Animal Laboratory Diagnosis, First Edition. Edited by J. Jill Heatley and Karen E. Russell.

Table 22.1 Selected species of terrestrial invertebrates included in this chapter or commonly found in captivity.

Common name	Scientific name
Chilean rose tarantula	*Grammostola rosea*
Mexican redknee tarantula	*Brachypelma smithi*
Goliath birdeater tarantula	*Theraphosa blondi*
Texas brown tarantula	*Aphonopelma hentzi*
Emperor scorpion	*Pandinus imperator*
Giant African millipede	*Archispirostreptus gigas*
Tiger centipede	*Scolopendra polymorpha*
Vietnamese centipede	*Scolopendra subspinipes*
Amazon giant centipede	*Scolopendra gigantea*
Honeybee	*Apis mellifera*
Madagascar hissing cockroach	*Gromphadorhina portentosa*
American cockroach	*Periplaneta americana*

The tubular heart lies along the dorsal midline of the opisthosoma and opens cranially and caudally into aortae and lateral vessels, which in turn give way to an extensively branching arterial system throughout the body (Figure 22.1) [8, 9]. There are no capillaries or veins; thus, the circulatory system is semi-open. Pumping of the heart causes pressure changes that draw the hemolymph back into the opisthosoma and back to the heart. Some of the fluid passes through the two pairs of book lungs for oxygenation prior to entering the heart. The book lungs are so named because they consist of many parallel thin lamellae than allow for passive diffusion and exchange of gases [10]. They are found in the cranial half of the ventral opisthosoma, and open through slits in the exoskeleton called spiracles.

Scorpion anatomy is similar to that of tarantulas, with several notable exceptions. The chelicerae are small and do not bear fangs. The pedipalps are modified into pincers for subduing and handling prey. There is no pedicel, and the prosoma and the segmented opisthosoma are broadly connected. The caudal aspect of the abdomen (also called the metasoma or tail) terminates in a telson segment containing a sting and venom glands. Ventrally and caudal to the last pair of walking legs is a pair of comb-like sensory structures called the pectines. Scorpions have four pairs of book lungs. The circulatory system has been described in detail [11, 12].

Myriapods include the millipedes (class Diplopoda) and centipedes (class Chilopoda), accounting for almost 13 000 species [13]. The body plan is long with many segments. In centipedes and millipedes, respectively, most segments have one and two pairs of walking legs attached to each. The head contains the eyes, a pair of antennae, and the mouthparts. In centipedes, it also contains a pair of forcipules, appendages that each bear a fang attached to a venom gland. Also unique to centipedes is a pair of anal legs attached to the most caudal segment. In general, millipedes have a heavily calcified exoskeleton and tubular shape, while centipedes are more dorsoventrally flattened.

Similar to snakes, the internal anatomy of myriapods is lengthened to fit their body form. Most organs and systems are long and tubular, including the dorsally located heart and the digestive system. Very few vessels are present, and hemolymph passes in and out of the heart through ostia to bathe the tissues in each body segment. Respiration occurs through a tubular trachea system of airways that allow gas exchange directly with the tissues. These tubular tracheae open to the environment through spiracles in each segment, and unlike insects, myriapods are unable to close the spiracles to preserve expiratory fluid loss.

Insects likely number greater than one million species, displaying enormous diversity in adaptation to almost

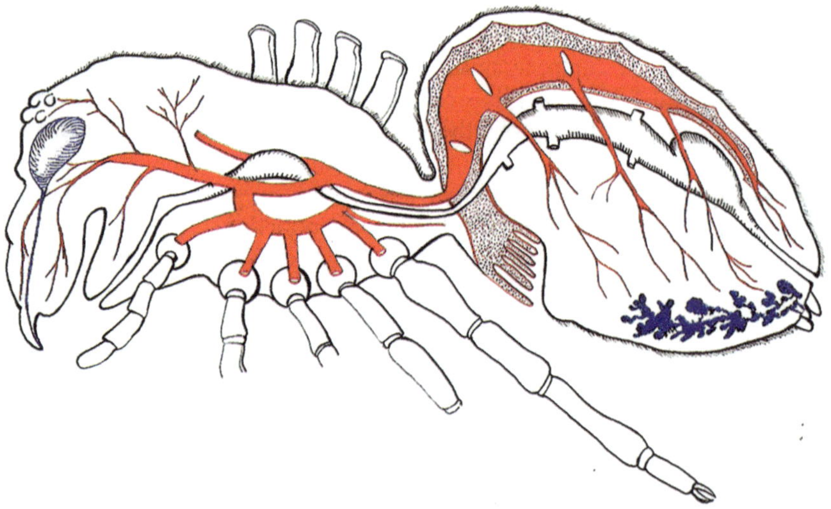

Figure 22.1 Diagram of the semi-open circulatory system anatomy of a spider. Note the location of the tubular heart along the dorsal midline of the opisthosoma (abdomen).

every ecological niche [13]. However, their basic anatomic plan varies little (Figure 22.2). The body consists of three regions: the head, thorax, and abdomen. The head contains the compound eyes, pair of antennae, and the mouthparts. The latter are often highly modified for sucking, piercing, cutting, sponging, or chewing, depending on a species' specialized feeding habits.

The thorax is further divided into three segments: the pro-, meso-, and metathorax. Each thoracic segment contains a pair of legs for a total of six, and the latter two each have a pair of wings, as well. The legs and wings may be modified for functions other than walking and flying, respectively. The abdomen is also subdivided into segments.

Insect circulatory systems are similar to those of myriapods, with a tubular heart in the dorsal half to third of the body and few vessels (Figure 22.2). However, there are some features that are unique to the insects. Many appendages have an associated accessory heart at their base to supply hemolymph to extremities. Additionally, the heart has the ability for periodic heartbeat reversal to prioritize hemolymph flow within the body [13]. Also similar to myriapods, insect hemolymph does not transport respiratory gases, based on an extensive tubular trachea system. However, a major difference between the two groups of animals is that insects are able to close their spiracles; this allows them to conserve body water, one of the key features of their adaptation to arid environments.

Sample Collection and Handling

Collection of hemolymph from arachnids is a relatively easy procedure. The two most common sites are the heart and the arthrodial membranes in the legs. The procedure for the latter site has been described [5, 14], but is not recommended by the author since it is difficult to obtain a sufficient amount in a reasonable time period. Inserting a needle into an arthrodial membrane may also stimulate autotomy of the appendage in an animal that is not anesthetized.

Intracardiac hemolymph collection is the preferred method. It allows for relatively large samples to be obtained rapidly. The procedure has been described in multiple sources [5, 15, 16]. The animal is placed on a secure, flat surface. The index finger applies gentle pressure to the carapace, while the thumb of the same hand stabilizes the caudal end of the opisthosoma in the tarantula or the base of the tail in scorpions. The free hand inserts a needle at a 45°–90° angle through the exoskeleton along the dorsal midline at the midpoint of the opisthosoma (Figure 22.3). Insertion of the needle is best done through an intersegmental membrane in scorpions. Due to the position of the heart, the bevel of the needle need not penetrate farther than just inside the exoskeleton.

For most specimens, a 26 gauge (g.) or finer needle is adequate. The exoskeleton of arachnids is inelastic, and leakage of hemolymph often occurs after removal of the

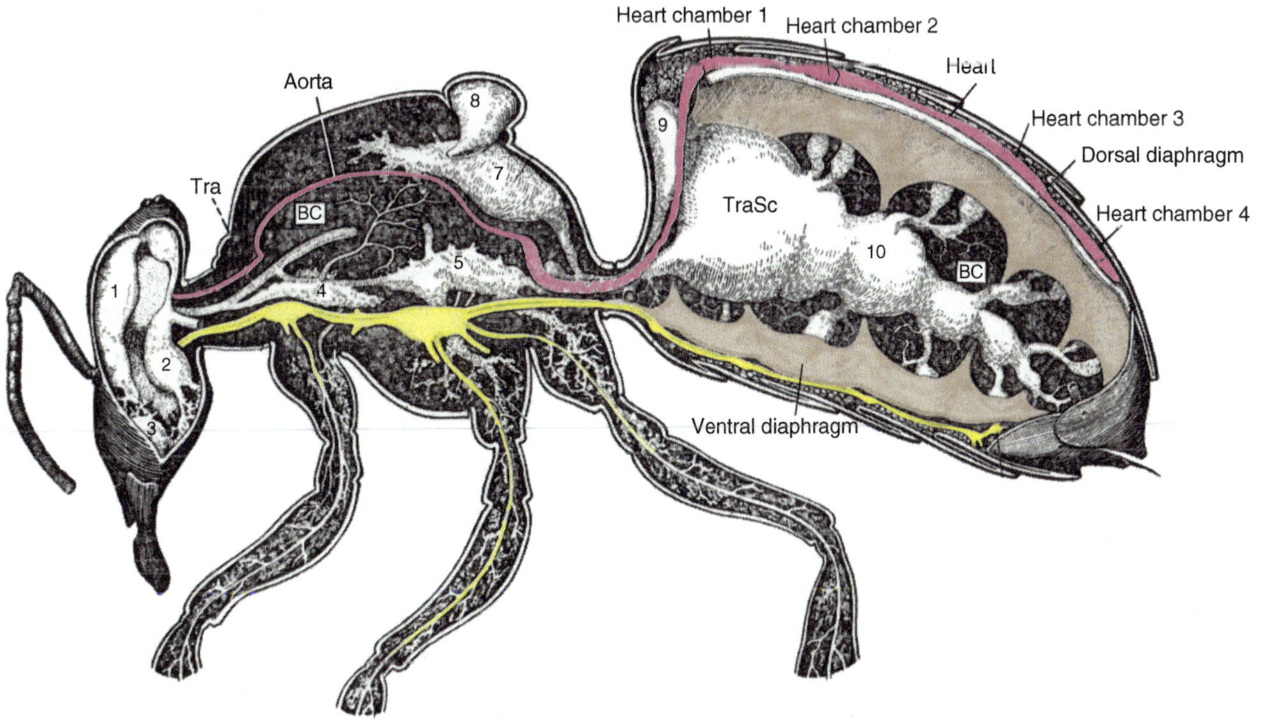

Figure 22.2 Diagram of the circulatory system of a honeybee (*Apis mellifera*).

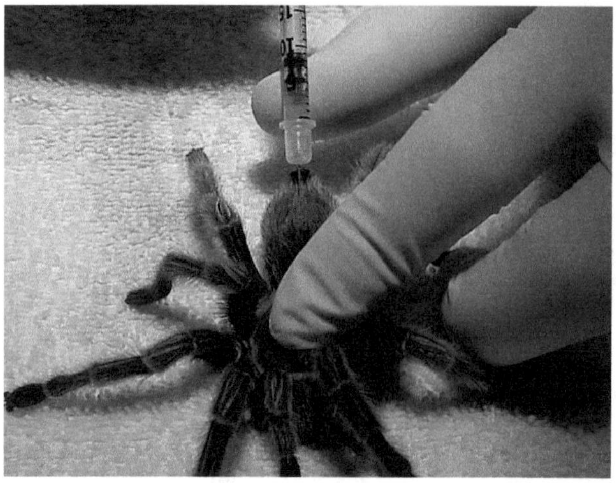

Figure 22.3 Example of intracardiac hemolymph collection from a subadult Chilean rose tarantula (*Grammostola rosea*).

needle. This can be stopped with judicious application of surgical glue. Some clinicians have reported that manual pressure also works, but this has not been the experience of the author. A 1 ml syringe is adequate, although up to 3 ml syringes can be used with the larger species, such as *Theraphosa blondi*.

Hemolymph comprises approximately 20% of the body weight of spiders [17]. The safe volume that can be collected from an arachnid is not known. In general, the rule of thumb is 1% of body weight, as in vertebrate species. However, the author has taken nearly 3% of body weight from individual tarantulas without causing obvious negative clinical or morphologic (e.g., lack of leg extension, shriveled opisthosoma) effects. The actual volume that can be removed from any individual animal will depend on its size. For arachnids, a source of fresh, accessible standing water should always be offered to an animal that has undergone hemolymph sampling. Animals will often drink soon after such a procedure, presumably to restore bodily fluid volume.

Whenever possible, it is recommended that hemolymph collection be performed with the patient under anesthesia. Several studies involving inhalant anesthetic use with tarantulas are available in the literature [18–20], as are descriptions for constructing anesthetic chambers [21, 22] or more direct administration of the gas [5, 23]. Anesthesia facilitates the procedure by decreasing error in the site and depth of needle insertion and amount of sample collected. It also reduces the probability of injury to either the handler or the patient. Arachnids present multiple hazards, including bites and pinches, urticating hairs (New World tarantulas), and envenomations. Though no tarantula envenomation has ever been confirmed to cause death [24], a number of scorpions are known to produce venom that can result in serious illness or fatality [25]. However, tarantulas possess relatively large fangs, and secondary infections from potential bacterial pathogens (e.g., *Aeromonas hydrophila, Staphylococcus aureus, Pseudomonas aeruginosa*) residing on their mouthparts are possible [16, 26].

A review of the pertinent literature reveals several typical methods for collection of hemolymph from honeybees. These methods may or may not involve prior euthanasia of the animals, depending on the situation (e.g., experience of the personnel, available equipment). Hemolymph is collected with a fine capillary tube or micropipette after one of the following: ventral flexion of the head and puncture of the neck membrane; puncture or incision of the thorax or abdomen; decapitation or removal of an appendage (i.e., wing or leg). Punctures are performed with a sterile pin or needle; however, the collection instrument may also be used as the method of puncture. A volume of 5–10 μl can be collected from individual animals, so pooling of samples from a number of bees would be necessary for chemistry analysis in most clinical settings.

Collection of hemolymph from other insect species and myriapods is similar to that in honeybees. One of the most common methods represented in the literature involves puncturing the intersegmental membranes, and either extracting hemolymph with a needle or allowing it to exude into a capillary or other type of tube. These punctures are usually performed in the area of the dorsal midline, so that hemolymph may be collected directly from the heart; however, collection from the body cavity may also occur. The other common method is to sharply incise an appendage, such as a leg or antenna, to allow the hemolymph to flow out of the body. Again, pooling of samples from a population may be necessary in clinical settings, as the actual volume that can be obtained from any individual animal is variable and often small.

It is recommended that anesthesia be employed for sampling of larger individuals, due to the same reasons as in arachnids. Centipedes move rapidly and can deliver painful bites; physical trauma and secondary infections are possible. Similar to tarantulas, larger centipedes (e.g., *Scolopendra* spp.) also have fangs of significant size that can deliver venom capable of deleterious effects on human health or fatality [27]. However, the clinician must also weigh the benefits of anesthesia for sample collection against the possible adverse effects it could cause in sample analyses results [20, 28, 29].

Sample Handling

Clotting of hemolymph cells, known as hemocytes, occurs extremely rapidly after collection. Though sodium citrate has been recommended as an anticoagulant for use with tarantulas [15], the author and others have not had success with it, heparin, or ethylenediaminetetraacetic acid (EDTA) [30]. Various solutions have been devised to prevent coagulation of invertebrate hemocytes [31], though none are available on a commercial basis nor practical in a clinical setting. An alternative is to preload the collection syringe with a known amount of 10% formalin, which also allows for determination of a total hemocyte count (THC) [30]. However, formalin may alter cellular morphology and make identification and detailed observations more difficult [30]. Due to the low cellularity of hemolymph, samples may be centrifuged at 800 × *g* for 10–20 min to concentrate the hemocytes. Direct smears of fresh hemolymph can be prepared, though drying may also alter cellular morphology and cause degranulation. Typical medical stain preparations can be used, including Wright-Giemsa, Diff-Quick, lactophenol cotton blue, Gomori methenamine silver (GMS), periodic acid-Schiff (PAS), Ziehl-Neelsen, and Gram stains [30].

For biochemical analysis, cell-free hemolymph is typically desired. If the hemocytes are allowed to coagulate, samples can be centrifuged in a manner similar to that for collection of plasma from vertebrate blood and the supernatant harvested. Alternatively, the clot may be removed with a sterile instrument.

The viability of invertebrate cell-free hemolymph samples after storage and the effects of temperature and time are not known. In general, it is recommended that biochemical analyses be performed as soon as possible after collection. If this is not possible, samples should be kept on ice or refrigerated until utilized for analysis. Storage at ultra-low temperatures (i.e., 70–80 °C) is also recommended for anything other than brief periods between sample collection and analysis.

Specific Analytes

Most reports of clinical pathology findings in arachnids are based on captive populations. Thus, data based on the "natural" state is usually unknown. The information on the analytes below (Tables 22.2 and 22.3) is based on available literature that is clinically relevant. Analyte not included either have little or no representation in the literature or minimal clinical application.

Hemogram

The nomenclature regarding hemocyte types in arthropods has historically been confusing, having been complicated by the various methods of sample preparation and cell description by early investigators [50]. However, a hemocyte classification system provided by Jones [51] and Price and Ratcliffe [52] is generally applicable to all arthropod taxa. This system includes the following six basic cell types: prohemocyte, plasmatocyte, granular hemocyte, cystocyte, spherule cell, and oenocytoid. Controversy still remains in relation to this subject, as other cell types have been described, such as the adipohemocyte, podocyte, cyanocyte, and vermiform cell. Also, some authors describe different types of granular hemocytes [50, 53]. Representative images of the various cell types, including light microscopic morphology and electron microscopic ultrastructure, are available elsewhere [50–63].

The functions of the various hemocyte types are not fully understood. In general, they are involved in cellular immune defenses (e.g., phagocytosis, nodule formation, encapsulation), initiation of humoral defenses, protein (e.g., hemocyanin) synthesis, clotting/wound repair, and material transport [63–68]. Also of note is that investigations into morphologic changes in hemocytes or changes in THC or hemocyte differential counts in response to injury or disease are poorly represented in the literature. For most invertebrate species, the overall hemolymph cellularity is extremely low in comparison to vertebrates and varies widely by taxa [50].

Hemocytopoiesis in spiders occurs in two places within the heart, the adventitia and myocardial cells of the inner wall [63]. Prohemocytes are the first to be produced; they then form the other cell types through a series of differentiations that change the intracellular organelles and other components [63]. Thus, all spider hemocytes have a common origin, but occur on a spectrum of functional and morphologic specialization. The hemocytes found in spiders include the prohemocyte, plasmatocyte, granular hemocyte, oenocytoid, cyanocyte, and possibly the cystocyte [50, 63]. Granulocytes are the most common type [69, 70].

In addition to the cell types listed above, spiders also have a unique, well-described type known as leberidocytes [63]. These cells are found in the hemolymph transiently during ecdysis [71, 72]. In the Haitian brown tarantula (*Phormictopus cancerides*), leberidocytes begin to appear in the hemolymph 10–12 days prior to, and reach a peak of 47% (range: 41%–60%) of the THC during molting; they are present for approximately a total of four weeks [72]. Leberidocytes start appearing in the hemolymph of *Eratigena [Tegenaria] atrica* four days before the molt, comprise 40% of the THC just before molting, and reach a peak of 63% of the THC just after molting; they are no longer present by the fifth day after ecdysis [71]. Leberidocytes contain large amounts of glycogen, though for what purpose is unknown [72].

When infection or injury occurs in a spider, hemocytes migrate to the etiologic agent or site [70]. Granulocytes are capable of phagocytosis and encapsulation, though likely their more important function is to produce and store antimicrobial peptides (e.g., acanthoscurrin,

Table 22.2 Hemolymph biochemical values for select terrestrial invertebrate species.

Species		Goliath birdeater tarantula [32] *Theraphosa blondi*	Chilean rose tarantula [32, 33] *Grammostola rosea*	Texas brown tarantula [34] *Aphonopelma hentzi* [35]	Texas brown tarantula [36] *Aphonopelma hentzi* [37]	Texas brown tarantula [38] *Aphonopelma hentzi* [35]	Mexican redknee tarantula [39] *Brachypelma smithi* Brazilian black tarantula *Grammostola pulchra* (data for both species combined)	Arizona hairy scorpion [40] *Hadrurus arizonensis*	Dune scorpion [40] *Smeringurus mesaensis*
Sample attributes		Male and female; subadult; captive	Subadult; unknown sex; captive	Unknown age and sex; captive	Female; adult; captive	Unknown sex and age; captive	Unknown sex and age; captive	Unknown age and sex; captive	Unknown age and sex; captive
Animal number *Sample number*		Male: 6 female: 5	12	5–20	20	4–28	unknown	3	3
Data format		Mean ± SD or median {10–90% quartiles} [range]	Mean ± SD or median {10–90% quartiles} [range]	Mean ± SE	Mean ± SE	Mean ± SD	Mean ± SD	Mean ± SE [range]	Mean ± SE [range]
Analyte	**Units, SI (conventional)**								
Glucose	mmol/l (mg/dl)	1.03 ± 0.12 [0.78–1.75] (18.6 ± 2.1) ([14–31.5])	0.97 {0.77–1.54} [0.75–1.69] (17.5 {13.9–27.8}) ([13.–30.5]) [32]				1.39 ± 0.56 (25 ± 10)		
Uric acid	μmol/l (mg/dl)	11.90 {5.95–19.03} [5.95–20.82] 0.2 {0.1–0.32}) ([0.1–0.35])	7.14 {0–17.84} [0–41.64] (0.12 {0–0.3}) ([0–0.7]) [32]						
Urea	mmol/l (mg/dl)	1.07 {0.36–2.43} [0.36–8.21] (3 {1–6.8}) ([1–23])	0.36 {0.18–0.50] [0.18–0.71] (1 {0.5–1.4}) ([0.5–2]) [32]						
Protein	g/l (g/dl)	41 {8–47} [8–50] (4.1 {0.8–4.7}) ([0.8–5])	64 {37–72} [32–73] (6.4 {3.7–7.2}) [3.2–7.3]) [32]	56.89 ± 2.45 (5.69 ± 0.25)	53.44 ± 3.12 (5.34 ± 0.31)		70 ± 10 (7 ± 1)		
Albumin	g/l (g/dl)	0 {0–1.5} [0–2] (0 {0–0.15}) ([0–0.2])	0.2 {0–1.5} [0–5] (0.02 {0–0.15}) ([0–0.5]) [32]						
Aspartate aminotransferase	(IU/l)	4.4 ± 1.7 [2–7.5]	5.7 {2.1–34.7} [2–41.5] [32]						
Creatinine phosphokinase	(IU/l)	17 {2.4–28.8} [2–29]	25.7 ± 7.5 [8–36] [32]						
Calcium	mmol/l (mg/dl)	2.98 ± 0.43 [2.2–3.6] (11.9 ± 1.7) ([8.8–14.4])	4.23 ± 0.45 [3.33–4.98] (16.9 ± 1.8) ([13.3–19.9]) [32]	3.94 ± 0.13 (15.76 ± 0.52)	3.91 ± 0.11 (15.64 ± 0.44)	4.3 ± 0.2 (17.2 ± 0.8)	4.5 ± 0.75 (18 ± 3)	9.8 ± 0.69 [8.8–10.7] (39.2 ± 2.76) ([35.2–42.8]	8.1 ± 0.94 [6–10] (32.4 ± 3.76) ([24–40])

Chinese scorpion [41] *Mesobuthus martensii*	Giant forest scorpion [42] *Heterometrus swammerdami*	Giant forest scorpion [43] *Heterometrus fulvipes*	Common emperor scorpion [38] *Pandinus imperator*	Common emperor scorpion [39] *Pandinus imperator*	Millipede [44] *Pachydesmus crassiscutis*	Kalahari millipede [45] *Triaenostreptus triodus*	Kalahari millipede [45] *Triaenostreptus triodus*	New Zealand giant centipede [46] *Cormocephalus rubriceps*	American cockroach [47, 48] *Periplaneta americana*
Unknown age and sex; wild and captive	Unknown age, sex, status	Male, female; adult; captive	Unknown sex and age; captive	Unknown sex and age; captive	Adult; wild; unknown sex	Male, female; adult; wild	Male, female; adult; captive	Unknown sex and age; wild	Male; adult; captive [48] male, female; adult; captive [47]
Unknown	Unknown	Unknown male: *9–16*, female: *9–20*	4–12	Unknown	7–18	Male: 9–11 female: 13	11–40 of each sex	Unknown	7–10 [48] 144 of each sex [47] *48 (each pooled from 3 individuals) for each sex* [47]
Mean ± SE	[range]	Mean ± SD	Mean ± SD	Mean ± SD	Mean ± SE	Mean ± SD	Mean ± SD	Mean ± SE	Mean ± SD [48] Mean [47]
				1.22 ± 0.56 (22 ± 10)				6 ± 1 (108 ± 18)	
				35.69 ± 23.79 (0.6 ± 0.4)					Male: 1076.6 (18.1) [47] female: 1576.2 (26.5) [47]
		Male: 75.45 ± 6.95 (7.55 ± 0.70) female: 71.76 ± 9.88 (7.18 ± 0.99) combined average: 73.48 ± 8.6 (7.35 ± 0.86)		50 ± 34 (5 ± 3.4)		Male: 59.5 ± 11.9 (5.95 ± 1.19) female: 45.1 ± 13.1 (4.51 ± 1.31)	Male: 38.8 ± 15.5 (3.88 ± 1.55) female: 63.8 ± 19.6 (6.38 ± 1.96)	42.5 ± 9.3 (4.25 ± 0.93)	
6.3 ± 0.3 (25.2 ± 1.2)	[5–10] ([20–40])	Male: 6.68 ± 1.36 (26.72 ± 5.44) female: 5.52 ± 2.24 (22.08 ± 8.96) combined: 6.08 ± 1.07 (24.32 ± 4.28)	4.1 ± 0.7 (16.4 ± 2.8)	4.5 ± 1 (18 ± 4)				4.8 ± 0.4 (19.2 ± 1.6)	3.7 ± 0.3 (14.8 ± 1.2)

(*Continued*)

Table 22.2 (Continued)

Species		Goliath birdeater tarantula [32] *Theraphosa blondi*	Chilean rose tarantula [32, 33] *Grammostola rosea*	Texas brown tarantula [34] *Aphonopelma hentzi* [35]	Texas brown tarantula [36] *Aphonopelma hentzi* [37]	Texas brown tarantula [38] *Aphonopelma hentzi* [35]	Mexican redknee tarantula [39] *Brachypelma smithi* Brazilian black tarantula *Grammostola pulchra* (data for both species combined)	Arizona hairy scorpion [40] *Hadrurus arizonensis*	Dune scorpion [40] *Smeringurus mesaensis*
Sample attributes		Male and female; subadult; captive	Subadult; unknown sex; captive	Unknown age and sex; captive	Female; adult; captive	Unknown sex and age; captive	Unknown sex and age; captive	Unknown age and sex; captive	Unknown age and sex; captive
Animal number *Sample number*		Male: 6 female: 5	12	5–20	20	4–28	unknown	3	3
Data format		Mean ± SD or median {10–90% quartiles} [range]	Mean ± SD or median {10–90% quartiles} [range]	Mean ± SE	Mean ± SE	Mean ± SD	Mean ± SD	Mean ± SE [range]	Mean ± SE [range]
Phosphorus	mmol/l (mg/dl)	0.65 ± 0.19 [0.36–1] (2 ± 0.6) ([1.1–3.1])	0.39 ± 0.13 [0.23–0.68] (1.2 ± 0.4) ([0.7–2.1]) [32]				0.26 ± 0.23 (0.8 ± 0.7)		
Sodium	mmol/l (=mEq/l)	190 ± 14.3 [170–218]	172.8 ± 33.3 [115–206] [32]	190.8 ± 6.1	188.30 ± 7.43	188.5 ± 4.4	245 ± 20	353 ± 13.8 [330–386]	332 ± 23.8 [295–390]
Potassium	mmol/l (=mEq/l)	2 ± 0.4 [1.6–2.8]	2 ± 0.5 [1.1–2.8] [32]	1.9 ± 0.03	1.42 ± 0.04	2.5 ± 0.4	2.5 ± 0.5	11.2 ± 0.24 [10.8–11.8]	9.2 ± 2.2 [5.6–14.4]
Chloride	mmol/l (=mEq/l)			242.3 ± 2.6	241.84 ± 9.01	215.6 ± 6.6		344 ± 18.4 [318–389]	306 ± 8.6 [299–327]
Magnesium	mmol/l (mg/dl)			3.95 ± 0.19 (9.61 ± 0.46)	4.01 ± 0.05 (9.76 ± 0.12)	0.4 ± 0.1 (0.97 ± 0.24)		1.7 ± 0.16 [1.4–2.1] (4.14 ± 0.39) ([3.41–5.11])	1.8 ± 0.53 [0.8–3.2] (4.38 ± 1.29) ([1.95–7.79])
Osmolality	mOsm/L		359.79 ± 18.57 [33]	477 ± 7.2	482.41 ± 5.41				

Chinese scorpion [41] *Mesobuthus martensii*	**Giant forest scorpion [42] *Heterometrus swammerdami***	**Giant forest scorpion [43] *Heterometrus fulvipes***	**Common emperor scorpion [38] *Pandinus imperator***	**Common emperor scorpion [39] *Pandinus imperator***	**Millipede [44] *Pachydesmus crassiscutis***	**Kalahari millipede [45] *Triaenostreptus triodus***	**Kalahari millipede [45] *Triaenostreptus triodus***	**New Zealand giant centipede [46] *Cormocephalus rubriceps***	**American cockroach [47, 48] *Periplaneta americana***
Unknown age and sex; wild and captive	**Unknown age, sex, status**	**Male, female; adult; captive**	**Unknown sex and age; captive**	**Unknown sex and age; captive**	**Adult; wild; unknown sex**	**Male, female; adult; wild**	**Male, female; adult; captive**	**Unknown sex and age; wild**	**Male; adult; captive [48] male, female; adult; captive [47]**
Unknown	**Unknown**	**Unknown male: *9–16*, female: *9–20***	**4–12**	**Unknown**	**7–18**	**Male: 9–11 female: 13**	**11–40 of each sex**	**Unknown**	**7–10 [48] 144 of each sex [47] *48 (each pooled from 3 individuals) for each sex* [47]**
Mean ± SE	**[range]**	**Mean ± SD**	**Mean ± SD**	**Mean ± SD**	**Mean ± SE**	**Mean ± SD**	**Mean ± SD**	**Mean ± SE**	**Mean ± SD [48] Mean [47]**
				0.13 ± 0.16 (0.4 ± 0.5)					
284.7 ± 5	[150–335]	Male: 221.7 ± 52.5 female: 197.8 ± 34.7 combined: 209.7 ± 44.6	230.5 ± 3.4	234 ± 13	66 ± 2.9	Male: 130 ± 11 female: 132 ± 11	Male: 121 ± 12 female: 119 ± 12	214.7 ± 10.9	132 ± 7 [48]
6.8 ± 0.8	[0.5–3]	Male: 1.4 ± 0.83 female: 1.35 ± 0.84 combined: 1.37 ± 0.83	2.9 ± 0.2	4.2 ± 1.3	5.7 ± 0.5	Male: 7 ± 0.9 female: 6.4 ± 0.9	Male: 7 ± 2.6 female: 7 ± 1.6	4.9 ± 0.7	8.7 ± 0.7 [48]
266	[150–450]	Male: 251.4 ± 44.3 female: 277.1 ± 63.1 combined: 266.5 ± 56.1	219.2 ± 3.3		38 ± 2.9	Male: 86 ± 10 female: 87 ± 11	Male: 90 ± 10 female: 87 ± 8	112.9 ± 11.1	107 ± 4 [48]
1.5 ± 0.3 (3.65 ± 0.73)	[5–25] ([12.17–60.83])	Male: 10.08 ± 3.35 (24.53 ± 8.15) female: 10.83 ± 3.16 (26.35 ± 7.69) combined: 10.43 ± 3.27 (25.38 ± 7.96)	1.1 ± 0.1 (2.68 ± 0.24)					1.6 ± 0.1 (3.89 ± 0.24)	4.7 ± 1 (11.44 ± 2.43) [48]
558.7 ± 4.9					165 ± 1.58	Male: 269 ± 22 female: 277 ± 14	Male: 290 ± 31 female: 292 ± 20	418.2	

Table 22.3 Hemolymph gases, pH, and electrolyte values for select terrestrial invertebrate species.

Analyte	Units, SI (conventional)	Goliath birdeater tarantula [32] *Theraphosa blondi*	Chilean rose tarantula [20] *Grammostola rosea*	Texas brown tarantula [38] *Aphonopelma hentzi* [35]	Texas brown tarantula [49] *A. hentzi* [35]	Mexican redknee tarantula [39] *Brachypelma smithi* Brazilian black tarantula[a] *Grammostola pulchra* (data for both species combined)	Emperor scorpion [38] *Pandinus imperator*
Sample attributes		6 Male, 5 female, subadult, captive; anesthesia with 5% isoflurane in oxygen	12 Subadult, unknown sex, captive; R: resting with no anesthesia, A: anesthesia with 5% sevoflurane in oxygen	5 Unknown sex and age; captive	4–7 Captive adult females, variable temperatures	Unknown number, sex and age; captive	5 Unknown sex and age; captive
Data format		Mean ± SD or median {10–90% quartiles} [range]	Mean ± SD or median [range]	Mean ± SD	Mean ± SD	Mean ± SD	Mean ± SD
Sodium	mmol/l (=mEq/l)		210.75 ± 11.33 [194.5–231.2]				
Potassium	mmol/l (=mEq/l)		3.93 ± 0.57 [3.3–4.96]				
Chloride	mmol/l (=mEq/l)		180.42 ± 11.01 [165.3–200.4]				
Ionized calcium	mmol/l (=mEq/l)	1.8 {1.67–2.27} [1.66–2.34]	1.79 ± 0.13 [1.62–2.02]			2.4 ± 0.1	
Ionized magnesium	mmol/l (=mEq/l)		R: 0.49 [0.25–0.68] A: 0.61 [0.33–0.66]				
pH		7.44 ± 0.05 [7.38–7.53]	7.480 ± 0.069 [7.303–7.570]	7.64 ± 0.03	15 C: 7.672 ± 0.032 20 C: 7.582 ± 0.037 25 C: 7.568 ± 0.018 30 C: 7.528 ± 0.026	7.28 ± 0.03	7.49 ± 0.07
pO_2	mm Hg	200 {147.8–348} [147–372]	R: 168.5 [90.3–178.8] A: 198.85 [142.1–210.9]				
PCO_2	mm Hg	20.3 ± 3.9 [15–28.8]	14.14 ± 3.85 [9.6–23.1]	7.46 ± 1.09	15 C: 6.97 ± 0.52 20 C: 10.05 ± 1.65 25 C: 10.60 ± 0.53 30 C: 14.09 ± 0.76		19.67 ± 2.94
TCO_2	mmol/l (=mEq/l)	14.5 ± 2.6 [10–18]	10.73 ± 1.35 [8.4–12.6]	9.24 ± 0.95	15 C: 10.68 ± 1.20 20 C: 14.71 ± 1.93 25 C: 11.19 ± 1.08 30 C: 12.52 ± 1.60	13 ± 3	18.19 ± 2.68
HCO_3	mmol/l (=mEq/l)	13.8 ± 2.7 [9.2–17.6]	10.31 ± 1.24 [8.1–12.1]	8.95 ± 0.91		12 ± 2.5	17.41 ± 2.61
Base excess	mmol/l (=mEq/l)		R: −13.11 ± 1.14 [−14.5–11.1] A: −14.11 ± 1.09 [−15.4–11.9]				
Oxygen saturation (sO_2)	%	100 {99–100} [99–100]					

[a] Data combined for these species.

gomesin) in their intracytoplasmic granules [66, 70, 73, 74]. Plasmatocytes are also involved in phagocytosis and encapsulation, while their other role is producing clotting factors and initiating the clotting cascade [66]. Cyanocytes produce hemocyanin protein, which besides its role in the respiratory system, also functions as part of the innate immune defenses (e.g., antimicrobial molecules, phenoloxidase system) [63, 66].

Scorpions hemocytes originate in two structures: the supraneural gland, which forms part of the wall of the supraneural artery within the ventral aspect of the mesosoma, and the lateral lymphoid glands, connected to the diaphragm in the anteroventral aspect of the mesosoma [75]. The scorpion hemocyte population consists of prohemocytes, plasmatocytes, granular hemoctyes, cystocytes, spherulocytes, and adipohemocytes [63]. A cell termed coagulocyte has also been described [56–58]. Cyanocytes are likely present; however, this particular hemocyte type has not yet been described in any scorpion species. [63]

Myriapod hemolymph contains prohemocytes, granular hemocytes (two forms), and plasmatocytes, with the latter two being the most common and second most common types, respectively [50]. Spherulocytes and coagulocytes may be present in some taxa, while discoid hemocytes, adipohemocytes, and oenocytoids are infrequently encountered [50]. The latter hemocyte type is thought to be involved ecdysis in some unknown capacity [50]. In general, chilopods have higher THCs than diplopods, but the number of circulating hemocytes may also depend on diet and environmental conditions [50, 76]. Non-sterile injury increases the THC of millipedes, though details are not available in the report describing this [76]. Hematopoiesis occurs in tissue along the dorsal blood vessel or heart [77].

Significant changes in hemocytes numbers occur during the molting cycle of the millipede *Thyropygus poseidon*, as measured during premolt (approximately five days before ecdysis), fresh molt (approximately 10 h after ecdysis), postmolt (approximately five days after ecdysis), and intermolt periods [77]. Granulocytes are at their highest mean differential count (34%) during the intermolt period, and are relatively stable (20%–25%) during the rest of the cycle. Plasmatocytes are at their highest during post- and intermolt (31%–35%) and lowest during premolt (7%). Cystocytes are also at their lowest during premolt (9%), but highest during fresh and postmolt (31%–40%). Prohemocytes and spherulocytes peak during fresh molt (10%) and premolt (63%), respectively. Adipohemocytes remain low (<3%) at all periods of the cycle. The THC also varies with the periods of the molting cycle, with higher values during pre- and postmolt (38 000 and 47 000/μl, respectively) than during intermolt and fresh molt (16 000 and 23 000/μl, respectively). All the values presented here regarding *Thy. poseidon* are estimations.

Insect hemocytes have been studied in greater detail than those of the other arthropod taxa presented here. Specifically, attempts have been made to parse their roles within the immune defenses, with the primary type being the granular hemocytes, plasmatocytes, and oenocytoids [64, 65, 68]. Which of the former two types is the most populous varies by taxa [68]. Both granular hemocytes and plasmatocytes are involved in phagocytosis and nodule formation of small infectious agents or particles, as well as encapsulation of protozoans, metazoans, parasites, and eggs and larvae of parasitic wasps [64]. Nodule formation involves multicellular hemocytic aggregates, while encapsulation includes multiple layers of hemocytes that may be organized or random [65]. Melanization may also occur as part of encapsulation in some taxa [64], and oenocytoids likely play a role in this phenomenon [68]. In many species, the cellular immune response increases in potency with development, either due to greater immune competence or number of circulating hemocytes [64, 78]. In addition to cellular defenses, hemocytes play many roles in the humoral defenses of insects, the details of which are reviewed elsewhere [64, 65, 68].

Changes in hemocyte morphology, differentials, or THC in response to infectious, parasitic, chemical, or traumatic insult vary by the nature of the condition and species of insect [79]. Several examples of this are available in cockroaches. In the German cockroach (*Blattella germanica*), natural infection with *Aspergillus flavus* causes hemocytes to respond by phagocytosis and encapsulation, but not nodule formation [80]. Compared to uninfected individuals, infected animals had marked decreases in prohemocytes and increases in granular hemocytes (30% vs. 0% and 8% vs. 45%, respectively). American cockroaches (*Periplaneta americana*), when injected with various bacteria, viral particles, *Saccharomyces cerevisiae* yeast, unfixed and formalin fixed sheep erythrocytes, nonbiological particles, and saline (controls), demonstrate various hemocytic reactions [81]. Plasmatocytes generally make up greater than 50% of the hemocyte population, and along with adipohemocytes are the primary cells involved in phagocytosis. Granular hemocytes and prohemocytes have a lesser role in phagocytosis. None of the bacteria are observed to be phagocytized, while the rest of the particles are and eventually become encompassed by nodule formation. (The authors report that the result is nodule formation, though the description of the structures is more similar to encapsulation.) Except for those surrounding the viral particles, all the nodules accumulate melanin. Compared to the saline controls, injection with any of the particles causes the

THC to more than double, significantly increases the plasmatocyte proportion, and increases the absolute numbers of adipohemocytes, granular hemocytes, and cystocytes. Finally, hemocytes of the death's head cockroach (*Blaberus craniifer*) show bactericidal activity against certain species of bacteria and not others in vitro [82]. When present, bactericidal activity of the hemocytes is exclusively due to phagocytosis.

Hematopoiesis in insects usually occurs in multiple organs, the number and location of which vary depending on taxa [68, 78]. Price and Ratcliffe [52] suggest that the lineage relationship of the various hemocyte types is fairly straightforward, and that they are all different developmental and/or functional stages of one cell type. However, the actual lineage relationships among the hemocyte types are likely more complicated, and various scenarios have been reported [65, 78].

Biochemical Panel

Enzymes

Arachnids lack tissue that is analogous to the liver, the primary tissue source of aspartate aminotransferase (AST) in vertebrate species. However, as stated above, arachnids possess striated muscle similar to that in vertebrates. This musculature is likely the tissue source for AST and creatine kinase activity in the hemolymph. Changes in the activity of either enzyme in hemolymph as a response to inflammation of or injury to muscle tissue have not been demonstrated for invertebrates.

Carbohydrates

Glucose is the primary carbohydrate in arachnid hemolymph [69]. Arachnids have low but measurable concentrations of hemolymph glucose, consistent with their low metabolic rates. In the curly hair tarantula (*Brachypelma albopilosum*), hemolymph glucose concentration varies by both age and sex [83]. Males exhibit significant increases in hemolymph glucose with each molt, whereas females do not exhibit changes during development. Also, males have a higher concentration of hemolymph glucose than females in the final juvenile, subadult, and adult life stages.

In honeybees, the predominant sugar in hemolymph is trehalose, with lesser concentrations of fructose and glucose [84–86]. Sucrose may also be present in relatively small concentrations [84]. Hemolymph sugars in honeybees are extremely high compared to many other insects; they are the primary source of energy for the high metabolic rates during activity (i.e., flight) [87]. As the metabolic rate increases, so do the hemolymph levels of trehalose, fructose, and glucose, until at the highest metabolic rates, trehalose actually decreases [87]. This is because the fat body that synthesizes trehalose cannot meet consumption demands.

Many factors may influence hemolymph sugar concentrations in honeybees. Patterns associated with the lunar phases have been described, with significant increases in trehalose and glucose during full and new moon stages [88]. Anesthesia with carbon dioxide causes reductions of greater than 80% in fructose and trehalose and greater than 50% in glucose, while cooling to 4 °C is associated with reductions of somewhat less magnitude [86]. As might be expected, decreased hemolymph sugar concentrations are also seen during starvation, but recover to normal levels within 10 min after feeding [86]. When stressed, honeybee total sugar levels in hemolymph can increase by greater than 30% [86].

Parasitic disease can also affect honeybee sugar concentrations in hemolymph. Two studies have examined the effect of the microsporidian parasite *Nosema ceranae*, with somewhat contradictory results. Mayack and Naug [89] found that infected foraging bees had decreased levels of trehalose, while glucose levels were static compared to those for uninfected bees (fructose was not included in the analysis). Aliferis et al. [90] reported that infected worker bees had decreased levels of fructose, increased levels of glucose, and trehalose levels were static relative to healthy bees. The differences may be explained by the different energetic states of the bees used in each study (foraging vs. in the hive) [90]. However, the authors of both studies concluded that *N. ceranae* causes significant energetic stress on individual bees, with likely resultant behavioral changes that have repercussions for the entire hive.

In worker honeybees infected with another detrimental parasite, the mite *Varroa destructor*, the amount of parasitism (i.e., the number of mites on an individual bee) was found to be inversely proportional to the amount of carbohydrates in homogenized abdominal tissue [91]. Since the fat body resides in the abdomen and is the central site of energy storage and synthesis [92], this relationship may be a factor in the morbidity and mortality associated with *V. destructor* infection.

Nitrogenous Waste Products

The primary excretory products of arachnids are guanine, adenine, hypoxanthine, and uric acid [69]. The presence of urea nitrogen in hemolymph is likely a result of oxidation of ingested amino acids, as in vertebrate species. However, the low concentrations of both uric acid and urea nitrogen in arachnid hemolymph suggest that they are not the chief excretory products. Interestingly, urea nitrogen concentration increases during dehydration in a manner similar to sodium and total protein [32].

In myriapods, ammonia and uric acid are the primary nitrogenous end products, with ammonia being the more abundant of the two substances [93, 94]. In centipedes, uric acid concentrations in the hemolymph are relatively high [94].

Uric acid is a major nitrogenous waste product in insects; in contrast to myriapods, the hemolymph concentration is usually relatively low [95]. Like many analytes within circulating hemolymph, the concentration is influence by a variety of factors, such as nutritional state, daily light and activity cycles, stage of development, and parasitism [95].

Electrolytes and Osmolality

The sodium concentration for arachnids is typically higher than would be expected in most vertebrate species, and can exceed the upper limit of measurement (often 180 mmol/l) of many in-clinic chemistry analyzers. Therefore, dilution of hemolymph samples prior to analysis may be indicated. A loose trend of higher sodium concentrations in xeric versus mesic species may exist. Little information regarding chloride concentrations in arachnids is available, but this analyte likely exhibits trends in parallel with sodium as it does in vertebrate species. Potassium concentrations for many tarantulas are lower than those reported for most vertebrate species, while those for *Pandinus imperator* are similar to vertebrate reference intervals. All three of these electrolytes are regulated by the anal excretory system (Malpighian tubules and stercoral pocket). However, a second regulatory system for spiders is present in the coxal glands. Coxal glands are present at the base of the walking legs and secrete fluid during feeding, though secretion can occur at other times in response to ion imbalances [96, 97]. Sodium, chloride, and potassium concentrations all increase in hemolymph and anal excretory and coxal gland products during dehydration [32, 96, 97]. Thus, measurement of these analytes, particularly sodium, may be a valuable diagnostic tool, since hypovolemia in arachnids does not manifest in morphologic changes until the condition is severe [5, 16].

The concentration of arachnid osmolality is much greater than that expected in vertebrate species. Since measurement of osmolality is not performed commonly in clinical settings, it can be estimated by a calculation using sodium (Na) and potassium (K) concentrations. For tarantulas, the formula is $2 \times (Na + K)$, which has been shown to have the best agreement with measured values for osmolality [33]. Osmolality has been shown to increase during dehydration in spiders [97], but marked osmoregulation has also been demonstrated [98]. Therefore, the ability to use osmolality as a diagnostic tool is questionable. It is useful in determining and choosing solutions for fluid therapy for arachnids. The commercial product that most closely matches hemolymph values is Normosol®-M with 5% dextrose (363 mOsmol/l), though the author has not used this product in a clinical setting. The next closest commercial product is physiologic (0.9%) saline (308 mmol/l), which has been successfully used in tarantulas [5, 32]. The use of lactated Ringer's solution and Hartmann's solution without clinical problems has also been reported [5]. Formulations for producing parenteral fluid solutions based on hemolymph ionic compositions are also available (Box 22.1) [34, 39].

Box 22.1 Formulas for Arachnid Parenteral Fluid Solutions [34, 39]

Formula	Ingredient	Amount
Formula 1	Normosol-R,	500 ml
	7.2% saline	50 ml
	10% calcium gluconate	0.85 ml
Formula 2	0.9% saline	500 ml
	7.2% saline	45 ml
	10% calcium glucone	0.85 ml
Formula 3	Sodium chloride	11.1 g/l
	Potassium chloride	0.15 g/l
	Magnesium chloride	0.81 g/l
	Calcium chloride	0.59 g/l
	Disodium phosphate	0.27 g/l

Osmolality has been studied more extensively in scorpions. Various species have been shown to experience increased hemolymph osmolality with desiccation [99–105]. Changes in osmolality may correlate with ion concentration changes in one or more of sodium, chloride, and potassium [104]. However, differences do exist. Scorpion species that are adapted to xeric environments tend to have better osmoregulation and are more affected by decreases in relative humidity than temperature increases when compared to species adapted to mesic environments [104, 105]. Higher temperatures and lower relative humidities can cause desiccation and hemolymph osmolality increases in mesic species [105]. Differences based on phylogeny and sex also exist, with females better able to regulate their hemolymph osmolality than males [99–101]. This latter finding is based on the fact that female scorpions have a larger hepatopancreas than males, which acts as a water reservoir in conditions conducive to desiccation [99–101]. Sex differences in hemolymph osmoregulation may also occur in spiders, as many species exhibit significant sexual dimorphism in regard to body size.

Similar to arachnids, the major contributions to the total osmolar concentration in the hemolymph of myriapods are sodium and chloride [106, 107]. A general trend by taxa has been identified, with lower hemolymph osmolality in diplopods than chilopods, though individual variation is high [108]. Millipede hemolymph osmolality has been relatively well studied, especially in regard to dehydration/desiccation. Millipedes are partially able to osmoregulate in response to water loss, though differences exist by species, sex, and speed of dehydration [44, 98, 103]. In contrast, the ability of centipedes to osmoregulate appears to be minimal [98].

In insects, hemolymph components that contribute to the total osmolar concentration can vary greatly by taxa [107]. The order Lepidoptera (butterflies and moths) and free amino acids, order Phasmida (stick insects) and magnesium and chloride, and order Blattodea (cockroaches) and sodium and chloride are examples of insect groups with their respective hemolymph constituents that provide the greatest osmotic effects. The ability to osmoregulate also likely varies between insect taxa, though cockroaches seem to be adept at it [109–111]. This strong osmoregulation effect is most likely due to removal of sodium and chloride from the hemolymph [109, 111, 112], though water storage within the body, such as in the salivary sacs, may also be contributory [113].

Proteins

The primary protein in arachnid hemolymph is the respiratory molecule hemocyanin, comprising 80% of the total [69]. Hemocyanin is analogous to the hemoglobin molecule of vertebrate species, with notable exceptions. Hemocyanin is freely dissolved in the hemolymph rather than bound within specialized cells; as a result, it is found in a much lower concentration than that of hemoglobin [69]. The molecule contains two central copper ions, which are much less efficient at binding oxygen than iron atoms [69], thus contributing to the low metabolic rate of arachnids. These copper atoms associated with hemocyanin molecules are also responsible for the blue color of hemolymph, and the intensity of the coloration varies directly with the amount of bound oxygen. The copper atoms present in and the resulting blue coloration of hemolymph may adversely affect colorimetric methods of protein concentration determination.

Hemolymph protein levels vary by age, but not sex, in the tarantula *B. albopilosum* [83]. Both males and females show significant increases in protein until the final (subadult) instar. During the subadult and adult life stages, the hemolymph protein concentrations are similar to those found in other theraphosid species [32, 34, 39].

Individual amino acid concentrations have been determined for a number of spider species [114]. A majority of these species have proline as the most prevalent, or one of the most prevalent, amino acids in hemolymph. This suggests that proline could have unspecified roles as an energy source or in osmoregulation, similar to some insects [115, 116]. Much less information is available regarding amino acids in scorpion species. However, in contrast to spiders, the hemolymph of the scorpion *Heterometrus (Palamnaeus) bengalensis* contains no proline, except for during the final few stages of the ecdysis cycle [117].

Protein and amino acid hemolymph concentrations have been reported for different myriapod species [45, 46, 106, 108, 118, 119]. In at least one millipede species, *Orthoporus ornatus*, protein concentration varies seasonally [106]. Protein and amino acid concentrations also have been demonstrated to vary by sex and living condition. Wild-caught males of the millipede *Jonespeltis splendidus* have twice the concentration of free amino acids as females [118]. For the millipede *Triaenostreptus triodus*, wild-caught males have significantly greater protein concentrations than females, while the reverse is true after the animals are held under laboratory conditions for two to three months [45].

Hemolymph protein in honeybees is affected by different diets in laboratory settings [120]. Bee protein levels are also affected by infection with *V. destructor*. The mites cause a significant decrease in the hemolymph total protein accumulation up to 30 days after emergence in worker bees [121]. This may in turn have physiologic consequences that affect colony survival, such as overwintering in temperate regions [121]. Mite infection also causes a decrease in protein amounts in homogenized tissues of the head and abdomen of bees, but not in the thorax [91]. The difference between the body segments may be explained by the use of certain amino acids (e.g., proline) for flight metabolism [115]. Desiccation has been shown to be associated with significant total protein and amino acid decreases in hemolymph of domestic and feral honeybees [122], an example of the role of organic molecules (e.g., amino acids) in osmoregulation of hemolymph in insects [107, 123].

When the amino acids of honeybees are evaluated, proline is predominant [90, 115, 124], similar to many other insect species [116, 123]. Although sugars are the primary source of energy for bees, proline may play some role as an energy source utilized during flight [115]. The amount of amino acids in hemolymph is somewhat dependent on honeybee caste, as well as life stage and age [124]. Workers have lower concentrations of all amino acids than queens and drones, and differences in some individual amino acid concentrations exist between the latter two castes. Queen bees experience a significant increase in amino acid concentrations with the onset of egg laying, while workers and drones reach a maximum level at approximately five days of age with subsequent gradual tapering.

Protein and amino acid concentrations in insect hemolymph are affected by many internal (e.g., growth phase, molting, disease) and external (e.g., diet, toxins) factors [95]. Generally, insects have high levels of amino acids in their hemolymph, and in many species proline is predominant [95, 123]. Amino acid concentrations for the cockroach species *Blaberus discoidalis* and *P. americana* are available [125–127]. Proline may have a significant physiologic role as an energy source in *P. americana*, as 50%–60% decreases in hemolymph concentration occur after forced activity or electrical stimulation in the animals [128]. The role of proline as an energy source has been shown in other insect species [95, 115].

Calcium

Total calcium concentrations in arachnids are generally greater than values expected in mammals, but similar to those found in female birds and reptiles undergoing reproductive activity (i.e., oogenesis). Arachnids possess striated muscles, and calcium is required for proper function of myocytes [32], as well as other biologic processes. The ionized calcium concentration is typically higher than that of vertebrate species. This is likely a consequence of the fact that arachnids do not have significant amounts of a binding protein such as albumin [32]. Without a skeletal system or other calcified tissues, the relatively low levels of phosphorus in arachnids are probably adequate for its many other physiologic roles.

Among terrestrial arthropod species, millipedes have the highest body content of calcium, primarily due to their heavily calcified exoskeleton [129]. It has been shown that they have relatively high concentrations of calcium circulating in their hemolymph [106].

Vitamins

The concentration of vitamin D in *The. blondi* hemolymph is significantly lower than would be expected in the blood of vertebrate species [130]. It is unknown if the vitamin D is synthesized by the spiders or obtained from their prey. In either case, the metabolic role of the compound or its possible conversion to 1,25-dihydroxyvitamin D has yet to be determined.

Vitamin concentrations in the hemolymph of other terrestrial invertebrates have not been investigated. Most studies are focused on whole-body amounts of vitamins in invertebrates that would be fed to predators in captive situations [131, 132].

Blood Gases and pH

Tarantulas and scorpions in general are "sit and wait" predators, and respiratory gas exchange is conducted via simple diffusion. This lifestyle correlates well with their low metabolic rates. On the basis of resting oxygen consumption rates, their metabolism is a fifth of the average vertebrate poikilotherm and a hundredth of the average homeotherm of similar size [10]. At rest, the spiracles are mostly closed; this leaves an opening size of approximately 0.23 mm^2 for all four book lungs of a 15 g tarantula, for example [10]. In the recovery period after significant activity, the spiracles retract to allow for a total opening size of 6 mm^2, vastly increasing oxygen consumption [10]. Thus, samples could be affected if an animal is active in avoiding capture or struggles against restraint prior to hemolymph collection.

As diffusion is the method of gas exchange in arachnids, sampling for hemolymph gases performed with animals under inhalant anesthesia is likely to skew measurements due to the increased oxygen concentrations to which the animals are exposed. More studies involving unanesthetized animals at various levels of activity are needed.

Almost no insect species contain any oxygen-carrying molecule in their hemolymph, due to the extensive tracheal system that supplies oxygen directly to the tissues [95]. Interestingly, myriapods have a similar tracheal system, but have also been shown to contain hemocyanin in their hemolymph [95, 133]. The significance of the coexistence of these two oxygen transport systems is unknown.

The range of hemolymph pH in arachnids is typically found to be narrow, and values are similar to those of vertebrate species. However, significant changes occur. During activity, arachnids rapidly convert from aerobic to anaerobic metabolism, with a subsequent increase in lactate production and decrease in pH [38, 134]. Also, both spiders and scorpions have been shown to experience an inverse relationship between temperature and pH due to increases in partial pressure of carbon dioxide [49, 135].

References

1 Genersch, E. (2010). Honey bee pathology: current threats to honey bees and beekeeping. *Applied Microbiology and Biotechnology* 87 (1): 87–97.

2 vanEngelsdorp, D. and Meixner, M.D. (2010). A historical review of managed honey bee populations in Europe and the United States and the factors that may affect them. *Journal of Invertebrate Pathology* 103: S80–S95.

3 Pizzi, R. (2008). Disease management in ex-situ invertebrate conservation programs. In: *Zoo and Wild Animal Medicine Current Therapy*, vol. 6 (ed. M.E. Fowler and R.E. Miller), 88–96. Saunders.

4 Pizzi, R. (2009). Veterinarians and taxonomic chauvinism: the dilemna of parasite conservation. *Journal of Exotic Pet Medicine* 18 (4): 279–282.

5 Pizzi, R. (2012). Spiders. In: *Invertebrate Medicine*, 2e (ed. G.A. Lewbart), 187–221. Wiley.

6 Platnick, N. I. 2013. The World Spider Catalog, Version 13.5. American Museum of Natural History, online at http://research.amnh.org/iz/spiders/catalog. DOI: 10.5531/db.iz.0001.

7 Frye, F.L. (2012). Scorpions. In: *Invertebrate Medicine*, 2e (ed. G.A. Lewbart), 223–234. Wiley.

8 Huckstorf, K., Kosok, G., Seryfarth, E.A., and Wirkner, C.S. (2013). The hemolymph vascular system in *Cupiennius salei* (Araneae: Ctenidae). *Zoologischer Anzeiger* 252 (1): 76–87.

9 Pohlmann, A., Moller, M., Decker, H., and Schreiber, W.G. (2007). MRI of tarantulas: morphological and

perfusion imaging. *Magnetic Resonance Imaging* 25 (1): 129–135.
10 Paul, R.J. (1992). Gas exchange, circulation, and evergy metabolism in arachnids. In: *Physiological Adaptations in Vertebrates* (ed. S.C. Wood, R.E. Weber, A.R. Hargens and R.W. Millard), 169–197. Dekker.
11 Klubmann-Fricke, B.J., Prendini, L., and Wirkner, C.S. (2012). Evolutionary morphology of the hemolymph vascular system in scorpions: a character analysis. *Arthropod Structure & Development* 41 (6): 545–560.
12 Wirkner, C.S. and Prendini, L. (2007). Comparative morphology of the hemolymph vascular system in scorpions – a survey using corrosion casting, microCT, and 3D-reconstruction. *Journal of Morphology* 68 (5): 401–413.
13 Ruppert, E.E., Fox, R.S., and Barnes, R.D. (2004). *Invertebrate Zoology: A Functional Evolutionary Approach*, 7e. Brooks/Cole.
14 Johnson-Delaney, C.J. (1998). Invertebrates. In: *Exotic Companion Medicine Handbook* (ed. C.J. Johnson-Delaney), 1–26. Zoological Education Network.
15 Visigalli, G. (2004). Guide to hemolymph transfusion in giant spiders. *Exotic DVM Magazine* 5 (6): 42–43.
16 Zachariah, T.T. and Mitchell, M.A. (2008). Invertebrate medicine and surgery. In: *Manual of Exotic Pet Practice* (ed. T.N. Tully and M.A. Mitchell), 11–38. Saunders.
17 Stewart, D.M. and Martin, A.W. (1970). Blood and fluid balance of the common tarantula, *Dugesiella hentzi*. *Zeitschrift für Vergleichende Physiologie* 70 (3): 223–246.
18 Dombrowski, D.S., De Voe, R.S., and Lewbart, G.A. (2013). Comparison of isoflurane and carbon dioxide anesthesia of rose-haired tarantulas (*Grammostola rosea*). *Zoo Biology* 32 (1): 101–103.
19 Zachariah, T.T., Mitchell, M.A., Guichard, C.M., and Singh, R.S. (2009). Isoflurane anesthesia of goliath birdeater spiders (*Theraphosa blondi*) and Chilean rose spiders (*Grammostola rosea*). *Journal of Zoo and Wildlife Medicine* 40 (2): 347–349.
20 Zachariah, T.T., Mitchell, M.A., Watson, M.K. et al. (2014). Effects of sevoflurane anesthesia on righting reflex and hemolymph gas analysis variables for Chilean rose tarantulas (*Grammostola rosea*). *American Journal of Veterinary Research* 75 (6): 521–526.
21 Applebee, K.A. and Cooper, J.E. (1989). An anaesthetic or euthanasia chamber for small animals. *Animal Technology* 40 (1): 39–43.
22 Melidone, R. and Mayer, J. (2005). How to build an invertebrate surgery chamber. *Exotic DVM Magazine* 7 (5): 8–10.
23 O'Brien, M. (2008). Invertebrate anesthesia. In: *Anaesthesia of Exotic Pets* (ed. L. Longley), 279–295. Saunders.
24 Escoubas, P. and Rash, L. (2004). Tarantulas: eight-legged pharmacists and combinatorial chemists. *Toxicon* 43 (5): 555–574.
25 Peterson, M.E. (2008). Toxic exotics. *Veterinary Clinics of North America: Exotic Animal Practice* 11 (2): 375–387.
26 McCoy, R.H. and Clapper, D.R. (1979). The oral flora of the South Texas tarantula, *Dugesiella anax* (Araneae: Theraphosidae). *Journal of Medical Entomology* 16 (5): 450–451.
27 Ozsarac, M., Karcioglu, O., Ayrik, C. et al. (2004). Acute coronary ischemia following centipede envenomation: case report and review of literature. *Wilderness & Environmental Medicine* 15 (2): 109–112.
28 Matthews, J.R. and Downer, R.G.H. (1973). Hyperglyceamia induced by anaesthesia in the American cockroach, *Periplaneta americana* L. *Canadian Journal of Zoology* 51 (3): 395–397.
29 Matthews, J.R., Downer, R.G.H., and Morrison, P.E. (1976). Estimation of glucose in the haemolymph of the American cockroach, *Periplaneta americana*. *Comparative Biochemistry and Physiology Part A: Physiology* 53 (2): 165–168.
30 Van Wettere, A. and Lewbart, G.A. (2007). Cytologic diagnosis of diseases of invertebrates. *The Veterinary Clinics of North America. Exotic Animal Practice* 10 (1): 235–254.
31 Ratcliffe, N.A., Mead, G.P., and Renwrantz, L.R. (1986). Insect haemocyte separation – an essential prerequisite to progress in understanding insect cellular immunity. In: *Immunity in Invertebrates* (ed. M. Brehelin), 3–10. Springer-Verlag.
32 Zachariah, T.T., Mitchell, M.A., Guichard, C.M., and Singh, R. (2007). Hemolymph biochemistry reference ranges for wild-caught goliath birdeater spiders (*Theraphosa blondi*) and Chilean rose spiders (*Grammostola rosea*). *Journal of Zoo and Wildlife Medicine* 38 (2): 245–251.
33 Zachariah TT, Mitchell MA, Langan JN, Acierno MJ. Hemolymph osmolality of the Chilean rose spider (Grammostola rosea). Proceedings of the Association of Reptile and Amphibian Veterinarians 17th Annual Conference, 2010, p. 117.
34 Schartau, W. and Leidescher, T. (1983). Composition of the hemolymph of the tarantula *Eurypelma californicum*. *Journal of Comparative Physiology B: Biochemical, Systemic, and Environmental Physiology* 152 (1): 73–77.
35 Nentwig, W. (2012). The species referred to as *Eurypelma californicum* (Theraphosidae) in more than 100 publications is likely to be *Aphonopelma hentzi*. *Journal of Arachnology* 40 (1): 128–130.
36 Punzo, F. (1989). Composition of the hemolymph of mygalomorph spiders (Orthognatha). *Comparative Biochemistry and Physiology. Part A, Physiology* 93 (4): 757–760.
37 Hamilton, C.A., Hendrixson, B.E., and Bond, J.E. (2016). Taxonomic revision of the tarantula genus

Aphonopelma Pocock, 1901 (Araneae, Mygalomorphae, Theraphosidae) within the United States. *ZooKeys* 560: 1–340. https://doi.org/10.3897/zookeys.560.6264.

38 Paul, R.J., Pfeffer-Seidl, A., Efinger, R. et al. (1994). Gas transport in the hemolymph of arachnids. II. Carbon dioxide transport and acid-base balance. *Journal of Experimental Biology* 188 (1): 47–63.

39 Wellehan J, De Voe R. Clinical aspects of terrestrial invertebrates. Proceedings of the invertebrate medicine wet lab, American Association of Zoo Veterinarians 39th Annual Conference, 2007.

40 Bowerman, R.F. (1976). Ion concentrations and pH of the hemolymph of the scorpions *Hadrurus arizonensis* and *Paruroctonus mesaensis*. *Comparative Biochemistry and Physiology Part A: Physiology* 54 (3): 331–333.

41 Kimura, Y., Terakawa, S., Hsu, K., and Ji, Y.-H. (1988). Ionic composition of the haemolymph of a Chinese scorpion, *Buthus martensi*. *Comparative Biochemistry and Physiology Part A: Physiology* 91 (2): 323–325.

42 Padmanabhanaidu, B. (1962). Ionic composition of the blood of scorpion. I. Some organic and inorganic constituents of the blood. *Current Science* 31 (1): 21.

43 Padmanabhanaidu, B. (1966). Ionic composition of the blood and the blood volume of the scorpion, *Heterometrus fulvipes*. *Comparative Biochemistry and Physiology* 17 (1): 157–166.

44 Woodring, J.P. (1974). Effects of rapid and slow dehydration on the hemolymph osmolarity and Na^+-K^+ concentration in the millipede *Pachydesmus crassicutis*. *Comparative Biochemistry and Physiology Part A: Physiology* 49 (1): 115–119.

45 Marcus, E.R., Baransky, M., de Kooker, G.M., and Know, C.M. (1987). Haemolymph composition of the Kalahari millipede, *Triaenostreptus triodus* (Attems). *Comparative Biochemistry and Physiology Part A: Physiology* 87 (3): 603–606.

46 Bedford, J.J. and Leader, J.P. (1975). The composition of the haemolymph of the New Zealand centipede, *Cormocephalus rubriceps* (Newport). *Comparative Biochemistry and Physiology Part A: Physiology* 50 (3): 561–564.

47 Hilliard, S.D. and Butz, A. (1969). Daily fluctuations in the concentrations of total sugar and uric acid in the hemolymph of *Periplaneta americana*. *Annals of the Entomological Society of America* 62 (1): 71–74.

48 Weidler, D.J. and Sieck, G.C. (1977). A study of ion binding in the hemolymph of *Periplaneta americana*. *Comparative Biochemistry and Physiology Part A: Physiology* 56 (1): 11–14.

49 Loewe, R. and de Eggert, H.B. (1979). Blood gas analysis and acid-base status in the hemolymph of a spider (*Eurypelma californicum*) – influence of temperature. *Journal of Comparative Physiology* 134 (4): 331–338.

50 Xylander, W.E.R. (2009). Hemocytes in Myriapoda (Arthropoda): a review. *Invertebrate Survival Journal* 6 (2): 114–124.

51 Jones, C.J. (1962). Current concepts concerning insect hemocytes. *American Zoologist* 2 (2): 209–246.

52 Price, C.D. and Ratcliffe, N.A. (1974). A reappraisal of insect haemocyte classification by the examination of blood from fifteen insect orders. *Zeitschrift für Zellforschung und Mikroskopische Anatomie* 147 (4): 537–549.

53 Soares, T., Cavalcanti, M.G.S., Ferreira, F.R.B. et al. (2013). Ultrastructural characterization of the hemocytes of *Lasiodora* sp. (Koch, 1850) (Araneae: Theraphosidae). *Micron* 48: 11–16.

54 Hilken, G., Brockmann, C., and Nevermann, L. (2003). Hemocytes of the centipede *Scutigera coleoptrata* (Chilopoda, Notostigmophora) with notes on their interactions with the tracheae. *Journal of Morphology* 257 (2): 181–189.

55 Nevermann, L., Xylander, W.E.R., and Seifert, G. (1991). The hemocytes of the centipede *Lithobius forficatus* (Chilopoda, Lithobiomorpha). *Zoomorphology* 110 (6): 317–327.

56 Patil, A.E. and Shah, U.H. (2011). Types of hemocytes in scorpion *Mesobuthus tamulus tamulus*. *The Bioscan* 6 (4): 597–599.

57 Patil, A.E. and Shah, U.H. (2012). Hemocytes in scorpion – *Heterometrus xanthopus*. *The Bioscan* 7 (1): 139–141.

58 Patil, A.E. and Shah, U.H. (2012). Ultrastructural studies of hemocytes in scorpion, *Heterometrus xanthopus*. *The Bioscan* 7: 491–493.

59 Rajulu, G.S. (1971). A study of haemocytes in a centipede *Scolopendra morsitans* (Chilopoda: Myriapoda). *Cytologia* 36 (3): 515–521.

60 Ravindranath, M.H. (1973). The hemocytes of a millipede, *Thyropygus poseidon*. *Journal of Morphology* 141 (3): 257–268.

61 Ravindranath, M.H. (1974). The hemocytes of a scorpion *Palamnaeus swammerdami*. *Journal of Morphology* 144 (1): 1–9.

62 Sherman, R.G. (1973). Ultrastructurally different hemocytes in a spider. *Canadian Journal of Zoology* 51 (11): 1155–1159.

63 Sherman, R.G. (1981). Chelicerates. In: *Invertebrate Blood Cells*, vol. 2 (ed. N.A. Ratcliffe and A.F. Rowley), 355–384. Academic Press.

64 Gillespie, J.P., Kanost, M.R., and Trenczek, T. (1997). Biological mediators of insect immunity. *Annual Review of Entomology* 42: 611–643.

65 Lavine, M.D. and Strand, M.R. (2002). Insect hemocytes and their role in immunity. *Insect Biochemistry and Molecular Biology* 32 (10): 1295–1309.

66 Kuhn-Nentwig, L. and Nentwig, W. (2013). The immune system of spiders. In: *Spider Ecophysiology* (ed. W. Nentwig), 81–91. Springer-Verlag.

67 Nevermann, L., Kaiser, H.E., and Xylander, W.E.R. (1996). Microbial induced hemocytic immune reactions in chilopods. *In Vivo* 10 (2): 161–168.

68 Strand, M.R. (2008). The insect cellular immune response. *Insect Science* 15 (1): 1–14.

69 Foelix, R.F. (2011). *Biology of Spiders*, 3e. Oxford University Press.

70 Fukuzawa, A.H., Vellutini, B.C., Lorenzini, D.M. et al. (2008). The role of hemocytes in the immunity of the spider *Acanthoscurria gomesiana*. *Developmental & Comparative Immunology* 32 (6): 716–725.

71 Browning, H.C. (1942). The integument and moult cycle of *Tegenaria atrica* (Araneae). *Proceedings of the Royal Society of London B: Biological Sciences* 131 (862): 65–86.

72 Deevey, G.B. (1941). The blood cells of the Haitian tarantula and their relation to the moulting cycle. *Journal of Morphology* 68 (3): 457–491.

73 Lorenzini, D.M., Silva, P.I., Fogaca, A.C. et al. (2003). Acanthoscurrin: a novel glycine-rich antimicrobial peptide constitutively expressed in the hemocytes of the spider *Acanthoscurria gomesiana*. *Developmental & Comparative Immunology* 27 (9): 781–791.

74 Silva, P.I., Daffre, S., and Bulet, P. (2000). Isolation and characterization of gomesin, an 18-residue cysteine-rich defense peptide from the spider *Acanthoscurria gomesiana* hemocytes with sequence similarities to horseshoe crab antimicrobial peptides of the tachyplesin family. *Journal of Biological Chemistry* 275 (43): 33464–33470.

75 Farley, R.D. (1984). The ultrastructure of hemocytopoietic organs in the desert scorpion, *Paruroctonus*. *Tissue and Cell* 16 (4): 577–588.

76 Xylander WER. Immune defense reactions of Myriapoda – a brief presentation of recent results. Proceedings of the 8th International Congress of Myriapodology, 1992, pp. 101–110.

77 Ravindranath, M.H. (1974). Changes in the population of circulating hemocytes during molt cycle phases of the millipede, *Thyrpygus poseidon*. *Physiological Zoology* 47 (4): 252–260.

78 Lackie, A.M. (1988). Haemocyte behavior. In: *Advances in Insect Phsyiology*, vol. 21 (ed. P. Evans and V.B. Wigglesworth), 85–178. Academic Press.

79 Wittig, G. (1962). The pathology of insect blood cells: a review. *American Zoologist* 2 (2): 257–273.

80 Kulshrestha, V. and Pathak, S.C. (1997). Aspergillosis in German cockroach *Blatella germanica* (L.) (Blattoidea: Blattellidae). *Mycopathology* 139 (2): 75–78.

81 Ryan, M. and Nicholas, W.L. (1972). The reaction of the cockroach *Periplaneta americana* to the injection of foreign particulate material. *Journal of Invertebrate Pathology* 19 (3): 299–307.

82 Anderson, R.S., Homes, B., and Good, R.A. (1973). *In vitro* bactericidal capacity of *Blaberus craniifer* hemocytes. *Journal of Invertebrate Pathology* 22 (1): 127–135.

83 Trabalon, M. and Blais, C. (2012). Juvenile development, ecdysteroids and hemolymph level of metabolites in the spider *Brachypelma albopilosum* (Theraphosidae). *Journal of Experimental Zoology* 317 (4): 236–247.

84 Alumont, E., Lensky, Y., and Holstein, P. (1969). Sugars and trehalase in the reproductive organs and hemolymph of the queen and drone honey bees (*Apis mellifica* L. var. *ligustica* spin.). *Comparative Biochemistry and Physiology* 28 (3): 1419–1425.

85 Arslan, A., Standifer, L.N., and Don, H. (1986). Carbohydrates in honey bee hemolymph. *Comparative Biochemistry and Physiology Part B: Comparative Biochemistry* 84 (3): 363–367.

86 Woodring, J., Boulden, M., Das, S., and Gade, G. (1993). Studies on blood sugar homeostasis in the honeybee (*Apis mellifera*, L.). *Journal of Insect Physiology* 39 (1): 89–97.

87 Blatt, J. and Roces, F. (2001). Haemolymph sugar levels in foraging honeybees (*Apis mellifera carnica*): dependence on metabolic rate and *in vivo* measurement of maximal rates of trehalose synthesis. *Journal of Experimental Biology* 204 (15): 2709–2716.

88 Mohssine, E.H., Bounias, M., and Counuet, J.M. (1990). Lunar phase influence on the glycemia of worker honeybees. *Chronobiology* 17 (3): 201–207.

89 Mayack, C. and Naug, D. (2010). Parasitic infection leads to decline in hemolymph sugar levels in honeybee foragers. *Journal of Insect Physiology* 56 (11): 1572–1575.

90 Aliferis, K.A., Copley, T., and Jabaji, S. (2012). Gas chromatography-mass spectrometry metabolite profiling of worker honey bee (*Apis mellifera* L.) hemolymph for the study of *Nosema ceranae* infection. *Journal of Insect Physiology* 58 (10): 1349–1359.

91 Bowen-Walker, P.L. and Gunn, A. (2001). The effect of the ectoparasitic mite, *Varroa destructor* on adult worker honeybee (*Apis mellifera*) emergence weights, water, protein, carbohydrate, and lipid levels. *Entomologia Experimentalis et Applicata* 101 (3): 207–217.

92 Arrese, E.L. and Soulages, J.L. (2010). Insect fat body: energy, metabolism, and regulation. *Annual Review of Entomology* 55: 207–225.

93 Bennett, D.S. (1971). Nitrogen excretion in the diplopod *Cylindroiulus londinensis*. *Comparative Biochemistry and Physiology Part A: Physiology* 39 (4): 611–624.

94 Lewis, J.G.E. (1981). *The Biology of Centipedes*. Cambridge University Press.

95 Mullins, D.E. (2013). Chemistry and physiology of the hemolymph. In: *Comprehensive Insect Physiology, Biochemistry and Pharmacology, Volume 3: Integument, Respiration and Circulation* (ed. G.A. Kerkut and L.I. Gilbert), 355–400. Pergamon Press.

96 Butt, A.G. and Taylor, H.H. (1991). The function of spider coxal organs: effects of feeding and salt-loading on *Porrhothele antipodiana* (Mygalomorpha: Dipluridae). *Journal of Experimental Biology* 158 (1): 439–461.

97 Butt, A.G. and Taylor, H.H. (1995). Regulatory responses of the coxal organs and the anal excretory system to dehydration and feeding in the spider *Porrhothele antipodiana* (Mygalomorpha: Dipluridae). *Journal of Experimental Biology* 198 (5): 1137–1149.

98 Riddle, W.A. (1985). Hemolymph osmoregulation in several myriapods and arachnids. *Comparative Biochemistry and Physiology Part A: Physiology* 80 (3): 313–323.

99 Gefen, E. (2008). Sexual dimorphism in desiccation responses of the sand scorpion *Smeringurus mesaensis* (Vaejovidae). *Journal of Insect Physiology* 54 (5): 798–805.

100 Gefen, E. and Ar, A. (2004). Comparative water relations of four species of scorpions in Israel: evidence for phylogenetic differences. *Journal of Experimental Biology* 207 (6): 1017–1025.

101 Gefen, E. and Ar, A. (2005). The effect of desiccation on water management and compartmentalisation in scorpions: the hepatopancreas as a water reservoir. *Journal of Experimental Biology* 208 (10): 1887–1894.

102 Punzo, F. (1991). The effects of temperature and moisture on survival capacity, cuticular permeability, hemolymph osmoregulation and metabolism in the scorpion, *Centruroides hentzi* (banks) (Scorpiones, Buthidae). *Comparative Biochemistry and Physiology Part A: Physiology* 100 (4): 833–837.

103 Riddle, W.A., Crawford, C.S., and Zeitone, A.M. (1976). Patterns of hemolymph osmoregulation in three desert arthropods. *Journal of Comparative Physiology* 112 (3): 295–305.

104 Robertson, H.G., Nicolson, S.W., and Louw, G.N. (1982). Osmoregulation and temperature effects on water loss and oxygen consumption in two species of African scorpion. *Comparative Biochemistry and Physiology Part A: Physiology* 71 (4): 605–609.

105 Warburg, M.R., Goldenberg, S., and Ben-Horin, A. (1980). Thermal effect on evaporative water loss and haemolymph osmolarity in scorpions at low and high humidities. *Comparative Biochemistry and Physiology Part A: Physiology* 67 (1): 47–57.

106 Pugach, S. and Crawford, C.S. (1978). Seasonal changes in hemolymph amino acids, proteins, and inorganic ions of a desert millipede *Orthoporus ornatus* (Girard) (Diplopda: Spirostreptidae). *Canadian Journal of Zoology* 56 (6): 1460–1465.

107 Sutcliffe, D.W. (1963). The chemical composition of haemolymph in insects and some other arthropods, in relation to their phylogeny. *Comparative Biochemistry and Physiology* 9 (2): 121–135.

108 Xylander, W.E.R. (2009). Physico-chemical properties of haemolymph of Chilopoda and Diplopoda (Myriapoda, Arthropoda): protein content, pH, osmolarity. *Soil Organisms* 81 (3): 431–439.

109 Edney, E.B. (1968). The effect of water loss on the haemolymph of *Arenivaga* sp. and *Periplaneta americana*. *Comparative Biochemistry and Physiology* 25 (1): 149–158.

110 Laird, T.B. and Winston, P.W. (1975). Water and osmotic pressure regulation in the cockroach, *Leucophaea maderae*. *Journal of Insect Physiology* 21 (5): 1055–1060.

111 Wall, B.J. (1970). Effects of dehydration and rehydration on *Periplaneta americana*. *Journal of Insect Physiology* 16 (6): 1027–1042.

112 Hyatt, A.D. and Marshall, A.T. (1977). Sequestration of haemolymph sodium and potassium by fat body in the water-stressed cockroach *Periplaneta americana*. *Journal of Insect Physiology* 23 (11): 1437–1441.

113 Laird, T.B., Winston, P.W., and Braukman, M. (1972). Water storage in the cockroach *Leucophaea maderae* F. *Naturwissenschaften* 59 (11): 515–516.

114 Tillinghast, E.K. and Townley, M.A. (2008). Free amino acids in spider hemolymph. *Comparative Biochemistry and Physiology Part B: Biochemistry and Molecular Biology* 151 (3): 286–295.

115 Micheu, S., Crailsheim, K., and Leonhard, B. (2000). Importance of proline and other amino acids during honeybee flight. *Amino Acids* 18 (2): 157–175.

116 Woodring, J.P. and Blakeney, E.W. (1980). The role of free amino acids in osmoregulation of cricket blood (*Acheta domesticus*). *Journal of Insect Physiology* 26 (9): 613–618.

117 Kumar, R. (1976). Changes in the free amino acid pattern of haemolymph of the common Indian scorpion *Palamnaeus bengalensis* during moulting. *Experientia* 32 (7): 880–881.

118 Nair, V.S.K. and Prabhu, V.K.K. (1971). On the free amino acids in the haemolymph of a millipede. *Comparative Biochemistry and Physiology Part B: Comparative Biochemistry* 38 (1): 1–4.

119 Rajulu, G.S. (1970). A comparative study of the free amino acids in the haemolymph of a millipede, *Spirostreptus asthenes*, and a centipede *Ethmostigmus spinosus* (Myriapoda). *Comparative Biochemistry and Physiology* 37 (3): 339–344.

120 Cremonez, T.M., De Jong, D., and Bitondi, M.M.G. (1998). Quantification of hemolymph proteins as a fast method for testing protein diets for honey bees (hymenoptera: Apidae). *Journal of Economic Entomology* 91 (6): 1284–1289.

121 Amdam, G.V., Hartfelder, K., Norberg, K. et al. (2004). Altered physiology in worker honey bees (hymenoptera: Apidae) infested with the mite *Varroa destructor* (Acari: Varroidae): a factor in colony loss during overwintering? *Journal of Economic Entomology* 97 (3): 741–747.

122 Atmowidjojo, A.H., Erickson, E.H., Wheeler, D.E., and Cohen, A.C. (1999). Regulation of hemolymph osmolality in feral and domestic honeybees, *Apis mellifera* L. (hymenoptera: Apidae). *Comparative*

Biochemistry and Physiology Part A: Molecular & Integrative Physiology 122 (2): 227–233.
123 Florkin, M. and Jeuniaux, C. (1974). Hemolymph: composition. In: *The Physiology of Insecta*, 2e, vol. 5 (ed. M. Rockstein), 255–307. Academic Press.
124 Hrassnigg, N., Leonhard, B., and Crailsheim, K. (2003). Free amino acids in the haemolymph of honey bee queens (*Apis mellifera* L.). *Amino Acids* 24 (1–2): 205–121.
125 Irving, S.N., Wilson, R.G., and Osborne, M.P. (1979). Studies on L-glutamate in insect haemolymph. III. Amino acid analysis of the haemolymph of various arthropods. *Physiological Entomology* 4 (3): 231–240.
126 Sowa, S.M. and Keeley, L.L. (1996). Free amino acids in the hemolymph of the cockroach, *Blaberus discoidalis. Comparative Biochemistry and Physiology Part A: Physiology* 113 (2): 131–134.
127 Stevens, T.M. (1961). Free amino acids in the hemolymph of the American cockroach, *Periplaneta americana* L. *Comparative Biochemistry and Physiology* 3 (4): 304–309.
128 Holden, J.S. (1973). Free amino acid levels in the cockroach, *Periplaneta americana. The Journal of Physiology* 232 (2): 61P–62P.
129 Reichle, D.E., Shanks, M.H., and Crossley, D.A. (1969). Calcium, potassium, and sodium content of forest floor arthropods. *Annals of the Entomological Society of America* 62 (1): 57–62.
130 Zachariah, T.T. and Mitchell, M.A. (2009). Vitamin D_3 in the hemolymph of goliath birdeater spiders (*Theraphosa blondi*). *Journal of Zoo and Wildlife Medicine* 40 (2): 344–346.
131 Finke, M.D. (2002). Complete nutrient composition of commercially raised invertebrates used as food for insectivores. *Zoo Biology* 21 (3): 269–285.
132 Oonincx, D.G. and Dierenfeld, E.S. (2012). An investigation into the chemical composition of alternative invertebrate prey. *Zoo Biology* 31 (1): 40–54.
133 Jaenicke, E., Decker, H., Gebauer, W. et al. (1999). Identification, structure, and properties of hemocyanins from diplopod Myriapoda. *Journal of Biological Chemistry* 274 (41): 29071–29074.
134 Paul, R.J., Bihlmayer, S., Colmorgen, M., and Zahler, S. (1994). The open circulatory system of spiders (*Eurypelma californicum, Pholcus phalangoides*): a survey of functional morphology and physiology. *Physiological Zoology* 67 (6): 1360–1382.
135 Dejours, P. and Ar, A. (1991). Temperature and starvation affect the hemolymph acid-base balance of the xeric yellow scorpion, *Leiurus quinquestriatus. Journal of Comparative Physiology B* 161 (4): 407–412.

23

Laboratory Diagnostics for Birds

Shane Raidal BVSc (Syd), PhD (Syd), FACVSc (Avian Health), DECZM (Wildlife Health)

Department of Veterinary Pathobiology, School of Animal & Veterinary Sciences, Charles Sturt University, Wagga Wagga, New South Wales, Australia

Introduction

In recent years, there has been a massive expansion in expertise in the fields of Avian and Exotic Medicine with many texts now available on these subjects, some in multiple editions, and a wide range of journals dedicated to the topic. Specialist avian and exotic diagnostic laboratories now exist to service the precise needs of well-informed avian practitioners. To the classically trained veterinary diagnostician, the provision of avian-specific laboratory expertise can be daunting when one considers that at more than 9000 extant bird species, the number of potentially unique avian patients is approximately twice that of mammals. Birds have a massive range of morphologic, physiologic, and functional adaptations as well as variation in body mass and athletic capacity. Comparatively very little is known about the nuances of individual species, let alone subtle differences that might be present in animals of differing age, health status, or reproductive status [1–3]. Furthermore, in ill health, the vast majority of birds express only subtle and nonspecific clinical signs, particularly in the early stages of a disease process. Thus, laboratory testing plays a very important role in avian health assessment and should focus on detecting and characterizing organ system derangement and the pathophysiological mechanisms, as well as helping detect specific etiologies. General tests such as hematology and plasma protein electrophoresis are invaluable for assessing both innate immune responses and alterations in the erythron, which can provide information on chronicity and severity of disease as well as providing baseline prognostic indications of recovery.

Hematology

As in other animals, analysis of blood samples is a cornerstone of avian diagnostics, and interpretation of results must consider the high metabolic rate of birds and the rapid turnover of erythrocytes. Birds are capable of responding rapidly to alterations in blood volume by redistributing fluids, recruiting immature erythrocytes, and synthesizing total plasma protein at a rate twice that of mammals [4–6]. Clinicopathologic derangements such as anemia and hypoproteinemia can occur quickly, particularly when disease processes target the hematopoietic system and liver. The hematologic response to disease depends on its inciting cause, the magnitude and duration of the disease process, the bird's metabolism, and the bird's ability to respond to a particular challenge [7, 8]. Accordingly, interpretation of results is most helpful when the characteristics of a particular species, both in health and in response to disease, are established. These basic facts are not known for the majority of avian species, and care should be taken when extrapolating knowledge obtained from sibling or distantly related species. Sometimes, the best comparison can be made with data collected from the same animal during times of normality (annual health examinations provide opportunities to collect such information). Serial sampling is also valuable for assessing response to therapy and prognosis in individual patients.

Collection of a high-quality venous blood sample, particularly from the smallest birds, can be intimidating for the inexperienced clinician. However, even from the smallest birds, blood can be collected from superficial veins that can be readily visualized through thin avian skin, and the most appropriate for venipuncture will depend on the size and anatomy of the species and the required sample volume. More species-specific detailed information on blood collection can be found elsewhere [8]. Nevertheless, the size and gauge of the needle as well as the size and volume of the syringe should be appropriate for the vessel and the volume of blood to be collected, although blood can be collected directly into hematocrit tubes. Needles must be removed from syringes before blood is expelled into blood collection tubes and with few notable exceptions, the preferred anticoagulant for

Exotic Animal Laboratory Diagnosis, First Edition. Edited by J. Jill Heatley and Karen E. Russell.

routine assessment of avian blood cell morphology is ethylenediaminetetraacetic acid (EDTA). However, EDTA-induced hemolysis reliably destroys blood samples from corvids and megapodes and has been reported in a number of other species [9]. In those birds that exhibit such hemolysis, heparin can be used but is not otherwise recommended as a routine anticoagulant for avian blood because it results in extensive clumping of all cell types and inaccurate cell counts [9, 10]. Citrate should be avoided as it may result in increased cell lysis, and whole blood samples in lithium heparin or EDTA should be stored at 4 °C and evaluated within 12 h for best results [11].

Modern hematology analyzers that have revolutionized the rapid and detailed analysis of mammalian blood samples are generally unreliable for avian blood samples, mainly because of their nucleated erythrocytes and thrombocytes [12, 13]. Accordingly, most diagnostic laboratories perform manual cell counts using a variety of techniques [7–9].

Arterial blood samples are rarely required from clinical patients but can be important in research settings when blood gases are to be measured [14]. Arterial blood samples are best analyzed immediately. In anesthetized medium-sized bird species, single arterial samples can be obtained from the carotid artery, which runs either as a paired or as a single fused vessel embedded among the hypaxial muscles of the neck. Occasionally, the brachial artery can be accessed accidentally during venous collection at this site, or the brachial artery can be cannulated in larger birds [15–17].

Plasma and Serum Analyses

When used in conjunction with other clinical and laboratory information, plasma biochemistries are useful for detecting diseases of the alimentary, hepatic, renal, respiratory, cardiovascular, hematopoietic, endocrine, or immune systems. While in-house and point-of-care analyzers can provide rapid results, few of these analyzers are completely reliable without routine maintenance and quality control, and cautious practitioners should be aware of their deficiencies [18, 19]; the dilution of small volumes of plasma to extend the number of tests that can be done is not recommended [20]. Hemolyzed samples caused by improper collection or storage of blood samples can significantly interfere with many hematologic analyses [21, 22].

Compared to the widespread use of bilirubin in mammalian clinical pathology, the lack of a simple enzymatic technique to detect and quantify plasma biliverdin is probably the single most important deficit in diagnostic capacity for assessing hepatic function in birds. Bilirubin assays provide no useful clinical information, and the very low bilirubin concentrations sometimes detected in avian plasma are invariably caused by bacterial enzymatic reduction of biliverdin in the intestine. Biliverdinaemia can occur with increased turnover of red-blood cells such as in hemolytic anemia or with liver disease and unlike unconjugated bilirubin. Water-soluble biliverdin is relatively non-toxic and is readily excreted in bile and urine, where it can cause a visible biliverdinuria. Routine urinalyses and dipstick tests do not detect biliverdin.

The physiological enterohepatic cycling of serum bile acids provides a clinically useful assessment of liver function, and elevations of serum bile acids can be observed with liver failure or cholestasis. However, these acids should be measured after a set period of fasting to minimize the effects of physiological postprandial elevations in normal birds [19, 20, 23–25]. Elevated bile acid levels had the highest association with confirmed hepatic disease, followed by high concentrations of alpha2-globulins, aspartate aminotransferase (AST), lactate dehydrogenase (LDH), and alpha1-globulins [26]. However, compared to dye or galactose clearance assays, measurement of serum bile acid concentration is an insensitive measure of hepatic function [27]. Measurement of plasma alanine aminotransferase (ALT) and AST can provide useful clinical information, but these are cytosolic enzymes with wide tissue distributions including liver, muscle, and kidney. ALT has a longer half-life than AST, and so will remain elevated in plasma for longer after tissue insult [28–31]. When used in conjunction with plasma creatinine kinase (CK) concentrations, AST can provide some assessment of hepatic disease, but the shorter half-life of CK can result in relative elevations in AST or ALT after a single muscle insult, so this empirical ratio should not be used as a sole screening test to evaluate hepatocellular injury [26]. Severe hepatocellular damage must occur to release mitochondrially bound glutamyl dehydrogenase (GLDH) into the plasma, where it has a short half-life, and elevations are thus of limited clinical value [30, 32].

Plasma alkaline phosphatase (ALP) concentrations reflect both skeletal bone and biliary system activity in mammals, but have little value in diagnosis of hepatocellular dysfunction in birds as it is primarily concentrated in the kidney and is rarely elevated with hepatic disease. As in mammals, gamma-glutamyltransferase (GGT) appears to be a relatively specific induced enzyme of the biliary tract that can be used to assess cholestasis [33–36].

Iron Storage Disease

Along with hepatic biopsy and histopathology, additional serum parameters relating to iron metabolism may be used to diagnose iron storage disease in susceptible avian species [37, 38]. These include total iron concentration, total iron-binding capacity and the derived transferrin saturation, ferritin, ceruloplasmin, and haptoglobin concentrations [30, 39]. The relatively recent discovery of hepcidin, a protein principally produced in hepatocytes, as a key regulator of iron absorption and release is likely to provide an improved understanding of the pathogenesis of iron storage disease in birds [40–45]. Hepcidin is released rapidly into the circulation in response to increased serum iron and to the presence of inflammatory cytokine IL-6; thus, chronic inflammation, through constant stimulation of hepcidin release, contributes to anemia of chronic disease [46, 47]. Hepcidin inhibits the function of ferroportin molecules on the surface of enterocytes, macrophages, and hepatocytes, leading to decreased intestinal iron absorption and release from reticuloendothelial stores. Mammals with hemochromatosis all have abnormally decreased hepcidin, or an abnormal lack of hepcidin response to elevated serum iron [48, 49]. Hepcidin is highly conserved in vertebrates and has direct antimicrobial activity, a feature that may provide insights into its original evolutionary function [50, 51], and recently developed assays capable of measuring circulating plasma hepcidin in a range of vertebrates should be suitable for avian samples [52].

Avian carbohydrate metabolism and blood glucose are principally controlled by glucagon, particularly in granivorous birds with a tendency toward a low insulin:glucose molar ratio (I : G) regardless of the absolute concentrations of insulin and glucose [53–57]. With stress such as handling and restraint, they readily exhibit significant hyperglycemia (>30 mmol/l) [58] which can exceed the renal threshold for glucose; thus, birds can have mild glu cosuria with stress hypoglycemia [57]. Serum glucose concentrations >40 mmol/l have been considered as diagnostic for diabetes mellitus [36, 59, 60] with some birds also having ketonuria but rarely ketosis. Beta hydroxybutyrate (BOHB), a ketone commonly used to assess diabetes mellitus and lipid catabolism in mammals, is less reliable in birds. While elevated serum BOHB may occur in birds that are fasting [53, 54, 61] and/or with the exertion effects of migration, it is not a reliable indicator of diabetes mellitus. This may be caused by the lipid-preserving effects of adequate or elevated absolute insulin concentrations in the face of hyperglucagonemia.

The Avian Renal System and Uric Acid

Birds are predominantly uricotelic, and clinicopathologic assessments of the renal system must consider that the kidneys, the intestinal tract, the salt glands, the skin, and the respiratory tract as well as the energy status might all contribute to avian osmoregulation and nitrogenous waste excretion [62, 63]. Dietary considerations are also important [64], with the enhanced protein catabolism of carnivorous birds causing postprandial elevations and otherwise higher reference blood uric acid ranges in raptors and penguins [23, 39] Postrenal modification of urine is a major reason why urinalysis has limited value in assessing renal concentration ability in avian patients [65]. While uric acid is synthesized almost entirely in the liver, it is actively secreted into the lumen by tubular renal epithelial cells, and the glomerular filtration rate (GFR) of reptilian type nephrons (RTNs) can be dramatically reduced under the stimulation of arginine vasotocin in response to dehydration, thus shutting off nephrons with the least capacity to concentrate urine. Since all collecting ducts from both reptilian and mammalian-type nephrons pass through the medullary cones, urine can be concentrated to some extent, regardless of which nephron it originated from, at the risk of intratubular uric acid precipitation. In otherwise normal birds, dehydration usually does not notably elevate blood uric acid concentrations until GFR decreases to the point that uric acid cannot be flushed through the nephron.

Serology

Serological tests rely on the demonstration of antigen-specific antibody, and while most of the currently available serodiagnostic capability is geared toward tests for infectious diseases [66–73], future tests for antibodies against environmental allergens may become important in the diagnostic work-up of hypersensitivities. Antibody titers must be interpreted along with the history, clinical signs, and the known pathogenesis and epidemiology of the disease being assessed. Serological assays are best used alongside antigen- and DNA-based diagnostic assays, especially in flock diagnosis, and in some circumstances, serology is much more valuable than high-sensitivity tests such as the polymerase chain reaction (PCR) [74, 75]. This is particularly true when there is sufficient irrelevant genetic variation to produce variable PCR results. Also, an endemically infected flock typically might have a higher seroprevalence than antigen or DNA excretion prevalence, particularly when the infectious agent is one that is excreted only for a short period, intermittently, or at low concentrations post infection. For example, if seropositivity is associated with freedom from disease [71] or, alternatively, with continuing persistent infection, then those animals can be either retained or separated, respectively.

Serology of *beak and feather disease virus* (BFDV) infection can be done by hemagglutination inhibition (HI), ELISA, or blocking-ELISA (bELISA) and is useful for detecting BFDV-infected flocks or seroconversion in individual birds [71, 76]. A high-plasma HI antibody titer (>1:320) in an adult bird is a good indicator that it does not have chronic PBFD, and PCR-negative birds are 12 times more likely to have antibody than PCR-positive birds [71]. Nestlings with incubating infection or acute disease may have low and declining antibody titers. The HI test can be done on serum, plasma, or whole blood collected onto filter paper [77].

Antigen Tests

Pathogen-specific antigens released into the blood or excreted in feces, feathers, and urine can be detected using a range of laboratory and or patient-side test kits [65, 78–81], and the potential for cross-reactions with environmental or contaminating antigens needs to be considered particularly for bacterial and fungal agents in fecal samples or oropharyngeal secretions. Problems with low sensitivity such as for galactomannan released from invasive *Aspergillus* spp. which can be detected in plasma or serum by ELISA [82] can be surmounted if the results are compared with ancillary tests.

PCR and DNA-based Diagnostic Tests

The use of PCR is becoming increasingly common in avian diagnostics for sex determination and pathogen detection. The technique is highly sensitive and is likely to remain one of the most powerful and reliable diagnostic methods available, provided that clinicians and laboratories understand what information is being provided by an individual PCR test result. Numerous risks for error exist in sample collection, handling, and processing as well as in the technique itself [83]. Most of these relate to the highly sensitive nature of the procedure, since PCR massively amplifies DNA, thus compounding the effects of contamination which can occur both at sample collection and within the laboratory. Laboratories should have dedicated rooms with controlled air and traffic flow as well as stringent hygiene control to minimize this possibility. Other steps such as co-amplification of housekeeping genes, culture, or parallel antigen testing using immunologic methods can be valuable controls to validate test results [84].

The term PCR is often used to summarize a wide range of laboratory techniques. The process for detecting RNA transcripts such as viral or host mRNA expression typically involves an initial step called reverse transcription in which the enzyme reverse transcriptase converts the target RNA molecule in the template to DNA, which the DNA polymerase can then copy. (The abbreviation RT-PCR is often used for reverse-transcription PCR to detect RNA as well as for real-time PCR, which are two different laboratory procedures. Confusingly, combinations of the two also exist.) [85] The advent of real-time PCR machines has greatly enhanced the analyses that can be done on a single sample, including better quantification assessment of pathogen load as well as automated detection of subtle gene variations using techniques such as high-resolution melt analysis which relies on the ability of the fluorescently labeled probe used in the test to bind to target amplicons [86–89].

Not all PCR tests are the same or comparable between laboratories, even when identical primer sequences and buffer optimization are used [90]. Different laboratories can produce discrepant results because they may use dissimilar template extraction procedures or primer annealing and extension conditions or cycles. Amplicons are then often used for downstream applications such as DNA sequencing or used as a template for a further amplification cycle such as a nested PCR, a technique that can detect target sequences in samples heavily contaminated with inhibitory material such as feces or large amounts of interfering genes [91]. Often the visualization of an amplicon of expected size in an agarose gel is all that is required for a positive PCR test result, and on rare occasions, other genes can be amplified nonspecifically to give a false positive result. Sometimes, the identity of an organism or gene sequence cannot be confirmed simply by the size of an amplicon, and further steps such as DNA sequencing are needed to make the diagnosis; this can also identify genetic variants of pathogens in disease outbreaks or for DNA-fingerprinting of an individual animal to determine paternity or genetic relatedness [92]. The latter can be an extremely important research tool for managing endangered species but is becoming more frequently requested for insurance and proof of ownership.

When multiple gene sequences of interest or of different pathogens are to be detected in a single sample type, laboratories may use a multiplex PCR to amplify all target sequences in the same reaction and to minimize assay time and consumables [93–95]. However, this may result in a decrease in the limits of detection for each individual target sequence.

Specificity and Sensitivity of PCR Tests

The elegant simplicity of PCR and its presumed high sensitivity is something of a fable. PCR tests have a *theoretical* ability to amplify a single copy of a gene when conditions are perfect and inhibiting factors are absent, but the *limits of detection* of a specific test must not be confused with the *sensitivity* of that test. Hemagglutination Assay (HA)testing for beak and feather disease virus (BFDV) has a higher limit of detection than PCR, but in routine testing PCR is more sensitive [71]. Sensitivity for the same assay can vary depending on the specific question being asked. Is the animal infected? Or, does it have disease? Or, is it recovering from infection? Where primers are highly specific to a site only present in the pathogen of interest, the resulting amplicon is proof that the pathogen is present in the sample but not necessarily that it is replicating. Again, the specificity of an individual PCR test might also depend greatly on the nature of the primers and the amplification conditions. For example, a generic trichomonad primer set is often used erroneously to detect the presence of *Trichomonas gallinae* when, in fact, these primers are now known to amplify DNA from many more species and genera of parabasalid parasites [96]. Similar false positive results can occur with hemoparasite detection [97].

False positive PCR results do occur [71], and one of the greatest procedural risks in PCR is contamination of the template with target DNA. This can come from either unintended contamination of samples with environmental material, principally during sample collection and handling, or by contamination of the template in the laboratory with PCR product from previous reactions [83]. Contamination from these sources is a very real concern, and great care should be taken to avoid it. Most molecular laboratories are aware of these issues and use negative controls from template preparation to facilitate product visualization or quantification. For most PCR protocols, the collection of tissues protected from environmental contamination (blood) is ideal, so long as these tissues are appropriate for the question being asked. While rarer than false positives, false negative results in PCR do occur for various reasons, and the clinician needs to be sure that the sample collected was appropriate tissue or adequate in volume. Occasionally, the concentration of target material is so low relative to the DNA content of the host tissue (such as with some hemoparasites) that it is extraordinarily difficult to provide enough pathogen DNA for a PCR without overwhelming the reaction with host DNA [98].

References

1 Bailey, T.A., Wernery, U., Howlett, J. et al. (1998). Age-related plasma chemistry findings in the buff-crested bustard (Eupodotis ruficrista gindiana). *J. Vet. Med. B Infect. Dis. Vet. Public Health* 45 (10): 635–640.

2 Hernandez, M. and Margalida, A. (2010). Hematology and blood chemistry reference values and age-related changes in wild bearded vultures (Gypaetus barbatus). *J. Wildl. Dis.* 46 (2): 390–400.

3 Deviche, P., Greiner, E.C. et al. (2001). Seasonal and age-related changes in blood parasite prevalence in Dark-eyed Juncos (Junco hyemalis, Aves, Passeriformes). *J. Exp. Zool.* 289 (7): 456–466.

4 Finnegan, M.V., Daniel, G.B., and Ramsay, E.C. (1997). Evaluation of whole blood transfusions in domestic pigeons (Columba livia). *J. Avian Med. Surg.* 11 (1): 7–14.

5 Ploucha, J.M., Scott, J.B., and Ringer, R.K. (1981). Vascular and hematologic effects of hemorrhage in the chicken. *Am. J. Physiol.* 240 (1): H9–H17.

6 Schindler, S.L. and Gildersleeve, R.P. (1987). Comparison of recovery from hemorrhage in birds and mammals. *Comp. Biochem. Physiol. Physiol.* 87 (3): 533–542.

7 Campbell, T.W. (2007). *Avian and Exotic Animal Hematology and Cytology*. Wiley-Blackwell.

8 Clark, P., Boardman, W. et al. (2009). *Atlas of Avian Haematology*. London: Blackwell.

9 Campbell, TW (2004). Hematology of birds. Veterinary Hematology and Clinical Chemistry. M. A. Thrall, Lippincott, Williams and Wilkins.

10 Robertson, G.W. and Maxwell, M.H. (1990). Modified staining techniques for avian blood-cells. *Br. Poult. Sci.* 31 (4): 881–886.

11 Harr, K.E., Raskin, R.E., and Heard, D.J. (2005). Temporal effects of 3 commonly used anticoagulants on hematologic and biochemical variables in blood samples from macaws and Burmese pythons. *Vet. Clin. Pathol.* 34 (4): 383–388.

12 Lilliehook, I., Wall, H., Tauson, R., and Tvedten, H. (2004). Differential leukocyte counts determined in chicken blood using the Cell-Dyn 3500. *Vet. Clin. Pathol.* 33 (3): 133–138.

13 Seliger, C., Schaerer, B., Kohn, M. et al. (2011). A rapid high-precision flow cytometry based technique for total white blood cell counting in chickens. *Vet. Immunol. Immunopathol.* 145 (1–2): 86–99.

14 Jaensch, S.M., Cullen, L. et al. (2000). Assessment of liver function in galahs (*Eolophus roseicapillus*) after partial hepatectomy: a comparison of plasma enzyme concentrations, serum bile acid levels, and galactose clearance tests. *J. Avian Med. Surg.* 14 (3): 164–171.

15 Desmarchelier, M., Rondenay, Y. et al. (2007). Monitoring of the ventilatory status of anesthetized birds of prey by using end-tidal carbon dioxide measured with a microstream capnometer. *J. Zoo Wildl. Med.* 38 (1): 1–6.

16 Powell, F.L., Shams, H. et al. (2004). Breathing in thin air: acclimatization to altitude in ducks. *Respir. Physiol. Neurobiol.* 144 (2-3): 225–235.

17 Scott, G.R. and Milsom, W.K. (2007). Control of breathing and adaptation to high altitude in the bar-headed goose. *Am. J. Phys. Regul. Integr. Comp. Phys.* 293 (1): R379–R391.

18 Acierno, M.J., Mitchell, M.A. et al. (2009). Evaluation of the agreement among three handheld blood glucose meters and a laboratory blood analyzer for measurement of blood glucose concentration in Hispaniolan Amazon parrots (Amazona ventralis). *Am. J. Vet. Res.* 70 (2): 172–175.
19 Greenacre, C.B., Flatland, B. et al. (2008). Comparison of avian biochemical test results with abaxis vetscan and hitachi 911 analyzers. *J. Avian Med. Surg.* 22 (4): 291–299.
20 Waldoch, J., Wack, R. et al. (2009). Avian plasma chemistry analysis using diluted samples. *J. Zoo Wildl. Med.* 40 (4): 667–674.
21 Cray, C., Rodriguez, M. et al. (2007). Protein electrophoresis of psittacine plasma. *Vet. Clin. Pathol.* 36 (1): 64–72.
22 Roman, Y., Bomsel-Demontoy, M.C. et al. (2009). Effect of hemolysis on plasma protein levels and plasma electrophoresis in birds. *J. Wildl. Dis.* 45 (1): 73–80.
23 Cray, C., Stremme, D.W. et al. (2010). Postprandial biochemistry changes in penguins (Spheniscus demersus) including hyperuricemia. *J. Zoo Wildl. Med.* 41 (2): 325–326.
24 Howlett, J.C., Holzer, W. et al. (1999). Serum bile acids in captive bustards. *Zentralbl. Veterinarmed. B* 46 (10): 701–705.
25 McDonald, D.L., Jaensch, S. et al. (2010). Health and Nutritional Status of Wild Australian Psittacine Birds: An Evaluation of Plasma and Hepatic Mineral Levels, Plasma Biochemical Values, and Fecal Microflora. *J. Avian Med. Surg.* 24 (4): 288–298.
26 Cray, C., Gautier, D. et al. (2008). Changes in clinical enzyme activity and bile acid levels in psittacine birds with altered liver function and disease. *J. Avian Med. Surg.* 22 (1): 17–24.
27 Jaensch, S.M., Cullen, L. et al. (2000). Assessment of liver function in chickens using galactose and indocyanine green clearances. *Avian Pathol.* 29 (2): 109–116.
28 Hanley, C.S., Thomas, N.J. et al. (2005). Exertional myopathy in whooping cranes (Grus americana) with prognostic guidelines. *J. Zoo Wildl. Med.* 36 (3): 489–497.
29 Calabuig, C.P., Ferrer, M. et al. (2010). Blood chemistry of wild Brazilian Coscoroba Swans during molt. *J. Wildl. Dis.* 46 (2): 591–595.
30 Samour, J., Naldo, J. et al. (2010). Hematologic and plasma biochemical reference values in Indian peafowl (Pavo cristatus). *J. Avian Med. Surg.* 24 (2): 99–106.
31 Gelli, D., Ferrari, V. et al. (2009). Serum Biochemistry and Electrophoretic Patterns in the Eurasian Buzzard (Buteo buteo): Reference Values. *J. Wildl. Dis.* 45 (3): 828–833.
32 Szabo, Z., Beregi, A. et al. (2010). Hematologic and plasma biochemistry values in white storks (Ciconia ciconia). *J. Zoo Wildl. Med.* 41 (1): 17–21.
33 Lumeij, J.T. (1987). Avian clinical pathology – general-considerations. *Vet. Q.* 9 (3): 249–254.
34 Lumeij, J.T. and Westerhof, I. (1987). Blood-chemistry for the diagnosis of hepatobiliary disease in birds - a review. *Vet. Q.* 9 (3): 255–261.
35 Katavolos, P., Staempfli, S. et al. (2007). The effect of lead poisoning on hematologic and biochemical values in trumpeter swans and Canada geese. *Vet. Clin. Pathol.* 36 (4): 341–347.
36 Phalen, D.N., Falcon, M. et al. (2007). Endocrine pancreatic insufficiency secondary to chronic herpesvirus pancreatitis in a cockatiel (Nymphicus hollandicus). *J. Avian Med. and Surg.* 21 (2): 140–145.
37 Gosselin, S.J. and Kramer, L.W. (1983). Pathophysiology of excessive iron storage in mynah birds. *J. Am. Vet. Med. Assoc.* 183 (11): 1238–1240.
38 Crissey, S.D., Ward, A.M. et al. (2000). Hepatic iron accumulation over time in European starlings (Sturnus vulgaris) fed two levels of iron. *J. Zoo Wildl. Med.* 31 (4): 491–496.
39 Helmick, K.E., Kendrick, E.L. et al. (2011). Diet manipulation as treatment for elevated serum iron parameters in captive raggiana bird of paradise (Paradisaea raggiana). *J. Zoo Wildl. Med.* 42 (3): 460–467.
40 Hugman, A. (2006). Hepcidin: an important new regulator of iron homeostasis. *Clin. Lab. Haematol.* 28 (2): 75–83.
41 Gkouvatsos, K., Papanikolaou, G. et al. (2012). Regulation of iron transport and the role of transferrin. *Biochim. Biophys. Acta.* 1820 (3): 188–202.
42 Anderson, G.J., Frazer, D.M. et al. (2009). Iron absorption and metabolism. *Curr. Opin. Gastroenterol.* 25 (2): 129–135.
43 Zhang, A.S. and Enns, C.A. (2009). Molecular mechanisms of normal iron homeostasis. *Hematology Am. Soc. Hematol. Educ. Program* 2009: 207–214.
44 Fu, Y.M., Li, S.P. et al. (2007). Identification and expression analysis of hepcidin-like cDNAs from pigeon (Columba livia). *Mol. Cell. Biochem.* 305 (1-2): 191–197.
45 Fleming, M.D. (2008). The regulation of hepcidin and its effects on systemic and cellular iron metabolism. *Hematology Am. Soc. Hematol. Educ. Program* 2008 (1): 151–158.
46 Raj, D.S. (2009). Role of interleukin-6 in the anemia of chronic disease. *Semin. Arthritis Rheum.* 38 (5): 382–388.
47 Ganz, T. and Nemeth, E. (2009). Iron sequestration and anemia of inflammation. *Semin. Hematol.* 46 (4): 387–393.
48 Brissot, P., Troadec, M.B. et al. (2008). Current approach to hemochromatosis. *Blood Rev.* 22 (4): 195–210.
49 Stremmel, W., Karner, M. et al. (2007). Liver and iron metabolism–a comprehensive hypothesis for the pathogenesis of genetic hemochromatosis. *Z. Gastroenterol.* 45 (1): 71–75.

50 Hilton, K.B. and Lambert, L.A. (2008). Molecular evolution and characterization of hepcidin gene products in vertebrates. *Gene* 415 (1-2): 40–48.

51 Pan, C.Y., Chow, T.Y. et al. (2010). Antimicrobial peptides of an anti-lipopolysaccharide factor, epinecidin-1, and hepcidin reduce the lethality of Riemerella anatipestifer sepsis in ducks. *Peptides* 31 (5): 806–815.

52 Malyszko, J. (2009). Hepcidin assays: ironing out some details. *Clin. J. Am. Soc. Nephrol.* 4 (6): 1015–1016.

53 Bernard, S.F., Orvoine, J. et al. (2003). Glucose regulates lipid metabolism in fasting king penguins. *Am. J. Phys. Regul. Integr. Comp. Phys.* 285 (2): R313–R320.

54 Bernard, S.F., Thil, M.A. et al. (2003). Lipolytic and metabolic response to glucagon in fasting king penguins: phase II vs. phase III. *Am. J. Phys. Regul. Integr. Comp. Phys.* 284 (2): R444–R454.

55 Sweazea, K.L., McMurtry, J.P. et al. (2006). Inhibition of lipolysis does not affect insulin sensitivity to glucose uptake in the mourning dove. *Comp. Biochem. Physiol. B Biochem. Mol. Biol.* 144 (3): 387–394.

56 Desmarchelier, M. and Langlois, I. (2008). Diabetes mellitus in a nanday conure (Nandayus nanday). *J. Avian Med. Surg.* 22 (3): 246–254.

57 Braun, E.J. and Sweazea, K.L. (2008). Glucose regulation in birds. *Comp. Biochem. Physiol. Biochem. Mol. Biol.* 151 (1): 1–9.

58 Fudge, A.M. (2000). *Laboratory Medicine, Avian and Exotic Pets.* Saunders.

59 Gancz, A.Y., Wellehan, J.F.X. et al. (2007). Diabetes mellitus concurrent with hepatic haemosiderosis in two macaws (Ara severa, Ara militaris). *Avian Pathol.* 36 (4): 331–332.

60 Pilny, A.A. and Luong, R. (2005). Diabetes mellitus in a chestnut-fronted macaw (Ara severa). *J. Avian Med. Surg.* 19 (4): 297–302.

61 Cockrem, J.F., Potter, M.A. et al. (2006). Corticosterone in relation to body mass in Adelie penguins (Pygoscelis adeliae) affected by unusual sea ice conditions at Ross Island, Antarctica. *Gen. Comp. Endocrinol.* 149 (3): 244–252.

62 Roxburgh, L. and Pinshow, B. (2002). Ammonotely in a passerine nectarivore: the influence of renal and post-renal modification on nitrogenous waste product excretion. *J. Exp. Biol.* 205 (12): 1735–1745.

63 McWhorter, T.J., Powers, D.R. et al. (2003). Are hummingbirds facultatively ammonotelic? Nitrogen excretion and requirements as a function of body size. *Physiol. Biochem. Zool.* 76 (5): 731–743.

64 Gartrell, B.D., Raidal, S.R. et al. (2003). Renal disease in captive swift parrots (*Lathamus discolor*): The effect of diet on plasma uric acid concentrations. *J. Avian Med. Surg.* 17 (4): 206–212.

65 Kondiah, K., Albertyn, J. et al. (2005). Beak and feather disease virus haemagglutinating activity using erythrocytes from African Grey parrots and Brown-headed parrots. *Onderstepoort J. Vet. Res.* 72 (3): 263–265.

66 Lierz, M., Hafez, H.M. et al. (2009). Anatomical distribution of avian bornavirus in parrots, its occurrence in clinically healthy birds and ABV-antibody detection. *Avian Pathol.* 38 (6): 491–496.

67 Phalen, D.N. (2002). Virus neutralization assays used in exotic bird medicine. *Semin. Avian Exot. Pet. Med.* 11 (1): 19–24.

68 Scott, A.N., Beckett, A. et al. (2006). Serological diagnosis of goose circovirus infections. *Avian Pathol.* 35 (6): 495–499.

69 Cray, C., Zielezienski-Roberts, K. et al. (2005). Serologic diagnosis of Sarcocystosis in Psittacine birds: 16 cases. *J. Avian Med. Surg.* 19 (3): 208–215.

70 Phalen, D.N. (2001). The use of serologic assays in avian medicine. *Semin. Avian Exot. Pet. Med.* 10 (2): 77–89.

71 Khalesi, B., Bonne, N. et al. (2005). A comparison of haemagglutination, haemagglutination inhibition and PCR for the detection of psittacine beak and feather disease virus infection and a comparison of isolates obtained from loriids. *J. Gen. Virol.* 86: 3039–3046.

72 de Kloet, A.H., Kerski, A. et al. (2011). Diagnosis of Avian bornavirus infection in psittaciformes by serum antibody detection and reverse transcription polymerase chain reaction assay using feather calami. *J. Vet. Diagn. Investig.* 23 (3): 421–429.

73 Sullivan, H., Linz, G. et al. (2006). West Nile virus antibody prevalence in red-winged blackbirds (Agelaius phoeniceus) from North Dakota, USA (2003-2004). *Vector Borne Zoonotic Dis.* 6 (3): 305–309.

74 Phalen, D.N., Wilson, V.G. et al. (1997). Prevalence of neutralizing antibody and virus shedding in psittacine birds infected with avian polyomavirus. *J. Avian Med. Surg.* 11 (2): 98–104.

75 Phalen, D.N., Radabaugh, C.S. et al. (2000). Viremia, virus shedding, and antibody response during natural avian polyomavirus infection in parrots. *J. Am. Vet. Med. Assoc.* 217 (1): 32–36.

76 Shearer, P.L., Sharp, M. et al. (2009). A blocking ELISA for the detection of antibodies to psittacine beak and feather disease virus (BFDV). *J. Virol. Methods* 158 (1-2): 136–140.

77 Riddoch, P.A., Raidal, S.R. et al. (1996). Psittacine circovirus antibody detection and an update on the methods for diagnosis of psittacine beak and feather disease. *Aust. Vet. Pract.* 26 (3): 134–136.

78 Cattoli, G., Drago, A. et al. (2004). Comparison of three rapid detection systems for type A influenza virus on tracheal swabs of experimentally and naturally infected birds. *Avian Pathol.* 33 (4): 432–437.

79 Robbin, L., Barker, I. et al. (2003). Rapid Antigen-Capture Assay To Detect West Nile Virus in Dead Corvids. *Emerg. Infect. Dis.* 9 (11): 1406–1410.

80 Sanada, N. and Sanada, Y. (2000). The sensitivities of various erythrocytes in a haemagglutination assay for the detection of psittacine beak and feather disease virus. *J. Vet. Med. B Infect. Dis. Vet. Public Health* 47 (6): 441–443.

81 Vanrompay, D., Van Nerom, A. et al. (1994). Evaluation of five immunoassays for detection of Chlamydia psittaci in cloacal and conjunctival specimens from turkeys. *J. Clin. Microbiol.* 32 (6): 1470–1474.

82 Cray, C., Watson, T. et al. (2009). Application of galactomannan analysis and protein electrophoresis in the diagnosis of aspergillosis in avian species. *J. Zoo Wildl. Med.* 40: 64–70.

83 Bonne, N.P., Clark, P. et al. (2008). Elimination of false-positive polymerase chain reaction results resulting from hole punch carryover contamination. *J. Vet. Diagn. Investig.* 20 (1): 60–63.

84 Saggese, M.D., Tizard, I. et al. (2010). Comparison of sampling methods, culture, acid-fast stain, and polymerase chain reaction assay for the diagnosis of mycobacteriosis in ring-neck doves (Streptopelia risoria). *J. Avian Med. Surg.* 24 (4): 263–271.

85 Wang, W., Ren, P. et al. (2009). Design of multiplexed detection assays for identification of avian influenza a virus subtypes pathogenic to humans by SmartCycler real-time reverse transcription-PCR. *J. Clin. Microbiol.* 47 (1): 86–92.

86 Marek, A., Gunes, A. et al. (2010). Classification of fowl adenoviruses by use of phylogenetic analysis and high-resolution melting-curve analysis of the hexon L1 gene region. *J. Virol. Methods* 170 (1-2): 147–154.

87 Steer, P.A., O'Rourke, D. et al. (2011). Application of high-resolution melting curve analysis for typing of fowl adenoviruses in field cases of inclusion body hepatitis. *Aust. Vet. J.* 89 (5): 184–192.

88 Rebelo, A.R., Parker, L. et al. (2011). Use of high-resolution melting curve analysis to identify Mycoplasma species commonly isolated from ruminant, avian, and canine samples. *J. Vet. Diagn. Investig.* 23 (5): 932–936.

89 Mitchell, S.L., Wolff, B.J. et al. (2009). Genotyping of Chlamydophila psittaci by real-time PCR and high-resolution melt analysis. *J. Clin. Microbiol.* 47 (1): 175–181.

90 Olsen, G. and Speer, B. (2009). Laboratory reporting accuracy of polymerase chain reaction testing for psittacine beak and feather disease virus. *J. Avian Med. Surg.* 23 (3): 194–198.

91 Tomasek, O., Kubicek, O. et al. (2008). Comparison of three template preparation methods for routine detection of beak and feather disease virus and avian polyomavirus with single and nested polymerase chain reaction in clinical specimens. *Avian Pathol.* 37 (2): 145–149.

92 Murphy, S., Legge, S. et al. (2003). The breeding biology of palm cockatoos (Probosciger aterrimus): a case of a slow life history. *J. Zool.* 261: 327–339.

93 Loa, C.C., Lin, T.L. et al. (2006). Differential detection of turkey coronavirus, infectious bronchitis virus, and bovine coronavirus by a multiplex polymerase chain reaction. *J. Virol. Methods* 131 (1): 86–91.

94 Freick, M., Muller, H. et al. (2008). Rapid detection of pigeon herpesvirus, fowl adenovirus and pigeon circovirus in young racing pigeons by multiplex PCR. *J. Virol. Methods* 148 (1-2): 226–231.

95 Messmer, T.O., Skelton, S.K. et al. (1997). Application of a nested, multiplex PCR to psittacosis outbreaks. *J. Clin. Microbiol.* 35 (8): 2043–2046.

96 Felleisen, R.S. (1997). Comparative sequence analysis of 5.8S rRNA genes and internal transcribed spacer (ITS) regions of trichomonadid protozoa. *Parasitology* 115 (Pt 2): 111–119.

97 Cosgrove, C.L., Day, K.P. et al. (2006). Coamplification of Leucocytozoon by PCR diagnostic tests for avian malaria: a cautionary note. *J. Parasitol.* 92 (6): 1362–1365.

98 Sehgal, R.N.M., Jones, H.I. et al. (2001). Host specificity and incidence of Trypanosoma in some African rainforest birds: a molecular approach. *Mol. Ecol.* 10 (9): 2319–2327.

24

Raptors

Michael P. Jones DVM, DABVP[1] and John Chitty MRCVS[2]

[1] *Avian and Zoological Medicine, College of Veterinary Medicine, The University of Tennessee, Knoxville, Tennessee, USA*
[2] *Anton Vets, Andover, Hants, UK*

Introduction

Clinical pathology and diagnostic testing in birds of prey is one of the most important aspects of the medical management of these species, especially in free-ranging birds of prey. Wild birds of prey are often missing a key element of the clinical exam, as little history is available to indicate why they presented to the veterinarian. To overcome this problem, the clinician should have a thorough understanding of clinical pathology in nondomestic avian species, and more specifically, in birds of prey. This chapter will provide the tools necessary to put the pieces of the clinical puzzle together to accurately evaluate the patient, discriminate between health and various disease conditions, and monitor the severity and clinical progression of diseases characterized by changes in hematology and biochemical analyses.

Species

Raptors are a multiphyletic group of predator birds further characterized by hooked bills and often sharp talons. Prey species range from mammals to invertebrates. The chapter will concentrate on raptors indigenous to North America (Table 24.1). However, raptor veterinarians are commonly exposed to species from around the world as these species are often kept in captivity in zoological parks, raptor education centers, raptor propagation centers, and by falconers. Raptor species commonly presented to veterinarians for assessment and care include eagles, falcons, hawks, kites, osprey, and vultures.

Restraint

Chemical restraint is rarely necessary for sample collection in raptors [32]. If the animal is unstable, in a critical state, or the clinician is inexperienced in sampling smaller species, then mask induction of anesthesia using isoflurane or sevoflurane may be required. Isoflurane anesthesia significantly reduced the packed cell volume (PCV) and protein concentrations in samples from American kestrels (*Falco sparverius*), and caused changes in many other analytes [52]. However, with the exception of increased potassium and decreased uric acid concentrations, effects were due to serial sample dilution rather than anesthesia, with the anesthetized bird's cardiovascular system being less able to compensate for serial samples [52]. Inform the laboratory, and be aware that if samples are taken under anesthesia, it will affect interpretation. Transportation of the bird may also induce a stress leukogram, with differing responses between different species and between trained and untrained birds [163]. Manual restraint normally requires one handler. However, for larger species – eagles, Old World vultures – two handlers may be required.

Materials

For most raptor species, venipuncture is achieved using 23 g., 5/8″ needles. However, in chicks and small species, 25 g. needles may be required. For jugular venipuncture of large eagles and vultures, 1″ needles may be required. 1–5 ml syringes and butterfly catheters may facilitate sample collection. Samples for routine tests should be taken into heparin tubes. For electrolyte analysis, the sample should either be tested immediately or placed into heparin gel tubes that are spun as soon as practicable, as potassium may change quickly in some raptor species [142]. For less commonly used tests, contact the testing laboratory prior to sampling to ascertain requirements for sample storage and transport. Two to four air-dried smears should be made immediately from blood not exposed to anticoagulant. This enables the hematologist to assess cellular morphologic changes without any anticoagulant effects and

Exotic Animal Laboratory Diagnosis, First Edition. Edited by J. Jill Heatley and Karen E. Russell.

Table 24.1 Common North American raptors.

Common name	Scientific name	Subspecies and comments
American kestrel	*Falco sparverius*	Widespread throughout North America, except arctic tundra [225]
Aplomado falcon	*Falco femoralis*	Southwest US (reintroduced), Central and South America [221, 225]
Bald eagle	*Haliaeetus leucocephalus*	*H l leucocephalus* – Southern US to Mexico *H l alascanus* – Northwest US, Canada and Alaska [221, 225] Interbreeding occurs between subspecies in US
Barn owl	*Tyto alba*	US except for northern states [220]
Black vulture	*Coragyps atratus*	Southern US
Broad-winged hawk	*Buteo platypterus*	Eastern US
California condor	*Gymnogyps californianus*	Western US (California, Arizona)
Cooper's hawk	*Accipiter cooperi*	Continental North America [221]
Crested caracara	*Caracara plancus*	Central Florida, coastal Texas, Western Louisiana and South central Arizona [225]
Ferruginous hawk	*Buteo regalis*	Great Basin east to western Great Plains, north to Canada, south to Arizona and New Mexico [225]
Great horned owl	*Bubo virginianus*	
Golden eagle	*Aquila chrysaetos*	Western US, Alaska, Canada, Northeastern US; winter in southern states [225]
Gyrfalcon	*Falco rusticolus*	Arctic regions, Canada and barely into Northern US [225]
Harris' hawk	*Parabuteo unicinctus*	Only member of the genus *Parbuteo*; Southwestern US; desert regions of southern and central Arizona, Southern New Mexico, and Southern Texas [225]
Merlin	*Falco columbarius*	*F. c. columbarius* (Taiga) – breed in boreal forests from Alaska to Newfoundland; winters in southern US and southward [225] Prairie merlin *F. c. richardsoni* – Northern Great Plains; winter there and southward [225] Black merlin *F. c. suckleyi* – Pacific northwest regions; some move southward in winter [225]
Mississippi kite	*Ictinia mississippiensis*	Breeds from North Carolina and northern Florida west to Kansas, southeastern Colorado, and Texas and north along Mississippi River to southern Illinois and Indiana, and west to Arizona [225]
North American goshawk	*Accipiter gentilis*	Breeds in forests of Northern US south in Appalachian Mountains to West Virginia, throughout Canada and Alaska, and in forested Western mountains [225]
Northern harrier	*Circus cyaneus*	Breeds throughout northern and central US and Canada [225]
Osprey	*Pandion haliaetus*	Continental North America [220]
Peregrine falcon	*Falco peregrinus*	*F. p. tundrius* (Tundra peregrine) – Breed on Arctic tundra from western Alaska to Greenland; migrate south to Latin America for winter [225] *F. p. anatum* (Anatum peregrine) – Breed in subarctic Alaska and Canada and throughout the Western US [225] *F. p. pealei* (Peale's peregrine) – Breed in Aleutian Islands and along the Pacific Northwest coast from British Columbia south to Oregon [225]
Prairie falcon	*Falco mexicanus*	Western US and southern Canada [225]
Red-shouldered hawk	*Buteo lineatus*	Several "races" of *B lineatus* [225]: *B l lineatus* – Eastern birds *B l alleni* – Northern Florida *B l exitmus* – South Florida *B l texanus* – Texas *B l elegans* – California Borders between races are not distinct

Table 24.1 (Continued)

Common name	Scientific name	Subspecies and comments
Red-tailed hawk	*Buteo jamaicensis*	Continental North America Several "races" and subspecies exist [135]: *B. j. borealis* – Eastern red-tailed hawk; range from Great Plains east of the Rocky Mountains and from central Canada south to Gulf coast and northern Florida [135, 225] *B j calurus* – Western red-tailed hawk; Rocky Mountains westward [225] *B j fuertesi* – Fuertes' red-tailed hawk; Oklahoma and Texas on the Great Plains, Arizona and New Mexico southward [135, 225] *B j Kriderii* – Krider's red-tailed hawk; breeds in southwest central Canada and adjacent US states; winters in North American prairie regions [135] *B j harlani* – Harlan's; Alaska and Northwestern Canada, winters in Great Plains region of US [135, 225] *B j umbrinus* – Florida red-tailed hawk [225] *B j alascensis* – Alaska red-tailed hawk [135] Additional subspecies exist out of North America
Rough-legged hawk	*Buteo lagopus*	Breeds on Arctic tundra and mixed tundra-boreal forest from western Alaska to Newfoundland [225]
Screech owl	*Megascops* sp. (Formerly *Otus* sp) [8]	*Megascops asio* – Eastern screech owl; Plains east to the Atlantic, southern Canada to Texas [220] *Megascops kennecoti* – Western screech owl; West from the Plains to Pacific, Pacific Northwest south to Mexican border [220]
Sharp shinned hawk	*Accipiter striatus*	Breeds in forests of eastern, northern, and mountainous western North America. Winters throughout US except northern Great Plains, and farther south [225]
Swainson's hawk	*Buteo swainsoni*	Breeds on prairies and open areas of western North America from southern Canada to south Texas and central California; majority of population migrates to south America while some stay in southern California, south Texas, and south Florida [225]
Swallow-tailed kite	*Elanoides forficatus*	Florida, along Gulf coast west to eastern Texas and Atlantic coast to South Carolina; entire population migrates to South America during the winter [225]
Turkey vulture	*Cathartes aura*	All of US; extends into southern Canada [225]

also provides a "safety net" should the blood sample be damaged in transit to the laboratory. Microtainer tubes are often used; blood is placed in the tube after the needle is removed from the syringe to avoid hemolysis. Calculation of safe blood volumes that may be collected for sampling appears similar to other non-aquatic avian species, with one species indicating circulating blood volume to be approximately 6%–7% body weight [14].

Venipuncture Sites

Jugular Vein

The right jugular vein is preferable for use, as the left jugular vein is much smaller in most raptors (Figure 24.1). The bird should be restrained or anesthetized, and the neck extended. Parting of the feathers reveals the vein, easily visualized through the skin and found medial to the trachea, under a large apterium. Placement of a digit at the base of the neck raises the vein. This approach allows for large volumes to be taken easily and is the first choice for venipuncture sites in raptors. Hemostasis is relatively simple, although large subcutaneous hematomas may form if the venipuncture site is not attended properly. Hematoma formation may preclude further use of this vein until the hematoma has resolved, which, depending upon size and animal health, often takes only 24–48 h. Restraint for this approach may be stressful to sensitive or dyspneic birds. This method may prove more difficult for left-handed individuals, although the left jugular may be used in larger species. For left-handed practitioners, an approach over the head and toward the heart may be more practical, as someone else provides raptor restraint. In larger raptors such as eagles, vultures, or female gyrfalcons, the muscular neck can be hard to extend. Struggling of the raptor during venipuncture may result in laceration of the vein and fatal subcutaneous hemorrhage. Death following jugular venipuncture in raptors is rare but may be more likely to occur based on preexisting coagulopathy.

Superficial Ulnar/Basilic Vein

The bird is restrained or anesthetized and placed in dorsal recumbency. One wing is extended, and the vein visualized (Figure 24.2). The phlebotomist raises the vein with his/her free hand by applying slight pressure proximal to the anconeal joint along the vein; this method is

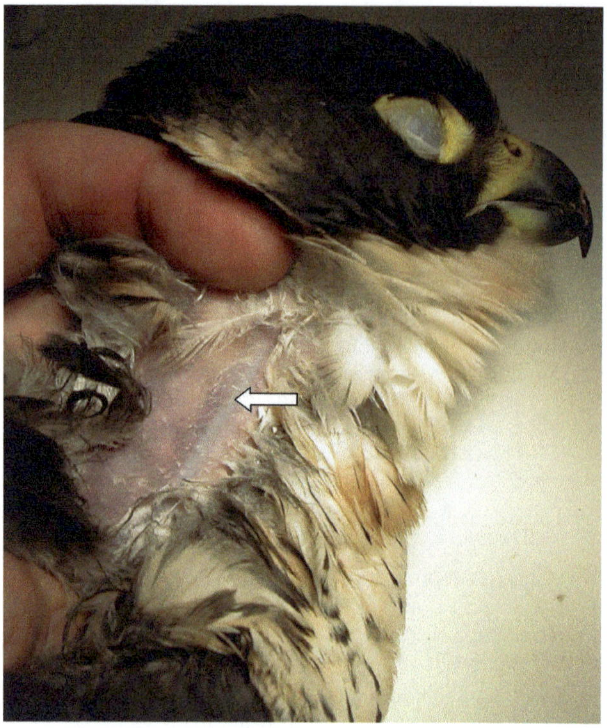

Figure 24.1 Location of the right jugular vein (white arrow) in a peregrine falcon. *Source:* © John Chitty, BVetMed, CertZooMed, MRCVS. Reproduced from the BSAVA Manual of Raptors, Pigeons and Passerine Birds with permission.

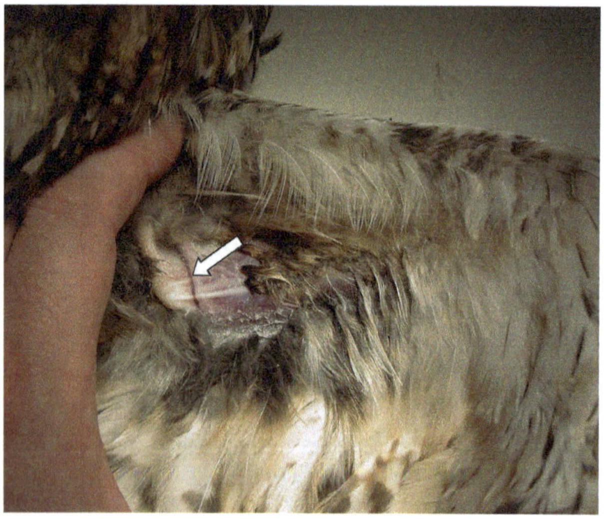

Figure 24.2 Location of the basilic vein (white arrow) as it crosses the proximal radius and ulna of the left wing in a tawny owl (*Strix aluco*). *Source:* © John Chitty, BVetMed, CertZooMed, MRCVS. Reproduced from the BSAVA Manual of Raptors, Pigeons and Passerine Birds with permission.

easier for left-handed individuals. Blood is drawn from the more distal aspect of the vein as it courses superficially over the ulna. Restraint for this method, especially in the larger species, and placing and maintaining an intravenous catheter for repeated sampling from this vein is relatively easy.

However, as a more fragile vein, large volumes may be more challenging to obtain, especially in smaller birds. Hemostasis may also be more challenging at this vein. To facilitate lowering blood pressure to allow hemostasis, replace the bird in its carrier or bay for calming, rather than prolonging handling. Unlike jugular venipuncture, ulnar vein hemorrhage is unlikely to be fatal and is easily visualized. Nonetheless, small losses may cause a lot of mess and distress to falconers. A drop of tissue glue may also facilitate hemostasis. Occasionally, a hematoma may form along with a slight wing drop that may last a day or two.

Superficial Plantar Metatarsal/Caudal Tibial Vein/Medial Metatarsal Vein

The bird is restrained, and the leg extended (Figure 24.3). The phlebotomist can then raise the vein by encircling the tibiotarsus with their free hand. Chicks can be left in a "sitting" position with feet in front of them to minimize restraint. However, in adults the leg must be fixed to avoid phlebotomist injury. The vein is superficial and simple to visualize and raise. Restraint (above) is easy especially in juveniles and chicks. It is an excellent site for catheter placement in chicks; however, in large raptors, owing to the proximity of the talons, there inherent risk of injury to the phlebotomist. This site is most useful in vultures that have less powerful talons (North American species; *Gyps* species; smaller Old World species). However, the concern of uric acid contamination of samples from urine excreted onto the legs in vultures dictates that the venipuncture site be thoroughly cleaned prior to sample collection. Hemostasis difficulties are similar to those described when using the superficial ulnar/basilica vein. Tissue glue may be applied or a light dressing applied after sampling.

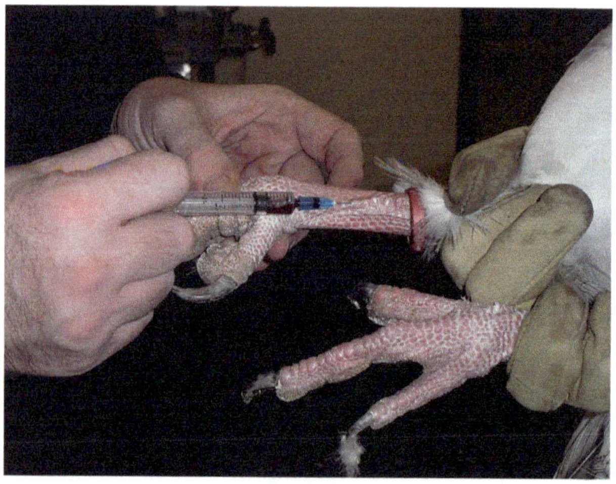

Figure 24.3 Use of the medial metatarsal vein for venipuncture in a white-headed vulture. *Source:* Courtesy Hawk Conservancy Trust. Reproduced from the BSAVA Manual of Raptors, Pigeons and Passerine Birds with permission.

Talon Clip

The talon or nail clip is considered inappropriate and inhumane in all species. Usually, only a small sample, often contaminated with uric acid, is obtained. Samples for hematologic analysis and cells counts obtained are poorly representative of patient health based on sampling of the capillary bed. This method is likely to cause excessive pain and damage to structures vital to the raptor's hunting ability.

Occipital Sinus

This approach may be used for sampling chicks, allowing larger volumes of blood than peripheral veins, or from anesthetized raptors slated for euthanasia. The approach is through the occipital sinus, as the bill is folded toward the breast to allow dorsal cervical extension. Entry into the spinal canal resulting in contamination with cerebrospinal fluid is likely.

Sample Handling and Storage

Studies specific to changes on raptor hematological variables based on handling and storage appear nonextant. However, in raptor determinations of reference data, both EDTA and heparin anticoagulants have been used [107, 198]. The sooner the CBC can be determined after sample collection, the better; and extremes of temperature are to be avoided. EDTA or lithium heparin both appear acceptable for CBC analysis of most raptors in the short term. Based on cellular staining artifact of heparin, most pathologists prefer EDTA.

Hemolysis and Lipemia

Artifactual changes in biochemical analyte values based on hemolysis and or lipemia can make interpretation of chemistry test results difficult. Venipuncture technique, delayed sample handling/separation of cells from plasma or serum (especially true with serum samples), hemolytic anemia, and lipemia may cause hemolysis within a sample. Hemolysis interferes with biochemistry results based on several mechanisms including increased absorbance and color interference, inhibition of chemical reactions, and release of analytes (aspartate aminotransferase and potassium) from red blood cells [87]. Hemolysis may cause falsely increased bile acids (spectrophotometric analysis), lactate dehydrogenase (LDH), creatine kinase (CK), alkaline phosphatase (ALP), and potassium [71]. Lipemia may be a result of postprandial sampling, reproductive activity in females, or various diseases (i.e., endocrinopathies, pancreatic disease, hepatic disease, or idiopathic hyperlipidemia) and interferes with chemistry tests that use color to measure analytes. Bile acids (spectrophotometric analysis), all liver enzymes including alkaline phosphatase, total bilirubin, hemoglobin, proteins, electrolytes, glucose, calcium, phosphorus, and uric acid may be falsely increased depending upon the severity of lipidemia [71, 87]. The effects of hemolysis and lipemia may vary based upon the type of chemistry analyzer used (i.e., wet or dry-chemistry analyzer) and the degree of hemolysis or lipemia in the sample. Do not use plasma or serum samples with marked or severe hemolysis for biochemical analysis. However, the biochemical generalizations above have not been specifically investigated or proved in raptor species.

Storage of Samples for Biochemical Analysis

The method of storage for plasma prior to analysis may have a significant impact on the concentration of several metabolites, and measurement of analytes in plasma should be made as quickly as possible without freezing the sample [21]. The effects of centrifuging whole blood within 1 h of collection, separating the plasma from blood cells, and keeping the sample at 4 °C for up to four days or below −20 °C for an unlimited time on samples taken from black kites (*Milvus milvus*) and red foxes *(Vulpes vulpes*) were evaluated [21]. Storing plasma samples at 4 °C for four days had no effect on the concentrations of cholesterol, glucose, triglycerides, urea, and uric acid, but concentration of triglycerides and glucose were underestimated, and concentrations of urea were overestimated in samples frozen at −20 °C for 30 days [21]. Samples stored at −20 °C for 15 days exhibited similar trends, but the differences were not significant. In raptors, if sample analysis cannot be performed soon after acquiring them, and they must be frozen, the effect of freezing and the time kept frozen on the metabolites of interest should be evaluated to correct analyte estimates [21].

Complete Blood Count

Hematology

The morphology of the cells red and white blood cells is similar to other avian species with most variability in the appearance of the eosinophil, which is important given the need to distinguish this cell from the similar heterophil. Your consulting hematologist should be familiar with cells in raptor and owl species. In addition, consistency of cytological staining and counting method is necessary to ensure consistent results and an accurate ability to interpret results. Hematologic reference data for various raptor species are presented in Tables 24.2–24.4.

Red Cell Parameters

These are similar to those assessed in other avian species in terms of parameters measured, methods of measurement, and interpretation of variation from the normal. Changes may be changes associated with age or sex. In

Table 24.2 Hematologic reference data for vultures and eagles.

Analyte	Species	Black vulture [214] (Coragyps atratus)	Griffon Ħ ⊙ vulture (*Gyps fulvus*) [170]	Egyptian Ħ ⊙ vulture (*Neophron percnopterus*) [170]	African white-backed vulture (*Gyps africanus*) [159]Ħ	California condor (*Gymnogyps californianus*) [53] Ħ	Spanish imperial eagle (*Aquila adalberti*) [170] Ħ ⊙	Golden eagle (*Aquila chrysaetos*) [16] Ħ ⊙	Bald eagle (*Haliaeetus leucocephalus*) [16, 107, 147]
	Data Type n = Units	Mean ± SD N = 7 ♀, 5 ⊙ Ħ, 53 Ơ	Mean ± SD N = 12	Mean ± SD N = 5	Mean ± SD N =21	Mean N = 17 (6 m-5y)Ơ N = 12 ⊙ > 5y	Mean ± SD N =12	Mean ± SD N =21 – 52	Mean ± SD N =21
PCV %		49.5 ± 6.1 ♀ 39.4 ± 6.9 ⊙ Ħ 31.9 ± 3.2 Ơ	45.5 ± 3.4	42.5 ± 3.6	44.3 ± 4.79	41.9 ± 2.5 Ơ 44.0 ± 2.5 ⊙	43.7 ± 3.6	42.1 ± 3.7	32 ± 4 [16] 44 ± 4 [107] 42.8 ± 4.3 [147]
Red cell count	**X 10^{12}/l**		2.63 ± 0.32	2.30 ± 0.44	2.55 ± 0.22		2.41 ± 0.15	2.56 ± 0.54	3.31 ± 0.36 [107]
Hemoglobin	**g/dl**		15.1 ± 1.9	13.7 ± 1.2	196.6 ± 16.83		13.6 ± 1.4	13.8 ± 1.3	11.83 ± 1.85 [16]
mean cellular hemoglobin (MCHC)	**Pg**		55.3 ± 6.7 (33.2 ± 2.5)	60.2 ± 6.3 (32.2 ± 0.4)	(39.3 ± 1.53)		56.7 ± 4.2 (31.3 ± 1.4)	44.0 ± 12.7 (32.8 ± 0.3)	(37.4 ± 5.4) [16]
Mean cell volume			170.0 ± 15.5	187.7 ± 21.7	196.7 ± 5.55		179.5 ± 10.5	168.2 ± 18.6	
White cell count	**X10^9/l (%)**		13.19 ± 7.32	16.03 ± 4.19	16.71 ± 1.63	19.8 ± 7.6 Ơ 15.7 ± 4.4 ⊙	14.87 ± 6.3	12.32 ± 7.95	17.21 ± 7.96 [16] 12.7 ± 5.0 [107] 13.0 ± 4.5 [147]
Heterophil	**X10^9/l (%)**		7.04 ± 5.02 (40.67 ± 10.52)	11.95 ± 2.2 69.75 ± 13.5	13.7 ± 6.11	8.6 ± 3.2 Ơ 10.7 ± 3	10.57 ± 5.03 (60.57 ± 13.1)	3.87 ± 1.98 (58.83 ± 9.75)	7.59 ± 3.82 (44 ± 11) [16] 10.03 ± 1.40 (79.0 ± 11) [107] 8.5 ± 3.2 (65.8 ± 14.4) [147]
Lymphocyte	**X10^9/l (%)**		5.02 ± 2.7 (40.67 ± 10.52)	4.90 ± 2.47 (27.25 ± 12.7)	1.02 ± 1.91	9.2 ± 6.5 Ơ 3.6 ± 0.3	4.8 ± 2.07 (30.79 ± 11.27)	2.29 ± 0.11 (34.17 ± 5.8)	6.75 ± 3.86 (38 ± 10) [16] 2.03 ± 1.14 (16.0 ± 9.0) [107] 2.8 ± 1.9 (22.4 ± 12.4) [147]
Monocyte	**X10^9/l (%)**		0.06 ± 0.07 (0.57 ± 0.53)	0.08 ± 0.09 (0.50 ± 0.58)	1.57 ± 1.04	0.7 ± 0.6 Ơ 0.5 ± 0.5	0.29 ± 0.17 (1.28 ± 0.71)	0.27 ± 0.23 (4.34 ± 4.16)	0.67 ± 0.43 (4 ± 2) [16] 0.13 ± 0.13 (1.0 ± 1.0) [107] 0.4 ± 0.5 (3.2 ± 3.4) [147]
Eosinophil	**X10^9/l (%)**		0.51 ± 1.19 (0.86 ± 1.57)	0.36 ± 0.16 (2.0 ± 0.82)	0.75 ± 0.71	0.8 ± 5.8 Ơ 0.8 ± 1.2	1.08 ± 0.36 (6.94 ± 2.92)	0.17 ± 0.10 (2.33 ± 1.15)	2.19 ± 1.60 (13 ± 6) [16] 0.25 ± 0.38 (2.0 ± 3.0) [107] 7.2 ± 7.2 (1.3 ± 1.6) [147]
Basophil	**X10^9/l (%)**		0	0.09 ± 0.11 (0.40 ± 0.54)	0	0.3 ± 0.3 Ơ 0.2 ± 0.3	0	0.20 ± 0.03 (0.20 ± 0.45)	0 [107] 0.2 ± 0.2 (1.3 ± 1.6) 147

Table 24.3 Hematologic reference intervals for falcons and owls.

Analyte	Species	Saker falcon (*Falco cherrug*) [34]	Peregrine falcon (*Falco peregrinus*) [34]	Gyrfalcon (*Falco rusticolus*) [34]	Lanner falcon (*Falco biarmicus*) [34]	Merlin (*Falco columbarius*) [34]	Eurasian eagle [34] owl (*Bubo bubo*)	Barn owl (Tyto alba) [204] H ʘ
	Data Type n = Units	Range N = 234	Range N = 127	Range N = 53	Range N = 42	Range N = 33	Range N = 20	Mean ± SD N = 31
PCV	**%**	38–49	37–53		37–53	39–51	36–52	46.2 ± 4
Red cell count	**X 10^{12}/l**	2.54–3.96	2.95–3.94		2.63–3.98	2.84–4.1	1.65–2.35	3.2 ± 0.4
Hemoglobin	**g/dl**	11.5–16.5	11.8–18.8		12.2–17.1	13.2–17.9	10.7–18.0	107 ± 15
Mean cellular hemoglobin (MCHC)	**Pg**	41.4–45.4 (30.4–34.9)	40–48.4 (31.9–35.2)		42.3–48.8 (31.7–35.3)	36–45.9 (34–36)	64.6–76 (32.5–37.6)	
Mean cell Volume		124–147	118–146		127–150	105–130	189–204	
White cell count	**X10^9/l (%)**	3.8–11.5	3.3–11		3.5–11	4–9.5	3.5–12.1	13.7 ± 2.7
Heterophil	**X10^9/l (%)**	2.6–5.85 (61.68 ± 11.16)	1.4–8.55 (60.95 ± 12.01)	2.31–8.85 (60.42 ± 14.68)	1.65–8.8	3.2–4.03	2.2–9.23	7.8 ± 2.0 (56.5 ± 11.5)
Lymphocyte	**X10^9/l (%)**	0.8–4.25 (31.11 ± 11.46)	1.1–3.3 (32 ± 11.81)	0.48–2.36 (34.37 ± 14.23)	1.1–5.13	1.2–1.56	1.5–5.07	5.5 ± 1.9 (40.3 ± 10.9)
Monocyte	**X10^9/l (%)**	0–0.8 (4.72 ± 3.02)	0.1–0.86 (6.23 ± 3.65)	0.03–0.90 (4.73 ± 3.67)	0–0.9	0–0.5	0–0.48	0.3 ± 0.3 (1.8 ± 2.1)
Eosinophil	**X10^9/l (%)**	0–0.2 (1.12)	0–0.3 (0.52)		0–0.2	0–0.15	0–0.48	0.1 ± 0.1 (1 ± 1)
Basophil	**X10^9/l (%)**	0–0.45 (0.40)	0–0.6 (0.26)		0–0.45	0–0.15	0–0.48	0.1 ± 0.1 (0.6 ± 0.5)

Table 24.4 Hematologic data for harriers and hawks.

Species		Montagu's harrier (*Circus pygargus*) [133]♀♂†	Northern goshawk (*Accipiter gentilis*) [34]	Ferruginous hawk (*Buteo regalis*) [34]	Red-tailed hawk (*Buteo jamaicensis*) [34]	Harris' hawk (*Parabuteo unicinctus*) [34]
Analyte	n = Data Type Units	mean ± SD N = 37 for PCV; N = 14 for the remainder of the hematologic data	Range N = 43	Range N = 18	Range N = 15	Range N = 53
PCV %		33 ± 4	43–53	37–48	35–53	40–55
Red cell count	**X 10^{12}/l**	2.05 ± 0.03	2.6–3.48	2.41–3.59	2.3–3.5	2.63–3.5
Hemoglobin	**g/dl**	12.75 ± 0.98	12.1–17.7	10.7–16.6	12.3–17.5	12.1–17.5
Mean cellular hemoglobin (MCHC)	**Pg**	63.22 ± 7.41	44.5–51.6 (30.5–34.3)	46–57.4 (29.7–34.5)	43–50.4 (31.2–35.0)	45.4–51.1 (30.1–33.0)
Mean cell volume		165.88 ± 25.44	141–156	150–178	123–175	121–171
White cell count	**X10^9/l (%)**	22.69 ± 9.64	4–11	4.5–6.8	3.4–7.5	4.8–10
Heterophil	**X10^9/l (%)**	7.09 ± 4.34	3.5–6.97	1.89–3.76	1.9–3.5	2.3–6.71
Lymphocyte	**X10^9/l (%)**	11.41 ± 3.73	0.3–3.1	1.38–1.93	1.3–2.1	0.6–2.36
Monocyte	**X10^9/l (%)**	0.58 ± 0.35	0–0.1	0.24–1.15	012–1.2	0.2–1.49
Eosinophil	**X10^9/l (%)**	3.63 ± 2.59	0–0.65	0.3–0.7	0.1–0.9	0–0.75
Basophil	**X10^9/l (%)**		0–0.35	0.15–0.6	0–0.5	0–1.55

All data presented as reference range unless denoted † for mean ± SD.

bearded vultures (*Gypaetus barbatus*) and African white-backed vultures (*Gyps africanus*), increased red cell and white cell counts, PCV, and hemoglobin concentration were found in adult birds compared to nestlings [95]. However, red blood cell size decreased in adult birds, reflecting the presence of fewer juvenile cells [95]. No apparent differences in PCV and RBC were found in captive American kestrels with respect to lighting regimens, breeding experience, age, or sex [197]. The PCV of raptors may fluctuate naturally, by as much as 18% in American kestrels [178]. The PCV of wild American kestrels was higher in winter than in spring and fall [101]. Diurnal variation of the PCV and red blood cell count (significantly higher in the morning than in the evening (9 a.m. PCV 42.2% ± 4.71; 9 p.m. PCV 37.7% ± 4.78) also occurs in red-tailed hawks (*Buteo jamaicensis*) [180].

Blood Parasites

Many species of parasite are found in the blood cells of raptors, especially wild and or juvenile birds (Figure 24.4) [171]. *Leucocytozoon, Hemoproteus, Babesia,* and *Plasmodium* species may all be found in circulating blood cells. With the exception of *Plasmodium* spp., these are rarely regarded as pathogenic unless present in large numbers, found in an immunocompromised host (usually a young bird or one with concurrent disease), or there are clinical signs compatible with and referable to hemoparasite infection.

Coagulation Parameters

Coagulation parameters in avian species are difficult to assess based on lack of species-specific reagents. In raptors, the thrombocyte count and morphology can also be considered. A lowered thrombocyte count or recruitment of thrombocytes into an inflammatory response may adversely affect the bird's ability to coagulate. Thrombocytes should be assessed on a fresh blood smear as clumping of these cells may result in a lowered automated count. The most common coagulopathies in raptors relate to hepatic disease and coumarol toxicosis (especially secondary). In owls with secondary anticoagulant rodenticides toxicity, pre-test coagulation times ranged from 0.25 to 3.35 min (0.75 ± 0.10; mean ± SE) [145]. Coagulation times measured three days after treatment for owls that survived were considered within normal range (0.83 ± 0.17; mean ± SE) [145].

White Cell Parameters

The white cell hemogram (leukogram) must interpreted by an experienced hematologist that understands and recognizes species differences in cell morphology;

morphologic changes in cells may indicate inflammation [37]. Cell counts should be reported as absolute counts and as percentage differentials to allow interpretation of relative changes in the leukogram [114]. If the leukogram is interpreted "in house," the clinician must have access to references for cell identification and interpretation of cellular changes [25–27, 38, 88].

Staining preferences and methods vary between laboratories and hematologists: Consistency in staining method is key for consistent interpretation. In the practice laboratory, simple highly repeatable staining methods, for example, differential/Diff-Quik (Polysciences, Pennsylvania, United States) are recommended.

Cell identification, interpretation of counts, and alterations for raptors are similar to those for other avian species [16, 111]. Most raptor species will have higher numbers of heterophils than lymphocytes, though the ratio may be reversed in normal owls [111]. In African white-backed vultures (*G. africanus*), higher white cell counts occurred in nestlings, which might represent stress-related effects [159]. White blood cell total counts over 30 000 cells/dl are often associated with serious disease in raptors such as infection with *Mycobacterium* spp., *Aspergillus* spp., or West Nile virus and indicate a guarded prognosis and the need for aggressive diagnosis and therapy. A stress leukogram, with increased heterophils and monocytes and decreased lymphocytes and eosinophils, has been documented in raptors due to transport and change of environment [163]. Eosinopenia in raptors may be difficult evaluate, as there are normally low numbers of this cell. The stress leukogram may be difficult to distinguish from an inflammatory hemogram, and both may occur simultaneously; however, generally there will not be a monocytosis, and the heterophils will lack toxic change in a stress leukogram.

Heterophil

The heterophil is the avian equivalent of the mammalian neutrophil and is linked with acute and continuing inflammatory reactions. The granules are characteristically rod-shaped but vary in color depending on the species and staining method [Figures 24.5, 24.6, 24.7, 24.8, 24.10] [26]. *Heteropenia* may occur in toxemia/septicemia, bone marrow "exhaustion" and sequestration of heterophils, debility, and viral infections, and it may be related to poor nutritional management in non-owl species if accompanied by eosinopenia [26, 27, 94]. The heterophil count may be inversely related to the eosinophil count in raptors, and an eosinophilia is often accompanied by heteropenia [111]. *Heterophilia* occurs in most inflammatory and infectious responses when the host is able to mount an inflammatory response. The heterophil count will often reflect the severity of the inflammatory response. Toxicosis, neoplasia, and a stress leukogram

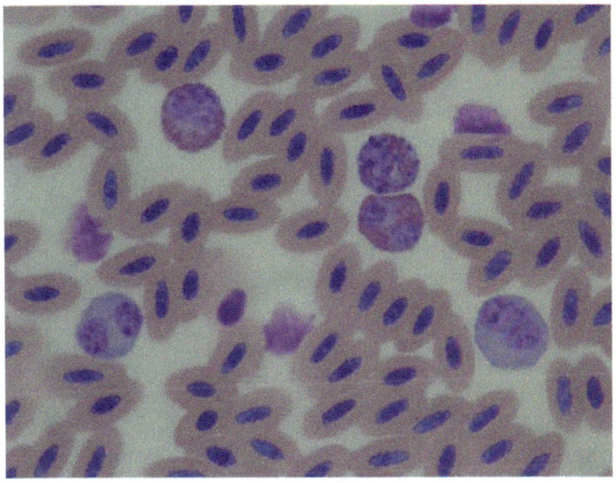

Figure 24.4 Hemoparasites. Species: Harris hawk; Magnification: x1000; Stain: Diff Quick.

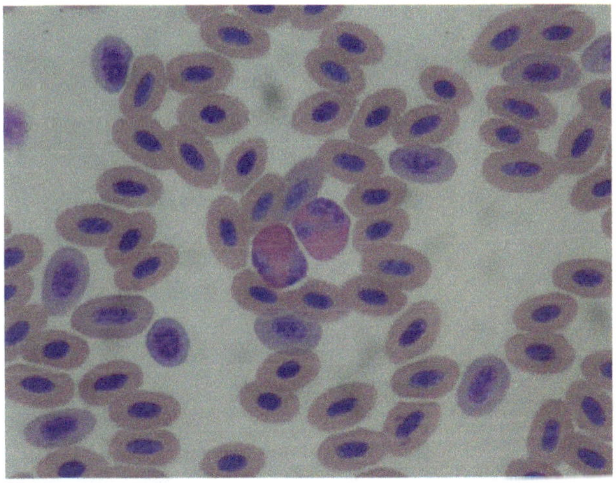

Figure 24.5 Comparison of raptor heterophil (left) and eosinophil (right); note the smaller more rounded granulation of the eosinophil. Species: Harris hawk; Magnification: x1000; Stain: Diff Quick.

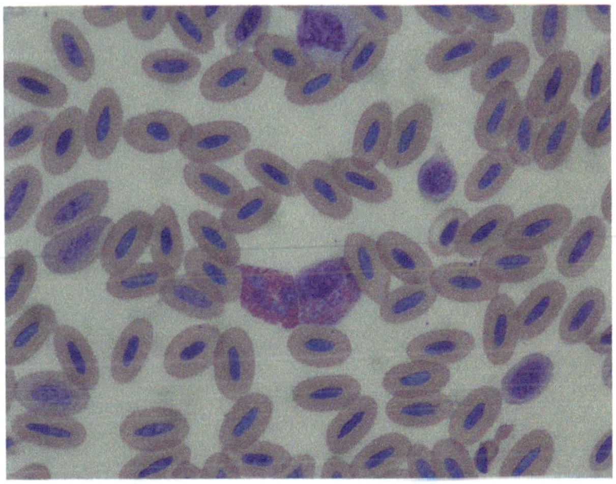

Figure 24.6 Raptor heterophil (middle left) and juvenile heterophil with toxic granulation (middle right). A monocyte (upper middle) and multiple stages of immature RBC are also shown. Species: Harris hawk; Magnification: x1000; Stain: Diff Quick.

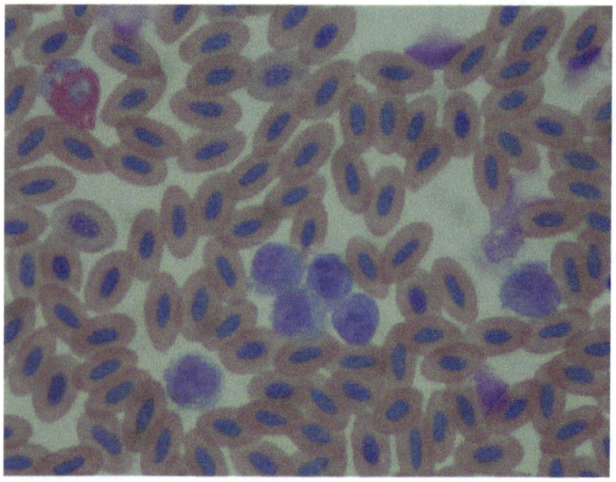

Figure 24.7 WBC raptor heterophils. Species: Harris hawk; Magnification: x1000; Stain: Diff Quick.

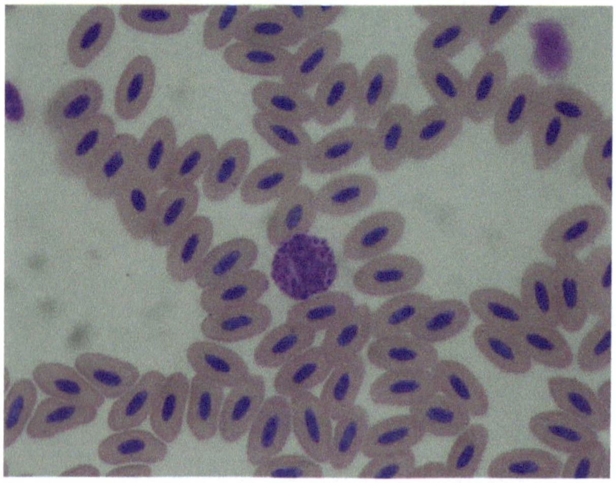

Figure 24.8 WBC raptor eosinophils. Species: Harris hawk; Magnification: x1000; Stain: Diff Quick.

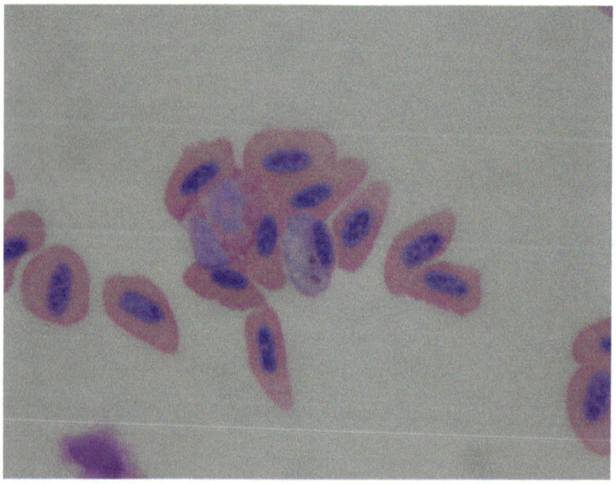

Figure 24.9 WBC raptor mono/lymph thrombocyte. Species: Harris hawk; Magnification: x1000; Stain: Diff Quick.

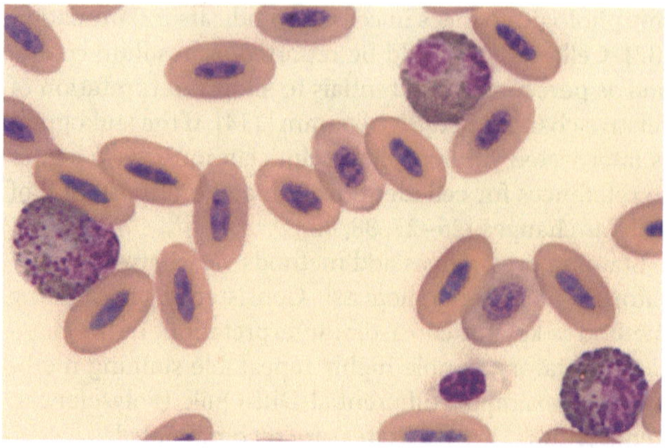

Figure 24.10 Toxic heterophils (upper left, lower right) in the blood smear of a turkey vulture (*Cathartes aura*) that suffered from osteomyelitis.

are also associated with heterophilia. A normal or decreased heterophil count does not exclude an inflammatory process, and assessment of cell morphology is of great importance. Heterophil *toxicity* is characterized by cytoplasmic basophilia, vacuole formation, nuclear degeneration (including chromatin clumping), and degranulation or fusing of granules [26]. It occurs in inflammatory disease as a response to infectious agents and may allow distinction between responses to infection from purely inflammatory disorders (e.g., trauma). A *Left shift* is a release of immature heterophils (band cells) from bone marrow in response to an overwhelming need and carries a guarded prognosis. A left shift has been documented to occur in raptors with mycobacterial disease [206].

Lymphocyte

Lymphocytes are the second most common leukocyte in most raptors after the heterophils; they have a round nucleus with little cytoplasm (Table 24.9). They can be distinguished from the similar thrombocyte by a higher nucleus:cytoplasm ratio and a round as opposed to an ovoid shape [26]. In most raptors, the heterophil is the most common leukocyte, except in most owls (exception Tytonidae spp.), in which the lymphocyte appears to be the most common cell type [111]. *Lymphopenia* is common in raptors. A relative lymphopenia occurs in the presence of heterophilia, while an absolute lymphopenia may occur in certain viral conditions, stress, chronic disease, and in any condition causing bone marrow suppression. *Lymphocytosis* is unusual but may be seen in some inflammatory conditions, and rarely in lymphoproliferative disease. *Reactive lymphocytes* indicate an inflammatory reaction, usually to an infectious agent. In this author's experience, such a finding is rarely found with heterophilia. The finding of reactive lymphocytes does not convey information on diagnosis or prognosis.

Monocyte

Monocytes are large cells that similar to their mammalian equivalent (Figures 24.4, 24.8, 24.9). In the healthy raptor, numbers in the bloodstream are low. *Monocytosis* is associated with chronic inflammatory responses, with increased numbers typifying such infections as aspergillosis and mycobacteriosis. Reactive monocytes may also be found in chronic bacterial disease.

Eosinophil

The eosinophil varies in appearance depending on the species and is morphologically distinguished from the heterophil [134]. Avian eosinophils are characterized by their round, usually red-orange granules, and light blue cytoplasm in Romanowsky-stained blood smears; however, raptor eosinophils may occasionally possess rod-shaped granules, and tinctorial properties may vary even between species [134]. Cytoplasmic staining characteristics and granule shape (rod or round) vary between species. In general, the granules are brighter staining and more numerous than those of the heterophil [26]. Eosinophils are a common cell type in healthy raptors, accounting for 10%–35% of the total white cell count [111, 124]. *Eosinopenia* is challenging to interpret, as finding few to no eosinophils in a sample is common. However, eosinopenia with heteropenia may be linked to poor nutritional management [94]. Severe stress or corticoid administration may cause an eosinopenia [124]. *Eosinophilia* occurs based on the role of the eosinophil in regulating/modulating mast cell activity, that is, in inflammatory conditions of mast cell-rich tissues, especially skin, gastrointestinal tract, lung, and reproductive tract. These include, but are not limited to, parasitic and pox viral infections [111, 114, 151]. Eosinophilia is rare in avian species other than raptors [124]. Toxic changes in eosinophils are also recorded in raptors [94]).

Basophil

The appearance of the basophil is similar to that in other avian species, and their role is likely similar to that in mammals. Numbers of basophils in raptors are usually low or absent. *Basophilia* may occur in inflammatory conditions, particularly in the respiratory tract, based on tissue damage, in conjunction with eosinophilia in intestinal parasitism [25, 111]. A basophil role in hypersensitivity reactions has also been proposed.

Biochemical Panel

Biochemical assays provide insight into the patient's metabolic status, and reference ranges or intervals have been established for a number of birds of prey. For those species without biochemical data, the use of reference ranges for species of a similar genus may be acceptable. Reference ranges for a number of analytes in various raptor species are available in Tables 24.5–24.7.

Many raptor biochemical parameters are influenced by various factors including environment, prey availability, nutritional status, photoperiod, temperature, age, sex, and so on [75, 178, 179, 184, 194, 224]. A study of circadian rhythm on 15 measured blood chemistry values in common buzzards (*Buteo buteo*) and eagle owls (*Bubo bubo*) over a 24 h period found that glucose, uric acid, urea, calcium, and triglyceride had significant diurnal rhythms in both species, while phosphorous, cholesterol, and cholinesterase only varied significantly in buzzards, and albumin: globulin and amylase exhibited diurnal variation exclusively in the eagle owls [75]. Glutamic oxaloacetic transaminase (GOT) (aspartate aminotransferase), albumin, globulin, total protein, and creatinine lacked diurnal variation in either species [75].

Liver Enzymes and Function Tests

The use of hepatic enzyme activity to evaluate liver health or disease in raptors can be difficult because no single enzyme currently assayed arises solely from the liver. Increased hepatic enzyme activities represent hepatocellular damage/leakage, but do not indicate specific etiologies or the degree of liver function compromise. For example, chronic or end-stage liver disease may only minimally increase or even decrease enzyme activity. Interpretation of enzyme activity changes is most accurate when used in conjunction with other tests that evaluate liver function (i.e., bile acids) or directly evaluate hepatic morphology (i.e., hepatic biopsy and histopathology). Additionally, hepatic enzyme activity may be affected by artifactual changes based on sample handling, hemolysis, and lipemia; the extent of this effect has not been specifically studied in raptors.

Aspartate Aminotransferase (AST)

AST is a cytosolic enzyme found in various tissues including liver, heart, kidney, skeletal muscle, and brain. Increased activities of this enzyme may indicate skeletal muscle injury or hepatocellular damage, while decreased concentrations may indicate loss of hepatocellular mass [72]. Despite this lack of specificity, AST is the most appropriate enzyme to evaluate the health of the patient's liver, especially when paired with CK activity, as increased CK activity is indicative of only skeletal muscle damage. AST activities appear to be lower in young raptors compared to adults [111]. In one study, AST activity increased dramatically, peaked on day three, and then returned toward baseline following liver damage (biopsy) in free-ranging raptors [128].

Table 24.5 Biochemical reference ranges for selected hawk, kite, and harrier species.

Species		**Common Buzzard [34, 76] (*Buteo buteo*)**	**Red-tailed hawk [6, 102, 149, 200, 205] (*Buteo jamaicensis*)**	**Harris' hawk [34, 205] (*Parabuteo unicinctus*)**	**Northern goshawk [34, 203] (*Accipiter gentilis*)**	**Montagu's harrier [133] (*Circus pygargus*)**	**Marsh harrier [34, 125] (*Circus aeruginosus*)**	**Black kite [34] (*Milvus migrans*)**
N		**40 Ħ prerelease [76]**	**4 [102] 7 [149] 20 [205] 10 ⊙ Ħ, anesthetized [6] 52⅄ [200]**	**9**	**6–7 [203]**	**32-33 ⅄Ọ̇**	**13, 9♂,4 ♀ ⊙ Ħ**	
Data format		**Range [34] Mean±SD [76]**	**Mean SD [205]**					
Analyte (Abbreviation)	**Units, SI (Conventional)**		**Range [102] Mean SEM [149] Mean SEM [200]**	**Range [34] Mean± SD [205]**	**Mean± SD**	**Mean± SD**	**Mean± SD**	**Range**
Albumin	g/l (g/dl)	5–14 [34] (0.5–1.40) 14.59 ± 1.081 (1.459 ± 0.108) [76] 1.52 ± 0.254 (15.230 ± 2.545 Ӟ [76]	13.4 ± 4.1 (1.34 ± 0.41) [6] 13.0 ± 0.4 (1.3 ± 0.04) [200] 22 ± 5 (2.2 ± 0.5)Ӟ [205]	13.9–17 [34] (1.39–1.7) [34] 20.0 ± 4.0 (2.0 ± 0.4) [205]	8.8–12.4 [34] (0.88–1.24)			6–23 (0.6–2.3)
A:G Ratio			1.2 ± 0.3 [205]	0.46–0.55 [34] 1.4 ± 0.6 [205]	0.4–0.57 [34]			
Alanine aminotransferase (ALT)	U/l (U/l)	0.5–58 [34] 40.4 ± 8.909 [76]	31 ± 5 [6] 38 ± 4.1 [200]		0–44 [34]		41.48 ± 16.94 [125] 35.10 ± 18.15 [125] 18–58 (GPT) [34]	35–60 (GPT) [34]
Alkaline phosphatase (ALP)	U/l (U/l)	35–86 [34] 89.8 ± 27.8 [76]	53 ± 18 [6] 27 ± 1.6 [200]2 45–90	20–96 [34]	15.6–87.5 [34]	1242.45 ± 213		20–100 [34]
Aspartate (AST) aminotransferase	U/l (U/l)	0.5–27 (GOT) [34] 330.9 ± 72.478 [76]	303 ± 22 [6] 113–180 [102] 327 ± 17 [200]	160–348 (GOT) [34]	176–409 [34] 0–31 (GOT) [34] 615 ± 135 [203]		♂310.67 ± 128.5 [125] ♀ 256.40 ± 117.2 [125] 140–440 (GOT) [34]	100–200 [33]
Total bilirubin	µmol/l (mg/dl)	0.684 ± 0.393 (0.040 ± 0.023) [76]	2.736 ± 1.368 (0.16 ± 0.08) [6] 8.55–10.26 (0.5–0.6) [102]					
Blood urea nitrogen (BUN)	mmol/l mg/dl	4.405 ± 1.166 (12.340 ± 3.268) [76]	1.66 ± 0.167 (4.67 ± 0.47) [6] 1.25 ± 0.1 (5.0 ± 0.4) [200]			2.29 ± 1.72 (6.414 ± 4.82)	♂1.97 ± 1.210 (5.52 ± 3.39) [125] ♀2.64 ± 1.428 (7.42 ± 4.00) [125]	
Calcium	mmol/l (mg/dl)	2–2.8 (8–11.2) [34] 2.556 ± 0.218 (10.238 ± 0.874) [76]	1.68–2.5 (8.4–10.0) [102]	2.1–2.66 [34] (8.4–10.64)	2.15–2.69 [34] (8.6–10.76)	2.07 ± 0.3 (8.28 ± 1.2)	♂2.31 ± 0.172 (9.25 ± 0.69) [125] ♀2.48 ± 0.32 (9.95 ± 1.31) [125]	1.8–2.7 [34] (7.2–10.8)

Cholesterol	mmol/l (mg/dl)	4.977 ± 0.746 (192.2 ± 28.836) [76]	2.58–3.87 (100–150) [102] 4.94 ± 0.155 (191 ± 6.0) [200]	6.6–13.1 [34] (254.82–505.8)	4–11.5 [34] (154.44–444.0)	6.08 ± 1.06 (234.75 ± 40.92)	♂15.24 ± 4.656 (588.58 ± 179.78) [125] ♀11.924 ± 3.27 (460.41 ± 126.31) [125]	
Chloride	mmol/l (mEq/l)		125 ± 3 [6]		120 ± 3.4 [203]			
Creatinine	µmol/l (mg/dl)	13.61 ± 8.04 (0.154 ± 0.091) [76]	44.2–106.08 (0.5–1.2) [102]	20.0–59 [34] (0.226–0.667)				
Creatine kinase (CK)	U/l (U/l)	1604.10 ± 649.109 [76]	1124 ± 251 [6] 1948 ± 429 [200]	224–650 [34]	218–775 [34] 3763 ± 1683.8 [203]		643.34 ± 482.30 [125]♂ ♀504.23 ± 189.30 [125]	
Globulin	g/l (g/dl)		24.0 ± 1.0 (2.4 ± 0.1)	21–29.4 [34] (2.1–2.94)	18–29.2 [34] (1.8–29.2)			
Glucose	mmol/l (mg/dl)	19.82 ± 2.51 (357.10 ± 45.217) [76]	19.58 ± 0.88 (356 ± 16) [6] 17.16–22.66 (312–412) [102] 23.32 ± 0.506 (424 ± 9.2) [200]	12.2–15.7 [34] (219.82–282.88)	11.5–15.9 [34] (207.21–286.48) 27.52 ± 5.47 (496 ± 98.6) [203]		♂18.56 ± 2.287 (334.43 ± 41.22) [125] ♀ 17.584 ± 0.288 (316.84 ± 5.20) [125]	
Gamma-glutamyl transferase (GGT)	U/l (U/l)			2–6.9 [34] (2–6.9)	3–7.6 [34] (3–7.6)			
Lactate (LDH) dehydrogenase	U/l (U/l)	2008.40 ± 314.614 (2008.40 ± 314.614) [76]	470–775 [102] 798 ± 107 [200]	160–563 [34] (160–563)	120–906 [34] (120–906)			
Magnesium	mmol/l (mEq/l; mg/dl)	1.159 ± 0.168 (2.319 ± 0.337) [76]			3.8 ± 0.34 (1.9 ± 0.17) [203]			
Phosphorus	mmol /l (mg/dl)	0.652 ± 0.464 (2.020 ± 1.438) [75]	1.013 ± 0.161 (3.14 ± 0.5) [6] 0.58–1.32 (1.8–4.1) [102]	0.8–2.14 [34] (2.47–6.627)	0.8–1.97 [34] (2.477–13.77)	2.09 ± 0.46 (6.47 ± 1.425)		
Potassium	mmol/l (mEq/l)		2.42 ± 0.73 [6]	0.8–2.3 [34] (0.8–2.3)	2.94 ± 1.245 [203]			
Sodium	mmol/l (mEq/l)			155–171 [34] (155–171)	143 ± 2.6 [203]			
Total protein	g/l (g/dl)	33–50 (3.3–5.0) [34] 38.450 ± 5.909 (3.84 ± 0.59) [75]	41.6 ± 6.9(4.16 ± 0.69) [6] 33–45 (3.3–4.5) [102] 36 ± 10.0 (3.5 ± 1.0) [200] 46 ± 10.1(4.6 ± 1.0)ɜ̈ [205]	31–45.7 (3.1–4.57) [34] 37 ± 5.0(3.7 ± 0.5) ɜ̈ [205]	26.3–42 [34] (2.63–4.2)	26.18 ± 2.81 (2.618 ± 0.281)	40.4 ± 8.8 (4.04 ± 0.88) [125]♂ 46.1 ± 16.8 (4.61 ± 1.7) [125]♀ 31–58 [34] (31–58)	30–41 [34] (3.0–4.1)
Triglycerides	mmol/l (mg/dl)	1.314 ± 0.592 (116.40 ± 52.50) [76]				1.84 ± 0.84 (162.97 ± 74.40)		
Uric acid	µmol/l (mg/dl)	448.122 ± 322.560 (7.534 ± 5.429) [76]	644.76 ± 303.35 (10.84 ± 5.1 [postprandial]) [6] 446.1–1058.7(7.5–17.8) [102] 493.68 ± 83.23 (8.3 ± 1.4) [200]	533–785 [34] (8.96–13.2)			♂ 383.65 ± 102.31 (6.45 ± 1.72) [125] ♀475.84 ± 269.444 (8.00 ± 4.53) [125]	

(*Continued*)

Table 24.5 (Continued)

Species		Common Buzzard [34, 76] (*Buteo buteo*)	Red-tailed hawk [6, 102, 149, 200, 205] (*Buteo jamaicensis*)	Harris' hawk [34, 205] (*Parabuteo unicinctus*)	Northern goshawk [34, 203] (*Accipiter gentilis*)	Montagu's harrier [133] (*Circus pygargus*)	Marsh harrier [34, 125] (*Circus aeruginosus*)	Black kite [34] (*Milvus migrans*)
N		40 Ħ prerelease [76]	4 [102] 7 [149] 20 [205] 10 ⊙ Ħ, anesthetized [6] 52ϡ [200]	9	6–7 [203]	32-33 ϡȮ	13, 9♂,4 ♀ ⊙ Ħ	
Data format		Range [34] Mean±SD [76]	Mean SD [205]					
Analyte (Abbreviation)	**Units, SI (Conventional)**		**Range [102] Mean SEM [149] Mean SEM [200]**	**Range [34] Mean± SD [205]**	**Mean± SD**	**Mean± SD**	**Mean± SD**	**Range**
Prealbumin	g/l (g/dl)	1.469 ± 1.751 (0.146 ± 0.175) [76]	17 ± 3.0 (0.17 ± 0.3) [205]	0.8 ± 1.0 (0.08 ± 0.1) [205]				
α_1-globulin		5.939 ± 1.258 (0.593 ± 0.125) [76]	29 ± 2.0 (0.29 ± 0.2) [205]	5.1 ± 4.0 (0.51 ± 0.4) [205]				
α_2-globulin		4.742 ± 2.360 (0.4742 ± 0.236) [76]	6.6 ± 1.0 (0.66 ± 0.1) [205]	5.1 ± 1.0 (0.51 ± 0.1) [205]				
β-globulin		7.525 ± 1.607 (0.752 ± 0.160) [76]	7.7 ± 3.0 (0.77 ± 0.3) [205]	4.3 ± 1.0 (0.43 ± 0.1) [205]				
γ-globulin		3.685 ± 1.75 (0.368 ± 0.175) [76]	4.8 ± 4.0 (0.48 ± 0.4) [205]	1.7 ± 1.0 (0.17 ± 0.1) [205]				
Amylase	U/l (U/l)	626.93 ± 414.19 [76]						
Lipase	U/l (U/l)	26.370 ± 5.144 [76]						
Insulin	pmol /l (μIU/ml)		26.39 ± 2.08 (3.8 ± 0.30) [149]					
Glucagon	ng/l (pg/ml)		198 ± 7.3 [149]					
Insulin:glucagon			0.4399 ± 0.0514 [149]					
Cholinesterase (CHE)	μmol/ml/min		0.66 ± 0.03 [200]					
Acetylcholinesterase (AChE)			0.14 ± 0.01 [200]					
Butyrylcholinesterase (BChE)			0.52 ± 0.02 [200]	Ξe				

KEY –Ȝ – Values determined by electrophoresis.

Table 24.6 Biochemical reference ranges for selected falcon and hybrid falcon species.

	Species	Peregrine falcon [34, 123, 131, 141] (*Falco peregrinus*)	American kestrel (*Falco sparverius*) [52, 200]	Gyrfalcon [130, 160] (*Falco rusticolus*) Ħ	Merlin [34] (*Falco columbarius*)	Saker falcon [34, 129] (*Falco cherrug*) Ħ	Lanner falcon [34] (*Falco biarmicus*)	Gyr x peregrine hybrid [34, 131]	Gyr x saker hybrid [34, 131]
	Data format	[34] Range [123] Mean ± SD [131, 141]95% CI	[52] Mean ± SD [200] Mean ± SEM	[130] 95% CI [160] Mean ± SD [Range]	Range	95% CI	Range 95% CI	Range 95% CI	Range 95% CI
	N, attributes	[123] nestling [141] 79 [131] 127♀ 1–3 y	29–18♀ 11♂ [52] ☞ 91	[52, 130] ♀ 162 67(20 ♂ 47♀)	N ♂,4 ♀	234	N	N	N
Analyte (abbreviation)	**Units, SI (conventional)**								
Albumin	g/l (g/dl)	12.5 ± 0.60 (1.25 ± 0.06) [123] 6.9–14.8 (0.69–1.48) [131] 12.7–22.4 (1.27–2.24) [141]	10 ± 2.0 (1 ± 0.2) [52] 9.0–0.2 (0.9–0.02) [200]	6.6–16.8 (0.66–1.68) [130]	8.6–16.1	5.2–15.0 (0.52–1.5)	9.6–16 [34]	6.8–14.3 (0.68–1.43) [131]	8.0–17.8 (0.8–1.78) [131]
A:G Ratio	na	0.8 ± 0.03 [123] 0.8–2.4	0.9 ± 0.4 [200]		0.47–0.58 [34]		0.44–0.57 [34]		
Alanine aminotransferase (ALT)	U/l (U/l)	29–90 [34] 124 ± 69 [131]	52 ± 3.4 [200] 41 ± 33.3 [52]	32–589 [130]		36–55 [34] 29–362 [129]		29–429 [131]	28–393 [131]
Alkaline phosphatase (ALP)	U/l (U/l)	31–121 [34] 135–596 [131] 31–121	242 ± 12 [200] 232 ± 71.7 [52]	3–982 [130]	54–310 [34]	285–450 [34] 86–842	180–510 [34]	116–705 [131]	67–879 [131]
Aspartate aminotransferase (AST)	U/l (U/l)	34–162 [34] 107 ± 71 [131]	98 ± 7.6[f] [200] 77 ± 29.2 [52]	44–471 [130]	50–125 [34]	45–95 [34] 40–358 [129]	30–118 [34]	44–469 [131]	40–544 [131]
Bile acids	µmol/l (µg/dl)	5–69 (2.04–28.16) [141]		35.40 ± 14.06; [5.41–68] [160] (14.46 ± 5.74 [2.20–27.77]) [160]		20–90 (8.16–36.76) [34] 1.7–13.3 (0.69–5.43) [34]			
Bilirubin (total)	µmol/l (mg/dl)	3.5–14.0 (0.205–0.818) [131]	6.84 ± 5.13 (0.4 ± 0.3) [52]						
Blood urea nitrogen (BUN)	mmol /l mg/dl	3.5 ± 2.1 (9.80 ± 5.88) [131] 0.34–9.0 (1.09–25.21) [131] 0.8–3.9 (2.24–10.92) [141]	2.142 ± 0.78 (6.0 ± 2.2) [52] 2.64 ± 0.142 (7.4 ± 0.4) [201]	0–9.5 (0–26.6) [130]		0.5–2.6 (1.4–7.28) [34] 0–8.3 (0–23.24) [129]	1.3–2.7 (3.64–7.56) [34]	0.3–7.8 (0.84–21.85) [131]	0–9.5 (0–26.61) [131]

(*Continued*)

Table 24.6 (Continued)

Analyte (abbreviation)	Species / Data format / N, attributes / Units, SI (conventional)	Peregrine falcon [34, 123, 131, 141] (*Falco peregrinus*)	American kestrel (*Falco sparverius*) [52, 200]	Gyrfalcon [130, 160] (*Falco rusticolus*) Ħ	Merlin [34] (*Falco columbarius*)	Saker falcon [34, 129] (*Falco cherrug*) Ħ	Lanner falcon [34] (*Falco biarmicus*)	Gyr x peregrine hybrid [34, 131]	Gyr x saker hybrid [34, 131]
	Data format	[34] Range [123] Mean ± SD [131, 141]95% CI	[52] Mean ± SD [200] Mean ± SEM	[130] 95% CI [160] Mean ± SD [Range]	Range	95% CI	Range 95% CI	Range 95% CI	Range 95% CI
	N, attributes	[123] nestling [141] 79 [131] 127♀ 1–3 y	29–18♀ 11♂ [52] ☞ 91	[52, 130] ♀ 162 67(20 ♂ 47♀)	N ♂,4 ♀	234	N	N	N
Analyte (abbreviation)	**Units, SI (conventional)**								
Calcium	mmol/l (mg/dl)	1.94–2.54 (7.76–10.16 [131] 1.97–2.46 (7.88–9.84; corrected for protein) [141]	1.77 ± 0.2 (7.1 ± 0.8) 1.97 ± 0.025 (7.9 ± 0.1)	1.98–3.48 (7.92–13.92)	2–2.45 (8–9.8) [34]	2.15–2.61 (8.6–10.44) [34] 1.97–2.77 (7.88–11.08) [129]	2.07–2.45 (8.28–9.8) [34]	1.88–2.58 (7.52–10.32) [131]	1.95–3.12 (7.8–12.48) [131]
Cholesterol	mmol/l (mg/dl)	3.18–9.07 (122.77–350.19)	5.93 ± 1.75 (229 ± 67.6) [52] 7.17 ± 0.19) (277 ± 7.7)	3.42–7.12 (132.04–274.9)	3–7.8 (115.83–301.15) [34]	4.5–8.6 (173.74–332.04) [34] 3.43–7.53 (132.43–291.11) [129]	3–8.8 (115.83–339.8) [34]	3.06–7.71 (118.14–286.1) [131]	2.77–10.05 (106.95–388.03) [131]
Chloride	mmol/l (mEq/l)	109–132 [131] 114–131	108 ± 33 [52]	117–144		114–125 [129]		114–159 [131]	114–163 [131]
Creatinine	μmol/l (mg/dl)	12–64 (0.135–0.72) [131]	26.52 ± 8.84 (0.3 ± 0.1) [52]	14–73 (0.15–0.82)	16–50 (0.18–0.56) [34]	23–75 (0.26–0.85) [34] 11–64 (0.12–0.72) [130]	37–75 (0.42–0.85) [34]	16–73 (0.34–0.82) [131]	13–75 (0.14–0.85) [131]
Creatine kinase (CK)	U/l (U/l)	120–442	1739 ± 733.7 [52] 891 ± 37		521–807 [34]	355–651 [34]	350–650 [34]		
Glutamate dehydrogenase (GLDH)	U/l (U/l)	<8							
Globulin	g/l (g/dl)		12 ± 4.0 (1.2 ± 0.4) [52] 22.0 ± 1.0 (2.2 ± 0.1)		17.2–25 (1.72–2.5) [34]	18–28 (1.8–2.8) [34]	21.2–21.8 (2.12–2.18) [34]		
Glucose	mmol/l (mg/dl)	17.9–28.7(322.52–517.11) [131] 16.5–22 (297.23–396.39)	16.92 ± 2.19 (305 ± 39.5) [52] 23.75 ± 0.371 (428 ± 6.7)	17.4–23.9 (313.51–430.63)	9–12 (162.16–216.2) [34]	12–14 (216.21–252.25) [34] 17.0–25.4 (306.30–457.65) [129]	11–15 (198.2–270.27) [34]	18.2–26.3 (327–473.87) [131]	17.8–26.1 (0.98–470.27) [131]

Gamma-glutamyl transferase (GGT)	U/l (U/l)	0–3				0.8–5.9 [34]			
Iron	μmol/l (μg/dl)	9.84–17.17 (59.94–95.86) [131]		10.75–32.53 (60.02–181.63)					
Lactate dehydrogenase (LDH)	U/l (U/l)	721–3899 [131] 108–2650	798 ± 28	870–3871	320–630 [34]	551–765 [34] 664–3852 [129]	434–897 [34]	544–3595 [131]	622–3720 [131]
Magnesium	mmol/l (mg/dl)	0.61 ± 0.11 (1.48 ± 0.26)		0.34–1.21 (0.87–2.94)		0.47–1.01 (1.14–2.48)		0.43–0.83 (1.04–2.02) [131]	0.41–1.10 (0.99–2.67) [131]
Phosphorus	mmol/l (mg/dl)	0.87–1.88 (2.64–5.82) [131] 0.55–1.53 (1.70–4.73) [141]	0.96 ± 0.29 (3 ± 0.9) [52] 0.77 ± 0.032 (2.4 ± 0.1)	0.45–2.89 (1.4–8.95)		0.81–2.08 (2.51–6.44) [129]		0.66–2.21 (2.04–6.84) [131]	0.78–2.38 (2.41–7.37) [131]
Potassium	mmol/l (mEq/l)	1.8–5.1 [131]	2.2 ± 0.7 [52] 6.9 ± 0	1.9–4.9 [130]	1–1.8 [34]	0.8–2.3 [34] 1.6–4.7 [129]	1–2.1 [34]	1.6–4.7 [131]	1.8–4.9 [131]
Sodium	mmol/l (mEq/l)	147–175 [131] 150–170	158 ± 3.2 [52] 158 ± 0.6 [200]	125–178 [130]	155–170 [34]	154–161 [34]	152–164 [34]	135–199 [131]	146–195 [131]
Total protein	g/l (g/dl)	37.9 ± 1.8) (3.79 ± 0.18) [123] 16.0–38.9 (1.6–3.89) [131] 24–39 (2.4–3.9) [141]	22.0 ± 4.0 (2.2 ± 0.4) [52] 31 ± 1.0 (3.1 ± 0.1) [200]	4.5–46.2 (0.45–4.62) [130]	27.5–39 (2.75–3.9) [34]	27–366 (2.7–36.6) [34] 6.85–44.6 (0.685–4.46) [129]	33–42 (3.3–4.2) [34]	4.7–40.2 (0.47–4.02) [131]	5.0–46.7 (0.5–4.67) [131]
Triglycerides	mmol/l (mg/dl)	0.37–1.41 (32.77–124.89) [131]		10.51–1.65 (45.17–146.14) [130]		0.48–2.31 (42.51–204.60) [129]		0.66–1.86 (58.45–164.74) [131]	0.55–2.03 (48.71–179.80) [131]
Uric acid	μmol/l (mg/dl)	170–1250 (2.85–21.01) [131] 253–995 (4.25–16.73) [141]	535.32 ± 344 98 (9.0 ± 5.8) [52] 1100.38 ± 65 42 (18.5 ± 1.1) [200]	80–690 (1.34–11.6) [130]	174–800 (2.92–13.44) [34]	320–785 (5.37–13.2) [34] 110–1260 (1.84–21.2) [129]		120–1740 (2.02–29.25) [131]	100–1180 (1.68–19.83) [131]
Prealbumin	g/l (g/dl)	3.1 ± 0.4 (0.31 ± 0.04) [123]							
α-1		2.3 ± 0.2 (0.23 ± 0.02) [123]							
α-2		1.6 ± 0.2 (0.16 ± 0.02) [123]							
β		10.2 ± 0.5 (1.02 ± 0.05) [123]							
γ		6.0 ± 0.8 (0.60 ± 0.08) [122]							
Amylase	U/l (U/l)	3–834 [131]							
Cholinesterase (CHE)	IU/l	1184.00 ± 74.99 [123]							
Cholinesterase (CHE)	μmol/ml/min		1.9 ± 0.05 [200]						
Acetylcholinesterase (AChE)			1.6 ± 0.05 [200]						
Butyrylcholinesterase (BChE)			0.26 ± 0.01 [200]						

Table 24.7 Biochemical reference data for select eagle species.

	Species	Bald eagle [50, 104, 144, 148, 205] (*Haliaeetus leucocephalus*)	Golden eagle [161, 170] (*Aquila chrysaetos*) ₪	Tawny eagle [34] (*Aquila rapax*)	White-tailed sea eagle [34] (*Haliaeetus albicilla*)	Spanish imperial eagle [74, 170] (*Aquila adalberti*)
	Data	Mean ± SEM [50, 148] Mean ± SD [104, 144, 205] [Reference interval] [104]	Mean ± SEM [161] Mean ± SD [170]	Range	Range	Mean ± SD, 12 (6 ♂ 6 ♀) Ħ ₪
	N, Attributes	41 (23 ♂ 18 ♀) Ħ, ₪t [104] 42–151 Ó, 35–45 d [144] 14 convalescing (9 ♂, 5 ♀) [148] 46 [205] 20 [50]	21 (12 ♂ 9 ♀) [161] 5 [170]			12 (6 ♂ 6 ♀) Ħ ₪
Analyte (abbreviation)	**Units (SI) (conventional)**					
Albumin	g/l (g/dl)	15.7 ± 2.6; 11.09–20.5 (1.57 ± 0.26; 1.09–2.05) Ӛ [102] 14.8 ± 4.3 (1.48 ± 0.43) [144] 16.0 ± 2.0 (1.6 ± 0.2) Ӛ [205]	20.46 ± 0.79 (2.05 ± 0.08) [161] 9.5 ± 0.8 (0.95 ± 0.08) [170]	11.1–13.5 (1.11–1.35) [34]		10.7 ± 2.5 (1.07 ± 0.25) [74] 12.95 ± 2.44 (1.30 ± 0.24) [170]
A:G Ratio	na	0.98 ± 0.21; 0.57–1.59 [104] 1.0 ± 0.3 [205]	0.84 ± 0.08 [173]	0.44–0.55 [34]		0.97 ± 0.28 [74] 1.9 ± 0.3 [170]
Alanine aminotransferase (ALT)	U/l (U/l)	17.11 ± 7.41 [144]	28.21 ± 2.36 [161] 13.9 ± 4.4 [170]		0–30 [34]	12.1 ± 3.6 [74]
Alkaline phosphatase (ALP)	U/l (U/l)	147.57 ± 51.96 [104]	67.31 ± 5.29 [161] 86.2 ± 62.7 [170]	17.1–69.7 [34]	7–76 [34]	91.7 ± 54.3 [74]
Aspartate aminotransferase (AST)	U/l (U/l)	352 ± 171; 131–956 [104] 132.73 ± 48.04 [144]	293.24 ± 18.96 [161] 62.6 ± 7.2 [170]		30–160 [34]	93.1 ± 32.8 [76] 278 ± 65 [72]
Bile acids	µmol/l (µg/dl)					36.5 ± 3.2 (14.3 ± 1.3) [74]
Bilirubin	µmol/l (mg/dl)	21.375 ± 18.13 (1.24 ± 1.06) [144]				
Blood urea nitrogen (BUN)	mmol/l (mg/dl)	4.78 ± 3.85 (13.41 ± 10.79) [144]	2.74 ± 0.17 (7.67 ± 0.47) [161]	0.8–2.7 (2.24–7.556) [34]		
Calcium	mmol/l (mg/dl)	2.325 ± 0.125; 2.05–2.6 (9.3 ± 0.5; 8.2–10.4) [104] 2.34 ± 0.556 (9.39 ± 2.24) [144]	2.37 ± 0.24 (9.48 ± 0.96) [161] 2.7 ± 0.2 (9.08 ± 0.05) [170]	2.21–2.66 (8.84–10.64) [34]		2.2 ± 0.1 (8.8 ± 0.4) [170] 2.96 ± 0.42 (11.9 ± 1.7) [74]

Cholesterol	mmol/l (mg/dl)		2.14 ± 0.09 (82.62 ± 3.47) [161] 4.8 ± 0.3 (185.33 ± 11.58) [169]	7.9–10.7 (305.01–413.13) [34]		5.8 ± 0.7 (223.93 ± 27.03) [173] 5.39 ± 0.56 (208 ± 22) [74]
Chloride	mmol/l (mEq/l)	104.98 ± 10.11 [144]	107.4 ± 4.0 [170]	114–123 [34]		104.3 ± 5.5 [170]
Creatinine	mmol/l (mg/dl)		53.27 ± 3.87 (0.60 ± 0.04) [161]	31–59 (0.35–0.66) [34]		81.4 ± 29.2 (0.92 ± 0.33) [170]
Creatine kinase (CK)	U/l (U/l)	714 ± 421; 190–1797 [104] 1268.71 ± 557.69 [144]	411.29 ± 58.37 [161] 150 ± 73 [170]			213 ± 116 [170] 288 ± 119 [74]
Globulin	g/l (g/dl)	3.6 ± 0.8; 1.9–5.9 (0.36 ± 0.08; 0.19–0.59) [104]		25.3–28.4 (2.53–2.84) [34]		
Glucose	mmol/l (mg/dl)	17.538 ± 2.331; 13.59–23.92 (316 ± 42; 245–431) [104] 12.38 ± 1.52 (223.03 ± 27.37) [144]	16.42 ± 0.73 (295.85 ± 13.15) [161] 16.8 ± 1.6 (302.70 ± 28.82) [170]	10.2–14.5 (183.78–261.26) [34]		19.5 ± 3.1 (351.35 ± 55.85) [170] 15.5 ± 1.0 (279 ± 18) [74]
Gamma-glutamyl transferase (GGT)	U/l (U/l)			1.0–2.7 [34]		
Lactate dehydrogenase (LDH)	U/l (U/l)	2547.63 ± 965.22 [144]	1209.89 ± 21.73 [161] 471 ± 132 [170]	211–369 [34]		394 ± 113 [170] 713 ± 166 [74]
Magnesium	mmol/l (mEq/l; mg/dl)		0.88 ± 0.21 (2.14 ± 0.51) [170]			0.67 ± 0.04 (1.62 ± 0.09) [170]
Phosphorus	mmol /l (mg/dl)	2.04 ± 0.42 (6.31 ± 1.3) [144]	1.73 ± 0.08 (5.35 ± 0.247) [161] 4.7 ± 0.4 (14.55 ± 1.23) [170]			5.8 ± 0.5 (17.96 ± 1.54) [169] 1.5 ± 0.31 (4.64 ± 0.96) [74]
Potassium	mmol/l (mEq/l)	4.28 ± 1.82 [144]	2.2 ± 0.9 [170]	1.5–3.1 [34]		1.8 ± 0.4 [170] 3.4 ± 1.2 [74]
Sodium	mmol/l (mEq/l)	135.85 ± 11.13 [144]	162 ± 7.8 170	153–157 [34]		159.5 ± 4.6 [173] 154 ± 5 [74]
Total protein	g/l (g/dl)	34.0 ± 5.0; 22–46 (3.4 ± 0.5; 2.2–4.6) [104] 32.8 ± 9.8 (3.28 ± 0.98) [144] 35 ± 5.0 (3.5 ± 0.53) [205]	49.76 ± 1.35 (4.98 ± 0.135) [161] 33 ± 2 (3.3 ± 0.2) [170]	29–41.4 (2.9–4.14) [34]	28–45 (2.8–4.5) [34]	38 ± 4 (3.8 ± 0.4) [170] 36 ± 3.29 (3.6 ± 0.33) [74]
Triglycerides	mmol/l (mg/dl)		2.04 ± 0.08 (180.6 ± 7.08) [161] 0.64 ± 0.17 (56.68 ± 15.06) [170]			0.75 ± 0.18 (66.43 ± 15.94) [170] 2.36 ± 1.02 (209 ± 90) [74]
Uric acid	μmol/l (mg/dl)	327.14 ± 202.23; 107.06–910.04 (5.5 ± 3.4; 1.8–15.3) [104] 800.61 ± 349.74 (13.46 ± 5.88) [144]	457.67 ± 97.46 (7.69 ± 1.63) [161] 345 ± 147 (5.8 ± 2.47) [170]	413–576 (6.94–9.68) [34]		223 ± 114 (3.74 ± 1.91) [170] 183 ± 106 (3.07 ± 1.78) [74]

(Continued)

Table 24.7 (Continued)

	Species	Bald eagle [50, 104, 144, 148, 205] (*Haliaeetus leucocephalus*)	Golden eagle [161, 170] (*Aquila chrysaetos*) ₪	Tawny eagle [34] (*Aquila rapax*)	White-tailed sea eagle [34] (*Haliaeetus albicilla*)	Spanish imperial eagle [74, 170] (*Aquila adalberti*)
	Data	**Mean ± SEM [50, 148] Mean ± SD [104, 144, 205] [Reference interval] [104]**	**Mean ± SEM [161] Mean ± SD [170]**	**Range**	**Range**	**Mean ± SD, 12 (6 ♂ 6 ♀) Ħ ₪**
	N, Attributes	**41 (23 ♂ 18 ♀) Ħ, ₪t [104] 42–151 Ó, 35–45 d [144] 14 convalescing (9 ♂, 5 ♀) [148] 46 [205] 20 [50]**	**21 (12 ♂ 9 ♀) [161] 5 [170]**			**12 (6 ♂ 6 ♀) Ħ ₪**
Analyte (abbreviation)	**Units (SI) (conventional)**					
Prealbumin	g/l (g/dl)	0.7 ± 0.9; 0–2.9 (0.07 ± 0.09; 0–0.29) 104 1.4 ± 1.0 (0.14 ± 0.1) 205	5.1 ± 0.7 (0.51 ± 0.07)			7.1 ± 1.8 (0.71 ± 0.018) 170 8.97 ± 0.95 (0.9 ± 0.10) 74
α-globulin	g/l (g/dl)		4.5 ± 1.2 (0.45 ± 0.012) [170]			7.1 ± 3.1 (0.71 ± 0.31) [170]
α-1 globulin	g/l (g/dl)	1.4 ± 0.4; 0.6–2.1 (0.14 ± 0.04; 0.06–0.21) [104] 4.3 ± 2.0 (0.43 ± 0.2) [205]				
α-2 globulin	g/l (g/dl)	4.7 ± 0.8; 3.2–0.68 (0.47 ± 0.08; 0.32–0.068) [104] 4.9 ± 2.0 (0.49 ± 0.2) [205]				
β-globulin	g/l (g/dl)	7.0 ± 1.9; 4.2–13.9 (0.70 ± 0.19; 0.42–1.39) [104] 5.4 ± 2.0 (0.54 ± 0.2) [206]	10.3 ± 1.39 (1.03 ± 0.14) [170]			9.2 ± 3.0 (0.92 ± 0.30) [170] 4.35 ± 1.03 (0.44 ± 0.10) [74]
γ-globulin	g/l (g/dl)	3.6 ± 0.8; 1.9–5.9 (0.36 ± 0.08;0.19–0.59) 104 3.4 ± 1.0 (0.34 ± 0.1) [205]	2.3 ± 0.4 (0.23 ± 0.04) [170]			2.9 ± 0.4 (0.29 ± 0.04) [170] 1.78 ± 0.51 (0.18 ± 0.05) [74]
Amylase	(U/l)					545 ± 242 [170]
Insulin	pmol/l (μIU/ml; mU/l; μg/ml))	9.86 ± 37.78 (1.42 ± 5.44; μIU m/l) [148]				
Glucagon	ng/l (pg/ml)	534 ± 53.9 [148]				
Insulin:glucagon		0.1823 ± 0.0235 [148]				
Cholinesterase	IU/l	663 ± 32[a] 1290 ± 310 [144]				1241 ± 319 [74]

ȝ electrophoresis.

Alanine Aminotransferase (ALT)

ALT is a cytosolic enzyme found in several tissues (liver, kidney, heart, skeletal muscle, lung, and intestine) [96, 136] in birds that is not a useful indicator of liver damage in avian species. Seasonal variation in ALT may occur in raptors independent of reproductive activity [111].

Alkaline Phosphatase (ALP)

ALP occurs in several tissues including kidney, intestine (duodenum), and liver (biliary epithelium) and is associated with osteoblastic activity in bone [87]. Young raptors, or those with nutritional or secondary nutritional hyperparathyroidism, have increased enzyme activity [111]. ALP concentrations gradually increased following liver biopsy in free-ranging raptors [128].

Glutamate Dehydrogenase (GLDH)

Although considered the most specific enzyme indicator of liver disease, GLDH has low sensitivity in avian species [72, 96]. Activity of GLDH increased dramatically and peaked on day three following liver biopsy in wild raptors [128].

Lactate Dehydrogenase

Activities of lactate dehydrogense (LDH) are neither sensitive nor specific for liver disease in birds and occurs in most tissues including skeletal muscle, cardiac muscle, liver, bone, and kidney. Activity of LDH has been used to evaluate muscle fitness or damage in raptors. Following flight training, baseline and peak plasma activities of LDH and CK in red-tailed hawks were affected by flight status in flight-trained, untrained, and disabled raptors [118]. In most hawks, LDH peaked 24 h post exercise and declined gradually during the subsequent 48 h [118]. Hawks that were flight-trained had the lowest basal LDH activity of the groups with a 9% decrease in LDH activity 24 h post exercise, while LDH activity was greater in untrained (156%) and disabled (63%) birds 24 h post exercise [118].

Bile Acids

Values for plasma or serum bile acids (BA) are more useful than hepatic enzymes for evaluating liver function as a sensitive and specific indicator of liver disease/dysfunction. A fast of 12–24 h is recommended prior to BA testing based on varying crop emptying times in raptors [87]. A postprandial rise in BAs in peregrine falcons suggest that blood samples should be obtained following a 24 h fast to avoid postprandial increased concentrations which may complicate interpretation. Normal plasma BA values in peregrine falcons (*Falco peregrinus*), gyrfalcons (*Falco rusticolus*), and saker falcons (*Falco cherrug*) are presented in Table 24.6.

Bilirubin and Biliverdin

Bile pigments, such as bilirubin and biliverdin, are of minimal diagnostic use in birds, which lack significant levels of hepatic biliverdin reductase for conversion of biliverdin to bilirubin [87, 152, 212]. Bacteria within the GI tract may produce biliverdin reductase and convert biliverdin to bilirubin, which can then be absorbed from the GI tract [87]. Bilirubin occurs only in scant concentrations, and biliverdin is undetectable in avian (chicken) plasma [72].

Muscle Enzymes

Creatine Kinase (CK)

CK is found in skeletal muscles, cardiac muscle, smooth muscle of the gastrointestinal tract, and the brain. Increased plasma concentrations of CK in birds of prey are associated with trauma (including surgical intervention), excessive exercise, intramuscular injections, capture myopathy, myositis, nutritional myopathies (i.e., vitamin E/selenium deficiency), ischemia, seizures, hyperthermia, hypothermia, heavy metal toxicity, and sample hemolysis [87, 223]. Concentrations of CK peak within 6–12 h following muscle damage or necrosis, then return to baseline concentrations 72–96 h post insult [87, 137, 223]. LDH and CK have been used as diagnostic indicators of muscle fitness and damage in mammals and has been studied in birds of prey. The effect of exercise on plasma activity of CK in red-tailed hawks was evaluated following a standardized flight training session. Baseline and peak enzyme activity of CK were affected by flight status (trained, untrained, and disabled hawks) [118]. LDH and CK peaked 24 h post exercise and declined during the next 48 h [118]. Hawks that were flight-trained demonstrated a slight decrease in LDH activity (9%) below the baseline and a moderate increase in CK activity (57%) above baseline compared to disabled and untrained hawks [118]. In the latter, LDH and CK concentrations increased 63 and 1450%, respectively, in disabled birds and increased 156% and 731%, respectively, in untrained hawks 24 h after exercise [118]. Activities of up to 1000 mg/dl may be considered normal in flight-trained raptors [31, 118].

Lactate

Lactate is produced during high-energy exercise and muscle exertion and has been used as a measure of fitness and performance in raptors, especially those that are being rehabilitated for release [31, 80]. Blood lactate concentrations were measured for 10 min following a standardized indoor flight exercise regimen in red-tailed hawks, rough-legged hawks (*Buteo lagopus*), and great horned owls (*Bubo virginianus*) to determine if lactate concentrations post exercise indicated flight fitness and if blood lactate and post-exercise respiratory rate were correlated [31]. Blood lactate concentrations peaked at 100–120 mg/dl post exercise and gradually decreased to or below preflight lactate concentrations of 50–80 mg/dl within 10 min in well-conditioned raptors [31]. In unconditioned raptors, lactate concentrations peaked at greater than 200 mg/dl 2 min after exercise, and recovery was not complete for 15 min post exercise [31]. Furthermore, in the well-conditioned raptors, 10 min lactate concentrations (30–50 mg/dl) reflected basal lactate concentration indicative of recovery from exercise [31].

Renal Analytes

Blood Urea Nitrogen (BUN)

BUN concentrations are typically low to undetectable in raptors by most laboratory methods used for avian species. In well-hydrated birds, most of the urea is excreted, whereas most urea is reabsorbed in dehydrated birds [96]. Because urea concentrations in avian plasma are often <2 mg/dl, its usefulness for assessing renal or hepatic disease in raptors is questionable [167]. Prudence dictates evaluation of trends in BUN concentrations rather than a single value. Increased BUN concentrations may indicate prerenal insufficiency (hemorrhage, diarrhea, dehydration), postrenal insufficiency following excessive intake of protein, or a normal postprandial increase [223]. In peregrine falcons (*F. peregrinus*), postprandial increases in plasma uric acid and urea concentrations may occur for up to 15 h following a meal [139]. Peak concentrations of urea (up to 3.1 mmol/l; 1.31 mg/dl) were noted 8 h postprandially [139].

Creatinine

Creatinine is of little value when assessing renal function in birds. Increased creatinine concentrations have not been associated with renal disease in raptors. In peregrine falcons, postprandial creatinine concentrations did not increase significantly from baseline [4, 139].

Uric Acid (UA)

Raptors are uricotelic, and UA is the major end product of protein catabolism. UA is produced in the liver and is mainly secreted in the proximal convoluted tubule in the healthy raptor and excreted along with the urates and feces in the stool independent of hydration. A small amount (~10%) undergoes glomerular filtration [167]. In some species, UA may be retropulsed into the rectum and ceca, where it can be broken down by bacteria into volatile fatty acids and ammonia [19, 87]. The fatty acids are absorbed by the GI tract (ceca in those species with ceca), and the ammonia is involved in the production of glutamine [19]; however, the extent to which this occurs in raptors is questionable. In bald eagles (*Haliaeetus leucocephalus*) the retropulsion of urine into the lower GI tract does not occur to the extent that it does in Galliformes, Psittaciformes, and other avian species [106].

Conditions marked by increased UA concentrations in raptors include renal disease (if renal function is impaired ≥70%), severe dehydration, high-protein diets, starvation, severe tissue damage and necrosis, heavy metal (lead) toxicosis, urinary obstruction, nephritis, nephrocalcinosis, hypovitaminosis-A-induced damage to renal tubular epithelium, and ovulation [136, 139, 167, 223]. Falconry birds undergoing weight management may experience increased UA concentrations until their weight is brought to a more normal state [111]. Administration of nephrotoxic drugs (i.e., aminoglycosides) may also cause hyperuricemia in raptors [10, 62]. Marked postprandial increases in UA occur and can be quite high in birds of prey. A significant postprandial increase in plasma UA concentrations was observed in peregrine falcons with peak concentrations (up to 1881 µmol/l [31.62 mg/dl]) occurring 3 to 8 h postprandially [139]. Concentrations may be increased for up to 15 h following a meal in peregrine falcons [139]. This author (MPJ) has noted a postprandial increase in UA concentrations up to 34.2 mg/dl (2034 µmol/l) approximately 12 h following a meal in a bald eagle. Interestingly, this physiologic hyperuricemia does not result in articular or visceral gout even though postprandial increases are similar to birds, with hyperuricemia associated with gout [111, 139]; however, persistent increases in UA should be further evaluated. Assess renal function in peregrine falcons and other raptors after a 24 h fast to differentiate between postprandial increases in UA and urea or renal induced hyperuricemia [139]. Since UA is produced in the liver, hypouricemia may suggest hepatic insufficiency [96].

Cardiac and Gastrointestinal Biomarkers

Biomarkers specific for cardiac and gastrointestinal disease of raptors have been minimally investigated and reference data yet to be reported. However cardiac disease is not uncommon among raptor species [12, 40, 117]. In a case of Cardiomyopathy and Right-sided Congestive Heart Failure in a Red-tailed Hawk (Buteo jamaicensis) cardiotroponins levels given as range of normal animals [clinical case], measured in plasma via iSTAT (0.00 [0.03]) and serum via ELISA (0.01-0.14 [0.40]), although higher than those of normal animals were considered normal or nondiagnostic.

Pancreas

Insulin and Glucagon – Carbohydrate metabolism may be more insulin dependent in raptors than in other omnivorous or granivorous avian species [149, 218]. Carbohydrates are a small percentage (2%) of the diet of raptors; the remainder of the diet consists primarily of fats (2%–28%) and proteins (17%–20%) [110]. Insulin, glucagon, and Insulin: Glucagon (I/G) ratios in red-tailed hawks fasted for 24h [149] and in bald eagles [148] are reported. In red-tailed hawks, plasma concentrations (mean ± SE) of insulin, glucagon, and I/G ratios prior to administration of 40ml of either saline, 10% amino acid solution, 20% fatty acid solution, or 50ml of saline blended with one whole mouse were 3.8 ± 0.30 μUnits/ml, 198 ± 7.3 pg/ml, and 0.4399 ± 0.0514, respectively [149]. In another study in fasted bald eagles [148], plasma insulin concentrations ranged from 64 to 245 pg/ml (1.42–5.44 μUnits/ml) (132 ± 10.7 pg/ml) and appeared to be higher in males, plasma glucagon concentrations ranged from 229 to 1239 pg/ml (534 ± 53.9) and tended to be higher in females, and plasma I:G varied from 0.0389 to 0.4691 mg/dl (0.1823 ± 0.0235) and appeared to be lowest in female eagles [148].

Decreased insulin concentrations are likely associated with diabetes mellitus or refeeding syndrome in birds [89]. Acute or chronic infectious diseases such as avian influenza [82], Chlamydia [150], mycobacteriosis [206] herpesvirus [226] adenovirus [193], and West Nile virus [59] can affect pancreatic morphology and function. Diabetes is rare in raptors; however, spontaneously occurring diabetes mellitus has been reported in a red-tailed hawk with generalized weakness, polyuria, and polydipsia [218]. Antemortem samples revealed a serum glucose concentration of 54.3 mmol/l (978.37 mg/dl) and glucosuria [218].

Exocrine Function

The exocrine portion of the pancreas secretes a collection of digestive enzymes that include trypsinogen, chymotrypsinogen, carboxypeptidases A, B, and C, deoxyribonucleases, ribonucleases, elastases, amylase, and lipase. These enzymes may also be detected in egested pellets from birds of prey given their unique gastrointestinal physiology of "casting" up indigestible food items in the form of a pellet [127].

Amylase – Amylase degrades carbohydrates, particularly starches, within the gastrointestinal tract [116]. Sources of amylase include the pancreas, liver (biliary system), and the small intestine [61, 96]. Hydration of food in the crop may assist digestion of foods with pancreatic amylase once it reaches the duodenum [116]. The little information available describes normal values of amylase in raptors (Tables 24.5–24.8). Plasma amylase concentrations are likely highly variable in raptors, and the degree to which amylases exists in avian saliva is unknown. Amylase ranges in red-tailed hawks are higher than suggested as normal in parrots [76]. Increased amylase concentrations may also indicate enteritis. Pancreatic biopsy is necessary to confirm pancreatic disease.

Lipase – Lipase breaks down dietary fats (triglycerides, phospholipids, cholesterol, cholesterol esters, terpenes, and carotenoids) into fatty acids, monosaccharides, and lysophospholipids [116]. Emulsification of fats is achieved through the combined activity of BAs, pancreatic lipase, phospholipase, and esterases within the lumen of the small intestine [116]. Although reference ranges for lipase in raptor species are available (Tables 24.5–24.7), no correlation between lipase activity and pancreatic disease has been documented. Evaluation of lipase concentrations are difficult based on dramatic differences in nutrient content of prey [13].

Glucose

Insulin, not glucagon, appears to be the primary moderator of carbohydrate metabolism and glucose concentrations in raptors, and raptors appear to be able to maintain blood glucose concentrations during fasting for longer periods than granivorous species [218]. Hyperglycemia has been reported in a red-tailed hawk with diabetes [218]. Insulin concentrations should be measured in any raptor with persistently and markedly increased glucose concentrations. Stress-related hyperglycemia may occur in raptors that recently enter captivity based on endogenous glucocorticoids. Lipemia and hemolysis can artifactually increase measured blood glucose concentrations in avian species, but this has not been specifically studied in raptors. Hypoglycemia may result from hepatic insufficiency, decreased food intake accompanied by continued strenuous exercise, starvation, septicemia, malabsorption and maldigestion, and artifactually from bacterial contamination. Carbohydrate absorption tests (xylene or glucose challenge) may be of benefit to rule out malabsorptive or maldigestive diseases [87]. Seizures based on hypoglycemia may occur in raptors when glucose concentrations fall below 80 mg/dl [111].

Lipids

Cholesterol

Cholesterol is not diagnostic for a specific disease. However, age, sex, diet, lack of exercise, and hypercholesterolemia may contribute to the development of atherosclerosis, which occurs in Falconiformes and Accipitriformes [60, 105, 196]. In black kites, plasma lipid and lipoprotein concentrations change with diet, which may benefit long-term management of raptors susceptible to atherosclerosis [60].

Triglycerides

Triglyceride intake facilitates absorption of fat-soluble vitamins and is the densest dietary energy source available [116]. Triglycerides are stored in adipose tissue to provide an energy source when food intake is limited [116]. It is unknown whether increased triglyceride

Table 24.8 Biochemical reference intervals for select owl species.

	Species	Great horned owl [5, 205] (*Bubo virginianus*)	Northern eagle owl [34, 75] (*Bubo bubo*)	Tawny owl [34, 198] (*Strix aluco*)	Barn owl [34, 204, 205] (*Tyto alba*)	Barred owl [205] (*Strix varia*)	Screech owl [205] (*Megascops asio*)
	Data format	**Mean ± SD**	**Range, Mean ± SD**	**Range [Min-Max] Mean ± SD**	**Mean ± SD**	**Mean ± SD**	**Mean ± SD**
	N, Attributes	**10–11**	**6 [75], Ħ**	**8 or *other* ₪ Ħ**	**12 [205] 42₪ [204]**	**4**	**7**
Analyte (abbreviation)	**Units SI (conventional)**						
Albumin	g/l (g/dl)	12.7 ±0.35 (1.27 ± 0.035) [5] 19 ± 2.0 (1.9 ± 0.2) [205]	11.1–13.5 (1.11–1.35) [34]	15.3–26.9 (1.53–2.69 [bromcresol green]) [198] 14.3 ± 3.3 (1.43 ± 0.33 [ӭ]) [198] 10.9–16.7 (1.09–1.67 [ӭ]) [198]	21.0 ± 4.0 (2.1 ± 0.4 ӭ) [205]	22.0 ± 3.0 (2.2 ± 0.3 ӭ) [205]	22.0 ± 5.0 (2.2 ± 0.5 ӭ) [205]
A:G Ratio	na	0.7 ± 0.2 [205]	0.65 ± 0.03 [75]		1.5 ± 0.6 [205]	0.7 ± 0.3 [205]	1.6 ± 0.7 [205]
Alanine aminotransferase (ALT)	U/l (U/l)	39 ± 14 [5]		32.5–40 [34] 5–87 [198]			
Alkaline phosphatase (ALP)	U/l (U/l)	31.0 ± 7.0 [5]		42.2–215 [34] 184–1459 [198]	358 ± 197 [204]		
Aspartate aminotransferase (AST)	U/l (U/l)	287 ± 65 [5]		23.5–103.5 [34] 214–368 [198]	272 ± 43 [204]		
Bile ac.ds	µmol/l (µg/dl)				43 ± 18 (17.56 ± 7.35) [204]		
Bilirubin	µmol/l (mg/dl)	(0.07 ± 0.06) [5]					
Blood urea nitrogen (BUN)	mmol/l (mg/dl)		5.58 ± 0.357 (16.40 ± 1.00) [75]	1.5–3.05 (4.20–8.54) [198]			
Calcium	mmol/l (mg/dl)	2.54 (10.19) [5]	2.16–2.61 (8.64–10.44) [34] 2.31 ± 0.045 (9.25 ± 0.18) [75]	2.3–3.08 (9.2–12.32) [198]	2.2–2.6 (8–10.4) [34]		
Cholesterol	mmol /l (mg/dl)		3.9–7.1 (150.58–274.13) [75]				
Chloride	mmol /l (mEq/l)	122 [5]					
Creatin:ne	mmol /l (mg/dl)		31–49 (0.35–0.55) [34]	18.6–61 (0.210–0.69) [198]			
Creatine kinase (CK)	U/l (U/l)	977 ± 407 [5]		2–344 [198]	2228 ± 578 [204]		

Glutamate (GLDH) dehydrogenase	U/l (U/l)				7.5 ± 2.5 [204]		
Globulin	g/l (g/dl)		18.7–22.4 (1.87–2.24) [34]	13.3–32.6 (1.33–3.26) [198]			
Glucose	mmol /l (mg/dl)	19.78 (356) [5]	13.5–21.7 (243.24–391) [34] 22.41 ± 0.49 (403.80 ± 8.80) [75]	18.8–21.8 (338.73–392.79) [198]			
Gamma-glutamyl transferase (GGT)	U/l (U/l)			4–77 [198]	9.5 ± 4.7 [204]		
Lactate dehydrogenase (LDH)	U/l (U/l)				1702 ± 475 [204]		
Phosphorus	mmol /l (mg/dl)	1.38 (4.3) [5]		1.13–4.10 (3.49–12.69) [198]			
Total protein	g/l (g/dl)	43.0 (4.33) [5] 47 ± 4.0 (4.7 ± 0.4) [205]		45.8 ± 13.9 (4.58 ± 1.39 Ab) [198] 53.0 ± 17.2 (5.30 ± 1.72 [refractometry]) [198]	30.6 ± 5.3 (3.06 ± 0.53) [204] 32 (3.2) [34]	55 ± 5.0 (5.5 ± 0.5) [205]	41.0 ± 10.0 (4.1 ± 1.0) [205]
Triglycerides	mmol /l (mg/dl)		3.8 ± 1.18 (337.50 ± 105.10) [75]				
Uric acid	µmol/l (mg/dl)	814 087 ± 642 038 (13.7 ± 10.8) [205]	713.76 ± 130.85 (12.00 ± 2.20) [75]	282–632 (4.74–10.62) [198]	428 ± 102 (7.2 ± 1.71) [204]		
Prealbumin	g/l (g/dl)	0.1 ± 0.2 (0.01 ± 0.02) [205]		2.6–7.8 (0.26–0.78) [198]	0.4 ± 1.0 (0.04 ± 0.1) [205]	0.1 ± 3.0 (0.01 ± 0.3) [205]	2.0 ± 2.0 (0.2 ± 0.2) [205]
α-1 globulin	g/l (g/dl)	7.5 ± 2.0 (0.75 ± 0.2) [205]		1.2–3.0 (0.12–0.3) [198]	4.4 ± 3.0 (0.44 ± 0.3) [205]	6.6 ± 3.0 (0.66 ± 0.3) [205]	2.2 ± 5.0 (0.22 ± 0.5) [205]
α-2 globulin	g/l (g/dl)	5.4 ± 1.0 (0.54 ± 0.1) [205]		1.3–3.1 (0.13–0.31) [198]	2.2 ± 2.0 (0.22 ± 0.2) [205]	6.8 ± 1.0 (0.68 ± 0.1) [205]	2.9 ± 1.0 (0.29 ± 0.1) [205]
β-globulin	g/l (g/dl)	11.0 ± 4.0 (1.1 ± 0.4) [205]		6.4–20.6 (0.64–2.06) [198]	7.2 ± 2.0 (0.72 ± 0.2) [205]	15.0 ± 4.0 (1.5 ± 0.4) [205]	5.85 ± 2.0 (0.58 ± 0.2) [205]
γ-globulin	g/l (g/dl)	4.1 ± 2.0 (0.41 ± 0.2) [205]		1.9–7.2 (0.19–0.72) [198]	2.7 ± 1.0 (0.27 ± 0.1) [205]	4.6 ± 2.0 (0.46 ± 0.2) [205]	5.8 ± 4.0 (0.58 ± 0.4) [205]
Amylase	U/l		491.70 ± 21.0 [75]		563 ± 114		

Table 24.9 Biochemical reference data for selected vulture and condor species.

Analyte (abbreviation)	Species	Black vulture [205, 214] (*Coragyps atratus*)	Turkey vulture [29, 205]	Bearded vulture[a] [95] (*Gypaetus barbatus*) ⅄	Egyptian ₪ vulture [51, 170] (*Neophron percnopterus*)	White-backed vultures [159] (*Gyps africanus*) Ħ	Griffon vulture [170] (*Gyps ₪ fulvus*) Ħ	California condor [53] Ħ (*Gymogyps californianus*)	Andean condor [210] (*Vultur gryphus*)
	Data N	7 [205], ₪5 Ħ 5 ⅄ [214]	2, [29]	21 Ó (< 105 d), 12 ₪	[51] 2–8, [170] 5 Ħ	(95% CI) 14 Ħ, 25 Ħ	12	26–50 (≥6 mo)	12 Ħ 14–19 ⅄
Albumin	g/l (g/dl)	19.0 ± 2.0 (1.9 ± 0.2) ӟ [205]	23.0 ± 4.0 ӟ (2.3 ± 0.4)		15.3 ± 1.4 (1.53 ± 0.014) [170]	11.69 ± 1.06; (10.31–13.19) (1.16 ± 0.10; 1.03–1.32)	17.7 ± 4.4 (1.77 ± 0.44)	10.4 ± 1.3 (1.04 ± 0.13)	12 ± 2.8 (1.2 ± 0.28)Ħ 35 ± 8.1 (3.5 ± 0.81)⅄
A:G Ratio		1.1 ± 0.3 [205]	1.2 ± 0.4		0.87 ± 0.29 [170]		0.76 ± 0.29	0.49 ± 0.08	
Alanine aminotransferase (ALT)	U/l (U/l)	89.3 ± 138.5Ħ 14.4 ± 10.4⅄			6.6 ± 4.9 [170] 16 ± 12 [51]	35.51 ± 1.99; 9.233–144.45	11.4 ± 6.1		
Alkaline phosphatase (ALP)	U/l (U/l)	122.2 ± 48.7Ħ 78.4 ± 14.4⅄		658.52 ± 395.71 Ó 59.86 ± 25.83₪	65.8 ± 24.5 [170] 83 ± 36 [51]		108.1 ± 114.3	82.6 ± 64.2	277.5 ± 107.5Ħ 227.9 ± 74.5⅄
Aspartate aminotransferase (AST)	U/l (U/l)	99.9 ± 95.9Ħ 223.0 ± 53.5⅄		110.19 ± 33.50 Ó 170.3 ± 59.33₪	64.9 ± 7.2 [170] 128 ± 52 [51]	1620.92 ± 2.24; 238–6160	118.5 ± 25.7	17.52 ± 17.2	13 ± 3.98Ħ 12.6 ± 5.03⅄
Bile acids	µmol/l (µg/dl)							8.83 ± 7.52 (3.61 ± 3.07)	
Blood urea nitrogen (BUN)	mmol/l mg/dl	1.64 ± 0.75 (4.6 ± 2.1)Ħ 10.6 ± 6.8 (3.78 ± 2.42)⅄		6.31 ± 3.17 Ó (17.68 ± 8.88) Ó 4.24 ± 1.80 (11.98 ± 5.06) ₪	1.117 ± 0.71 1.5 (3.12 ± 2.01)) [170] 1.3 ± 0.7 (3.64 ± 1.96) [51]	3.21 ± 1.01; 1.18–5.23) (8.99 ± 2.83; 3.30–14.64)	1.315 ± 0.755 (3.68 ± 2.11)		
Calcium	mmol/l (mg/dl)	2.85 ± 0.475 (11.4 ± 1.9)Ħ 1.97 ± 0.17 (7.9 ± 0.7)⅄		2.42 ± 0.3 Ó (9.68 ± 1.20) 2.41 ± 0.16 (9.64 ± 0.67) ₪	2.7 ± 0.4 (10.8 ± 1.6) [170]	1.71 ± 0.77; 1.49–1.93 (6.8 ± 3.08; 5.96–7.72)	3.5 ± 0.9 (14 ± 3.6)	2.1 ± 0.12 (8.40 ± 0.48)	2.07 ± 0.42 (8.3 ± 1.68)Ħ 2.07 ± 0.29 (8.3 ± 1.19)⅄
Cholesterol	mmol/l (mg/dl)	4.39 ± 0.74 (169.5 ± 28.8)Ħ 5.31 ± 1.06 (205.4 ± 41.0)⅄		6.19 ± 1.62 Ó (239.23 ± 62.58) 5.12 ± 1.49 (198.03 ± 57.58) ₪	7.9 ± 0.8 (305.02 ± 30.88) [170] 8.6 ± 0.6 (332.04 ± 23.16)		5.1 ± 1.1 (196.9 ± 42.47)	5.3 ± 0.8 (204.7 ± 29.0)	
Chloride	mmol/l (mEq/l)	118.3⅄			100.5 ± 4.5 [170]		98.2 ± 12.2	117.1 ± 1.6	

Creatinine	mmol/l (mg/dl)			17.68 ± 15.91 Ó (0.20 ± 0.18) 0.25131.83 ± 11.49 (0.25 ± 0.13) ₪	44.3 ± 26.6 (0.50 ± 0.30) [170] 30.94 ± 4.42 (0.35 ± 0.05) [51]				
Creatine kinase (CK)	U/l (U/l)			2645 ± 933.74 Ó 1254.1 ± 585.88₪	401 ± 47 [170]	287.47 ± 137.00; 112.85–596.15	274 ± 251	224.0 ± 140.3	143 ± 48.5[Ħ] 160.8 ± 145.3[ˀ]
Globulin	g/l					21.78 ± 1.14; 16.76–28.30) (2.170.11; 1.67–2.83)		21.4 ± 4.6 (2.14 ± 0.46)	31 ± 8.2 (3.1 ± 0.82)[Ħ] 24 ± 6.6 (2.4 ± 0.66)[ˀ]
Glucose	mmol/l (mg/dl)	18.67 ± 1.56 (336.5 ± 28.1)[Ħ] 19.33 ± 3.45 (348.4 ± 62.2)[ˀ]		13.82 ± 3.06 (249.09 ± 55.26) Ó 13.80 ± 2.51 (248.74 ± 45.23) ₪	17.7 ± 4.2 (318.91 ± 75.67) [170] 15.7 ± 1.6 (282.88 ± 28.82) [51]		16.2 ± 2.5 (291.9 ± 45.04)	16.0 ± 2.0 (288.8 ± 35.3)	
Lactate dehydrogenase (LDH)	U/l (U/l)	513.5 ± 183.1[Ħ] 1066.0 ± 228.1[ˀ]		3099.48 ± 1437.47 Ó 1170.4 ± 386.04₪	629 ± 398 [170] 628 ± 105 [51]		254 ± 153	148.4 ± 43.5	
Magnesium	mmol/l (mEq/ l; mg/dl)			0.88 ± 0.26 (1.77 ± 0.53) Ó 1.275 ± 0.26 (2.55 ± 0.52) ₪	0.75 ± 0.08 (1.52 ± 0.16) [170]		0.79 ± 0.13 (1.58 ± 0.26)		1 ± 0.23 (2.0 ± 0.47)[Ħ] 0.75 ± 0.18 (1.5 ± 0.37)[ˀ]
Phosphorus	mmol/l (mg/dl)	0.87 ± 0.83 (2.7 ± 2.6)[Ħ] 0.323 ± 0.096 (1.0 ± 0.3)[ˀ]		2.08 ± 0.66 (6.46 ± 2.05) Ó 0.91 ± 0.27 (2.83 ± 0.84) ₪	7.3 ± 1.6 (22.60 ± 4.95) [170]		4.3 ± 1.1 (13.31 ± 3.40)	1.14 ± 0.6 (3.54 ± 1.85)	1.32 ± 0.46 (4.1 ± 1.45)[Ħ] 1.22 ± 0.35 (3.8 ± 1.11)[ˀ]
Potassium	mmol/l (mEq/l)	0.8[ˀ]			1.6 ± 0.3	1.41 ± 0.61; 1.16–1.67	2.1 ± 0.9	3.2 ± 0.5	
Sodium	mmol/l (mEq/l)	154.6[ˀ]			151.6 ± 4.7	153.70 ± 12.17; 148.59–158.87[g,ˀ]	154.9 ± 6.7	147.2 ± 3.6	
Total protein	g/l (g/dl)	37.0 ± 6.0 (3.7 ± 0.6 Ӭ]) [205] 22 ± 10 (2.2 ± 1.0)[Ħ]	44.0 ± 7.0 (4.4 ± 0.7 Ӭ])	36 ± 4.9 Ó Ѣ (3.60 ± 0.49) 39.8 ± 4.5 (3.98 ± 0.45) Ѣ ₪	39 ± 7 3.9(0.7±) 43 ± 7 (4.3 ± 0.7) [51]	34.96 ± 3.75; 33.30–36.54) (3.5 ± 0.37; 3.33–3.65)[ˀ]	39 ± 8 (3.9 ± 0.8)	32.5 ± 2.9 (3.25 ± 0.29)	43 ± 10 (4.3 ± 1.0)[Ħ] 35 ± 8.1 (3.5 ± 0.81)[ˀ]
Triglycerides	mmol/ l (mg/dl)	0.76 ± 0.39 (67.7 ± 34.6)		1.72 ± 0.76 Ó (152.54 ± 67.51) 0.57 ± 0.22 (50.53 ± 19.64) ₪	1.33 ± 0.43 (117.8 ± 38.08) 1.21 ± 0.56 (108 ± 50) [51]		1.10 ± 0.47 (97.43 ± 41.63)		
Uric acid	μmol/l (mg/dl)	(14.9 ± 8.6)[Ħ] 618.59 ± 356.88(10.4 ± 6.0)[ˀ]		286.1 ± 96.95 Ó (4.81 ± 1.63) 207.58 ± 116.58 (3.49 ± 1.96)₪	230 ± 159 (3.86 ± 2.67)	650 ± 30; 580–714 (10.92 ± 0.50; 9.75–12.00)[ˀ]	328 ± 167 (5.51 ± 2.80)	439.56 ± 309.9 (7.39 ± 5.21)	

(Continued)

Table 24.9 (Continued)

Analyte (abbreviation)	Units, SI (conventional)	Black vulture [205, 214] (*Coragyps atratus*)	Turkey vulture [29, 205]	Bearded vulture[a] [95] (*Gypaetus barbatus*) ⱻ	Egyptian ₪ vulture [51, 170] (*Neophron percnopterus*)	White-backed vultures [159] (*Gyps africanus*) Ħ	Griffon vulture [170] (*Gyps* ₪ *fulvus*) Ħ	California condor [53] Ħ (*Gymogyps californianus*)	Andean condor [210] (*Vultur gryphus*)
	Data N	7 [205], ₪5 Ħ 5 ⱻ [214]	2, [29]	21 Ó (< 105 d), 12 ₪	[51] 2–8, [170] 5 Ħ	(95% CI) 14 Ħ, 25 Ħ	12	26–50 (≥6 mo)	12 Ħ 14–19 ⱻ
Prealbumin	g/l (g/dl)	6.0 ± 1.0 (0.60 ± 0.1) [205]	0.4 ± 0.8 (0.04 ± 0.08)		4.5 ± 1.5 (0.45 ± 0.15)		1.7 ± 2.4 (0.17 ± 0.24)		
α-globulin	g/l (g/dl)				8.9 ± 3.6 (0.89 ± 0.36) [170]		8.3 ± 2.5 (0.83 ± 0.25)		
α1-globulin	g/l (g/dl)	2.9 ± 1.0 (0.29 ± 0.1) [205]	3.7 ± 1.0 (0.37 ± 0.1)						
α2-globulin	g/l (g/dl)	4.5 ± 2.0 (0.45 ± 0.2) [205]	5.8 ± 1.0 (0.58 ± 0.1)						
β-globulin	g/l (g/dl)	6.8 ± 3.0 (0.68 ± 0.3) [205]	5.2 ± 2.0 (0.52 ± 0.2)		5.5 ± 1.4 (0.55 ± 0.14) [170]		11.7 ± 4.0 (1.17 ± 0.4)		
γ-globulin	g/l (g/dl)	3.6 ± 2.0 (0.36 ± 0.2) [205]	5.9 ± 2.0 (0.59 ± 0.2)		6.0 ± 1.4 (0.6 ± 0.14) [170]		5.8 ± 3.4 (0.58 ± 0.34)		
Amylase	U/l (U/l)			1179.22 ± 421.06 Ó 745.9 ± 250.22₪					
Lipase	U/l (U/l)			62.22 ± 54.26 Ó 955.1 ± 221.38₪					
Lead	μmol/l (μg/dl)		< 2.0 [29]					<0.29 (<6.0)	
Zinc	μmol/l (μg/dl)							22.0 ± 9.7 (144.1 ± 63.6)	

Data presented as mean ± SD unless otherwise noted.
Free-living ⱻ, Captive Ħ, Ӟ electrophoresis, Biuret Ꮑ, Adult ₪, Juvenile Ó.
[a] Total protein from plasma samples; remaining analytes from serum samples [95].

concentrations in birds are associated with diseases such as diabetes mellitus, hypothyroidism, or cardiac disease as in humans and other mammals. Interpretation of appropriate triglyceride concentrations for birds is challenging. Intra-and interspecies variations exist and are further complicated by age, sex, activity (i.e., sedentary or migratory), diet, season, reproduction and hormones, diet intake, disease, nutritive value of prey items, and geographic location [30, 63, 191].

Electrolytes

Important plasma electrolytes to measure include sodium, chloride, potassium, and bicarbonate. Magnesium should be considered when evaluating calcium homeostasis imbalances. Electrolytes are necessary for maintaining osmotic pressure, electroneutrality, and fluid balance within the body. They should be evaluated with a complete understanding of the patient's hydration status, appetite and thirst, concurrent medical therapy, and disease processes that may alter electrolyte concentrations within the body [87]. In general, electrolyte and acid–base status remain to be thoroughly investigated in raptor species.

Sodium

Sodium, the major extracellular electrolyte, is interpreted along with the patient's hydration status. Plasma sodium concentrations are primarily under renal control. Nasal salt secretions also appear in many raptor species and contain sodium, potassium, chloride, and calcium [22]. However, the extent to which they control blood sodium concentrations, or control osmolality as in seabirds is undetermined [96]. Hypernatremia is indicative of several conditions including dehydration, decreased water uptake, water loss, salt poisoning, and dehydration of the blood sample itself [96]. Hyponatremia may occur as a result of diarrhea, kidney disease/failure, psychogenic polydipsia (over hydration), excessive intravenous fluid administration [70], and artifact based on lipemia or hyperproteinemia [96].

Potassium

Potassium, the primary intracellular cation, is interpreted along with the patient's acid–base status. Hyperkalemia indicates conditions that cause acidosis (metabolic or respiratory), renal disease/failure, severe tissue damage, adrenal gland disease, dehydration, and hemolytic anemia [7, 96]. Hypokalemia is indicative of chronic diarrhea or vomiting, starvation, sample handling (i.e., allowing whole blood samples to sit before separating and removing plasma), diuresis, and artifactually due to lipemia or hyperproteinemia [70, 96]. However, with the exception of the effect of sample handling on potassium, most of these other conditions and their effect upon potassium in birds of prey, which is lower than in most mammals, remain unstudied. It is particularly noteworthy that the effect of hemolysis upon potassium concentrations of raptor blood has not been investigated.

Chloride

Chloride, the primary extracellular anion, typically has concentrations which follow changes in sodium. Hyperchloremia may indicate dehydration but is uncommon in birds [96]. Interpretation of hypochloremia may be difficult, but may occur as a result of regurgitation/vomiting (loss of gastric fluid), kidney disease, or congestive heart failure. Most of these generalization related to changes in chloride have not been specifically investigated in raptors; one should also note that pellet egestion occurs daily in these species without a known change in sodium or other ions.

Proteins

Most plasma proteins are synthesized in the liver, with the exception of immunoglobulins (produced by lymphocytes and plasma cells) and protein hormones. Total protein, albumin, and globulins are commonly reported on biochemical profiles of raptors. Total protein is determined by either Biuret analysis or a refractometer. Values determined by a refractometer may be inaccurate in avian species based on high glucose concentrations in the blood and other compounds such as chromagens and lipids [87]. Protein electrophoresis detects albumin and the globulins (α_1 α_2, β, and Υ globulins) and, when combined with other screening tests such as the CBC and serum or plasma biochemical analysis, may be a useful diagnostic aid in the detection of various inflammatory diseases, in monitoring response to therapy, and as a prognostic indicator [43, 205]. Species, assay, and laboratory-specific data are required to best assess protein electrophoresis (EPH) results [43].

Reports differ regarding use serum or plasma for EPH. One report suggests plasma for EPH because serum does not contain fibrinogen, a β protein and an important marker of acute inflammation [186]. Plasma is also preferred in raptors because samples collected in serum separator tubes without anticoagulant are likely to lose their fluidity, making analysis difficult [205]. Furthermore, total plasma protein averages 1.7 mg/dl greater than that of serum based on the presence of fibrinogen, an acute phase protein and indicator of acute inflammation [205]. In EPH of falcons, serum was used because fibrinogen in plasma samples can obscure EPH results in the beta- and gamma-globulin regions, and heparin may interfere with BCG dye [100, 120, 138, 207].

Protein electrophoretic patterns differ significantly between genera, but not based on sex or taxonomic group [44, 120, 123, 146, 205]. Healthy raptor EPH may differ from Psittaciformes based on having low to negligible prealbumin fractions, and a high-amplitude monoclonal α-1-globulin fraction that shoulders off the albumin peak [43, 205]; Alpha-1 concentrations can reach 1.08 g/dl or 27% of the total protein concentration in raptors [43]. In addition, while β- and γ-globulin fractions were similar to those of psittacines, the α-2-globulins fraction was greater in raptors compared to psittacines [43, 205]. Serum EPH of healthy and *Aspergillus*-infected falcons (peregrine falcons, gyrfalcons (*F. rusticolus*), saker falcons (*F. cherrug*), red-naped shaheens (*Falco pelegrinoides babylonicus*), and gyr-hybrid falcons) found no differences in A:G ratios or protein fractions based on species or sex [120]. However, albumin concentrations determined by the BCG method, total albumin concentrations (albumin + prealbumin), and prealbumin were higher in the healthy group [120].

Wing-tip edema and necrosis syndrome (WTONS) has been described in raptors in the United Kingdom and the Middle East [64]. Frost/cold damage has been proposed as the cause of WTONS. However, serum EPH initially reveals increased α-globulins with decreased ß- and γ-globulin concentrations and decreased albumin [33]. While inflammation is the primary lesion in frost damage [222], the electrophoretogram typically shows increased α_1-, α_2-, and ß-globulin fractions and decreased albumin [18]. A specific protein rise in the early stages suggests a more specific inflammatory cause than frost/cold damage. As the disease progresses, all globulin fractions increase, resulting in a polyclonal gammopathy.

Recently, a fatal syndrome of wasting, weight loss, green mutes, and sudden death has been described in falcons in the United Arab Emirates characterized by the presence of amyloid in most organs including the liver, spleen, kidney, and adrenal glands [45, 86, 190]. The liver is considered the primary target organ in falcons, although joints are the primary target organ in chickens [86, 122]. The amyloid was histochemically identified as amyloid A (AA), which is often associated with chronic inflammatory or infectious diseases (e.g., aspergillosis, pododermatitis, tuberculosis, parasitic infections, poxvirus, or visceral gout) [23, 86, 190]. Serum amyloid A (SAA) is an acute phase protein (APP) which is produced in the liver as part of the acute phase response initiated by infection, inflammation, stress, and neoplasia [45]. SAA is found within the β-globulin fractions along with transferrin, fibrinogen, and C-reactive protein. As such, protein EPH or detection of specific APP may be a useful prognostic indicator of inflammation in birds [23, 45]. A semi-quantitative serum test for falcon serum amyloid A (f-SAA) has been developed [86]. SAA was measured in healthy falcons and falcons having noninflammatory or inflammatory/infectious diseases [23]. Healthy falcons' SAA ranged from 0.1 to 6.8 mg/l (mean ± SD; 3.4 ± 1.4 mg/l), from 0.8 to 8.5 mg/l (mean ± SD; 4.0 ± 3.1 mg/l) in falcons with noninflammatory disease, and from 2.3 to 137.5 mg/l (mean ± SD; 47.7 ± 29.7 mg/l) in falcons with inflammatory disease [23]. Concentrations of SAA reflected the severity of inflammation and were deemed suitable for real-time monitoring of inflammatory disease and response to therapy [23].

Blood Gases and Acid–Base Balance

The use of acid–base status to assess raptor patients is underused, most likely because little information is available that describes normal acid–base status in birds of prey. Heparinized venous blood samples are commonly used [7], although arterial samples are accessible in larger birds from the deep radial artery as it crosses the elbow or as it courses distally between the radius and ulna. The pH, PCO_2 and HCO_3 are assessed. Arterial blood samples of awake, but restrained red-tailed hawks revealed PaO2 = 108.0 Torr, PaCO2 = 27.0 Torr, and pH = 7.489 [119].

Vitamins, Minerals, Heavy Metals, and Toxins

Vitamins

Determination of blood vitamin concentrations in raptors may be of value in clinical syndromes where specific vitamin deficiencies are included in the differential list. Thiamine and vitamin E are the main vitamins which have been determined for these species. In juvenile Northern Goshawks (*Accipiter gentilis*) showing signs of thiamine deficiency and a response to thiamine therapy, blood concentrations of thiamine ranged from 2.2 to 6.0 μg/l [28]. Concentrations of plasma thiamine in healthy free-ranging and captive Northern goshawks were between 45.1 and 200 μg/l [28]. For thiamine analysis, collect samples into EDTA. Because vitamin E is fat-soluble, blood concentration may be less useful and poorly reflective of tissue concentrations/stores. Plasma concentrations of α-tocopherol vary with diet, thus implying that such measurement will correlate well with current dietary intake [192]. Mean concentrations of vitamin E in falcons (mixed species and hybrids) were 27.5 ± 8.7 mg/l (range 16.7–46.1 mg/l) [192]. Serum α-tocopherol concentrations determined in 29 adult raptors representing 11 species fed an identical commercial diet supplemented with α-tocopherol acetate to supply 925 or 1364 IU vitamin E/kg diet dry matter (DM) [24] were (mean ± SE) for Andean condors (*Vultur gryphus*) (38.1 ± 38 μg/ml), an Audubon's caracara (*Polyborus plancus*) (129 μg/ml), bald eagles (40.4 ± 17.2 μg/ml), cinereous vultures (*Aegypius monachus*) (16.6 ± 2.2 μg/ml), golden eagles (*Aquila chrysaetos*) (51.5 ± 8.5 and 126.6 ± 16.5 μg/ml), a great horned owl (48.4 μg/ml), Griffon vultures (*Gyps fulvus*) (15.1 ± 2.2 μg/ml), king vultures (*Sarcoramphus papa*) (43.7 ± 3.6 μg/ml), snowy owls (*Nyctea scandiaca*) (21.6 ± 1.4 μg/ml), turkey vultures (*Cathartes aura*) (103.1 ± 19.4 μg/ml), and white-tailed sea eagles (*Haliaeetus albicilla*) (670.8 ± 94.6 μg/ml) [24]. White-tailed sea eagles had significantly higher serum α-tocopherol concentrations than all other species examined [24]. Samples for α-tocopherol should be taken into lithium heparin and plasma separated as soon as possible. Plasma should be frozen if not examined immediately.

Minerals

Phosphorus

Phosphorus occurs as an organic form, which is found primarily in the liver and skeletal muscle, and as inorganic phosphorus. Phosphorus, which is under the control of parathyroid hormone (PTH), is involved in many metabolic processes within the body including combining with calcium to form hydroxyapatite required for healthy beak and bone structure [87]. Most clinical assays for phosphorus measure the inorganic form in plasma or serum. Increased phosphorus concentrations are not significant findings in birds with renal disease. Increased phosphorus concentrations are more indicative of sample hemolysis, musculoskeletal disorders, damage to intestinal mucosa, or are iatrogenic (dietary supplementation) [87]. Decreased phosphorus concentrations in birds of prey are most likely based on decreased dietary intake or associated with refeeding syndrome based on the effects of insulin on plasma phosphorus, potassium, magnesium, and electrolytes.

Calcium – Total, Ionized, and Free

Most calcium resides in bony tissue, which acts as a storehouse should the need arise to correct calcium imbalances in the blood. The remaining small percentage is available for metabolic processes, normal neuromuscular function, and coagulation. Calcium occurs in three forms; a free, ionized, biologically active form (approximately 50%), a form bound to anions such as phosphate, citrate, and bicarbonate (approximately 10%), and a portion which is bound primarily by albumin and alpha and beta-globulins (approximately 40%). PTH, calcitonin, vitamin D3, and estrogen regulate physiologic metabolism of calcium in birds.

Most assays measure total calcium concentrations in serum or plasma; however, ionized calcium can be measured separately and should be performed if total calcium concentrations are abnormal. Total body calcium should be interpreted with an understanding of the plasma protein (in particular, hypoalbuminemia) concentrations. An adjustment formula for plasma calcium concentrations in peregrine falcons is [140]:

$$\text{Adjusted}\,Ca^{2+}(\text{mmol/l}) = Ca^{2+}(\text{mmol/l}) - 0.02\,\text{Total protein}(\text{g/l}) + 0.67$$

However, the use of adjusted calcium is not reliable, and ionized calcium concentrations, although poorly documented in raptor literature, are likely a better indication of calcium homeostasis.

Hypercalcemia commonly occurs during egg production in female avian species, most likely the result of increased concentrations of circulating carrier proteins. However, oversupplementation with vitamin/mineral supplements, lipemia, hemolysis, and bacterial contamination of the blood sample may also create hypercalcemia. Hypocalcemia may result from disease conditions that affect plasma protein (particularly albumin) concentrations such as hepatic insufficiency, protein-losing enteropathies, starvation, and chronic infectious diseases. Hypocalcemia as a result of secondary nutritional hyperparathyroidism may occur in both young chicks and adult raptors fed diets with inadequate calcium [104].

Determination of iron concentrations in birds of prey has not been fully investigated. When submitting samples for iron concentrations, the anticoagulant or tube used must not contain iron, EDTA, oxalate, or citrate that bind iron and falsely decrease reported concentrations [87]. Hemosiderosis and hemochromatosis based on excessive dietary intake of iron has not been described in in raptors. However, hemosiderosis associated with infectious disease has been reported in raptors infected with West Nile virus and *Pasteurella multocida* [59, 153]. Lead poisoning in captive Andean condors and trematode infection (*Bothriogaster variolaris*) in snail kites (*Rostrhamus sociabilis plumbeus*) has also been associated with hemosiderosis [39, 165].

Heavy Metals

Lead Toxicosis

Lead intoxication can occur in any raptor and is commonly reported in bald eagles, golden eagles, and California condors (*Gymnogyps californianus*), which appear less tolerant than other species [29, 46, 73, 108, 112, 164, 175, 176]. Turkey vultures were deemed especially susceptible to lead intoxication in one study; however, recent studies suggest that turkey vultures are more tolerant to lead poisoning than other raptor species [67, 165, 182]. Raptors likely vary in their sensitivity to lead toxicosis based on factors including nutritional status, amount of lead ingested, rate of passage through the gastrointestinal tract, genetic predisposition, and lead availability [108, 165]. Lead toxicosis, especially chronic exposure, occurs in free-ranging raptors from ingestion of spent lead, prey/carrion injured or killed by lead ammunition, and lead-based fishing tackle. Hunting seasons increase the incidence and prevalence of lead intoxication of raptors. Lead-intoxication-based retained lead fragments in joint spaces occur in humans who suffer from gunshot wounds and may also occur in raptors [166, 181]. Lead fragments lodged in muscle are of little toxic consequence. Lead disrupts many physiologic processes within the nervous, hematopoietic, musculoskeletal, and urinary systems [79]. Raptors ability to egest a "casting" or "pellet" of indigestible food may facilitate removal of lead pellets or fragments from the crop, proventriculus, or ventriculus.

Diagnosis of lead toxicosis is based on clinical signs, hematology and biochemical analyses, radiography, toxicologic analysis, and postmortem evaluation. Clinical signs of lead toxicosis in raptors include depression, anorexia, crop stasis, weight loss, paresis or paralysis, blindness, and seizures [67, 108]. A hypochromic regenerative anemia arising from the premature destruction and decreased production of red blood cells is a common finding in birds with lead toxicosis [11, 20]. Red blood cells may contain cytoplasmic vacuoles and basophilic stippling (hemoglobin precipitation) [68]. In red-tailed hawks exposed to 0.82 mg Pb/kg body weight for three weeks, reduction in hematocrit or hemoglobin concentration was not evident; however, decreased hematocrit and hemoglobin was evident in hawks exposed to increased doses for 11 weeks [175]. Biochemical parameters that may be altered in cases of lead intoxication include increased activities of CK, LDH, and AST and increased concentrations of total protein and UA [54, 68].

Blood lead concentrations can rise within days of exposure to lead [29]. Thus, blood and tissue lead analysis may be useful evaluate a bird suffering from lead toxicosis; however, antesmortem measurement of tissue concentrations is not routine. Submit whole blood samples in heparinized tubes, because most lead is found in RBCs [68]. Although atomic absorption spectrophotometry is the most sensitive method for blood lead analysis, the LeadCare Analyzer (LeadCare Blood Lead Testing System, ESA Inc., Masachussets, United States), a point-of-care blood lead testing system, can provide similar results compared to spectrophotometry [176, 189]. Important disadvantages of the Lead Care System include expense and an inability to measure blood lead concentrations greater than 65 mg/dl (0.65 ppm) [189].

Lead toxicity should be suspected based on blood concentrations greater than 20 μg/dl (0.2 ppm) and consistent clinical signs. Based on the frequency of lead poisoning in bald eagles, these birds should be treated if blood lead concentrations are 20 μg/dl even if clinical signs are not readily apparent [176]. Although blood concentrations greater than 50 μg/dl are diagnostic, clinical signs may occur with blood lead concentrations as low as 15 μg/dl (0.15 ppm) [11, 20, 54, 67, 68, 187]. Blood lead concentrations of 20–50 μg/dl suggest subclinical exposure, concentrations >100 μg/dl are associated with toxic exposure and clinical signs (muscle wasting, weakness, anemia, weight loss, biliverdinuria, and muscle incoordination), and concentrations >500 μg/dl are compatible with death [67] [112]. In free-flying turkey vultures exposed to lead from big game hunting, blood lead concentrations ≤10 μg/dl were consistent with exposure to environmental background sources of lead, and concentrations ≥10 μg/dl indicated exposure to a point source of lead such as ingestion of lead fragments. These values were based upon another study [35] that found blood lead concentrations in control turkey vultures, bald eagles, and prerelease California condors in captivity were <2 μg/dl, <10 μg/dl, and <4 μg/dl, respectively. Increased protoporphyrin concentrations (EPP) associated with lead poisoning have been reported in some species of birds of prey [12]. Decreased delta-aminolevulinic acid dehydratase (ALAD) activity may be detected in raptors but may not correlate well with clinical signs or even presence of disease [29, 66–68, 77, 97, 98, 165]. For example, while decreased ALAD is a sensitive indicator of lead exposure, it can remain depressed over an extended time even in healthy raptors [66].

Mercury

Mercury is a heavy metal that occurs naturally within the environment (soil, air and water), but is also introduced, typically in aquatic systems, through sewage, industrial waste, and seeds coated with fungicide containing mercury [69]. Mercury occurs in two forms, an organic most toxic form, methylmercury (MeHg), and an inorganic nontoxic form, [Hg(II)], which can be converted to methylmercury by aquatic bacteria [185]. Raptors and other birds in an aquatic environment may be exposed to mercury through foraging behavior and movement within the contaminated ecosystem. Agricultural use of alkyl mercury as a fungicide for seeds has resulted in exposure of upland raptors [36]. Juvenile raptors of species such as ospreys (*Pandion haliaetus*), bald eagles, and others that depend upon prey from aquatic environments may be more likely to show clinical signs, and have highest risk

for methylmercury toxicity during hatching and fledging as seen in other aquatic bird species [1].

Definitive diagnosis of mercury toxicity can be difficult because there is no set value for residual mercury in tissues to indicate mercury toxicity for most avian species. In goshawks [15], subtle histologic changes in the kidneys with >100 mg/kg indicate that some species may be more refractory to mercury damage. A complete necropsy and other laboratory diagnostic tests are required to confirm the diagnosis of mercury toxicity as birds accumulate and tolerate varying concentrations of mercury. Mercury monitoring methods involve the use of eggs, liver and kidney tissue, whole blood, and feathers [93]. Whole blood mercury values have 1:1 correlation with liver MeHg [92]. Methyl mercury content of newly grown feathers of young birds correlates with blood concentrations at the time of feather growth [93]. In ospreys, no relationship of Hg concentration in primary feathers and the sequence of feather molt was attributed to the irregular and protracted molting pattern of osprey [99]. Histologic lesions of mercury toxicity have been documented in numerous organs in egrets but not in raptors [199].

Toxins

Organochlorines

The use of insecticide organochlorines such as dichlorodiphenyltrichloroethane (DDT) has been banned in the United States since 1972; however, its use in other countries for arthropod control continues [93]. Organochlorines bioaccumulate in the environment, and predatory species such as raptors are particularly vulnerable to intoxication [93]. The devastating effects of DDT and its breakdown product, dichlorodiphenyldichloroethylene (DDE), on raptor populations, especially peregrine falcons and bald eagles, is well documented. Historically, monitoring pesticides has required measuring organochlorine residue in eggs or necropsy specimens. However, several studies suggest the use of plasma for monitoring local exposure and long-term residue trends in raptor populations [42, 58, 91, 103]. DDE residues in plasma are highly correlated with brain DDE, exposure rate, and the amount of DDE in eggs of free-ranging birds of prey [91].

Insecticides and Pesticides

Organophosphates and Carbamates

Incidental inhalation, ingestion, or contact with environmental or household toxins such as organophosphates (OP) (dichlorvos, malathion, parathion, etc.), carbamates (carbaryl, carbofuran, etc.), and pyrethrins can occur in free-ranging and captive birds of prey. Pyrethrins and carbamates (e.g., 5% Sevin) can be used safely to control ectoparasites on raptors; however, excessive preening resulting in ingestion or inhalation can result in a dose-related intoxication [54]. Free-ranging raptors are likely to become intoxicated by consuming or scavenging prey species exposed to these toxins. OPs and carbamates inhibit acetylcholinesterase (AChE) and prevent hydrolysis of acetylcholine, which results in massive stimulation of cholinergic receptors and cholinergic crisis [81, 176] Organophosphates bind to AChE, resulting in a stable, unreactive enzyme that can be reactivated only at a slow rate [57, 81]. In contrast, carbamates attach to AChE and undergo the formation of the carbamylated enzyme and then the decarbamylation of the inhibited AChE with the generation of free, active enzyme. The difference between OPs and carbamates is ultimately the rate of dephosphorylation or decarbamylation [57, 81]. The rate of dephosphorylation is slow with organophosphates such that AChE is thought to be irreversibly inhibited [57]. Birds are more susceptible to AChE (AChEI) than mammals [11, 68, 187] Antemortem diagnosis of OP or carbamate toxicosis depends upon investigation for acetylcholinesterase activity in whole blood. Samples collected for analysis should be frozen to avoid rapid metabolism of AChEI which could result in false negative results. wWhole blood from an unexposed bird should be included to serve as a control [54]. Activities of <1000 IU/l AchE in avian plasma are considered diagnostic [11, 68]. Consult your state or other veterinary diagnostic laboratory before collecting or submitting samples for AChEI analysis.

Rodenticide Toxicoses

Free-ranging and captive birds of prey may be exposed to anticoagulant rodenticides. First-generation anticoagulant rodenticides (FGARs) such as warfarin or diphacinone are less toxic than second-generation anticoagulant rodenticides (SGARs) such as brodifacoum, and require multiple or large-dose ingestion or a longer period of exposure [11, 68]. In contrast, brodifacoum toxicity requires only a single dose [201]. Rodenticide toxicity has been reported in numerous species of raptors worldwide and typically occurs following consumption of poisoned prey (rodents) [3, 55, 56, 90, 121, 156–158, 173, 174, 176, 201, 217]. Anticoagulant rodenticides interfere with vitamin K_1 metabolism by preventing the reduction of vitamin K1 epoxide, resulting in a decrease in reduced vitamin K_1. [155, 158] Interference with vitamin K_1 metabolism leads to abnormal synthesis of the vitamin K-dependent clotting factors (II, VII, IX, and X).

In mammals, a diagnosis of rodenticide toxicity is based upon history of exposure, clinical signs, hematologic signs consistent with rodenticide toxicity, and laboratory diagnostic tests (fibrin degradation products [FDPs], prothrombin time, partial thromboplastin time, thrombin time, and measuring residues of rodenticides in blood and tissues [liver]) [155, 176]. A prolonged prothrombin time [PT], partial thromboplastin, or thrombin time with normal fibrinogen, FDPs, and platelet count is diagnostic. However, antemortem testing for rodenticide toxicity remains challenging in avian species based on variability of clotting factors (may lack factors XI, XII, and prekallikrein of the intrinsic pathway between birds and mammals), few laboratories offer PT testing in birds, lack of validation studies for use of heterologous or mammalian thromboplastin in birds, and the large blood volume required to perform these tests [142, 158, 208]. Commercially available tests for avian coagulation are lacking, and tests performed with mammalian thromboplastin provide inaccurate results [158]. Assay of PT has been validated for use in Japanese quail (*Coturnix japonica*) and barn owls [219]. Mean PT for barn owl chicks (age 40–55 days) was 21.4 s. The toxicity and potential risk of diphacinone was assessed in eastern screech owls (*Megascops asio*) using PT and Russell's viper venom times (RVVT) [174]. This report determined that four sham-dosed control screech owls had PTs ranging from 11.9 to 14.4 s and RVVTs from 20.9 to 23.6 s [174]. Observation of clotting times may be useful in assessing potential for anticoagulant toxicity. Place 0.1–0.2 ml of blood in a serum collection tube and monitor by inversion for clotting every 30 s [158]. Blood collected from normal raptors should clot within 5 min, while bird birds suffering from anticoagulant rodenticide toxicity may lack evidence of clot formation for several hours [158].

Hormones – Thyroid, Adrenal, and Reproductive Hormones

Thyroid and Parathyroid

Thyroid testing (stimulation test) is limited in avian medicine based on the expense of thyroid stimulating hormone (TSH). T4 concentrations (determined by radioimmunoassay) without TSH stimulation testing are unlikely to confirm a diagnosis of hyper- or hypothyroidism in birds. Serum rather than plasma is preferred for determination of hormone concentrations based on historical reference ranges from mammals; plasma samples can be submitted to most laboratories. Contact the laboratory for their preference prior to submission to ensure they can provide reference values based on plasma and for birds of prey. Thyroid diseases including goiter, neoplasia (rare in avian species), and cyst formation have been described in several species of bird of prey [9, 65, 85, 188, 216]. No raptor has presented with clinical signs typical of hypo- or hyperthyroidism. Hypothyroidism may play a role in feather abnormalities and "pinching off syndrome" in white-tailed sea eagles [154]. Diseases associated with the parathyroid glands such as nutritional secondary hypothyroidism have been described in birds of prey fed diets with inappropriate calcium:phosphorus [5, 41, 83, 209].

Adrenal Glands

The medullary (chromaffin) cells produce epinephrine and norepinephrine, while the cortical cells produce corticosterone and aldosterone. The functions of the latter two hormones are similar to those in mammalian species except that corticosterone has both glucocorticoid and mineralocorticoid activities in birds [115, 172]. Aldosterone maintains sodium and other electrolyte balance, while corticosterone regulates electrolyte balance and carbohydrate and lipid metabolism. Corticosterone concentrations are modulated by adrenocorticotrophic hormone (ACTH) release from the pituitary gland in response to corticotropin releasing factor from the hypothalamus [49, 115]. Baseline and post-ACTH corticosterone concentrations in bald eagles and Andean condors have been reported [229] (Table 24.7). Cushing's disease has not been reported in birds of prey; however, stress from recent capture, handling, fear, prolonged hospitalization, temperature extremes, food and water deprivation, and chronic infectious diseases (aspergillosis, tuberculosis) likely increase corticosterone concentrations in blood [49, 115, 172]. In raptors, adrenal cortical carcinoma and lesions associated with West Nile virus infections have been described [84, 228].

Reproductive Hormones

In female birds of prey, two developed ovaries and two oviducts may occur. The ovaries produce estrogens, progesterone, and androgens. Follicular development and estrogen secretion is stimulated by follicle stimulating hormone (FSH) from the pituitary gland. Estrogen facilitates development of secondary sex characteristics, the brood patch, female plumage characteristics, the oviduct, deposition of calcium in the medullary bone in preparation for eggshell formation, behavioral characteristics such as nest building, and widening of the pelvic canal to allow egg passage [115]. In male birds of prey, the testes produce testosterone, which facilitates development of the male sexual and behavioral characteristics and plumage color. Development of the testes and production of spermatozoa is influences by FSH, while testosterone production is influenced by the effect of luteinizing hormone (LH) on the interstitial cells. Steroid hormone concentrations can be determined from plasma, feces, and saliva in avian species. Hormone concentrations can change based on the time of year, photoperiod and nesting and breeding activity, temperature extremes, and environmental toxin exposure. The effect of DDT, its metabolite, and hormone disruptors (estrogen and androgen mimics) are well documented in raptor literature [17].

Harris' hawks are unique among raptors in that the young of previous years, or even unrelated birds (most commonly males), will exhibit helping behavior and cooperatively provide food to the alpha birds to assist in the feeding of the young of the current breeding cycle [47]. Plasma concentrations of progesterone and prolactin were determined by radioimmunoassay in free-ranging adult breeders, adult-plumaged helpers, and juvenile-plumaged Harris' hawks during the nesting cycle [215]. Progesterone concentrations did not differ between males and female; however, progesterone concentrations were the highest (2–4 ng/ml) in adult females prior to egg laying [215]. In females during nest building, the mean progesterone in breeding birds was twice that of adult or juvenile-plumaged birds [215]. Prolactin concentrations varied significantly with sex and role in cooperative breeding and were significantly increased in breeding females during nest building (14.1 ng/ml), in breeding males (8.4 ng/ml), and in females (25.5 ng/ml) during incubation [215]. Interestingly, prolactin concentrations dropped immediately after the eggs hatched in male and female breeders (5.6 ng/ml and 7.3 ng/ml, respectively) but rose significantly in the adult-plumaged male helper hawks (mean 9.1 ng/ml) during the nestling and fledgling stage [215]. Increased prolactin concentrations were associated with increased helping behavior and food provided to the adult breeders [215].

Urinalysis

Urinalysis may have some uses in raptor medicine. The physical appearance of raptor urine is similar to other bird species with a white, insoluble urate component and a clear watery component. However, the liquid component is normally more profuse and watery than in herbivorous or granivorous birds. Yellow coloration of the urine is not a sign of ill health. However, the urate component should be white. Urine may be collected and separated from the expelled mute by aspiration into a syringe and centrifugation. Conventional dipstick tests may be used; however, the effects of fecal mixing in the cloaca must be considered. Traces of blood, protein, glucose, and leucocytes can be associated with disease of the reproductive, gastrointestinal, or urinary tracts. Endoscopic catheterization of a ureter per cloacum can facilitate collection of a small volume of urine to confirm a dipstick glucose concentration, but requires prolonged anesthesia. Raptor urine tends to be mildly acidic to neutral pH [211]. In falcon urine, protein concentrations declined after 24 h. However, urine stability allowed a 24-h delay in testing without significant effect on results. Fasting or feeding did not appear to impact urinalysis results [211]. Urinalysis results from clinically healthy falcons are presented in Table 24.10.

Table 24.10 Urinalysis values of clinically healthy falcons (n = 78) by Dipstick method [211].

Analyte	Number positive	Number negative	Range
Blood	43	33	
Bilirubin	45	31	
Protein	16	60	
Nitrite	2	74	
Ketones	0	76	
Ascorbic acid	16	60	
Glucose	10	66	
pH			5–7
Density			1005–1030
Leucocytes	12	64	

Serology and PCR for Raptors (Table 24.11)

Aspergillosis

Aspergillus serology is available commercially for use in raptors. This indirect ELISA was developed for falcons, while specific tests for use in owls have also been developed [2]. The test is directed against *Aspergillus fumigatus*, the most common organism isolated in raptor aspergillosis. However, this organism is fairly ubiquitous in the environment, so positive serology may exist in the absence of clinical disease. Similarly, false negative results may occur if fungal growth is restricted to more immunologically protected sites such as tracheal lumen if another *Aspergillus* spp. or other fungal organism is causative, or in the immunosuppressed animal. Paired serology should become antibody-positive within a week of exposure. *Aspergillus* serology may be of limited value in the diagnosis of aspergillosis, but may be most useful in developing a prognosis and monitoring the host immune response to disease in affected individual raptors [48]. Agar gel diffusion tests for *Aspergillus* appropriate for dogs are not suitable for use in raptors.

Mycoplasma

Mycoplasma species appear common in birds of prey, are uncommonly referable to clinical signs, and are proposed as commensals [132]. While these organisms may be

Table 24.11 Select diagnostic tests and laboratory information of use in raptor species.

Test or service	Samples and test information	Laboratory information
Aspergillus	Antibodies detected by ELISA, Protein electrophoresis, Galactomannan (antigen)	Avian and Wildlife Laboratory, University of Miami, Miller School of Medicine, Division of Comparative Pathology 1600 NW 10th Ave, RMSB 7101A, Miami, FL 33136, Phone: (305) 243–6700; Fax: (305) 243–6662 Website: www.cpl.med.miami.edu/avian-and-wildlife/about-us-avian
CBC and Chemistry Panels	See specimen submission form	
DNA Sexing		
Thyroid (T4)		
Acute phase proteins (Serum amyloid A [SAA], C-reactive protein [CRP], haptoglobin [P])		
Anticoagulant and Rodenticide Screen	Includes brodifacoum, diphacinone, warfarin, others (liquid & solid)	Cornell University, College of Veterinary Medicine, Animal health Diagnostic Center. It33aca, New York 14853–6401 P33one: (607) 253–3900 Fax: (607) 253–3943 Email: diagcenter@cornell.edu Website: ahdc.vet.cornell.edu/sects/serol
Avian Influenza	Antibody AGID, PCR	
Avian Virus Isolation	Tissues, tracheal and cloacal swabs	
West Nile virus (WNV)	PCR, serum neutralization, and isolation	
Avian virus isolation	Tissue culture	University of Georgia College of Veterinary Medicine Infectious Diseases Laboratory 110 Riverbend Road, Riverbend North, Room 150, University of Georgia, Athens, GA 30602 Phone: (706) 542–8092; Fax (706) 583–0843; Lab: (706) 542–5812; Email: idllab@uga.edu Website: www.vet.uga.edu/idl or www.idl-uga.com
Chlamydia	DNA probe, antibody by IFA, Elementary body agglutination	
Immunohistochemistry	See specimen submission form	
West Nile virus	Antibody titer, immunohistochemistry, in situ hybridization	
Acetylcholinesterase	See specimen submission form	Louisiana State University, School of Veterinary Medicine, Louisiana Animal Disease Diagnostic Laboratory, 1909 Skip Bertman Dr., Room 159, Baton Rouge, LA 70803, Phone: (222) 578-9777l; Fax: (222) 578–9784; Email: svmweb@vetmed.lsu.edu Website:www.vetmed.lsu.edu/laddl/index.33tml
Anticoagulants		
Chlorinate hydrocarbons, Organophosphates		
Heavy Metal (lead, copper, zinc)		

Avian DNA Sexing Aspergillus Galactomannan CBC & biochemistry testing Consultation Services heavy Metals (lead and zinc) Cytology, histopathology, and Necropsy services	See specimen submission form Antibody detection Antigen detection See specimen submission form	ANTECH Diagnostics® Corporate 33eadquarters 17672-B Cowan Avenue, Irvine, CA 92614 Phone: ANTECH East 1-(800) 872–1001; ANTECH West 1-(800) 745–4725; ANTECH Canada 1-(800) 341–3440; ANTECH Test Express 1-(888) 397–8378; Email: info@antechdiagnostics.com Website: www.antechdiagnostics.com/main/33ome.aspx IDEXX Laboratories Inc. United States: One IDEXX Drive, Westbrook, Maine 04092 Europe Headquarters: IDEXX Europe B.V., Scorpius 60 Building F, 33oofddorp, 2132 LR, The Netherlands Website: www.idexx.com
Specialty Avian, Exotic, Wildlife, and Zoological Species Necropsy, cytology and histopathology services	Contact laboratory for submission requirements	Zoo/Exotic Pathology Service 2825 KOVR Drive, West Sacramento, CA 95605 Phone: (916) 725–5100; Fax: (916) 725–6155 Email: DReavill@zooexotic.com or totvogel@gmail.com Drs. Drury Reavill and Robert Schmidt Website: www.zooexotic.com Northwest Zoo Path 654 W. Main Street, Monroe, WA 98272 Phone: (360) 794–0630; Fax: (360) 794–4312 Email: mikeg@zoopath.com or zoopath1@gmail.com Dr. Michael Garner Website: www.zoopath.com

isolated and identified using culture and/or PCR technology, serology would seem of little use given their ubiquitous nature and lack of pathogenicity in birds of prey.

West Nile Virus

Wild birds are primary hosts for the West Nile virus (WNV), and many raptor species have been documented as infected [143]. Ornithophilic mosquito species, in particular *Culex pipiens*, are responsible for bird-to-bird transmission of WNV. WNV antibodies are detected by serum neutralization. Detection of WNV may be accomplished by PCR, immunohistochemistry [228] of affected tissues, in situ hybridization of affected formalin fixed tissues, and virus isolation. Two studies have described the use of the VecTest antigen-capture assay (Medical Analysis Systems, Ventura, California, United States) to detect WNV from oral and tissue swabs in both live and deceased birds of prey [162, 202]. While a combination of serologic and oral swab testing increases the sensitivity of clinic-admitted raptor surveillance almost twofold, the oral VecTest alone was poorly sensitive for most raptors other than small samples of American kestrels [162, 202].

Avian Influenza

A commercially available blocking enzyme-linked immunosorbent assay (b-ELISA) (FlockChek AI MultiS-Screen Ab Test, IDEXX, Westbrook, ME) used to test for serologic evidence of exposure to avian influenza is applicable to raptors [177]. A survey of asymptomatic raptors indicated exposure to influenza A viruses in bald eagles, but rarely among other raptor species known to prey upon or scavenge aquatic avian species [78, 177]. Similarly, real-time reverse transcription PCR (rRT-PCR) used to evaluate cloacal swabs from raptors presented to wildlife rehabilitation centers in the United States found mixed infections with H1N1 and H2N1 subtypes in a bald eagle.

Rabies

A study of raptors in California revealed no serological evidence of rabies virus, indicating these species were of little importance in the epidemiology of rabies [195]. However, seroconversion was detected by passive hemagglutination in a great horned owl 27 days after it was fed the remains of an experimentally infected rabid spotted skunk (*Spilogale putorius*) skunk [109]. The owl was able to suppress the infection until it received 2 mg of dexamethasone intramuscularly 66 days after being fed the carcass daily for 10 days [109]. Rabies virus was detected by fluorescent antibody staining of oral swabs, corneal impression smears, mouse inoculation, and transmission electron microscopy [109]. No clinical signs of rabies infection were observed in the owl [109].

Herpes Virus

Raptors and owls may be in infected with herpesvirus. Owl herpesvirus (OHV) and falcon herpesvirus (FHV) are closely related to pigeon herpesvirus (PHV), and the most common route of infection is ingestion of infected pigeons. Diagnosis of herpes viruses in raptors is determined by presence of consistent clinical signs, histologic lesions, serologic identification, electron microscopy, and virus isolation from infected tissues (FHV – liver, spleen, intestine or bone marrow; OHV – liver, spleen, bone marrow, bursa or thymus) [168, 183]. PCR of infected tissues or tracheal/pharyngeal swabs for herpes virus may be performed [168, 213]; however, genetic typing may be necessary to identify specific herpes viruses. Serology may be appropriate to assess exposure in birds surviving an outbreak.

Trichomonas

Trichomonas gallinae infection is common in many species of raptors including hawks, eagles, falcons, and owls, based on consumption of infected columbiformes, and debilitation or immunosuppression. Diagnosis is made by wet preparation from oral or pharyngeal lesions, mounted in warmed saline and examined soon after sampling to prevent false negative results. Swabs may also be taken from lesions or from the pharynx to assess carriage of the organism in asymptomatic birds and submitted for PCR. Culture of the organism from lesions is also possible [169]. Cross-reactivity between different *Trichomonas* species and a commercially available diagnostic test InPouch TF (BioMed Diagnostics Inc., Oregon, United States) designed for detection of *Tritrichomonas fetus* has been used to diagnose and monitor a *Trichomonas vaginalis*-like infection in a bald eagle [113]. Based on increased sensitivity and reliability compared to wet mount microscopy, this test may be preferred for surveillance of *Trichomonas* sp., especially in asymptomatic raptors [113, 227].

Gender Determination

Standard DNA sexing techniques appear applicable to raptors [126] as the Z and W chromosome products appear to be differentiable using normal techniques. Blood, oropharyngeal swabs, freshly plucked body feathers, and even eggshells may be used for sex determination. Prior to submission of samples, the laboratory should be contacted as they may require specific submission or handling techniques for the samples. Where immediate results are needed, or raptor health is of concern, endoscopic sexing is recommended.

References

1 Ackerman, J.T., Eagles-Smith, C.A., and Herzog, M.P. (2011). Bird mercury concentrations change rapidly as chicks age: toxicological risk is highest at hatching and fledging. *Environ. Sci. Technol.* 45 (12): 5418–5425.

2 Aguilar, R.F. and Redig, P.T. (1995). Diagnosis and treatment of avian aspergillosis. In: *Current Veterinary Therapy, Small Animal Practice XII* (ed. J.D. Bonagura and R. Kirk), 1294–1299. Philadelphia: WB Saunders, Co.

3 Albert, C.A., Wilson, L.K., Minaeau, P. et al. (2010). Anticoagulant rodenticides in three owl species from western Canada, 1988-2003. *Arch. Environ. Contam. Toxicol.* 58: 451–459.

4 Allen, J. (1988). Avian clinical chemistries. In: *Exotic Animals* (ed. E.R. Jacobson and G.V. Kollias), 143–157. New York: Churchill Livingstone.

5 Altman, R.B. (1982). Disorders of the skeletal system. In: *Diseases of Cage and Aviary Birds*, 2e (ed. M.L. Petrak), 383–384. Philadelphia: Lea & Febiger.

6 Altman, R.B., Clubb, S.L., Dorrestein, G.M. et al. (1997). Appendix I hematology/biochemical reference ranges. In: *Avian Medicine and Surgery* (ed. R.B. Altman, S.L. Clubb and G.M. Dorrestein), 1004–1023. Philadelphia: WB Saunders.

7 Bailey, T.A. (2008). Biochemistry. In: *Avian Medicine*, 2e (ed. J. Samour), 52–62. Philadelphia: Mosby Elsevier.

8 Banks, R.C., Cicero, C., Dunn, J.L. et al. (2003). Forty-fourth supplement to the American Ornithologists' Union check-list of North American birds. *Auk* 120 (3): 923–931.

9 Bates, G., Tucker, R.L., Ford, S., and Mattix, M.E. (1999). Thyroid adenocarcinoma in a bald eagle (*Haliaeetus leucocephalus*). *J. Zoo Wildl. Med.* 30: 439–442.

10 Bauck, L.A. and Haigh, J.C. (1984). Toxicity of gentamicin in great horned owls (*Bubo virginianus*). *J. Zoo Anim. Med.* 15 (2): 64–66.

11 Bauk, L. and LaBonde, J. (1997). Toxic diseases. In: *Avian Medicine and Surgery* (ed. R.B. Altman, S.L. Clubb, G.M. Dorrestein, et al.), 604–613. Philadelphia: WB Saunders, Co.

12 Beyer, W.N., Spann, J.W., Sileo, L. et al. (1988). Lead poisoning in six captive avian species. *Arch. Environ. Contam. Toxicol.* 19: 121–130.

13 Bird, D.M., Ho, S.K., and Paré, D. (1982). Nutritive values of three common prey items of the American kestrel. *Comp. Biochem. Physiol.* 73A (3): 513–515.

14 Bond, C.F. and Gilbert, P.W. (1958). Comparative study of blood volume in representative aquatic and non-aquatic birds. *Am. J. Physiol.* 194: 519–521.

15 Borg, K., Erne, K., Hanko, E. et al. (1970). Experimental secondary methyl mercury poisoning in the goshawk (*Accipiter g. gentilis* L). *Environ. Pollut.* 1: 91–104.

16 Bowerman, W.W., Stickle, J.E., Sikarskie, J.G. et al. (2000). Hematology and serum chemistries of nestling bald eagles (*Haliaeetus leucocephalus*) in the lower peninsula of MI, USA. *Chemosphere* 41: 1575–1579.

17 Bowerman, W.W., Best, D.A., Giesy, O.P. et al. (2003). Associations between regional differences in polychlorinated biphenyls and dichlorodiphenyldichloroethylene in blood of nestling bald eagles and reproductive productivity. *Environ. Toxicol. Chem.* 22: 371–376.

18 Brailovskii, S.A. and Ledentsov, Y.K. (1959). The action of low temperature and ionizing radiation on the serum proteins and protein fractions. *Bull. Exp. Biol. Med.* 48 (5): 1365–1367.

19 Braun, E.J. and Campbell, C.E. (1989). Uric acid decomposition in the lower gastrointestinal tract. *J. Exp. Zool. Suppl.* 7: 70–74.

20 Brown, T.P. and Julian, R.J. (2003). Other toxins and poisons. In: *Diseases of Poultry* (ed. Y.M. Saif, H.J. Barnes, J.R. Glisson, et al.), 1133–1159. Ames: Iowa State University Press.

21 Bustamante, J. and Travaini, A. (1994). Effect of keeping plasma frozen at -20°C on the concentration of blood metabolites. *Comp. Biochem. Physiol.* 107A (4): 661–664.

22 Cade, T.J. and Greenwald, L. (1966). Nasal salt secretion in falconiform birds. *Condor* 68: 338–350.

23 Caliendo, V., McKinney, P., Bailey, T. et al. (2013). Serum amyloid a as an indicator of health status in falcons. *J. Avian Med. Surg.* 27 (2): 83–89.

24 Calle, P.P., Dierenfeld, E.S., and Robert, M.E. (1989). Serum α-tocopherol in raptors fed vitamin E-supplemented diets. *J. Zoo Wildl. Med.* 20 (1): 62–67.

25 Campbell, T. (1994). Hematology. In: *Avian Medicine: Principles and Applications* (ed. B.R. Ritchie, G.J. Harrison and L.R. Harrison), 199–222. Lake Worth, FL: Wingers Publishing, Inc.

26 Campbell, T. and Ellis, C. (2007). *Avian and Exotic Animal Hematology and Cytology*, 3e, 76–77. Ames: Blackwell Publishing.

27 Campbell, T.W., Smith, S.A., and Zimmerman, K.L. (2010). Hematology of waterfowl and raptors. In: *Schalm's Veterinary Hematology*, 6e, 978–979. Ames: Blackwell Publishing.

28 Carnarius, M., Hafez, H.M., Henning, A. et al. (2008). Clinical signs and diagnosis of thiamine deficiency in juvenile goshawks (*Accipiter gentilis*). *Vet. Rec.* 163: 215–217.

29 Carpenter, J.W., Pattee, O.H., Fritts, S.H. et al. (2003). Experimental lead poisoning in Turkey vultures (*Cathartes aura*). *J. Wildl. Dis.* 39 (1): 96–104.

30 Casado, E., Balbontin, J., and Ferrer, M. (2002). Plasma chemistry in booted eagle (*Hieraaetus pennatus*)

during breeding season. *Comp. Biochem. Physiol. A* 131: 2233–2241.

31 Chaplin, S.B., Mueller, L.R., and Degernes, L.A. (1993). Physiological assessment of flight conditioning of rehabilitated raptors. In: *Raptor Biomedicine* (ed. P.T. Redig, J.E. Cooper and D. Remple), 167–173. Minneapolis, MN: University of Minnesota Press.

32 Chitty, J.R. (2008a). Basic techniques. In: *British Small Animal Veterinary Medical Association Manual of Raptors, Pigeons and Passerine Birds* (ed. J. Chitty and M. Lierz), 62–72. Gloucester UK: BSAVA.

33 Chitty, J.R. (2008b). Raptors: feather and skin diseases. In: *British Small Animal Veterinary Medical Association Manual of Raptors, Pigeons and Passerine Birds* (ed. J. Chitty and M. Lierz), 270–277. Gloucester: British Small Animal Veterinary Association.

34 Chitty, J.R. and Lierz, M. (2008c). Appendix 3-laboratory reference ranges. In: *British Small Animal Veterinary Association Manual of Raptors, Pigeons and Passerine Birds* (ed. J. Chitty and M. Lierz), 394–397. Gloucester UK: BSAVA.

35 Church, M.E., Gwiazda, R., Risebrough, R.W. et al. (2006). Ammunition is the principal source of lead accumulated by California condors reintroduced to the wild. *Environ. Sci. Technol.* 40 (19): 6143–6150.

36 Clark, A.J. and Scheuhammer, A.M. (2003). Lead poisoning in upland-foraging birds of prey in Canada. *Ecotoxicology* 12 (1–4): 23–30.

37 Clark, P. and Raidal, S. (2009). Hematological indicators of inflammation exhibited by Australian Falconiformes. *Comp. Clin. Pathol.* 18: 1–6.

38 Clark, P., Boardman, W., and Raidal, S. (2009). *Atlas of Clinical Avian Hematology*. Oxford, UK: Wiley-Blackwell.

39 Cole, R.A., Thomas, N.J., and Roderick, C.L. (1995). *Bothrigaster vanolans* (Trematoda: Cycloelidae) infection in two Florida snail kites (*Rostrhamus sociabilis plumbeus*). *J. Wildl. Dis.* 31 (4): 576–578.

40 Cooper, J.E. and Pomerance, A. (1982). Cardiac lesions in birds of prey. *J. Comp. Pathol.* 92: 161–168.

41 Cooper, J.E. (1985). *Veterinary Aspect of Captive Birds of Prey, 2nd Edition with 1985 Supplements*. Saul, Gloucestershire: Standfast Press.

42 Court, G.S., Gates, C.C., Boag, D.A. et al. (1990). A toxicological assessment of peregrine falcons *Falco peregrinus tundrius* breeding in the Keewatin District of the Northwest Territories, Canada. *Can. Field-Nat.* 104: 255–272.

43 Cray, C. and Tatum, L.M. (1998). Applications of protein electrophoresis in avian diagnostics. *J. Avian Med. Surg.* 12 (1): 4–10.

44 Cray, C., Rodriguez, M., and Zaias, J. (2007). Protein electrophoresis of psittacine plasma. *Vet. Clin. Pathol.* 36: 64–72.

45 Cray, C., Zaias, J., and Altman, N.H. (2009). Acute phase response in animals: a review. *Comp. Med.* 59 (6): 517–526.

46 Custer, T.W., Franson, J.C., and Pattee, O.H. (1984). Tissue lead distribution and hematologic effects in American kestrels (*Falco sparverius*) fed biologically incorporated lead. *J. Wildl. Dis.* 20 (1): 39–43.

47 Dawson, J.W. and Mannan, R.W. (1991a). Dominance hierarchies and helper contributions in Harris' hawks. *Auk* 108: 649–660.

48 Deem, S.L. (2003). Fungal diseases of birds of prey. *Vet. Clin. North Am. Exot. Anim. Pract.* 6: 363–376.

49 de Matos, R. (2008). Adrenal steroid metabolism in birds: anatomy, physiology, and clinical considerations. *Vet. Clin. North Am. Exot. Anim. Pract.* 11 (1): 15–23.

50 Dieter, M.P. and Wiemeyer, S.N. (1978). Six different plasma enzymes in bald eagles (*Haliaeetus leucocephalus*) and their usefulness in pathological diagnosis. *Comp. Biochem. Physiol.* 61: 153–155.

51 Dobado-Berrios, P.M., Tella, J.L., Ceballos, O. et al. (1998). Effects of age and captivity on plasma chemistry values of the Egyptian vulture. *Condor* 100: 719–725.

52 Dressen, D., Wimsatt, J., and Burkhard, M.J. (1999). The effects of isoflurane anesthesia on hematologic and plasma biochemical values of American kestrels (*Falco sparverius*). *J. Avian Med. Surg.* 13 (3): 173–179.

53 Dujowich, M., Mazet, J.K., and Zuba, J.R. (2005). Hematologic and biochemical reference ranges for captive California condors (*Gymnogyps californianus*). *J. Zoo Wildl. Med.* 36 (4): 590–597.

54 Dumonceaux, G. and Harrison, G.J. (1994). Toxins. In: *Avian Medicine: Principles and Applications* (ed. B.W. Ritchie, G.J. Harrison and L.R. Harrison), 1030–1052. Lake Worth, FL: Winger Publishing, Inc.

55 Eason, C.T. and Spurr, E.B. (1995). Review of the toxicity and impact of brodifacoum to non-target wildlife in New Zealand. *N. Z. J. Zool.* 22: 371–379.

56 Eason, C.T., Murphy, E.C., Wright, G.R.G. et al. (2002). Assessment of risks of brodifacoum to non-target birds and mammals in New Zealand. *Ecotoxicology* 11: 35–48.

57 Ecobichon, D.J. (2001). Mechanisms of toxicity. In: *Casarett & Doull's Toxicology: The Basic Science of Poisons*, 6e (ed. C.D. Klaassen), 763–810. New York: McGraw-Hill.

58 Elliot, J.E. and Shutt, L. (1993). Monitoring organochlorines in blood of sharp-shinned hawks *Accipiter striatus* migrating through the Great Lakes. *Environ. Toxicol. Chem.* 12: 241–250.

59 Ellis, A.E., Mead, D.G., Allison, A.B. et al. (2007). Pathology and epidemiology of natural West Nile viral infection of raptors in Georgia. *J. Wildl. Dis.* 43 (2): 214–223.

60 Facon, C., Beaufrère, H., Gaborit, C. et al. (2014). Cluster of atherosclerosis in a captive population of

black kites (*Milvus migrans* subsp.) in France and effect of nutrition on the plasma lipid profile. *Avian Dis.* 58 (1): 176–182.

61 Farner, D.S. (1943). Biliary amylase in the domestic fowl. *Biol. Bull.* 84 (3): 240–243.

62 Fernández-Repollet, E., Rowley, J., and Schwartz, A. (1982). Renal damage in gentamicin-treated lanner falcons. *J. Am. Vet. Med. Assoc.* 181 (11): 1392–1394.

63 Ferrer, M. and Dobado-Berrios, P. (1998). Factors affecting plasma chemistry values of the Spanish imperial eagle, *Aquila adalberti*. *Comp. Biochem. Physiol. A.* 120: 209–217.

64 Forbes, N.A. and Harcourt-Brown, N.H. (1991). Wing tip edema and dry gangrene of raptors. *Vet. Rec.* 128 (24): 575.

65 Forbes, N.A., Cooper, J.E., and Higgins, R.J. (2000). Neoplasms in birds of prey. In: *Raptor Biomedicine III* (ed. J.T. Lumeij, J.D. Remple, P.T. Redig, et al.), 127–146. Lake Worth, FL: Zoological Education Network.

66 Franson, J.C., Sileo, L., Pattee, O.H. et al. (1983). Effects of chronic dietary lead in American kestrels (*Falco sparverius*). *J. Wildl. Dis.* 19: 110–113.

67 Franson, J.C. (1996). Interpretation of tissue lead residues in birds other than waterfowl. In: *Environmental Contaminants in Wildlife* (ed. W.N. Beyer, G.H. Heinz and A.W. Redmon-Norwood), 265–279. Boca Raton, FL: CRC Lewis Publishers.

68 Frazier, D.L. (2000). Avian toxicology. In: *Manual of Avian Medicine* (ed. G.H. Olsen and S.E. Orosz), 228–263. Philadelphia: Mosby, Inc.

69 Friend, M. and Franson, J.C. (1999). *Field Manual of Wildlife Diseases – General Field Procedures and Diseases of Birds*, 337–340. Washington D.C.: U.S. Department of the Interior U.S. Geological Survey.

70 Fudge, A.M. (1997). Avian clinical pathology – hematology and chemistry. In: *Avian Medicine and Surgery* (ed. R. Altman, S. Clubb, G. Dorrestein, et al.), 142–157. Philadelphia: WB Saunders Co.

71 Fudge, A.M. (2000a). Avian blood sampling and artifact considerations. In: *Laboratory Medicine: Avian and Exotic Pets* (ed. A.M. Fudge), 1–8. Philadelphia: WB Saunders Co.

72 Fudge, A.M. (2000b). Avian liver and gastrointestinal testing. In: *Laboratory Medicine: Avian and Exotic Pets* (ed. A.M. Fudge), 47–55. Philadelphia: WB Saunders Co.

73 Garcia-Fernandez, A.J., Martinez-Lopez, E., Romero, D. et al. (2005). High Levels of Blood Lead in Griffon Vultures (Gyps fulvus) from Cazorla Natural Park (Southern Spain). *Environ. Toxicol.* 20 (4): 459–463.

74 García-Montijano, M., Garcia, A., Lemus, J.A. et al. (2002). Blood chemistry, protein electrophoresis, and hematologic values of captive Spanish imperial eagles (*Aquila adalberti*). *J. Zoo Wildl. Med.* 33 (2): 112–117.

75 García-Rodríguez, T., Ferrer, M., Recio, F. et al. (1987). Circadian rhythms of determined blood chemistry values in buzzards and eagle owls. *Comp. Biochem. Physiol.* 88A (4): 663–669.

76 Gelli, D., Ferrari, V., Franceschini, F. et al. (2009). Serum biochemistry and electrophoretic patterns in the Eurasian buzzard (*Buteo buteo*): reference values. *J. Wildl. Dis.* 45 (3): 828–833.

77 Gómez-Ramírez, P., Martínez-López, E., María-Mojica, P. et al. (2011). Blood lead levels and δ-ALAD inhibition in nestlings of Eurasian eagle owl (*Bubo bubo*) to assess lead exposure associated to an abandoned mining area. *Ecotoxicology* 20: 131–138.

78 Goyal, S.M., Jindal, N., Chander, Y. et al. (2010). Isolation of mixed subtypes of influenza a virus from a bald eagle (*Haliaeetus leucocephalus*). *Virol. J.* 7: 174.

79 Goyer, R.A. and Clarkson, T.W. (2001). Toxic effects of metals. In: *Casarett & Doull's Toxicology: The Basic Science of Poisons*, 6e, 811–867. New York: McGraw-Hill.

80 Greene, D.M., Engelmann, M., and Steck, T.R. (2004). An assessment of cage flight as an exercise method for raptors. *J. Raptor Res.* 38 (2): 125–132.

81 Gregus, Z. and Klaassen, C.D. (2001). Mechanisms of toxicity. In: *Casarett & Doull's Toxicology: The Basic Science of Poisons*, 6e (ed. C.D. Klaassen), 35–81. New York: McGraw-Hill.

82 Hall, J.S., Ip, H.S., Franson, C. et al. (2009). Experimental infection of a North American raptor, American kestrel (Falco sparverius), with highly pathogenic avian influenza virus (H5N1). *PLoS One* 4 (10): e7555.

83 Halliwell, W.H., Graham, D.L., and Ward, P. (1973). Nutritional diseases of birds-of-prey. *J. Zoo Anim. Med.* 4 (3): 18–20.

84 Halliwell, W.H. and Graham, D.L. (1978). Neoplasm in birds of prey. In: *Zoo and Wild Animal Medicine* (ed. M.E. Fowler), 286. Philadelphia: WB Saunders, Co.

85 Hamerton AE. 1943. Proceedings of the Zoological Society of London 112: 149.

86 Hampel, M.R., Kinne, J., Wernery, U. et al. (2009). Increasing fatal AA amyloidosis in hunting falcons and how to identify the risk: a report from the United Arab Emirates. *Amyloid* 16 (3): 122–132.

87 Harr, K.E. (2006). Diagnostic value of biochemistry. In: *Clinical Avian Medicine Vol. II* (ed. G.J. Harrison and T.L. Lightfoot), 611–629. Palm Beach, FL: Spix Publishing Inc.

88 Hawkey, C. and Dennett, T. (1989). *A Colour Atlas of Comparative Veterinary Haematology*. London, UK: Wolfe.

89 Hazelwood, R.L. (2000). Pancreas. In: *Sturkie's Avian Physiology*, 5e (ed. G. Causey Whittow), 539–555. San Diego: Academic Press.

90 Hegdal, P.L. and Colvin, B.A. (1988). Potential hazard to eastern screech-owls and other raptors of brodifacoum bait used for vole control in orchards. *Environ. Toxicol. Chem.* 7 (3): 245–260.
91 Henny, C.J. and Meeker, D.L. (1981). An evaluation of blood plasma for monitoring DDE in birds of prey. *Environ. Pollut. (Series A)* 25: 291–304.
92 Henny, C.J., Hill, E.F., Hoffman, F.J. et al. (2002). Nineteenth century mercury: hazard to wading birds and cormorants of the Carson River, Nevada. *Ecotoxicology* 11: 213–231.
93 Henny, C.J. and Elliott, J.E. (2007). Toxicology. In: *Raptor Research and Management Techniques* (ed. D.M. Bird and K.L. Bildstein), 329–350. Blaine, WA: Hancock House Publishers.
94 Hernández, M., Martin, S., and Forés, P. (1990). Clinical hematology and blood chemistry values for the common buzzard (*Buteo buteo*). *J. Raptor Res.* 24: 113–119.
95 Hernández, M. and Margalida, A. (2010). Hematology and blood chemistry reference values and age-related changes in wild bearded vultures (*Gypaetus barbatus*). *J. Wildl. Dis.* 46 (2): 390–400.
96 Hochleithner, M. (1994). Biochemistries. In: *Avian Medicine and Surgery: Principles and Applications* (ed. B.W. Ritchie, G.J. Harrison and L. Harrison), 223–245. Lake Worth, FL: Wingers Publishing.
97 Hoffman, D.J., Pattee, O.H., Wiemeyer, S.N. et al. (1981). Effects of lead shot ingestion on delta-aminolevulinic acid dehydratase activity, hemoglobin concentration, and serum chemistry in bald eagles. *J. Wildl. Dis.* 17: 423–431.
98 Hoffman, D.J., Franson, J.C., Pattee, O.H. et al. (1985). Biochemical and hematological effects of lead ingestion in nestling American kestrels (*Falco sparverius*). *Comp. Biochem. Physiol.* 80C: 431–439.
99 Hopkins, W.A., Hopkins, L.B., Unrine, J.M. et al. (2007). Mercury concentrations in tissues of osprey from the Carolinas, USA. *J. Wildl. Manag.* 71 (6): 1819–1829.
100 Hrubec, T.C., Whichard, J.M., Larsen, C.T. et al. (2002). Plasma versus serum: specific difference in biochemical analyte values. *J. Avian Med. Surg.* 16 (2): 101–105.
101 Hunter, S.R. and Powers, L.R. (1980). Raptor hematocrit values. *Condor* 82: 226–227.
102 Ivins, G.K., Weddle, W.H., and Halliwell, W.H. (1986). Hematology and serum chemistries in birds of prey. In: *Zoo and Wildlife Medicine*, 2e (ed. M.E. Fowler), 434–437. Philadelphia: WB Saunders.
103 Jarman, W.M., Burns, S.A., Mattox, W.G. et al. (1994). Organochlorine compounds in the plasma of peregrine falcons and gyrfalcons nesting in Greenland. *Arctic* 47: 334–340.
104 Jones, M.P. (2008). Raptors: raptors: paediatrics and behavioural development and disorders. In: *British Small Animal Veterinary Medical Association Manual of Raptors, Pigeons and Passerine Birds* (ed. J. Chitty and M. Lierz), 250–259. Gloucester: British Small Animal Veterinary Association.
105 Jones, M.P. (2013). Vascular diseases in birds of prey. *J. Exotic. Pet. Med.* 22 (4): 348–357.
106 Jones, M.P., Morandi, F., Wall, J.S. et al. (2013). Distribution of 2-deoxy-2-fluoro-d-glucose in the coelom of healthy bald eagles (*Haliaeetus leucocephalus*). *Am. J. Vet. Res.* 74 (3): 426–432.
107 Jones, M.P., Arheart, K., and Cray, C. (2014). Reference intervals, longitudinal analyses, and index of individuality of commonly measured laboratory variables in captive bald eagles (*Haliaeetus leucocephalus*). *J. Avian Med. Surg.* 28 (2): 118–126.
108 Jones, R. (2008). Raptors: systemic and non-infectious diseases. In: *British Small Animal Veterinary Medical Association Manual of Raptors, Pigeons and Passerine Birds* (ed. J. Chitty and M. Lierz), 284–298. Gloucester: British Small Animal Veterinary Association.
109 Jorgenson, R.D., Gough, P.M., and Graham, D.L. (1976). Experimental rabies in a great horned owl. *J. Wildl. Dis.* 12 (3): 444–447.
110 Joseph, V. (1998). Emergency care of raptors. *Vet. Clin. North Am. Exot. Anim. Pract.* 1 (1): 77–98.
111 Joseph, V. (1999). Raptor hematology and chemistry evaluation. *Vet. Clin. North Am. Exot. Anim. Pract.* 2 (3): 689–699.
112 Kelly, T.R. and Johnson, C.K. (2011). Lead exposure in free-flying Turkey vulture is associated with big game hunting in California. *PLoS One* 6 (4): e15350.
113 Kelly-Clark, W.K., McBurney, S., Forzán, M.J. et al. (2013). Detection and characterization of a *Trichomonas* isolate from a rehabilitated bald eagle (*Haliaeetus leucocephalus*). *J. Zoo Wildl. Med.* 44 (4): 1123–1126.
114 Kerr, M.G. (2002). *Veterinary Laboratory Medicine*, 2e. Oxford UK: Blackwell.
115 Keymer, I.F. and Samour, J. (2008). Endocrine disorders. In: *Avian Medicine* (ed. J. Samour), 302–308. Philadelphia: Mosby Elsevier.
116 Klasing, K.C. (1998). *Comparative Avian Nutrition*. New York: CAB International.
117 Knafo, S.E., Rapoport, G., Williams, J. et al. (2011). Cardiomyopathy and right-sided congestive heart failure in a red-tailed hawk (*Buteo jamaicensis*). *J. Avian Med. Surg.* 25 (1): 32–39.
118 Knuth, S.T. and Chaplin, S.B. (1994). The effect of exercise on plasma activities of lactate dehydrogenase and creatine kinase in red –tailed hawks (*Buteo jamaicensis*). *J. Raptor Res.* 28 (1): 27–33.
119 Kollias, G.V. and McLeish, I. (1978). Effects of ketamine hydrochloride in red-tailed hawks (*Buteo jamaicensis*) I – arterial blood gas and acid base.

Comp. Biochem. Physiol. C: Comp. Pharmacol. 60C: 57–59.

120 Kummrow, M., Silvanose, C., Di Somma, A. et al. (2012). Serum protein electrophoresis by using high-resolution agarose gel in clinically healthy and *Aspergillus* species-infected falcons. *J. Avian Med. Surg.* 26 (4): 213–220.

121 Lambert, O., Pouliquen, H., Larhantec, M. et al. (2007). Exposure of raptors and waterbirds to anticoagulant rodenticides (difenacoum, bromadiolone, coumatetralyl, coumafen, brodifacoum): epidemiological survey in Loire Atlantique (France). *Bull. Environ. Contam. Toxicol.* 79: 91–94.

122 Landmann, W.J.M., Sletten, K., Koch, C.A. et al. (1996). Chicken joint amyloid protein is of type AA: characterization of the amyloid protein. *Scand. J. Immunol.* 43: 210–230.

123 Lanzarot, M.I., Montesinos, A., San Andrés, M.I. et al. (2001). Hematological, protein electrophoresis and cholinesterase values of free-living nestling peregrine falcons in Spain. *J. Wildl. Dis.* 37 (1): 172–177.

124 Latimer, K.S. and Bienzle, D. (2010). Determination and interpretation of the avian leukogram. In: *Schalm's Veterinary Hematology*, 6e (ed. D.J. Weiss and K.J. Wardrop), 345–357. Ames: Blackwell Publishing Ltd.

125 Lavin, S., Cuenca, R., and Marco, I. (1992). Hematology and blood chemistry of the marsh harrier (*Circus aeruginosus*). *Comp. Biochem. Physiol.* 103A (3): 493–495.

126 Leppert, L., Zadorozhny, T.V., Belthoff, J.R. et al. (2006). Sex identification in four owl species from Idaho: DNA and morphometrics. *J. Raptor Res.* 40 (4): 291–294.

127 Leprince, P., Dandrifosse, G., and Schoffeniels, E. (1979). The digestive enzymes and acidity of the pellets regurgitated in raptors. *Biochem. Syst. Ecol.* 7: 223–227.

128 Lierz, M., Ewringmann, A., and Gobel, T. (1998). Blood chemical parameters for wild raptor patients and their changes after liver biopsy [in German]. *Berl. Munch. Tierarztl. Wochenschr.* 111 (7–8): 295–301.

129 Lierz, M. (2002). Blood chemistry values of the Saker falcon (*Falco cherrug*). *Tierärtztl. Prax.* 30: 368–388.

130 Lierz, M. (2003). Plasma chemistry reference values for gyrfalcons (*Falco rusticolus*). *Vet. Rec.* 153: 182–183.

131 Lierz, M. and Hafez, H.M. (2006). Plasma chemistry reference values in hybrid falcons in relation to their species of origin. *Vet. Rec.* 159: 79–82.

132 Lierz, M., Hagen, N., Hernandez-Divers, S.J., and Hafez, H.M. (2008). Occurrence of mycoplasmas in free-ranging birds of prey in Germany. *J. Wildl. Dis.* 44 (4): 845–850.

133 Limiñana, R., López-Olvera, J.R., Gallardo, M. et al. (2009). Blood chemistry and hematologic values in free-living nestlings of Montagu's harriers (*Circus pygargus*) in a natural habitat. *J. Zoo Wildl. Med.* 40 (4): 687–695.

134 Lind, P.J., Wolff, P.L., Petrini, K.R. et al. (1990). Morphology of the eosinophil in raptors. *J. Assoc. Avian Vet.* 4 (1): 33–39.

135 Lish, J.W. and Voelker, W.G. (1986). Field identification aspects of some red-tailed hawk subspecies. *Am. Birds* 40 (2): 197–202.

136 Lumeij, J.T. and Westerhof, I. (1987). Blood chemistry for the evaluation of hepatobiliary disease in birds; a review. In: *A Contribution to Clinical Investigative Methods for Birds with Special Reference to the Racing Pigeon (Columbia livia domestica)* (ed. J.T. Lumeij), 36–43. Utrecht: University of Utrecht.

137 Lumeij, J.T., Meidam, M., and Wolfswinkel, J. (1988). Enzyme activities in tissues and elimination half-lives of homologous muscle and liver enzymes in the racing pigeon (*Columbia livia domestica*). *Avian Pathol.* 17: 851–864.

138 Lumeij, J.T., Bruinje, J.J., and Kwant, M.M. (1990). Comparison of different methods of measuring protein and albumin in pigeon sera. *Avian Pathol.* 19 (2): 255–261.

139 Lumeij, J.T. and Remple, J.D. (1991). Plasma urea, creatinine, and uric acid concentrations in relation to feeding in peregrine falcons (*Falco peregrinus*). *Avian Pathol.* 20: 79–83.

140 Lumeij, J.T., Remple, J.D., and Riddle, K.E. (1993). Relationship of plasma total protein and albumin to total calcium in peregrine falcons (*Falco peregrinus*). *Avian Pathol.* 22 (1): 183–188.

141 Lumeij, J.T., Remple, J.D., Remple, C.J. et al. (1998). Plasma chemistry in peregrine falcons (*Falco peregrinus*): reference values and physiological variations of importance for interpretation. *Avian Pathol.* 27: 129–132.

142 Lumeij, J.T. (2008). Avian clinical biochemistry. In: *Clinical Biochemistry of Domestic Animals*, 6e (ed. J.J. Kaneko, J.W. Harvey and M.L. Bruss), 839–872. Burlington, MA: Academic Press.

143 McLean, R.G. and Ubico, S.R. (2007). Arboviruses in birds. In: *Infectious Diseases of Wild Birds* (ed. N.J. Thomas, D. Bruce Hunter and C.T. Atkinson), 17–62. Ames, IA: Blackwell Publishing Ltd.

144 Mealey, B., Parks, G.M., and Pages, C.M. (2004). Serum chemistry values for nestling bald eagles (*Haliaeetus leucocephalus*) in Florida bay, Everglades National Park. *J. Raptor Res.* 38 (1): 96–100.

145 Mendenhall, V.M. and Pank, L.F. (1980). Secondary poisoning of owls by anticoagulant rodenticides. *Wildl. Soc. Bull.* 8 (4): 311–315.

146 Melillo, A. (2013). Applications of serum protein electrophoresis in exotic pet medicine. *Vet. Clin. Exot. Anim.* 16: 211–225.

147 Miller, M.R., Wayland, M.E., and Bortolotti, G.R. (2001). Hemograms for and nutritional condition of migrant bald eagles tested for exposure to lead. *J. Wildl. Dis.* 37 (3): 481–488.

148 Minick, M.C. and Duke, G.E. (1991). Simultaneous determinations of plasma insulin, glucose and glucagon levels in fasting, previously stressed but convalescing bald eagles, *Haliaeetus leucocephalus linnaeus. Comp. Biochem. Physiol.* 99A (3): 307–311.

149 Minick, M.C., Duke, G.E., Fishman, S.W. et al. (1996). Effects of intragastric nutrients upon simultaneously determined plasma insulin, glucagon, insulin/glucagon ratios and glucose in red-tailed hawks, *Buteo jamaicensis* Gmelin. *Comp. Biochem. Physiol.* 113 (2): 173–179.

150 Mirandé, L.A., Howerth, E.W., and Poston, R.P. (1992). Chlamydiosis in a red-tailed hawk (*Buteo jamaicensis*). *J. Wildl. Dis.* 28 (2): 284–287.

151 Mitchell, E.B. and Johns, J. (2008). Avian hematology and related disorders. *Vet. Clin. Exot. Anim.* 11: 501–522.

152 Mizobe, M., Kondo, F., Kumamoto, K. et al. (1997). High-performance liquid chromatographic analysis of bilirubin and biliverdin from jaundiced broilers. *J. Vet. Med. Sci.* 59 (8): 677–680.

153 Morishita, T.Y., Lowenstine, L.J., Dwight, C. et al. (1997). Lesions associated with Pasteurella multocida infection in raptors. *Avian Dis.* 41 (1): 203–213.

154 Müller, K., Altenkamp, R., Brunnberg, L. et al. (2007). Pinching-off syndrome in free-ranging white-tailed sea eagles (*Haliaeetus albicilla*) in Europe: frequency and geographic distribution of a generalized feather abnormality. *J. Avian Med. Surg.* 21 (2): 103–109.

155 Murphy, M.J. and Gerken, D.F. (1989). The anticoagulant rodenticides. In: *Current Veterinary Therapy X: Small Animal Practice* (ed. R.W. Kirk), 143–146. Philadelphia: WB Saunders, Co.

156 Murray, M. and Tseng, F. (2008). Diagnosis and treatment of secondary anticoagulant rodenticide Toxicosis in a red-tailed hawk (*Buteo jamaicensis*). *J. Avian Med. Surg.* 22 (1): 41–46.

157 Murray, M. (2011). Anticoagulant rodenticide exposure and toxicosis in four species of birds of prey presented to a wildlife clinic in Massachusetts, 2006-2010. *J. Zoo Wildl. Med.* 42 (1): 88–97.

158 Murray M. 2013. Presenting problem: Anticoagulant rodenticide toxicosis in free-living birds of prey. LafeberVet.com website. August 5, 2013. Available at http://www.lafebervet.com/emergency-medicine/birds/presenting-problem-antidoagulant-rodenticide-toxicosis-in-free-living-birds-of-prey.

159 Naidoo, V., Diekmann, M., Wolters, K. et al. (2008). Establishment of selected baseline blood chemistry and hematologic parameters in captive and wild-caught African white-backed vultures (*Gyps africanus*). *J. Wildl. Dis.* 44 (3): 649–654.

160 Naldo, J.L., Samour, J., and Sakkir, M. (2012). Plasma bile acids reference value in the gyr falcon (*Falco rusticolus*). *Comp. Clin. Pathol.* 21: 953–955.

161 Nazifi, S., Nabinejad, A., and Sepehrimanesh, M. (2008). Haematology and serum biochemistry of golden eagles (*Aquila chrysaetos*) in Iran. *Comp. Clin. Pathol.* 17: 197–201.

162 Nemeth, N., Kratz, G., Edwards, E. et al. (2007). Surveillance for West Nile virus in clinic-admitted raptors, Colorado. *Emerg. Infect. Dis.* 13 (2): 305.

163 Parga, M., Pendl, H., and Forbes, N. (2001). The effect of transport on hematologic parameters in trained and untrained Harris's hawks (*Parabuteo unicinctus*) and Peregrine falcons (*Falco peregrinus*). *J. Avian Med. Surg.* 15 (3): 162–169.

164 Pattee, O.H., Bloom, P.H., Scott, J.M. et al. (1990). Lead hazards within the range of the California condor. *Condor* 92: 931–937.

165 Pattee, O.H., Carpenter, J.W., Fritts, S.H. et al. (2006). Lead poisoning in captive Andean condors (*Vulture gryphus*). *J. Wildl. Dis.* 42 (4): 772–779.

166 Peh, W.C.G. and Reinus, W.R. (1995). Lead arthropathy: a cause of delayed onset lead poising. *Skelet. Radiol.* 24: 357–360.

167 Phalen, D.N. (2000). Avian Renal Disorders. In: *Laboratory Medicine: Avian and Exotic Pets* (ed. A.M. Fudge), 61–68. Philadelphia: WB Saunders, Co.

168 Pinkerton, M.E., Wellehan, J.F.X., Johnson, A.J. et al. (2008). Columbid herpesvirus-1 in two Cooper's hawks (*Accipiter cooperii*) with fatal inclusion body disease. *J. Wildl. Dis.* 44 (3): 622–628.

169 Pokras, M.A., Wheeldon, E.B., and Sedgwick, C.J. (1993). Trichomoniasis in owls: report on a number of cases and a survey of the literature. In: *Raptor Biomedicine* (ed. P.T. Redig, J.E. Cooper, J.D. Remple and D.B. Hunter), 88–91. Univ Minnesota.

170 Polo, F.J., Celdran, J.F., Peinado, V.I. et al. (1992). Hematological values for four species of bird of prey. *Condor* 94: 1000–1013.

171 Powers, L., Pokras, M., Rio, K. et al. (1994). Hematology and occurrence of hemoparasites in migrating sharp-shinned hawks (*Accipiter striatus*) during fall migration. *J. Raptor Res.* 28 (3): 178–185.

172 Rae, M. (2000). Avian endocrine disorders. In: *Laboratory Medicine: Avian and Exotic Pets* (ed. A.M. Fudge), 76–89. Philadelphia: WB Saunders, Co.

173 Rattner, B.A., Horak, K.E., Warner, S.E. et al. (2011). Acute toxicity, histopathology, and coagulopathy in American kestrels (Falco sparverius) following

administration of the rodenticide diphacinone. *Environ. Toxicol. Chem.* 30 (5): 1213–1222.

174 Rattner, B.A., Horak, K.E., Lazarus, R.S. et al. (2012). Assessment of toxicity and potential risk of the anticoagulant rodenticide diphacinone using eastern screech owls (*Megascops asio*). *Ecotoxicology* 21: 832–846.

175 Redig, P.T., Lawler, E.M., Schwartz, S. et al. (1991). Effects of chronic exposure to sublethal concentrations of lead acetate on heme synthesis and immune function in red-tailed hawks. *Arch. Environ. Contam. Toxicol.* 21: 72–77.

176 Redig, P.T. and Arent, L.R. (2008). Raptor toxicology. *Vet. Clin. Exot. Anim.* 11: 261–282.

177 Redig, P.T. and Goyal, S.M. (2012). Serologic evidence of exposure of raptors to influenza a virus. *Avian Dis.* 56 (2): 411–413.

178 Rehder, N.B., Bird, D.M., and Lague, P.C. (1982). Variations in blood packed cell volume of captive American kestrels. *Comp. Biochem. Physiol.* 72A (1): 105–109.

179 Rehder, N.B. and Bird, D.M. (1983). Annual profiles of blood packed cell volumes of captive American kestrels. *Can. J. Zool.* 61 (11): 2550–2555.

180 Rehder, N.B., Bird, D.M., Lague, P.C., and MacKay, C. (1982). Variation in selected hematological parameters of captive red-tailed hawks. *J. Wildl. Dis.* 18 (1): 105–109.

181 Rehman, M.A., Umer, M., Sepah, Y.J. et al. (2007). Bullet-induced synovitis as a cause of secondary osteoarthritis of the hip join: a case report and review of literature. *J. Med. Case Rep.* 1: 171.

182 Reiser, M.H. and Temple, S.A. (1981). Effects of chronic lead ingestion on birds of prey. In: *Recent Advances in the Study of Raptor Diseases* (ed. J.E. Cooper and A.G. Greenwood), 21–25. West Yorkshire: Chiron Publications Ltd.

183 Ritchie, B.W. (1995). Herpesviridae. In: *Avian Viruses: Function and Control*, 171–222. Lake Worth, FL: Wingers Publishing.

184 Rodríguez, A., Negro, J.J., and Figuerola, J. (2011). Sources of variation for nutritional condition indices of the plasma of migratory lesser kestrels in the breeding grounds. *Comp. Biochem. Physiol., Part A Mol. Integr. Physiol.* 160: 453–460.

185 Rolfhus, K.R., Hall, B.D., Monson, B.A. et al. (2011). Assessment of mercury bioaccumulation within the pelagic food web of lakes in the western Great Lakes region. *Ecotoxicology* 20 (7): 1520–1529.

186 Rosenthal, K.L. (2000). Avian protein disorders. In: *Laboratory Medicine: Avian and Exotic Pets* (ed. A.M. Fudge), 171–173. Philadelphia: WB Saunders, Co.

187 Rupley, A.E. (1997). *Manual of Avian Practice*, 301–309. Philadelphia: WB Saunders.

188 Samour, J.H., Naldo, J.L., Wernery, U. et al. (2001). Thyroid cystadenocarcinoma in a saker falcon (*Falco cherrug*). *Vet. Rec.* 149: 277–278.

189 Samour, J.H. and Naldo, J. (2002). Diagnosis and therapeutic management of lead toxicosis in falcons in Saudi Arabia. *J. Avian Med. Surg.* 16 (1): 16–20.

190 Samour, J. (2006). Management of raptors. In: *Clinical Avian Medicine Vol II* (ed. G.J. Harrison and T.L. Lightfoot), 948–954. Palm Beach, FL: Spix Publishing.

191 Sarasola, J.H., Negro, J.J., and Travaini, A. (2004). Nutritional condition and serum biochemistry for free living Swainson's hawks wintering in Central Argentina. *Comp. Biochem. Physiol., Part A Mol. Integr. Physiol.* 137: 697–701.

192 Schink, B., Hafez, H.M., and Lierz, M. (2008). Alpha-tocopherol in captive falcons: reference values and dietary impact. *J. Avian Med. Surg.* 22 (2): 99–102.

193 Mm, S., Oaks, J.L., Rotstein, D. et al. (2005). Characterization of a new species of adenovirus in falcons. *J. Clin. Microbiol.* 43 (7): 3402–3413.

194 Shapiro, C.J. and Weathers, W.W. (1981). Metabolic and behavioral responses of American kestrels to food deprivation. *Comp. Biochem. Physiol.* 68A: 111–114.

195 Shannon, L.M., Poulton, J., Emmons, R.W. et al. (1988). Serological survey for rabies antibodies in raptors from California. *J. Wildl. Dis.* 24 (2): 264–267.

196 Shrubsole-Cockwill, A., Wojnarowicz, C., and Parker, D. (2008). Atherosclerosis and ischemic cardiomyopathy in a captive, adult red-tailed hawk (*Buteo jamaicensis*). *Avian Dis.* 52: 537–539.

197 Snyder, J.E., Bird, D.M., and Lague, P.C. (1981). Variations in selected parameters in the blood of captive American kestrels. In: *Recent Advances in the Study of Raptor Diseases* (ed. J.E. Cooper and A.G. Greenwood), 178. West Yorkshire, UK: Chiron.

198 Spagnolo, V., Crippa, V., Marzia, A. et al. (2008). Hematologic, biochemical, and protein electrophoretic values in captive tawny owls (*Strix aluco*). *Vet. Clin. Pathol.* 37 (2): 225–228.

199 Spalding, M.G., Frederick, P.C., McGill, H.C. et al. (2000). Histologic, neurologic, and immunologic effects of methylmercury in captive great egrets. *J. Wildl. Dis.* 36 (3): 423–435.

200 Stein, R.W., Yamamoto, J.T., Fry, D.M. et al. (1998). Comparative hematology and plasma biochemistry of red-tailed hawks and American kestrels wintering in California. *J. Raptor Res.* 32 (2): 163–169.

201 Stone, W.B., Okoniewski, J.C., and Stedelin, J.R. (2003). Anticoagulant rodenticides and raptors: recent findings from New York, 1998-2001. *Bull. Environ. Contam. Toxicol.* 70: 34–40.

202 Stone, W.B., Okoniewski, J.C., Therrien, J.E. et al. (2004). VecTest as diagnostic and surveillance tool for West Nile virus in dead birds. *Emerg. Infect. Dis.* 10 (12): 2175–2181.

203 Stout, J.D., Brinker, D.F., Driscoll, C.P. et al. (2010). Serum biochemistry values, plasma mineral levels, and whole blood heavy metal measurements in wild northern goshawks (*Accipter gentilis*). *J. Zoo Wildl. Med.* 41 (4): 649–655.

204 Szabo, Z., Klein, A., and Jakab, C. (2014). Hematologic and plasma biochemistry reference intervals of healthy adult barn owls (*Tyto alba*). *Avian Dis.* 58: 228–231.

205 Tatum, L.M., Zaias, J., Mealey, B.K. et al. (2000). Protein electrophoresis as a diagnostic indicator and prognostic tool in raptor medicine. *J. Zoo Wildl. Med.* 31 (4): 497–502.

206 Tell, L.A., Ferrell, S.T., and Gibbons, P.M. (2004). Avian Mycobacteriosis in free-living raptors in 107. California: 6 cases (1997-2001). *J. Avian Med. Surg.* 18 (1): 30–40.

207 Thomas, J.S. (2000). Protein electrophoresis. In: *Schalm's Veterinary Hematology*, 5e (ed. B.F. Felmann, J.G. Zinkl and N.C. Jain), 899–903. Baltimore, MD: Lippincott Williams & Wilkins.

208 Thomson, A.E., Squires, E.J., and Gentry, P.A. (2002). Assessment of factor V, VII and X activities, the key coagulant proteins of the tissue factor pathway in poultry plasma. *Br. Poult. Sci.* 43 (2): 313–321.

209 Toyoda, T., Ochia, K., Komatsu, M. et al. (2004). Nutritional secondary hyperparathyroidism and osteodystrophia fibrosa in a Hodgson's hawk-eagle (*Spizaetus nipalensis*). *Avian. Pathol.* 33 (1): 9–12.

210 Toro, H., Pavéz, E.F., Gough, R.E. et al. (1997). Serum chemistry and antibody status to some avian pathogens of free-living and captive condors (*Vultur gryphus*) of Central Chile. *Avian. Pathol.* 26: 339–345.

211 Tschopp, R., Bailey, T., Di Somma, A. et al. (2007). Urinalysis as a noninvasive health screening procedure in Falconidae. *J. Avian Med. Surg.* 21 (1): 8–12.

212 Vajro, P., Thaler, M.M., and Blankaert, N. (1995). Bile pigment composition and bilirubin esterification in the developing chick. *Pediatr. Res.* 38 (3): 349–355

213 VanDevanter, D.R., Warrener, P., Bennett, L. et al. (1996). Detection and analysis of diverse herpesviral species by consensus primer PCR. *J. Clin. Microbiol.* 34 (7): 1666–1671.

214 Villegas, A., Sanchez, J.M., Costillo, E. et al. (2002). Blood chemistry and haematocrit of the black vulture (*Aegypius monarchus*). *Comp. Biochem. Physiol., Part A Mol. Integr. Physiol.* 132: 489–497.

215 Vleck, C.M., Mays, N.A., Dawson, J.W. et al. (1991). Hormonal correlates of parental and helping behavior in cooperatively breeding Harris' hawks (*Parabuteo unicinctus*). *Auk* 108: 638–648.

216 Wadsworth, P.F. and Jones, D.M. (1979). Some abnormalities of the thyroid gland in non-domesticated birds. *Avian Pathol.* 8: 279–284.

217 Walker, L.A., Turk, A., Long, S.M. et al. (2008). Second generation anticoagulant rodenticides in tawny owls (*Strix aluco*) from great Britain. *Sci. Total Environ.* 392 (1): 93–98.

218 Wallner-Pendleton, E.A., Rogers, D., and Epple, A. (1993). Diabetes mellitus in a red-tailed hawk (*Buteo jamaicensis*). *Avian Pathol.* 22: 631–635.

219 Webster KH. 2009.Validation of prothrombin time (PT) assay for assessment of brodifacoum exposure in Japanese quail and barn owls. (Master's thesis). Retrieved from Simon Fraser University Library Research Repository. Available at http://summit.sfu.ca/item/9810.

220 Weidensaul, S. (1989). *North American Birds of Prey*. New York: WH Smith Publishers.

221 Weidensaul, S. (1996). *Raptors, the Birds of Prey: An Almanac of Hawks, Eagles, and Falcons of the World*. Hong Kong: Lyons and Burford, Publishers.

222 Wellehan, J.F.X. (2003). Frostbite in birds: pathophysiology and treatment. *Compend. Contin. Educ.* 25 (10): 776–781.

223 Wernery, R., Wernery, U., Kinne, J., and Samour, J. (2004). *Colour Atlas of Falcon Medicine*. Hannover: Schlütersche Verlagsgesellschaft mbH & Co.

224 Westlake, G.E., Martin, P.A., Stanley, P.I. et al. (1983). Control enzyme levels in the plasma, brain and liver from wild birds and mammals in Britain. *Comp. Biochem. Physiol. C* 76: 15–24.

225 Wheeler, B.K. and Clark, W.S. (1995). *A Photographic Guide to North American Raptors*. London: Academic Press.

226 Wheler, C.L. (1993). Herpesvirus disease in raptors: a review of the literature. In: *Raptor Biomedicine* (ed. P.T. Redig, J.E. Cooper, et al.), 103–107. Minneapolis: University of Minnesota Press.

227 Willette, M., Ponder, J., Cruz-Martinez, L. et al. (2009). Management of select bacterial and parasitic conditions of raptors. *Vet. Clin. North Am. Exot. Anim. Pract.* 12 (3): 491–517. Review Article.

228 Wünschmann, A., Shivers, J., Bender, J. et al. (2005). Pathologic and immunohistochemical findings in goshawks (*Accipiter gentilis*) and great horned owls (*Bubo virginianus*) naturally infected with West Nile virus. *Avian Dis.* 49 (2): 252–259.

229 Zenoble, R.D., Kemppainen, R.J., Young, D.W. et al. (1985). Effect of ACTH on plasma corticosterone and cortisol in eagles and condors. *J. Am. Vet. Med. Assoc.* 187: 1119–1120.

25

Psittaciformes

Thomas N. Tully, Jr., DVM, MS, DABVP (Avian), DECZM (Avian)

Department of Veterinary Clinical Sciences, Louisiana State University School of Veterinary Medicine, Baton Rouge, Louisiana, USA

Introduction

A cornerstone to assessing parrot health is clinical pathologic testing and the ability critically assess diagnostic results. The large number of parrot species dictates that many available diagnostic tests have not been validated for all species. Moreover, many published reference ranges have been compiled from specific instrumentation and clinical cases where the age and medical history are unknown. Clinical case circumstances are unlikely to be similar to those parameters in which the reference range was established. Veterinarians must understand that the assessment of diagnostic test result values rely on many factors (e.g., history, clinical presentation, complicating disease factors, husbandry, nutrition, sex, reproductive status, and environment). Therefore, reference ranges, whether gleaned from publication or provided by diagnostic laboratories, seldom provide a definitive answer. Utilizing clinical pathology to aid in the assessment of parrot health is considered a standard of care in avian medicine. It has been stated that many birds do not express clinical signs until late in the disease process, and the signs they do show may be subtle and nonspecific [1]. While the clinical signs may be subtle and nonspecific, the astute bird owner will recognize the abnormalities and present the bird for a medical evaluation. It is often through diagnostic testing that the magnitude of the illness is determined. An African gray parrot that may be slightly depressed can have a total white cell count of 75 000 when the expected range is 8000–15 000. The importance of using clinical pathology for the successful treatment of psittacine patients cannot be underestimated. Diagnostic tests can also confirm disease conditions which birds may suffer.

Species

The popularity of parrots as pets, use as exhibit animals in zoological collections, and the ever-increasing need for conservation efforts has resulted in a rapid advancement of health-care related to these species. The avian order Psittaciformes consists of approximately 372 species with 3 "super" families, Psittacoidea (true parrots), Cacatuoidea (cockatoos), and Strigopoidea (New Zealand parrots) [2]. The greatest diversity and concentration of Psittaciformes are in the tropical/subtropical continental ecosystems. These birds are characterized by zygodactyl feet and curved bills. Psittaciformes have been maintained as pets and have been an integral part of diverse cultures throughout the world for many centuries (Figure 25.1). They are one of the most common bird groups maintained as pets and zoological exhibit animals in many countries [3]. The destruction of breeding habitat and illegal trade has resulted in many psittacine species being listed as threated or endangered by the Convention on International Trade in Endangered Species (CITES). For many veterinarians treating psittacine species, the parrot species presented for care are more easily defined (Table 25.1). Restrictions on wild bird importation in the United States and Europe, the ease of captive reproduction, and popularity of the

Exotic Animal Laboratory Diagnosis, First Edition. Edited by J. Jill Heatley and Karen E. Russell.

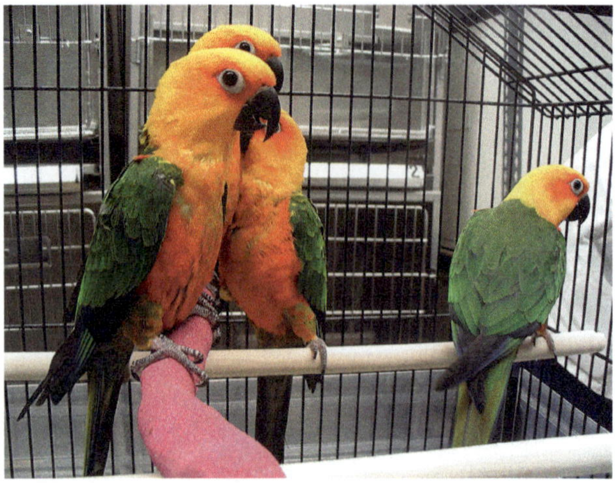

Figure 25.1 Parrots are common pets due to their beauty, companionship qualities, and intelligence.

species as a pet each contribute to these changes. Smaller species numbers being treated allows the scientific community to concentrate their efforts when developing diagnostic testing parameters that allow for a more precise interpretation of results by the veterinary practitioner.

Sample Collection

As with many animal patients that are presented to veterinary clinics, parrot species are often nervous and stressed. Abnormal physiologic responses by these patients can adversely affect laboratory results [4]. Increased endogenous corticosteroid concentrations and adrenocortical stress can cause a transient leukocytosis, heterophilia, lymphopenia, and eosinopenia [4, 5]. The increased adrenocortical stress can be exacerbated by placement in a travel cage, travel, interaction with other animals in a waiting room, and restraint prior to collection of the sample to be submitted for diagnostic testing [4]. The veterinarian must critically assess the patient prior to collection of diagnostic samples for its ability to withstand the stress of restraint. It is of no benefit to the diagnostic process if the patient dies during the sample collection procedure. When assessing the need to perform a diagnostic test, one should remember that diagnostic tests are used confirm diagnoses, not make diagnoses.

Successful phlebotomy is based on one's confidence, proper positioning of the patient, exposure of the vein, and appropriate equipment. Reduced stress to the patient restraint decreases adverse consequences to sick birds and provides more accurate test results. Since a one-handed "draw" technique is recommended for parrot blood collection, a $3\,cm^3$ syringe and a 26–25 gauge (g.) needle is the equipment of choice for birds that weigh >50 g. For birds that weigh <50 g, a $1\,cm^3$ syringe with a 26–25 g. needle is recommended since the plunger of the syringe will not significantly bend if 0.4 ml of blood is collected. The needle hub should be snugly affixed to the syringe to prevent air aspiration into the sample. The numbers of the syringe barrel should face the phlebotomist to allow observance of collection of the safe maximum amount of blood and to avoid overcollection in small psittacine patients. The bevel of the needle may be facing up or down. The thin (6–8 cell layers) pliable skin of psittacine species combined with vessel mobility and

Table 25.1 Overview of parrot species commonly presented to veterinary hospitals and areas of origin.

Common name	Scientific name	Geographic origin
Budgerigar	*Melopsittacus undulatus*	Australia
Ring-necked parakeet	*Psittacula spp.*	Africa, Indochina, Malaysia
Cockatiel	*Nymphicus hollandicus*	Australia
Cockatoo	*Cacatua* spp.	Australia
Macaw	*Ara* spp.	South & Central America
African gray	*Psittacus* spp.	Central Africa
Lovebirds	*Agapornis* spp.	Africa
Lories	*Eos* spp.	Indonesia
Lorikeets	*Trichoglossus* spp.	Australia
Parrotlet	*Forpus* spp.	Mexico, Central and South America
Amazon	*Amazona* spp.	Mexico, Central and South America
Conure	*Aratinga* spp.	Central, South America, Brazil
Quaker or Monk	*Myiopsitta monachus*	Paraguay, Uruguay, Argentina

strong elastic tunica adventitia dictate that the vein be visualized in most of these species prior to attempting venipuncture. Unless the vein is visualized, it is nearly impossible to collect blood from a parrot using a blind technique. Depending on the phlebotomist's preference, the needle can be bent to obtain a better angle of approach to the vein for insertion into the vessel lumen.

Restraint

The avian veterinarian and/or veterinary technician should become proficient at collection of diagnostic samples (e.g., blood) from the unanesthetized parrot patient. Parrot species <150 g, can be held in the non-dominant hand while using the other to collect blood (Figure 25.2). For larger parrots, cockatoos, and macaws, an associate is required to restrain the bird for the phlebotomist (Figure 25.3). Sedation of avian patients prior to handling may reduce the stress involved with collection of diagnostic samples. For macaws and large cockatoos, intranasal sedation has been advocated to reduce stress on the patient, and intranasal administration of midazolam (1–2 mg/kg) and combined with butorphanol (1–2 mg/kg) may be administered if deep sedation is required [6]. Midazolam sedation can be reversed with flumazenil (0.05–0.1 mg/kg INas, IV or IM) [6]. The effects of this intranasal sedation technique on blood parameters have not been determined. General anesthesia of parrots should be restricted to cases in which the patient's health would be compromised if not anesthetized, in rare instances; anesthesia may be required for the extremely fractious, stressed large parrot patient. Anesthetics most commonly used in birds are the inhalational and include sevoflurane and isoflurane; induction via face mask is common. Intubation is not generally recommended unless procedures are expected to last greater than 20 min, which should not be the case for just sample collection.

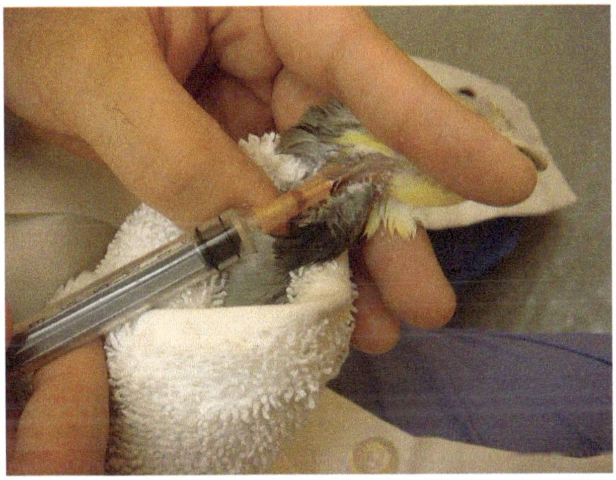

Figure 25.2 A one-handed blood collection technique being performed on a budgerigar.

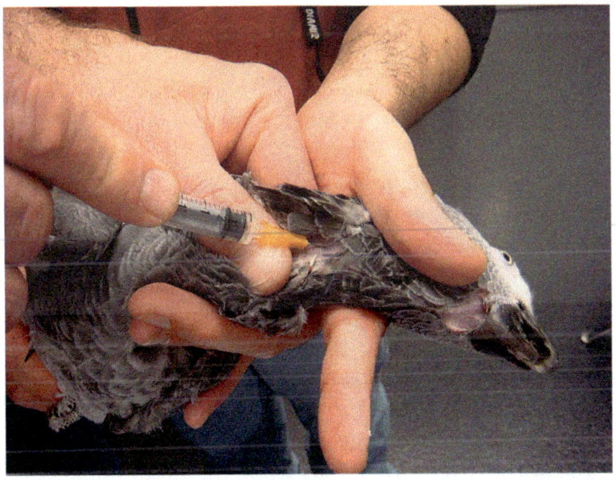

Figure 25.3 Collection of blood from a larger psittacine patient requires assistance.

Sample Site Options

Approaches to three venipuncture sites most often used for collection of blood from parrot species, the right jugular vein, the basilic vein, and the median metatarsal vein, are described below. Although recommended, these are not the only veins where blood can be collected. If there is a vein not listed that is easy to access, that location should be considered for obtaining the blood sample. Clipping a claw allows one to "milk" blood from the vascular capillary bed and has been used in the past for acquiring blood samples from psittacine patients. Blood collected from a clipped claw is only useful for providing samples for genetically or "DNA" sexing a bird. Blood test (e.g., complete blood count, plasma chemistry panel) results are severely compromised when claw blood is used, reducing a veterinarian's ability to properly assess the patient. Silver nitrate sticks are recommended for hemostasis of bleeding parrot claws.

Jugular Vein

The author prefers collecting blood from all psittacine patients from the right jugular vein. Although there are differing techniques of directing the needle toward the body or toward the head, the author prefers directing the needle toward the head when accessing this vein (Figure 25.4). The forefinger and middle finger are used in a scissors hold under the head while the thumb holds off the vein and provides a stable base to rest the barrel of the syringe as the needle is inserted into the vein. Negative pressure is achieved by pulling slightly on the plunger of the syringe as the needle enters the skin directly over the vein. Once blood enters, the hub of the needle insertion ceases, and a slow continuous draw is

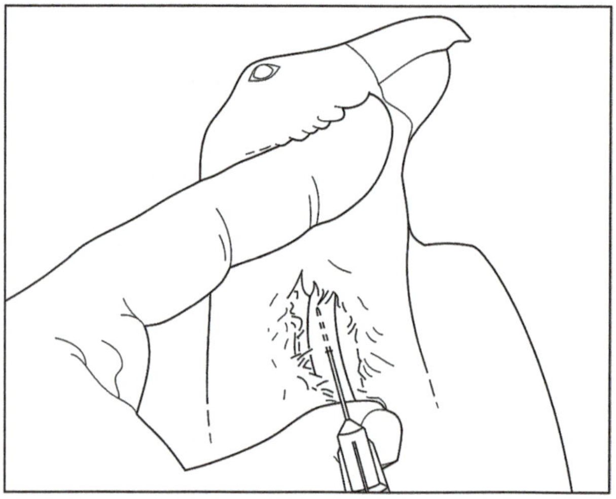

Figure 25.4 The location of choice to collect blood from most psittacine species is the right jugular vein.

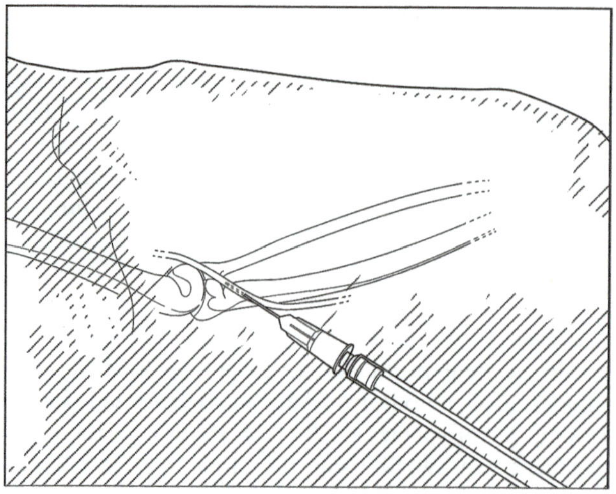

Figure 25.5 Blood collection from the basilic vein.

placed on the plunger until the desired amount of blood is obtained. The needle is then removed from the vein, and digital pressure is placed on the vein for 45–60 s. The left jugular vein may be used but is universally smaller in all parrot species. Left jugular venipuncture is also challenging based on parrot positioning for phlebotomists that are right-hand dominant. Collection of blood from the left jugular vein requires the parrot's beak to face into the hand holding the bird. Successful collection of blood from a parrot's left jugular vein requires practice, experience, and patience.

Basilic Vein

Collection of blood from the basilic vein that courses over the proximal aspect of the ulna toward the humerus requires a more parallel approach of the needle. With the bird held in dorsal recumbency, the wing is extended to expose the ventral surface. The feathers at the distal ulna are moistened with an alcohol-soaked cotton ball and swept away to expose the venipuncture site. The forefinger and middle finger are used to hold off the vein at the mid humerus while the thumb rests near the proximal radius and ulna (Figure 25.5). Rest the barrel of the syringe on the thumb as the needle is inserted, almost parallel, into the basilic vein as it courses dorsally over the ulna toward the humerus. Negative pressure is maintained on the syringe from the time the needle enters the skin until blood is observed in the hub of the needle. Once blood is observed, slow negative pressure is maintained until the required amount is withdrawn. This vein tends to collapse if excess pressure is placed on the plunger. If blood stops flowing, release pressure from the plunger, and look for subsequent blood flow into the barrel of the syringe. In some birds, "milking" the vein may be required, via repeated aspiration and release of the plunger. After the needle is removed, digital pressure should remain on the venipuncture site for at least 1 to 2 min. Despite sufficient digital pressure, hematoma formation routinely occurs in this exposed area. Pet bird owners should be informed of the likelihood of hematoma formation after blood has been collected from the basilic vein.

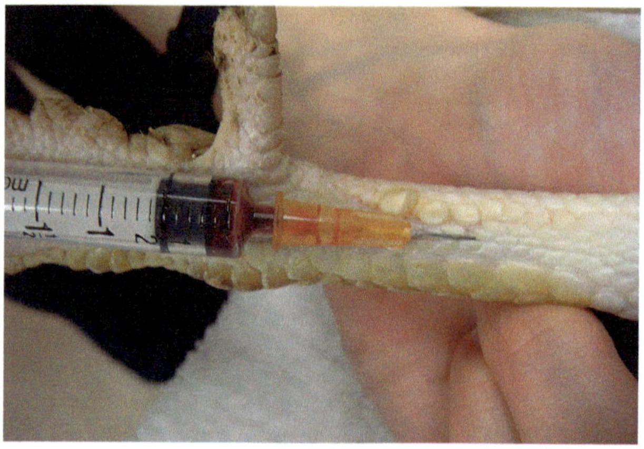

Figure 25.6 Blood collection from the medial metatarsal vein.

Medial Metatarsal Vein

The medial metatarsal vein is the blood collection site of last resort in most parrot species, as the short tarsometatarsal bone creates challenges in access and stabilization of the syringe for a one-handed draw technique (Figure 25.6). This difficulty is exacerbated in the conscious bird. However, in larger parrots, the median metatarsal vein can be used for catheter placement. With the leg extended, the forefinger and middle finger hold off the vessel at the distal tibiotarsus while the thumb holds the foot against the palm of the hand. As the syringe barrel rests on the thumb, the needle is inserted at a parallel angle over the vessel into the lumen. Using the same technique described for the basilic vein, blood is collected, after which the needle withdrawn, and digital pressure placed on the venipuncture site. If needed, a piece of cotton ball can be taped to the leg for hemostasis.

Sample Handling

For Psittaciforme blood collection, plastic pediatric blood collection tubes, which minimize sample overdilution, are the product of choice. When injecting blood into the tubes, the cap must be removed from the tube and the needle from the syringe. Slowly introduce the blood along the inside of the container, after which the cap is placed on the pediatric blood tube before it is slowly rotated back and forth 3 or 4 times to adequately mix the anticoagulant and blood. Avian whole blood is susceptible to osmotic changes in purple-topped tubes that contain ethylenediaminetetraacetic acid (EDTA), especially erythrocytes [7]. If the whole blood is maintained in the purple-topped tubes >24 h, the avian erythrocytes have a tendency to swell [7]. Whole blood samples placed in EDTA miniature collection tubes are suitable for complete blood counts, blood lead analysis, and fibrinogen assays. Dark green-topped miniature blood collection tubes contain the anticoagulant heparin. Whole blood placed in the heparin collection tubes can be used for complete blood counts, blood lead analysis, and gene-based diagnostic testing (e.g., viral, DNA sexing) [7]. Plasma obtained from centrifuging the heparin tube can be used to obtain chemistry analysis, plasma zinc concentrations, or antibody titers for viral and bacterial diseases. For smaller psittacine patients, heparinized capillary tubes, with large internal diameters, aid in obtaining the maximum amount of plasma from a small blood sample [7]. Whole blood in capillary tubes is only useful in determining the packed cell volume of the patient.

Prior to submitting samples to a clinical pathology laboratory, obtain all information regarding collection, sample transfer, sample storage, packaging, and shipment from a laboratory representative. To submit blood samples to an outside diagnostic laboratory, tubes and slides must be shipped according to the standards of that facility. All tubes should be properly labeled, double-packaged, and placed in a tightly sealed container with ice packs and filler (e.g., foam peanuts) to prevent shifting or breakage. Diagnostic samples are often shipped with improper labels and/or packaging, resulting in null results. Proper handling, labeling, packaging, and shipping are just as important as the initial collection of the diagnostic sample.

Many factors can adversely affect the interpretation of parrot blood samples submitted for hematologic testing Lipemic blood samples have been associated with ovulation, hepatic disorders, and reproductive tract disease [7]. Parrot health and previous treatment can affect diagnostic test results. If possible, collection of blood samples should occur before any treatment is administered to the patient. Interpretive caution is required for the dehydrated parrot, since the absolute cell counts and biochemical analytes may have increased concentrations compared to actual [7]. Treatment for hypocalcemic conditions and heavy metal toxicosis prior to blood collection for specific diagnostic tests for those disease conditions will reduce the reliability of the results. Exogenous administration of corticosteroids and intramuscular injections of drugs (e.g., enrofloxacin, vitamin A–D_3) will cause elevations in nonspecific enzyme activities, including aspartate aminotransferase (AST), lactate dehydrogenase (LDH), and creatine kinase (CK) [7, 8].

Complete Blood Count

The complete blood count is arguably the most important diagnostic test offered to assess the health of psittacine patients. A complete blood count will assess the bird's red and white blood cells, fibrinogen, and whether hemoparasites are present. The complete blood count can be accomplished in the veterinary clinic or submitted to an outside diagnostic laboratory. If the technical staff is proficient, running the complete blood count in-house is preferable to outsourcing the test because time needed to transport the sample can be saved.

For an in-house complete blood count, the blood film preparation is the first priority. Results gained from the blood film include a differential white cell count, white and red cell morphology, and thrombocyte and hemoparasite evaluation. Blood smears can be made from a fresh drop of blood from the tip of a syringe or a drop of blood from an EDTA tube that had been collected 2 to 3 h earlier and should be immediately fixed [9].

Erythrocytes

The avian erythrocyte is elliptical, nucleated, and much larger than mammalian erythrocytes [10]. Most Psittaciforme erythrocytes range from 130 to 180 fl [10]. Of circulating red blood cells, 2%–10% are immature red cells or reticulocytes [1]. Reticulocytes and polychromatic cells increase based on the parrot's active regenerative erythrocytic response to anemia (Figure 25.7). In the normal parrot, polychromatic cells are usually identified at 1%–5% in circulating blood [10]. Mild (1+) anisocytosis, variability in cell size, is a routine erythrocyte finding in pet birds. Poikilocytosis,

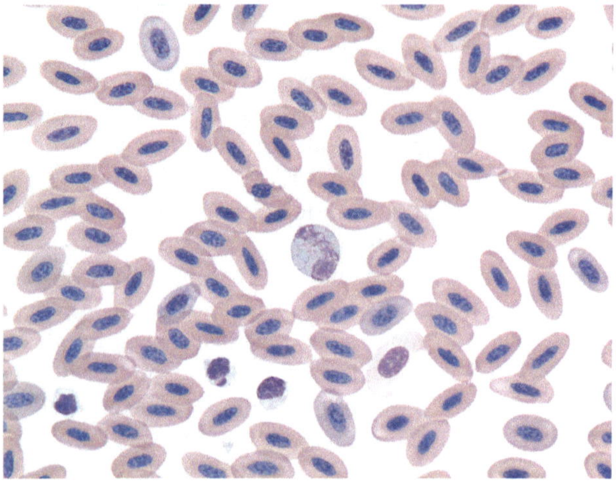

Figure 25.7 Cockatiel: Regenerative response to anemia is indicated by the increased amount of polychromasia. The leukocyte in the lower left is a normal lymphocyte, in the upper center is a heterophil, and to the right is an eosinophil. Original magnification 1000×, Wright-Giemsa.

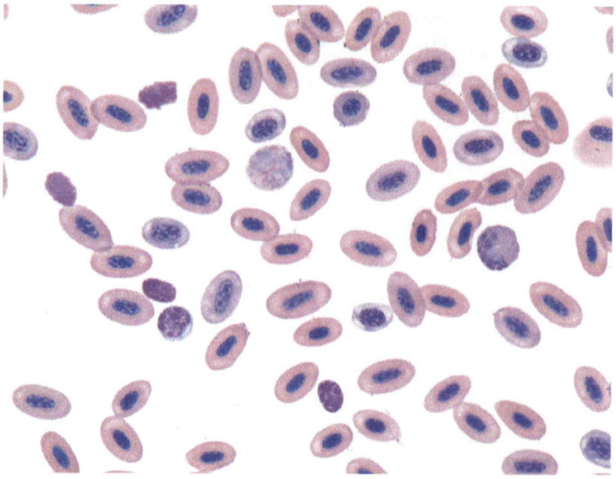

Figure 25.8 Cockatoo: From left to right are a thrombocyte, a heterophil, and a basophil. Original magnification 1000×, Wright-Giemsa.

a variability in cell shape, may be associated with septicemia, anemia, or simply a preparation artifact [10]. Lead toxicosis has been implicated as an underlying cause of erythrocytic ballooning. Erythrocytic ballooning refers to bulges noted in the normal oval shape of the erythrocyte often accompanied by areas of hypochromasia [10].

The packed cell volume (PCV) is commonly used to estimate the percentage or volume of erythrocytes in a blood sample. Use of hematocrit tubes and centrifugation remains the gold standard for this analyte, although other methods are available. The PCV and the total red blood cell count are used to determine the mean corpuscular volume (MCV), mean corpuscular hemoglobin (MCH), and mean corpuscular hemoglobin concentration (MCHC). The calculation for the MCV, fl = (PCV × 10)/RBC, expresses the average volume of individual erythrocytes [9]. The calculation for the MCH, pg = (Hb × 10)/RBC, expresses the average hemoglobin content of a single erythrocyte [9]. The calculation for the MCHC, g/l = (Hb × 100)/PCV, expresses the volume within the erythrocyte occupied by hemoglobin [9].

Total Red Blood Cell Count

The total red blood cell count can be determined through automated or manual methods. The manual method used to determine total red blood cell counts for psittacine species is the same as that recommended for other avian species.

Hemoglobin (Hb)

Hemoglobin estimation in Psittaciformes is complicated by the presence of nucleated red blood cells. Avian red blood cells must be lysed to release the hemoglobin for measurement, and the remaining nuclei within the sample must be removed to obtain reliable results. However, nuclear centrifugation for removal may remove attached hemoglobin, causing a falsely low colorimetric reading [9]. To obtain better hemoglobin results, a calibration graph using commercially available hemoglobin standards n = may be made to express hemoglobin as oxyhemoglobin [9]. Hemoglobin can then be estimated from oxyhemoglobin using a commercially available hemoglobinometer [9]. Commercial laboratory testing is also available for hemoglobin.

Thrombocytes

Mature thrombocytes are small oval cells with a pyknotic nucleus and colorless cytoplasm in mature cells (Figure 25.8). These cells participate in blood coagulation and tend to clump in blood films similar to platelets in mammalian species [1, 11]. Reactive thrombocytes, characterized by blebbing, or enlargement of the cytoplasm, may be associated with phagocytic defense function [7]. Thrombocytes are usually counted when a blood film is being scanned to determine a differential white blood cell count [7, 9]. Thrombocyte clumping will adversely affect the ability to accurately count these cells. To estimate the absolute number of thrombocytes: [9] (Number thrombocytes counted per 40 × field/100) × WBC = thrombocytes × 10^9 /l.

Leukocytes

The total white blood cell count and differential analysis of white blood cells within the peripheral blood of Psittaciformes is one of the best diagnostic tests to

Table 25.2 Hematologic reference ranges in selected psittacine species [5, 12, 13].

		Budgerigar	Cockatiel
Animals sampled		1542	9267
Data		Mean [Range]	Mean [Range]
White blood cell count (WBC)	$\times 10^{9}/l = (\times 10^{3}/\mu l)$	6.7 [3–10]	8.0 [5–11]
Heterophils	Proportion of 1.0 (%)	56.7 [40–68]	59.4 [46–72]
Lymphocytes	Proportion of 1.0 (%)	31.7 [22–60]	42.4 [26–60]
Monocytes	Proportion of 1.0 (%)	6.18 [1–13]	0.05 [0–1]
Eosinophils	Proportion of 1.0 (%)	3 [1–6]	0.61 [0–2]
Basophils	Proportion of 1.0 (%)	0.48 [0–2]	0.12 [0–1]
Hematocrit	Proportion of 1.0 (%)	51.45 [43.4–56.1]	52.63 [41.4—58.9]
Hemoglobin	g/l (g/dl)	14.7 [12.42–16.89]	12.15 [10.2–14.7]
Red blood cell (RBC) count	$\times 10^{12}/l = (\times 10^{3}/\mu l)$	4.32 [3.77–4.6]	3.93 [3.1–4.4]
Mean corpuscular volume (MCV)	μm^3 = fl	121.5 [116–127]	135.9 [126–142]
Mean corpuscular hemoglobin (MCH)	Pg/cell	26.1 [23.1–30.89]	31 [26.4–35.8]
Mean corpuscular hemoglobin concentration (MCHC)	g/dl	21.79 [19.8–23.9]	22.68 [20.45–25.2]

determine the health status of the patient. When assessing the differential white blood cell count, one can assess the patient's general condition (Table 25.2). Conditions that affect the accuracy of a total leukocyte count include presence of preparation artifacts, counting methodology, whole blood transit time, and sampling methods. These tests are offered through commercial laboratories and can be manually determined similar to those techniques used for other avian species. The leukocyte cell types identified in Psittaciformes blood are similar to those described for other avian species. These cell types include the heterophil (primary granulocyte), eosinophil, thrombocyte, basophil, monocyte, and lymphocyte. Changes in the leukogram of parrots may reflect stress, the many causes of inflammation, or stem from immunosuppression or neoplasia. Extreme leukocytosis (> 100 000/μl) may be associated with avian chlamydiosis, chronic inflammatory disease, and or hematopoietic neoplasms [10, 14].

As with many animal patients that are presented to veterinary clinics, parrot species are often nervous and stressed. Abnormal physiologic responses by these patients can adversely affect laboratory results [7]. Increased endogenous corticosteroid concentrations and adrenocortical stress can cause a transient leukocytosis, heterophilia, lymphopenia, and eosinopenia [7, 15, 16]. The increased adrenocortical stress can be exacerbated by placement in a travel cage, travel, interaction with other animals in a waiting room, and restraint prior to collection of the sample to be submitted for diagnostic testing [7]. An increase in relative and absolute numbers of immature leukocytes is referred to as a left shift. Causes of a left shift in parrots include stress, corticosteroid administration, and acute inflammatory processes (e.g., mycobacteriosis, aspergillosis, avian chlamydiosis, and severe tissue necrosis) [10]. Toxic heterophils, leukocyte degranulation, and reactive lymphocytes are often detected in birds suffering from septic conditions associated with either bacterial or viral infections.

Heterophils

Heterophils are the most common granulocyte in many parrot species (Figures 25.8–25.11). Increased heterophil counts (heterophilia) most often occur based on inflammation or stress through the presence of endogenous adrenal hormones. Inflammation is often associated with increases in circulating heterophils within the blood of companion avian species. The inflammatory process may or may not be not be specifically associated with infectious disease. Noninfectious inflammatory processes and some metabolic disease may elicit an increase of the heterophil cell numbers in parrot species [17]. Moreover, young Psittaciformes may have a physiological normal heterophila [18, 19]. True heteropenia or a low heterophil count is an uncommon finding in parrot differential blood counts. As with other avian species, a true heteropenic condition, may be related to a

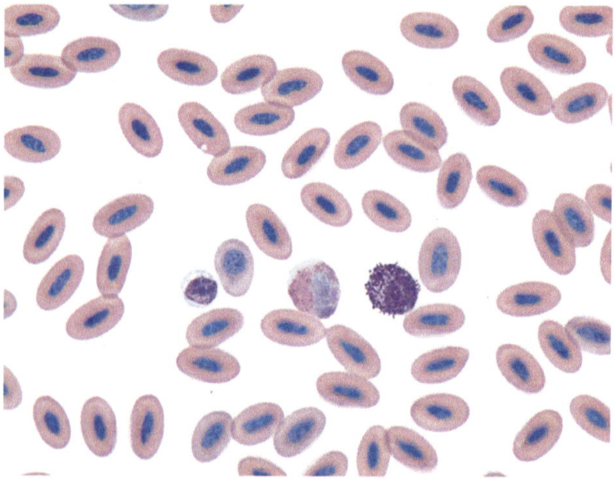

Figure 25.9 Macaw: One lymphocyte and two heterophils are shown, with mild polychromasia noted in the background. Original magnification 1000×, Wright-Giemsa.

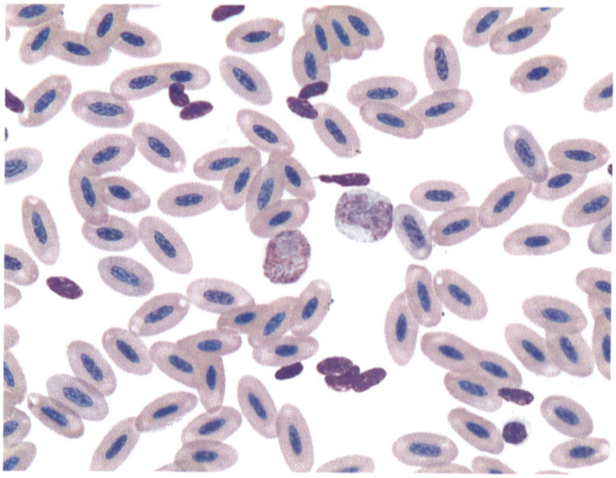

Figure 25.11 African gray: From left to right are one monocyte, eosinophil, and heterophil among normal erythrocytes. Original magnification 1000×, Wright-Giemsa.

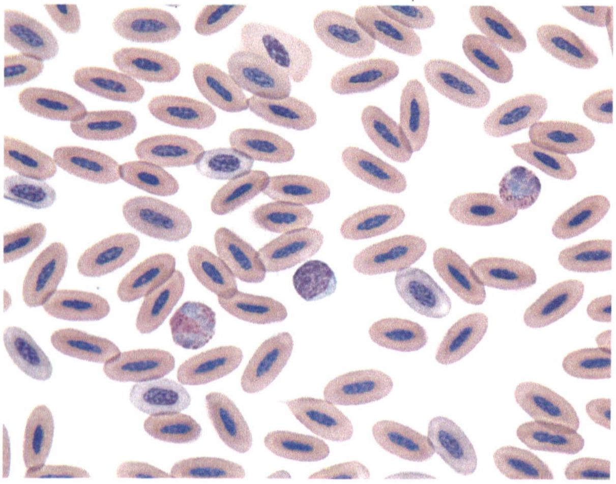

Figure 25.10 Budgerigar: Example of one heterophil (center) and one monocyte (right). There are several free nuclei from ruptured cells in this field. Original magnification 1000×, Wright-Giemsa.

severe septicemia associated with a bacterial infection. African gray parrots infected with circovirus will develop a clinical condition in which severe heteropenia is observed.

Lymphocytes

Lymphocytes are of similar form in parrots as in mammals (Figures 25.7 and 25.9). An increase in the absolute or relative lymphocyte count often corresponds to a significant immune stimulus [18]. Lymphocytosis in Psittaciformes has been associated with viral infections (e.g., psittacine herpesvirus, psittacine circovirus) but may be variable if the patient has concurrent diseases (e.g., avian chlamydiosis). In Amazon parrots, the lymphocyte may be the predominate white blood cell in a differential count, comprising over 50% of white cells [10]. Although an inverse heterophil-to-lymphocyte ratio may be of concern, as discussed it is considered a normal finding in some parrot species. Conversely, smudging artifact can also cause an elevation in the relative lymphocyte count [10]. Causes of low lymphocyte counts in parrots relative to other avian species are presumed to be similar.

Monocytes

Monocytes are of similar form in parrots as mammals (Figures 25.10 and 25.11).Chronic inflammation is the primary underlying factor of increased circulating monocytes in Psittaciformes. Marked monocytosis often occurs in parrots diagnosed with aspergillosis, avian chlamydiosis, or mycobacteriosis [11]. Other clinical presentations that result in an increased monocyte count include chronic granulomatous or histiocytic inflammation and suspected, treatment-responsive avian chlamydiosis cases [5].

Eosinophils

Eosinophils are often present in low numbers in the healthy parrot leukocyte count. True eosinophilia and an interpretation of this condition is controversial for companion avian species. Eosinophil granules of Psittaciformes may poorly or variably uptake color based on species and choice of stain (Figures 25.12, 25.13, 25.14, and 25.15). True Eosinophilia is an uncommon finding in parrot species and has not been confirmed to correlate to parasitism. Reports of parrot species (e.g., cockatiel) with eosinophils and parasitism are based on single case studies and do not reflect scientific validation of this condition [12]. Differentials for high absolute or

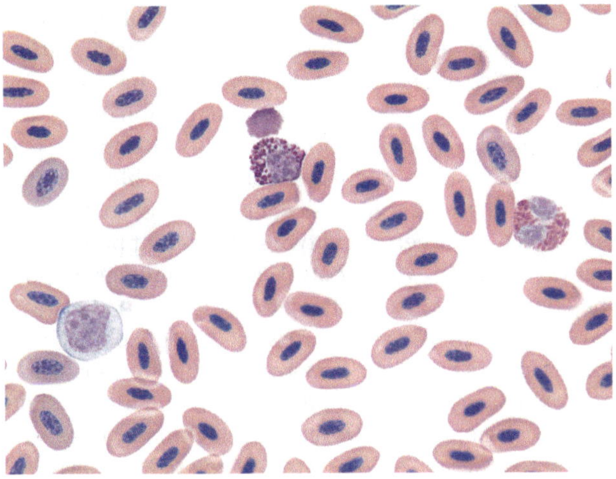

Figure 25.12 Budgerigar: Example of an eosinophil with variably blue to purple granules. Original magnification 1000×, Wright-Giemsa.

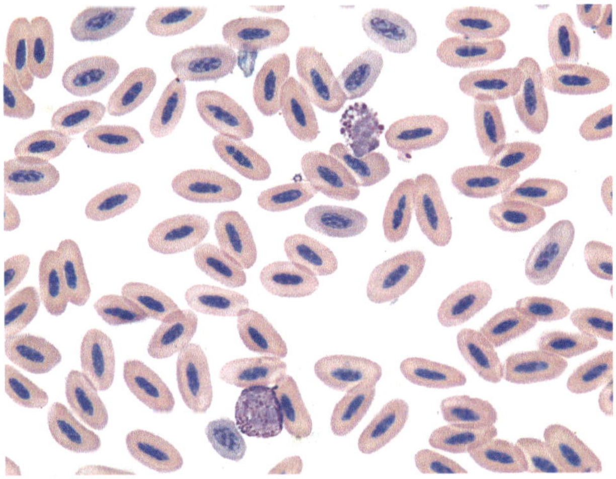

Figure 25.13 Budgerigar: Color of granules within leukocytes can vary based on stain chosen. This is an eosinophil from the same individual as shown in Figure 25.7, but this blood smear was stained with Diff-Quik. Original magnification 1000×.

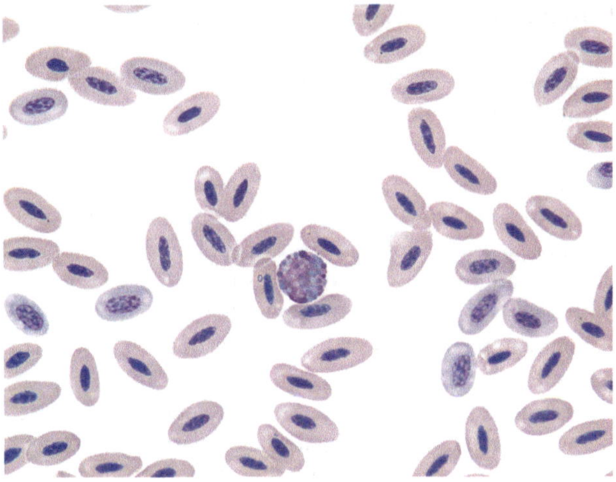

Figure 25.14 Eclectus: The leukocyte at the top of the field is an eosinophil, and the leukocyte at the lower portion of the field is a basophil. Original magnification 1000×, Wright-Giemsa.

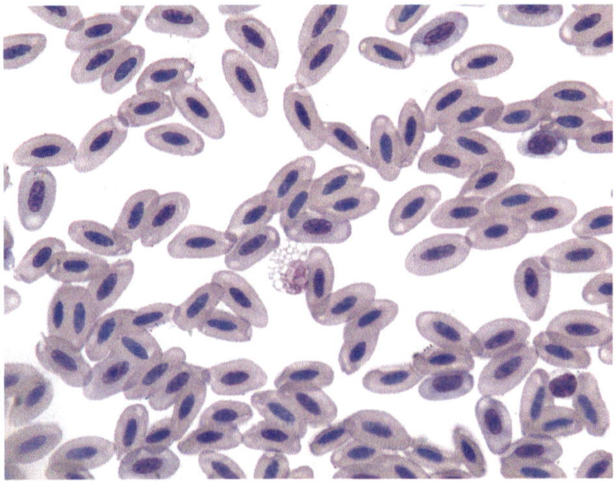

Figure 25.15 Lovebird: Example of an eosinophil with lavender-blue granules. In different psittacine species, eosinophil granules range from pink to blue to very poorly staining. Original magnification 1000×, Wright-Giemsa.

relative eosinophil counts from companion avian species must include laboratory error based on the ease of mistaking heterophils for eosinophils [18].

Basophils

Basophils are uncommon in most healthy parrots, but relatively increased numbers of basophils are found in some conure species and the spectacled Amazon parrot [18]. Transient basophilia has been associated with trauma (e.g., self-mutilation, blunt force, postsurgical) in parrot species [18]. Avian chlamydiosis has been implicated as an underlying cause of basophilia diagnosed in budgerigars, cockatiels, and Amazon parrots [20].

Leukemia

Although uncommon in Psittaciformes, leukemia has been diagnosed in budgerigars, Amazon parrots, and macaws [18, 21]. Based on case review, lymphocytic leukemia is diagnosed more often in the smaller parrot species, while macaws are predisposed to granulocytic leukemia [18]. Leukocytosis alone does not confirm a diagnosis of leukemia, as many disease processes can result in white blood cell increase. Leukemia should be a top differential disease diagnosis when the leukocyte count is significantly increased and there are a large number of "blast-like" cells in the peripheral blood [18, 21]. Leukemia in pet birds is considered rare, but when diagnosed, Amazon parrots frequently have lymphocytic leukemia while macaws develop granulocytic leukemia [10]. Leukemia is diagnosed when the leukocyte count is greatly increased and a large number of blast-like cells are identified in the blood [11].

Hemoparasites

For companion parrot species, blood parasites are rarely diagnosed. Psittaciformes are susceptible to blood parasites but are rarely exposed to infected vectors associated with disease transmission. Parrots that live in their native habitat can be infected with a number of the blood-borne parasites. Birds that are housed in North American outdoor aviaries may also be exposed and infected with hemoparasites. Most hemoparasites of parrots lack clinical import and rarely cause morbidity or mortality. For most parrots with hemoparasitism, treatment is based on the patient's health status and may be forgone unless there are overt clinical signs that can be directly correlated to the disease condition. For most parrot cases in which blood parasites have been identified, treatment is often based on the patient's health status while infected. Treatment is seldom recommended for hemoparasites infecting parrot species unless there are overt clinical signs that can be directly correlated to the disease condition.

Hemoparasites may often be recognized upon review of the blood smear of an infected patient. Schizonts of *Plasmodium* spp. occur within the cytoplasm of the erythrocytes; they are lateral or polar to the nucleus, and do not distort the cell [21]. *Plasmodium* spp. have been identified in wild-caught cockatoo species. The gametocytes of *Haemoproteus* spp. may also be observed within the erythrocytes [21]. The *Haemoproteus* spp. organism takes up most of the cytoplasm space within the erythrocyte but does not distort the cell. The *Haemoproteus* spp. gametocytes have a distinct shape, central nucleus, and yellow, black, brown, and purple granular pigment [21]. Conures, white cockatoos, and macaws have been diagnosed with hemoproteus parasitism [18]. *Leukocytozoon* spp. have been identified in parrot species captured in the wild and those maintained in outdoor aviaries. The gametocyte of this intracellular parasite is found in the cytoplasm of the erythrocyte or leukocyte and distorts the shape of the cell. Two extracellular blood parasites have been identified in wild-caught parrot species, *Trypanosoma avium* and microfilaria of filaroid nematodes [5]. For images of hemoparasites in avian species, refer to Chapters 24 (on raptors) and 28 (on passerines) of this text.

Hemostasis

The little scientific information on avian hemostasis appears to be, for the most part, similar between species. The thrombocyte is the corresponding cell to the mammalian platelet. The clotting pathways and specific clotting factors have not been validated but appear to be similar to mammals [22]. Therefore, information provided in other avian chapters can be used for Psittaciformes in regard to the coagulation panel for determining a patient's clotting ability. Relatively few articles have been published on parrot blood types [23–25]. There is a general understanding that differences occur between blood types of different parrot species [21]. Clinical evidence and scientific findings support the conclusion that an initial blood transfusion between parrot species is safe. "Cross-matching" donor and patient parrots prior to performing a blood transfusion by mixing a sample of blood from each on a glass slide can be attempted. However, this technique does not appear to accurately predict transfusion reaction in avian species [26]. Scientific studies of parrots have confirmed that autologous (patient's own blood) and homologous (blood from the same species) blood transfusions provide the most effective and long-lasting therapeutic options when whole blood is needed [1, 14]. Heterologous (blood from a different avian species) blood transfusions are not an effective treatment option for parrots, with the transfused blood staying in circulation for a relatively short period of time when compared to the autologous and homologous blood products [1, 14].

Biochemical Panel

The plasma biochemistry panel is an important diagnostic test for Psittaciformes that aids in determining the overall health of a patient, as it is for other animal species (Table 25.3). A thorough understanding of the case and examination of the patient will often direct the clinician to abnormalities that may exist on the biochemical panel. Two important reasons to run a biochemical panel on an avian patient are to (1) establish an analyte baseline for future reference and (2) determine the magnitude of disease through the parameters measured by the panel. The following description of the biochemical panel will review body system analytes as they correspond to the parrot patient. For most avian chemistry evaluations, lithium heparin is the preferred anticoagulant for the blood sample [27].

Liver Enzymes and Associated Analytes

On the basis of studies of parrot species, a variety of enzyme concentrations correlate with liver pathology (Table 25.4) [28, 29]. When analyzing the biochemistry panel for liver-specific enzyme correlation to disease, consider physiologic factors that may affect the results. Conditions that may increase liver enzyme activities of nonspecific analytes include muscle trauma, anorexia, and patient stress [28]. Specific analytes, such as

Table 25.3 Biochemical reference ranges of selected psittacine species [5, 12, 13].

Analyte (abbreviation)	Units, SI [conventional]	Budgerigar	Cockatiel
Data format		**Mean [Range]**	**Mean [Range]**
Animals sampled		**1542**	**9267**
Alanine (ALT) aminotransferase	U/l = (IU/l)		4.5 [0–9]
Gamma-glutamyl transferase (GGT)	U/l = (IU/l)	5 [1–10]	3 [0–5]
Alkaline (ALP) phosphatase	U/l = (IU/l)	68.3 [24–96]	51.1 [12–100]
Lactate (LDH) dehydrogenase	U/l = (IU/l)	251.7 [156–384]	255 [122–378]
Bile acids	Mmol/l	81.1 [32–117]	75.8 [44–108]
CK U/l	U/l = (IU/l)	235.0 [117–368]	269.1 [160–420]
AST U/l	U/l = (IU/l)	262.3 [156–375]	244.6 [128–396]
Creatinine	mmol/l (mg/dl)		0.25 [0.1–0.4]
Uric acid	mmol/l (mg/dl)	512.1 [285.5–764.9] (8.61[4.8–13])	419.3 [202.2–648.3] (7.05 [3.4–11])
Calcium	mmol/l (mg/dl)	2.31 [2.00–2.80] (9.27 [8.0–11.2])	2.30 [2.05–2.71] (9.2 [8.2–10.9])
Inorganic phosphorus	mmol/l (mg/dl)		4 [3.2–4.8]
Amylase	U/l	437.3 [302–560]	360.7 [113–870]
Glucose	mmol/l (mg/dl)	18.31 [11.99–25.31] (329.8 [216–456])	18.10 [12.66–24.42] (326.1 [228–440])
Cholesterol	mmol/l (mg/dl)	4.68 [3.10–5.95] (181.1 [120–230])	(3.92 [2.33–5.17]) (151.7 [90–200])
Sodium	mmol/l = (mEq/l)		142.5 [130–155]
Potassium	mmol/l = (mEq/l)		3.5 [2.5–4.5]
Total protein	g/l (g/dl)	28.3 [21–43] (2.8 [2.1–4.3])	29 [21–47.9] (2.9 [2.1–4.8])
Albumin	g/l (g/dl)	11.1 [9–12] (1.1 [0.9–1.2])	14.5 [8–18] (1.5 [0.8–1.8])
Globulin	g/l (g/dl)	11 [7–15] (1.1 [0.7–1.5])	28 [21–38] (2.78 [2.1–3.8])
Albumin by EPH	g/l (g/dl)		1.25 [0.7–1.8]
Alpha-1 globulin EPH	g/l (g/dl)		0.225 [0.05–0.4]
Alpha-2 globulin EPH	g/l (g/dl)		0.245 [0.05–0.44]
Beta globulin EPH	g/l (g/dl)		0.395 [0.21–0.58]
Gamma globulin EPH	g/l (g/dl)		0.27 [0.11–0.43]
Albumin:globulin	g/l (g/dl)		2.9 [1.5–4.3]

gamma-glutamyl transferase (GGT), are highly specific for liver tissue, but of low sensitivity and therefore have not proved beneficial for routine assessment of liver disease [30]. Since most of the enzymes associated with the liver also occur in muscle, one generally assesses the muscle-specific CK activities in conjunction with the nonspecific liver enzymes, particularly LDH. The absence of an increased CK activity and a simultaneous rise in LDH suggests liver damage [30]. Sample hemolysis could also produce similar results.

The primary bile pigment produced from destruction of erythrocytes in avian species is biliverdin [28]. Parrots diagnosed with liver disease often have green/yellowish green urates based on biliverdin pigment (biliverdinuria). Cholestasis and liver failure are thought to contribute to increased concentrations of biliverdin in birds. However, a commercial biliverdin diagnostic test remains unavailable. Rapid hepatic uptake of biliverdin in chickens suggests that hepatic evaluation via this analyte is not beneficial for Psittaciformes [29]. Bile acids plasma assays are accepted to assess liver function in birds [13, 28]. Although plasma bile acid concentrations increase after eating, these concentrations decrease rapidly in parrot species [31]. Therefore, single-point bile acid assays of diagnostic relevance can be performed on parrot species regardless of fasting status. Plasma bile acid assays do not determine the etiology underlying liver disease but provide useful information regarding decreased liver function. Bile duct hyperplasia and severe hepatic fibrosis have been associated with a substantial increase of the plasma bile acid concentration in parrots [28]. However, increased concentrations of

Table 25.4 Utility of select analytes in assessment of liver disease in psittacine species.

Analyte (abbreviation)	Activities
Creatine kinase (CK)	Present in skeletal, cardiac, and smooth muscle; absent in liver
Alanine aminotransferase (ALT)	Present in many tissues, including liver
Lactate dehydrogenase (LDH)	Present in many tissues, including liver
Γ-glutamyltransferase(GGT)	Low activity in the avian liver
Aspartate aminotransferase (AST)	Present in skeletal, cardiac, and smooth muscle, and liver tissue
Alkaline phosphatase (ALP)	Present in cell membranes of the liver (biliary epithelium), kidney, intestine, and bone (osteoblasts)
Glutamate dehydrogenase (GDH)	Most specific enzyme for avian liver damage, with relatively low sensitivity

plasma bile acid may not be detectable in cases of peracute to acute hepatitis.

Ammonia is derived through the hydrolysis of glutamine in the intestinal tract and from the effect of bacterial proteases, ureases, and amine oxidases on digested food in the colon [32]. In birds, ammonia is converted to less toxic uric acid in the liver [32]. Increased ammonia concentrations have been associated with hepatic encephalopathy in mammalian patients, but this correlation does not appear to be evident in parrot species [33, 34]. Fasting ammonia concentrations in parrots ranged from 36 to 274 μM/l, much higher than those reported for mammals [33, 34]. However, up to 4× increases in ammonia concentrations in parrots diagnosed with liver failure have been anecdotally reported [32].

Muscle Enzymes

CK and AST are enzymes present in all muscle types and allow for excellent evaluation of muscle damage through plasma biochemical analysis. Trauma, muscle necrosis from intramuscular injections, and cachexia (muscle wasting) are common clinical presentations from which muscle enzyme concentrations will significantly increase.

Renal Analytes

The lack of bladder and cloacal anatomy of birds dictate that few renal analytes are of diagnostic value to the veterinarian treating parrot species. The most useful renal analyte to assess renal disease in parrots is uric acid. Uric acid is the major nitrogenous waste by product in avian urine [35]. The majority of uric acid enters the urine through proximal tubule secretion, while 10% is filtered through the glomeruli [36]. Uric acid secretion is largely unaffected by the glomerular filtration rate until it cannot flow through the tubules, in severe states of dehydration [37]. Birds in renal failure often do not show clinical signs or increases in blood uric acid concentrations until death is imminent. Currently, there are no other biochemical analytes that have proved useful in consistently determining renal function in Psittaciformes, including urea, creatinine, proteins, and plasma electrolytes.

Pancreas

Exocrine

For many analytes that are used to determine pancreatic health in mammalian species, there has been no validation in Psittaciformes, including amylase and lipase [32]. Amylase and lipase are cytosolic enzymes generated from the pancreas, liver, and small intestine (amylase) and from the pancreas and small intestine lipase [38]. Anecdotal clinical reports state that there may be increased amylase concentrations associated with acute pancreatitis and proventricular dilatation disease [39].

Glucose and Endocrine Pancreas

Diabetes mellitus does occur in psittacine species. The common clinical signs of diabetes mellitus in psittacine species include polyuria, polydipsia, glucosuria, ketonuria, and a persistent hyperglycemia [40]. While serum insulin and plasma glucagon concentrations have been measured in psittacine species, commonly veterinary practitioners diagnose diabetes mellitus in psittacine species through plasma glucose concentrations and urine ketone assessment. Assays to determine serum insulin and plasma glucagon concentrations are generally not available to the veterinary practitioner.

The major glucose regulating hormone in parrots is glucagon, which is secreted by the A cells of the pancreas. The plasma glucagon concentrations in birds are 1–4 ng/ml [41]. Glucagon secretion is increased by hypoglycemia, amino acids, and acetylcholine and inhibited by glucose and insulin [41]. Insulin is secreted by the pancreatic islet B cells [40]. As opposed to their mammalian counterparts, glucose is thought to be a primary stimulator of insulin in avian species [41]. Thus, diabetes mellitus in granivorous birds, including parrots, is likely caused by a glucagon excess, not an insulin deficiency [40]. Normal blood glucose concentrations in healthy birds range from 250 to 500 mg/dl [40]. Since there may be transient cases of hyperglycemia, the patient should be retested after a 24–48 h rest period. Differing underlying etiologies of diabetes mellitus between species and individuals within a species are likely, based on the variable insulin and glucagon results reported from parrot patients [40]. Histopathologic assessment of a pancreatic sample collected from an avian patient will provide the most useful information regarding pancreatic disease at this time [38].

Gastrointestinal Biomarkers

At this time, no specific gastrointestinal analytes have been determined for parrots, and few current analytes are useful. Diagnostic testing utilized for the gastrointestinal tract of Psittaciformes involves both primary (e.g., cytology, culture) and secondary (e.g., CBC, plasma biochemical analysis) investigations. More involved testing of the upper gastrointestinal tract includes hematology evaluations (CBC, plasma biochemistry panel, histopathologic evaluation of a harvested tissue sample, and serologic and blood testing for specific disease conditions). Secondary tests are useful in determining a more generalized pathologic condition and in some cases definitively identifying the causative disease. A CBC is beneficial to evaluate the magnitude of inflammation that may be present through elevations in the total leukocyte count. If necrosis and pathology affect skeletal and smooth muscle of the GI tract, the plasma biochemical panel will have enzyme elevations of CK, LDH, and AST. If GI bleeding is suspected by the presence of melena, this condition can be confirmed using a standard laboratory fecal occult test. Gastrointestinal bleeding can be associated with heavy metal toxicosis.

Cardiac Biomarkers

In Psittaciformes, the evaluation of the cardiac disease through clinical pathology testing is primarily confined to the CBC and plasma biochemical analysis. If there is inflammation associated with heart disease as a consequence of a bacterial or fungal infection, leukocytosis may result [30]. Viral or a severe bacterial septicemic condition may result in a leukopenia [19]. Biochemical analytes that may be increased by cardiac disease include CK (cardiac muscle damage), AST, ALT, GDH (hepatocellular damage based on congestive heart failure), hypocalcemia (cardiac arrhythmias), hyperuricemia (pericardial gout), and increased cholesterol (atherosclerosis) [19]. Cardiac troponins have received minimal diagnostic investigation in parrots. Other diagnostic testing to evaluate cardiac health involves imaging modalities, pulse oximetry, and electrocardiography [42].

Lipids and Lipoproteins

In Psittaciformes, cholesterol is an excellent biochemical analyte to evaluate reproductively active female parrots. Prior to and during egg laying, the female bird will often have increased cholesterol concentrations [32]. Increased cholesterol plasma concentrations and lipemic blood samples have been associated with various disease conditions including hypothyroidism, diabetes mellitus, hyperadrenocorticism, pancreatitis, or a primary lipid/lipoprotein disorder [32]. A lipemic blood sample falsely increases all liver enzymes, ALP, hemoglobin, bile acids, glucose, calcium, and phosphorus [32]. Biochemical assays that measure cholesterol provide values of total cholesterol which consists of both free cholesterol and cholesterol esters [38]. Cholesterol concentrations reported for birds apparently range from 180 to 250 mg/dl [20]. Reported causes of hypercholesterolemia in parrot species include hypothyroidism, diabetes mellitus, atherosclerosis, and high-fat diets [43]. Increased plasma cholesterol concentrations and an accompanying lipemia have been described in Amazon parrots, macaws, and rose-breasted cockatoos with hepatic lipidosis [38, 43]. Decreased plasma cholesterol concentrations have been diagnosed in birds with hepatic disease, aflatoxicosis, decreased dietary intake of fat, E. *coli* infections, endotoxemia, and spirochetosis [38, 43]. Triglyceride concentrations in Psittaciformes vary depending on climate, hormone influence, gender, and diet [38]. Increased triglyceride plasma concentrations in parrots have been associated with starvation, egg peritonitis, estrogen injections, and physical activity [38, 43].

Electrolytes, Acid Base

To best assess plasma electrolytes of a psittacine patient, all aspects of the bird's condition should be known, including appetite, hydration status, overall health, and current treatment [38]. As in other species, sodium and potassium are the major intra- and extracellular cations, respectively, and chloride is the major extracellular anion. Sodium is controlled by the kidneys, adrenal glands, and salt glands. Increased sodium concentrations are associated with increased sodium ingestion, increased water loss, decreased water intake, and salt poisoning [38]. Dehydration of the blood sample may result in artificial increases in hypernatremia, while hyperlipemia and hyperproteinemia may cause a false reduction in sodium concentrations [43]. Hyponatremia in Psittaciformes is related to diarrhea, renal disease, overhydration, and liver disease [20]. Chloride concentrations are correlated to sodium and bicarbonate concentrations [38]. Low plasma concentrations of chloride occur in parrots suffering regurgitation, renal disease, congestive heart failure, and water retention [38]. Hyperkalemia may be caused by metabolic or respiratory acidosis, renal failure, hypoadrenocorticism, severe tissue damage/necrosis, dehydration, and hemolytic anemia [38]. Hypokalemia can result from decreased dietary intake, increased loss through GI tract (e.g., vomiting, diarrhea), and by allowing the blood sample to remain at room temperature for too long [43].

Acid Base

Increased bicarbonate concentrations signal metabolic acidosis, while decreased concentrations indicate metabolic acidosis [44]. Many diagnostic laboratories measure total CO_2 concentrations as indicators of bicarbonate concentrations, since approximately 90% of the CO_2 present in plasma is in the form of bicarbonate [38]. Increased anion gap may indicate metabolic or respiratory acidosis and is calculated by subtracting anions from cations [38, 44]. During patient acidosis, intracellular potassium leaves the cell and hydrogen ions enter. Rapid treatment of the acidotic patient may result in potassium returning into the cell, which may create a potentially life-threatening hypokalemic state [38].

Blood Proteins

In small mammal medicine (e.g., dogs and cats), measuring total solids on plasma from centrifuged EDTA whole blood using a refractometer gives a reasonable estimation of total protein [29]. However, in avian species, the total protein concentrations measured by a refractometer are influenced by high concentrations of light-refractive compounds in the plasma, including chromagens, lipids, and glucose [43]. The greater concentrations of light-refractive compounds adversely affect the true total protein measurement of avian species when using a refractometer. Therefore, the Biuret analysis of total protein in which peptide bonds are reacted with cupric ions to form a colored product measured spectrophotometrically at 540 nm is recommended. Today, most diagnostic laboratories and in-house serum chemistry analyzers (Abaxis) provide accurate total protein readings [43]. For parrot species that have lower blood glucose concentrations, the refractometer may provide a rapid assessment of total protein but should never be used as the sole measure to determine this analyte. In cases of hyperproteinemia, dehydration should always be a considered a primary differential diagnosis. In budgerigars, myelosis, a chronic lymphoproliferative disease, has also been associated with hyperproteinemia [43]. Advanced age has been recognized as a cause of increase protein concentrations in parrot species [45, 46].

Serum protein electrophoresis evaluates serum protein distribution by electrophoresis and has been promoted, in companion avian medicine, as a basic diagnostic test to aid in specific disease diagnosis. Serum protein electrophoresis is not a new or novel test and is well established in veterinary medicine. No other clinical discipline (e.g., canine, feline, equine) views serum protein electrophoresis as a basis diagnostic test; rather, it is considered as one which may be used in very specific cases. This test is very nonspecific in its assessment of a patient's general condition; in most cases, the same information can be found in the complete blood count and plasma chemistry panel results. There have also been studies that show the ineffectiveness of serum protein electrophoresis as a diagnostic test for parrot species [27, 47, 48]. For psittacine species, there is no difference in interpretation of serum protein electrophoresis results from that of other avian groups.

Other than the coagulation proteins, which are removed through clot separation, serum proteins include all plasma proteins [27]. With the exception of immunoglobulins and protein hormones, most plasma proteins are synthesized in the liver [43]. Knowledge of the location of protein formation often aids in the diagnostic assessment of patient protein concentrations. There is usually a very small difference (0.1–0.2 g/dl) between most avian plasma and serum protein concentrations [27]. Lithium heparin is an acceptable anticoagulant for avian plasma electrophoresis evaluation [27]. For clinical diagnostic purposes, plasma proteins are divided into two fractions, albumin and globulins. Prealbumin, measured electrophoretically, has been described in some parrot species with the only known function being the transport of thyroid hormones [27, 43, 47–49]. In the healthy bird, the greatest protein fraction comprises albumin [43]. Of the proteins, albumin most influences colloidal osmotic pressure, and is involved with acid–base homeostasis and transport of small molecules (e.g., mineral, hormones, vitamins, and fatty acids) [27].

The globulin fraction of the total protein analyte contains alpha, beta, and gamma components. Alpha globulins, acute phase proteins, often increase with inflammatory disease, and include many transport proteins. The beta globulins are also acute phase proteins and contain carrier proteins, C-reactive protein, complement, ferritin, and fibrinogen [27]. Most of the immunoglobulins (IgM, IgA, and some IgG) are found in the beta-2 globulin fraction [27, 49]. In birds, the gamma globulin concentration contains the majority of the immunoglobulins.

Fibrinogen in parrots is an acute reactive inflammatory protein that can be a more sensitive indicator of inflammation than the complete blood count [1, 10]. Increased fibrinogen concentrations in the peripheral blood can correlate to infections and inflammation [17]. It also appears that reproductively active female birds may have an increased concentration of fibrinogen. The most accurate fibrinogen analysis from an avian patient is performed on a fresh high-quality blood sample [11].

Blood Gases

Measuring blood gases (pCO_2, pO_2, and pH) is not practical for the majority of veterinarians that treat birds. Blood gas measurement is not practical for psittacine species for two main reasons: (1) most practices do not have the necessary equipment required to properly run the sample "in-house," and (2) most parrot patients cannot withstand the blood loss required to run multiple samples. Owing to the difficulty of obtaining arterial blood from a parrot, if blood gases are analyzed, it is performed on venous blood. The avian sample should be analyzed as soon as possible because the nucleated avian erythrocyte consumes oxygen 7–10× faster than their mammalian counterpart [43]. Collect the sample in precooled syringes, bring it immediately to the analyzer, and place it on ice. Since measuring blood gases in psittacine patients is not practicable, there has been little advancement through scientific research in this area. However, reference values have been established for budgerigars: (pH 7.334–7.489; pCO_2 30.6–43.2 mmHg) [43].

Vitamins, Minerals and Metals, and Toxins

Calcium

The biologically active, freely diffusible fraction of calcium is called ionized or free [43]. Calcium regulation in birds is occurs through interaction with parathyroid hormone, active vitamin D, magnesium, and calcitonin [43]. In avian species, a general reference range of 1.0–1.3 mmol/l has been established for ionized calcium by the University of California Davis School of Veterinary Medicine [43]. Total calcium concentrations of parrots are usually measured by most diagnostic laboratories. Calcium measurements and hormonal interaction of calcium in psittacine species mimics that of other avian species. Blood sample quality is very important in obtaining accurate total calcium results from a diagnostic laboratory. Total calcium results are adversely affected if the blood sample develops hemolysis, is lipemic, is a whole blood sample, or contains bacterial contamination [25]. When a female parrot is hormonally active to lay eggs, the total calcium concentrations will be significantly increased in preparation for egg shell formation within the uterus.

True hypocalcemic tetany may occur most frequently in African gray parrots (*Psittacus erithacus*) [50]. Many theories attempt to explain this disease syndrome in African gray parrots from calcium-poor diets to low vitamin D concentrations. Low magnesium concentrations in African gray parrots diagnosed with hypocalcemic tetany may affect their ability to properly assimilate calcium stores from within their body. Although uncommon in pet parrot species, hypocalcemia may occur more commonly in hens that are prolific egg layers without calcium supplementation, older (>10 years) Amazon parrots, and cockatiels [51].

Iron

No commercially available diagnostic assays currently determine plasma iron concentrations in Psittaciformes. Hepatic biopsy is recommended for birds in which liver disease (e.g., hemochromatosis or hemosiderosis) is suspected [28]. These diseases appear to more commonly affect parrot species originating from low-iron environments or with frugivorous or nectivorous diets.

Phosphorus

Phosphorus concentrations in psittacine species are measured and assessed similar to other avian species. Hydroxyapatite in the beak and bone is comprised of a complex of inorganic phosphate and calcium [50]. Phosphorus is an important component in many physiologic systems of birds. In parrots, phosphorus concentrations and renal disease do not correlate [29, 50].

Magnesium

Recent correlation of magnesium with the disease syndrome of hypocalcemic tetany in African gray parrots has been reported. Although many factors are associated with this disease condition, hypomagnesemia may also be involved. Low serum magnesium concentrations may affect the parrot's ability to mobilize calcium reserves from bone. Two recent articles describe this physiologic correlation and provide serum magnesium reference ranges for psittacine species [44, 52].

Vitamin A

Maintenance dietary requirements of cockatiels (*Nymphicus hollandicus*) are 2000–4000 IU/kg, but concentrations <10 000 IU/kg do not significantly influence plasma concentrations [51]. Birds maintained on sufficient dietary concentrations of vitamin A may not develop clinical signs of disease associated with deficiency until they have been fed a poor-quality diet for 18 months [36]. Dietary vitamin A can be adequately provided from 2.4 mg/kg beta-carotene in cockatiels [22]. Approximately 10% of the >500 carotenoids have provitamin A activity. Liver biopsies are recommended to measure vitamin A concentrations in psittacine species since it contains approximately 90% of the total-body vitamin A [53]. Adequate vitamin A storage concentrations in the liver are considered to be 2–5 IU vitamin A/g liver [53]. Plasma vitamin A (retinol concentration for 167 sampled parrots was (mean ± standard deviation) 0.471 ± 0.209 μg/ml) [54]. However, concentrations of retinol differed significantly among groups based on relatively low concentrations in Pesquet's parrots (*Psittrichas fulgidus*). Thus, circulating concentrations of vitamins A in psittacine birds may depend significantly on subfamily and genera, and as in other species may poorly reflect total-body vitamin status [54]. The interpretation of laboratory data for vitamin A (international units, IU) and for provitamin (retinol equivalents (RE)) and equivalencies are as follows [55]:

0.6 μg ß – carotene is equivalent to 1 IU provitamin A activity

1 RE = 1 μg retinol = 6 μg ß – carotene or 12 μg of other provitamin A carotenoids

1 RE = 3.33 IU retinol = 1.818 IU vitamin A palmitate = 10 IU ß – carotene

Vitamin D

This vitamin is composed of a group of closely related compounds that have antirachitic activity and can be obtained from the diet or the sun's effect on the body [55]. Intestinal absorption and mobilization of calcium and phosphorus is improved the physiologic modification of vitamin D_3 into the hormone 1,25-dihydroxyvitamin D_3 [55]. It has been proposed that the vitamin D dietary requirement for poultry (200 IU/kg) is suitable for reproductively active African gray parrots [55].

Vitamin E

Tocopherols and tocotrienols in the forms of α, β, δ, and γ are the components of vitamin E [55]. The highest concentration of vitamin E activity is found in α-tocopherol [55]. However, analysis for the vitamin E concentration in a parrot's blood may not reflect body α-tocopherol concentrations [22]. Deficiencies of vitamin E in avian species result in neuromuscular and vascular disease and poor reproductive success [55]. Plasma or serum vitamin E concentrations determined for 115 captive parrots had mean α-tocopherol concentrations of 13.05 ± 6.60 μg/ml. Relatively low concentrations occurred in Pesquet's parrots (*Psittrichas fulgidus*) and high concentrations in hyacinth macaws (*Anodorhynchus hyacinthinus*). Thus, circulating concentrations of vitamin E in psittacine birds may depend significantly on subfamily and genera [54].

Vitamin K

Vitamin K is an integral part of the clotting process. A dietary deficiency of vitamin K has also been implicated in the mortality of some species of fig parrots (*Opopsitta* spp.) from cerebral hemorrhage [53]. Daily supplementation of 300 μg/bird of vitamin K_1 is suggested as a preventive measure [53].

Metals

Lead

Lead is the likely most common ingested toxin diagnosed in pet psittacine species. The most common clinical signs associated with lead toxicosis are neurologic (e.g., ataxia), nonregenerative anemia, and gastrointestinal/renal (e.g., diarrhea, hematuria). Lead toxicosis is implicated as causative of erythrocytic ballooning, a bulging of the normal oval erythrocyte shape accompanied by hypochromasia [14]. Radiographic images of the parrot suspected to be intoxicated by lead can be obtained, to look for a foreign body within the gastrointestinal track but may not be diagnostic and are not specific for lead toxicosis. Some sources of lead readily ingestible by parrots may not be evident on radiographic images, (e.g., lead-impregnated paint chips). This author took postmortem radiographic images of an Amazon parrot that ingested an entire lead fishing weight, and no metal was detected within the gastrointestinal tract. The same parrot had blood lead concentrations at the top of the toxic range. *Diagnosis of lead toxicosis in a psittacine patient should only come after blood lead concentrations are determined.* For blood lead concentrations, inquire what anticoagulant is recommended for the sample. Just 0.5 ml of whole blood may prove adequate for analysis. The most useful tissues to submit, either through biopsy or necropsy sampling, are the liver and kidney. Lead is a nonessential element; thus, lead concentrations should be less than the wet weight concentration expressed as parts per million, 0.2 in the body (or blood), and 2 in the liver and kidney [56]. Tissue concentrations at necropsy of >6 ppm indicate lead poisoning, while the lower concentrations indicate lead exposure which may or may not be related to clinical disease [56].

Zinc

Zinc toxicity in parrot species has been a significant health concern for the last 20 years. Although zinc is an essential mineral, overexposure through ingestion of zinc objects (e.g., toys) or zinc-impregnated water (e.g., dew drops from cage wire) will cause clinical disease. Radiographic evaluation, hematology, and analysis of whole blood, plasma, or serum are required to make a definitive diagnosis of zinc toxicity. It must be remembered that glass or all-plastic syringes and blood collection tubes with royal blue stoppers are recommended to collect the samples for zinc toxicology analysis [56]. Toxic zinc concentrations in parrot species are >14 ppm [56, 57] For analyzing necropsy tissue samples, the recommended tissue samples include the liver, kidney, and pancreas [56]. The pancreas often contains the highest concentration of zinc concentrations in both normal birds and those that have died of zinc toxicosis [56]. Normal zinc concentrations in cockatiel tissue samples are pancreas 26 ppm, liver 22 ppm, and kidney 18 ppm [56] To assess the live patient for zinc toxicosis, nonhemolyzed plasma collected with an all-plastic syringe may be placed in a plastic Microtainer® with a plastic stopper (lithium heparin anticoagulant), or in a serum tube with a royal blue stopper and no contact with rubber [4, 7, 54]. *Parrots may suffer from heavy metal toxicosis with no evidence of a metallic foreign body present either through radiographic imaging or endoscopic evaluation of the GI tract.*

Other Toxicants

In psittacine species, in particular those that are maintained as companion pets, there are a number of toxins from which exposure may occur. Fortunately the exposure to these toxicants is rare, with the exception of the inhaled toxin polytetrafluoroethylene (PTFE) from Teflon-coated cookware. Diagnosis of PTFE toxicosis can only be made through history of exposure and postmortem lesions characterized by severe pulmonary congestion and hemorrhage [56]. With most bird toys and cage furniture products being manufactured in countries outside of the United States, there has been an increase in the incidence of both lead and other trace element toxicosis, especially cadmium. Bird toys and cage furniture manufacturers have no oversight in construction and material used. Therefore, it is prudent to consider all possible differential diagnoses when a parrot patient presents with clinical disease signs consistent with heavy metal toxicosis (e.g., neurologic, gastrointestinal, nonregenerative anemia).

Hormones

Although some diseases are associated with hormonal influence in psittacine species, associated diagnostic testing, known treatment regimens, as well as scientifically generated normal concentrations of these hormones are relatively unknown. Most current knowledge relating to avian hormones has been established through scientific investigations involving chickens and ducks. Hormones produced by the pituitary gland, including gonadotropins (e.g., follicular stimulating hormone (FSH), luteinizing hormone (LH), and thyroid stimulating hormone (TSH)) follow a similar development process in parrot species as in other birds. In psittacine species, the most common pituitary disease presentation is neoplasia (adenomas and carcinomas) [58]. Pituitary adenomas and carcinomas have been diagnosed primarily in budgerigars and to a lesser extent in cockatiels and lovebirds [59]. Pituitary tumors are difficult to diagnose antemortem and are often associated with nonspecific central neurologic clinical signs including head tremors, torticollis, and ataxia. Despite studies published on the baseline plasma corticosterone and post-adrenocorticotropic hormone (ACTH) stimulation plasma corticosterone concentrations, these are seldom used in the clinical setting. Naturally occurring hyperadrenocorticism or hypoadrenocorticism remain unreported in birds [59]. Adrenal disease has been reported relatively often in psittacine species during necropsy examination, although the clinical manifestations of this condition are routinely benign when an external physical evaluation of a patient's health is being performed.

Thyroid hormone production in avian species is similar to that found in mammals [40]. TSH acts by boosting the uptake of iodide and production of thyroglobulin by the follicular cells of the thyroid gland and promoting the hydrolysis of thyroglobulin by the follicular cells, thereby releasing T_4 and T_3 [40]. T_4 acts as a negative feedback mechanism on the production and release of TSH. While both T_3 and T_4 are released from the thyroid tissue, the majority of T_3 is created by peripheral deiodination of T_4 by 5′-deiodinase [40]. The ratio of serum T_3 and T_4 depends on species, but their potencies are equivalent between avian groups [40]. Clinical signs associated with thyroid disease include feather growth, color and structure abnormalities, egg quality, and reproduction. One case report describes naturally occurring hypothyroidism in a scarlet macaw with clinical signs similar to those caused by experimental thyroidectomy of birds [40]. The most common disease associated with the thyroid gland in psittacine species is goiter [40]. Budgerigars historically have been the primary psittacine species in which goiter has been diagnosed, although others may be diagnosed with this disease. Affected budgerigars may have been fed a diet deficient in iodine, resulting in thyroid gland hypertrophy. Treatment and prevention of goiter in psittacine species, in particular budgerigars, is through the addition of 0.3% Lugol's iodine to the drinking water [59]. Diagnosing hypothyroidism in avian species is difficult, as normal T_4 concentrations may be below the detectable limits of the test [59]. Moreover, T_4 concentrations in mammals and birds are influenced by external stressors (e.g., handling and food intake) [60]. Therefore, no definitive diagnosis should ever be made on the basis of one T_4 test result. The diagnosis of hypothyroidism should be based on a confirmatory thyroid stimulation test (Table 25.5) [61]. Both bovine and human thyroid stimulating products have been used in psittacine species and have been found to substantially increase T_4 concentrations after administration [61]. Thyroid neoplasms occurring in psittacine species include thymomas, adenomas, and carcinomas. Thyroid neoplasms may be evident in affected birds from swelling in the upper cervical region. Although African gray parrots may have clinical signs consistent with hypocalcemia syndrome and may

Table 25.5 Recommended procedure for TSH stimulation test in psittacine birds [59].

1) Collect blood concentration for baseline T_4 concentration.
2) Administer suggested dose of TSH intramuscularly at the rate of 1.0 IU/kg.
3) Collect a blood sample 6 h later for a post–TSH T4 concentration (normal parrot serum T4 concentration should at least double after administration of TSH).

be diagnosed with parathyroid hyperplasia, the multifactorial nature of this disease makes this finding of minimal clinical import.

Urinalysis

For psittacine and other avian species, the preferred clinical method to collect urine is from a voided sample on an impermeable surface (e.g., plastic). Because urine of avian species is exposed to fecal material in the cloaca, diagnostically valid urine analytes are limited to ketones, glucose, and renal casts. If the urine glucose concentrations correspond to evidence of ketones and increased blood glucose, then an appropriate assessment of the patient can be made. Diabetes mellitus, a rare disease of companion psittacine species, will result in a patient having increased blood and urine glucose, with ketones in the urine sample. With current testing technology, again only ketones, glucose, and renal casts are of clinical diagnostic relevance in a psittacine urinary evaluation. To evaluate renal pathology and renal function in parrot species, an endoscopic renal biopsy is recommended.

Serology and PCR Testing

Serology measures antibody produced by the bird against a disease antigen from the serum or plasma [62]. The antibodies measured in the serum or plasma are commonly IgM (acute phase antibody) and IgG (chronic phase antibody). For all diagnostic tests, one must critically assess to assure it conforms to scientific standards and evaluation. However, for many emerging diseases and advancing technologies, some companies and individuals may take advantage of veterinarians' desire to have diagnostic tests, even without validation. It is highly recommended to use a diagnostic laboratory which is licensed, inspected, and accredited by a respected national diagnostic laboratory oversight association. PCR technology has developed over the last 15 years to become a known and desired testing technology for infectious disease that affects psittacine species. This testing technology identifies antigenic DNA or RNA from the sample collected and is very sensitive. However, PCR samples are easily contaminated in the laboratory, and positive results do not distinguish between true infection, contamination, or exposure.

Many diseases affect psittacine birds in which serologic and/or PCR testing methodologies are available to diagnose infectious diseases. These infectious diseases include psittacine beak and feather disease, avian polyomavirus, avian bornavirus, avian chlamydiosis, and paramyxovirus. Veterinarians should use an accredited diagnostic laboratory that caters to the companion exotic practitioner, and must understand the diagnostic test they are requesting and what the results mean. Only through knowledge of the diagnostic tests offered will the veterinarian be able to distinguish between results that are true or false.

References

1 Degernes, L.A., Crdosier, M.L., Harrison, L.D. et al. (1999). Autologous, homologous, and heterologous red blood cell transfusions in cockatiels (*Nymphicus hollandicus*). *J. Avian. Med. Surg.* 13: 2–9.

2 Joseph, L., Toon, A., Schirtzinger, E.E. et al. (2012). A revised nomenclature and classification for family-group taxa of parrots (Psittaciformes). *Zootaxa* 3205: 26–40.

3 Boehrer, B. (2004). *Parrot culture.* Philadelphia, PA: Philadelphia University Press.

4 Campbell, T.W. and Ellis, C.K. (2007). *Avian & Exotic animal hematology & cytology*, 3e. Blackwell Pub Professional: Ames, IA.

5 Clark, P., Boardman, W., and Raidal, S. (2009). *Atlas of clinical hematology*, 130–138. Ames, IA: Wiley-Blackwell.

6 Mans C, Sladky KK. Intranasal sedation in avian patients. www.vetmed.wisc.edu/alumni/2012/intranasal-sedation-in-parrots/ accessed July 24, 2012

7 Fudge, A.M. (2000). Avian blood sampling and artifact considerations. In: *Laboratory medicine: avian & exotic pets* (ed. A.M. Fudge), 1–8. Philadelphia, PA: WB Saunders.

8 Maxwell, M.H. (1993). Avian blood leukocyte response to stress. *World Poult. Sci. J.* 49: 34–43.

9 Samour, J. (2006). Diagnostic value of hematology. In: *Clinical avian medicine*, vol. II (ed. G.J. Harrison and T.L. Lightfoot), 587–610. Palm Beach, FL: Spix Publishing.

10 Fudge, A.M. (2000). Avian complete blood count. In: *Laboratory medicine: avian & exotic pets* (ed. A.M. Fudge), 9–18. Philadelphia, PA: WB Saunders.

11 Campbell, T.W. (1994). Hematology. In: *Avian medicine: principles and application* (ed. B.W. Ritchie, G.J. Harrison and L.R. Harrison), 176–198. Lake Worth, FL: Wingers Pub.

12 Fudge AM, McEntee L. Giardiasis: diagnosis syndromes. Proc Assoc Avian Vet Conf, Miami, FL pp 155-164, 1986

13 Hoefer, H.L. (1994). Bile acid testing in psittacine birds. *Semin. Avian. Exotic. Pet Med.* 3: 33–37.

14 Degernes, L.A., Harrison, L.D., Smith, D.W. et al. (1999). Autologous, homologous, and heterologous red blood cell transfusions in conures of the genus Aratinga. *J. Avian. Med. Surg.* 13: 10–14.

15 Clark, P., Boardman, W.S.J., and Raidal, S.R. (2009). *Collection and handling of blood samples, in: atlas of clinical avian hematology. Ames, IA*, 7. Wiley-Blackwell.

16 Lucas, A.M. and Pennington, E.M. (1958). The statistical reliability of differential counts of chicken blood. *Poult. Sci.* 37: 544–549.

17 Hawkey, C.M. and Hart, M.G. (1988). An analysis of the incidence of hyperfibrinogenemia in birds with bacterial infections. *Avian Pathol.* 17: 515–517.

18 Fudge, A.M. and Joseph, V. (2000). Disorders of the avian leukocyte. In: *Laboratory medicine: avian & exotic pets* (ed. A.M. Fudge), 19–27. Philadelphia, PA: WB Saunders.

19 Strunk, A. and Wilson, G.H. (2003). Avian cardiology. *Vet. Clin. North Am. Exot. Anim. Pract.* 6: 1–28.

20 Fudge, A.M. (1997). Avian clinical pathology, hematology, and chemistry. In: *Avian medicine and surgery* (ed. R.B. Altman, S.L. Clubb, G.M. Dorrestein and K. Quesenberry), 142–157. Philadelphia, PA: WB Saunders.

21 Hammond, E.E., Guzman, D.S., Garner, M.M. et al. (2010). Long term treatment of chronic lymphocytic leukemia in a green-winged macaw (*Ara chloroptera*). *J. Avian. Med. Surg.* 24 (4): 330–338.

22 Spruling, N.W. (1982). Comparative physiology of blood clotting. *Comp. Biochem. Physiol. A* 71: 219–230.

23 Hohenhaus, A.E. (2004). Importance of blood groups and blood group antibodies in companion animals. *Transfus. Med. Rev.* 18 (2): 117–126.

24 Matsumoto, K. and Okada, I. (1961). Blood group systems in the chicken. *Jpn. J. Genet.* 36: 257–267.

25 Shaw S, Tully TN, Nevarez J. Avian transfusion medicine. Comp Cont Edu cpvetlearn.com/Media/PublicationsArticle/PV?209_Shaw.pdf accessed Sept 17, 2012

26 Altman RB. Heterologous blood transfusion in avian species. Proc Assoc Avian Vet Conf, San Diego, CA pp 7-8, 1982

27 Lumeij, J.T. (1987). The diagnostic value of plasma proteins and non-protein nitrogen substances in birds. *Vet. Q.* 9: 262–268.

28 Fudge, A.M. (2000). Avian liver and gastrointestinal testing. In: *Laboratory medicine: avian & exotic pets* (ed. A.M. Fudge), 47–55. Philadelphia, PA: WB Saunders.

29 Lumeij, J.T. (1997). Avian Clinical biochemistry. In: *Clinical biochemistry of domestic animals* (ed. J.J. Kaneko), 857–883. San Diego, CA: Academic Press.

30 Isaza, R., Buergelt, C., and Kollias, G.V. (1992). Bacteremia and vegetative endocarditis associated with a heart murmur in a blue and gold macaw. *Avian Dis.* 36: 1112–1116.

31 Flammer K. Serum bile acids in psittacine brids. Proc Assoc Avian Vet Conf, Reno, NV pp 9-12, 1994

32 Harr, K.E. (2006). Diagnostic value of biochemistry. In: *Clinical avian medicine*, vol. II (ed. G.J. Harrison and T.L. Lightfoot), 611–629. Palm Beach, FL: Spix Publishing.

33 Lumeij JT, Peccati C. (1993): Suspected hepatoencephalopathy in an African grey parrot. 2nd Euro Conf Assoc Avian Vet, Utrecht, The Netherlands pp 558–564.

34 Potter, K., Conner, T., and Galliara, A.M. (1983). Cholangiocarcinoma in a yellow-faced Amazon parrot (Amazona xanthops). *Avian Dis.* 27: 556–596.

35 Wideman, R.F. (1988). Avian kidney anatomy and physiology. *CRC Critical Rev. Poult. Biol.* 1: 133–176.

36 Phalen, D.N. (2000). Avian renal disorders. In: *Laboratory medicine: avian & exotic pets* (ed. A.M. Fudge), 61–68. Philadelphia, PA: WB Saunders.

37 Lumeij, J.T. (1994). Nephrology. In: *Avian medicine: principles and application* (ed. B.W. Ritchie, G.J. Harrison and L.R. Harrison), 538–555. Lake Worth, FL: Wingers Pub.

38 Jones, M.P. (1999). Avian clinical pathology. *Vet. Clin. North Am. Exot. Anim. Pract.* 2: 663–687.

39 Speer BL: A clinical look at the avian pancreas in health and disease. Proc Assoc Avian Vet Conf, St. Paul, MN pp 57–64, 1998

40 Rae, M. (2000). Avian endocrine disorders. In: *Laboratory medicine: avian & exotic pets* (ed. A.M. Fudge), 76–89. Philadelphia, PA: WB Saunders.

41 Hazelwood, R.L. and Meyer, D.C. (1996). Pancreas and pineal. In: *Avian physiology*, 4e (ed. P.D. Sturkie), 494–504. New York, NY: Springer-Verlag.

42 Feltrer Y, Strike T, Routh A, Gaze D, Shave R. Point-of-care cardiac troponin I in non-domestic species: a feasibility study.

43 Hochleithner, M. (1994). Biochemistries. In: *Avian Medicine: principles and application* (ed. B.W. Ritchie, G.J. Harrison and L.R. Harrison), 223–245. Lake Worth, FL: Wingers Pub.

44 Kirchgessner, M.S., Tully, T.N. Jr., Nevarez, J. et al. (2012). Magnesium therapy in a hypocalcemic African grey parrot (Psittacus erithacus). *J. Avian Med. Surg.* 26 (1): 17–21.

45 Clubb, S.L., Schubot, R.M., and Joyner, K. (1991). Hemotologic and serum biochemical references intervals in juvenile cockatoos. *J. Assoc. Avian. Vet.* 5 (1): 16–26.

46 Clubb, S.L., Schubot, R.M., and Joyner, K. (1990). Hemotologic and serum biochemical references intervals in juvenile eclectus parrots (*Electus roratus*). *J. Assoc. Avian. Vet.* 4 (4): 218–225.

47 Rosenthal, K.L., Johnston, M.S., and Shofer, F.S. (2005). Assessment of the reliability of plasma electrophoresis in birds. *Am. J. Vet. Res.* 66 (3): 375–378.

48 Rosenthal, K.L., Johnston, M.S., Shofer, F.S., and Poppenga, R.H. (2005). Psittacine plasma

concentrations of elements: daily fluctuations and clinical implications. *J. Vet. Dian. Invest.* 17 (3): 239–244.

49 (a) Vanderheyden, N. (1994). Evaluation and interpretation of the avian hemogram. *Semin. Avian Exot. Pet Med.* 3 (1): 5–13. (b) Werner LL, Reavill DR. The diagnostic utility of serum protein electrophoresis. *Vet. Clin. North Am. Exot. Anim. Pract.* 2(3):651–662, 1994.

50 Fudge, A.M. (2000). Avian metabolic disorders. In: *Laboratory medicine: avian & exotic pets* (ed. A.M. Fudge), 56–60. Philadelphia, PA: WB Saunders.

51 Koutsos EA, Klosing KC. Vitamin A nutrition in cockatiels. Proc Joint Nutri Symp. Antwerp, Belgium, p 141, 2002

52 de Carvalho, F.M., Gaunt, S.D., Kearney, M.T. et al. (2009). Reference intervals of plasma calcium, phosphorus, and magnesium for African grey parrots (*Psittacus erithacus*) and Hispaniolan parrots (*Amazona ventralis*). *J. Zoo Wildl. Med.* 40 (4): 675–679.

53 McDowell, L.R. (2000). *Vitamins in animal and human nutrition*. Ames, IA: Iowa State University Press.

54 Torregrossa, A.M., Puschner, B., Tell, L. et al. (2005 Sep). Circulating concentrations of vitamins a and E in captive psittacine birds. *J. Avian Med. Surg.* 19 (3): 225–229.

55 McDonald, D. (2006). Nutritional considerations Sect 1: Nutrition and dietary supplementation. In: *Clinical avian medicine*, vol. I (ed. G.J. Harrison and T.L. Lightfoot), 86–108. Palm Beach, FL: Spix Publishing.

56 Sigurdson, C.J. and Franson, J.C. (2000). Avian toxicologic diagnosis. In: *Laboratory Medicine: avian & exotic pets* (ed. A.M. Fudge), 174–192. Philadelphia, PA: WB Saunders.

57 Howard, B.R. (1992). Health risk of housing small psittacines in galvanized wire mesh cages. *J. Am. Vet. Med. Assoc.* 200: 1667–1674.

58 Leach, M.W. (1992). A survey of neoplasia in pet birds. *Semin. Avian Exot. Pet Med.* 1 (2): 65–72.

59 Rupley, A.E. (1997). *Manual of avian medicine in practice*, 298. Philadelphia, PA: W.B. Saunders.

60 Lumeij, J.T. (1994). Avian clinical enzymology. *Semin. Avian Exotic Pet Med.* 3: 14–24.

61 Lothrop, C.D., Loomis, M.R., and Olsen, J.H. (1985). Thyrotropin stimulation test for evaluation of thyroid function in psittacine birds. *J. Am. Vet. Med. Assoc.* 186: 47–48.

62 Phalen, D.W. (2000). Avian viral diagnostics. In: *Laboratory medicine: avian & exotic pets* (ed. A.M. Fudge), 111–123. Philadelphia, PA: WB Saunders.

26

Galliformes

Jennifer R. Cook DVM, MS, DACVP (Clinical Pathology)[1] *and J. Jill Heatley DVM, MS, DABVP (Avian, Reptilian, Amphibian), DACZM*[2]

[1] *Idexx Laboratories, Inc., Bloomfield Hills, Michigan, USA*
[2] *Department of Small Animal Clinical Sciences, College of Veterinary Medicine & Biomedical Sciences, Texas A&M University, College Station, Texas, USA*

Introduction

Clinical pathology data are a critical part of diagnostic and medical management for individual companion animals, which many Galliformes have become. Similarly, clinicopathologic data are of immense importance within the poultry industry for surveillance of herd health. In the research setting, the chicken is considered the premier nonmammalian research model and is used for vaccine development and study of metabolism, oncology, genetics, evolution, nutrition, immunology, and virology. The tremendous amount of information in the literature regarding the effects of husbandry and research-based permutations on hematologic data and health/growth statistics is beyond the scope of this text. Further, this information is not always directly applicable to the establishment of normal reference intervals or the study of clinicopathologic data in naturally occurring disease processes. For many traditional clinicopathologic parameters used in mammals, clinical significance and utility in gallinaceous species is not established. Moreover, many potentially useful parameters lack validated methodologies or reference intervals. Clinicopathologic data is dependent on methodology, signalment, seasonality, husbandry, and many other internal and external parameters. Because laboratory-specific, methodology-specific, and population-specific reference intervals are typically lacking, clinicians must make inferences based on the reference data available. To that end, we provide this chapter as a clinical summary of available, pertinent literature for Galliformes. With this summary, we strive to encapsulate the relevant literature useful to the clinician for diagnostic and health assessment purposes, which is mainly based on the domestic chicken, *Gallus gallus*.

Species

The Galliformes are an order of heavy-bodied ground-feeding birds that includes junglefowl (chicken), turkey, grouse, New and Old World quail and ptarmigan, partridge, pheasant, chachalaca, guinea fowl, peafowl, and the Cracidae (Guan and curassow) (Table 26.1). Historically, buttonquails (Turnicidae) were considered Galliformes, but they are now known to be shorebirds adapted to an inland lifestyle. The earliest Galliforme-like fossils hail from the late Cretaceous with fossils dating to approximately 85 million years ago. This group of about 300 species is found in essentially all of the world's continents, although they rarely inhabit islands unless introduced by humans. Galliformes are important as seed dispersers and predators in the ecosystems they inhabit and are often reared by humans for their meat and eggs, for recreational hunting, or for display. The red jungle fowl (chicken), common turkey, peafowl, and helmeted guinea fowl have been domesticated for centuries. Most of the information in this chapter is drawn from the vast extant available literature in chickens. However, when possible, we have also included comments and information for other Galliformes.

Sample Collection

As with other species, the benefit of obtaining blood, urine, or other clinical pathology samples (e.g., fine needle aspirates of bone marrow, body cavity effusions, or mass lesions) must be weighed against the possible detrimental effects of handling, restraint, and sedation, especially for patients with respiratory or hemostatic difficulty. Adequate hemostasis after venipuncture is

Exotic Animal Laboratory Diagnosis, First Edition. Edited by J. Jill Heatley and Karen E. Russell.

Table 26.1 Galliforme species maintained as pets, or for display, game, or food production.

Common name	Specific and scientific name	Family	Native geographic range
Chachalaca	Ortalis vetula	Cracidae	Southern US to Central America
Guan	White-crested guan *Penelope pileata* *Chamaepetes* spp.		Mexico to South America
Curassow	Great curassow *Crax rubra*		Mexico to tropical South America
Turkey	*Meleagridis gallopavo*	Meleagrididae	North America[a]
Guinea Fowl	*Agelastes, Numida, Guttera, Acryllium* spp. Helemeted guinea fowl, *Numida meleagris*	Numididae	Africa[a]
Quail	Japanese quail *Coturnix coturnix* Bobwhite Quail *Colinus virginianus*	Phasianidae	Mainly North America[a]
Rock ptarmigan	*Lagopus muta*		Worldwide northern climes
Chicken	Red Jungle Fowl *Gallus gallus* Domestic Chicken *G. gallus (domesticus)*		India, China, Malaysia, Philippines[a]
Pheasant	*Phasianus colchicas*		Eurasia, Africa, SE Asia[b]
Peafowl	*Pavo cristatus, Pavo muticus, Afropavo congensis*		Asiatic, African
Partridge	Gray partridge *Perdix perdix*		Holarctic
Grouse	Ruffled grouse – *Bonasa umbellus* American woodcock – *Philohela minor* Sage grouse – *Centrocercus urophasianus* Sharp-tailed grouse – *Pediocetes phasianellus*	Tetraonidae	North America, Europe[b]

[a] Domesticated.
[b] Some species introduced worldwide or widely.

particularly important in the domestic chicken prior to return to the flock to avoid cannibalism, which may be more likely in young birds [1]. Sampling site may affect some hematologic parameters in Galliformes. In the Japanese quail, hemoglobin and packed cell volume (PCV) were highest in samples obtained from the medial metatarsal veins, followed in descending order by samples obtained from the brachial vein, jugular vein, and the heart [2].

Restraint

In most Galliformes, blood may be collected using only manual restraint. However, analgesia, sedation, or even anesthesia may be necessary in fractious or large patients, which may be dangerous to themselves or others [3, 4]. Avian anesthesia is beyond the scope of this chapter, but excellent reviews exist. Common drug choices include midazolam, butorphanol, and isoflurane; use of local anesthetics may also be considered [5, 6]. Adequate fasting to ensure crop emptying is recommended prior to venipuncture attempt.

Venipuncture Sites

Appropriate venipuncture sites in pet Galliformes include the medial metatarsal vein, the jugular vein, and the ulnar or wing vein. Alternative venipuncture sites of historical or research import, or limited to use for collection of large samples prior to euthanasia or to facilitate euthanasia under anesthesia, include the retroorbital sinus, the occipital sinus, toenail clip, and cardiocentesis [7]. In a study of sampling sites of the Japanese quail, cardiac sampling was considered traumatic, resulted in many side effects, and was not recommended for use in ongoing experiments [2]. Nerve damage indicates that samples obtained via toenail clip are painful. Further problems with this collection method include small sample size unrepresentative of peripheral circulation, and also likely contamination of the sample with uric acid [8, 9]. As gallinaceous species are ground-dwelling, walking birds prone to bumblefoot, pain, and continued site contamination from the environment sampling these sites are of further concern. As they are inappropriate for use in companion species, these sites of venipuncture for Galliformes will not be further discussed. Additional references are available for sampling of the chicken repeatedly or for laboratory purposes [1, 10].

Medial Tarsometatarsal Veins

The medial metatarsal veins can provide reasonably sized samples from many Galliformes. Above the hock (tibiotarsal/tarsometatarsal joint), this vein is surrounded by muscles, which reduces the risk of hematoma formation but may obscure visualization [1]. Below the hock, occlusion may be necessary, as scalation may hinder direct visualization of the vein. Minimal subcutaneous tissue surrounds this vein at the mid-tibiotarsus, and skin scales limit local tissue expansion. Thus, external bleeding post venipuncture is common at the more distal site. The chicken is placed in lateral recumbency to sample the medial aspect of the ventral leg. Adequate patient restraint and a shallow angle of approach (10–30°) are necessary. The author generally prefers a 1 ml syringe and a 26 or 25 gauge (g.) needle for blood collection from this vein. To limit post-venipuncture blood loss, facilitate clotting, and limit contamination of this site, application of a short-term bandage after sampling is recommended of the more distal sampling site.

Jugular Vein

Galliformes have both right and left jugular veins, although the left is usually approximately 30% the size of the right. Thus, the right jugular vein is preferred for venipuncture; however, the left may also be used. Complications or hindrances which may arise with venipuncture at this site include hematoma formation; a full crop or esophagus which hinders visualization of the vein(s) and makes the patient more likely to regurgitate or aspirate; and also the proximity of air sacs, into which blood may enter during or post venipuncture, causing the patient to cough or sneeze blood post venipuncture. In the authors' experience, most of these complications are rare in the healthy chicken, and with appropriate experience, restraint, and collection equipment, this site is most likely to yield the best sample with the least effort and time. The patient is generally restrained in left lateral recumbency to approach the large right jugular vein. In a study of collection that found hematologic differences based on sampling site in the Japanese quail, jugular venipuncture exhibited the least sample variability [2]. The relatively mobile, superficial vein is stabilized by extending the neck until it is straight and positioning the keel so that the patient is in lateral recumbency. The vein courses posterior to the trachea and anterior to the esophagus. Alcohol application allows feathers to flatten along the featherless tract to allow visualization of the vein through the skin. The vein may be entered at a shallow angle (10°–20°) from either the cranial or caudal aspect; occluding the vein may or may not be necessary. Needle and syringe choice depend on patient size, operator preference, and sample size needed. 23–26 g. needles, winged infusion sets and 1–5 ml syringes or vacutainers are appropriate options; [11] a 3 ml syringe with a 20 gauge needle can be used to collect 1.5 ml of blood [12].

Wing Veins

Based on the confluence of veins at the ventral aspect of the wing near the anconeal joint, numerous names are used somewhat interchangeably for the veins of the wing. These include the basilic vein, brachial vein, and the cutaneous or recurrent ulnar vein. With the aid of alcohol to wet down and sweep away feathers, the vein can be visualized as it courses along the ventral aspect of the wing between the biceps and triceps muscles. The vein may be accessed at multiple sites along its path, including at the bifurcation and as it traverses the radius and ulna proximal to the anconeal joint. Despite its ease of visualization, successful venipuncture of the wing vein involves many challenges. A lack of subcutaneous tissues, the local motion of the joint, and the tendency of the patient to move during venipuncture all make this site prone to hematoma formation. Failure to collect a reasonably sized sample in smaller species from this vein is not uncommon. In companion Galliformes, the author prefers to reserve use of these veins for catheterization and administration of fluids and medications. Should venipuncture be attempted, heavy sedation and analgesia, or anesthesia, are recommended. Patient positioning preferred by the author is dorsal recumbency with the wing outstretched but not hyperextended. The patient may also be held vertically against the restrainer's body in field settings. The vein is best visualized with alcohol applied to the local area. Needle and syringe choice depend on patient size, operator preference, and sample size needed. Local anatomy and the angle at which this vein courses make approach at a shallow angle (10°–20°) necessary [1]. Small-gauge needles (25 or 26 g.) with 1 ml syringes or 25 g. winged infusion sets provide better chance of reasonable sample size collection in patients weighing 1.5 kg or less. Placement of the nondominant hand on the wing bones or feathers stabilizes the collection site. The dominant hand can then rest on the nondominant hand for stabilization during venipuncture. The needle, bevel up, is directed toward the patient to enter the vein as the vein courses over the ulna or proximal to the humeroradial joint. Placement of light pressure to the site after sample collection is recommended to facilitate hemostasis [8, 9, 12–17].

Bone Marrow Collection

Bone marrow collection may be performed antemortem from the medial proximal tibiotarsus, just distal to the femoral-tibiotarsal (knee) joint. After aseptic preparation and skin incision, a Jamshidi™ biopsy-aspiration needle with stylet is advanced into the marrow cavity, the stylet is removed, and a 6 or 12 ml syringe is attached for positive pressure aspiration [18].

Blood and Sample Volume

Domestic poultry have a relatively small percentage of blood volume of 6.0%–7.5% compared to other birds based on body weight [1]. Wider blood volume ranges have been reported for the chicken (49–149 ml/kg) [8, 9]. Blood volume of the white Holland turkey hen is 7.2%

body weight [19]. Blood/plasma volumes, respectively, of the ring-necked pheasant, given as ml/100 g bodyweight, are 6.7/4.5 in males and 4.8/3.2 in females [20]. Blood and plasma volumes of the Japanese quail vary based on age and sex. Blood/plasma volumes of young unsexed, male adult, female adult laying, and female adult non-laying quail were determined as 83.2/59.1, 74.2/47.3, 71.2/47.3, and 67.6/42.9 ml/kg of bodyweight, respectively [21]. Blood and plasma volumes of many other Galliformes remain uninvestigated but should be assumed similarly low in most, based on the ground-dwelling nature and minimal flight capabilities of many of these heavy-bodied species. In the healthy domestic chicken, 7.5 ml/kg of body weight should be the maximum blood volume withdrawn in a single collection, and a minimum of 14 days should be allowed for hematologic parameter recovery [1]. Fortunately, most standard clinicopathologic tests have much lesser requirements.

In the research setting, a single collection of 2% bodyweight may be tolerated by the domestic chicken if warm isotonic fluids are administered to offset volume loss [1]. Chickens have remarkable regenerative capacity and can return to a normal hematocrit three days after depletion of 30% of total blood volume [22]. In juvenile and adult quail (*Coturnix coturnix japonica*), with and without replacement of blood volume by saline, recovery of total peripheral erythrocyte mass and total peripheral leukocyte mass occurred within 72 h post phlebotomy [23, 24]. In guinea fowl, *Numida meleagris galeata*, subjected to removal of 30% of blood volume, RBC, PCV, and MCHC decreased significantly but were fully restored by the 4th week post blood sampling [25].

Sample Handling

Anticoagulant Options

For the chicken complete blood count (CBC), ethylenediaminetetraacetic acid (EDTA) tubes may be used [8, 9]. However, If CBC and biochemistry panel are desired with a small volume of blood, lithium heparin is the preferred anticoagulant to maximize sample size. For Brush turkeys *(Alectura lathami*), black and other curassows (*Crax alector*), and guans, blood may clot or lyse with EDTA, therefore heparin- or citrate-based anticoagulants are recommended for these species. Blood smears for differential leukocyte count and morphology should be made promptly after blood collection, preferably from blood that has not been anticoagulated. Prolonged exposure (>30 min) to anticoagulants may distort the cellular morphology of leukocytes, erythrocytes, and thrombocytes, and may compromise adequate staining [26–28]. Lithium heparin anticoagulated blood was considered more reliable in one study for i-STAT® analysis than fresh whole blood, which tended to produce cartridge errors [9]. Most biochemistry analyses can be performed on plasma or serum. Lithium heparin is preferred; other anticoagulants such as EDTA, sodium heparin, and sodium citrate may interfere with biochemical analyses [29]. Use of citrate and oxalate containing anticoagulants are not recommended for use in chickens or guinea fowl samples based on hemolysis and reduced PCV [30].

Because chicken blood has potential use as a biological flocculant, preservation at room temperature in nonsterile conditions to prevent clot formation, degradation, and hydrogen sulfide production has been investigated [31]. Of the three chemicals investigated, potassium EDTA was superior and prevented coagulation for four days at room temperature with less production of toxic gas. Blood treated with potassium oxalate or potassium citrate produced dangerous amounts of toxic gas and could only prevent coagulation without refrigeration for about one day. Thus, although further studies are indicated, for hematologic purposes, potassium EDTA shows promise in Galliformes for preservation of samples shipped without refrigeration.

Sample Storage

Based on the extensive study of chicken health as a food animal, studies of blood storage are extant. For other species, much less information is available. However, for many biochemical parameters, the optimum sample (plasma vs. serum) and data regarding the stability of the analyte under various storage conditions (refrigeration, freezing) are lacking. Therefore, in clinical practice or in assessment of species where the effects of storage has not been evaluated, for biochemical analyses, blood should be spun and plasma- or serum-separated quickly to reduce errors associated with hemolysis or prolonged exposure to erythrocytes. Storage *may* affect the following parameters in Galliformes: bile acids, bilirubin, lactate dehydrogenase (LDH), creatine kinase (CK), alkaline phosphatase (ALP), potassium, calcium, phosphorous, albumin, fibrin, and glucose [26]. Alternatively, for biochemical and hormone analysis, blood may be placed in plastic tubes, allowed to clot at 20 °C for 4 h, and then serum-separated and stored at −20 °C until analysis performed [16].

Leukogram and erythron parameters of chicken and turkey blood stored using different anticoagulants, temperatures, and times have been evaluated (Table 26.2). In summary, storage of chicken blood samples at 4 °C would give reliable results for parameters studied within 30 h of collection, and for 72 h if leukogram and mean corpuscular volume (MCV) need not be evaluated. Storage at 29 °C would be reliable for 12 h (or up to 18 h without evaluation of MCV). Storage at 37 °C would be reliable

Table 26.2 Effect of storage of chicken blood with the anticoagulant sodium EDTA [32].

Parameter	Storage time (h)	Storage temperature (°C)	Change
Packed cell volume	18	29, 37	Increase
	72	4	None
Leukocytes	18	29, 37	Decrease
	30	4	
Mean cell volume	12	29, 37	Increase
	30	4	
Erythrocytes, hemoglobin	48	37	Decrease
	72	4, 29	None

for 9 h, up to 12 h without evaluation of mean corpuscular hemoglobin concentration (MCHC), and up to 18 h without evaluation of MCV [32]. Although leukocytes were not assessed, findings were otherwise similar for turkey blood stored at 4, 24, and 33 °C [33].

In chickens, heparinized plasma is considered a more reliable sample for assessment of biochemical analytes, based on the ability to separate plasma from the cellular elements of blood immediately with centrifugation [34]. In the single supportive study, paired blood samples were either heparinized for immediate centrifugation and plasma harvest, or allowed to clot for 90 min prior to serum separation. Differences occurred in 9 of the 17 analytes examined. Plasma had higher concentrations of albumin, potassium, and chloride and an increased albumin to globulin (A/G) ratio. Serum had higher concentrations or activities of total protein, calculated globulin, CK, calcium, magnesium, and phosphorous. Bile acids, AST, LDH, uric acid, glucose, cholesterol, and sodium did not differ significantly based on sample type. However, some studies have also had reasonable biochemical results with chicken serum by allowing clot formation to occur at 4 °C, which likely minimizes the biochemical changes attributable to blood cell metabolism [16]. Standing blood for short periods of time (up to approximately 2 h) should not cause in vitro hypoglycemia, because avian erythrocytes use fatty acids, not glucose, as the main energy source [35]. For chicken blood samples, hemolysis can decrease glucose, albumin, and CPK values and increase uric acid and phosphorous concentrations [34, 36].

Specific Analytes

Complete Blood Count

Hematologic values of apparently healthy Galliformes are provided in Tables 26.3 and 26.4.

Erythrocytes

Packed cell volume (PCV) may be determined using standard centrifuge methodologies (2500 rpm, 3 to 5 min) [11]. Calculation of hematocrit (HCT) is not generally recommended for use in Galliformes; however, HCT of chickens determined by the i-STAT does have good correlation with PCV determined by centrifugation [51]. Hemoglobin of Galliformes may be determined via the hemoglobinometer, the cyanmethemoglobin method, or by the spectrophotometer [15, 16, 52].

Cell Morphology

Chicken erythrocytes are typical avian red blood cells. They are approximately 12 × 8 μm ovals with homogenous orange-red cytoplasm and an oval central nucleus containing condensed chromatin and indistinct nucleoli. Young, polychromatophilic erythrocytes are commonly observed in healthy Galliformes (1+, or 1%–5% of all erythrocytes) based on the relatively short life span (25–45 days) of avian erythrocytes [53]. Polychromatophils are often the same size and shape as mature erythrocytes with medium blue to purple homogenous cytoplasm and less condensed, patchy chromatin. Younger polychromatophils are shorter and rounder, while still retaining a definite ovoid shape. Immature erythrocytic precursors (rubricytes, prorubricytes, and rubriblasts) are round with condensed to patchy chromatin and small to moderate amounts of deep blue cytoplasm. These cells are distinguished from lymphocytes based on more abundant cytoplasm and darker, less smooth chromatin. Estimation of polychromasia on a peripheral blood smear will underestimate reticulocytosis; not all reticulocytes appear polychromatophilic [29]. Reticulocytosis is best evaluated with a supravital stain, such as new methylene blue, that stains cytoplasmic aggregates of reticulin (retained RNA from immature cells) dark blue. Reticulin should encircle at least half of the nucleus for a cell to be considered a reticulocyte [54]. Polychromasia or more accurately, reticulocytosis, of greater than 5%–10% indicates a regenerative response to anemia [29]. Saline replacement of blood volume following hemorrhage in adult and juvenile quail (*C. coturnix japonica*), increased total numbers and differential percentages of circulating reticulocytes at 72 h post phlebotomy above the reticulocyte values of phlebotomized quail receiving no saline [24]. Poikilocytosis is rarely observed in birds, but could indicate severe systemic infections that have damaged bone marrow or preparation artifact.

In the healthy Galliforme, red blood cell parameters are affected by age, sex, reproductive activity, diet, species, and sometimes by breed or strain. Neonates and young juvenile chickens have a physiologic anemia, with a direct correlation of age and PCV occurring in animals

Table 26.3 Hematologic data for healthy chickens (*Gallus gallus domesticus*).

Breed		**Ross [16] Ross, Cobb [12]**	**Nigerian [15, 37] Normal, frizzled, and naked-necked**	**Thai [11]**	**White leghorns [27, 38]**	**Bangladesh [39]**	**Kashmir [40]**	**Bantam [41] C: Cochin or P: Polish**	**Astra S [42]**	
Attributes		**♂ 13 mo [16] ♀ 25–36 wk [12]**	**♂♀ 20 wk [15]**	**♂♀**	**♂ 4–6 mo [38] ♀ young adult [27]**	**6–12 mo**	**Adult**	**♂, 40 wk**	**1 wk**	**18 wk**
Sample size		**5 [16], 165 [12]**	**60 [15]**	**12**	**[38] 14, [27] 20**	**20♂, 20♀**	**30♂ 55 ♀**	**8 Each breed**	**10♂ 10 ♀**	**10♂ 10♀**
Sample number		**30 [16]**		**60**	**[38] 37**					
Data format										
Analyte (abbreviation)	**Units SI (US)**	**Mean ± SD [range]**	**Mean ± SE**	**Mean**	**[38] Mean ± SE [range] [38] Mean ± SD [range]**	**Mean ± SE**		**Mean ± SE**	**Mean ± SD [range]**	**Mean ± SD [range]**
Erythrocyte count (RBC)	$\times 10^{12}$/l (=10^{6}/μl)		♂ 4.26 ± 0.05 ♀ 3.49 ± 0.05	2.39		♂ 3.37 ± 0.30 ♀ 2.48 ± 0.25	♂ 3.20 ± 0.07 ♀ 2.98 ± 0.08	C: 3.12 ± 0.10 P: 3.29 ± 0.10	♂ 1.79 ± 0.15 [1.64–2.0] ♀ 2.17 ± 0.19 [1.91–2.32)	♂ 3.06 ± 0.12 [2.82–3.41] ♀ 2.49 ± 0.12 [2.38–2.52]
Hemoglobin (HgB)	mmol/l (g/dl)	[43] 6.76 ± 0.74 [10.9 ± 1.2] [44] 5.52 ± 0.50 [4.53–6.52) [8.9 ± 0.8 [7.3–10.5)]	♂ 7.90 ± 0.08 [12.73 ± 0.13] ♀ 6.55 ± 0.11 [10.56 ± 0.17]	8.88	[38] 7.57 ± 0.06 [6.70 ± 8.75] (12.2 ± 0.1 [10.8–14.1])	♂ 5.88 ± 0.24 [9.48 ± 0.38] ♀ 5.14 ± 0.24 [8.29 ± 0.39]	♂ 8.20 ± 0.24 [13.21 ± 0.39] ♀ 7.03 ± 0.12 [11.32 ± 0.19]	C: 8.63 ± 0.06 [13.9 ± 0.10] P: 7.79 ± 0.48 [12.56 ± 0.30]	♂ 4.84 ± 0.37 [4.53–5.59] [7.8 ± 0.6 [7.3–9.0] ♀ 5.59 ± 0.31 [5.28–6.21] [9.0 ± 0.5 [8.5–10.0]	♂ 8.75 ± 0.50 [7.94–9.56] (14.1 ± 0.8 [12.8–15.4] ♀ 5.77 ± 0.31 [5.40–6.23] [9.3 ± 0.5 [8.7–10.1)]
Packed cell volume (PCV)	l/l (%)	[43] 0.383 ± 0.030 [38.3 ± 3.0] [44] 0.261 ± 0.024 (0.213–0.308) [26.1 ± 2.4 (21.3–30.8)]	♂ 0.381 ± 0.004 [38.07 ± 0.41] ♀ 0.313 ± 0.005 [31.33 ± 0.51]	31.87		♂ 0.331 ± 0.007 [33.05 ± 0.69] ♀ 0.312 ± 0.006 [31.20 ± 0.62]	♂ 0.407 ± 0.005 [40.70 ± 0.51] ♀ 0.352 ± 0.006 [35.21 ± 0.61]	C: 0.404 ± 0.011 [40.38 ± 1.10] P: 0.413 ± 0.009 [41.25 ± 0.90]	♂ 0.259 ± 0.008 (0.250–0.270) [25.9 ± 0.8 (25.0–27.0)] ♀ 0.280 ± 0.009 (0.260–0.290) [28.0 ± 0.9 (26.0–29.0)]	♂ 0.316 ± 0.002 [0.29–0.34] [31.6 ± 1.9 (29.0–34.0)] ♀ 0.296 ± 0.002 (0.270–0.310) [29.6 ± 1.7 (27.0–31.0)]
Mean corpuscular volume (MCV)	fl		♂ 89.48 ± 0.82 ♀ 90.01 ± 1.22	137.61		♂ 99.22 ± 9.26 ♀ 128.55 ± 13.57	♂ 127.18 ± 2.68 ♀ 118.15 ± 76	C: 124.30 ± 2.25 P: 116.98 ± 0.64		
Mean corpuscular hemoglobin concentration (MCHC)	g/l (g/dl)		♂ 335.1 ± 3.60 (33.51 ± 0.36) ♀ 337.3 ± 1.80 (33.73 ± 0.18)	291.0 (29.10)		♂ 286.5 ± 8.60 (28.65 ± 0.86) ♀ 265.8 ± 13.3 (26.58 ± 1.33)	♂ 324.5 ± 5.70 (32.45 ± 0.57) ♀ 321.4 ± 3.90 (32.14 ± 0.39)	C: 325.7 ± 9.40 (32.57 ± 0.94) P: 305.7 ± 9.20 (30.57 ± 0.92)		
White blood cell count (WBC)	$\times 10^{9}$/l (=$\times 10^{3}$/μl)	[43] 29.772 ± 19.745	♂ 5.633 ± 0.038 ♀ 5.573 ± 0.031	12.100	[27] 25.413 ± 5.784 (14.375–36.750)	♂ 19.13 ± 0.43 ♀ 20.68 ± 0.54	♂ 16.80 ± 0.47 ♀ 22.20 ± 0.37	C: 19.13 ± 0.50 P: 18.5 ± 0.50	♂ 7.8 ± 1.6 (6.0–10.0) ♀ 7.7 ± 1.8 (5.0–9.5)	♂ 17.2 ± 1.5 (16.5–21.0) ♀ 21.5 ± 2.4 (18.5–25.5)

Heterophils	$\times 10^9$/l (=$\times 10^3$/μl)			[27] 4.242 ± 1.383 (1.951–6.983)	♂ 4.36 ± 0.20 ♀ 4.01 ± 0.12	♂ 5.47 ± 0.10 ♀ 5.87 ± 0.10	C: 5.50 ± 0.13 P: 4.97 ± 0.11	♂ 1.12 ± 0.16 (0.94–1.40) ♀ 1.21 ± 0.16 (1.08–1.23)	♂ 3.96 ± 0.17 (3.78–4.13) ♀ 4.59 ± 0.54 (4.09–5.16)
Band heterophils	$\times 10^9$/l (=$\times 10^3$/μl)			[27] 0.114 ± 0.157 (0–0.520)					
Eosinophils				[27] 0.717 ± 0.459 (0–1.563)	♂ 0.60 ± 0.14 ♀ 0.37 ± 0.11	♂ 0.95 ± 0.04 ♀ 1.94 ± 0.06	C: 0.14 ± 0.04 P: 0.14 ± 0.06	♂ 0.13 ± 0.04 (0.8–0.16) ♀ 0.08 ± 0	♂ 0.23 ± 0.10 (0.17–0.34) ♀ 0.43 ± 0
Eos ± hetero	$\times 10^9$/l (=$\times 10^3$/μl)	[43] 11.136 ± 6.975							
Basophils	$\times 10^9$/l (=$\times 10^3$/μl)			0.530 ± 0.482 (0–2.000) [27]	♂ 0.19 ± 0.00 ♀ 0.18 ± 0.08	♂ 0.34 ± 0.03 ♀ 0.71 ± 0.05	C: 0.29 ± 0.06 P: 0.44 ± 0.06	♂ 0.10 ± 0.04 (0.08–0.16) ♀ 0.13 ± 0.04 (0.08–0.15)	♂ 0.29 ± 0.10 (0.17–0.34) ♀ 0.36 ± 0.12 (0.21–0.43)
Lymphocytes	$\times 10^9$/l (=$\times 10^3$/μl)	[43] 17.112 ± 13.647		[27] 18.013 ± 5.274 (10.118–27.946)	♂ 11.86 ± 0.55 ♀ 14.60 ± 0.18	♂ 8.21 ± 0.14 ♀ 11.14 ± 0.16	C: 12.84 ± 0.10 P: 12.90 ± 0.11	♂ 6.32 ± 0.16 (6.16–6.47) ♀ 6.19 ± 0.19 (6.01–6.39)	♂ 12.38 ± 0.17 (12.21–12.56) ♀ 15.70 ± 0.65 (15.05–16.34)
Monocytes	$\times 10^9$/l (=$\times 10^3$/μl)	[43] 1.524 ± 4.292		[27] 1.782 ± 0.709 (0.431–2.876)	♂ 0.32 ± 0.09 ♀ 0.57 ± 0.0.16	♂1.83 ± 0.06 ♀ 2.42 ± 0.08	C: 0.52 ± 0.08 P: 0.39 ± 0.02	♂ 0.13 ± 0.04 (0.08–0.16) ♀ 0.10 ± 0.04 (0.08–0.15)	♂ 0.40 ± 0.10 (0.34–0.51) ♀ 0.43 ± 0.22 (0.22–0.65)
Band heterophils	%			[27] 0.5 ± 0.6 (0–2)					
Heterophils	%		16.92	17.3 ± 6.2 (7–32) [27]	♂ 22.8 ± 1.06 ♀ 19.4 ± 0.60	♂ 32.55 ± 0.61 ♀ 26.32 ± 0.46	C: 28.75 ± 0.70 P: 26.88 ± 0.60	♂ 14.33 ± 2.08 (12–18) ♀ 15.66 ± 2.08 (14–16)	♂ 23.0 ± 1.0 (22–24) 21.33 ± ♀ 2.51 (19–24)
H : L	Ratio						*C: 0.43 ± 0.30 P: 0.39 ± 0.2*		
Eosinophils	%		3.90	[27] 2.8 ± 1.6 (0–6)	♂ 3.15 ± 0.75 ♀ 1.80 ± 0.52	♂ 5.67 ± 0.24 ♀ 8.69 ± 0.26	C: 0.75 ± 0.20 P: 0.75 ± 0.30	♂ 1.66 ± 0.57 (1–2) ♀ 1.0 ± 0 (1)	♂ 1.33 ± 0.57 (1–2) ♀ 2.0 ± 0 (2)
Basophils	%		2.23	[27] 2.3 ± 2.1 (0–8)	♂ 1.0 ± 0.00 ♀ 0.85 ± 0.37	♂ 2.05 ± 0.18 ♀ 3.19 ± 0.23	C: 1.50 ± 0.30 P: 2.38 ± 0.30	♂ 1.33 ± 0.57 (1–2) ♀ 1.66 ± 0.57 (1–2)	♂ 1.66 ± 0.57 (1–2) ♀ 1.66 ± 0.57 (1–2)
Lymphocytes	%		73.13	[27] 70.1 ± 7.2 (57–82)	♂ 62.0 ± 2.85 ♀ 70.6 ± 0.88	♂ 48.87 ± 0.81 ♀ 49.98 ± 0.72	C: 67.13 ± 0.50 P: 69.73 ± 0.60	♂ 81.0 ± 2.0 (79–83) ♀ 80.33 ± 2.51 (78–83)	♂ 72.0 ± 1.0 (71–73) ♀ 73.0 ± 3.0 (70–76)
Monocytes	%		3.68	7.1 ± 2.8 (3–13)	♂ 1.65 ± 0.49 ♀ 2.75 ± 0.79	♂ 10.90 ± 0.35 ♀ 10.85 ± 0.36	C: 2.75 ± 0.40 P: 2.13 ± 0.10	♂ 1.66 ± 0.57 (1–2) ♀ 1.33 ± 0.57 (1–2)	♂ 2.33 ± 0.57 (2–3) ♀ 2.0 ± 1.0 (1–3)
Erythrocyte length	μm					♂ 13.86 ± 0.11 ♀ 12.78 ± 0.09			
Erythrocyte width	μm					♂ 8.37 ± 0.09 ♀ 7.86 ± 0.07			

Table 26.4 Hematologic reference data for select Galliforme species.

Analyte (abbreviation)	Units, SI (US)	Blue peafowl, Indian peafowl *Pavo cristatus* [45, 46]	Guinea fowl *Numida meleagris* [47]	Ring-necked pheasant *Phasianus colchicus* [48–50]
Sample size, attributes		**6♀ 6♂ 1 yr [46]** **41♂ 28♀ 1–3 yr [45]**	**49♂ 40♀ Adult**	**8, 102 d [49]** **15♂, 15♀, 1 yr [50]** **23, 4–12 wk [48]**
Data format		**Mean ± SD [46]** **Mean ± SD (range) [45]**	**Mean ± SE**	**Mean ± SD [49, 50]** **Mean ± SE (range) [48]**
Total leukocyte (WBC)	$\times10^9$/l (=$\times10^3$/μl)	9.52 ± 3.54 [3.80–18.90] [45]	♂ 22.2 ± 17.10 ♀ 21.42 ± 18.37	18.125 ± 3.870 [49] ♂ 28.529 ± 3.378 ♀ 27.824 ± 3.096 [50] 41.6 ± 2.6 (21–63.5) [48]
Heterophil	$\times10^9$/l (=$\times10^3$/μl)	4.52 ± 2.29 [1.01–13.20] [45]	♂ 3.70 ± 0.58 ♀ 3.34 ± 0.49	5.56 ± 2.317 [49] ♂ 11.726 ± 7.621 ♀ 13.372 ± 6.023 [50] [48] 6.24 ± 0.62 (4.16–8.74)
Lymphocyte	$\times10^9$/l (=$\times10^3$/μl)	4.68 ± 1.94 [1.27–10.20] [45]	♂ 17.85 ± 0.90 ♀ 17.16 ± 1.11	[49] 10.225 ± 3.157 [49] [50] ♂ 11.917 ± 1.754 ♀ 7.875 ± 1.190 [48] 27.87 ± 0.79 (25.0–31.2)
H : L ratio				♂ 1.14 ± 0.75 ♀ 2.12 ± 1.07 [50]
Monocyte	$\times10^9$/l (=$\times10^3$/μl)	[46] 0.08 ± 0.13 [0–0.50] [45]	♂ 0.224 ± 0.036 ♀ 0.150 ± 0.036	0.651 ± 0.551 [49] ♂ 2.048 ± 0.595 ♀ 1.271 ± 0.230 [50]
Eosinophil	$\times10^9$/l (=$\times10^3$/μl)	[46] 0.16 ± 0.16 [0–0.74] [45]	♂ 0.493 ± 0.047 ♀ 0.493 ± 0.056	[49] 0.555 ± 0.996 [50] ♂ 1.173 ± 0.326 ♀ 1.285 ± 0.183
Basophil	$\times10^9$/l (=$\times10^3$/μl)	[46] 0.07 ± 0.09 [0–0.40] [45]	♂ 0.246 ± 0.019 ♀ 0.193 ± 0.017	1.075 ± 0.740 [49] [50] ♂ 2.472 ± 0.583 ♀ 5.258 ± 1.079 [50] [48] 5.37 ± 1.5 (0.83–10.82)
Hematocrit	l/l (%)	♂ 0.251 ± 0.016 [25.1 ± 1.6] [46] ♀ 0.269 ± 0.057 [26.9 ± 5.7] [46] 0.381 ± 0.030 (0.320–0.460) [45] [38.1 ± 3.0 {32.0–46.0)] [45]	♂ 0.408 ± 0.006 [40.8 ± 0.66] ♀ 0.381 ± 0.005 [38.1 ± 0.48]	[49] 0.332 ± 0.025 [33.2 ± 2.5] [50] ♂ 0.435 ± 0.013 [43.5 ± 1.3] ♀ 0.387 ± 0.010 [38.7–1.0] 0.34 ± 0.004 (0.32–0.40) [34.0 ± 0.4(32.0–4.0)] [48]
Hemoglobin	mmol/l (g/dl)	♂ 7.39 ± 0.60 [11.90 ± 0.96] [46] ♀ 7.22 ± 0.37 [11.63 ± 0.60] [46] 8.61 ± 0.78 (7.20–11.11) [45] [13.87 ± 1.26 (11.60–17.90)] [45]	♂ 8.81 ± 0.34 [14.2 ± 0.54] ♀ 7.70 ± 0.18 [12.4 ± 0.29]	[49] 9.58 ± 0.79 [15.43 ± 1.27] [50] ♂ 9.90 ± 0.67 [15.96 ± 1.08] ♀ 10.39 ± 0.66 [16.74 ± 1.07] [48] 10.2 ± 0.2 (8.9–11.7) [16.4 ± 0.3 (14.4–18.9)]
Red blood cell (RBC)	$\times10^{12}$/l (=$\times10^6$/μl)	♂ 1.397 ± 0.085 [46] ♀ 1.593 ± 0.049 [46] [46] 2.25 ± 0.28 [1.79–3.51] [45]	♂ 2.65 ± 0.09 ♀ 2.44 ± 0.10	2.530 ± 0.336 [49] ♂ 2.72 ± 0.129 ♀ 2.37 ± 0.122 [50] 3.10 ± 0.07 (2.57–3.87) [48]
Mean corpuscular hemoglobin concentration (MCHC)	g/l (g/dl)	♂ 473.7 ± 17.9[47.37 ± 01.79] ♀ 433.3 ± 29.7[43.33 ± 2.97] [46] 363.2 ± 10.5 (341–389) [36.32 ± 1.05 (34.10–38.90)] [45]	♂ 343 ± 8.1 [34.3 ± 0.81] ♀ 324 ± 6.7 [32.4 ± 0.67]	[48] 474 ± 50 (430–500) [47.4 ± 0.5 (43–50)]
MCV	fl	♂179.70 ± 2.89 ♀168.70 ± 2.29[46] 170.46 ± 13.58 [131.0–196.8] [45]	♂ 155.4 ± 4.24 ♀ 161.8 ± 5.42	[48] 112.0 ± 2.0 (94–131)
Thrombocytes	$\times10^9$/l (=$\times10^3$/μl)	♂ 28.33 ± 1.53 30.00 ± 1.00 [46] 31.60 ± 10.73 [15.4–69.20] [45]		

less than six months of age [55, 56] (Table 26.5). As chicks progress from hatch through 35 weeks of age, red blood cell count (RBC), hemoglobin concentration (Hb) and PCV increase, while MCV and MCHC do not [42, 57, 58]. Male chickens tend to have higher mean values for PCV, Hb, RBC, and RBC length and width [15, 39, 40, 42, 59]. Males overtook females in RBC, HCT, and Hb at 7, 12, and 16 weeks of age, respectively [42]. Egg-producing chickens have higher RBC counts at the time of peak production [60]. Hematocrit may vary by breed/strain of chicken. In Egyptian chickens, the naked-necked variety had a higher hematocrit than heterozygous or normally feathered chickens [61]. However, no hematologic parameter differences were found among four different broiler strains [57]. In chickens, PCV positively correlates with colloid osmotic pressure (COP) [62].

Dietary supplementation of and drug administration to Galliformes may change RBC parameters. Dietary supplementation of broiler chickens living at high altitude with vitamin E and selenium increased RBC, PCV, and Hb [63]. Dietary copper supplementation up to 150 mg/kg can increase RBC, hemoglobin, and PCV [64]. Cobalt supplementation increases Hb, RBC, and PCV of chickens via increased erythropoietin. However, chickens consuming excessive cobalt are vulnerable to reduced growth and polycythemia, which increases blood viscosity and causes cardiac hypertrophy. Cobalt toxicity, exacerbated by low iron and complicated by high altitude, is also linked in chickens to pulmonary hypertension, which may result in increased RBC, Hb, PCV, and MCV in the ascitic chicken [65]. Hens with dietary supplementation of sesame seeds had increases in RBC, Hb, PCV, MCHC, and decreased MCV [43]. Alternatively, high-cholesterol diets depress erythrocyte parameters of chickens [66]. The anticoccidial drug artemisinin has a dose-dependent suppressive effect on RBC and hematocrit [67].

The effect of disease upon RBC parameters of chickens has been relatively well studied. Polycythemia is rare in chickens and is usually based on hemoconcentration (dehydration) or hypoxia secondary to respiratory disease or rearing at high altitude. Egg-producing chickens have higher RBC counts at time of peak production [60]. Erythroleukemias of Galliformes are rarely reported [29]. As in other species, pathologic anemia is categorized as regenerative (hemorrhage, hemolysis) or non-regenerative. Regenerative anemia is marked by anisocytosis and at least 2+ polychromasia [54]. Microcytic, hypochromic anemia should raise concern for chronic blood loss from parasites or iron-deficient diets. Macrocytic hypochromic anemia indicates regeneration, such as response to hemolysis from zinc or lead toxicities, *Plasmodium* infection, or dietary rapeseed meal [54, 68]. Non-regenerative anemia is typically normocytic and normochromic and may be caused by chronic (inflammatory) disease; toxins (chemotherapeutics, aflatoxin, ochratoxin, chronic lead exposure);

Table 26.5 Effect of age on PCV (%) of juvenile chickens [42, 55–57].

Breed	Leghorn [55]	Broiler [56]	Ross [57]	Astra [42]	Astra [42]
Sample size age	100	100	20	10 ♂	10 ♀
1 d			28.28 ± 0.7	25.6 ± 0.51 [25–27]	26.3 ± 0.57 [25–28]
3 d	29 [23–36]	33.8 [26–42]			
7 d	30 [25–37]	36.0 [29–43]	29 ± 0.84	25.9 ± 0.8 [25–27]	28.0 ± 0.9 [26–29]
14 d	31 [26–38]	37.4 [33–41]	29 ± 0.84	29.1 + 2.0 [27–31]	29.6 ± 1.3 [28–31]
21 d	32 [28–37]	36.2 [32–40]	29.57 ± 0.1	27.8 ± 1.1 [27–30]	29.8 ± 1.0 [28–31]
28 d	36 [31–41]	37.4 [33–42]	30.14 ± 0.46	27.3 ± 1.0 [26–28]	28.0 ± 1.7 [26–30]
35 d	34 [30–40]	37.2 [33–42]	31 ± 0.82	28.1 ± 1.8 [26–30]	28.8 ± 0.9 [28–30]
42 d		36.2 [31–41]	31.71 ± 1.32	27.6 ± 1.6 [29–30]	28.1 ± 1.1 [28–30]
49 d		33.6 [28–40]	32.43 ± 1.06	28.0 ± 0.8 [27–29]	28.1 ± 1.9 [25–30]
56 d			35.43 ± 0.84	27.5 ± 1.3 [27–29]	28.3 ± 1.9 [25–31.1]
9 wk				28.1 ± 1.3 [26–30]	28.1 ± 0.4 [27–29]
10 wk				29.0 ± 1.5 [27–30]	28.1 ± 1.3 [26–30]
12 wk				32.3 ± 1.9 [29–34]	29.5 ± 1.2 [28–31]
14 wk				31.6 + 1.9 [29–34]	29.6 ± 1.7 [27–31]
16 wk				38.5 ± 1.7 [38–40]	29.8 ± 1.2 [28–31]
18 wk				42.3 ± 1.5 [41–44]	29.8 ± 1.2 [27–31]

Data given as Mean ± SE [Range].

diets that are too high in protein or calcium [29]; nutritional deficiencies (protein, iron, folate, vitamin A); neoplasia; hypothyroidism; or, nephropathy causing lack of erythropoietin [54].

In the chicken, heat stress decreases PCV and hemoglobin, based on physiologic hemodilution to protect and maintain intravascular volume during extracellular water loss [13]. Chickens with stunting syndrome have decreased RBC, Hb, and PCV values, attributed to malabsorption of nutrients. In chickens with induced aflatoxicosis, increased RBC and hematocrit occurred in hens, and a decreased RBC was observed in broiler chicks [69]. Hens with lymphoid leukemia (avian leukosis) exhibited increased RBC, Hb, PCV, and MCHC but a decrease in MCV [43]. Ancillary clinicopathologic testing in the workup of anemia may include the slide agglutination test; blood culture, serology, or polymerase chain reaction (PCR) for infectious agents; toxin screens; or, aspiration or biopsy of liver, spleen, and bone marrow.

Hemoparasites

Free-living and captive Galliformes may suffer a variety of hemoparasitic infections including *Plasmodium* spp., *Leucocytozoon* spp., *Hemoproteus* spp., *Trypanosoma* spp., and microfilaria [70–72]. Clinical disease and mortality appear more common in captive, domesticated, or semi-domesticated species. Disease in domestic fowl may be severe, as indicated by anemia, lethargy, and other attendant nonspecific clinical signs. Infection is seldom clinical in free-living Galliformes [73]. Although a rare finding in avian species, trypanosomiasis was historically considered more common in Galliformes from Europe [74]. Chickens experimentally infected with *Plasmodium juxtanucleare* had increased total leukocytes and basophils and decreased thrombocytes, but lacked changes in erythrocyte parameters. Both erythrocytes and thrombocytes were infected [75]. Diagnosis of hemoparasitic infection may be made by microscopic observation of the blood smear with visual parasite identification. Low levels of infection may also be diagnosed via PCR.

Thrombocyte Morphology and Abnormalities

Thrombocytes are similar size to lymphocytes or smaller, with a more condensed, dark chromatin, a more irregularly shaped nucleus, and clear to pale blue/purple cytoplasm (Figures 26.1–26.3). Thrombocytes may easily be confused with lymphocytes, but the latter tend to be slightly larger and rounder, have a higher N:C ratio, slightly lighter chromatin and darker cytoplasm, and do not cluster [29]. Thrombocytes may have small numbers of small pink cytoplasmic granules and small clear vacuoles, and they will frequently form large clumps at the feathered edge and small clumps within the monolayer of the blood smear [29]. Because of their tendency to cluster, thrombocytes are difficult to enumerate by manual or automated methods, and the clinician must often settle for thrombocyte estimation. Estimates are based on manual peripheral blood smear evaluation, with 1–2 per 1000× oil immersion field being considered acceptable. Total thrombocyte counts can be made with a Neubauer chamber, or can be estimated by averaging the number of thrombocytes counted in five different 1000× oil immersion fields within the monolayer [76]. Multiplying this number by 3500 results in the estimated thrombocyte count per microliter [77].

Thrombocytopenia of the chicken may be caused by viral infection, bacterial sepsis, disseminated intravascular coagulation (DIC), or neoplasia [29, 35]. In chickens, Newcastle disease virus and infectious chicken anemia virus cause damage to thrombopoietic precursors in bone marrow, leading to thrombocytopenia. In experimental Newcastle infection, thrombocytopenia of 50% of prior values occurred three days post infection. Avian influenza causes thrombocytopenia via consumption and DIC [77]. Chicken anemia virus targets hematopoietic precursors and lymphocytes in the thymus and results in aplastic anemia, thrombocytopenia, hemorrhage, leukopenia, immunosuppression, and thymus depletion in chicks one to two weeks of age [78]. Thrombocytopenia may occur in cases of Galliforme leukemia [54, 68].

Hemostasis

Chickens have an intact tissue factor (extrinsic) pathway, using tissue factor (FIII), FVII, FX, FV, calcium, and phospholipid surfaces in activating prothrombin (FII) to thrombin [79]. The extrinsic system is more active than the intrinsic in chickens (Table 26.6). Antithrombin III of the chicken is synthesized in hepatocytes, binds heparin, and inhibits thrombin and factor Xa [80]. Methodologies for determination of hemostasis analytes are many, and the results are not interchangeable [80, 82, 83, 90, 91]. Considerable sequence differences between avian and mammalian clotting factors dictate that chicken reagents (avian brain thromboplastin) are best used to assay clotting times. Lipemia may interfere with some prothrombin time (PT) assays [82]. The clinician should ensure that either a specific, same-methodology reference range is consulted, or that normal animal samples are sent for simultaneous assessment with the patient sample [76]. Citrated plasma is the preferred sample for hemostasis testing; for some assays, sodium EDTA has also been used [52, 92]. Freezing plasma at −20 °C may affect PT; therefore, freezing at a minimum of −70 °C or storage at 4 °C for up to 4 h prior to testing is recommended if storage prior to assay is required [52, 79, 81–83, 92].

Table 26.6 Coagulation parameters of poultry [52, 80–84].

Analyte	Units	Domestic chicken (*Gallus gallus domesticus*)	Leghorns			Domestic turkey (*Meleagridis gallapavo*)		Japanese quail *Coturnix japonica*[f] [84]
Subject attributes		Cockerels, capons, pullets	2 wk ♂♀	Adult	White broiler hens, cockerels ♀♂, 6–34 wk	White 2–24 mo	White, 1–24 mo	Adult, 22 wk
Anticoagulant Sample		Plasma		NaEDTA or Na-citrate Frozen plasma	Na-citrate Frozen plasma	Na-citrate Refrigerated plasma		Na-citrate Frozen plasma
Data format		Mean [range][a] [81]	[Range][b] [52]	Mean±SD[c] [80]	[Range][d] [82]	Mean± SE (95% CI)[e] [83]		Median (5th–95th percentile)
Sample size		77 (WBT) 57 (PT)	21	6	36	60	50	21
Whole blood clotting time	seconds	Cockerels: 306 [75–1021] Pullets: 552 [<60–2340] Capons: 270 [<60–450]						
Prothrombin time (PT) CBT	s	13.2 [9.0–16.5]	[16.8–25.4]		[20.0–30.0]	13.02 ± 0.170 (10.39–15.64)	12.40 ± 0.111 (11.03–13.77)	12.7 (10.85–15.39)
(PT) RVV						16.64 ± 0.295 (12.08–21.21)	12.56 ± 0.272 (9.04–16.07)	
Antithrombin III	mg/l (mg/dl)			143 ± 24 (14.3 ± 2.4)				
Bleeding time	min		Comb: 4.47 ± 0.422 Wattle: 2.5 ± 0.151 [85]					

[a] Biggs and Macfarlane technique (1962) for PT; chicken brain thromboplastin (CBT) [86].
[b] Thrombotimer 1 assay for PT (Teknimex, Mexico City) [52].
[c] ATIII measured by amidolytic assay, human alpha-thrombin and chromogenic substrate S-2238 [80].
[d] Stored at −20 °C; PT on Fibrometer (Becton Dickson Company, Cockeysville, MD); Coag-a-mate XM (Organon Teknika, Durham, NC) inconsistent results with lipemia [87].
[e] Stored 4 °C up to 4 h; plasma added to calcium chloride, chicken brain thromboplastin preserved in phenol saline. PT measured manually (Quick, 1945) [88].
[f] Chicken brain thromboplastin (CBT) method thawed frozen plasma at −80 °C); PT via Start 4® Hemostasis Analyzer (Diagnostica Stago Inc.) [89].

General differentials for coagulopathies in Galliformes include liver insufficiency, septicemia/DIC, vitamin K deficiency, rodenticide toxicity, and feed contaminants such as aflatoxin and ochratoxin A [29, 93]. Prothrombin times (PT) were prolonged, but thrombocyte counts were not affected in chickens experimentally infected with infectious bursal disease virus [52]. Dietary lipid affects PT, fibrinogen concentration, and thrombocyte aggregation via platelet PGE_2 in chickens [76]. Dietary intake of peach palm oil results in a more favorable LDL:HDL and haemostatic pattern in broiler chickens compared to palm oil, corn oil or beef tallow. In hens and broiler chicks exposed to aflatoxin, an increased PT was the most sensitive measured clinicopathologic indicator of toxicosis [69]. Other mycotoxins (ochratoxin and T-2 toxin) have similarly been shown to increase PT in chickens [93].

Blood Types

Chickens have multiple blood group systems that are autosomal and co-dominant, with multiple alleles in each group and at least 28 different blood group antigens [44, 53, 94]. However, chickens lack preformed alloantibodies; therefore, first-time transfusion can be accomplished using a donor of a different species, although same-species donation or use of a hemoglobin containing colloid (Oxyglobin, BioPure, Cambridge, Massachusetts) is preferable in order to minimize hemolysis [54]. Ideally, cross-matching is performed before each transfusion. A procedure for avian cross-matching has been described [53]. Blood transfusion may be indicated in severely or acutely anemic patients for whom the potential benefit outweighs the stress of the procedure and the risk of adverse reactions. Transfusion technique using fresh donor avian blood (blood storage is not described) or oxyglobin is similar as for mammals [53]. Independently segregating blood group factors A, B, and C have been described for ring-necked pheasants (*Phasianus colchicus*) [95].

Leukogram

Romanowsky-type stains (Wright-Giemsa, DiffQuik®) are appropriate for routine blood smear evaluation of the chicken. A staining technique for better differentiation of heterophil and eosinophil granules has been described but is not widely used [96]. Counting of white cells may be performed with a hemocytometer using eosinophil or Natt and Herrick's stains and methodologies. Several automated flow cytometry-based techniques have been published for the determination of the white blood cell count (WBC), RBC, and differentials but are not routinely available to the veterinary practitioner [97]. However, given the inability to differentiate white blood cells, expense, sample preparation requirements, and poor correlations with traditional cell counting techniques, manual white blood cell counting remains the preferred method for clinical practice [11, 15, 27–29, 98–101]. WBC estimates may be made from a well-made, fresh peripheral blood smear with an even distribution of leukocytes [28]. One averages the number of leukocytes in ten different 400 magnification fields and multiplies this number by 1500–2000. Although this method is the least reliable WBC counting technique, it should be considered along with observation of the blood smear in general, as an adjunct diagnostic while awaiting laboratory results.

Leukocytes counts of chickens have a diurnal rhythm that is age dependent [102]. Chickens have multiphasic leukocyte development from hatch to 16 weeks, with an initial increase and then a leveling off of WBC around eight weeks, concomitant with an initial decrease and subsequent rise of the heterophil to lymphocyte (H:L) ratio to a final range of approximately 0.2–0.3 [42]. Sex and strain do not appear to clinically influence this initial WBC development, but differences may be seen as early as 12 weeks [57, 58]. Female Galliformes tend toward higher total leukocyte counts than males [39, 40].

Leukocytosis (increased WBC) is common in chickens and may signal inflammation of several etiologies. Total WBC of chicks affected by vitamin E/selenium deficiency increased more than twofold, reflective of inflammation associated with myocyte necrosis [103]. Chickens with dietary supplementation of sesame seed or olive oil had an increased WBC count [43, 66]. Leukopenia (decreased WBC) may be artifactual based on lysis of leukocytes from heavy-handed smearing of fragile leukocytes from aged/standing or leukemic blood samples [68]. Thus, blood smears are best made immediately and examined in-house from blood that has not been exposed to anticoagulants, prior to sending samples to a laboratory. Severe inflammation can cause peripheral leukocyte depletion, and careful examination of heterophils for left shifts and toxic changes (see morphology, below), should be pursued as supporting evidence. Experimental ochratoxicosis produced leukopenia at higher doses [104].

Heterophil to Lymphocyte Ratio

The heterophil to lymphocyte ratio (H:L) has been used to assess stress response, immunocompetency, and inflammation in chickens [78, 105]. A biphasic H:L response may occur in chickens, whereby after an initial increase based on mild to moderate stress, the H:L ratio may depress in extreme stress based on the development of heteropenia. In experimentally induced acute inflammation, the resultant H:L increase lasted approximately 7 days and then returned to baseline by 14 days [27, 106]. Both cortisol and lipopolysaccharide (LPS) can increase the H:L ratio (normally 1:4) and stimulate release of heterophilic precursors from bone marrow [107].Therefore, the use of the H:L ratio as a sole indicator of the stress response is not recommended [105]. An automated heterophil count is more sensitive than the H:L ratio or manual methods of WBC differential determination to detect experimental corticosteroid-induced stress response [108]. Heat stress and crowding increases the H:L ratio of domestic chickens [13, 109]. Vitamin-E-enhanced diets increase the H:L ratio, likely based on increased cellular phagocytic function and decreased cutaneous basophil hypersensitivity response [110]. An increased H:L ratio was observed in white Leghorn hens selected for low productivity, poor survivability, cannibalism, and aggression. Based on immune status and social behavior, low survivability groups had less stress resistance as evidence by the higher H:L ratio. Thus, in chickens, selection for desired phenotypic traits may alter hematologic and immunologic characteristics [111]. The H:L increased to 0.81 in 6-8 week old broiler chicks subjected to overcrowding in both summer and rainy seasons [112].

Lymphocytes

Most chickens are lymphocyte dominant, with the exception of the California gray chicken [27]. Lymphocytes are similar to mammalian in appearance and are smaller than granulocytes and monocytes (Figures 26.1 and 26.4). They are round with high nuclear:cytoplasmic (N:C) ratios and small amounts of medium blue cytoplasm that may contain small numbers of focal pink/purple granules. Nuclei are round with clumped to condensed chromatin. These cells are slightly larger, have darker cytoplasm, and less condensed chromatin than thrombocytes. Reactive lymphocytes are slightly larger with increased amounts of dark blue cytoplasm and may have a pale Golgi zone. These may occur secondary to increased antigenic stimulation such as viral disease [54]. An automated flow cytometric technique using monoclonal antibodies can differentiate chicken lymphocytes from thrombocytes [113].

Lymphocytosis in Galliformes may be caused by lymphoproliferative disease, increased antigenic/inflammatory stimulation (including vaccination), or epinephrine release (physiologic lymphocytosis) [29]. Chickens fed high oleic-acid-rich oil diets for six weeks had an increased lymphocyte percentage attributed to the immunostimulatory properties of olive oil [66]. Hens with lymphoid leukemia (avian leukosis) had an increased WBC (55 000/μl vs. 23 000/μl in controls), increased lymphocyte percentage (80% vs. 60%), and lower percentages of other leukocytes. RBC, Hb, PCV, MCHC were increased, but MCV was decreased. Toxic heterophils were present (2+), and bone marrow was hypercellular [43]. Normocytic, normochromic anemia, and thrombocytopenia may occur in cases of leukemia [54, 68]. Marek's disease, an alphaherpes virus, causes lymphoproliferation in multiple tissues [114]. Retroviruses in chickens can cause leukemia [29]. Bone marrow aspirate cytology and/or core biopsy is recommended in cases of suspected lymphoproliferative disease, when CBC results are supportive but inconclusive. Experimental infection with Newcastle's disease causes lymphocytosis [77].

Lymphopenia may be caused by stress (glucocorticoids), viral infection, or bone marrow synthetic failure/pancytopenia [35]. Heat stress decreases the lymphocyte count [13]. Experimentally administered lipopolysaccharide (LPS) causes lymphocyte apoptosis and necrosis [107]. Experimental ochratoxicosis and infection with avian reovirus and *Mycoplasma* spp. have also caused lymphopenia [104, 106, 115]. Selection for phenotypic traits may unwittingly alter lymphocyte counts. In white Leghorn hens selected for poor production, low survivability, cannibalism, and aggression, fewer lymphocytes and lower CD4:CD8 ratios were observed [111]. Vitamin E/selenium deficiency decreases lymphocyte counts [103].

Heterophils

Heterophils are round with pale cytoplasm that is filled with numerous, small, rod-shaped, pink to orange granules that may obscure nuclear detail. Nuclei are bilobed to trilobed with patchy, clumped chromatin (Figures 26.3–26.5). Identifying left shifts in avian heterophils is challenging based on intense heterophil granulation. Normal chicken heterophil nuclei also have fewer nuclear lobules than mammalian neutrophils. A heterophil mean nuclear score is a more objective quantification of heterophil nuclear lobulation to identify band heterophils and more immature, non-segmented forms (heterophilic myelocytes and metamyelocytes). Unstained blood smears are fixed in methanol for 5–10 min and then stained with Gill's #2 hematoxylin, which will stain only the nuclei, not cytoplasmic granules. One-hundred consecutive heterophil nuclei are graded quantitatively based on total absence of lobulation, slight indentation, and number of lobes [27]. As in other species, left-shifted

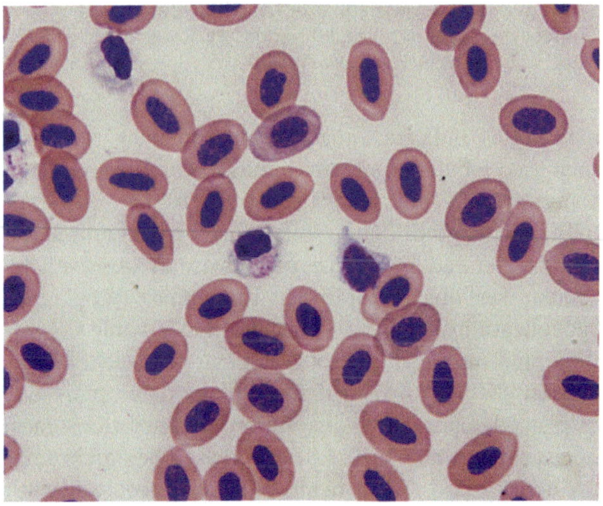

Figure 26.1 Thrombocyte (left) and lymphocyte (right) from the blood smear of a chicken (*Gallus gallus*). Note the small fuchia granules and increased density of nucleus within in the thrombocyte.

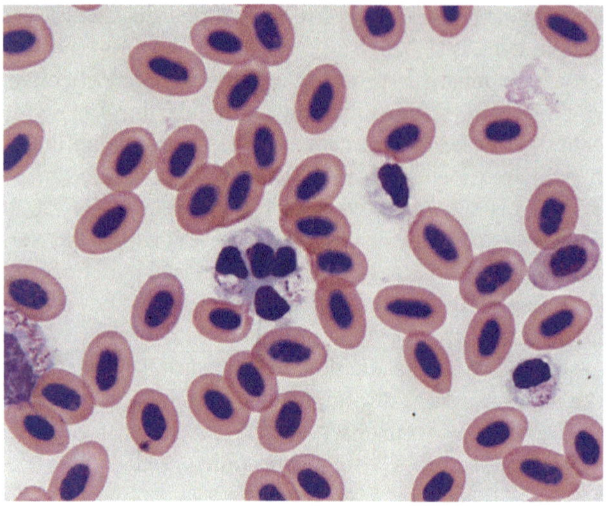

Figure 26.2 Thrombocyte clump and free thrombocytes from the blood smear of a chicken (*Gallus gallus*).

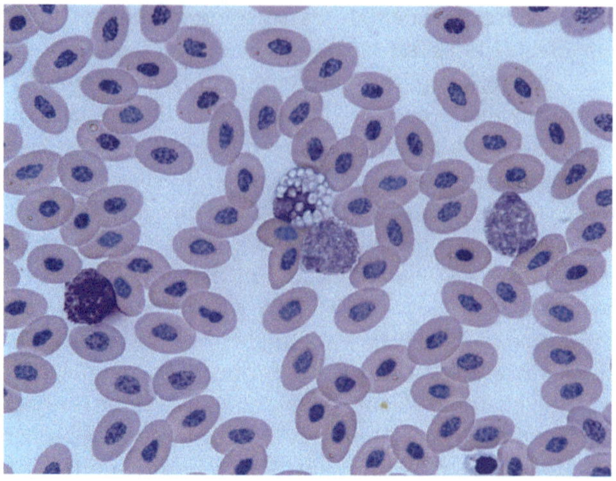

Figure 26.3 Cells from the blood smear of a turkey (*Gallus gallus*). From left to right: basophils, eosinophil (upper larger granules), heterophil, thrombocyte (lower right), and another heterophil (upper right).

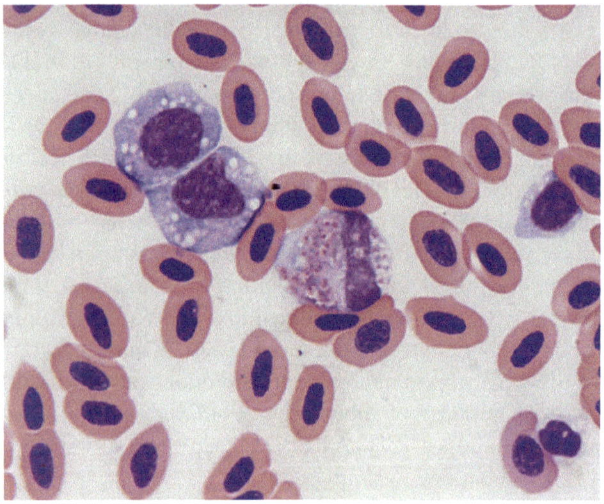

Figure 26.4 Monocytes (left), toxic band heterophil (center), lymphocyte (upper right), and thrombocyte (lower left) from the blood smear of a chicken (*Gallus gallus*).

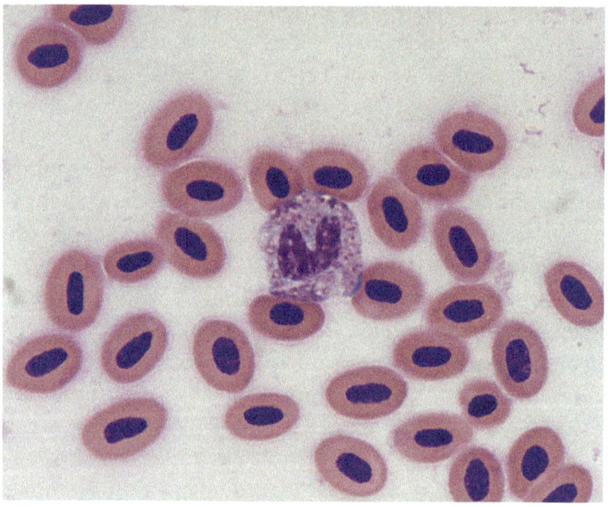

Figure 26.5 Toxic band heterophil from the blood smear of a chicken (*Gallus gallus*).

heterophils indicate an acute inflammatory response. Increased lobulation of heterophils in chickens has been experimentally induced by heat stress [105].

Toxic change of heterophils caused by inflammation and accelerated bone marrow release is observed by cellular swelling, cytoplasmic basophilia, cytoplasmic vacuolization/degranulation, abnormal granule coloration (blue-purple), fusion of granules, and nuclear degeneration [35, 54]. Ultrastructurally, toxic heterophils may display edema, granule dissolution, retained ribosomes, nuclear membrane blebs, and decreased heterochromatin density [27]. Toxic heterophils are associated with acute inflammation and severe diseases such as sepsis, viremia, mycosis, and necrosis, and are associated with poor prognosis [54, 88]. Hens with lymphoid leukemia (avian leukosis) had toxic heterophils (2+) [43].

As previously noted, heterophilia may be based on stress response (epinephrine or cortisol mediated) or other causes of an inflammatory leukogram such as infectious, toxic, neoplastic, or traumatic etiologies. In experimentally induced acute inflammation in chickens, heterophilia peaked within one day, left-shift peaked at 12–24h and lasted three days, and toxic change also occurred. Heterophil hypersegmentation (right shift) then occurred from day four to day seven. All values returned to baseline by 14 days [27, 106]. Administration of hydrocortisone and adrenocorticotropic hormone (ACTH) produced heterophilia in chickens, along with other changes expected in a stress leukogram. Chickens often have cortisol-mediated stress leukograms secondary to capture, handling, caging, housing conditions (crowding stress or heat stress), and social interactions [13, 106, 109]. Heterophilia was observed in white Leghorn hens selected for low productivity, poor survivability, cannibalism, and aggression [111]. Male Galliformes often have higher heterophil percentages than females [39, 40]. Viral and bacterial infections (Avian influenza, Avian reovirus, *Mycoplasma* spp.) may also cause heterophilia [77, 106, 115]. Non-infectious diseases such as stunting syndrome and vitamin E and selenium deficiency have also been associated with increased heterophil counts [103, 116].

Heteropenia may result from sepsis/endotoxemia, viral infections, myelophthisis, or bone marrow toxicity/suppression based on pharmaceuticals [29, 35]. Heteropenia of chickens appears less commonly reported than in other avian species and may be a poor prognostic sign. Experimental Newcastle disease infection of chickens caused transient heteropenia followed by heterophilia [77].

Monocytes

Monocytes are round with moderate amounts of medium blue to blue-gray cytoplasm that may contain small, discrete, clear vacuoles or small pink granules (Figures 26.4, 26.6). Nuclei may be round, oval, or amoeboid/polymorphic. When nuclei are round to slightly ovoid, distinguishing monocytes from lymphocytes may be challenging. Monocytes are generally larger with slightly more ovoid nuclei and less condensed chromatin [54]. Higher relative counts of monocytes in healthy female chickens, compared to males may be observed [39, 40].

Monocytosis may be caused by acute inflammation and by chronic diseases in the chicken, including bacterial infections (e.g., Mycobacteriosis, chlamydiosis), mycoses,

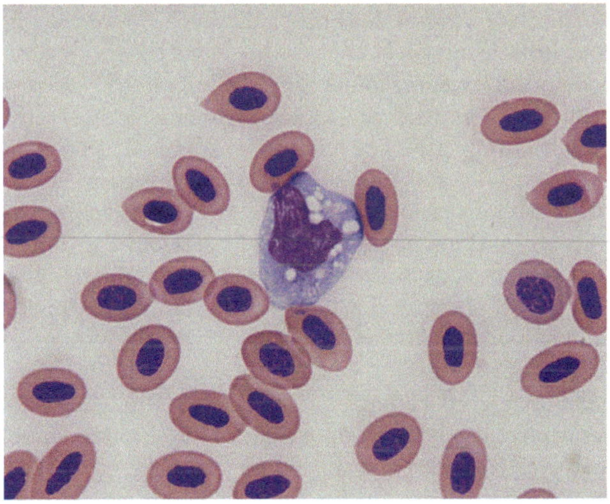

Figure 26.6 Monocyte from the blood smear of a chicken (*Gallus gallus*).

zinc deficiency, foreign bodies, or tissue necrosis [17, 29, 35, 106]. The link between zinc deficiency and monocytosis may be due to reduced alimentary epithelial integrity [17]. On the basis of experimental studies, monocytes are the fourth most sensitive cell indicator of the ACTH and cortisol-mediated stress response, behind heterophils, eosinophils, and lymphocytes [117]. Monocytosis may occur quite early in the inflammatory process of chickens. In experimentally induced acute inflammation of the chicken, monocytosis peaked at two days and continued for only four days [27, 106]. Experimental avian influenza infection in four-week-old Leghorn chickens produced monocytosis within 60 h, while monocytosis occurs 6–10 days post experimental infection with virulent strains of Marek's disease virus [92, 118]. Other diseases in which monocytosis has been documented in chickens include vitamin E/selenium deficiency (twofold increase) and experimental *Mycoplasma* spp. infection [103, 106]. Increases in monocyte count may occur after severe heat stress in chickens [105]. Monocytopenia is difficult to assess based on the relatively low number of monocytes expected in circulation. Monocytopenia occurs in experimentally induced toxicosis of ochratoxin A (high dose) in chickens and paraquat in quail [29, 104]. Experimental Newcastle disease infection of chickens resulted in a 50% reduction of monocytes and a monocytopenia at three days post infection [77].

Eosinophils

Eosinophils are round and are of similar size as heterophils but have a pale blue cytoplasm [119] (Figure 26.3). They typically contain bilobed nuclei. In the domestic fowl, common quail, guinea fowl, and turkey, cytoplasmic granules are spherical and homogenous in color [119]. Eosinophilia seems to result from the accumulation of older cells in circulation rather than from addition of cells recently released from bone marrow [120]. On the basis of multiple experiments in chickens, eosinophils likely do not serve the same role functional role in Galliformes as in mammals [119].

Sex, diurnal rhythm, strain, and age appear to have little effect on eosinophils in the chicken, and glucocorticoid administration does not affect percentages in circulation [108, 120]. However, eosinophilia was one of many changes observed in white Leghorn hens selected for low productivity, poor survivability, cannibalism, and aggression [111]. As a cell with low percentages in the peripheral circulation of normal Galliformes, eosinopenia is rarely diagnosed and likely is of little clinical consequence. Experimental *Mycoplasma* spp. infection in young chickens did produce a relative eosinopenia at one month post infection which resolved by 13 months after infection, and severe heat stress may cause decreased percentages of circulating eosinophils [105, 106, 121].

In young chickens, the most dependable experimental model for induction of eosinophilia is multiple intraperitoneal injections of bovine serum albumin. Parasitism has been variably associated with eosinophilia. Infections with *Trichostrongylus tenuis* cecal threadworm, *Heterakis gallinarum*, and *Austrobilharzia variglandis* have produced eosinophilia in the domestic fowl and in other Galliformes. However, many other experimental infections with parasites in the domestic fowl have failed to produce an eosinophilia. Forced molt, *Pasteurella* vaccination, and aflatoxicosis in chickens, and malathion toxicosis in quail have been associated with eosinophilia [29, 105]. Blood smear evaluation for the presence of hemoparasites is warranted to further investigate potential parasitic causes of eosinophilia in the Galliforme.

Basophils

Basophils of Galliformes are similar to those of other avian species – round and slightly smaller than other granulocytes, with clear to pale purple cytoplasm and numerous small round dark purple cytoplasmic granules (Figure 26.3). Nuclei are round and centrally located with condensed chromatin. The function and diagnostic value of the basophil in domestic fowl remains unclear; however, experimental evidence in the domestic chicken suggests that this cell mediates early inflammation and intermediate hypersensitivity but does not contribute to delayed hypersensitivity. The cell may both degranulate early in the inflammatory process as well as have weak phagocytic capabilities [119].

Basophils may be more common in avian than in mammalian blood and are not uncommon in the domestic fowl, often equaling roughly half the number of eosinophils in circulation [119]. Age, sex, season, overcrowding stress, and species of Galliforme, but not diurnal rhythm, affect basophil numbers [112, 119]. In quail and turkeys, circulating basophils are rarer, with a ratio of one basophil per five eosinophils in circulation reported for the quail [119]. Newly hatched quails and turkeys have more circulating basophils than adults. Adult male quails may have more basophils than females [119]. In adult pheasants, circulating basophil numbers were highest from December through February and lowest from September through November [119]. In general, the association of disease states with basophilia or basopenia remains unclear and poorly studied. In the chicken, experimentally induced acute inflammation caused sporadic basopenia, but experimental administration of glucocorticoids did not affect basophil percentages [27, 106, 108]. Chickens undergoing experimental vitamin E/selenium deficiency and mycoplasmosis had decreased basophil counts [103, 106]. Chickens suffering stunting syndrome had increased basophils [116]. Severe heat stress in chickens resulted in lower basophil numbers and granule depletion of basophils [13, 105].

Biochemical Panel (Tables 26.7 and 26.8)

For Galliformes as in other birds, few biochemical analytes are thoroughly validated or studied [128]. Below we summarize clinically applicable knowledge for biochemical parameters specifically investigated in Galliformes. Generally, lithium heparinized plasma is preferred for biochemistry samples based on changes in serum attributed to clot formation and red cell metabolism, determined from a single study in chickens [34]. For additional details of sample handling related to the biochemical panel, please see sample collection and storage headings.

Liver Enzymes and Biomarkers

Diagnosis of liver disease in the chicken is challenging based on a lack of enzyme specificity or observable icterus. In the Galliforme, yellow plasma should not be misinterpreted as icterus, as birds do not produce bilirubin from biliverdin due to lack of the biliverdin reductase enzyme. Yellow plasma may occur secondarily to carotenoid ingestion. Increased liver enzyme activities are typically associated with cellular damage/necrosis for cytosolic leakage enzymes, or with cholestasis for membrane-associated induction enzymes, but these are not independent or mutually exclusive pathologies. Enzyme activities below reference intervals may be interpreted as normal for that animal, or evidence of reduced hepatic mass or function. Hepatobiliary disease may be present when enzyme activities fall within reference intervals, and conversely, increased liver enzymes (indicating damage/necrosis) are not reflective of overall liver function or prognosis [35, 68]. Here we discuss enzymes and bile acids that have been used to assess liver health in the chicken. Proteins, lipids, and other biochemical parameters that may also be used to assess liver function are discussed under their respective headings.

Aspartate aminotransferase (AST, SGOT) is a cytosolic leakage enzyme that is sensitive but not specific for hepatocellular damage/necrosis. Abundant AST occurs in the chicken heart, liver, skeletal muscle, kidney, and brain [8]. Increased activities are interpreted as liver or muscle origin, and thus should be interpreted with CK [35]. In chickens with inherited muscular dystrophy, stunting syndrome, and vitamin E/selenium deficiency AST increases as evidence of liver and muscle necrosis and fibrosis [8, 103, 116]. Recent intramuscular injections should be taken into consideration when evaluating AST and other muscle-derived enzymes [68]. In laying hens, increased activities of plasma AST in pre-peak vesus peak egg production were attributed to increased feed and increased hepatic workload in pre-peak hens [129]. In chickens fed oregano, sage, rosemary, and pepper extract as an organic growth promoter and antimicrobial agent, AST showed a twofold increase [130].

Table 26.7 Biochemical reference data for the domestic fowl, *Gallus gallus*.

Analyte (abbreviation)	Units, SI (conventional)	Ross [193][194] Ross & Cobb [12]	Nigerian [15] Normal, frizzled, and naked-necked	Brown pullets [122]	White Leghorn [38] Leghorn [123] White Leghorn, White plymouth rock [124]	Bantam [41] C:Cochin P: Polish	Native Kashmir [40]
Sample attributes		♂ 13 mo [16] ♀ 25–36 wk [12]	♂♀ 20 wk	♀ 5–9 wk	♂4–6 mo [38] ♀ 3–27 wk [123] ♀♂6 mo [124]	♂ 40 wk	
Animal number ***Sample number***		5, *30* [16] 165 [12]	30♂, 30♀	80	6–14, *13–40* [38] 20 [123] 30 [124]	8 each breed	♂24, ♀32
Data format		Mean ± SD [range]	Mean ± SD	Mean ± SD	Mean ± SE [range] [38] [range] [123] mean ± SD [124]	Mean ± SE	Mean ± SE
Glucose	mmol/l (mg/dl)	12.1 ± 1.3 [16, 125] (218 ± 23.7) 12.99 0.76 [12] 11.48–16.71 [234 ± 13.7 (207–301)]	♂ 3.99 ± 0.003 [71.87 ± 0.77] ♀ 3.27 ± 0.06 [58.83 ± 1.03]		13.32 ± 0.11 [11.11–14.04) [240 ± 2 (200–253)] [38]		♂ 12.64 ± 0.34 (227.83 ± 6.07) ♀ 12.62 ± 0.27 [227.43 ± 4.93]
Albumin	g/l (g/dl)	15.0 ± 2.0 (1.5 ± 0.2) [16]	♂ 36.27 ± 0.38 (3.63 ± 0.04) ♀ 30.03 ± 0.39 (3.00 ± 0.04)			CB: 23.7 ± 7.0 (2.37 ± 0.70) CB: 24.4 ± 1.0 (2.44 ± 0.10)	♂ 17.8 ± 0.6 (1.78 ± 0.06) ♀ 22.0 ± 0.7 (2.20 ± 0.07 g/dl)
A:G	(Ratio)					CB: 1.39 ± 0.15 PB: 1.19 ± 0.12	
Alanine Aminotransferase (ALT)	(IU/l)	24.6 ± 55.4 [16]			13 ± 7 [124]		
Aspartate Aminotransferase (AST)	(IU/l)	261.2 ± 151.8 [16]			171 ± 59 [124]		
Alkaline Phosphatase (ALP)	(IU/l)	352.8 ± 98.7 [16]			4 m: 420 ± 30 (280–620) [38] 5 m: 130 ± 10 (60–210) [38]		♂ 69.9 ± 4.8 ♀ 78.9 ± 6.0
Bilirubin (Total, TBIL)	µmol/l (mg/dl)	5.13 ± 1.7 [16] (0.3 ± 0.1)					
Calcium (Ca)	mmol/l [mg/dl]	3.8 ± 0.2 [15.2 ± 0.8] [16]		2.1 ± 0.09 [8.4 ± 0.36]	2.55 ± 0.03 (2.28–2.78) [38] [10.2 ± 0.1 (9.1–11.1)] [38] Venous 3.25–4.24 [123] [13.0–16.96] Arterial 2.99–4.15 [123] [11.96 ± 16.60]		♂ 2.70 ± 0.13 [10.79 ± 0.50] ♀ 3.00 ± 0.12 [12.01 ± 0.47]
Cholesterol	mmol/l (mEq/l)	3.76 ± 0.52 (145.0 ± 20.0)] [16]	♂ 4.56 ± 0.04 (176.23 ± 1.71) ♀ 3.74 ± 0.06 (144.23 ± 2.20)			CB: 6.95 ± 0.20 (268.15 ± 7.6) PB: 7.29 ± 0.24 (281.50 ± 9.30)	♂ 3.01 ± 0.13 (116.33 ± 4.90) ♀ 3.65 ± 0.14 (141.02 ± 5.36)
Creatinine	µmol/l (mg/dl)		♂ 136.1 ± 1.8 (1.54 ± 0.02) ♀114.0 ± 1.8 (1.29 ± 0.02)				♂136.1 ± 15.0 (1.54 ± 0.17) ♀143.2 ± 7.07 (1.62 ± 0.08)

(Continued)

Table 26.7 (Continued)

Analyte (abbreviation)	Units, SI (conventional)	Ross [193][194] Ross & Cobb [12]	Nigerian [15] Normal, frizzled, and naked-necked	Brown pullets [122]	White Leghorn [38] Leghorn [123] White Leghorn, White plymouth rock [124]	Bantam [41] C:Cochin P: Polish	Native Kashmir [40]
Sample attributes		♂ 13 mo [16] ♀ 25–36 wk [12]	♂♀ 20 wk	♀ 5–9 wk	♂4–6 mo [38] ♀ 3–27 wk [123] ♀♂6 mo [124]	♂ 40 wk	
Animal number ***Sample number***		5, *30* [16] 165 [12]	30♂, 30♀	80	6–14, *13–40* [38] 20 [123] 30 [124]	8 each breed	♂24, ♀32
Data format		Mean ± SD [range]	Mean ± SD	Mean ± SD	Mean ± SE [range] [38] [range] [123] mean ± SD [124]	Mean ± SE	Mean ± SE
Creatine Phosphokinase (CPK)	(IU/l)	3242.5 ± 1954.8] [16]					
Globulin	g/l (g/dl)	37.0 ± 4.0 (3.7 ± 0.4)] [16]	♂ 24.27 ± 0.30 (2.43 ± 0.03) ♀ 19.97 ± 0.32 (2.00 ± 0.03)			CB: 19.5 ± 1.6 (1.95 ± 0.16) PB: 21.3 ± 1.2 (2.13 ± 0.12)	♂ 21.5 ± 1.7 (2.15 ± 0.17) ♀ 27.9 ± 1.4 (2.79 ± 0.14)
Lactate Dehydrogenase (LDH)	(IU/l)	694.7 ± 511.7 [16]			[18] 447 ± 171		
Magnesium (Mg)	mmol/l (mg/dl)			0.9 ± 0.2 (2.19 ± 0.49)			
Phosphorous (P)	mmol/l [mg/dl]	1.16 ± 0.323 [3.6 ± 1.0] [16]		2.0 ± 0.15 [6.19 ± 0.46]	0.81 ± 0.03 (0.48–1.16) [38] [2.5 ± 0.1 (1.5–3.6)] [38]		♂ 1.35 ± 0.06 [4.19 ± 0.20] ♀ 1.53 ± 0.10 [4.74 ± 0.30]
Potassium (K)	mmol/l (=mEq/l)	4.8 ± 0.9 [16] 4.9 ± 0.4 (4.0–6.0)[12]		4.6 ± 0.2	3.8 ± 0.1 (3.1–4.6) [38]	CB: 4.72 ± 0.07 PB: 4.85 ± 0.04	
Protein (total)	g/l (g/dl)	52.0 ± 6.0 (5.2 ± 0.6) [16]				CB: 43.5 ± 1.0 (4.35 ± 0.10) PB: 45.6 ± 0 (4.56 ± 0)	♂ 39.9 ± 1.8 (3.99 ± 0.18) ♀ 49.7 ± 1.6 (4.97 ± 0.16)
Sorbitol dehydrogenase (SDH)	(IU/l)	17.5 ± 16.3 [16]					
Triglyceride	mmol/l (mg/dl)	0.86 ± 0.26 (76.3 ± 23.3) [16]					
Sodium (Na)	mmol/l (=mEq/l)	159.0 ± 7.3 [16] 147.1 ± 2.8 (141–157) [12]		110 ± 7.8	152 ± 1 (140–161) [38]	CB: 139.68 ± 0.89 PB: 4.72 ± 0.07	
Urea	mmol/l (mg/dl)		♂ 12.10 ± 0.15 (33.90 ± 0.41) ♀ 10.08 ± 0.17 (28.23 ± 0.49)				

Table 26.8 Biochemical reference data for select Galliforme species.

Analyte (abbreviation)		Broiler and white Leghorn Chickens *Gallus gallus* [126]	Blue peafowl, Indian peafowl *Pavo critatus* [45, 46]	Ring-necked pheasants *Phasianus colchicus* [48–50]	Red-legged partridges *Alectoris rufa* [48]	Bronze turkeys *Meleagris gallopavo* [127]
Sample size attributes		**20♂ Broilers (MB) 20♀ Broilers (FB) 20♂ Leghorns (ML) 42 d**	**6♂ 6♀ 1 yr [46] 41♂, 28♀, 1–3 yr [45]**	**8, 102 d [49] 10♂ 10♀ 5 wk [50] 24 4–12 wk [48]**	**N:20, 4–12 wk**	**N:15♀, 1 yr**
Data format	**Units, SI (US)**	**Mean ± SD**	**Mean ± SD [range]**	**Mean ± SD**	**Mean ± SE [range]**	**Mean ± SD**
Albumin	g/l (g/dl)	MB: 13.7 ± 1.4 (1.37 ± 0.14) FB: 14.2 ± 0.08 (1.42 ± 0.008) ML: 13.9 ± 1.9 (1.39 ± 0.19)	♂ 17.60 ± 3.40 [46] (1.76 ± 0.34) [46] ♀ 21.37 ± 0.50 (2.14 ± 0.05) 20.3 ± 2.7 [13.3–24.7] (2.03 ± 0.27 [1.33–2.47]) [45]	19.6 ± 4.7 (1.96 ± 0.47) [49] ♂ 19.3 ± 4.2 (1.93 ± 0.42) [50] ♀ 18.4 ± 1.9 (1.84 ± 0.19) [50] 18.1 ± 0.4 [15.1–22.7] (1.81 ± 0.04 [1.51–2.27]) [48]	18.2 ± 0.4 [16.3–23.0] [1.82 ± 0.04 [1.63–2.30])	18 ± 6.0 (1.8 ± 0.6)
Alkaline phosphatase (ALP)	U/l (units/l)		♂ 140.33 ±97.96 ♀ 29.00 ± 2.00 [46] (290 ± 95 [130–467]) [45]			
Alanine aminotransferase (ALT)	U/l (units/l)		♂ 2.67 ± 0.62 [46] ♀ 9.33 ± 3.65 1.7 ± 1.7 (0–7.2) [45]			
Aspartate aminotransferase (AST)	U/l (units/l)	MB: 254 ± 293 FB: 199 ± 21 ML: 183 ± 12	♂ 106.67 ± 7.23 [46] ♀ 137.00 ± 42.04 [46] 124 ± 38 [19–222] [45]			332 ± 204
Amylase	U/l (units/l)		♂ 635.67 ± 40.25 [46] ♀ 644.33 ± 5.51 (1810 ± 300 (1193–2617))			
Bile acids	μmol/l (ug/ml)		♂ 30.33 ± 15.50 [46] (12.39 ± 6.33) ♀ 57.33 ± 5.13 (23.42 ± 2.10) 51.1 ± 18.0 (22.0–90.0) ((20.9 ± 7.4 (9.0–36.8)) [45]			
Calcium (Ca)	mmol/l (mg/dl)	MB: 2.73 ± 0.13 (10.92 ± 0.52) FB: 2.76 ± 0.10 (11.04 ± 0.40) ML: 2.73 ± 0.25 (10.92 ± 1.00)	*ionized Ca:* [46] ♂ 1.39 ± 0.01 (5.56 ± 0.04) ♀ 1.42 ± 0.05 (5.68 ± 0.20) 3.35 ± 0.30 (2.90–4.30) (13.4 ± 1.20 [11.6–17.2]) [45]	2.63 ± 0.02 (2.45–2.75) [48](10.52 ± 0.08 (9.80–11.00)) [48]	2.71 ± 0.03 (2.45–2.90) (10.84 ± 0.12 (9.80–11.60))	
Chloride (Cl)	mmol/l (=mEq/l)	MB: 112 ± 1.5 FB: 112 ± 2.1 ML: 109 ± 2.5	♂ 102.00 ± 0.01 [46] ♀ 102.67 ± 1.53	116.5 ± 0.7 (110–125) [48]	114.7 ± 0.7 (108–119)	

(Continued)

Table 26.8 (Continued)

Analyte (abbreviation)		Broiler and white Leghorn Chickens *Gallus gallus* [126]	Blue peafowl, Indian peafowl *Pavo critatus* [45, 46]	Ring-necked pheasants *Phasianus colchicus* [48–50]	Red-legged partridges *Alectoris rufa* [48]	Bronze turkeys *Meleagris gallopavo* [127]
Sample size attributes		20♂ Broilers (MB) 20♀ Broilers (FB) 20♂ Leghorns (ML) 42 d	6♂ 6♀ 1 yr [46] 41♂, 28♀, 1–3 yr [45]	8, 102 d [49] 10♂ 10♀ 5 wk [50] 24 4–12 wk [48]	N:20, 4–12 wk	N:15♀, 1 yr
Data format	**Units, SI (US)**	**Mean ± SD**	**Mean ± SD [range]**	**Mean ± SD**	**Mean ± SE [range]**	**Mean ± SD**
Cholesterol	mmol/l (mg/dl)	MB: 3.23 ± 0.31 (124.7 ± 12.0) FB: 3.13 ± 0.39 (120.8 ± 15.1) ML: 2.93 ± 0.51 (113.1 ± 19.7)	♂ 2.80 ± 0.63 (108.1 ± 24.3) [46] ♀ 4.07 ± 1.34 (157.1 ± 51.7) 3.80 ± 0.62 (2.66–5.48) (147 ± 24 [103–212]) [45]			
Creatine kinase (CK)	U/l (units/l)		♂ 1684.33 ± 233.43 ♀ 1508.67 ± 503.70 [46] 1482 ± 453 (830–3063) [45]			
Creatinine	μmol/l (mg/dl)	MB: 52.3 ± 5.7 (0.6 ± 0.1) FB: 52.1 ± 6.7 (0.6 ± 0.1) ML: 50.5 ± 8.6 (0.6 ± 0.1)	♂ 16.30 ± 5.03 [46] ♀ 22.23 ± 10.50 [46] 72.7 ± 18.2 (54.5–118.2) (0.8 ± 0.2 [0.6–1.3]) [45]			
Gamma-glutamyltransferase (GGT)	U/l (units/l)		♂ 2.33 ± 0.56 ♀ 2.33 ± 1.31 [46] 1.6 ± 2.3 (0–7.7) [45]	5.77 ± 1.63 [49] ♂ 5.24 ± 1.61 [50] ♀ 5.0 ± 1.15 [50]		5.3 ± 3.6
Glucose	mmol/l (mg/dl)	MB: 15.1 ± 1.3 (271.8 ± 23.4) FB: 14.7 ± 0.75 (264.6 ± 13.5) ML: 15.5 ± 1.0 (279.0 ± 18.0)	♂ 18.10 ± 0.63 [46] (325.8 ± 11.3) [46] ♀ 17.5 ± 1.42 (315.0 ± 25.6) 22.92 ± 2.44 (17.83–27.56) (413 ± 44 [321–496]) [45]	19.5 ± 0.3 (15.8–23.7) (351.0 ± 5.4 [284.4–426.6]) [48]	19.8 ± 0.3 (17.4–22.7) (356.4 ± 5.4 (313.2–408.6))	
Lactate dehydrogenase (LDH)	U/l (units/l)	MB: 966 ± 934 FB: 731 ± 304 ML: 358 ± 116	♂ 196.00 ± 57.06 [46] ♀ 137.00 ± 74.99 [46] 232 ± 77 (74–508) [45]			
Magnesium (Mg)	mmol/l (mg/dl)	MB: 1.03 ± 0.12 (2.51 ± 0.29) FB: 1.00 ± 0.08 (2.43 ± 0.19) ML: 0.95 ± 0.06 (2.31 ± 0.15)	♂ 0.62 ± 0.13 (1.51 ± 0.32) [46] ♀ 0.40 ± 0.02 (0.97 ± 0.05)	0.85 ± 0.03 (0.67–1.19) (2.07 ± 0.07 [1.63–2.90]) [48]	0.90 ± 0.03 (0.65–1.19) [2.19 ± 0.07 (1.58–2.90))	
Phosphorus (P)	mmol/l (mg/dl)	MB: 2.58 ± 0.23 (7.99 ± 0.71) FB: 2.63 ± 0.21 (8.14 ± 0.65) ML: 2.47 ± 0.34 (7.65 ± 1.05)	♂ 1.37 ± 0.24 (4.24 ± 0.74) [46] ♀ 1.67 ± 0.26 (5.17 ± 0.80) [46] 2.10 ± 0.68 (1.06–4.55) (6.5 ± 2.1 [3.3–14.1]) [45]	2.61 ± 0.05 (2.30–3.10) (8.08 ± 0.15 [7.12–9.60]) [48]	2.35 ± 0.07 (1.63–2.71) [7.28 ± 0.22 (5.05–7.46))	

Potassium (K)	mmol/l (=mEq/l)	MB: 4.74 ± 0.84 FB: 4.83 ± 0.79 ML: 4.41 ± 0.59	♂ 3.18 ± 0.03 [46] ♀ 3.89 ± 0.67	6.82 ± 0.26 (5.51–8.74) [48]	6.83 ± 0.21 (5.56–8.70)	
Sodium (Na)	mmol/l (=mEq/l)	MB: 150 ± 2.8 FB: 151 ± 2.7 ML: 148 ± 2.2	♂ 149.67 ± 0.58 [46] ♀ 150.00 ± 2.00	151.6 ± 0.5 (147–156) [48]	151.4 ± 0.8 (146–161)	
Total bilirubin	μmol/l (mg/dl)	MB: 2.60 ± 0.50 (0.15 ± 0.03) FB: 2.40 ± 0.75 (0.14 ± 0.04) ML: 2.55 ± 0.92 (0.15 ± 0.05)	♂ 3.40 ± 0.40 (0.20 ± 0.02) [46] ♀ 4.73 ± 0.78 (0.28 ± 0.05) 3.45 ± 1.72 (0–8.62) (0.2 ± 0.1 [0–0.5]) [45]			
Total protein	g/l (g/dl)	MB: 32.6 ± 2.3 (3.26 ± 0.23) FB: 34.2 ± 1.8 (3.42 ± 0.18) ML: 32.9 ± 1.7 (3.29 ± 0.17)	♂ 35.53 ± 4.68 (3.53 ± 0.47) [46] ♀ 49.30 ± 7.44 (4.93 ± 0.74) [46] 41.1 ± 6.2 (27.2–54.3) (4.11 ± 0.62 [2.72–5.43]) [45]	[43] 40.3 ± 3.6 (4.03 ± 0.36) [49] ♂ 40.2 ± 6.9 [4.02 ± 0.69) [50] ♀ 36.0 ± 3.4 [3.60 ± 0.34) [50] 35.0 ± 0.6 (30.7–42.4) [48] [3.50 ± 0.06 (3.07–4.24)) [48]	36.9 ± 0.8 (30.7–44.4) [3.69 ± 0.08 (3.07–4.44))	66 ± 15 (6.6 ± 1.5)
Urea	mmol/l (mg/dl)		♂ 0.27 ± 0.06 (0.76 ± 0.17) [46] ♀ 0.433 ± 0.153 (1.21 ± 0.43) 0.43 ± 0.43 (0–2.36) (1.2 ± 1.2 [0–6.6]) [45]			2.0 ± 0.4 (5.6 ± 1.0)
Uric acid	μmol/l (mg/dl)	MB: 380 ± 77 (6.4 ± 1.3) FB: 388 ± 70 (6.5 ± 1.2) ML: 325 ± 61 (5.5 ± 1.0)	♂ *163.33 ± 62.56 (2.75 ± 1.05)* [46] ♀ *213.67 ± 71.60 (3.59 ± 1.20)* [46] 178.4 ± 71.4 (29.7–362.8) (3.0 ± 1.2 (0.5–6.1)) [45]	419.9 ± 125.5 (7.06 ± 2.11) [49] ♂ 346.8 ± 52.3 (5.83 ± 0.88) [50] ♀ 330.7 ± 98.1 (5.56 ± 1.65) [50]		380.7 ± 184.4 (6.4 ± 3.1)

In Japanese quail undergoing experimental heat stress during egg production, control group plasma AST/SGOT activities were increased compared to those receiving vitamin E supplementation, suggesting a protective effect of this vitamin [131, 132].

Alanine aminotransferase (ALT, SGPT) and lactate dehydrogenase (LDH, LD) are non-liver-specific cytosolic leakage enzymes found in several tissues in chickens. Highest ALT activity occurs in the chicken kidney, but the heart, liver, skeletal muscle, lung, and intestine also have clinically relevant activities [35]. Increased ALT activity may occur secondary to hemolysis or carbon tetrachloride poisoning. The utility of urinary ALT as a marker of renal disease has not been evaluated [8]. Hemolysis or prior injections can increase LDH activity and ALT to a lesser extent. Compared to CK, LDH has a shorter half-life; in the absence of hemolysis, persistent LDH increase without CK increase is suggestive of liver rather than muscle damage. LDH may also show extensive variation based on apprehension and restraint of Galliformes [16]. In chickens with stunting syndrome, increased ALT suggests liver and intestinal damage [116]. Slightly decreased LDH activity occurred in six-month-old chickens compared to one-month-old chickens, but no such differences were detected in ALT or AST [124].

Glutamate dehydrogenase (GDH, GLDH) is a mitochondrial enzyme of liver, kidney, and brain tissue [8]. As renal sources are excreted via urine, increased blood GDH is the most specific enzyme for hepatocellular damage. However, GDH sensitivity for liver disease is low, as cytoplasmic damage and leakage alone will not cause increased enzyme activity [35, 68, 133]. Gamma-glutamyltransferase (GGT) is a mainly membrane-associated enzyme of the biliary and renal systems, and elevations may support a diagnosis of hepatobiliary disease, cholestasis, and/or biliary hyperplasia. This enzyme is more specific than sensitive and inconsistently rises in cases of hepatic disease. Thus, a finding within the reference interval should not rule out the presence of hepatobiliary disease [35, 133]. In laying hens, increased activity of plasma GGT in pre-peak versus peak egg production was attributed to increased feed and increased hepatic workload in pre-peak hens [129]. For chickens suffering experimentally induced ochratoxicosis or aflatoxicosis, increased GGT activity is considered evidence of hepatotoxicity [69, 134].

Bile Acids, Biliverdin, and Ammonia

Bile acids are produced in the liver from cholesterol and secreted via the biliary system into the intestine, where they are fecally excreted or reabsorbed in a cycle of enterohepatic circulation. Major bile acids in chickens include chenodeoxycholic acid, cholyltaurine (taurocholic acid), and glycolithocholic acid, with smaller amounts of allocholyltaurine, as determined by high-performance liquid chromatography and mass spectrometry [133, 135, 136]. Despite the adaptation of bile acid assays for multiple avian species including Galliformes, validation and appropriate species-specific reference intervals appear lacking [137]. Further complicating use and interpretation are varying methodologies with different units of measurement, as well as the interferences of hemolysis and lipemia [133]. Colorimetric methods do not require species-specific antibodies, are most widely used, and tend to produce higher results than radioimmunoassay (RIA) because a wider spectrum of bile acids is detected. However, their validity is questionable. Bile acid increases indicate reduced hepatic uptake function, reduced conjugation, or reduced secretion into the intestine. In avian species, increases in bile acids tend to carry a poor prognosis and are associated with severe conditions such as fibrosis, lipidosis, and biliary hyperplasia. Subnormal levels, although uncommon, indicate reduced substrate or hepatic synthesis. However, few, if any of these generalities regarding the diagnostic use of bile acids have been assessed in Galliformes [138]. Biliverdin and ammonia concentrations have not been evaluated as clinical markers of hepatobiliary disease, but their development would be useful to assess for the presence of cholestasis and hepatic insufficiency, respectively. Biliverdin is seldom detected in the plasma of normal chickens, presumably based on efficient hepatic uptake and the short half-life of this enzyme. Additionally, commercial assays for this enzyme remain unavailable. Green- or yellow-stained urates in excreta may indicate increases in circulating bile acids or bile pigments, or biliverdinuria. Bilirubin, while occasionally reported in the literature, is generally accepted as not present in Galliformes. The yellow coloration of skin or plasma, or the false finding of increased total bilirubin or icterus in standard laboratory assays, is likely attributable to carotenoid pigment coloration.

Muscle and Bone Enzymes

Creatine kinase (CK, CPK) is formed from creatine in skeletal muscle, cardiac muscle, and brain. This enzyme is a very sensitive and specific indicator of muscle damage. Because this enzyme may be degraded by bacterial action, subnormal values could indicate sample contamination. Extensive variation in CK may occur based on apprehension and restraint of subjects [16]. Prior injections and sample hemolysis may also increase CK activity in chicken blood samples [34]. In cases of experimental vitamin E/selenium deficiency, ALT, AST and CK were increased indicating liver and muscle necrosis and fibrosis [103]. Aside from skeletal muscle, AST is also an important marker of liver disease or damage in Galliformes; more information is provided in the section "Liver Enzymes and Biomarkers." Also originating from liver and muscle, but with a shorter half-life than CK, is lactate dehydrogenase (LDH).

Alkaline phosphatase (ALP, ALKP, SAP, AP) is a membrane-associated enzyme with renal, intestinal, and liver activity [35]. In birds, ALP has more bone- and eggshell-related activity than hepatobiliary activity, and thus is not a useful marker of cholestasis. Increases in ALP activity are associated with increased osteoblastic activity, including growth, fractures, rickets, nutritional secondary hyperparathyroidism, osteomyelitis, and ovulation [8]. ALP rises in chickens with stunting syndrome [116]. In white Leghorn chickens, plasma ALP in animals older than five months of age was lower than the activity in animals four months of age [38].

Renal Analytes

In Galliformes, urea is produced from amino acid degradation in the liver, but lack of clinically significant amounts may hinder detection renal or liver insufficiency. Creatinine and BUN may be undetectable, or may increase to detectable concentrations based on prerenal dehydration or renal disease [133]. Creatinine is formed in muscle tissue from creatine phosphate and is not a reliable indicator of renal disease in birds. Additionally, the assay may be falsely increased by the reaction of nonspecific chromogens. Serum/plasma urea nitrogen (BUN) increase may be most useful in detecting dehydration/reduced glomerular filtration rate (GFR), as urea filtered by the glomerulus is reabsorbed instead of the normal pathway of excretion. However, in most healthy birds, BUN is at or below the level of detection for most assays. BUN and creatinine concentrations increase dehydrated pigeons, but similiar studies have not been performed in gallinaceous birds [9, 35]. In African chickens, males have higher mean values for creatinine than females [15, 59].

The major end product of nitrogen metabolism (60%–80%) in birds is uric acid, which is produced in the liver and actively secreted in kidney tubules independent of the state of hydration or urine flow rate [9]. Uric acid is assayed via enzymatic or chromatographic methods, or by capillary electrophoresis [139]. Plasma uric acid concentrations are neither sensitive nor specific for renal function or detection of renal disease in Galliformes. Hyperuricemia is often insensitive, occurring only in late-stage renal disease. Hyperuricemia can also be nonspecific, developing in cases of severe dehydration (prerenal) or postprandially in carnivorous or omnivorous species [35].

Experimental models or renal intoxication or dietary supplementation have produced variable results regarding renal analytes of Galliformes. Experimental administration of the nephrotoxin ochratoxin A in chickens was associated with increased plasma creatinine, uric acid, and potassium concentrations, but lower BUN concentrations. Renal enlargement with edema and tubular necrosis was found histologically. Significant hypoalbuminemia may have been based on renal protein loss or hepatic insufficiency [134, 140]. Serum uric acid and urea were increased (<2X controls) in chickens fed oregano, sage, rosemary, and pepper extract as an organic growth promoter and antimicrobial agent, suggesting renal impairment at higher doses. The effect on uric acid was dose dependent [130]. Ancillary diagnostics for evaluation of renal disease include urinalysis, imaging, and the gold standard, renal biopsy.

Pancreas

Chickens have higher glucose concentrations than mammals, and assay methodology must have an upper limit of detection which exceeds the range of the species at hand. Granivorous birds have higher pancreatic glucagon than insulin activity; thus, pancreatic compromise may induce hypoglycemia rather than diabetes mellitus [133]. Other differentials for hypoglycemia in Galliformes are similar to those of companion mammals and include sepsis, functional/synthetic liver failure, starvation, and paraneoplastic syndromes. In chicken samples, hemolysis results in decreased glucose concentration, but serum harvest after 90 min of RBC contact for clot formation does not result in hypoglycemia relative to plasma. Glucagon is the major lipolytic hormone in birds [141]. Plasma insulin concentrations and dynamics of insulin secretion are similar in chickens and mammals [142, 143]. Research has shown breed/strain differences in insulin and insulin receptor concentrations, suggesting that different genetic strains have insulin resistance and may serve as research models [144]. Plasma and serum glucose, insulin, and glucagon concentrations in poultry have been determined (Table 26.9), but only glucose values are routinely determined in clinical practice.

In Galliformes, hyperglycemia may result from endogenous or exogenous glucocorticoids. Heat stress causes a cortisol-mediated hyperglycemia [13]. Studies of African chickens have shown males to have higher mean values for glucose [15, 59]. For commercial hens, post-peak (egg) production chickens had lower glucose concentrations that pre-peak animals, but the significance of this finding was not evaluated [12].

In the chicken, pancreatic lipase and several lipases of triglyceride metabolism have been sequenced and are comparable with their mammalian counterparts [147, 148]. Little information exists about the utility of amylase and lipase as diagnostic tools for pancreatic disease in Galliformes [35]. Pancreatic amylase, trypsin, and chymotrypsin increase with age of the chicken, vary in concentration based on breed, and are associated with body weight (it was hypothesized that the breed-related differential enzyme concentrations may affect the growth

Table 26.9 Hormone values for the domestic chicken, *Gallus gallus domesticus*.

Analyte (abbreviation)	Units	Ross [16]	Rhode Island Red [145]	Ross [86]	Nouzilly[a] Beltsville[b] [143, 146]
Attributes		♂ 13 mo	♀ T4–53 wk T3–25 wk	♂ 28–42 d	
Sample number; animal number		5; S:30	10	30	5–10
Data format		Mean ± SD	Mean ± SE	Range	Mean ± SE
Insulin	pmol/l (ng/dl)				[a]Fasted: 1.03 ± 0.17 (0.60 ± 0.10) [b]Fasted: 1.20 ± 0.57 (0.70 ± 0.33) [a]Fed: 3.22 ± 0.72 (1.87 ± 0.42) [b]Fed: 3.73 ± 0.74 (2.17 ± 0.43)
Thyroxine (T4)	nmol/l (μg/dl)	16.7 ± 2.6 (1.3 ± 0.2)	1.9 ± 0.6 (0.15 ± 0.05)	28d: 16–38 (1.24–2.95) 35d: 18–42 (1.40–3.26) 42d: 24–38 (1.86–2.95)	
Triiodothyronine (T3)	nmol/l (μg/dl)	1278.2 ± 366.5 (83.0 ± 23.8)	3.65 ± 0.231 (0.237 ± 0.015)	28d: 1.2–2.0 (0.08–0.13) 35d: 1.3–2.3 (0.08–0.15) 42d: 1.8–3.9 (0.12–0.25)	
Corticosterone	nmol/l (μg/dl)	23.12 ± 2.89 (0.8 ± 0.1)			

rate) [149]. Amylase was increased in chickens with stunting syndrome, suggesting pancreatic damage [116]. Serum lipase activity increased twofold in chickens fed oregano, sage, rosemary, and pepper extract (fed as an organic growth promoter and antimicrobial agent), compared with control chickens [130].

Gastrointestinal Biomarkers

Little in the literature supports diagnosis of gastrointestinal (GI) disease in chickens via clinicopathologic means. Immunoreactive cells and nerve fibers for glucagon, gastric inhibitory peptide (GIP; a glucagon-family hormone that stimulates pancreatic beta cells to release insulin), and gastrin releasing peptide (GRP; stimulates pancreatic release of digestive enzymes) are located in the intestine of chickens [150]. Carbohydrate absorption tests (such as xylose) might suggest gastrointestinal disease, but these tests have not been validated for the Galliforme [133].

Cardiac Biomarkers

Troponins C, I, and T occur in the chicken. A troponin with specialized metal binding capacity has been found only in the avian breast muscles of the Craciformes and Galliformes [151]. This T-troponin may facilitate the explosive but short flights of these species [152]. Troponins in hatchling chickens are relatively increased [range of means, 5.74–8.35 ng/ml] likely based on an embryonic isoform, but then decrease to concentrations consistent with those of humans [mean < 0.2 ng/ml] by three weeks of age [153, 154]. Serum Troponin T (range, mean ± SD, given in ng/ml) was significantly higher in young ascitic broiler chickens (0.05–7.6, 1.10 ± 1.168) than in age-matched healthy broilers (0.02–1.10, 0.2 ± 0.247) [153]. As ascitic syndrome in broiler chickens is associated with right-sided cardiac failure, these findings suggest that troponins may be useful in the diagnosis of cardiac disease in Galliformes.

Lipids

Sex and egg production affect cholesterol concentrations in the chicken. During egg production, females may have higher concentrations of circulating cholesterol, very low density lipoproteins (VLDL), low density lipoproteins (LDL), apolipoprotein B, and triglycerides, which travel from the liver to the ovary for inclusion into the egg yolk. Thus, lipemia may be physiologically normal during egg formation [40, 133, 155]. However, likely based on breed and reproductive cycle, African cocks had higher mean values of cholesterol than females [15, 59]. Lipids and lipoproteins continue to be intensively studied in the Galliforme as models of atherosclerosis and for the study of nutrition as food animals. As in humans, dietary intake affects plasma lipids and lipoproteins of chickens. High dietary cholesterol intake (1%) increased serum cholesterol, LDL, VLDL, and triacylglycerol, and decreased serum HDL concentrations in chickens in only six weeks [66]. Hypercholesterolemia in chickens has also been caused by a high-lysine diet (4%–5%) and copper deficiency [156, 157]. Dietary copper supplementation decreases serum cholesterol concentrations in chickens [64]. Serum cholesterol and LDLs are increased in chickens with femoral head separation disorder [158]. Ochratoxicosis decreases serum triglyceride and cholesterol concentrations in young broiler chicks and hens, likely owing to hepatotoxicity [69].

Electrolytes (Tables 26.7, 26.8, and 26.10)

Electrolytes should be interpreted with knowledge of the patient's hydration status and any possible disease states that may predispose to gastrointestinal or renal electrolyte loss. In Galliformes, direct potentiometry is preferred to indirect potentiometry or flame photometry determination of electrolytes, because the latter may underestimate sodium of chloride based on physiologic or pathogenic hyperlipidemia or hyperproteinemia [35, 159]. However, even in direct potentiometry, discrepancies may occur, likely based on the relative instability of potassium in chicken blood [133]. Poor correlation between potassium measured in whole blood immediately via the i-STAT and a standard chemistry analyzer has been reported [51]. Therefore, plasma is best separated from erythrocytes directly after centrifugation of blood for laboratory analysis of electrolytes [133]. Values may be affected by sample type, handling, storage, degradation, and methodology. Values for blood plasma and urinary electrolytes for Galliformes are provided in Tables 26.7, 26.8, 26.10, and 26.12.

Serum or plasma electrolyte concentrations of the Galliforme may be affected by water intake, hydration status, dietary intake, acid base status, free water retention by the kidney (including edematous disorders such as congestive heart failure, cirrhosis, and nephrotic syndrome), tissue necrosis, aldosterone activity, and sensible and insensible hypertonic, isotonic, and hypotonic fluid losses (which are usually based on GI or renal loss). Most of these effects are assumed to occur and have not been specifically investigated for Galliformes. Finally, the clinician must recall that blood electrolyte concentrations may not reflect total body stores (this is common for potassium, which is mainly intracellular).

Both infectious and non-infectious diseases, as well as physiological processes, affect electrolyte balance in the Galliforme. Heat stress may decrease sodium and potassium concentrations in chickens [13]. Young pheasants (*P. colchicus*) and partridges (*Alectoris rufa*) with *Spironucleus* infection, which decreases intestinal absorption, had lower plasma sodium and chloride concentrations. In commercial egg-producing hens, post-peak production animals had higher sodium concentrations than pre-peak animals [12]. Diet affects electrolytes in the chicken and other Galliformes. Experimentally decreased protein in the diet decreased plasma sodium, chloride, and potassium concentrations in broiler chickens [160]. Decreasing dietary concentrations of sodium and chloride reduced blood pH, pCO_2, and bicarbonate, but increased plasma potassium [161]. A high-calcium diet increased serum calcium but reduced concentrations of phosphorous and potassium in one study [122]. Dietary vitamin D deficiency creates a reversible, uncompensated hyperchloremic metabolic acidosis in the chicken. The ensuing type II renal tubular acidosis, with increasing tubular loss of bicarbonate, further decreases production of the biologically active form of vitamin D. Acidosis also contributes to calciuria and phosphaturia, further perpetuating hypocalcemia and hypophosphatemia from insufficient vitamin D. Nutritional secondary hyperparathyroidism is the end result [162].

Blood Proteins

Serum or plasma proteins may be measured by, in order of increasing accuracy, refractometry, dye binding (bromocresol green/BCG), Biuret method, or electrophoresis [34, 133, 163, 164]. These methods do not produce interchangeable results. Species differences of protein fraction mobility on electrophoresis, based on differing amino acid sequences and charge distribution, dictate use of species-specific controls. Serial electrophoresis measurements of albumin and globulins can be used to gauge response to treatment in individual animals. Fibrinogen in chicken plasma may be measured by the heat precipitation method as an indicator of inflammation [9, 165]. In chickens and turkeys, refractometry is more comparable to the Biuret method of total protein determination than for other avian species [9, 133, 165, 166]. Plasma protein has increased concentrations (up to 1 g/dl) compared to serum, based on the presence of fibrinogen and other clotting factors in plasma [9, 35]. As in other species, albumin is the largest protein fraction [9]. Values for blood proteins of Galliformes are provided in Tables 26.7 and 26.8.

Ovotransferrin, a 65-kD hepatic acute phase protein also produced in the oviduct, chondrocytes, fibroblasts, and neural cells, can be measured by a non-species-specific plasma spectrophotometric competitive enzyme immunoassay (EIA) [167]. A component of egg white, ovotransferrin is an iron transport protein with antimicrobial and immunostimulatory properties that enhance heterophil and macrophage function [168]. In chickens, serum ovotransferrin was increased at seven days in an experimental model of inflammation, and in those infected with bacteria and viruses [169]. In a model of experimental acute inflammation, ovotransferrin increased at 16 h, peaked at three days, and returned to baseline by 10 days.

Chickens have lower total protein concentrations and serum colloid osmotic pressure than those of mammals [62].

Reproduction, sex, age, breed, and diet affect total protein and colloid osmotic pressure in the chicken. Egg formation is characterized by slightly increased albumin and globulin-spectrum egg-yolk proteins (lipoproteins and vitellogenin) under the influence of estrogen. Together, these may cause a physiologic hyperproteinemia and decreased A/G ratio [9, 35, 133]. Higher total protein based on albumin may also occur in females [40]. Reproductively active females may have higher fibrinogen concentrations [68]. Calculated serum colloid osmotic pressure is higher in adult males than adult females based on differences in alpha1-globulin and albumin concentrations. In chickens, PCV positively correlates with COP [62]. In contrast, African chicken males have higher mean values for albumin and globulin than females [15, 59]. Naked neck and feathered Egyptian male chickens also had higher total protein, albumin, and globulin concentrations than females of the same strain. Hematocrit, total protein, and globulin also differ by strain of chicken; homozygous naked neck chickens had higher values than heterozygous or homozygous feathered [61]. Chickens fed high-oleic-acid-rich oil (olive oil 5%) diets for six weeks had increased total globulin and gamma globulin fractions [66].

Pathologic, rather than physiologic, hyperproteinemia may signal dehydration (normal A/G ratio), inflammation (fungal disease such as aspergillus, chlamydiosis, tuberculosis, and egg-yolk peritonitis), or a lymphoproliferative disorder [35]. Differential diagnoses for hypoalbuminemia are similar to those in mammals and include maldigestion, malabsorption, liver synthetic failure, protein-losing enteropathy, protein-losing nephropathy, dermal lesions, and hemorrhage. Albumin decreases slightly (with concurrent globulin increase and decreased A/G ratio) in cases of inflammatory disease [9, 133]. Stunting syndrome is characterized by decreased total serum protein, A/G ratio, hypoalbuminemia, and hyperglobulinemia, consistent with inflammation and decreased digestion and absorption of dietary proteins [116]. Experimental ochratoxicosis (21-day exposure) decreased serum total protein, albumin, and globulin concentrations in young chicks, likely based on hepatotoxicity [134]. In hens suffering from aflatoxicosis, decreased total plasma protein, albumin, and beta-globulins, but increased gamma-globulins, occurred likely based on hepatotoxicity, although renal loss could not be ruled out [69]. Experimental Avian reovirus infection produced hyperglobulinemia in chickens [115].

Blood Gases, pH, and Lactate

Blood gas samples should be collected in pre-cooled syringes, stored on ice, and assayed as quickly as possible to prevent metabolism of oxygen by nucleated RBCs, which will metabolize oxygen several times faster than anucleate mammalian erythrocytes [9]. Unlike blood gas values, ionized calcium, and hematocrit, there is poor correlation between potassium measured on the i-STAT analyzer and a standard chemistry analyzer. Base excess (BE) was the only other parameter with poor correlation [51]. Heat stress may lower pCO_2 and HCO_3, consistent with respiratory alkalosis [13]. Bicarbonate is believed to decrease secondary to increased chloride, which has an acidifying action in response to respiratory alkalosis [13]. Chicken embryos raised at high altitude (2.9 km) showed higher hemoglobin concentrations and lower arterial p_aO_2 when compared with embryos raised at sea level. Additionally, lower venous blood pH and higher venous pCO_2 were noted; these changes likely represent increased oxygen unloading from hemoglobin [170].

On the i-STAT, HCO_3, TCO_2, Hb, and sO_2 are calculated. These parameters as well as the measured parameters (pH, arterial pO_2, pCO_2, Na, iCa, and PCV) had good correlation with those measured by traditional laboratory equipment on the same blood samples (Table 26.10) [51]. For commercial hens, post-peak (egg) production animals had higher pH and BE values and lower pCO_2 concentrations than pre-peak animals, but the significance of these data is unclear and may be affected by different strains/husbandry status [12]. A high-calcium diet causes metabolic alkalosis with increased blood pH, HCO_3, BE, and lower p_aO_2, p_aCO_2, and s_aO_2 in the chicken. Serum calcium was increased, sodium, magnesium, and chloride were unchanged, and phosphorous and potassium were reduced. Urinary excretion of calcium and chloride was enhanced, while urinary excretion of sodium, magnesium, and phosphorus was reduced. Urinary pH was also increased above controls [122].

Vitamins, Minerals, Metals, and Toxins

Iron, TIBC, and Ferritin

Several cases of acute death based on excessive iron storage (hepatic hemosiderosis) progressing to hemochromatosis (characterized by hepatic fibrosis, necrosis, and nodular regeneration) are reported for the curassow, a species with possible genetic predisposition for excessive tissue deposition of iron [133, 171]. Iron overload may be detected on a biochemical profile via increased hepatocellular enzymes (reflective of excessive iron storage and damage to this organ). Iron assay is rare in birds based on lack of testing antibodies and validation [133]. Avian ferritin is comprised of an H subunit with a ferroxidase moiety for iron incorporation, but lacks an associated L subunit as occurs in mammals. Chicken ferritin has stronger heme-binding activity than mammalian ferritins [89]. Dietary copper supplementation may raise serum iron and zinc concentrations [64].

Table 26.10 Blood gas and electrolyte values for the domestic chicken, *Gallus gallus domesticus*.

Analyte		Lohmann selected Leghorn, arterial i, C [51]	Ross, Cobb ♀ 25–36 wk[135] Ross ♂ 13 mo [16]	Brown pullet ♀ 5–9 wk [122]	White Leghorn ♂ 4–6 mo [38] [44] Leghorn 23–27 wk [123]	CB – Cochin Bantam; PB – Polish Bantam ♂ 40 wk [41]
Sample size		40	165 [12]; 5, S:30 [16]	80	14, S:33–39 [38]; 20 [123]	8 each breed
Data format	**Units**	**Mean ± SD**	**Mean ± SD**	**Mean ± SD**	**Mean ± SE (range)**	**Mean ± SE**
Sodium (Na)	mmol/l (=mEq/l)	C: 153.98 ± 4.475 i: 144.03 ± 4.491	141.6–152.6 [12] 159.0 ± 7.3	110.0 ± 7.8	152 ± 1 (140–161) [38]	CB: 139.68 ± 0.89 PB: 139.5 ± 0.61
Potassium (K)	mmol/l (=mEq/l)	C: 2.97 ± 0.688 i: 3.04 ± 0.573	4.1–5.7 [12] 4.8 ± 0.9 [16]	4.6 ± 0.2	3.8 ± 0.1 (3.1–4.6) [38]	CB: 4.72 ± 0.07 PB: 4.85 ± 0.04
Chloride (Cl)	mmol/l (=mEq/l)		104.2 ± 3.1 [16]	10.6 ± 0.06	117 ± 1 (106–124) [38]	
Ionized calcium	mmol/l (mEq/l)	C: 1.23 ± 0.119 (2.46 ± 0.238) i: 1.17 ± 0.146 (2.34 ± 0.292)	1.20–1.73 (2.40–3.46) [12]		Venous 1.26–1.58 (2.52–3.16) [123] Arterial 1.19–1.48 (2.38–2.96) [123]	
pH		C: 7.54 ± 0.089 i: 7.58 ± 0.116	7.28–7.57 [12]	7.42 ± 0.001		
pCO_2	mmHg	C: 25.39 ± 8.389 i: 25.50 ± 7.365	25.9–49.5 [12]	39.2 ± 0.7		
pO_2	mmHg	C: 275.95 ± 97.53 i: 313.10 ± 137.6	32.0–60.5 [12]	85.7 ± 0.7		
HCO_3	mmHg	C: 24.74 ± 2.522 i: 23.16 ± 4.308	18.9–30.3 [12]	25.3 ± 0.5		
TCO_2	mmol/l (=mEq/l)	C: 20.75 ± 3.504 i: 23.90 ± 4.494	19.9–31.5 [12]			
Base Excess	mmol/l (=mEq/l)	C: 0.17 ± 3.004 i: 2.01 ± 5.385	−6.8–7.2 [12]	2.25 ± 0.43		
Oxygen (sO2) Saturation	%		70.6–93.3 [12]	86.6 ± 0.6		

S = Animal number i,C = analyte values from paired arterial samples via i-STAT (i) or conventional methods (C): pH, pCO_2, pO_2, HCO_3, tCO_2, BE, sO_2 via Rapidlap 800, Bayer, Zurich, Switzerland; Na, K, Cl via serum Cobas Integra, Roche Diagnostics, Rotkreuz, Switzerland; ionized calcium via serum, Nova CRT 8 electrolyte analyzer, Nova Biomedical, Waltham MA.

Experimentally feeding high levels of zinc was shown to decrease iron absorption and decrease liver and bone concentrations of iron [172, 173].

Calcium and Phosphorous

Values for blood and plasma concentrations of calcium and phosphorous of galliformes are provided in Tables 26.7, 26.8, and 26.10. Lipemia, hyperproteinemia, hemolysis, or bacterial contamination of blood can falsely increase calcium. Hypercalcemia may be physiologic during egg laying. Thus, reference ranges for calcium may be higher in oviparous females and in those suffering from egg binding and egg-yolk coelomitis [133]. Aberrations in diet, albumin, vitamin D, or parathyroid hormone (primary or secondary renal or nutritional disorders) may influence calcium concentrations [35]. Common dye binding assays can be affected by these physiologic changes and artifacts [68]. Measurement of blood calcium may not be reflective of total body stores; conversely, a normal concentration does not rule out nutritional deficiency [68]. A study of 20 normal laying hens showed slightly higher (average 0.22 mmol/l) ionized calcium concentrations in venous blood in comparison with arterial blood. Additionally, there were parallel shifts in total and ionized calcium concentrations depending on the stage of cycle, with maximal concentrations 3–6 h after oviposition and minimal concentrations 18–21 h after oviposition [123]. In this research, blood samples were stored at 4 °C for 4 h before analysis.

The finding of acute hypocalcemia is supportive of a diagnosis of calcium tetany for hens in high egg production. The i-STAT handheld clinical analyzer is validated, has good interassay correlation with standard chemistry analyzers, and is effective in detecting hypocalcemic chickens on the basis of low ionized calcium measurement [51, 174]. Chickens affected by calcium tetany also suffered uncompensated metabolic acidosis (decreased pH and HCO_3^- and normal pCO_2). Sudden death syndrome, similar to calcium tetany but without hypocalcemia, may instead be associated with hypernatremia or hypokalemia [12, 174].

Hyperphosphatemia may occur secondary to hemolysis, intestinal necrosis, decreased GFR, renal failure, or hypoparathyroidism. Glucocorticoid therapy may cause hypophosphatemia. Phosphorous is an unreliable indicator of renal insufficiency, and values vary widely depending on reproductive status and urine volume. Aberrations may be seen in metabolic bone disease [35, 68]. Hypocalcemia and hyperphosphatemia were noted in experimentally induced cases of hypoxia, causing pulmonary hypertension, right-sided congestive heart failure, and ascites of chickens. The authors attributed the electrolyte abnormalities to redistribution within the heart under the influence of catecholamines [175]. Chickens fed high-cholesterol diets for six weeks had decreased calcium and phosphorous but increased magnesium concentrations [66].

Vitamins

Because Galliformes are an important food source in the developed and developing world, minimum dietary requirements for vitamins and minerals and experimentally induced vitamin deficiencies have received significant scientific attention, particularly in poultry. Values for select plasma vitamin concentration of Gallformes are provided in Table 26.11. For example, plasma selenium and glutathione peroxidase were decreased in experimental vitamin E/selenium deficiency of chickens, which was associated with sterile inflammation and myocyte necrosis [103]. Experimental

Table 26.11 Select plasma vitamins of select Galliformes.

		Domestic chicken *Gallus gallus* [176, 177]	Domestic chicken *G. gallus* [178]	Red-legged partridge *Alectoris rufa* [179, 180]
Attributes		Laying ♀, 20–28 wk control (Ø) flax (f), sunflower (s) seed 4–8 wk dietary supplement *8–12 mo laying ♀ White Leghorn × Rhode Island Red*	Ross 308 ♂ broilers, Control Ø, or dietary supplement of vitamins C, E, or C & E	
Sample size, Data format		25, Range of 4–8 week means *5–11, Mean ± SEM*	12, Mean ± SE	Adult captive controls 12 ♀, 12 ♂
Analyte (abbreviation)	Units			
Vitamin A (Retinol)	µmol/l (µg/dl)	Ø 0.3433–0.52 (9.83–14.89) f 0.2800–1.0467 (8.02–29.99) s 0.3333–1.1667 (9.55–33.43)	Ø 2.816 ± 0.154 (80.70 ± 4.40) C 2.405 ± 0.165 (68.90 ± 4.72) E 2.06 ± 0.126 (59.11 ± 3.61) C&E 2.184 ± 0.207 (62.58 ± 5.92)	Retinol (µM) 10.53 ± 0.33
β-carotene	µmol/l (µg/dl)		Ø 0.8231 ± 0.004 (44.25 ± 4.35) C 0.8591 ± 0.080 (46.19 ± 4.30) E 1.100 ± 0.067 (59.11 ± 3.61) C&E 0.830 ± 0.105 (44.51 ± 5.65)	
Vitamin C (ascorbic acid)	µmol/l (mg/dl)	Ø 601.9–908.5 (10.6–15.0) f 624.6–863.1 (11.0–15.2) s 601.9–851.7 (10.6–15.0)	Ø 1393.4 ± 42 (24.58±0.74[a]) C 1502 ± 80.1 (26.46±1.41[a]) E 1413 ± 46.56 (24.89±0.82[a]) C&E 1384 ± 57.35 (24.39 ± 1.01[a])	
Vitamin D	pmol/ml	*Heavy shell 0.82 ± 0.05* *Light shell 0.76 ± 0.09* *Magnum 0.70 ± 0.07* *Shell gland 0.78 ± 0.08* *High-calcium diet – 0.86 ± 0.14* *Medium calcium diet – 1.37±0.12*		
Vitamin E (Tocopherol)	µmol/l (mg/dl)	Ø 65.57–73.84 (2.91–3.18) f 69.20–92.88 (2.98–4.00) s 93.11–126.6 (4.01–5.45)	Ø 20.9 ± 2.3 (0.90 ± 0.1) C 18.81 ± 1.7 (0.81 ± 0.08) E 127 ± 26.2 (5.47 ± 1.13) C&E 95.2 ± 21.4 (4.10± 0.92)	Tocopherol (µM) 8.61 ± 0.76

[a] Given as µg/dl in source, suspect typographical error, transcribed as mg/dl.

vitamin D deficiency for four weeks resulted in reversible hypocalcemia and hyperchloremic metabolic acidosis of chickens [162]. Experimental vitamin A deficiency for only eight weeks produced hypothyroidism in young Leghorn chicks [181]. While numerous specific minimum dietary vitamin requirements have been determined for chickens, turkeys, and Japanese quail, minimal information is available for acceptable or deficient plasma values [182]. Vitamins most likely to be deficient in the omnivorous diet of the chicken turkey and quail are A, D, and E [182]. While the chicken, turkey, and Japanese quail produce vitamin C endogenously, the willow ptarmigan chick suffers a syndrome reminiscent of scurvy without dietary provision of vitamin C [182]. Inadvertent dietary oversupplementation of breeding ring-necked pheasants *(P. colchicus)* resulted in numerous cranial deformities of chicks [183]. Effects of vitamin oversupplementation may be just as severe in other Galliformes.

In domestic female birds, vitamin D metabolites have been extensively studied as necessary for bone health and egg (shell) production. Circulating vitamin D metabolite concentrations for the domestic hen have been determined (Table 26.10). "Normal" values for these metabolites are few as vitamin D metabolism is complex and affected by many physiologic factors such as ultraviolet light exposure, diet, and estrogen concentrations. Plasma concentrations of 25(OH)D (calcifediol) and $1,25(OH)_2D_3$ (calcitriol), but not $24,25(OH)_2D_3$ (dihydroxycholecalciferol) fluctuate during the egg production cycle in hens [184]. Circulating $1,25(OH)_2D_3$ increases during the prelay period and at the onset of egg production, likely based on physiologic calcium deficiency induced by estrogens [184]. Plasma $1,25(OH)_2D_3$ concentrations peak during eggshell formation to facilitate calcification of medullary bone during egg production [184].

Toxins

Based on their use as food and food-producing animals, many experimental toxic effects have been studied in poultry. However, toxicosis appears relatively uncommon in poultry and other Galliformes compared to other avian species. Below, we have restricted our comments to those expected to create detectable clinicopathologic changes.

Mycotoxins

Aflatoxin is a primary liver toxicant in chickens, causing fatty degeneration and biliary hyperplasia. Aflatoxicosis is immunosuppressive, impairs leukocyte function, and reduces serum complement [78]. Experimental aflatoxicosis in laying chickens caused anemia, hyperglycemia, increased ALP activity, decreased BUN, and hyponatremia [87]. In hens and broiler chicks, aflatoxicosis caused slightly increased PT (both groups), increased RBC and hematocrit (hens), decreased RBC (chicks), decreased total plasma protein, albumin, and beta-globulins (hens), and increased gamma-globulins (hens). Increased PT was concluded to be the most sensitive indicator of toxicosis [69]. Other mycotoxins (ochratoxin and T-2 toxin) have been shown to increase PT in chickens [93]. Both aflatoxin and ochratoxin cause non-regenerative anemias (typically normocytic and normochromic) and coagulopathies in chickens [29, 93]. Ochratoxin A (produced by *Aspergillus* and *Penicillium*) causes hydropericardium, hepatitis, myocarditis, interstitial nephritis, and depletion of lymphocytes from lymphoid organs in the chicken [185]. Phagocytic activity and cell-mediated immune responses are also reduced [78]. Increased plasma concentrations of uric acid, creatinine, and potassium, but lower BUN concentrations, occurred in chickens suffering experimentally induced ochratoxicosis. Renal enlargement, edema, and tubular necrosis of the kidneys were documented on necropsy and histologic examination. Significant hypoalbuminemia may have been based on renal protein loss [134, 140]. In chickens, experimental ochratoxicosis produces leukopenia, lymphopenia, and monocytopenia at higher doses, without altering the heterophil count [104]. Assays for plasma Ochratoxin A and Aflatoxin B-1 are generally limited to research use [186, 187].

Heavy Metals

As ground-dwelling omnivorous birds, Galliformes may be attracted to shiny objects and suffer hardware disease and the attendant metal toxicities. However, clinically reported cases and attendant pathological changes in Galliformes appear rare. Lead assays should be performed on heparinized whole blood. EDTA may interfere with the assay, and plasma and serum are not suitable samples because lead is erythrocyte associated [8, 9]. Blood lead concentrations can be assayed in-house by ESA Leadcare II (ESA, Chelmsford, Massachusetts) [26]. Lead intoxication causes anemia that is typically regenerative, macrocytic, and hypochromic. Basophilic stippling is not a feature of avian lead toxicity; instead, erythrocytes may appear as swollen or ballooned (termed "D cells" due to their shape) [54, 68]. Erythrocytes may have shortened life spans and display nuclear pyknosis [54]. Natural lead intoxication of a flock of 20 laying hens showed highest lead concentrations in the kidney, liver, ovaries, and egg yolk. Blood lead concentrations positively correlated with yolk concentrations [188]. Zinc toxicity causes similar hematologic abnormalities. Zinc may impair iron absorption, causing a functional iron deficiency, resulting in hypochromasia, hemolysis, and ineffective erythropoiesis or regenerative anemia [54, 172, 173]. Zinc toxicity may have a more severe clinical manifestation in iron-deficient chicks [189].

Pesticides and Herbicides

Fipronil and imidacloprid, commonly used as insecticidal seed coatings, cause adverse effects in Galliformes [179, 180, 190]. Gallinaceous birds seem particularly sensitive to fipronil based on captive studies and field assessment [191]; in some Galliforme species, such as the red-legged partridge, these insecticides may be contributing to species decline [179, 180, 190]. Hematologic and biochemical changes associated with oral administration of up to 2.4 mg/kg imidacloprid for up to 28 days include decreased total leukocyte count, dose-dependent hypoglycemia, and increased serum glutamate oxaloacetate transaminase (SGOT, AST) activity [191]. In red-legged partridges (26 control, 27 exposed), many analytes were affected by fipronil-coated seed ingestion (mean ± SE of control/exposed): lutein (μM) 2.11 ± 0.17/1.66 ± 0.17, zeaxanthin (μM) 12.81 ± 1.07/7.57 ± 1.03, hematocrit (%) 42.9 ± 1.1/37.6 ± 1.3, albumin (g/l) 17.5 ± 0.4/15.5 ± 0.9, uric acid (mg/dl) 6.12 ± 0.48/17.3 ± 3.14, calcium (mg/dl) 13.1 ± 1.15/10.3 ± 0.56, magnesium (mg/dl) 3.17 ± 0.1/2.83 ± 0.13, total protein (g/l) 46.5 ± 1.2/40.2 ± 2.4, and triglycerides (mg/dl) 413 ± 89/202 ± 80 [191]. Monocytopenia has been noted in experimental toxicoses of the herbicide paraquat in quail [29].

Hormones

Chicken hormones vary with age, sex, time of day, season, temperature, diet, reproductive status, and handling stress [16, 192–195]. Reference data for select hormones of chickens are provided in Table 26.9.

Thyroid

The thyroid hormones of the chicken have similar growth and metabolic functions as their mammalian counterparts. In chickens, growth is controlled by growth hormone (GH), which stimulates insulin-like growth factor-1 (IGF-1) and triiodothyronine (T3) [141]. Both T3 and thyroxine (T4) rise from 28 to 42 days of age [86, 196]. Radioimmunoassays have been validated for T3 and T4 using avian serum [16, 145, 195]. In hens, the chemiluminescence immunoassay (CLIA) and an enzyme-linked immunosorbent assay (ELISA) are available for assay of avian serum thyroid hormones, but are comparable only in determination of free T4 (fT4).. Total T4 and T3 were comparatively higher, while fT3 was lower, via CLIA [193]. Autoimmune thyroiditis, with antibodies directed against the thyroglobulin molecule, occurs in obese-strain chickens and is linked to a defect in thyroidal uptake of dietary iodine. Antibodies can be detected via ELISA [197, 198]. Experimental vitamin A deficiency causes functional hypothyroidism in young chickens (see the section titled Vitamin). Clinically diagnosed thyroid dysfunction in non-research-purposed Galliformes appears to be rare, although histological abnormalities including neoplasia have been described in pheasant species [199, 200].

Corticosterone

In chickens, corticosterone, the dominant adrenal glucocorticoid, is controlled by negative feedback from corticosterone and thyroxine on the pituitary gland. A diurnal rhythm of corticosterone occurs in the chicken, turkey, and quail, with maximal plasma concentrations occurring at predawn or dawn [141, 201]. Radioimmunoassays have been validated for corticosterone using avian serum [16, 195, 202]. However, as neither clinical hypoadrenocorticism nor hyperadrenocorticism has been documented in Galliformes, these assays are largely relegated to research use.

Reproductive Hormones

Reproduction has been extensively studied in food-producing Galliformes such as the chicken, turkey, and Japanese quail. Many hormones are involved in avian reproduction, including gonadotropin-releasing hormone (GnRH), luteinizing hormone (LH), follicle stimulating hormone (FSH), testosterone, estradiol, progesterone, and prolactin [203, 204]. However, assays of these hormones are generally limited to research use, and clinical diagnostic use in the Galliforme appears rare. Use of GnRH agonist implants in quail appears to produce only short-term reductions in sex steroids and egg production [205].

Urinalysis

The avian kidney excretes nitrogenous wastes using ammonia, phosphate, and uric acid–urate buffer systems [206, 207]. Uric acid is synthesized in the liver (and in the kidney to a lesser extent) from purines and is actively secreted by proximal tubules [133]. Urinary uric acid is microscopically packaged into non-crystalline spheres (0.5–13 μm diameter) containing protein to avoid uric acid crystal obstruction of nephrons and ureters. Thus, liquid phase avian urine, within urate microspheres, has a higher protein concentration than mammalian urine. Albumin comprises approximately 60% of the many urinary proteins.

In the Galliforme, urinalysis is fraught with technical challenges and therefore is seldom preformed in clinical practice. Many Galliforme species are ground-dwelling birds that originate in tropical or arid environments requiring water conservation. Birds excrete nitrogenous wastes with protein in order to conserve water, as compared to the mammalian strategy that uses water for excretion and conserves protein [14]. Thus, urinary excreta of Galliformes are often pasty and dry with minimal liquid. Collection of urine is further complicated owing to the anatomically shared exit of urine and feces from the cloaca. Experimental techniques of urine collection include colostomy, ureteral cannulation, and ureteral exteriorization, but these require anesthesia and have complications [208]. In polyuric states, urine can be aspirated from a clean collection surface. In most instances in clinical practice, urine of the Galliforme may be contaminated with both reproductive tract and gastrointestinal tract materials.

Urinalysis (U/A) is indicated for full evaluation of the genitourinary system, for example, in states of polyuria, azotemia, uratemia, or if abnormal urates (e.g., green instead of normal white color) or genitourinary masses are present [133]. The liquid portion of urine should have a clear component with urine specific gravity lower than that of mammals (1.005–1.020). Urine is typically acidic in omnivores. Normal sediment may contain bacteria from fecal contamination, uric acid crystals that are needle shaped, uric acid microsphere precipitates, and squamous epithelial cells (if free-catch) [133]. Biliverdinuria is the pathologic equivalent of mammalian bilirubinuria and may be caused by fecal contamination, hemolytic anemia, or cholestasis. Unfortunately, commercial assays for biliverdin remain unavailable; thus, clinicians often arrive at the diagnosis by observing bright green feces, which may also be caused by diet constituents or anorexia. Urobilinogen dipstick test to confirm fecal contamination of the sample is not recommended for Galliformes, who are opportunistic carnivores. Hemoglobinuria may indicate intravascular hemolysis, which may occur secondary to lead toxicosis from backyard exposure to paint chips. Contamination of the sample with blood from the gastrointestinal or urogenital tracts may cause false positive results. Electrolyte fractional excretions can be performed on fresh or frozen (−20 °C) samples (Table 26.12) [122]. High-calcium diets in chickens enhance urinary excretion of calcium and chloride, reduce sodium, magnesium, and phosphate urinary excretion, and increase urinary pH [122].

Table 26.12 Urinary electrolyte concentrations for 16 female pullets, *Gallus gallus domesticus* [122].

Electrolyte	Excretion mmol/l (mEq/l); Mean ± SD
Calcium	3.36 ± 0.16 (6.72 ± 0.32)
Inorganic phosphorous	0.84 ± 0.16 (1.68 ± 0.32)
Sodium	18.73 ± 2.26 (18.73 ± 2.26)
Potassium	11.22 ± 1.65 (11.22 ± 1.65)
Magnesium	3.74 ± 0.01 (7.48 ± 0.02)
Chloride	2.61 ± 0.26 (2.61 ± 0.26)

Serology and PCR

Because commercial chicken flocks have specific requirements for interstate shipment and health assessment at slaughter, many PCR and serology assays are available for use in Galliformes. The validity and usefulness of these assays for Galliformes other than domestic poultry must be carefully evaluated by the clinician prior to sampling. Many options for testing are often available from a state or local diagnostic laboratory that specializes in poultry health. Contacting the laboratory regarding the appropriate sampling method and disease and species of interest is highly recommended prior to sampling. Results from species for which tests have not been validated may have regulatory consequences. A myriad of viral, bacterial, and other etiologic agents cause disease in chickens but are beyond the scope of this chapter. Many excellent texts are available for review of these diseases, for which the diagnostic options continue to expand [209–211]. As an example at the time of this writing, ELISA assays to assess exposure are commercially available for avian influenza, avian reovirus, chicken anemia virus, infectious bursal disease virus, Newcastle disease virus, avian encephalomyelitis virus, avian leukosis virus, avian rhinotracheitis, infectious bronchitis, infectious laryngotracheitis, Fowl Pox virus, reticuloendotheliosis, rotavirus, coccidiosis, *Mycoplasma* spp., *Bordetella avium*, *Pasteurella multocida* ("fowl cholera"), *Salmonella* spp., and *Escherichia coli*.

References

1 Kelly, L. and Alworth, L. (2013). Techniques for collecting blood from the domestic chicken. *Lab Animal* 42 (10): 359–361.

2 Arora, K. (2010). Differences in hemoglobin and packed cell volume in blood collected from different sites in Japanese quail (*Coturnix japonica*). *International Journal of Poultry Science* 9 (9): 828–830.

3 Campbell, T. and Ellis, C. (2013). *Avian and Exotic Animal Hematology and Cytology*. John Wiley & Sons.

4 Morishita, T. (2014). Chapter 18. Galliformes. In: *Fowler's Zoo and Wild Animal Medicine* (ed. R. Miller and M. Fowler), 143–155. Philadelphia PA: Elsevier Health Sciences.

5 Brandão, J., Cunha, A.F., Pypendop, B. et al. (2015). Cardiovascular tolerance of intravenous lidocaine in broiler chickens (*Gallus gallus domesticus*) anesthetized with isoflurane. *Veterinary Anaesthesia and Analgesia* 42 (4): 442–448.

6 Heard, D. (2014). Galliformes and columbiformes. In: *Zoo Animal and Wildlife Immobilization and Anesthesia*, 2e (ed. G. West, D. Heard and N. Caulkett), 473–480. Ames, Iowa: Wiley Blackwell.
7 Zimmermann, N. and Dhillon, A. (1985). Blood sampling from the venous occipital sinus of birds. *Poultry Science* 64 (10): 1859–1862.
8 Lumeij, J. and Westerhof, I. (1987). Blood chemistry for the diagnosis of hepatobiliary disease in birds. A review. *Veterinary Quarterly* 9 (3): 255–261.
9 Lumeij, J. (1987). The diagnostic value of plasma proteins and non-protein nitrogen substances in birds. *Veterinary Quarterly* 9 (3): 262–268.
10 Nordstrom, J. and Smith, A. (1970). Technique for multiple venipuncture blood sampling in the chicken. *Poultry Science* 49 (1): 329–330.
11 Orawan, C. and Aengwanich, W. (2007). Blood cell characteristics, hematological values and average daily gained weight of Thai indigenous, Thai indigenous crossbred, and boiler chickens. *Pakistan Journal of Biological Sciences* 10 (2): 302–309.
12 Martin, M., Wineland, M., and Barnes, H. (2010). Selected blood chemistry and gas reference ranges for broiler breeders using the i-STAT® handheld clinical analyzer. *Avian Diseases* 54 (3): 1016–1020.
13 Borges, S., Fischer da Silva, A., Majorka, A. et al. (2004). Physiological responses of broiler chickens to heat stress and dietary electrolyte balance (sodium plus potassium minus chloride, milliequivalents per kilogram). *Poultry Science* 83 (9): 1551–1558.
14 Janes, D. and Braun, E. (1997). Urinary protein excretion in red jungle fowl (*Gallus gallus*). *Comparative Biochemistry and Physiology Part A: Physiology* 118 (5): 1273–1275.
15 Peters, S., Gunn, H., Imumorin, I. et al. (2011). Haematological studies on frizzled and naked neck genotypes of Nigerian native chickens. *Tropical Animal Health and Production* 43 (3): 631–638.
16 Spano, J., Pedersoli, W., Kemppainen, R. et al. (1987). Baseline hematologic, endocrine, and clinical chemistry values in ducks and roosters. *Avian Diseases* 31 (4): 800–807.
17 Wight, P., Dewar, W., and Mackenzie, G. (1980). Monocytosis in experimental zinc deficiency of domestic birds. *Avian Pathology* 9 (1): 61–66.
18 Al-Sadi, H. and Hussein, E. (2010). Cytological evaluation of bone marrow in normal laying hens and those with lymphoid leukosis. *Veterinary World* 3 (11): 497–499.
19 McCartney, M. (1952). Total blood and corpuscular volume in turkey hens. *Poultry Science* 31 (1): 184–185.
20 Bond, C. and Gilbert, P. (1958). Comparative study of blood volume in representative aquatic and nonaquatic birds. *American Journal of Physiology - Legacy Content* 194 (3): 519–521.
21 Nirmalan, G. and Robinson, G. (1972). Effect of age, sex, and egg laying on the total erythrocyte volume (51CrO4 label) and the plasma volume (125I-serum albumin label) of Japanese quail. *Canadian Journal of Physiology and Pharmacology* 50 (1): 6–10.
22 Ploucha, J., Scott, J., and Ringer, R. (1981). Vascular and hematologic effects of hemorrhage in the chicken. *American Journal of Physiology* 240 (1): H9–H17.
23 Gildersleeve, R., Galvin, M., Thaxton, J., and McRee, D. (1985). Hematological response of Japanese quail to acute hemorrhagic stress. *Comparative Biochemistry and Physiology Part A: Physiology* 81 (2): 403–409.
24 Schindler, S., Gildersleeve, R., Thaxton, J., and McRee, D. (1987). Hematological response of hemorrhaged Japanese quail after blood volume replacement with saline. *Comparative Biochemistry and Physiology Part A: Physiology* 87 (4): 933–945.
25 Olayemi, F. (2009). Haematological changes in Guinea fowls (*Numida meleagris galeata*, Pallas) following haemorrhage. *International Journal of Poultry Science* 8 (11): 1093–1095.
26 Doneley, B. (2011). Clinical technique: techniques in the practice diagnostic laboratory – a review. *Journal of Exotic Pet Medicine* 20 (2): 117–123.
27 Latimer, K., Tang, K., Goodwin, M. et al. (1988). Leukocyte changes associated with acute inflammation in chickens. *Avian Diseases* 32 (4): 760.
28 Walberg, J. (2001). White blood cell counting techniques in birds. *Seminars in Avian and Exotic Pet Medicine* 10 (2): 72–76.
29 Irizaary-Rovira, A. (2004). Avian and reptilian clinical pathology (Avian hematology & biochemical analysis), Section XI. In: *Veterinary Clinical Pathology Secrets*, 282–313. St. Louis: Elsevier, Inc.
30 Uko, O. and Ataja, A. (1996). Effects of anticoagulants and storage (4° C) on packed cell volume (PCV) of Nigerian domestic fowl (*Gallus domesticus*) and guinea fowl (*Numida meleagris*). *British Poultry Science* 37 (5): 997–1002.
31 Garcia, R., Stein, S., and Piazza, G. (2014). Poultry Blood Preservation and the Impact of Preservation on Flocculant Activity. *Applied Engineering in Agriculture* 30 (3): 445–453.
32 Ihedioha, J., Idika, I., Ogamba, G., and Akam, C. (2008). Changes in the haematological values of avian blood samples stored at varying temperatures for a period of up to 72 hours. *Comparative Clinical Pathology* 17 (2): 73–79.
33 Hadzimusic, N., Katica, M., Muharemovic, Z., and Mušanovic, J. (2010). Effect of temperature storage on hematological parameters of avian turkey blood. *International Journal of Collaborative Research on Internal Medicine and Public Health* 2 (5): 158–166.
34 Hrubec, T., Whichard, J., Larsen, C., and Pierson, F. (2002). Plasma versus serum: specific differences in

biochemical analyte values. *Journal of Avian Medicine and Surgery* 16 (2): 101–105.

35 Jones, M. (1999). Avian clinical pathology. *Veterinary Clinics of North America: Exotics Animal Practice* 2 (3): 663–687.

36 Andreasen, J., Andreasen, C., Sonn, A., and Robeson, D. (1996). The effect of haemolysis on serum chemistry measurements in poultry. *Avian Pathology* 25 (3): 519–536.

37 MMereole, F. (1996). The study of haematologic parameters in the Nigerian local chicken. *Nigerian Journal of Animal Production* 23 (1): 94–97.

38 Beljan, J., Madley, T., Hellewell, A., and Hein, L. (1971). Determination of selected avian blood plasma chemistry values using the Technicon AutoAnalyzer;rM. *Poultry Science* 50 (1): 229–232.

39 Sharmin, M. and Myenuddin, M. (2004). Hematological values of the indigenous chickens. *Bangladesh Journal of Veterinary Medicine* 2 (2): 163–164.

40 Pampori, Z. and Iqbal, S. (2007). Haematology, serum chemistry and electrocardiographic evaluation in native chickens of Kashmir. *International Journal of Poultry Science* 6 (8): 578–582.

41 Sreekumar, K., Mejo, K., Jayavardhanan, K. et al. (2007). Certain haematobiochemical parameters of adult cochin and polish bantams. *Journal of Bombay Veterinary College* 15 (1–2): 70–73.

42 Krasnodebska-Depta, A. and Koncicki, A. (1999). Physiological values of hematological indices in chickens. *Polish Journal of Veterinary Sciences* 2 (4): 165–170.

43 Abdul-Rahman, S., Abdulmajeed, A., and Alkatan, M. (2009). Effect of sesame seeds on blood physiological and biochemical parameters in broiler breeder hens. *Iraqi Journal of Veterinary Sciences* 23 (1): 25–28.

44 Aksoy, F., Ertugrul, O., Atasoy, F. et al. (2000). A study on blood group alleles of Denizli fowl. *Turkish Journal of Veterinary and Animal Sciences* 24 (5): 431–434.

45 Samour, J., Naldo, J., Rahman, H., and Sakkir, M. (2010). Hematologic and plasma biochemical reference values in Indian peafowl (*Pavo cristatus*). *Journal of Avian Medicine and Surgery* 24 (2): 99–106.

46 Xiao-xia, X., Guo-hong, Q., Fu-min, Y. et al. (2015). Determination of blood physiological and biochemical values in blue peafowl. *Journal of Food and Nutritional Research* 3 (2): 104–108.

47 Nalubamba, K., Mudenda, N., and Masuku, M. (2010). Indices of health: clinical haematology and body weights of free-range Guinea fowl (*Numida meleagris*) from the southern province of Zambia. *International Journal of Poultry Science* 9 (12): 1083–1086.

48 Lloyd, S. and Gibson, J. (2006). Haematology and biochemistry in healthy young pheasants and red-legged partridges and effects of spironucleosis on these parameters. *Avian Pathology* 35 (4): 335–340.

49 Schmidt, E., Paulillo, A., Dittrich, R. et al. (2007). The effect of age on hematological and serum biochemical values on juvenile ring-necked pheasants (*Phasianus colchicus*). *International Journal of Poultry Science* 6 (6): 459–461.

50 Schmidt, E., Paulillo, A., Santin, E. et al. (2007). Hematological and serum chemistry values for the ring-necked pheasant (*Phasianus colchicus*). *International Journal of Poultry Science* 6 (2): 137–139.

51 Steinmetz, H., Vogt, R., Kastner, S. et al. (2007). Evaluation of the i-STAT portable clinical analyzer in chickens (*Gallus Gallus*). *Journal of Veterinary Diagnostic Investigation* 19 (4): 382–388.

52 Lima, A., Fehervari, T., Paasch, L., and Calderón, N. (2005). Haematological and histological findings in Leghorn chickens infected with infectious bursal disease virus strain 73668. *Acta Veterinaria Hungarica* 53 (4): 501–506.

53 Martinho, F. (2009). Indications and techniques for blood transfusion in birds. *Journal of Exotic Pet Medicine* 18 (2): 112–116.

54 Mitchell, E. and Johns, J. (2008). Avian hematology and related disorders. *Veterinary Clinics of North America: Exotic Animal Practice* 11 (3): 501–522.

55 Goodwin, M., Brown, J., Latimer, K., and Miller, S. (1991). Packed cell volume reference intervals to aid in the diagnosis of anemia and polycythemia in young leghorn chickens. *Avian Diseases* 35 (4): 820–823.

56 Goodwin, M., Davis, J., and Brown, J. (1992). Packed cell volume reference intervals to aid in the diagnosis of anemia and polycythemia in young broiler chickens. *Avian Diseases* 36 (2): 440–443.

57 Talebi, A., Asri-Rezael, S., Rozeh-Chai, R., and Sahraei, R. (2005). Comparative studies on haematological values of broiler strains (Ross, Cobb, Arbor-acres and Arian). *International Journal of Poultry Science* 4 (8): 573–579.

58 Král, I. and Suchý, P. (2000). Haematological studies in adolescent breeding cocks. *Acta Veterinaria Brno* 69 (3): 189–194.

59 Oyewale, J. (1987). Haematological studies on apparently healthy Nigerian domestic chickens (*Gallus domesticus*). *Bulletin of Animal Health and Production in Africa* 35 (2): 108–112.

60 Farahat, G., Abdel-Azim, A., and Osman, A. (2009). Breed differences and phenotypic correlations of antioxidant enzyme activities, some physiological parameters, and productive traits of chickens. *Egyptian Poultry Science* 29 (2): 623–644.

61 Galal, A., Abd El - Motaal, A., Ahmed, A., and Zaki, T. (2008). Productive performance and immune response of laying hens as affected by dietary propolis supplementation. *International Journal of Poultry Science* 7 (3): 272–278.

62 Peltonen, L. and Sankari, S. (2011). Ott's protein osmotic pressure of serum and interstitial fluid in chickens (*Gallus gallus*): effect of age and gender. *Journal of Experimental Biology* 214 (4): 599–606.

63 Biswas, A., Ahmed, M., Bharti, V., and Singh, S. (2011). Effect of antioxidants on physio-biochemical and hematological parameters in broiler chickens at high altitude. *Asian-Australasian Journal of Animal Sciences* 24 (2): 246–249.

64 Samanta, B., Ghosh, P., and Das, B.A. (2011). The effects of copper supplementation on the performance and hematological parameters of broiler chickens. *Asian-Australasian Journal of Animal Science* 24 (7): 1001–1006.

65 Diaz, G., Julian, R., and Squires, E. (1994). Cobalt-induced polycythaemia causing right ventricular hypertrophy and ascites in meat-type chickens. *Avian Pathology* 23 (1): 91–104.

66 Mandour, A., Hedaya, S., and Dowidar, Y. (1999). Usage of olive oil to alleviate the adverse effect of high dietary cholesterol on some biochemical and hematological traits in broiler chickens. *Assiut Veterinary Medical Journal* 41 (82): 72–87.

67 Shahbazfar, A., Mardjanmehr, S., Arab, H. et al. (2011). Effects of artemisinin in broiler chickens following chronic oral intake. *Tropical Animal Health and Production* 43 (4): 843–849.

68 Fudge, A. (1997). Avian clinical pathology – hematology and chemistry. In: *Avian Medicine and Surgery* (ed. R. Altman, S. Clubb, G. Dorrestein and K. Quesenbery), 142–147. Philadelphia: WB Saunders.

69 Fernandez, A., Verde, M., Gomez, J. et al. (1995). Changes in the prothrombin time, haematology and serum proteins during experimental aflatoxicosis in hens and broiler chickens. *Research in Veterinary Science* 58 (2): 119–122.

70 Bennett, G., Gabaldon, A., and Ulloa, G. (1982). Avian Haemoproteidae. 17. The haemoproteids of the avian family Cracidae (Galliformes); the guans, curassows and chachalacas. *Canadian Journal of Zoology* 60 (12): 3105–3112.

71 Bradley, R., Fedynich, A., and Lerich, S. (2004). Survey of hemoparasites in scaled quail from elephant mountain wildlife management area, Brewster County, Texas. *Texas Journal of Agriculture* 17: 18–22.

72 Fallis, A. and Jacobson, R. (1973). Haematozoa in domestic chickens and guinea fowl in Tanzania and transmission of Leucocytozoon neavei and Leucocytozoon schoutedeni. *The Journal of Protozoology* 20 (3): 438–442.

73 Gimba, F., Zakaria, A., Mugok, L. et al. (2014). Haemoparasites of domestic poultry and wild birds in Selangor, Malaysia. *Malaysian Journal of Veterinary Research* 5 (1): 43–51.

74 Kucera, J. (1 January 1982). Blood parasites of birds in Central Europe. 4. Trypanosoma, Atoxoplasma, microfilariae and other rare haematozoa. *Folia Parasitology* 29 (2): 107–113.

75 Silveira, P., DaMatta, R., and Dagosto, M. (2009). Hematological changes of chickens experimentally infected with *Plasmodium (Bennettinia) juxtanucleare*. *Veterinary Parasitology* 162 (3–4): 257–262.

76 Baldizán, G., Oviedo, M., Michelangeli, C., and Vargas, R. (2010). Effects of peach palm oil on performance, serum lipoproteins and haemostasis in broilers. *British Poultry Science* 51 (6): 784–790.

77 Calderón, N., Galindo-Muniz, F., Ortiz, M. et al. (2005). Thrombocytopenia in Newcastle disease: haematological evaluation and histological study of bone marrow. *Acta Veterinaria Hungarica* 53 (4): 507–513.

78 Hoerr, F. (2010). Clinical aspects of immunosuppression in poultry. *Avian Diseases* 5 (1): 2–15.

79 Johnson, S., Turrentine, M., and Swayne, D. (1985). Coagulation of plasma from the chicken (*Gallus domesticus*): Phospholipids influence clotting rates induced by components from Russell's viper venom. *Comparative Biochemistry and Physiology Part B: Comparative Biochemistry* 82 (4): 647–653.

80 Amrani, D., Mosesson, M., and Koide, T. (1985). Evidence that chicken antithrombin III is a developmentally regulated glycoprotein synthesized by hepatocytes. *Biochimica et Biophysica Acta (BBA) Molecular Cell Research* 847 (3): 324–334.

81 Stopforth, A. (1970). A study of coagulation mechanisms in domestic chickens. *Journal of Comparative Pathology* 80 (4): 525–533.

82 Thomson, A., Squires, E., and Gentry, P. (2002). Assessment of factor V, VII and X activities, the key coagulant proteins of the tissue factor pathway in poultry plasma. *British Poultry Science* 43 (2): 313–321.

83 Timms, L. (1977). The estimation of prothrombin time of chicken and turkey plasma using a phenol-saline thromboplastin or Russell viper venom. *British Veterinary Journal* 133 (6): 623–628.

84 Webster, K., Harr, K., Bennett, D. et al. (2015). Assessment of toxicity and coagulopathy of broadifacoum in Japanese quail and testing in wild owls. *Ecotoxicology* 24: 1087–1101.

85 Juarez-Estrada, M., Petrone Garcia, V., Valazco, X., and Tellez, G. (2001). Evaluation of the lee-white modified technique and three clotting time techniques in leghorn chicks. *Archivos de Medicina Veterinaria* 33 (1): 97–103.

86 Stojevic, Z., Milinkovic-Tur, S., and Curcija, K. (2000). Changes in thyroid hormone concentrations in chicken blood plasma during fattening. *Veterinarski Arhiv* 70 (1): 31–37.

87 Thapa, N., Muralimanohar, M., Balachandran, C., and Sarathchandra, G. (2009). Effects of aflatoxin mixed feed on haematobiochemical profile in layer chicken. *SAARC Journal of Agriculture* 7 (1): 85–90.

88 Thrall, M. (2004). *Veterinary Hematology and Clinical Chemistry*. Philadelphia: Lippincott Williams & Wilkins.

89 Watanabe, M., Yuge, M., Uda, A. et al. (2011). Structural and functional analyses of chicken liver ferritin. *Poultry Science* 90 (7): 1489–1495.

90 Doerr, J., Wyatt, R., and Hamilton, P. (1975). Investigation and standardization of prothrombin times in chickens. *Poultry Science* 54 (4): 969–980.

91 Quick, A. (1941). The prothrombin concentration in the blood of various species. *American Journal of Physiology* 132: 239–244.

92 Ramírez, G., Fehervari, T., Paasch, L., and Calderón, N. (2005). Haematological and histological findings in birds experimentally infected with highly pathogenic H5N2 avian influenza virus. *Acta Veterinaria Hungarica* 53 (4): 493–499.

93 Doerr, J., Huff, W., Tung, H. et al. (1974). A survey of T-2 toxin, ochratoxin, and aflatoxin for their effects on the coagulation of blood in young broiler chickens. *Poultry Science* 53 (5): 1728–1734.

94 Dietert, R., Golemboski, K., and Austic, R. (1994). Environment-immune interactions. *Poultry Science* 73 (7): 1062–1076.

95 Vohs, P. (1966). Blood group factors for analyzing pheasant populations. *Journal of Wildlife Management* 30 (4): 745–753.

96 Kass, L., Harrison, G., and Lindheimer, C. (2002). A new stain for identification of avian leukocytes. *Biotechnic and Histochemistry* 77 (4): 201–206.

97 Seliger, C., Schaerer, B., Kohn, M. et al. (2012). A rapid high-precision flow cytometry based technique for total white blood cell counting in chickens. *Veterinary Immunology and Immunopathology* 145 (1–2): 86–99.

98 Bowen, O., Dienglewicz, R., Wideman, R., and Erf, G. (2009). Altered monocyte and macrophage numbers in blood and organs of chickens injected i.v. with lipopolysaccharide. *Veterinary Immunology and Immunopathology* 131 (3–4): 200–210.

99 Clark, P., Boardman, W., and Raidal, S. (2009). *Atlas of Clinical Avian Hematology*. Oxford: Wiley-Blackwell.

100 De Boever, S., Croubels, S., Demeyere, K. et al. (2010). Flow cytometric differentiation of avian leukocytes and analysis of their intracellular cytokine expression. *Avian Pathology* 39 (1): 41–46.

101 Lilliehöök, I., Wall, H., Tauson, R., and Tvedten, H. (2004). Differential leukocyte counts determined in chicken blood using the Cell-Dyn 3500. *Veterinary Clinical Pathology* 33 (3): 133–138.

102 Karmakar, R. and Kundu, S. (1994). Variations in diurnal rhythm of leucocytes in white Leghorn chicks of two different ages. *Folia Biologica* 41 (2): 106–111.

103 Bartholomew, A., Latshaw, D., and Swayne, D. (1998). Changes in blood chemistry, hematology, and histology caused by a selenium/vitamin E deficiency and recovery in chicks. *Biological Trace Element Research* 62 (1): 7–16.

104 Chang, C., Huff, W., and Hamilton, P. (1979). A leucocytopenia induced in chickens by dietary ochratoxin A. *Poultry Science* 58 (3): 555–558.

105 Maxwell, M. (1993). Avian blood leucocyte responses to stress. *World's Poultry Science Journal* 49 (1): 34–43.

106 Branton, S., Lott, B., Deaton, J. et al. (1997). The effect of added complex carbohydrates or added dietary fiber on necrotic enteritis lesions in broiler chickens. *Poultry Science* 76 (1): 24–28.

107 Shini, S., Kaiser, P., Shini, A., and Bryden, W. (2008). Differential alterations in ultrastructural morphology of chicken heterophils and lymphocytes induced by corticosterone and lipopolysaccharide. *Veterinary Immunology and Immunopathology* 122 (1–2): 83–93.

108 Post, J., Rebel, J., and ter Huurne, A. (2003). Automated blood cell count: a sensitive and reliable method to study corticosterone-related stress in broilers. *Poultry Science* 82 (4): 591–595.

109 Campo, J. (2005). Effect of intermingling chicks and bird density on fear and stress responses in chickens. *Archiv fur Geflugelkunde* 69 (5): 199–205.

110 Boa-Amponsem, K., Price, S., Picard, M. et al. (2000). Vitamin E and immune responses of broiler pureline chickens. *Poultry Science* 79 (4): 466–470.

111 Cheng, H., Eicher, S., Chen, Y. et al. (2001). Effect of genetic selection for group productivity and longevity on immunological and hematological parameters of chickens. *Poultry Science* 80 (8): 1079–1086.

112 Karthiayini, K. and Philomina, P. (2008). Effect of overcrowding stress on haematological parameters of broiler chicken. *Indian Journal of Poultry Science* 43 (3): 313–316.

113 Bohls, R., Smith, R., Ferro, P. et al. (2006). The use of flow cytometry to discriminate avian lymphocytes from contaminating thrombocytes. *Developmental and Comparative Immunology* 30 (9): 843–850.

114 Carvallo, F., French, R., Gilbert-Marcheterre, K. et al. (2011). Mortality of one-week-old chickens during naturally occurring Marek's disease virus infection. *Veterinary Pathology* 48 (5): 993–998.

115 Singh, R., Agrawal, D., and Chauhan, R. (2005). Haemato-biochemical alterations in stunted chickens with experimental avian reovirus infection. *Indian Journal of Poultry Science* 40 (3): 296–298.

116 Rani, M., Ahmad, N., Prasad, P., and Sri, L.C. (2011). Hematological and biochemical changes of stunting syndrome in broiler chicken. *Veterinary World* 4 (3): 124–125.

117 Gray, H., Paradis, T., and Chang, P. (1989). Research note: physiological effects of adrenocorticotropic hormone and hydrocortisone in laying hens. *Poultry Science* 68 (12): 1710–1713.

118 Barrow, A., Burgess, S., Howes, K., and Nair, V. (2003). Monocytosis is associated with the onset of leukocyte and viral infiltration of the brain in chickens infected with the very virulent Marek's disease virus strain C 12/130. *Avian Pathology* 32 (2): 183–191.

119 Maxwell, M. and Robertson, G. (1995). The avian basophilic leukocyte: a review. *World's Poultry Science Journal* 51 (3): 307–325.

120 Maxwell, M. (1985). Nuclear Lobe Index in Avian Eosinophils. *Research in Veterinary Science* 38 (3): 361–363.

121 Maxwell, M., Hocking, P., and Robertson, G. (1992). Differential leucocyte responses to various degrees of food restriction in broilers, turkeys and ducks. *British Poultry Science* 33 (1): 177–187.

122 Guo, X., Huang, K., Chen, F. et al. (2008). High dietary calcium causes metabolic alkalosis in egg-type pullets. *Poultry Science* 87 (7): 1353–1357.

123 Kölling, K., Hofmeier, A., and Merkenschlager, M. (1992). Ionized calcium in blood of domestic fowl: dependence on ovulatory cycle. *Journal of Veterinary Medicine Series A* 39 (1–10): 115–120.

124 McDaniel, L. and Chute, H. (1961). Enzyme activity levels in chicken plasma. *American Journal of Veterinary Research* 22: 99–103.

125 Spano, J., Whitesides, J., Pedersoli, W., and Krista, L. (1988). Clinical chemistries by automated analysis in avian species. *Veterinary and Human Toxicology* 30 (Su. 1): 17.

126 Bowes, V., Julian, R., and Stirtzinger, T. (1989). Comparison of serum biochemical profiles of male broilers with female broilers and white leghorn chickens. *Canadian Journal of Veterinary Research* 53: 7–11.

127 Schmidt, E., Paulillo, A., Lapera, I. et al. (2010). Serum biochemical paramaters of female bronze turkeys (*Meleagris gallopavo*) during egg-laying season. *International Journal of Poultry Science* 9 (2): 177–179.

128 Harr, K. (2006). Diagnostic value of biochemistry. In: *Clinical Avian Medicine* (ed. G. Harrison and T. Lightfoot), 611–629. Palm Beach, Florida: Spix Publishing.

129 Goncalves, F., Ribeiro, E., Montagner, P. et al. (2010). Serum levels of liver enzymes in laying hens before and during the peak of egg production. *Acta Scientiae Veterinariae* 38 (3): 311–314.

130 Traesel, C., Wolkmer, P., Schmidt, C. et al. (2011). Serum biochemical profile and performance of broiler chickens fed diets containing essential oils and pepper. *Comparative Clinical Pathology* 20 (5): 453–460.

131 Kaya, S. (2007). Influence of different dietary vitamin E supplementation on some plasma components and egg production of laying Japanese quails during heat stress. *Medycyna Weterynaryjna* 63 (12): 1568–1571.

132 Scholtz, N., Halle, I., Flachowsky, G., and Sauerwein, H. (2009). Serum chemistry reference values in adult Japanese quail (*Coturnix coturnix japonica*) including sex-related differences. *Poultry Science* 88 (6): 1186–1190.

133 Harr, K. (2002). Clinical chemistry of companion avian species: a review. *Veterinary Clinical Pathology* 31 (3): 140–151.

134 Huff, W., Kubena, L., and Harvey, R. (1988). Progression of ochratoxicosis in broiler chickens. *Poultry Science* 67 (8): 1139–1146.

135 Elkin, R., Wood, K., and Hagey, L. (1990). Biliary bile acid profiles of domestic fowl as determined by high performance liquid chromatography and fast atom bombardment mass spectrometry. *Comparative Biochemistry and Physiology Part B: Comparative Biochemistry* 96 (1): 157–161.

136 Yeh, Y. and Hwang, D. (2001). High-performance liquid chromatographic determination for bile components in fish, chicken and duck. *Journal of Chromatography B, Biomedical Sciences and Applications* 751 (1): 1–8.

137 Crampton, D. and Wathen, L. (1990). HPLC assay for quantifying serum bile acids in several species. *Clinical Chemistry* 36 (12): 2142–2143.

138 Bromidge, E., Wells, J., and Wight, P. (1985). Elevated bile acids in the plasma of laying hens fed rapeseed meal. *Research in Veterinary Science* 39 (3): 378–382.

139 Matejcková, J., Tuma, P., Samcová, E., and Zemanová, Z. (2007). Determination of uric acid in plasma and allantoic fluid of chicken embryos by capillary electrophoresis. *Journal of Separation Science* 30 (12): 1947–1952.

140 Huff, W., Wyatt, R., and Hamilton, B. (1975). Nephrotoxicity of dietary ochratoxin A in broiler chickens. *Applied Microbiology* 30 (1): 48–51.

141 Scanes, C. (2009). Perspectives on the endocrinology of poultry growth and metabolism. *General and Comparative Endocrinology* 163 (1–2): 24–32.

142 Simon, J. and Rosselin, G. (1978). Effect of fasting, glucose, amino acids and food intake on in vivo insulin release in the chicken. *Hormone and Metabolic Research* 10 (2): 93–98.

143 Simon, J., Rideau, N., Taouis, M., and Dupont, J. (2011). Plasma insulin levels are rather similar in chicken and rat. *General and Comparative Endocrinology* 171 (3): 267–268.

144 Shiraishi, J., Yanagita, K., Fukumori, R. et al. (2011). Comparisons of insulin related parameters in commercial-type chicks: evidence for insulin resistance in broiler chicks. *Physiology and Behavior* 103 (2): 233–239.

145 Hoshino, S., Noda, M., Yamamoto, R., and Wakita, M. (1997). Radioimmunoassays for thyroid hormones in chicken serum. *Bulletin of the Faculty of Bioresources, Mie University, No.* 17: 1–5.

146 Sinsigalli, N.A., McMurtry, J.P., Cherry, J.A., and Siegel, P.B. (1987 May 1). Glucose tolerance, plasma insulin and immunoreactive glucagon in chickens selected for high and low body weight. *The Journal of nutrition.* 117 (5): 941–947.

147 Fendri, A., Frikha, F., Mosbah, H. et al. (2006). Biochemical characterization, cloning, and molecular modelling of chicken pancreatic lipase. *Archives of Biochemistry and Biophysics* 451 (2): 149–159.

148 Sato, K., Seol, H., and Kamada, T. (2010). Tissue distribution of lipase genes related to triglyceride metabolism in laying hens (*Gallus gallus*). *Comparative Biochemistry and Physiology Part B: Biochemistry and Molecular Biology* 156 (1): 62–66.

149 Kadhim, K., Zuki, A., Noordin, M. et al. (2011). Activities of amylase, trypsin, and chymotrypsin of pancreas and small intestinal contents in the red jungle fowl and broiler breed. *African Journal of Biotechnology* 10 (1): 108–115.

150 Pirone, A., Ding, B., Lenzi, C. et al. (2011). The small intestine of the adult New Hampshire chicken: an immunohistochemical study. *Anatomia, Histologia, Embryolgia* 40 (3): 163–168.

151 Esther, A., Iftach, S., and Esther, P. (1994). Troponin T of galliformes and craciformes. *FEBS Letters* 341: 308–311.

152 Jin, J. and Smillie, L. (1994). An unusual metal-binding cluster found exclusively in the avian breast muscle troponin T of Galliformes and Craciformes. *FEBS Letters* 341 (1): 135–140.

153 Maxwell, M., Robertson, G., and Moseley, D. (1994). Potential role of serum troponin T in cardiomyocyte injury in the broiler ascites syndrome. *British Poultry Science* 35 (5): 663–667.

154 Maxwell, M., Robertson, G., and Moseley, D. (1995). Serum troponin T concentrations in two strains of commercial broiler chickens aged one to 56 days. *Research in Veterinary Science* 58 (3): 244–247.

155 Kirchgessner, T., Heinzmann, C., Svenson, K. et al. (1987). Regulation of chicken apolipoprotein B: cloning, tissue distribution, and estrogen induction of mRNA. *Gene* 59 (2–3): 241–251.

156 Bakalli, R., Pesti, G., Ragland, W., and Konjufca, V. (1995). Dietary copper in excess of nutritional requirement reduces plasma and breast muscle cholesterol of chickens. *Poultry Science* 74 (2): 360–365.

157 Leszczynski, D. and Kummerow, F. (1982). Excess dietary lysine induces hypercholesterolemia in chickens. *Experientia* 38 (2): 266–267.

158 Durairaj, V., Okimoto, R., Rasaputra, K. et al. (2009). Histopathology and serum clinical chemistry evaluation of broilers with femoral head separation disorder. *Avian Diseases* 53 (1): 21–25.

159 Stockham, S. and Scott, M. (2008). *Fundamentals of Veterinary Clinical Pathology*. Ames, Iowa: Blackwell Publishing.

160 Giacobbo, F., Klosowski, E., Nunes, R. et al. (2014). Effect of different levels of crude protein and electrolyte balance on performance, blood parameters and bone characteristics for broiler chickens in phase of 36 to 42 days old. *Semina: Ciências Agrárias (Londrina)* 35 (4): 2175–2184.

161 Hamilton, R. and Thompson, B. (1980). Effects of sodium plus potassium to chloride ratio in practical-type diets on blood gas levels in three strains of white Leghorn hens and the relationship between acid-base balance and egg shell strength. *Poultry Science* 59 (6): 1294–1303.

162 Booth, B., Tsai, H., and Morris, R. (1977). Metabolic acidosis in the vitamin D-deficient chick. *Metabolism* 26 (10): 1099–1105.

163 Archer, F. and Battison, A. (1997). Differences in electrophoresis patterns between plasma albumins of the cockatiel (*Nymphicus hollandicus*) and the chicken (*Gallus gallus domesticus*). *Avian Pathology* 26 (4): 865–870.

164 Spano, J., Whitesides, J., Pedersoli, W. et al. (1988). Comparative albumin determinations in ducks, chickens, and turkeys by electrophoretic and dye-binding methods. *American Journal of Veterinary Research* 49 (3): 325–326.

165 Lumeij, J. and de Bruijne, J. (1985). Evaluation of the refractometric method for the determination of total protein in avian plasma or serum. *Avian Pathology* 14 (3): 441–444.

166 Andreasen, C., Latimer, K., Kircher, I., and Brown, J. (1989). Determination of chicken and turkey plasma and serum protein concentrations by refractometry and the biuret method. *Avian Diseases* 33 (1): 93–96.

167 Horrocks, N., Irene Tieleman, B., and Matson, K. (2011). A simple assay for measurement of ovotransferrin -- a marker of inflammation and infection in birds. *Methods in Ecology and Evolution* 2 (5): 518–526.

168 Giansanti, F., Leboffe, L., Pitari, G. et al. (2012). Physiological roles of ovotransferrin. *Biochimica et Biophysica Acta (BBA) - General Subjects* 1820 (3): 218–225.

169 Xie, H., Huff, G., Huff, W. et al. (2002). Identification of ovotransferrin as an acute phase protein in chickens. *Poultry Science* 81 (1): 112–120.

170 Wei, Z., Zhang, H., Jia, C. et al. (2007). Blood gas, hemoglobin, and growth of Tibetan chicken embryos incubated at high altitude. *Poultry Science* 86 (5): 904–908.

171 Candido, M., Silva, L., Moura, J. et al. (2011). Comparison of clinical parameters in captive Cracidae fed traditional and extruded diets. *Journal of Zoo and Wildlife Medicine* 42 (3): 437–443.

172 Pimentel, J., Cook, M., and Greger, J. (1992). Anemia induced by ingestion of excess zinc in chicks: importance of red blood cell turnover? *The Journal of Nutritional Biochemistry* 3 (3): 146–150.

173 Pimentel, J., Greger, J., Cook, M., and Stahl, J. (1992). Iron metabolism in chicks fed various levels of zinc and copper. *The Journal of Nutritional Biochemistry* 3 (3): 140–145.

174 Martin, M., Wineland, M., Fletcher, O., and Barnes, H. (2011). Selected blood chemistry values in mobility-impaired broiler breeder hens with suspected calcium tetany using the i-STAT® handheld clinical analyzer. *Avian Diseases* 55 (3): 340–345.

175 Yersin, A., Huff, W., Kubena, L. et al. (1992). Changes in hematological, blood gas, and serum biochemical variables in broilers during exposure to simulated high altitude. *Avian Diseases* 36 (2): 189–196.

176 Bar, A., Rosenberg, J., and Hurwitz, S. (1984). The lack of relationships between vitamin D3 metabolites and calcium-binding protein in the eggshell gland of laying birds. *Comparative Biochemistry and Physiology Part B: Comparative Biochemistry* 78 (1): 75–79.

177 Mohamed, S., Barri, M., Elbasheir, S. et al. (2015). The influence of feeding laying hens N-3 and N-6 fatty acids sources on blood antioxidants status: a comparative study. *Mediterranean Journal of Biosciences* 1 (1): 10–19.

178 Cinar, M., Yildrim, E., Yigit, A. et al. (2014). Effects of dietary supplementation with vitamin C and vitamin E and their combination on growth performance, some biochemical parameters, and oxidative stress induced by copper toxicity in broilers. *Biological Trace Element Research* 158 (2): 186–196.

179 Lopez-Antia, A., Ortiz-Santaliestra, M., Mougeot, F., and Mateo, R. (2013). Experimental exposure of red-legged partridges (*Alectoris rufa*) to seeds coated with imidacloprid, thiram and difenoconazole. *Ecotoxicology* 22 (1): 125–138.

180 Lopez-Antia, A., Ortiz-Santaliestra, M., Mougeot, F., and Mateo, R. (2015). Imidacloprid-treated seed ingestion has lethal effect on adult partridges and reduces both breeding investment and offspring immunity. *Environmental Research* 136: 97–107.

181 Nockels, C., Ewing, D., Phetteplace, H. et al. (1984). Hypothyroidism: an early sign of vitamin A deficiency in chickens. *The Journal of Nutrition* 114 (9): 1733–1736.

182 Klasing, K.C. (1988). Vitamins. In: *Comparative Avian Nutrition* (ed. K.C. Klasing), 277–329. New York: CABI Publishing.

183 Latshaw, J.D., Morishita, T.Y., Sarver, C.F., and Thilsted, J. (December 2004). Selenium toxicity in breeding ring-necked pheasants (*Phasianus colchicus*). *Avian Diseases* 48 (4): 935–939.

184 Dacke, C., Sugiyama, T., and Gay, C. Chapter 25: The role of hormones in the regulation of bone turnover and eggshell calcification. In: *Sturkie's Avian Physiology* (ed. C. Scanes), 557–558. Waltham MA: Elsevier.

185 Madhuri, D. and Verma, P. (2009). Effect of ochratoxin-A on pathology of hydropericardium syndrome in broiler chickens. *Indian Journal of Veterinary Pathology* 33 (1): 35–38.

186 Kawamura, O., Sato, S., Kajii, H. et al. (1989). A sensitive enzyme-linked immunosorbent assay of ochratoxin A based on monoclonal antibodies. *Toxicon* 27 (8): 887–897.

187 Lawellin, D., Grant, D., and Joyce, B. (1977). Enzyme-linked immunosorbent analysis for aflatoxin B1. *Applied and Environmental Microbiology* 34 (1): 94–96.

188 Trampel, D., Imerman, P., Carson, T. et al. (2003). Lead contamination of chicken eggs and tissues from a small farm flock. *Journal of Veterinary Diagnostic Investigation* 15 (5): 418–422.

189 Blalock, T. and Hill, C. (1988). Studies on the role of iron in zinc toxicity in chicks. *Biological Trace Element Research* 17 (1): 17–29.

190 Lopez-Antia, A., Ortiz-Santaliestra, M., Camarero, P. et al. (2015). Assessing the risk of fipronil-treated seed ingestion and associated adverse effects in the red-legged partridge. *Environmental Science & Technology* 49 (22): 13649–13657.

191 Balani, T., Agrawal, S., and Thaker, A. (2011). Hematological and biochemical changes due to short-term oral administration of imidacloprid. *Toxicology international* 18 (1): 2–4.

192 El-Slamony, A., Abdalla, E., Faddle, A. et al. (2015). Effect of supplementing selenium and zinc in diet on some sex hormones, productive, reproductive and physiological parameters of laying golden Montazah chickens during summer season. 1. The effect on females. *Egyptian Poultry Science Journal* 35 (3): 647–672.

193 Eshratkhah, B., Asad Zadeh, S., Forouzan, V. et al. (2010). Comparative study on the determination of serum thyroid hormones by two methods of immunoassay in broiler breeder poultry. *Comparative Clinical Pathology* 20 (4): 337–340.

194 Ngernsoungnern, P., Sartsoongnoen, N., Prakobsaeng, N. et al. (2012). Plasma leptin concentrations during the reproductive cycle in the native Thai chicken (*Gallus domesticus*). *Animal Reproduction Science* 136 (1): 115–120.

195 Zenoble, R., Kemppainen, R., Young, D., and Clubb, S. (1985). Endocrine responses of healthy parrots to

ACTH and thyroid stimulating hormone. *Journal of the American Veterinary Medical Association* 187 (11): 1116–1118.

196 Decuypere, E. and Kühn, E. (1988). Thyroid hormone physiology in galliformes: age and strain related changes in physiological control. *American Zoologist* 28 (2): 401–415.

197 Chan, C., Byfield, P., Chamption, B., and Himsworth, R. (1989). Selective autoimmune response to the chicken-specific structures of thyroglobulin in obese strain chickens. *Clinical and Experimental Immunology* 77 (1): 117–123.

198 Kofler, H., Kofler, R., Wolf, H. et al. (1984). Development of an enzyme-linked immunosorbent assay for the detection of autoantibodies against thyroglobulin in chickens. *Journal of Immunological Methods* 69 (2): 243–252.

199 Guadalupe Escorcia-Quintana, M., Leticia Calderon-Apodaca, N., and Garcia-Espinosa, G. (2008). Thyroid adenocarcinoma in a versicolor pheasant (*Phaisanus versicolor*). Case report. *Veterinaria Mexico* 39 (4): 435–441.

200 Wadsworth, P. and Jones, D. (1979). Some abnormalities of the thyroid gland in non-domesticated birds. *Avian Pathology* 8 (3): 279–284.

201 Carsia, R. (2014). Ch 26: Adrenals. In: *Sturkie's Avian Physiology* (ed. C.G. Scanes), 577–611. Waltham MA: Elsevier.

202 Hirschenhauser, K., Spreitzer, K., Lepschy, M. et al. (2012). Excreted corticosterone metabolites differ between two galliform species, Japanese quail and chicken, between sexes and between urine and faecal parts of droppings. *Journal of Ornithology* 153 (4): 1179–1188.

203 Ottinger, M. and Bakst, M. (1995). Endocrinology of the avian reproductive system. *Journal of Avian Medicine and Surgery* 9 (4): 242–250.

204 Silver, R. and Ball, G. (1989). Review: Brain, hormone and behavior interactions in avian reproduction: status and prospectus. *The Condor* 91 (4): 966–978.

205 Petritz, O., Guzman, D., Paul-Murphy, J. et al. (2013). Evaluation of the efficacy and safety of single administration of 4.7-mg deslorelin acetate implants on egg production and plasma sex hormones in Japanese quail (*Coturnix coturnix japonica*). *American Journal of Veterinary Research* 74 (2): 316–323.

206 Long, S. and Skadhauge, E. (1983). The role of urinary precipitates in the excretion of electrolytes and urate in the domestic fowl. *Journal of Experimental Biology* 104: 41–50.

207 Long, S. and Skadhauge, E. (1983). Renal acid excretion in the domestic fowl. *Journal of Experimental Biology* 104: 51–58.

208 Manangi, M., Clark, F., and Coon, C. (2007). Improved colostomy technique and excrement (urine) collection device for broilers and broiler breeder hens. *Poultry Science* 86 (4): 698–704.

209 Coles, B. (2000). Ch 12: Galliformes. In: *Avian Medicine* (ed. T. Tully, M. Lawton and G. Dorrestein), 266–295. Oxford, United Kingdom: Butterworth-Heinemann.

210 Greenacre, C. and Morishita, T. (2014). *Backyard Poultry Medicine and Surgery*. Hoboken: Wiley.

211 Miller, P. (2014). Newcastle disease in poultry (Avian pneumoencephalitis, exotic or velogenic Newcastle disease). In: *Merck Veterinary Manual* (ed. S. Aiello, M. Moses and M. Steigerwald). Merck Publishing Group https://www.merckvetmanual.com/poultry/newcastle-disease-and-other-paramyxovirus-infections/newcastle-disease-in-poultry.

27

Pigeons and Doves

Lauren Virginia Powers DVM, DABVP (Avian Practice) and DABVP (Exotic Companion Mammal Practice)[1] *and Devorah Marks Stowe DVM, DACVP (Clinical)*[2]

[1] *Avian and Exotic Pet Service, Carolina Veterinary Specialists, Huntersville, North Carolina, USA*
[2] *Clinical Pathology, North Carolina State University, Raleigh, North Carolina, USA*

Introduction

This chapter reviews the available literature for clinical pathology of columbiformes (pigeons and doves) (Table 27.1). The extensive use of the rock pigeon (*Columba livia*) in research, disease surveillance, aviculture, hobby, and food has provided the vast majority of reported data for *C. livia*. Fewer studies have focused on columbiformes in states of experimentally induced or naturally acquired disease. Even fewer studies have investigated the clinical pathology of free-ranging, endangered, or threatened columbiforme species [1, 2].

Species

The avian order Columbiformes includes two families, the family Columbidae (pigeons and doves), and the family Pteroclididae (sandgrouse). Within the family Columbidae, there are approximately 290 species. The terms "pigeon" and "dove" are used interchangeably, although the term "dove" is typically reserved for smaller species [3]. Pigeon domestication is the earliest known for any avian species. There are more than 800 domestic varieties of the rock pigeon (*C. livia*, referred to here as "pigeon"), and over 200 recognized breeds by the National Pigeon Association of the United States [4]. Worldwide, domestic pigeons comprise approximately 50% of birds in captivity, and global populations of feral pigeons are estimated as at least 500 million birds [4, 5].

The pigeon is a stout, hardy, medium-sized, long-lived bird [4]. The smallest living columbiforme species is the diamond dove (*Geopelia cuneata*) at 23–37 g, while the largest is the Victoria crowned pigeon at up to 3.0 kg in body weight. The homing (racing) pigeon is capable of high speed flights over remarkably long distances and returns to its roost after release, attributes ideal for racing [4]. At about two to three years of age, the racing pigeon reaches maximum physiologic performance, which remains high until about seven to nine years of age [6]. Pigeons are raised for a variety of purposes, including racing, show, research, and human consumption (squab) [4]. The pigeon is used as a model for human disease (e.g., atherosclerosis) and is used in environmental toxicologic and infectious disease surveillance studies.

Other columbiforme species are bred for public exhibits and private collections. Species commonly kept in zoos include the Victoria crowned pigeon (*Goura victoria*) and fruit doves. Examples of domestic doves kept in aviculture include the Chinese lace-necked dove (*Streptopelia chinensis*), diamond dove (*G. cuneata*), and the European ring-necked or ringed dove (*Streptopelia risoria*). Columbiforme species native to the United States include the mourning dove (*Zenaida macroura*), white-winged dove (*Columba asiatica*), band-tailed pigeon (*Columba fasciata*), white-crowned pigeon (*Columba leucocephala*), and Inca dove (*Scardafella inca*). Recent population declines have been observed in several native columbiforme species, including the mourning dove, which may be associated with exposure to environmental contaminants, overhunting, or habitat declines [7]. Pigeon species considered threatened or endangered include the Nicobar (*Caloenas nicobarica*), pheasant (*Otidiphaps nobilis*), common crowned (*Goura cristata*), Victoria crowned, and Scheepmaker's crowned (*Goura scheepmakeri*) pigeons [2].

Sample Collection

Handling and Restraint

Handling and restraint time should always be kept to a minimum in any avian species [8, 9]. Manual restraint is usually sufficient for sample collection in most

Exotic Animal Laboratory Diagnosis, First Edition. Edited by J. Jill Heatley and Karen E. Russell.

Table 27.1 Columbiformes commonly presented for veterinary care.

Common name(s)	Scientific name
Rock pigeon; rock dove; domestic pigeon; pigeon	*Columba livia*
Mourning dove	*Zenaida macroura*
Galapagos dove	*Zenaida galapagoensis*
European ring-necked; ringed dove	*Streptopelia risoria*
Eurasian collared dove	*Streptopelia decaocto*
Nigerian laughing dove	*Streptopelia senegalensis*
Chinese lace-necked dove	*Streptopelia chinensis*
Pink pigeon	*Columba mayen*
Wood pigeon	*Columba palumbus*
White-winged dove	*Columba asiatica*
Band-tailed pigeon	*Columba fasciata*
White-crowned pigeon	*Columba leucocephala*
Victoria crowned pigeon	*Goura victoria*
Common crowned pigeon	*Goura cristata*
Scheepmaker's crowned pigeon	*Goura scheepmakeri*
Peaceful dove	*Geopelia cuneata*
Diamond dove	*Geopelia cuneata*
Inca dove	*Scardafella inca*
Nicobar pigeon	*Caloenas nicobarica*
Pheasant pigeon	*Otidiphaps nobilis*

columbiformes. However, in timid species, injectable sedation or gas anesthesia may be used to facilitate sample collection. Appropriate fasting should be considered in columbiformes, as regurgitation is common in these species. During 3 h of handling in pigeons, the relative heterophil count more than doubled, and the relative lymphocyte count dropped. Creatine phosphokinase (CK) activity and glucose concentration increased, while uric acid concentration decreased [9].

Blood Volume and Sample Size Limitations

The blood volume of pigeons at 140–210 ml/kg body weight is among the highest of avian species of similar size, which may be an adaptation to a high oxygen demand from rigorous flight [10–13]. Most clinical references suggest not exceeding 1% body weight (10 ml/kg) for blood sample collection volumes in birds, particularly in clinically ill patients, and these guidelines should be followed when possible for pigeons [8, 14]. However, one study demonstrated that adverse effects were not seen in pigeons until 3% of body weight (30 ml/kg) was drawn, considerably more than chickens (2%) and crows and pheasants (1%) [15].

Sample Collection Sites

Veins commonly used in pigeons are the ulnar, brachial, and medial metatarsal veins [8, 13, 16, 17]. In pigeons, the jugular vein is obscured by the *plexus venosus intracutaneous collaris* [4, 8, 18] (Figures 27.1, 27.2, and 27.3). This plexus of anastamosing vessels runs from the head to the base of the neck and is divided dorsally into left and right sections [4]. This plexus is used for sexual display and thermoregulation [4]. Jugular venipuncture is not advised in pigeons based on the risk of life-threatening hemorrhage from this plexus. Vaccines should not be administered in this anatomical site, as deaths immediately following vaccination using oil-adjuvanted avian paramyxovirus-1 vaccines in this area have been reported in pigeons (Figure 27.4) [4, 18].

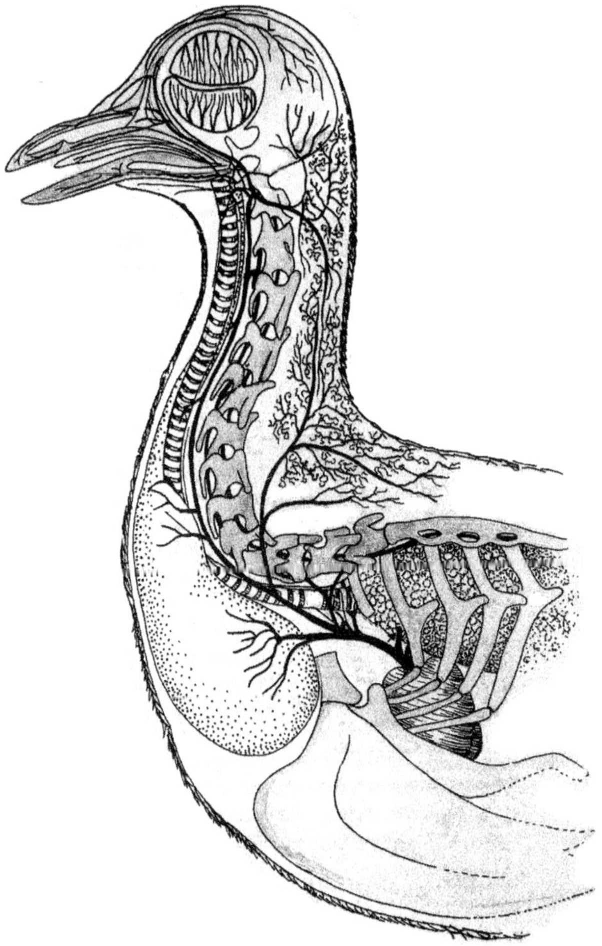

Figure 27.1 Illustration of the *plexus venosus intracutaneous collaris* in the pigeon, *Columba livia* [17]. *Source:* Figure adapted from Brückner 1987 and used with permission. 1 – *V. jugularis*; 2 – *V. cervicalis cutanea descendens*; 3 – *Vv. cutaneacolli*; 4 – *V. cervicalis cutanea ascendens*; 5 – *Plexus venosus subcutaneous collaris.*

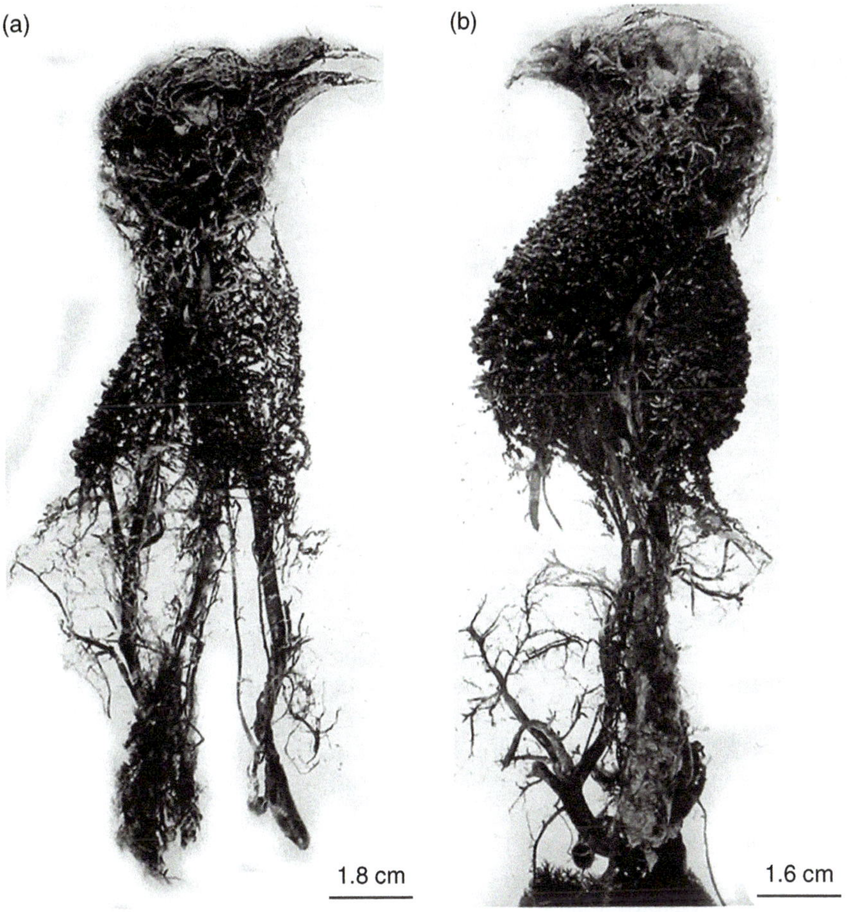

Figure 27.2 Latex casting of vascular structures including the *plexus venosus intracutaneous collaris* in the female (a) and male (b) pigeon (*Columba livia*). *Source:* Photo by Dorothea Brückner provided by Erhard F. Kaleta, Klinik für Vögel, Reptilien, Amphibien und Fische, Justus-Liebig-Universität Gießen, Germany.

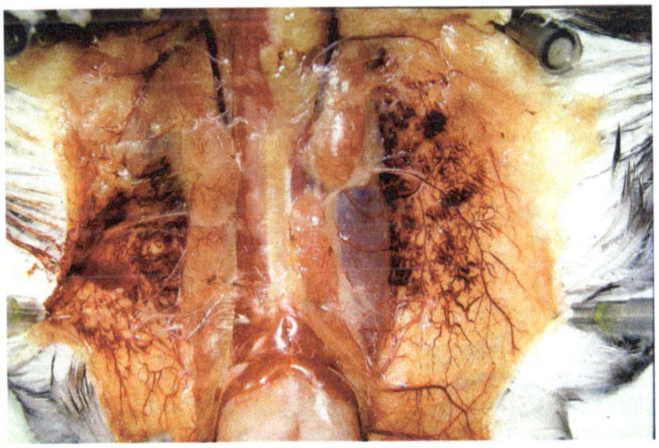

Figure 27.3 *Plexus venosus intracutaneous collaris* in the male pigeon, *Columba livia*, dorsal dissection. Because of the thin wall of the blood vessels, some extravasal blood is visible. *Source:* Photo by Dorothea Brückner provided by Erhard F. Kaleta, Klinik für Vögel, Reptilien, Amphibien und Fische, Justus-Liebig-Universität Gießen, Germany.

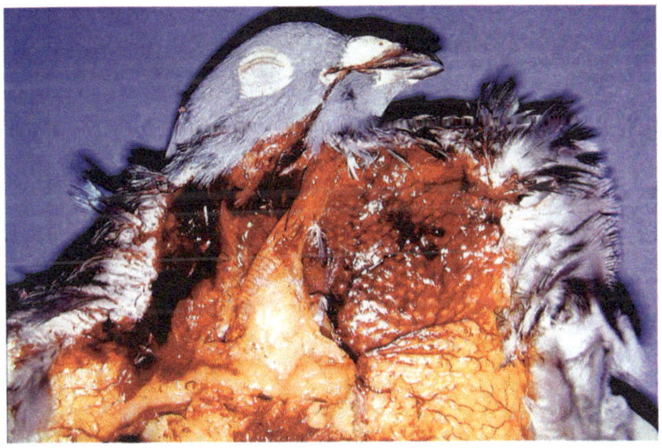

Figure 27.4 Apoplectiform death of a pigeon (*Columba livia*) from massive hemorrhage of the *plexus venosus intracutaneous collaris* after vaccination with an inactivated oil-adjuvanted avian paramyxovirus-1 vaccine paramedian to the cervical vertebral column. *Source:* Photo by Dorothea Brückner provided by Erhard F. Kaleta, Klinik für Vögel, Reptilien, Amphibien und Fische, Justus-Liebig-Universität Gießen, Germany.

Sample Handling

If hematology is performed, blood smears should be made as soon as possible to reduce undesired changes in cellular morphology [8]. If plasma or serum is to be harvested, the blood sample should be centrifuged immediately after collection [8]. In pigeon blood held at room temperature, plasma potassium concentration decreased by approximately 60% within 2 h, likely associated with a shift of potassium ions from the plasma into the erythrocytes [7, 8, 17].

Anticoagulants

For pigeon blood [19], disodium and dipotassium salts of ethylenediaminetetraacetic acid (EDTA) were superior to heparin (unstated salt) in delaying hemolysis, although hemolysis still occurred with both heparin and EDTA over time. In contrast, when sodium heparin, EDTA, trisodium citrate, and disodium oxalate were compared as anticoagulants for pigeon blood in a subsequent study [20], sodium heparin affected blood pH, hematocrit (HCT), osmolarity, and plasma protein concentrations the least.

Specific Analytes

Complete Blood Count (CBC)

Hematocrit (HCT, or Packed Cell Volume, PCV)

Age, sex, migration, geographical elevation, energy expenditure, parasitism, nutrition, genetics, and reproduction can strongly influence the HCT of pigeons [6, 16, 21–23]. The pigeon HCT is one of the highest of avian species studied [13, 24]. In pigeons, the maximum HCT occurs at two to three years of age and decreases linearly beginning at seven to nine years [6]. Molt, breeding activity, summer months, and a sedentary lifestyle are associated with a lower HCT in columbiformes [2, 6, 11, 16, 18, 25]. Egg laying (likely based on dehydration), free flight, and winter months are associated with higher HCT in columbiformes [2, 11, 18, 25].

Hemoglobin (Hb)

For powerful flight capabilities, Hb concentrations in flying pigeons are among the highest in birds of similar size and higher than those in ground-dwelling columbiformes [2, 13, 24, 26]. Adult pigeons have a higher Hb concentration than immature birds [23]. In feral pigeons, Hb concentration is highest during the winter [11, 23]. Male pigeons and ring-necked doves have higher Hb concentrations than females in all seasons [27].

Erythrocytes and Thrombocytes

Pigeons and doves have nucleated erythrocytes similar in appearance to other avian species, and morphologic changes that occur with disease are likely similar. The mean erythrocyte life span in pigeons was 17–25 days by Cr [28] labeling and 21 ± 3.4 days by iron kinetics [29]. In a separate study [30], the maximum erythrocyte life span as determined by radiochromium tagging in the adult pigeon was 35–45 days. The pigeon has among the highest RBC counts (erythrocyte number) of birds studied, which is likely attributable to flying activity [24, 26]. The RBC count of flying pigeon species is higher than ground-dwelling columbiformes [2]. Adult pigeons have higher RBC counts than immature birds, which may also be associated with flight [23]. Male pigeons have a higher RBC count than females throughout the year [11]. The RBC count is highest in the winter and lowest during the summer in pigeons [11]. The reticulocyte count in pigeons ranges from 4% to 12%, with no sex differences observed [13]. No studies investigating thrombocyte counts or morphology specific to columbiforme species were found by the authors.

Red Cell Indices

The mean corpuscular volume (MCV), mean corpuscular hemoglobin (MCH), and the mean corpuscular hemoglobin concentration (MCHC) can be calculated for pigeons and other birds using the same formulas as for mammals [1]. The most common erythrocyte parameters used to assess the health of the avian patient are HCT, Hb, MCV, and MCHC. MCH is higher in young birds [23]. Hematologic indices in young pigeons should approach adult values by about four weeks of age [31]. In feral pigeons, the MCV and the MCH were highest in the winter, possibly in preparation for reproduction [23]. The MCHC in the Nigerian laughing dove (*Streptopelia senegalensis*) was higher than that of the Nigerian duck (*Anas platyrhynchos*), possibly owing to flight activity [26].

Leukocytes

Lymphocytes are the predominant leukocyte in columbiformes, followed by heterophils (Table 27.2) [23, 32]. In feral pigeons, the WBC count was highest in the winter months [23]. Changes in leukocyte counts and morphology in varied physiologic conditions and states of health are similar to those seen in other avian species. In seropositive pigeons latently infected with *Chlamydia* spp., a decrease in the WBC count (36,670 ± 12 600/μl to 22,330 ± 9140/μl), a decrease in lymphocytes (50.03 ± 15.65 to 39.06 ± 17.71%), and an increase in monocytes (2.58 ± 1.78 to 12.53 ± 5.61%) occurred, possibly related to chronic immunostimulation [23].

Hemoparasites

Blood parasites are commonly observed on blood smear evaluation of wild columbiformes. About 1/3 of wild pigeons and doves had hemoparasites on blood smear evaluation. Common hemoparasites are *Hemoproteus* spp., *Plasmodium* spp., trypanosomes, microfilariae, and *Leukocytozoon* spp. [11, 33] *Hemoproteus* spp. infection pathogenicity is usually low unless the bird is immunocompromised. Clinical findings with *Hemoproteus* spp. infection can include anorexia, depression, hepatomegaly, splenomegaly, leukocytosis, and hemolytic anemia. Infected birds had increased alanine aminotransferase (ALT) and aspartate aminotransferase (AST) activities and a decrease in albumin concentration, possibly from damage caused by hepatic migration of the parasite [34].

Table 27.2 Hematologic reference data for some columbiforme species.

Analyte (abbreviation)	Units, SI (conventional)	Pigeon, or rock dove (*Columba livia*)		Nicobar pigeon [2] (*Caloenas nicobarica*)	Pheasant pigeon [2] (*Otidiphaps nobilis*)	Common crowned pigeon [2] (*Goura cristata*)	Victoria crowned pigeon [2] (*Goura victoria*)	Nigerian laughing dove [63,†] (*Streptopelia senegalensis*)
Data Format		Mean ± SD [Range]	Mean ± SD	Mean ± SD [Range]	Mean ± SD [Range]	Mean ± SD [Range]	Mean ± SD [Range]	Mean ± SD
Animals Sampled		Adult non-breeding unknown sex [1, 6, 24] n = 136–145 [6], 30 [1], 9 [24]	Male ♂, n = 15–20 [10] Female ♀, n = 15–25 [10, 16]	n = 16	n = 3	n = 9	n = 6	Male ♂ n = 14 Female ♀ n = 7
Hematocrit	%	61.1 ± 4.0 [50.7–68.8] [6] 49.3 ± 6.4 [17.65–58.51] [1] 50.2 ± 3.1 [24]	50.60 ± 1.02 ♂ 44.4 ± 1.09 Non-Laying ♀ 54.4 ± 1.027 Incubating ♀ 40.6 ± 1.327	50.7 ± 2.6 [45.0–56.0]	41.7 ± 9.0 [33.0–51.0]	34.3 ± 3.3 [30.0–39.5]	37.6 ± 3.8 [33.8–42.0]	43.58 ± 7.33 ♂ 44.57 ± 6.88 ♀
Hemoglobin	g/l (g/dl)	207 ± 21 [133–241] *(20.7 ± 0.21 [13.3–24.1])* [6] 156 ± 22 [120–192] *(15.6 ± 2.2 [12–19.2])* [1] 165 ± 16 (16.5 ± 1.6) [24]	169 ± 3.5 ♂ *(16.91 ± 0.35)* 132 ± 5.1 ♀ *(13.22 ± 0.51)*	170 ± 15 *(17.0 ± 1.5)* [127–197] *(12.7–19.7)*	139 ± 28 *(13.9 ± 2.8)* [114–170] *(11.4–17.0)*	108 ± 15 *(10.8 ± 1.5)* [82–127] *(8.2–12.7)*	126 ± 16 (12.6 ± 1.6) [106–147] *(10.6–14.7)*	148.60 ± 22.10 ♂ *(14.8 ± 2.21)* ♂ 157.80 ± 22.90 ♀ *(15.8 ± 2.29)* ♀
Erythrocytes (red blood cells; RBC)	$10^6/\mu l$	3.85 ± 0.53 [2.10–4.91] [6] 3.49 ± 0.92 [0.86–5.32] [1] 3.74 ± 0.5 [24]	2.64 ± 0.13 ♂ 2.28 ± 0.123 ♀	3.40 ± 0.47 [2.67–4.33]	2.6 ± 0.4 [2.26–3.00]	2.23 ± 0.35 [1.80–2.80]	2.31 ± 0.23 [1.95–2.60]	2.78 ± 0.44 ♂ 2.97 ± 0.24 ♀
Erythrocyte length	μm	12.7 ± 0.6 [11.1–15.6] [6]		13.90 ± 0.92 [12.4–5.9]	13.47 ± 0.77 [12.0–15.0]	14.11 ± 1.09 [12.0–17.1]	13.65 ± 0.69 [12.0–14.7]	
Erythrocyte width	μm	7.3 ± 0.5 [5.4–9.1] [6]		7.30 ± 0.42 [6.5–8.5]	7.59 ± 0.54 [6.5–8.6]	6.11 ± 0.73 [5.4–8.5]	8.15 ± 0.72 [6.9–8.2]	
Nucleus length	μm	7.0 ± 1.0 [4.0–9.4] [6]		6.62 ± 0.75 [5.1–8.6]	6.28 ± 0.75 [5.1–8.6]	6.11 ± 0.73 [4.9–8.2]	5.85 ± 0.69 [4.2–7.6]	
Nucleus width	μm	2.6 ± 0.4 [1.3–4.6] [6]		2.65 ± 0.75 [2.2–3.2]	2.90 ± 0.33 [2.3–3.6]	2.89 ± 0.27 [2.3–3.6]	2.87 ± 0.29 [2.3–3.4]	
Mean corpuscular volume (MCV)	fl	162 ± 25 [117–260] [6] 156.8 ± 698 [90.36–456] [1] 135.50 ± 14.74 [24]	181.36 ± 6.56 ♂ 220.66 ± 16.31♀	149.8 ± 16.5 [127.6–168.5]	153.7 ± 12.1 [146.0–170.0]	158.7 ± 14.7 [142.9–175.0]	166.9 ± 18.2 [134.6–178.3]	160.10 ± 36.52 ♂ 150.09 ± 18.42 ♀
Mean (MCH) corpuscular hemoglobin	Pg	45.9 ± 13.7 [30.65–91.9] [1] 44.39 ± 3.25 [24]	68.28 ± 2.91 ♂	50.0 ± 5.5 [41.3–57.6]	53.3 ± 3.1 [50.4–56.6]	50.8 ± 5.2 [44.2–57.3]	55.0 ± 7.3 [42.5–61.3]	55.06 ± 12.89 ♂ 53.12 ± 5.93 ♀
Mean (MCHC) corpuscular hemoglobin concentration	%	34 ± 3 [23–41] [6] 31.7 ± 5 [21.43–42.91] [1] 32.91 ± 2.04 [24]	33.45 ± 0.88 ♂ 30.37 ± 1.59 ♀	33.5 ± 1.8 [28.3–36.1]	33.6 ± 0.8 [33.1–34.5]	31.9 ± 4.3 [27.9–38.0]	32.6 ± 1.5 [31.1–15.0]	34.95 ± 5.37 ♂ 35.64 ± 4.28 ♀

(*Continued*)

Table 27.2 (Continued)

Analyte (abbreviation)	Units, SI (conventional)	Pigeon, or rock dove (*Columba livia*)		Nicobar pigeon [2] (*Caloenas nicobarica*)	Pheasant pigeon [2] (*Otidiphaps nobilis*)	Common crowned pigeon [2] (*Goura cristata*)	Victoria crowned pigeon [2] (*Goura victoria*)	Nigerian laughing dove [63,†] (*Streptopelia senegalensis*)
Data Format		Mean ± SD [Range]	Mean ± SD	Mean ± SD [Range]	Mean ± SD [Range]	Mean ± SD [Range]	Mean ± SD [Range]	Mean ± SD
Animals Sampled		Adult non-breeding unknown sex [1, 5, 24] n = 136–145 [6], 30 [1], 9 [24]	Male ♂, n = 15–20 [10] Female ♀, n = 15–25 [10, 16]	n = 16	n = 3	n = 9	n = 6	Male ♂ n = 14 Female ♀ n = 7
Leukocytes (white blood cells; WBC)	$10^3/mm^3$	9.7 ± 4.3 [1.63–29.2] [6] 11.46 ± 8.53 [1.10–40.26] [1]	12.81 ± 0.67 ♂ 11.69 ± 0.59 ♀	4.23 ± 1.92 [2.00–8.25]	6.91 ± 2.43 [4.12–8.62]	17.71 ± 4.87 [11.75–25.12]	10.85 ± 6.54 [5.13–20.75]	0.75 ± 0.28 ♂ 0.64 ± 0.26 ♀
Heterophils	%	55.4 ± 9.1 [28–71] [1]		52.2 ± 15.7 [42–71]	54.1 ± 11.4 [46–67]	66.0 ± 9.0 [55–78]	52.8 ± 12.0 [40–70]	
Lymphocytes	%	30.7 ± 6.6 [21–52] [1]		37.4 ± 9.9 [27–51]	42.5 ± 13.6 [27–51]	30.3 ± 8.4 [18–40]	44.6 ± 12.1 [27–58]	
Monocytes	%	3.7 ± 2.6 [0–12] [1]		21. ± 1.6 [1–5]	1.6 ± 0.8 [0–2]	1.0 ± 0.5 [0–2]	0.7 ± 0.8 [0–2]	
Eosinophils	%	7.3 ± 3.4 [2–16] [1]		2.7 ± 2.3 [1–9]	0.6 ± 1.1 [0–2]	24 ± 1.4 [1–5]	0.7 ± 0.8 [1–4]	
Basophils	%	3.0 ± 2.5 [0–11] [1]		0 [0]	1.2 ± 1.2 [0–2.5]	0.25 ± 0.5 [0–1]	0.3 ± 0.5 [0–1]	

Values reported as mean ± SD and/or [Range]; Φ Non-breeding adult unless otherwise noted.

Multiple species of Hemoproteus have been observed in numerous species, clinical differences remain unknown, but species may be PCR speciated and may be variably present based on bird species, age, and region [35, 36].

Hemoproteus multipigmentatus is endemic in the Galapagos dove (*Zenaida galapagoensis*) populations [37]. *H. multipigmentatus* can be distinguished from other subspecies by the presence of numerous small pigment granules in the mature gametocytes [37].

Pigeons are highly susceptible to *Plasmodium* spp., which can cause anorexia, depression, hemoglobinuria, biliverdinuria, and sudden death. Splenomegaly and hepatomegaly may be observed on postmortem exam. Anemia, leukocytosis, and lymphocytosis may be present in infected birds. *Leucocytozoon marchouxi* in a pink pigeon (*Columba mayen*) population was more prevalent and more likely to result in severe pathology in juvenile birds, with an overall prevalence rate of 18.3% [38]. Microfilariae are common in blood smears of avian species, and most are nonpathogenic to the host; columbiformes appear to be no exception to this generality.

Hemostasis, Blood Types, and Cross-Matching

Coagulation assays are more likely to be performed in the research setting than in the clinical setting for avian species. Coagulation assays in birds often include prothrombin time (PT) and activated partial thromboplastin time (APTT). Appropriate equipment and avian-specific reagents should be used if available. No published data specific to columbiforme species are available. To the best of the authors' knowledge, no studies have evaluated blood types and cross-matching in columbiformes.

Biochemical Panel

Liver Enzymes

Assessment of muscle enzymes such as creatine phosphokinase (CK) should be performed to differentiate causes of hepatic enzyme elevations in birds [39]. AST activity increased fourfold for 140 h, and ALT activity increased fivefold for 214 h after intramuscular (IM) injection of doxycycline in pigeons [8, 39]. The half-lives of ALT and AST are longer than for CK and lactate dehydrogenase (LDH) in pigeons [39, 40]. The mean elimination half-life of liver-derived AST and ALT in six pigeons was 7.66 ± 1.55 and 15.69 ± 1.70 h, respectively, while the mean elimination half-life of muscle-derived CK and liver-derived LDH were 3.07 ± 0.59 and 0.71 ± 0.10 h, respectively [40].

The most sensitive plasma enzyme indicator of liver disease in pigeons induced by administration of ethylene glycol or D-galactosamine was AST, followed by ALT, gamma-glutamyltransferase (GGT), and LDH [8, 39]. ALT activity increased sooner than LDH, and the relative increase in ALT activity was greater than for LDH and persisted longer despite the high concentrations of LDH in the liver. These findings relate to the enzyme elimination half-life of LDH, which is comparatively short [8, 39]. Aflatoxin B_1–induced hepatotoxicosis in pigeons increased activities of AST and ALT and LDH [41]. Activities of AST and ALT increased after IM administration of carprofen in pigeons, which caused myositis, myodegeneration, hepatic necrosis, and hepatic lipidosis [42].

The mitochondrial enzyme glutamate dehydrogenase (GDH, GMD, GLD, and GLDH) is a specific indicator of hepatocellular necrosis in the pigeon [39], but the short elimination half-life (0.68 ± 0.17 h)[40] and low sensitivity limit its clinical usefulness [8, 40]. Increased plasma GDH activity occurred only after extensive hepatic necrosis in pigeons [8, 39]. In racing pigeons, GGT specifically indicated induced liver disease, but was not as sensitive as AST [39]. Alkaline phosphatase (AP) is neither sensitive nor specific for the evaluation of liver damage in pigeon; no increased activity was associated with aflatoxin B_1-induced hepatotoxicosis [39]. The elimination half-life of GDH in the pigeon of 0.68 ± 0.17 h is shorter than AST (7.66 ± 1.55 h) or ALT (15.99 ± 1.70 h) but is similar to LDH (0.71 ± 0.10 h) [39].

Biliverdin, Bilirubin, and Plasma Bile Acids

Plasma bile acids and their salts are formed in the liver from cholesterol and are excreted in the intestines [8]. Continuous secretion of bile acids occurs in the pigeon, which does not possess a gall bladder [8]. Bile acids can be measured enzymatically (spectrophotometrically) or by radioimmunoassay (RIA) [28]. Heparin and hemoglobin can result in decreased spectrophotometric recovery of total bile acids [28]. However, values for RIA measurement of bile acids in columbiformes are not available.

A significant postprandial increase in total bile acids occurs in racing pigeons [28]. Pigeons' lack of gall bladder appears to cause no postprandial increase in bile acids in contrast to birds which possess a gall bladder [28]. Pigeon fasting bile acids was 35.4 ± 18.1 μmol /L, and the 1 h postprandial bile acids was 71.2 ± 16.5 μmol /L [28]. In pigeons, total plasma bile acids is a sensitive indicator of liver disease [28, 39, 41]. Experimentally induced liver disease in pigeons resulted in up to 10-fold increased concentrations of bile acids (100 to 800 μmol /L) [28]. In racing pigeons, a fasting bile acids of >70 μmol /L and postprandial bile acids >100 μ mol /L may indicate hepatobiliary disease [8, 28]. Sporadic, short-term elevations in total bilirubin, AST, ALT, GGT, and LDH activities were observed in pigeons with *Salmonella*-induced hepatitis [43].

Muscle Enzymes

Experimental muscle injury induced by IM injection of doxycycline resulted in increased activities of muscle tissue enzymes in pigeons [39]. The greatest increases occurred for CK, followed by LDH, AST, and ALT. Creatine phosphokinase activity increased after as little as 16 h after injury, but by 66 h, plasma activities had returned to reference intervals, likely based on the short elimination half-life of 3.07 ± 0.59 h. Increased ALT activity persisted for nine days after muscle injury because of its longer elimination half-life (7.66 ± 1.55 h) [39, 40].

Renal Analytes

Uric acid excretion in pigeons is 90% dependent on tubular secretion and is largely independent of urine flow rate and hydration status [44]. Plasma uric acid concentration is influenced by age, diet, and fasting; reproductive activity; and hydration status in pigeons [17]. Increased uric acid concentrations may occur with severe tissue necrosis or after a high-protein meal in pigeons [44, 45]. During reproduction, the concentration of uric acid increased in pigeons from beginning to mid-incubation, suggesting an increase in nitrogen metabolism during this period [31]. Uric acid concentrations increased 1.4-to 2-fold after three days of water deprivation, but values did not rise above reference intervals [44]. The plasma uric acid concentration in racing pigeons of 6.30 ± 0.50 mg/dL (375 ± 30 μmol/L) [17] was higher than that in white Carneau pigeons, a model for atherosclerosis, at 3.68 ± 0.22 mg/dL (219 ± 13 μmol/L) [46]. This discrepancy could be attributable to breed differences, methodology, or differences in fasting [17, 44]. Uric acid increases to 25.22 mg/dL (1500 μmol/L) in pigeons after long-distance and long-duration flights (5–22 h) [47, 48].

Although uric acid concentrations of > 15 mg/dL (>890 μmol/L) are suggestive of impaired renal function in birds, loss of 70%–75% or greater of renal function may be necessary cause increased uric acid concentrations [45]. Thus, increased concentrations of uric acid are likely a relatively late, poor, and nonspecific indicator of renal dysfunction in birds [45].

Urea (CH_4N_2O) and blood urea nitrogen (BUN) are related but inequivalent analytes. BUN refers solely to the nitrogen portion of urea and is often expressed as mg/dL, whereas urea is expressed in mmol/L. Urea is produced by the liver from protein metabolism. In pigeons, the formation of urea occurs mainly through arginolysis [8, 48]. Because birds are uricotelic, only small quantities of urea are present in the circulation at any given time [8, 44]. Urea is excreted by the kidney through glomerular filtration. Tubular resorption occurs and is dependent on hydration status [44]. In pigeons deprived of water for 48 h and then subjected to 50 °C heat for 2 to 3 h, serum BUN increased from 3.09 ± 2.66 mg/dL (1.10 ± 0.95 mmol /L) to 19.00 ± 6.91 mg/dL (6.78 ± 2.47 mmol/L) [49]. In a separate study of dehydration in pigeons, plasma urea concentration showed a 6.5- to 15.3-fold increase to significantly above reference intervals [44]. Strenuous, long-distance flight was associated with a fourfold increase in urea concentration in racing pigeons [47, 48].

Urea and BUN are widely considered to have little diagnostic value in birds, but because secretion is dependent upon the glomerular filtration rate (GFR), assessment may be a sensitive method for the detection of prerenal azotemia in pigeons [8]. Plasma concentrations of BUN are often below the limits of detection, and therefore assays may need to be modified to be of use in birds. In birds, creatine is excreted through renal tubular secretion by the kidney before conversion to creatinine [44]. Creatinine is widely believed to have low diagnostic value in birds. One study reported a 1.2- to 1.5-fold increase after dehydration, and values increased significantly above reference intervals in pigeons [44]. Although limited studies investigating creatinine in pigeons during states of dehydration and disease have been done, creatinine may be useful for detecting prerenal azotemia [8, 44].

N-acetyl-β-D-glucosaminidase (NAG) is a marker of acute gentamicin nephrotoxicity in pigeons [45]. Plasma concentrations of NAG paralleled increases in concentrations of uric acid and creatine, while urine creatine and NAG increased 50- to 60-fold. The assessment of urine NAG may provide a noninvasive method to assess birds such as pigeons for renal disease in free-ranging populations [45].

Pancreas

Exocrine Pancreas

Pancreatic enzymes in birds include amylase, lipase, trypsin, and chymotrypsin, which digest carbohydrates, fats, and proteins [32]. Plasma concentrations of amylase and lipase have only been evaluated in healthy adult pigeons [8, 32]. Plasma amylase and lipase concentrations were normal in a pigeon with exocrine pancreatic insufficiency [32]. Few reliable diagnostic tests for pancreatic function exist for birds such as pigeons. Consider surgical biopsy and histopathology to obtain a diagnosis of pancreatic disease [32].

Endocrine Pancreas

Glucose Birds maintain a higher plasma concentration of glucose compared with other vertebrates such as mammals; pigeons are no exception [6]. Plasma glucose concentrations vary in pigeons with breed, time of day, reproductive status, and activity [8, 17, 31, 50]. Courtship, mating and 72 h fasting can also cause increased glucose [8, 31, 50]. After an 80–90 min flight of 48 km, an increase in glucose occurred in racing pigeons [11]. In pigeons that flew 2–22 h for 113–620 km [47, 48], no changes in glucose or lactate were seen. The increase in lactate during short flights suggests carbohydrate use during the initial phase of the flight [8, 47, 48].

Insulin Glucagon rather than insulin regulates glucose in pigeons. Spontaneous diabetes mellitus, hallmarked by persistent hyperglycemia, occurs in the pigeon [8]. Studies of insulin or glucagon in columbiforme species have not been conducted.

Cardiac

No studies investigating analytes of cardiac function in columbiformes have been done to the best of the authors' knowledge.

Lipids

Lipids, particularly fatty acids, are the main source of energy for flight in pigeons, and concentrations of high-density lipoprotein (HDL) and cholesterol are generally higher in pigeons than in other avian species [8, 51]. Increased free fatty acids and decreased cholesterol occur after endurance flights in pigeons [47, 52]. During the reproductive cycle, plasma concentrations of cholesterol decrease during courtship and breeding and rise by mid-incubation of eggs, possibly associated with the production of crop milk in both sexes during this period [31].

Differences occur based on breed in the lipid metabolism of pigeons [53]. The white Carneau pigeon is predisposed to developing atherosclerosis, particularly on cholesterol-containing diets, and has been used extensively as a research model for this disease [53, 54]. Concentrations of cholesterol and triglycerides rise after introduction of diets containing cholesterol to both show racer and white Carneau pigeons. Hypercholesterolemia is associated with aortic atherosclerotic lesions in white Carneau pigeons [53]. Plasma cholesterol concentrations from young white Carneau and show racer pigeons consuming a cholesterol-free grain-based diet averaged about 300 mg/dL (7.77 mmol/L), approximately 200 mg/dL (5.18 mmol/L) as HDL and the remainder (100 mg/dL or 2.59 mmol/L) as low-density lipoproteins (LDL) [55]. Consumption of a cholesterol-containing diet increased plasma cholesterol concentrations in both breeds to greater than 2000 mg/dL (51.8 mmol/L) [55]. About 50% of this increase was LDL, the remainder being low-density lipoproteins (P-VLDL) [55].

Iron

Spontaneous disease associated with iron metabolism has not been reported in columbiformes. Iron concentrations in pigeons are comparable to other avian species, but may be higher in reproductively active hens [13, 17]. The total iron binding capacity (TIBC) was 209.5 ± 4.47 δg/dL (37.5 ± 0.8 µmol/L) using the Guanidine-ferrozine colorimetric method [17].

Osmolality and Electrolytes

Water consumption in pigeons is influenced by age, breed, body size, environmental temperature, and diet. Columbiformes sacrifice the strict regulation of electrolytes to survive a wide range of osmotic pressures for the sake of water conservation [49]. Thus, water deprivation results in increased plasma osmolality in pigeons. Plasma osmolality of racing pigeons increased from 311 ± 3.4 to 352 ± 3.7 mOsm(mmol)/kg H_2O after a 72 h fast [44, 49]. Osmolality in hydrated pigeons 334.73 ± 18.23 mOsm(mmol)/kg increased to 436.73 ± 28.54 mOsm(mmol)/kg in birds deprived of water for 48 h and exposed to 50 °C heat for 2 to 3 h.

Plasma concentrations [mEq(mmol)/L] of sodium, potassium, chloride, and calcium [163.36 ± 9.50, 3.37 ± 1.46, 113.55 ± 9.11, 8.82 ± 1.25 (162.9 ± 12.57mmol/L)], all increased to [218.45 ± 15.62, 4.74 ± 3.05, 162.91 ± 12.57, 11.83 ± 1.15 mg/dL (2.96 ± 0.29 mmol/L)] respectively [49]. Water deprivation for 65.4 h and exposure to heat of 40 °C increased plasma osmolality to 374.8 mOsm(mmol)/kg H_2O [56]. In hens, plasma sodium decreases soon after egg laying despite a small clutch size of two eggs [31]. Potassium is filtered and actively excreted by the kidneys in birds. Plasma potassium is strongly affected by hemolysis and extended blood storage in pigeons [7, 8, 17].

Blood Proteins

Plasma protein concentration can be affected by hydration status, nutritional status, physical activity, and reproductive activity in pigeons [31]. Water deprivation for 48 h followed by exposure to 50 °C temperature for 2 or 3 h caused increased total protein, albumin, and globulin in pigeons, although the albumin:globulin (A : G) ratio was unaffected [49].

Total Solids and Total Protein

When pigeon standards are used with the Biuret method for measuring plasma protein, values are comparable to human standards [57]. However, most commercial laboratories use human reagents, and clinicians should use reference intervals established using commonly available methods [8]. In practice, the refractometric method is often used to estimate total plasma protein. In pigeons, values obtained by refractometer, with and without temperature compensation, were higher than values obtained using the Biuret method [58]. The cause for this discrepancy may be based on other components of plasma such as chromagens, lipids, and glucose [8]. The refractometric method is not a reliable method for determination of plasma or serum protein in the pigeon and should only be used to estimate these values [8, 59].

Protein Electrophoresis

Protein electrophoresis provides the most accurate and reliable measurement of blood proteins in birds [24, 57].

Observed protein fractions in birds include prealbumin, albumin, and the α-,β-,and γ-globulins. In healthy pigeons, albumin is the largest protein fraction [8].The α- and β-globulins are acute phase proteins and include lipoproteins, transferrin, fibrinogen, complement, and others. The γ-globulin fraction includes the immunoglobulins and is often increased with inflammatory disease [8]. The plasma protein electrophoretic pattern in six non-breeding hens was total protein: 2.88 ± 0.24 g/dL (28.8 ± 2.4 g/L); albumin: 29.8 ± 2.0%; α-1 globulin: 30.6 ± 1.6%; α-2 globulin: 8.3 ± 1.2%; β-globulin: 20.4 ± 3.0%; γ-globulin: 11.5 ± 3.6% [16]. A prealbumin fraction was not detected [16]. Pigeons have a relatively high α-globulin concentration in comparison with ducks and turkeys, often up to a third of the total protein [51, 55]. This may be based on the presence of the apolipoprotein apo A-I associated with comparatively increased concentrations of HDL and cholesterol of pigeons [16, 51]. The α-globulin peak could be incorrectly interpreted to result from inflammation, because numerous positive acute phase proteins such α-1 antitrypsin and α-2 macroglobulin migrate in the α-globulin region in birds [51]. Increased concentrations of apo A-I could result from an adaptation of lipid metabolism in pigeons in which fatty acids are the primary energy source for long-distance flights [51, 55].

Albumin

Albumin concentration is lower in non-breeding pigeon hens than in females ducks or turkeys [16]. Albumin concentrations increase during nest building, possibly in association with vitellogenesis during pre-ovulation in hens [16].

Fibrinogen and Other Blood Proteins

The total protein concentration in pigeon plasma is higher than serum (by 0.174 g/dl [1.74 g/L]) based on fibrinogen in the plasma [8, 14, 58, 59]. Fibrinogen concentrations can increase above established normal reference intervals with bacterial infections in pigeons.

Blood Gases, pH, Lactate (Table 27.3)

Blood gases and blood lactate in pigeons in normal states and in response to changes in temperature, simulated altitude, and flight distance have been studied. However, no studies have evaluated blood gases and lactate in pigeons during disease states. Blood lactate increases with short flights, at simulated high altitudes in pigeons and flight in a wind tunnel [9.0 ± 2.7 mg/dL (1.0 ± 0.30 mmol/L) to 59.8 ± 21.4 mg/dL (6.64 ± 2.38 mmol/L)] [62–64]. Increased lactate during short flights suggests that carbohydrates are used in the initial phase of flight [8]. Long-distance flights were not associated with elevations in blood lactate [47], suggesting that lipids are the main source of energy during flight [8].

Blood gas reference intervals (central 95% of values) for 60 pigeons determined using a RapidLab 248 blood gas analyzer (Bayer Health Care, Mijdrecht, the Netherlands) at 37 °C were pH 7.48–7.60; pCO_2 24.5–30.8 mmHg; pO_2 58.2–71.2 mmHg; the calculated reference intervals for 42.1 °C (the mean core body temperature of the pigeons) were pH 7.41–7.51; pCO_2 30.4–39.0 mmHg; pO_2 83.4–100.3 mmHg [65].

Vitamins, Minerals, Metals, and Toxins

Calcium and Regulatory Hormones

Plasma concentrations of calcium vary with age, nutritional status, and reproductive status in pigeons. Total plasma calcium (tCa) concentration increases from 2.2 mmol/l in hens starting about four days prior to ovulation to over 5.0 mmol/l at the time of ovulation as a result of an increase in protein-bound calcium associated with the rise in circulating yolk protein. Ionized calcium (iCa) remains unchanged [8]. Plasma concentrations of calcium are lower in pigeons of both sexes during the feeding and brooding of the young, which may indicate a diversion of calcium toward the production of crop milk, which is rich in calcium (Table 27.3) [31].

Toxins

Heavy Metals Lead poisoning occurs in mourning doves and white-winged doves that ingest spent lead shot in areas where the birds are hunted [66, 67]. Blood lead concentrations of >2 ppm (20 µg/dl, or 0.97 µmol/L) are suggestive of, and > 5 ppm (50 µg/dL, or 2.42 µmol/L) diagnostic for, lead toxicosis in birds [68]. Studies have shown δ-aminolevulinic acid (δ-ALAD) to be a sensitive indicator of lead exposure in these pigeons and doves [67, 69, 70]. In humans, blood lead concentrations of 50–60 µg/dL (2.42–2.90 µmol/L) result in decreases in α-ALAD by about 75%, while in pigeons similar blood lead concentrations caused a decrease of about 90% [69]. Mourning doves that ingested lead shot had reduced activity of α-ALAD with 30.67 ± 8.8 units of activity for affected birds (6) compared to 230.88 ± 20.59 units of activity for all birds studied (35) [67]. A mild decrease in the HCT and a significant decrease in δ-ALAD activity were seen after oral administration of 5 mg/kg lead acetate over several weeks to pigeons [70]. Increased heterophil:leukocyte ratios and a decreased HCT occurred in mourning doves experimentally fed lead pellets [68]. Erythrocyte protoporphyrin, a biomarker of early lead exposure, was increased at blood lead concentrations of >50 µg/dL (2.42 µmol/L) in pigeons experimentally administered lead through contaminated soil [71]. Erythrocytic intranuclear inclusions have been observed by electron microscopy in pigeons with high blood lead concentrations [8]. No specific reports evaluating zinc toxicosis in columbiforme species were found in the literature.

Table 27.3 Biochemical analyte values for select columbiformes.

Analyte (abbreviation)	Units, SI (conventional)	Pigeon, or rock dove (*Columba livia*)	Nicobar pigeon [2] (*Caloenas nicobarica*)	Pheasant pigeon [2] (*Otidiphaps nobilis*)	Common crowned pigeon [2] (*Goura cristata*)	Victoria crowned pigeon [2] (*Goura victoria*)	Mourning dove [7] (*Zenaida macroura*)		Nigerian laughing dove [26] (*Streptopelia senegalensis*)
Animals sampled		n = 7–9 [24], 50–58 [8, 17] n = 30 [1] 105 [60] 16 [9] n = 134–145 [6], 20–24 [8] n = 50 [10]	16	3	9	6	♂ N = 86–97	♀ N = 86–91	N = 5–10 Non-breeding adults
Alanine aminotransferase (ALT)	U/l	4.2 ± 2.9 [2.0–20] {19–48} [60] 75.9 ± 64.3 [12.2–255] [1] 25 ± 1.6 [17] {19–48} [8]	9.72 ± 6.56 [2.38–19.4]	12.19 ± 4.91 [8.72–15.66]	7.16 ± 1.47 [6.06–10.31]	6.43 ± 2.42 [3.24–8.83]			
Albumin	g/l (g/dl)	9.4 ± 7 (0.94 ± 0.7) [31] 21.3 ± 3.25 (2.13 ± 0.33) [24] 17.5 ± 0.36 (1.75 ± 0.04) [17]					11.9 ± 0.2 (1.19 ± 0.02) [10–20 (1.00–2.00)] 12.1 ± 0.2 (1.21 ± 0.02) [9.0–17.0 (0.90–1.70)]	11.8 ± 0.1 (1.18 ± 0.01) [10.0–16.0 (1.00–1.60)] 12.2 ± 0.2 (1.22 ± 0.02) [10.0–17.0 (1.00–1.70)]	10.20 ± 4.20 (1.02 ± 0.42) [26]
Alkaline phosphatase (AP)	U/l	315 ± 172 [75.1–1234] [6] {160–780} [60] 367 ± 25 [17]	225.2 ± 195.0 [22.6–684.9]	490.5 ± 195.0 [267.1–626.0]	44.3 ± 22.6 [27.9–79.3]	22.4 ± 11.9 [11.3–41.5]			
Amylase	IU/l	480 {382–556} [3]							
Aspartate aminotransferase (AST)	U/l	49 ± 20 [15–134] {5–123} [60] 297.2 ± 177 [92.68–693.4] [1] 58.6 ± 2.5 [17] 40 ± 7.1 [29–54] [9] {45–123} [8]	123.0 ± 82.6 [40.1–265.3]	65.6 ± 9.51 [58.9–72.35]	54.08 ± 8.42 [41.16–64.34]	42.80 ± 11.92 [23.5–54.2]	227.53 ± 8.71 [81.00–663.00] 252.60 ± 11.37 [94.00–709.00]	245.44 ± 10.68 [93.00–757.00] 270.07 ± 11.10 [143.00–659.00]	
Bile acids, total	μg/ml (μmol/l)	{9.0–24.5 (22–60)} [60]							
Calcium, ionized	mmol/l (mg/dl)	{1.32–1.39 (5.28–5.56)} [8]							
Calcium, total	mmol/l (mg/dl)	2.1 ± 0.7 (8.40 ± 2.80) [0.9–4.0 (3.60–16.00)] [6] 2.3 ± 0.03 (9.20 ± 0.12) [17] {1.9–2.6 (7.60–10.40)} [8]	2.62 ± 0.55 (10.46 ± 2.2) [2.22–3.00 (8.89–12.02)]	4.05 ± 0.24 (16.19 ± 0.98) [3.87–4.22 (15.49–16.88)]	2.22 ± 0.12 (8.88 ± 0.46) [2.10–2.35 (8.40–9.40)]	2.42 ± 0.20 (9.68 ± 0.78) [2.25–2.70 (9.00–10.80)]	2.50 ± 0.02 (9.98 ± 0.09) [1.90–3.02 (7.60–12.10)] 2.37 ± 0.02 (9.47 ± 0.08) [1.80–2.88 (7.20–11.50)] [7]	2.44 ± 0.03 (9.74 ± 0.10) [1.60–3.00 (6.40–12.00)] 2.45 ± 0.05 (9.79 ± 0.21) [2.02 ± 6.28 (8.10–25.10)]	

(*Continued*)

Table 27.3 (Continued)

Analyte (abbreviation)	Units, SI (conventional)	Pigeon, or rock dove (*Columba livia*)	Nicobar pigeon [2] (*Caloenas nicobarica*)	Pheasant pigeon [2] (*Otidiphaps nobilis*)	Common crowned pigeon [2] (*Goura cristata*)	Victoria crowned pigeon [2] (*Goura victoria*)	Mourning dove [7] (*Zenaida macroura*)		Nigerian laughing dove [26] (*Streptopelia senegalensis*)
Animals sampled		**n = 7–9 [24], 50–58 [8, 17] n = 30 [1] 105 [60] 16 [9] n = 134–145 [6], 20–24 [8] n = 50 [10]**	**16**	**3**	**9**	**6**	**♂ N = 86–97**	**♀ N = 86–91**	**N = 5–10 Non-breeding adults**
Chloride	mmol/l (mEq/l)	97 ± 7 [81–128] [6] 117.1 ± 2.9 [24] 107 ± 0.5 [17] {101–113} [8]	100.5 ± 11.9 [86.2–126.8]	130.3 ± 12.6 [121.4–139.2]	101.1 ± 3.32 [96.4–106.8]	104.9 ± 4.34 [100.5–109.9]	113.21 ± 0.45 [104.00–137.00] 113.64 ± 0.33 [107.00–121.00]	112.20 ± 0.36 [101.00–119.00] 112.60 ± 0.42 [96.00–123.00]	
Cholesterol	mmol/l (mg/dl)	7.0 ± 1.7 (270 ± 65.6) [2.3–11.7 (88.3–452)] 6.48 ± 1.48 (250.3 ± 57.18) [0.59–8.98 (22.7–346.9)] [1]	11.10 ± 2.79 (428.6 ± 107.9) [7.66–15.19 (295.9–586.4)]	10.26 ± 4.45 (396.0 ± 171.9) [6.03–14.91 (232.7–575.6)] [2]	6.81 ± 1.53 (262.9 ± 59.2) [5.38–9.48 (207.7–366.1)]	6.30 ± 3.51 (243.2 ± 135.7) [4.49–12.46 (173.2–481.2)]	6.69 ± 0.13 (258.48 ± 4.88) [4.53–11.42 (175.00–441.00)] 6.00 ± 0.15 (231.79 ± 5.80) [3.16–14.24 (122.00–550.00)]	6.78 ± 0.17 (261.68 ± 6.40) [3.65–13.11 (141.00–506.00)] 6.19 ± 0.21 (239.11 ± 7.92) [2.18–12.56 (84.00–485.00)]	
Creatine phosphokinase (CPK)	U/l	89 ± 40 [19–306] [6] (110–480) [60] 203 ± 13.5 [17] 147 ± 64.8 [63–296] [9] {110–480} [8]	251.3 ± 168.3 [43.3–510.4] [2]	233.7 ± 213.1 [106.8–479.7] [2]	117.2 ± 51.9 [65.8–220.5] [2]	341.6 ± 235.2 [146.7–750.0]			
Creatinine	μmol/l (mg/dl)	36.24 ± 16.80 (0.41 ± 0.19) [1.41–64.53 (0.016–0.73)] [1] 28 ± 0.6 (0.32 ± 0.01) [17] {23–36 (0.26–0.41)} [8]	31.8 ± 13.3 (0.36 ± 0.15) [19.4–57.5 (0.22–0.65)]	33.6 ± 7.1 (0.38 ± 0.08) [26.5–39.8 (0.30–0.45)]	69.8 ± 13.3 (0.79 ± 0.15) [56.6–83.1 (0.64–0.94)]	68.1 ± 8.84 (0.77 ± 0.10) [58.3–79.6 (0.66–0.90)]			116.69 ± 64.53 (1.32 ± 0.73)
γ-glutamyltransferase (GGT)	U/l	{<1–3} [8]					8.24 ± 0.65 [5.00–48.00] 11.16 ± 0.40 [9.00–37.00]	8.71 ± 0.47 [5.00–29.00] 10.87 ± 0.31 [9.00–27.00]	
Globulin	g/l (g/dl)						15.6 ± 0.4 (1.56 ± 0.04) [11.0–34.0 (1.10–3.40)] 14.2 ± 0.3 (1.42 ± 0.03) [9.0–26.0 (0.90–2.60)]	15.2 ± 0.2 (1.52 ± 0.02) [10.0–20.0 (1.00–2.00)] 14.4 ± 0.3 (1.44 ± 0.03) [7.0–26.0 (0.70–2.60)]	6.70 ± 1.20 (0.67 ± 0.12)

Glucose	mmol/l (mg/dl)	18.4 ± 2.03 (332 ± 36.6) [11.7–24.7 (211–445)] 16.3 ± 5.28 (294 ± 95.1) [1.50–22.4 (27–404)] [1] 18.9 ± 2.59 (341.1 ± 46.6) [24] 16.6 ± 0.2 (299 ± 3.6) [17] 19.3 ± 1.62 (347 ± 29.2) [16.5–22.6 (298 – 407)] [9] {12.9–20.5 (232–369)} [8]	16.0 ± 1.93 (289.0 ± 34.7) [12.89–19.84 (232.2–357.4)]	19.67 ± 2.55 (354.4 ± 46.0) [17.07–22.2 (307.5–399.4)]	12.89 ± 0.92 (232.3–16.6) [11.17–13.86 (201.3–249.7)]	14.21 ± 2.33 (256.0 ± 41.9) [11.69–17.73 (210.7–319.4)]	26.53 ± 0.47 (477.96 ± 8.51) [19.48–36.80 (351.00–663.00)] 27.18 ± 0.50 (489.68 ± 9.04) R = [17.21–45.62 (310.00–822.00)]	25.91 ± 0.47 (466.87 ± 8.55) [18.87–39.85 (340.00–718.00)] 27.92 ± 0.65 (503.06 ± 11.78) 18.98–61.94 (342.00–1116.00)
Glutamate dehydrogenase (GDH)	U/l	{0–1} [60] {<8} [8]						
Iron	μmol/l (μg/dl)	29.2 ± 24.0 (163 ± 134) [8.36–94.9 (46.7–530)] 23 ± 2.1 (128 ± 11.7) [17] [49.6–65.5 (277–366)] [13]						
Lactate dehydrogenase (LDH)	U/l	99 ± 51 [42.7–329] {30–205} [60] 1069 ± 581 [500.6–2434] [1] 57 ± 3.2 [17] 44 ± 46.9 [6 – 172] [9] {30–205} [8]	584.0 ± 496.3 [172.9 – 1808]	101.3 ± 72.2 [50.2–152.4]	257.6 ± 131.4 [134.6–518.5]	219.5 ± 94.3 [126.8–344.1]	1040.27 ± 94.33 [445.00–8117.00] 905.35 ± 36.38 [312.00–1822.00]	1091.30 ± 104.57 [425.00–9168.00] 1175.26 ± 108.11 [320.00–8528.00]
Lactic acid	mmol/l (mg/dl)	1.81 ± 0.59 (16.3 ± 5.3) [24]						
Lipase	IU/l	2.3 {0–5} [8]						
Magnesium	mmol/l (mg/dl)	0.90 ± 0.16 (2.19 ± 0.39) [0.45–1.56 (1.09–3.80)] [6] 1.3 ± 0.03 (3.16 ± 0.07) [17]	1.03 ± 0.20 (2.63 ± 0.49) [0.94–1.22 (2.28–2.98)]	1.20 ± 0.11 (2.92 ± 0.27) [1.12–1.28 (2.73–3.11)]	0.84 ± 0.16 (2.04 ± 0.39) [0.67–1.10 (1.64–2.63)]	0.95 ± 0.18 (2.30 ± 0.44) [0.74–1.18 (1.81–2.86)]	1.05 ± 0.02 (2.55 ± 0.04) [0.78–1.48 (1.90–3.60)] 1.18 ± 0.01 (2.87 ± 0.03) [0.86–1.60 (2.10–3.90)]	1.02 ± 0.02 (2.48 ± 0.04) [0.70–1.40 (1.70–3.40)] 1.18 ± 0.01 (2.87 ± 0.03)] [0.86–1.52 (2.10–3.70)]
Osmolality	mmol/kg (mOsm/kg)	306 ± 0.9 [17] {297–317} [8]	313.0 ± 18.7 [295.0–346.0] [2	311.3 ± 10.0 [301.0–321.0] [2]	316.6 ± 8.5 [289.0–310.0] [2]	315.4 ± 8.5 [305.0–328.0]		
pCO_2	mmHg	43.0 ± 6.9 [24]						
pH		7.35 ± 0.006 [24]						

(*Continued*)

Table 27.3 (Continued)

Analyte (abbreviation)	Units, SI (conventional)	Pigeon, or rock dove (*Columba livia*)	Nicobar pigeon [2] (*Caloenas nicobarica*)	Pheasant pigeon [2] (*Otidiphaps nobilis*)	Common crowned pigeon [2] (*Goura cristata*)	Victoria crowned pigeon [2] (*Goura victoria*)	Mourning dove [7] (*Zenaida macroura*)		Nigerian laughing dove [26] (*Streptopelia senegalensis*)
Animals sampled		**n = 7–9 [24], 50–58 [8, 17] n = 30 [1] 105 [50] 16 [9] n = 134–145 [6], 20–24 [8] n = 50 [10]**	**16**	**3**	**9**	**6**	**♂ N = 86–97**	**♀ N = 86–91**	**N = 5–10 Non-breeding adults**
Phosphorus	mmol/l (mg/dl)	0.78 ± 0.39 (2.41 ± 1.21) [0.16–2.26 (0.50–7.00)] [6] 0.83 ± 0.04 (2.57 ± 0.12) [17] {0.57–1.33 (1.76–4.12)} [8]	13.64 ± 0.18 (42.22 ± 0.56) [13.51–13.76 (41.82– 42.61)]	13.68 ± 9.56 (42.35 ± 29.6) [6.91–20.45 (21.40–63.30)]	6.89 ± 1.06 (21.34 ± 3.27) [5.94–8.46 (18.40–26.20)]	5.65 ± 1.72 (17.48 ± 5.31) [4.13–8.04 (12.80–24.90)]	1.22 ± 0.04 (3.78 ± 0.12) [0.61–2.39 (1.90–7.40)] 2.39 ± 0.04 (3.89 ± 0.11) [0.68–2.71 (2.10–8.40)]	1.20 ± 0.03 (3.70 ± 0.10) [0.48–2.13 (1.50–6.60)] 1.25 ± 0.04 (3.87 ± 0.12) [0.68–2.62 (2.10–8.10)]	
pO_2	mmHg	49.7 ± 7.3 [24]							
Potassium	mmol/l (mEq/l)	2.0 ± 0.4 [1.0–4.0] [6] 4.1 ± 0.2 [31] 2.1 ± 0.2 [24] 4.4 ± 0.06 [17] {3.9–4.7} [8]					7.05 ± 0.20 [3.60–12.50] 7.78 ± 0.19 [4.00–14.90] [7]	6.76 ± 0.18 [3.90–13.00] 7.81 ± 0.18 [4.50–12.00]	50.58 ± 22.18 57.24 ± 21.89
Sedimentation rate [61]	mm 1 hr. mm 2 hr.	0.63 ± 0.48 [24] 1.3 ± 1.6 [24]							
Sodium	mmol/l (mEq/l)	122 ± 8 [95–152] [6] 156 ± 8 [31] 159.8 ± 3.7 [24] 145 ± 0.3 [17] {141–149} [8]					146.26 ± 0.37 [137.00–160.00] 144.00 ± 0.33 [137.00–154.00]	145.41 ± 0.31 [138.00–153.00] 143.43 ± 0.41 [125.00–156.00]	161.54 ± 54.59 174.69 ± 20.07
Total iron binding capacity (TIBC)	μmol/l (μg/dl)	37.5 ± 0.8 (210 ± 4.47) [17] 27.0–31.0 (151–173) [13]							
Total protein	g/l (g/dl)	31 ± 6 (3.1 ± 0.6) [21–59 (2.1–5.9)] [6] Ø♀♂ ***35*** 33.1 ± 3 (3.31 ± 0.3) [31] 98 ± 7 (9.8 ± 0.7) [85–110 (8.5–11)] [1] 26.57 ± 5.47 (2.66 ± 0.55) [24] 27 ± 0.4 (2.7 ± 0.04) [17] 31.3 ± 2 (3.13 ± 0.2) [27.6–35.5 (2.76–3.55)] [9] {21–35 (2.1–3.5)} [8]	32.6 ± 4.1 (3.26 ± 0.41) [26.2–37.7 (2.62–3.77)]	32.7 ± 7.5 (3.27 ± 0.75) [28.4–41.4 (2.84–4.14)]	44.6 ± 3.7 (4.46 ± 0.37) [38.7–49.3 (3.87–4.93)]	35.8 ± 4 (3.58 ± 0.40) [30.1–40.3 (3.01–4.03)]	27.5 ± 0.5 (2.75 ± 0.05) [21.0–51.0 (2.10–5.10)] 26.2 ± 0.4 (2.62 ± 0.04) [18.0–39.0 (1.80–3.90)]	26.8 ± 0.4 (2.68 ± 0.04) [20.0–35.0 (2.00–3.50)] 26.6 ± 0.5 (2.66 ± 0.05) [17.0–39.0 (1.70–3.90)]	16.80 ± 4.90 (1.68 ± 0.49)

Triglycerides	mmol/l (mg/dl)	2.5 ± 1.1 (221 ± 97) [1.1–4.8 (97–425)] 0.86 ± 0.08 (76 ± 7) [55] 5-month old 13.61 ± 7.53 (1204 ± 666) [55]5-month old	2.02 ± 0.62 (179.1 ± 55.1) [1.02–3.17 (90.3–280.1)]	8.46 ± 3.54 (748.9 ± 313.7) [4.37–10.52 (386.6–930.9)]	1.73 ± 1.27 (152.7 ± 112.0) [0.49–4.42 (43.7–391.3)]	1.60 ± 2.23 (141.8 ± 197.7) [0.43–5.59 (37.8–495.1)]			
Urea, blood urea nitrogen (BUN)	mmol/l (mg/dl)	0.23 ± 0.10 (0.64 ± 0.28) [0.17–0.70 (0.48–1.96)] [1] 6.41 ± 1.75 (17.95 ± 4.9) [3.57–10.53 (10–29.5)] [17] {0.4–0.7 (1.12–1.96)} [8]	2.09 ± 0.49 (5.86 ± 1.36) [1.43–29.6 (4.01–83.0)]	1.8 ± 0.17 (5.12 ± 0.48) [1.7–2.0 (4.70–5.64)]	3.03 ± 0.80 (8.49 ± 2.23) [1.86–4.47 (5.22–12.52)]	3.57 ± 0.83 (9.99 ± 2.32) [2.46–4.57 (6.88–12.79)]			3.43 ± 1.69 (9.61 ± 4.73) 3.36 ± 1.55 (9.41 ± 4.34)
Uric acid	μmol/l (mg/dl)	345 ± 107 (5.8 ± 1.8) [125–833 (2.10–14.0)] 375 ± 30 (6.30 ± 0.50) [17] 321 ± 101 (5.4 ± 1.7) [173–518 (2.9–8.7)] [9] {150–765 (2.52–12.86)} [8]	612 ± 159 (10.28 ± 2.67) [390–830 (6.56–13.96)]	779 ± 273 (13.10 ± 4.59) [466–968 (7.83–16.27)]	405 ± 275 (6.81 ± 4.62) [133–952 (2.24–16.00)]	413 ± 177 (6.94 ± 2.98) [216–717 (3.63–12.06)]	305 ± 10.7 (5.13 ± 0.18) [113–595 (1.90–10.00)]	308 ± 13.7 (5.17 ± 0.23) [89.2–791 (1.50–13.30)]	

Values given as mean ± SD [Range],{$P_{2.5} - P_{97.5}$} Median ***n* not covered in column header.**

Benzimidazoles Benzimidazole anthelmintics including fenbendazole and albendazole cause dose-dependent radiomimetic bone marrow suppression in avian species including pigeons. Marked leukopenia was observed in 87.5% of columbiformes treated with fenbendazole (50 or 100 mg/kg once daily for two to nine days) and 100% of columbiformes treated with albendazole (50 or 100 mg/kg once daily for two to nine days) [72]. Peripheral blood from surviving birds showed regenerative anemia, heteropenia, and scattered immature thromboblasts [73].

Mycotoxins Aflatoxin B_1 is a potent hepatotoxin and a common mycotoxin that affects birds [41]. In experimental aflatoxicosis with aflatoxin B_1 in pigeons, elevations in plasma activities of AST and ALT, AST, and LDH [41], and elevations in bile acids, AST, LDH, ALT, and CK activities were observed [74].

Environmental Contaminants Because feral pigeons are ubiquitous in urban environments, they are studied for secondary exposure to environmental pollutants and contaminants to assess the health risks to human and wildlife species. Experimental intramuscular carbofuran administration was associated with a drop in the RBC and Hb, along with heterophilia, eosinophilia, and lymphopenia in pigeons [75].

Hormones

Thyroid Hormones

Thyroxine (T_4) is the major secretory product of the thyroid gland, although triiodothyronine (T_3) is the principal metabolically active thyroid hormone in birds, and columbiformes are no exception [76]. Concentrations of circulating T_3 and T_4 vary according to time of day, season, reproductive status, and age in pigeons [76, 77]. The highest concentrations of T_4 were found in July at 2.07 μg/dL (26.6 nmol/L) and the lowest in September at 1.28 μg/dL (16.5 nmol/L) in adult pigeons of both sex in the Netherlands [76]. These values were similar to other avian species, which are generally much lower than values found in mammals [76]. No differences were seen in age or sex in this study [76]. The mean peak concentration in T_4 after intramuscular injection of 1.0 unit of bovine thyroid stimulating hormone (bTSH) was 13.21 μg/dL (170 nmol/L) and was seen at 24 h post injection [76]. High T_3 and low T_4 concentrations during the winter months in Finland were seen in pigeons in a separate study. For example, for birds kept outdoors, the mean plasma concentrations of T_3 and T_4 during the winter months were 222 ± 16 ng/dL (3.42 ± 0.25 nmol/L) and 0.418 ± 0.037 μg/dL (5.38 ± 0.48 nmol/L), respectively, as compared with during the summer months of 154 ± 7 ng/dL (2.37 ± 0.11 nmol/L) and 0.725 ± 0.068 μg/dL (9.33 ± 0.88 nmol/L), respectively [77].

Adrenal Hormones

In birds, corticosterone is the major glucocorticoid [78]. Baseline corticosterone concentrations varied in racing pigeons between <0.2 μg/dl (2 ng/mL, or 5.8 nmol/L) and 1.24 μg/dl (12.4 ng/mL, or 35.8 nmol/L) [78]. Higher circulating concentrations of corticosterone occur during the winter months in both indoor and outdoor pigeons in Finland [77]. For pigeons kept outdoors, the mean plasma concentration of corticosterone during the winter months was 9.39 ± 0.68 ng/mL (27.14 ± 1.97 nmol/L), as compared with during the summer months of 4.24 ± 0.48 ng/mL (12.25 ± 1.39 nmol/L) [77]. Corticosterone secretion in birds is regulated by adrenocorticotropic hormone (ACTH). Peak concentrations of corticosterone occurred at 90 min post injection in pigeons administered 125 μg ACTH intramuscularly [78]. The hypothalamic–pituitary–adrenal system in pigeons is more sensitive to suppression by glucocorticoids than in mammals, with the longest suppression observed after IV administration of dexamethasone when compared with cortisol and prednisolone [79].

Reproductive Hormones

The pigeon is a non-seasonal breeder [16, 80], and minimal changes occurred in luteinizing hormone (LH) and follicle stimulating hormone (FSH) in pigeons maintained indoors in Finland [80], although cold ambient temperatures decreased LH concentrations in another study [77]. Prolactin facilitates the production of crop milk in pigeons. Experimentally, prolactin concentration increased from July through November despite a lack of reproduction [80]. In ring-necked doves, plasma concentration of prolactin begins to decline four days after squab hatch, concomitant with the regression of production of crop milk [80].

Serology and PCR

Chlamydia psittaci

Most infected feral pigeons are asymptomatic, latent carriers of *C. psittaci* [81]. 52.6% of feral pigeons in a Madrid study were PCR positive via blood or cloacal swab for *C. psittaci* [82]. All *C. psittaci* genotypes can be transmitted to humans [81]. In Europe, more than 100 human cases associated with contact with feral pigeons have been reported [81, 83]. However, other reports suggest that pigeon strains have relatively low virulence and low zoonotic potential [84, 85]. Chlamydiae can be isolated from feces, cloacal swabs, or tissue impression smears and detected using special stains including Gimenez, Macchiavello, modified Ziehl-Neelsen or the direct immunofluorescence assay (DIF) or through PCR [81]. The nine genotypes of chlamydia (A to F, E/B, WC,

Table 27.4 Selected infectious disease diagnostics for use in columbiformes. Sample types listed from most to least preferable.

Bacterial isolation (culture)	Samples and test information	Laboratory
Chlamydia (*C. psittaci*)	Tissue, swabs, feces. Do not freeze samples.	United States Department of Agriculture **(USDA)**, Animal and Plant Health Inspection Service **(APHIS)**, National Veterinary Services Laboratories **(NVSL)**, P.O. Box 844, 1920 Dayton Avenue, Ames, Iowa 50010 Phone (515) 337-7514. Website: www.aphis.usda.gov/wps/portal/aphis/ourfocus/animalhealth?1dmy&urile=wcm%3apath%3a%2Faphis_content_library%2Fsa_our_focus%2Fsa_animal_health%2Fsa_lab_information_services%2Fsa_about_nvsl%2Fct_about_nvsl
Mycobacterium avium	Tissues and swabs	
	Fluid and fluid swabs	Diagnostic Center for Population and Animal Health **(DCPAH)**, Michigan State University, 4125 Beaumont Road, Lansing, MI 48910-8104. Phone (517) 353-1683. Website http://www.dcpah.msu.edu
Salmonella spp.	Culture (*Salmonella* spp.) and phage typing (e.g., for *Salmonella typhimurium*)	USDA, APHIS, NVSL
	Culture	Numerous commercial and state veterinary diagnostic laboratories
Special Stains	**Samples and Test Information**	**Laboratory**
M. avium	Acid-fast stain. Fluid and cultures	USDA, APHIS, NVSL
	Acid-fast stain	Numerous commercial and state veterinary diagnostic laboratories
Virus Isolation	**Samples and Test Information**	**Laboratory**
Avian Influenza Virus	Wet tissue and swab. Lab should be contacted for arrangements and further information. Dry swabs are not acceptable	USDA, APHIS, NVSL
Serology	**Samples and Test Information**	**Laboratory**
Chlamydia (*C. psittaci*)	Elementary Body Agglutination (EBA)	Infectious Diseases Laboratory **(IDL)**, 110 Riverbend Road, Riverbend North, Room 150, University of Georgia, Athens, GA 30602. Phone (706) 542-8092. Website www.idl-uga.com
	Immunofluorescence Assay (IFA)	
	Complement Fixation (CF). 2 ml serum minimum required	USDA, APHIS, NVSL
PCR	**Samples and Test Information**	**Laboratory**
Chlamydia (*C. psittaci*)	Choanal or cloacal swabs and whole blood	IDL
	Cloacal, pharyngeal, choanal swabs. Synthetic swabs and viral transport system advised.	DCPAH
M. avium	Cultures and fixed tissues containing lesions	USDA, APHIS, NVSL
	Swabs and tissue samples	Animal Genetics UK **(AGUK)**, P.O. Box 107, Truro, Cornwall, United Kingdom. TR1 2YR. Phone 01872 262737 (Country Code +44). Website http://animalgenetics.eu/
	Cloacal swabs, Whole blood, feces, tissues, and swabs	Veterinary Molecular Diagnostics (**VMD**). 5989 Meijer Drive, Suite 5, Milford, Ohio, 45150. Phone (513) 576-1808. Website http://www.vmdlabs.com/
Salmonella spp.	Swabs of excrement or cut tissue	IDL
Avian Paramyxovirus Serotype-1	Real-Time RT-PCR assay targeting the matrix gene	USDA, APHIS, NVSL

(*Continued*)

Table 27.4 (Continued)

PCR	Samples and Test Information	Laboratory
Pigeon circovirus (PiCV)	Whole blood in EDTA or ACD, frozen or fixed tissues Tissue sample frozen or in alcohol. Environmental swabs	Zoologix, Inc. – 9811 Owensmouth Avenue Suite 4, Chatsworth, CA 91311. Phone (818) 717-8880. Website http://www.zoologix.com AGUK VMD
Avian Influenza Virus	Wet swabs	USDA, APHIS, NVSL
	Oropharyngeal, cloacal swabs, and tissue. Synthetic swabs and virus transport systems advised	DCPAH
West Nile Virus	Brain	USDA, APHIS, NVSL
	Brain, spinal cord, CSF acceptable. Formalin fixed tissues can be tested	DCPAH

and M56) differ in their zoonotic potential, virulence traits, and host preference [81, 83]. Genotype B was the most common genotype identified in feral pigeons [83]. Isolation in tissue culture or in embryonated chicken eggs is still considered the gold standard and the preferred method by the World Organization for Animal Health (OIE) [81]. Complement fixation (CF), indirect immunofluorescence (DF), enzyme linked immunosorbent assay (ELISA), and microimmunofluorescence have been used in the detection of infection in pigeons [81]. Serovar B is considered host (pigeon) specific, and the most prevalent pigeon-associated serovar worldwide [21, 81, 85]. Serovar E is also commonly found in pigeons (Table 27.4) [21, 81].

Mycobacteriosis

Mycobacteriosis is a challenging disease to diagnose and treat in pigeons [86–88]. This chronic disease associated with granulomatous inflammation most often involves the liver, spleen, gastrointestinal tract, lung, or air sacs [87]. Mycobacteria are detectable in the feces using acid-fast stains such as Ziehl-Neelsen and Fite, if present in large numbers, and other acid-fast bacteria may be present [88]. Although bacterial culture is the definitive method for diagnosis [88], some mycobacterial species are difficult to grow and require prolonged incubation and enriched media [88]. Western blot serologic analysis has limited availability and requires species-specific reagents [87]. Single-amplification PCR was less sensitive for detection of mycobacterial infection than Ziehl-Neelsen staining on tissue samples, but nested PCR and real-time PCR assays may be more sensitive [88]. Although many columbiformes appear to have an increased prevalence and predisposition to mycobacteriosis, the domestic pigeon may be resistant to infection [86, 89]. Anemia and marked leukocytosis with heterophilia and monocytosis were seen in ring-necked doves experimentally infected with *Mycobacterium avium avium* [88]. Plasma protein electrophoresis was a sensitive indicator of infection in ring-necked doves, with increases in α-, β-, or γ-globulin concentrations associated decreased albumin concentration [88].

Salmonellosis

Salmonella enterica serotype *Typhimurium* causes paratyphoid in pigeons [84, 90]. *Salmonella* spp. can be isolated by culture and further characterized by serotype (e.g., agglutination O and H antisera) and phage type [90]. However, shedding may be intermittent, and culture requires selective media. Most *Salmonella*-inoculated pigeons developed polyuria and had renal pathology at necropsy; however, no changes in plasma concentrations of urea, uric acid, or creatine occurred [90].

Pigeon Paramyxovirus and Other Viral Diseases

Pigeon paramyxovirus serotype 1 (PPMV-1) affects columbiformes and can also infect poultry. The virus is widespread in racing pigeon populations worldwide and has also been isolated in wood pigeons (*Columba palumbus*) and Eurasian collared doves (*Streptopelia decaocto*) [91]. Experimental infection has also been induced in other columbiforme species such as the collared dove (*Streptopelia roseogrisea arabica*). In the United States, the virus is considered endemic, and periodic outbreaks occur. Commercial vaccines against PPMV-1 are available for pigeons.

Pigeon paramyxovirus infection can be associated with lymphocytic pancreatic inflammation and pancreatic necrosis, and changes in the reproductive and neurologic systems [91, 92]. Rapid diagnosis of PPMV-1 is made using a USDA-validated RT-PCR assay targeting the matrix gene. However, this standardized assay may miss some PPMV-1 subgroups [91]. A pigeon-specific probe improves detection of pigeon PPMV-1 (Table 27.4), suggesting that additional primers should be considered for the USDA surveillance plan [91].

PCR assays have also been developed for pigeon circovirus (PiCV), a virus that causes significant morbidity and mortality in young pigeons [84]. Serologic methods have been used to monitor other viral diseases in pigeons, such as West Nile virus, a flavivirus [93], and avian influenza virus (Table 27.4).

References

1 Khan, A., Ali, F., Saeed, M.Q. et al. (2011). A study on serum biochemistry and hematological profiling of blue rock pigeon (Columba livia) in Multan (Punjab, Pakistan). *Pak. J. Zool.* 43 (5): 1012–1014.

2 Peinado, V.I., Polo, F.J., Celdrán, J.F. et al. (1992). Hematology and plasma chemistry in endangered pigeons. *J. Zoo Wildl. Med.* 23 (1): 65–71.

3 Gibbs, D., Barnes, E., and Cox, J. (2001). *Pigeons and Doves: A Guide to the Pigeons and Doves of the World*, 13–15. Yale University Press.

4 Vogel, C., Gerlach, H., and Löffler, M. (1994). Columbiformes. In: *Avian Medicine: Principles and Application* (ed. B.W. Ritchie, G.J. Harrison and L.R. Harrison), 1200–1217. Winger's Publishing, Inc.

5 Johnston, R.F. and Janiga, M. (1995). *Heavy metals and other pollutants*, 239–246. Feral Pigeons. Oxford University Press.

6 Prinzinger, R. and Misovic, A. (2010). Age-correlation of blood values in the rock pigeon (Columba livia). *Comp. Biochem. Physiol. A* 156: 351–356.

7 Schulz, J.H., Mermudez, A.J., Tomlison, J.L. et al. (2000). Blood plasma chemistries from wild mourning doves held in captivity. *J. Wildl. Dis.* 36 (3): 541–545.

8 Lumeij, J.T. (2008). Avian Clinical Biochemistry. In: *Clinical Biochemistry of Domestic Animals*, 6e (ed. J.J. Kaneko, J.W. Harvey and M.L. Buss). Academic Press.

9 Scope, A., Filip, T., Gabler, C. et al. (2002). The influence of stress from transport and handling on hematologic and clinical chemistry blood parameters of racing pigeons (Columba livia domestica). *Avian Dis.* 46 (1): 224–229.

10 Gayathri, K.L. and Hedge, S.N. (1994). Sexual differences in blood values of the pigeons, Columba livia. *Comp. Biochem. Physiol.* 109B: 219–224.

11 Glomski, C.A. and Pica, A. (2011). *The Avian Erythrocyte: Its Phylogenetic Odyssey*, 227–237. Science Publishers.

12 Palomeque, J. and Planas, J. (1978). Blood volume in domestic pigeons. *Comp. Biochem. Physiol.* A59: 413–417.

13 Ramis, J. and Plamas, J. (1978). Iron metabolism in pigeons. *Q. J. Exp. Physiol.* 63: 383–393.

14 Lumeij, J.T. (1987). Avian clinical pathology. General considerations. *Vet. Quart.* 9 (3): 249–254.

15 Kovách, A.G., Szász, E., and Pilmayer, N. (1969). Mortality of various avian and mammalian species following blood loss. *Acta Physiol. Acad. Sci. Hung.* 35: 109–116.

16 Gayathri, K.L. and Hedge, S.N. (2006). Alteration in haematocrit values and plasma protein fractions during the breeding cycle of hens, Columba livia. *Anim. Reprod. Sci.* 91: 133–141.

17 Lumeij, J.T. and de Bruijne, J.J. (1985). Blood chemistry reference values in racing pigeons (Columba livia domestica). *Avian Pathol.* 14: 401–408.

18 Brückner D. Blutgefäßverlaufim Kopf – Und Halsbereich der Taube. PhD Thesis, Justus-Liebig-Universität Gießen, Germany. 1987.

19 Hattingh, J. and Smith, E.M. (1976). Anticoagulants for avian and reptilian blood: Heparin and EDTA. *Eur. J. Physiol.* 363: 267–269.

20 Fourie F.le R (1977). Effects of anticoagulants on the haematocrit, osmolarity, and pH of avian blood. *Poultry Sci.* 56: 1842–1846.

21 Anderson, A.A. (2005). Serotyping of US isolates of Chlamydophila psittaci from domestic and wild birds. *J. Vet. Diagn. Investig.* 17: 479–482.

22 Fair, J., Whitaker, S., and Pearson, B. (2007). Sources of variation in haematocrit in birds. *Ibis* 149: 535–552.

23 Pavlak, M., Vlahovic, K., Jercic, J. et al. (2005). Age, sexual and seasonal differences of haematological values and antibody status to Chlamydophila sp. in feral and racing pigeons (Columba livia forma domestica) from an urban environment (Zagreb, Croatia). *Eur. J. Wildl. Res.* 51: 271–276.

24 Balasch, J., Palomeque, J., Palacios, L. et al. (1974). Hematological values of some great flying and aquatic-diving birds. *Comp. Biochem. Physiol.* 49 (A): 137–145.

25 Kasprzak, M., Hetmanski, T., and Kulczykowska, E. (2006). Changes in hematological parameters in free-living pigeons(Columba livia f. urbana) during the breeding cycle. *J. Ornithol.* 147: 599–604.

26 Olayemi, F.O., Ojo, E.O., and Fagbohun, O.A. (2006). Haematological and plasma biochemical parameters of the Nigerian laughing dove (Streptopelia senegalensis) and the Nigerian duck (Anas platyrhynchos). *Vet. Arhiv.* 76 (2): 145–151.

27 Riddle, O. and Braucher, P.F. (1934). Hemoglobin and erythrocyte differences according to sex and season in doves and pigeons. *Am. J. Phys.* 108: 554–566.

28 Lumeij, J.T. (1991). Fasting and postprandial bile acid concentrations in racing pigeons (Columbia livia domestica) and mallards (Anas platyrhynchus). *J. Assoc. Avian Vet.* 5 (4): 197–200.
29 Kalomenopoulou, M. and Koliakos, G. (1989). Total body haematocrit iron kinetics and erythrocyte life span in pigeons. *Comp. Biochem. Physiol.* 92: 15–218.
30 Rodnan, G.P., Ebaugh, F.G., and Spivey Fox, M.R. (1957). The life span of the red blood cell and the red blood cell volume in the chicken, pigeon and duck as estimated by the use of Na2Cr51O4, with observations on red cell turnover rate in the mammal, bird and reptile. *Blood* 12 (4): 355–366.
31 Gayathri, K.L., Shenoy, K.B., and Hedge, S.N. (2004). Blood profile of pigeons (Columba livia) during growth and breeding. *Comp. Biochem. Physiol.* 138A: 187–192.
32 Amann, O., Visschers, M.J.M., Dorrestein, G.M. et al. (2006). Exocrine pancreatic insufficiency in pigeons. *Avian Pathol.* 35 (1): 58–62.
33 Akinpelu, A.I. (2008). Prevalence and intensity of blood parasites in wild pigeons and doves (Family: Columbidae) from Shasha Forest Reserve, Ile-Ife, Nigeria. *Asian J. Anim. Vet. Adv.* 3 (2): 109–114.
34 Borji, H., Moghaddas, E., Razmi, G.H. et al. (2011). Prevalence of pigeon haemosporidians and effect of infection on biochemical factors in Iran. *J. Parasit. Dis.* 35 (2): 199–201.
35 Godfrey, R.D., Pence, D.B., and Fedyrich, A.H. (1990). Effects of host and spatial factors on Haemoproteid community in mourning doves from Western Texas. *J. Wildl. Dis.* 26 (4): 435–441.
36 Lewis, J.C., Carpenter, J.W., and Morrison, J.A. (1975). Hemoprotozoa in mourning doves and other small birds of Western Oklahoma. *J. Wildl. Dis.* 11: 537–539.
37 Valkiūnas, G., Santiago-Alarcon, D., Levin, I.I. et al. (2010). A new Haemoproteus species (Haemosporida: Haemoproteidae) from the endemic Galapagos dove Zenaida galapagoensis, with remarks on the parasite distribution, vectors, and molecular diagnostics. *J. Parasitol.* 96 (4): 783–792.
38 Bunbury, N., Barton, E., Jones, C.G. et al. (2007). Avian blood parasites in an endangered columbid: Leucocytozoon marchouxi in the Mauritian pink pigeon Columba mayeri. *Parasitology* 134: 797–804.
39 Lumeij, J.T., Meidam, M., Wolfswinkel, J. et al. (1988). Changes in plasma chemistry after drug-induced liver disease or muscle necrosis in racing pigeons (Columba livia domestica). *Avian Pathol.* 17: 865–874.
40 Lumeij, J.T., de Bruijne, J.J., Slob, A. et al. (1988). Enzyme activities in tissues and elimination half-lives of homologous muscle and liver enzymes in the racing pigeon (Columba livia domestica). *Avian Pathol.* 17: 851–864.
41 Hadley, T.L., Grizzle, J., Rotstein, D.S. et al. (2010). Determination of an oral aflatoxin dose that acutely impairs hepatic function in domestic pigeons (Columba livia). *J. Avian Med. Surg.* 24 (3): 210–221.
42 Zollinger, T.J., Hoover, J.P., Payton, M.E. et al. (2011). Clinicopathologic, gross necropsy, and histologic findings after intramuscular injection of carprofen in a pigeon(Columba livia) model. *J. Avian Med. Surg.* 25 (3): 173–184.
43 Vereecken, M., De Herdt, P., Vanrobaeys, M. et al. (2001). Plasma biochemistry in pigeons experimentally infected with Salmonella. *Avian Dis.* 45: 467–472.
44 Lumeij, J.T. (1987). Plasma urea, creatinine and uric acid concentrations in response to dehydration in racing pigeons (Columba livia domestica). *Avian Pathol.* 16: 377–382.
45 Wismatt, J., Canon, N., Pearce, R.D. et al. (2009). Assessment of novel avian renal disease markers for the detection of experimental nephrotoxicosis in pigeons (Columba livia). *J. Zoo Wildl. Med.J Zoo Wildl Med* 40 (3): 487–494.
46 Wagner, W.D. (1978). Risk factors in pigeons genetically selected for increased atherosclerosis susceptibility. *Atherosclerosis* 31 (4): 453–463.
47 Bordel, R. and Haase, E. (1993). Effects of flight on blood parameters in homing pigeons. *J. Comp. Physiol. B.* 163: 219–224.
48 Bordel, R. and Haase, E. (2000). Influence of flight on protein catabolism, especially myofilament breakdown, in homing pigeons. *J. Comp. Physiol. B.* 170: 51–58.
49 Arad, Z., Horowitz, M., Eylath, U. et al. (1989). Osmoregulation and body fluid compartmentalization in dehydrated heat-exposed pigeons. *Am. J. Physiol.* 257 (26): R377–R382.
50 Lumeij JT. A Contribution to Clinical Investigative Methods for Birds, with Special Reference to the Racing Pigeon. PhD thesis, Utrecht University, Utrecht, The Netherlands, 1987.
51 Roman, Y., Bed'Hom, B., Guillot, A. et al. (2009). Identification of apolipoprotein A-I in the α-globulin fraction of avian plasma. *Vet. Clin. Pathol.* 38 (2): 206–212.
52 George, J.C., John, T.M., and Mitchell, M.A. (1989). Flight effects on plasma levels of lipid, glucagon and thyroid hormones in homing pigeons. *Horm. Met. Res.* 21 (10): 542–545.
53 Young, F. (1974). Serum lipids of young show racer and white Carneau pigeons fed a semipurified diet with or without cholesterol. *J. Nutr.* 104: 719–725.
54 Ray, R.M. and Young, F. (1978). Effect of dietary sucincreased and cholesterol on atherosclerosis, liver malate dehydrogenase and plasma lipoprotein lipase levels in pigeons. *J. Nutr.* 108: 944–953.
55 Barakat, H.A. and St. Clair, R.W. (1985). Characterization of plasma lipoproteins of grain- and cholesterol-fed white Carneau and show racer pigeons. *J. Lipid Res.* 26: 1252–1268.

56 Carmi, N., Pinshow, B., and Horowitz, M. (1994). Plasma volume conservation in pigeons: Effects of air temperature during dehydration. *Am. J. Physiol.* 36: R1449–R1453.

57 Lumeij, J.T., de Bruijne, J.J., and Kwant, M.M. (1990). Comparison of different methods of measuring protein and albumin in pigeon sera. *Avian Pathol.* 19: 255–261.

58 Lumeij, J.T. and Maclean, B. (1996). Total protein determination in pigeon plasma and serum: Comparison of refractometric methods with the biuret method. *J. Avian Med. Surg.* 10 (3): 150–152.

59 Lumeij, J.T. and de Bruijne, J.J. (1985). Evaluation of the refractometric method for the determination of total protein in avian plasma or serum. *Avian Pathol.* 14: 441–444.

60 Lumeij, J.T. and Wolfswinkel, J. (1988). Blood chemistry reference values for use in columbine hepatology. *Avian Pathol.* 17: 515–517.

61 George, J.C., John, T.M., and Koike, T.I. (1992). Flight effects on plasma levels of neurohypophysial hormones in homing pigeons. *Biol. Signal* 1 (3): 160–166.

62 Butler, P.J., West, N.H., and Jones, D.R. (1977). Respiratory and cardiovascular responses of the pigeon to sustained, level flight in a wind-tunnel. *J. Exp. Biol.* 71: 726.

63 Viswanathan, M., John, T.M., George, J.C. et al. (1987). Flight effects on plasma glucose, lactate, catecholamines and corticosterone in homing pigeons. *Horm. Metab. Res.* 19 (9): 400–402.

64 Weinstein, Y., Bernstein, M.H., Bickler, P.E. et al. (1985). Blood respiratory properties in pigeons at high altitudes: Effects of acclimation. *Am. J. Phys.* 249: R765–R775.

65 Schoemaker NJ, Kitslaar WJ. Venous blood gases in healthy racing pigeons. Proceedings of the Association of Avian Veterinarians Annual Conference, 2007, pp. 261–263.

66 Fedynich, A.M., Fredricks, T.B., and Benn, S. (2010). Lead concentrations of white-winged doves, Zenaida asiatica, collected in the lower Rio Grande Valley of Texas, USA. *Bull. Environ. Contam. Toxicol.* 85: 344–347.

67 Kendall, R.J. and Scanlon, P.F. (1982). Tissue lead concentrations and blood characteristics of mourning doves from southwestern Virginia. *Arch. Environ. Contam. Toxicol.* 11: 269–272.

68 Schulz, J.H., Millspaugh, J.J., Mermudez, A.J. et al. (2006). Acute lead toxicosis in mourning doves. *J. Wildl. Manag.* 70 (2): 413–421.

69 Elezai, I., Selimi, Q., Latai, K. et al. (2011). Metal bioaccumulation, enzymatic activity, total protein and hematology of feral pigeon (Columba livia), living in the courtyard of ferronickel smelter in Drenas. *J. Chem. Health Risks* 1 (1): 1–6.

70 Gonzalez, M. and Tejedor, M.C. (1992). δ-ALAD activity variations in red blood cells in response to lead accumulation in rock doves (Columba livia). *Bull. Environ. Contam. Toxicol.* 49: 527–534.

71 Bannon, D.T., Parsons, P.J., Centeno, J.A. et al. (2011). Lead and copper in pigeons (Columba livia) exposed to a small arms–range soil. *Arch. Environ. Contam. Toxicol.* 60: 351–360.

72 Howard, L.L., Papendick, R., Stalis, I.H. et al. (2002). Fenbendazole and albendazole toxicity in pigeons and doves. *J. Avian Med. Surg.* 16 (3): 203–210.

73 Gozalo, A.S., Schwiebert, R.S., and Lawson, G.W. (2006). Mortality associated with fenbendazole administration in pigeons (Columba livia). *J. Am. Assoc. Lab. Anim. Sci.* 45 (6): 63–66.

74 Grizzle, J., Hadley, T.L., Rotstein, D.S. et al. (2009). Effects of dietary milk thistle on blood parameters, liver pathology, and hepatobiliary scintigraphy in white Carneaux pigeons (Columba livia) challenged with B1aflatoxin. *J. Avian Med. Surg.* 23 (2): 114–124.

75 Sharma, L.L. and Saxena, P.N. (1998). Furadan SP50 induced haematological responses of blue-rock pigeon, Columba livia Gmelin. *Bull. Environ. Contam. Toxicol.* 61: 297–302.

76 Lumeij, J.T. and Westerhof, I. (1988). Clinical evaluation of thyroid function in racing pigeons (Columba livia domestica). *Avian Pathol.* 17: 63–70.

77 Rintamaki, H., Hissa, R., Etches, R.J. et al. (1986). Seasonal changes in some plasma hormones in pigeons: Diurnal variation under natural photoperiods with constant or seasonally changing ambient temperature. *Comp. Biochem. Physiol.* 84A (1): 33–38.

78 Lumeij, J.T., Boschma, Y., Mol, J. et al. (1987). Action of ACTH1-24 upon plasma corticosterone concentrations in racing pigeons (Columba livia domestica). *Avian Pathol.* 16: 199–204.

79 Westerhof, I., Van den Brom, W.E., Mol, J.A. et al. (1994). Sensitivity of the hypothalamic-pituitary-adrenal system of pigeons (Columba livia domestica) to suppression by dexamethasone, cortisol, and prednisolone. *Avian Dis.* 38: 435–445.

80 Saarela, S., Hissa, R., Etches, R. et al. (1986). Seasonal changes in some plasma hormones in pigeons from different environments. *Comp. Biochem. Physiol.* 84A (1): 25–31.

81 Magnino, S., Haag-Wackernagel, D., Ceigenfeind, I. et al. (2009). Chlamydial infections in feral pigeons in Europe: Review of data and focus on public health implications. *Vet. Microbiol.* 135: 54–67.

82 Vázquez, B., Esperón, F., Neves, E. et al. (2010). Screening for several potential pathogens in feral pigeons (Columba livia) in Madrid. *Acta Vet. Scand.* 52: 45–50.

83 Zweifel, D., Hoop, R., Sachse, K. et al. (2009). Prevalence of Chlamydophila psittaci in wild

birds — potential risk for domestic poultry, pet birds, and public health? *Eur. J. Wildl. Res.* 55: 575–581.

84 Cousquer, G. and Parsons, D. (2007). Veterinary care of the racing pigeon. *In Pract.* 29: 344–355.

85 Harlin, R. and Wade, L. (2009). Bacterial and parasitic diseases of Columbiformes. *Vet. Clin. North Am. Exot. Anim. Pract.* 12 (3): 453–473.

86 Bougiouklis, P., Brelou, G., Fragkiadaki, E. et al. (2005). Outbreak of avian mycobacteriosis in a flock of two-year-old domestic pigeons (Columba livia f. domestica). *Avian Dis.* 49: 442–445.

87 Gray, P.L., Saggese, M.D., Phalen, D.N. et al. (2008). Humoral response to Mycobacterium avium subsp. avium in naturally infected ring-neck doves (Streptopelia risoria). *Vet. Immunol. Immunop.* 125: 216–224.

88 Saggese, M.D., Tizard, I., and Phalen, D.N.J. (2010). Comparison of sampling methods, culture, acid-fast stain, and polymerase chain reaction assay for the diagnosis of mycobacteriosis in ring-neck doves (Streptopelia risoria). *Avian Med. Surg.* 24 (4): 263–271.

89 Witte, C.L., Hungerford, L.L., Papendick, R. et al. (2008). Investigation of characteristics and factors associated with avian mycobacteriosis in zoo birds. *J. Vet. Diagn. Investig.* 20: 186–196.

90 Kriz, P., Sisak, F., Slana, I. et al. (2011). Mycobacterium avium subsp. Avium and Salmonella enterica serotype Typhimurium var. Copenhagen phage type DT2 in pigeons. *Foodborne Pathog. Dis.* 8 (10): 1135–1137.

91 Kim, L.M., King DJ Gunzman, H. et al. (2008). Biological and phylogenetic characterization of pigeon paramyxovirus serotype 1 circulating in wild North American pigeons and doves. *J. Clin. Microbiol.* 46 (1): 3303–3310.

92 Al-Mulhim, I.A., Abu-Elzein, E.M.E., Gameel, A.A. et al. (2006). Comparative study on the clinico-pathological response of the collared dove (Streptopelia increasedogrisea arabica) and pigeons (Columba livia) to experimental infection with the pigeon paramyxovirus-1. *J. Anim. Vet. Adv.* 5 (5): 395–400.

93 Gibbs, S.E.J., Hoffman, D.M., Stark, L.M. et al. (2005). Persistence of antibodies to West Nile virus in naturally infected rock pigeons (Columba livia). *Clin. Diagn. Lab. Immun.* 12 (5): 665–667.

28

Passerine Birds

Kemba Marshall DVM, DABVP (Avian) [1] *and J. Jill Heatley DVM, MS, DABVP (Avian, Reptilian, Amphibian), DACZM* [2]

[1] *Purina Animal Nutrition Center, Gray Summit, Missouri, USA*
[2] *Department of Small Animal Clinical Sciences, College of Veterinary Medicine & Biomedical Sciences, Texas A&M University, College Station, Texas, USA*

Introduction

Clinical pathology may be used to evaluate the organ system health and function in passerine birds as in all animals. Hematologic and biochemical evaluation is a component of the minimum database for many species, but obtaining samples may be particularly challenging in passerine birds based on small sample size in these species. Additionally, clotting mechanisms of some within the Passeriformes are poorly understood. Assessment of values obtained either from hematologic, biochemical, or other testing maybe difficult based on lack of normative data. Sampling of other normal conspecifics or consulting previous baseline data may be invaluable for diagnostic purposes in these species. However, even minute samples may provide diagnostic information if handled and evaluated carefully. The aim of this chapter is to give practitioners an efficient text to increase knowledge of techniques to obtain diagnostics samples, increase comprehension of diagnostic tests, and provide test result interpretation for passerine birds.

Species

Passerine birds, known also as perching birds and songbirds, comprise approximately 60% of all bird species. Passeriformes are characterized by an anisodactyl foot to facilitate perching. Well-developed neopulmonic and paleopulmonic parabronchi provide highly efficient gas exchange, and fusion of the cranial thoracic air sacs results in a single median clavicular air sac. Of note also is that the right and left sinuses that lack connection [1]. Passeriformes range in size from the ~1.5 kg raven to species smaller than 5 g. Passerine birds are commonly maintained in captivity for their beautiful plumage, singing, and mimicry abilities. Songbirds are also studied in the laboratory and in the field to better understand neural plasticity, learning behavior, the speciation and radiation process and as bioindicators of infectious disease and environmental toxins [2]. The taxonomy of Passeriformes remains in flux owing to increasing discovery of genetic information leading to systematic reclassification. The term myna or mynah is often used in reference to any starling of the Indian subcontinent, regardless of taxonomic relationship. Similarly, the terms sparrow and finch are not taxonomically specific and include more than one family of birds. Table 28.1 [3] lists select passerine birds included in this chapter.

Sample Collection

Because of the diminutive and sometimes delicate nature of Passeriformes, special consideration should be given to the decision to collect blood or other samples for clinical pathology. To the best of our knowledge, only a single study of the cliff swallow, *Petrochelidon pyrrhonota,* has shown lower annual survivorship of blood-sampled birds versus those unsampled, which may have been based on factors in addition to blood collection such as species physiology, habitat, foraging style, and dispersal behavior [4, 5]. Multiple field studies have supported the concept that blood sampling of free-living Passeriformes has no significant impact on key indicators. These indicators include behavioral changes, survival rates, annual return rate or recapture probability, stopover duration during migration, body condition score, mass gain/loss, or reproduction [6, 7]. Thus, blood sampling of wild Passeriformes, following proper humane procedures and precautions, is not harmful [6, 7]. Nevertheless, the fact that any study found a statistically significant correlation between blood sampling and survival suggests that in

Exotic Animal Laboratory Diagnosis, First Edition. Edited by J. Jill Heatley and Karen E. Russell.

Table 28.1 Select Passerine birds commonly encountered by veterinarians or included in this chapter [3].

Family	Groups included	Common name	Scientific name
Corvidae	Vireos, shrikes, crows, ravens, jays	House crow Blue jay	*Corvus splendens* *Cyonocitta cristata*
Paridae	Titmice, chickadees, tits	Great tit Blue tit	*Parus major* *Cyanistes caeruleus*
Hirundinidae	Swallows, martins	Cliff swallow House martin	*Petrocheildon pyrrhonata* *Delichon urbica*
Pycnonotidae	Bulbuls	Red-vented bulbul	*Pycnonotus cafer*
Zosteropidae	White eyes	Japanese white-eye	*Zosterops japonicus*
Bombycillidae	Waxwings	Cedar waxwing	*Bombycilla cedrorum*
Troglodytidae	Wrens	Carolina wren	*Thryothorus ludovicianus*
Muscicapidae	Old World flycatchers, chats	Pied flycatcher	*Ficedula hypoleuca*
Turdidae	Thrushes, robins	American robin	*Turdus migratorius*
Sturnidae	Starlings	European starling Common myna(h)[a] Indian hill mynah	*Sturnus vulgaris* *Acridotheres tristis* *Gracula religiosa*
Mimidae	Mockingbirds, thrashers	Northern mockingbird	*Mimus polyglottos*
Ploceidae	Weavers	Baya weaver birds	*Ploecus phillipinus*
Estrildidae	Estrildid finches	Gouldian finch Zebra finch White-headed munia	*Chloebia gouldiae* *Taeniopygia guttata* *Lonchura maja*
Fringillidae	True finches	Canary Scarlet rosefinch Greenfinches	*Serinus canaria* *Carpodacus erythrinus* *Chloris spp.*
Passeridae Emberizidae	True sparrows American sparrows, buntings	Tree sparrow House sparrow Rufous-collared sparrow White-crowned sparrow White-throated sparrow	*Passer montanus* *Passer domesticus* *Zonotrichia capensis Zonotrichia leucophrys Zonotrichia albicollis*
Icteridae	Grackles, New World blackbirds, orioles, oropendolas	Red-winged blackbird Common grackle Boat-tailed grackle Western meadowlark	*Agelaius phoeniceus* *Quiscalus quiscali* *Quiscalus major* *Sturnella neglecta*
Cardinalidae	Cardinals, tanagers	Northern Cardinal Scarlet tanager Summer tanager Western tanager Rose-breasted grosbeak	*Cardinalis cardinalis* *Piranga olivacea* *Piranga rubra* *Piranga ludoviciana* *Pheucticus ludovicianus*

[a] The term myna or mynah is often used in reference to any starling of the Indian subcontinent, regardless of taxonomic relationship. Similarly, the terms sparrow and finch are not taxonomically specific and include more than one family of birds.

Passeriformes, blood sample volume and blood sampling techniques should be determined prior to sampling and adhered to in order to best protect avian welfare.

With a planned approach to first stabilize and then further evaluate the passerine patient, diagnostic clinicopathologic data can be obtained from even very small Passeriformes. From the blood smear, the differential white blood cell count (WBC), absolute white blood cell count, erythrocyte morphology, leukocyte morphology, and hemoparasite count can be determined. Red blood cell morphology may also be evaluated on the blood smear while the packed cell volume (PCV, hematocrit) and total solid concentrations are measured from microhematocrit tubes. Blood smear evaluations, PCV, and total solids measurement should be considered initial diagnostic tests. Compromised patients benefit from a warmed, oxygenated incubator and administration of warmed fluids prior to sample collection. Handling and sample collections from critically ill, unstable Passeriformes may result in pet death; this should be carefully explained to pet owners. Staggering tests over several days to allow for patient recovery and staging of sample collection in order of diagnostic priority must be considered to minimize patient stress and morbidity associated with sample collection.

Restraint for Venipuncture

Sedation and anesthesia are not required for venipuncture of passerine birds but should be considered depending on patient health status, venipuncturist experience, and anesthetic or sedative availability. Common anesthetic and analgesic choices in passerine birds include isoflurane, midazolam, and butorphanol [8, 9]. Fasting is typically unnecessary in these diminutive species, which lack a crop. As Passeriformes lack substantial amounts of subcutaneous tissue and are more prone to hematoma formation after venipuncture than mammals, firm, yet gentle pressure following venipuncture can help limit excessive hematoma formation [10]. Considerations and position specifics for each venipuncture site in Passeriformes are discussed later in this chapter.

Equipment

For patient safety, all collection materials should be prepared before the bird is restrained. A list of necessary samples should be written out and checked against necessary sampling materials to minimize time necessary for passerine physical restraint. Small-gauge needles and syringes, hematocrit tubes (plain or coated with anticoagulant), glass slides and/or cover slips, alcohol and cotton balls are the minimum to have prepared prior to attempting phlebotomy in the passerine. In general, use of smaller syringes and needles sizes will reduce the likelihood of patient trauma but also increased the likelihood of blood cell lysis and sampling clotting [6]. Small-gauge (27–25) needles and 0.2–3 ml syringes may be used for venipuncture in these species based on operator preference and species anatomy. Larger-volume syringes coupled with large-bore needles allow faster collection of large samples with less plunger motion. Other equipment for consideration should include small lancets, micro blood collection tubes, filter paper (for polymerase chain reaction (PCR) analyses), tissue glue, and replacement fluids. A heparin flush can be used to decrease the likelihood of sample clot formation. To "flush" a syringe, heparin is pulled into the syringe and then immediately pushed back into the bottle of heparin in one fluid motion. If droplets of sodium heparin remain, dilutional effects may occur, and analytical tests involving sodium and albumin may be altered. Microtainer tubes containing lithium heparin are the author's preference for receiving collected blood (BD Vacutainer Systems, New Jersey, United States). If collection volume is a concern, blood collected directly into microhematocrit tubes may be adequate for blood smears and to measure PCV and total protein concentration. The needle hub may contain enough blood for three microhematocrit tubes [11].

Sample, Blood, and Plasma Volumes

In the passerine patient, sample volumes should not exceed 1% of body weight and may need further reduction in the ill or injured passerine bird to ensure patient safety [11].Mean blood volume has been determined for the starling, *Sturnus vulgaris*, as 16.95 ± 2.5 ml/100 g of body weight [12]. During molt of captive Harris' sparrows, *Zonotrichia querula*, plasma osmolality, plasma volume, and blood volume increased, while hematocrit decreased by 6%. Erythrocyte numbers did not increase until molt was complete [13].

Collection Sites and Approaches

In Passeriformes, blood is most commonly collected from the brachial and jugular veins [7]. Methods described below are for right-handed venipuncturists and will likely require modification for left-handed individuals.

Jugular Vein

Jugular venipuncture allows collection of larger samples over a shorter time and more accurate control of blood sample volume. Additional benefits of jugular venipuncture include less likelihood of hematoma formation, and less equipment required for sample collection. Disadvantages include a more challenging collection technique and additional steps required for blood transfer and storage, making blood sample damage more likely [7]. A tuberculin or insulin syringe (1 ml or smaller) with a 26–28 gauge (g.) needle is recommended for venipuncture in small passerine birds. For larger birds like the red-winged black birds, a 3 ml syringe and 19 mm, 27.5 g. or 30 g. needle can be used [6].

The jugular vein and skin are thin but tough and mobile. Jugular venipuncture should not be pursued in these species if the vein cannot be directly visualized as it courses underneath the skin along the lateral aspect of the neck, posterior to the trachea and anterior to the cervical esophagus (Figure 28.1). Adequate restraint and immobilization are required for successful jugular venipuncture to avoid vein laceration. Multiple techniques have been described for techniques in which the same person restrains and obtains blood from these diminutive species. We have summarized these approaches, but for more detailed information consultation of the original references and obtaining training from an experienced individual is highly recommended.

The bird may be held in the left (or nondominant) hand with the head held gently between the index and

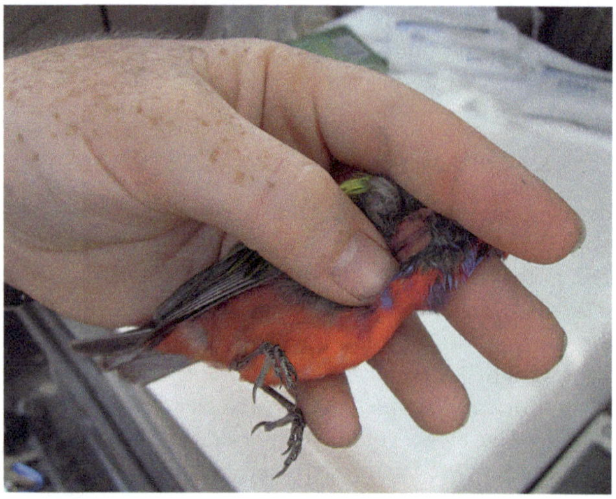

Figure 28.1 Lateral restraint for visualization of the right jugular vein of a male painted bunting, *Passerina ciris*.

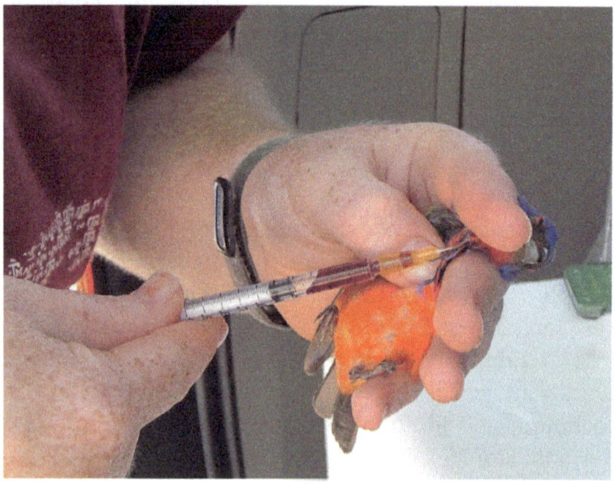

Figure 28.2 Restraint and jugular venipuncture of a male painted bunting, *Passerina ciris*.

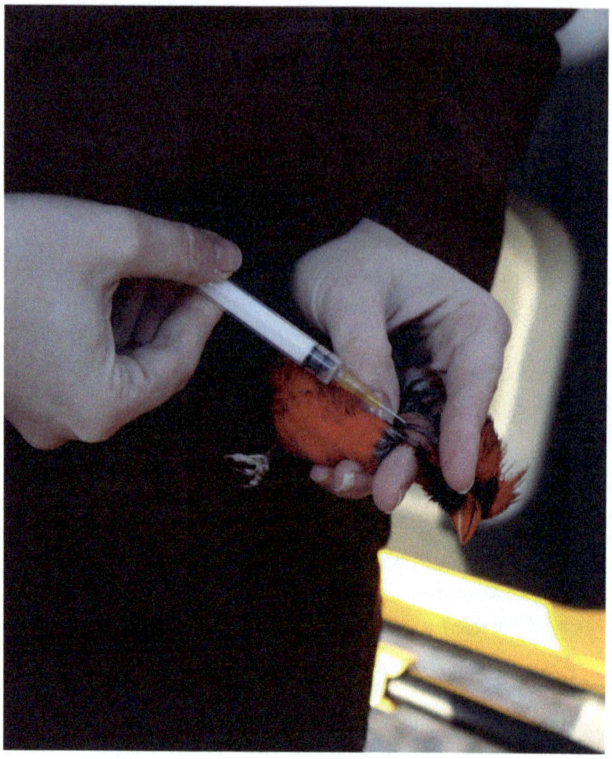

Figure 28.3 Jugular venipuncture of a male northern cardinal, *Cardinalis cardinalis*.

middle fingers. The body is held in left lateral recumbency within the palm with the legs tucked toward the body and the thumb resting either on the upward wing or more commonly the base or the neck/thoracic inlet (Figures 28.2–28.4). Alternatively, the bird can be held in the left hand with head between the index and middle fingers and the legs secured between the ring and pinky finger. The jugular vein is exposed by directing the right wing toward the tail (by pushing the carpus posteriorly) with the ring and small fingers [14]. Tension maintained between the thumb and fingers and a slight bend of the neck over the middle finger facilitates keeping the bird's neck immobile, maintaining feathers to the side of apteria to visualize the jugular vein, and allowing better fill of the jugular vein [7]. Restraint of the patient may be facilitated by slight cervical extension facilitated by holding the head between and extending the distal aspects of the middle and index fingers. The head position and body position may be modified in order to improve visualization, but a good general starting point is to have the body in lateral recumbency and the bill slightly more rotated toward the ground with a gentle bend in the neck over the forefinger.

Feathers are swept to the anterior and posterior aspects of the neck with alcohol. The needle is inserted shallowly, generally <0.25 cm. The syringe is held in the right hand, as the needle enters the vein at an acute angle of 15° from the skin. The syringe may be held overhand or underhand. The needle is best steadied by resting the syringe or needle bevel on the thumb of the left hand as it holds off the jugular vein at the thoracic inlet. Plunger aspiration may be performed via the ring finger if the syringe is held underhand or via thumb if the syringe is held overhand [6]. Should blood not immediately flow into the syringe upon aspiration, minor adjustments to facilitate blood flow may include slight backward or downward movement of the needle or needle rotation. After completing sample collection, the author recommends placing a small cotton ball at the site of venipuncture and holding it there for at least 30 s to facilitate hemostasis and absorb any residual alcohol or blood.

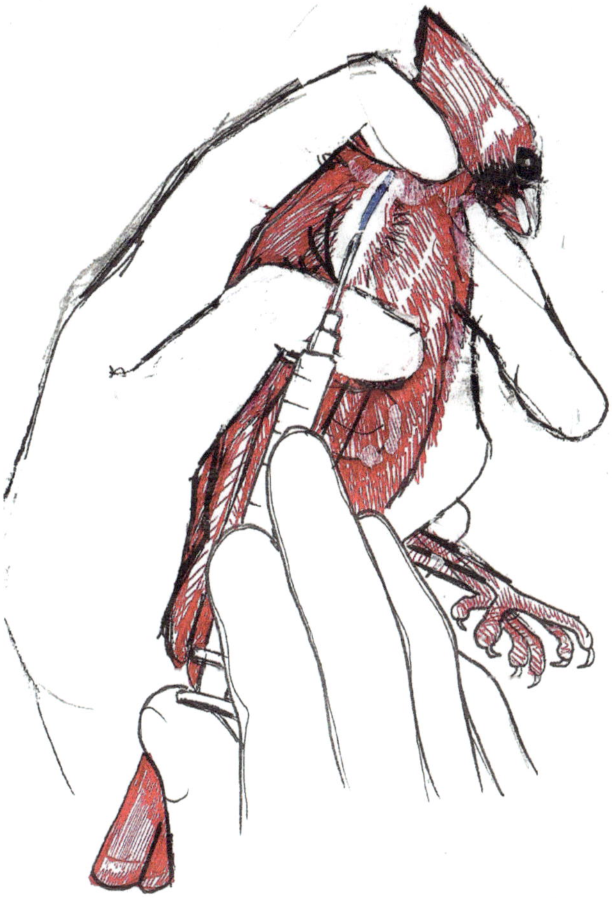

Figure 28.4 Approach to restraint and jugular venipuncture of a passerine bird, the northern cardinal, *Cardinalis cardinalis*. The bird is held laterally in the nondominant hand with the neck in extension. The head may be rotated slightly downward to avoid passerine aggression and to better visualize the jugular vein. Further syringe stabilization may be provided by placing the hub of the needle on the thumb, and positioning the thumb at the base of the neck to facilitate neck extension and jugular venous distension.

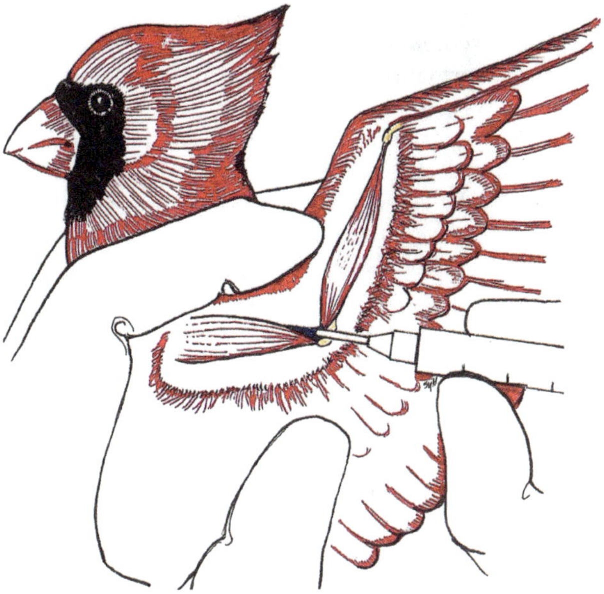

Figure 28.5 The sole venipuncturist approach for restraint and venipuncture of the ulnar vein, basilic, or wing vein of a Passeriforme requires training, skill, and preparation for adequate sample collection. The bander's hold and closed blood collection is demonstrated from the northern cardinal, *Cardinalis cardinalis*.

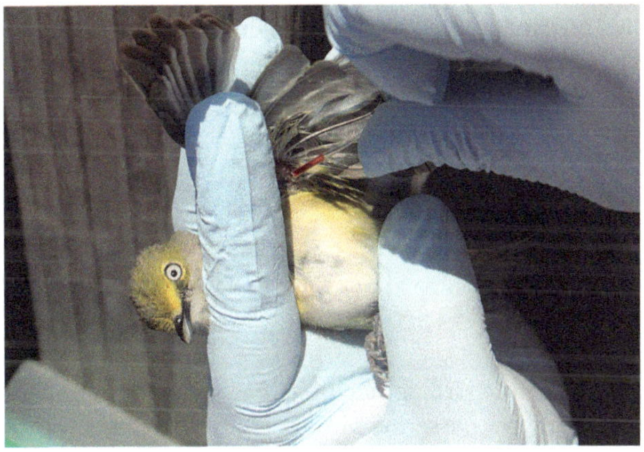

Figure 28.6 Open blood collection from the ulnar vein of a white eyed vireo, *Vireo griseus*, using the bander's hold and a hematocrit tube. *Source:* Image courtesy of Gabe Hamer, Texas A&M University.

Brachial Vein

The many advantages of blood draw from the brachial vein in Passeriformes make this a common option for blood collection from these species. This more peripheral venous site is technically easier to visualize and access, may have less severe consequences of poor sampling technique, requires less specialized technique and equipment (no syringe), and allows multiple attempts based on two sites of equal size for sampling in the two wings [7]. However, disadvantages of this site include a smaller expected sample size, an increased risk of hematoma formation, and increased sampling time and therefore patient handling time [7]. A "bander's grip" may be used for restraint of passerine birds to facilitate blood collection from the brachial vein [7] (Figures 28.5 and 28.6). Hold the bird in the nondominant hand, with head between the middle and index fingers. Rotate the body toward the thumb, tuck the legs under the body against the palm, and stabilize the bird with the base of the thumb. The left wing is then held in extension with the tips of index and middle fingers. The brachial vein is visible after feather flattening with 70% isopropyl alcohol. Venipuncture may be approached proximal or distal to the elbow joint; however, proximal puncture may allow increased blood volume collection [7]. Open collection with hematocrit tubes is commonly performed at this collection site.

Metatarsal Vein

This site of venipuncture is least commonly affected by hematoma formation in Passeriformes [7]. However, this small vein of passerine birds may be obscured based on leg scalation more distally or may be constricted based on frigid ambient temperatures. A 28–25 g. needle is recommended for 8–100 g passerine birds [7]. The needle is inserted bevel up, into the vein as it courses along the medial aspect of the lower leg. Samples obtained from this site as compared to cardiac puncture have increased plasma calcium, cholesterol, and hematocrit (Table 28.2) [15].

Unrecommended Sampling Sites

The toenail clip may be a quick and simple method of obtaining blood samples, but may result in sample contamination with tissue fluid, urates/fecal matter, tissue cells, or cellular debris. Toenail massage to facilitate blood flow changes the cell population of the blood sample. This method is painful to birds, may damage the nail bed, and is only recommended in case of emergency [10]. Cardiac puncture should not be used in birds which are not fully anesthetized (in preparation for euthanasia), based on high likelihood of causing patient mortality. This method is effective and efficient only when obtaining blood from a bird which is near death or freshly dead [7]. Blood samples obtained via cardiac puncture in Passeriformes give lower values for plasma calcium, cholesterol, and hematocrit than those obtained from the tibiotarsal vein (Table 28.2).

Sample Handling

Information regarding handling and storage of samples obtained from passerine birds is mainly anecdotal, with few prospective studies. However, based on small sample size, sample handling is of extreme importance in the diminutive species to ensure viable results from the first (and possibly only) sample obtained. Blood cell lysis has been associated with EDTA in some corvids including the jackdaw, *Corvus monedula*, and raven, *Corvus corax* [16]. Microtainers and microhematocrit tubes coated with dry lithium heparin reduce dilutional artifact concerns but cause staining and cellular artifact. Artifacts associated with heparin include blue coloration, poor leukocyte staining, and leukocyte clumping, which are reduced by excess heparin expulsion from the needle/syringe prior to blood draw [17]. The needle should be removed from the syringe before blood is placed into collection tubes. Ejecting blood through small-gauge needles may cause hemolysis and invalidation of hematologic and biochemical analysis results [18]. Blood collected into serum separator tubes should be spun down and refrigerated if analysis is not performed within a few hours of venipuncture. Blood smears should be stored in cardboard sleeves or plastic slide holders. Individual commercial labs should be contacted for shipping and handling instructions prior to mailing or courier pickup.

Specific Analytes

Complete Blood Count

Erythrocytes

Hematocrit or PCV is a measure of the relative volume of erythrocytes compared with the total blood volume. Hematocrit changes may reflect the concentration of or size of red blood cells [19]. Age, nutritional status, reproductive status, stage of molt, geographical elevation, season, and parasitism can all affect hematocrit [19, 20]. Because of the relatively short red blood cell (RBC) life span of these species, 1+ polychromasia is a common finding considered clinically acceptable in the healthy passerine birds (Figure 28.7). In nestling tree sparrows, *Passer montamus*, hematocrit increased with age from the late embryonic stage until fledging [21]. Females tend to have a relatively decreased hematocrit as estrogens inhibit and androgens stimulate erythropoiesis [20, 22]. In nestling pied flycatchers and blue tits, hematocrit is set by environmental conditions during the growth

Table 28.2 Comparative blood composition obtained from the tibiotarsal vein (TBT) or heart of the white-crowned sparrow *Zonotrichia leucophrys* from 50 paired samples [15].

Analyte	Calcium	(mEq/L)	Cholesterol	(mg/ml)	Hematocrit	(%)
Venipuncture site	TBT vein	Heart	TBT vein	Heart	TBT vein	Heart
Minimum	3.67	3.4	0.307	0.331	28	24
Maximum	89.56	71.3	5.259	5.704	66	57
Standard deviation	25.01	20.29	1.088	1.175	9.86	8.91
Average	21.59	18.05	1.078	1.049	46.8	40.7

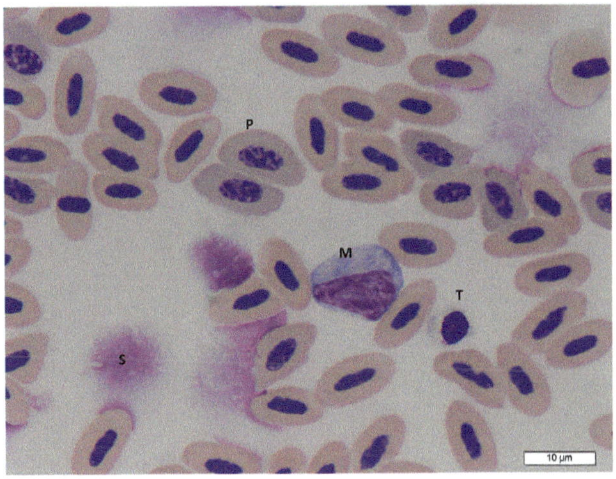

Figure 28.7 Blood smear from a northern cardinal, *Cardinalis cardinalis*, magnified 1000 × and stained with Elitech (formerly Wescor) methanolic Romanowsky stain. Mild 1+ polychromasia, typical in healthy passerine birds, is evident based on the polychromatophilic erythrocytes (P). Smudge cells (S) are evidence of poor smear preparation technique. A thrombocyte (T) and a monocyte (M) are also shown.

phase rather than by the hatch nest locale [23, 24]. Studies conflict regarding expected changes in RBC concentrations due to parasitism [25, 26]. In free-living Passeriformes, increased hematocrit is associated with readiness for migration and winter [27]. Increased hematocrit may increase oxygen transfer to tissues during times of increased work load, as has been demonstrated during migration and raising of young [28]. In species adapted to altitude, such as the Rosy finch, *Leucosticte arctoa*, increased O_2 affinity rather than increased HCT occurs. Increased HCT occurs because of short-term adjustments to hypoxia or cold, rather than adaptation to altitude [29].

Hemoparasites

Hemoparasites are commonly observed in the blood smears of captive and wild passerine birds but seldom have clinical significance. Most blood parasites are vector-transmitted protozoans living in tissues and in the peripheral blood of their hosts, consuming a variety of host metabolites and hemoglobin [30]. Hemoparasitism may be caused by *Hemoproteus* spp., *Leucocytozoon* spp., *Trypanosoma* spp., or microfilariae-producing species. In healthy populations of free-living Passeriformes, hemoparasite identification via light microscopy on blood smears is infrequent [27].

The neural parasite *Chandlerella quiscali* may cause marked host microfilaremia in the common grackle, *Quiscalus quiscula versicolor*, blue jay, *Cyanocitta cristata bromia*, brown-headed cowbird *Molothrus ater*, and starling, *Sturnus vulgaris*, but may also parasitize a variety of other avian hosts, some with lethal consequences [11]. Microfilariae from adult female nematodes may be underestimated as they appear in peripheral blood only at night [31]. Hemolytic anemia and attendant clinical signs, including death, presumably from infection with a nonhost-adapted species, have been reported [32]. Vector and fomite transmission of these parasites can occur. Additional passerine species affected include fringillid finches, magpies, sparrows, starlings, thrushes, wild tits, blue-faced parrot finches, and Old World warblers. Diagnosis is traditionally through identification of the intracellular parasite on a blood film; however, PCR although not yet commercially available, may be more sensitive and specific for detection of low levels of infection [32].

Atoxoplasma spp. are coccidian parasites with complex life cycles involving the reticuloendothelial and gastrointestinal systems that may cause morbidity and mortality in captive passerine birds. Atoxoplasmosis can affect many species of passerine birds including captive canaries, *S. canaria*, sparrows, finches, mynahs, starlings, thrushes, oropendolas, white eyes, and tanagers. In the live bird, diagnosis may be based on buffy coat or blood smear cytology, fecal wet mount and/or flotation, and by PCR testing of blood or feces [33]. Cytological examination of infected birds may allow identification of sporozoites within lymphocytes in peripheral blood films. *Atoxoplasma* spp. sporozoites are small (3–5 mm) and pale with round to oval eosinophilic intracytoplasmic inclusions that indent the lymphocyte nucleus, resulting in a characteristic crescent shape in Romanowsky-stained preparations [33].

Leukocytes

In general, the total white blood cell count in Passeriformes is often generalized as lower than expected in larger avian species. However, literature review reveals extensive total WBC variability in this diverse group of species. The larger *Corvus* spp. (crows) have reported WBC from $12.7–26.04 \times 10^3/mm^3$ [34]. The Gouldian finch, *Chloebia gouldii* [$7.51 \times 10^3/mm^3$], and the great tit, *Parus major* [$4.5 \times 10^3/mm^3$], have some of the lowest reported total leukocyte counts [34]. Total WBC and differentials for select Passeriforme species are given in Table 28.3. While evaluation of cellular ratios is commonplace in the study of free-living Passeriformes, leukocyte morphology has been minimally described in Passeriformes. The cell morphology of these species is assumed similar to that of other birds, but the nature of toxic change, left shift, and expected cellular dynamics in infection or trauma has received little attention in these species [34, 39].

Most Passeriformes are characterized by a low heterophil to lymphocyte ratio (H:L, 2:7) [39]. As in other species, many factors can affect the two primary white

Table 28.3 Hematologic reference data for select passerine species [35–37].

Analyte (abbreviation)	Unit SI (conventional)	Saffron finch, *Sicalis flaveola*	Gouldian finch *Erythrura gouldiae*	Double barred finch *Taeniopygia bichenovii*	Black-crested finch *Lophospingus pusillius*	Zebra finch *Taeniopygia guttata* [38]	Canary [35] *Serinus canaria*	Mynah *Acridotheres tristis*	Common crow [36, 37] *Corvus brachyrhynchos*
Data format		**Mean**	**Mean**	**Mean**	**Mean**	**Mean [range]**	**Mean**	**Range**	**Mean [Range]**
Leukocytes (WBC)	$\times 10^3/\mu L = (\times 10^9/L)$	10.51 (10.51)	9.846 (9.846)	9.846 (9.846)	10.20 (10.20)	19000 (1.9)	4–9 (4–9)	6–11 (6–11)	3.580 [36] 9.08 [0.0–17.16] [37]
Heterophils	$\times 10^3/\mu L = (\times 10^9/L)$	4.249 (4.249)	1.480 (1.480)	1.480 (1.480)	3.360 (3.360)	10 [4–23.6] (1 [0.4–2.4])		25–65 (0.25–0.65)	3.80[0.0–7.29] [37] (3.80[0.0–7.29]) [37]
	%						20–50 (0.2–0.5)		4.640 [37] (4.640)
Lymphocytes	$\times 10^3\ \mu L = (\times 10^9/L)$	5.529 (5.529)	6.583 (6.583)	6.583 (6.583)	8.770 (8.770)	57.4 [45.5–79.8] (5.7 [4.5–7.8])		20–60 (0.2–0.6)	3.84[0.0–8.73] [37]
	%						40–75 (0.4–0.75)		0.417 [37] (0.417) [37]
Monocytes	$\times 10^3/\mu L\ (\times 10^9/L)$	0.792 (0.792)	0.706 (0.706)	0.706 (0.706)	0.248 (0.248)	8.2 [1.4–16.9] (0.82 [0.14–1.7])		0–3 (0–0.3)	217 [0–528] [37] (217[0–528]) [37]
	%						0–1 (0–0.1)		2.494 [37] (2.494) [37]
Eosinophils	$\times 10^3/\mu L\ (\times 10^9/L)$	1.960 (1.960)	0.720 (0.720)	0.720 (0.720)	0.365 (0.365)	1.3 [0–8.1] (0.13 [0–0.8])		0–3 (0–0.3)	1215 [0–3588] [37] (12.16[0–35.88]) [37]
	%						0–1 (0–0.1)		
Basophils	$\times 10^9/L = (\times 10^3/\mu L)$					0.4 [0–4] (0.04 [0–0.4])		0–5 (0–0.5)	557 [37] 5.57 [37]
	%						0–1 (0–0.1)		43.5
Hematocrit (HCT)	% 0.01	47.7	50.4	50.4	50.8			2.4–4.0 (2.4–4.0)	0.43[0.30–0.56] [37] (43.3[30.2–56.3]) [37] 0.374 (37.4) [36]
Erythrocytes (RBC)	$\times 10^6/\mu L\ (\times 10^{12}/L)$	3.85 (3.85)					2.5–4.5 (2.5–4.5)		

blood cells, the lymphocyte and the heterophil [40]. Cellular changes as indicators of health in Passeriformes have perhaps best been studied in the great tit. In the great tit, handling stress increased heterophil counts 30–60 minutes after capture and decreased lymphocytes and eosinophil counts 60–120 minutes after capture. Accordingly, H:L also increased 60–120 minutes after capture. Thus, the stress leukogram occurs rapidly after handling of passerine birds [41]. Marked changes in this ratio, based on increase of heterophils and decrease of lymphocytes, have also occurred after capture in rufous-collared sparrows [35]. In nestling great tits, increased heterophil count, lymphocyte count, and H:L were associated with improved survival to fledging [42]. In adult great tits, migration survival is associated with decreased H:L and increased lymphocyte counts [43]. Free-living zebra finches have higher H:L and total leukocyte counts than aviary birds. However, differences were lessened by 10 days of captivity, likely based on the stress of acclimation [38]. The H:L ratio and white blood cell count were not affected by sex in the zebra finch [38].

In most Passeriformes, circulating monocyte, eosinophil, and basophil percentages are <10% [34]. However, species variability occurs, and assessing a blood sample from an apparently healthy conspecific for evaluation of WBC count and cell morphology may be more diagnostically appropriate for many lesser-known species than consultation of reference data. Reference images of monocytes, heterophils, eosinophils and basophils are found in Figures 28.9–28.11. Eosinophil counts may decrease based on captivity in some Passeriformes, such as the rufous-collared sparrows [44]. The scarlet rose finch, *Carpodacus erythrinus*, is an example of a basophilic species, with 42%–56% basophils normally in circulation, which may be further increased by *Hemoproteus* spp. infection [45].

Thrombocytes

Thrombocyte morphology of passerine birds is similar to that of other avian species (Figure 28.8). However, determinations of thrombocyte counts from apparently healthy passerine species appear rare [34]. Plateletcrit, defined as the percentage of platelets per blood volume, have reported mean ± SD values of (0.0059 ± 0.0027%), with platelet counts of ($11.87 \pm 5.67 \times 10^9$/l). A platelet distribution width of (6.15 ± 0.49%), and mean platelet volume ($5.20 \pm 0.72\,\mu m^3$) were derived from 31–36 apparently healthy great tit nestlings via automated analyzer [42]. These values should more properly be termed thrombocrit, thrombocyte count, and thrombocyte distribution width for Passeriformes. Reports of thrombocytopenia and thrombocytosis are also lacking in these species; the causes for these abnormalities are assumed to be similar to those in other animals.

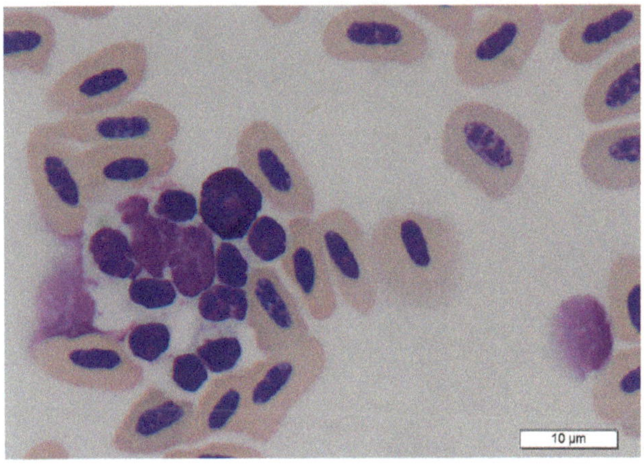

Figure 28.8 Blood smear from a northern cardinal, *Cardinalis cardinalis*, magnified 1000× and stained with Elitech (formerly Wescor) methanol-based Romanowsky stain. A thrombocyte clump is topped by a single basophil.

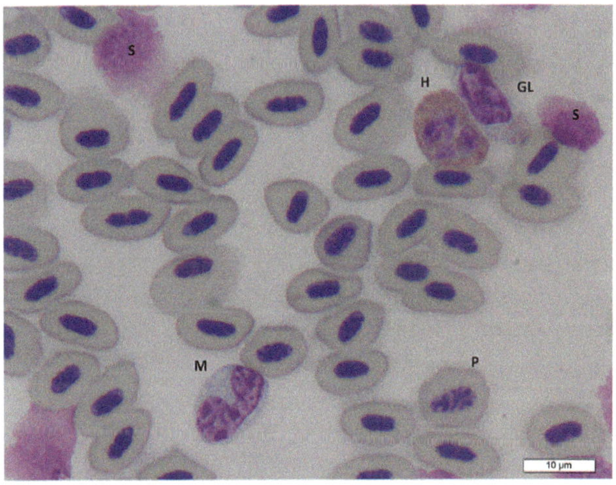

Figure 28.9 Blood smear from a northern cardinal, *Cardinalis cardinalis*, magnified 1000× and stained with Elitech (formerly Wescor) methanol-based Romanowsky stain. A monocyte (M), heterophil (H), polychromatophil (P), smudge cells (S), and a granular lymphocyte (GL) are shown.

Hemostasis

Hemostasis has received minimal study in passerine birds, but mechanisms and factors are thought the same as other avian species. No commercial assays are available to assess passerine hemostasis. However, whole blood clotting times are likely most applicable for clinical use in these species. Hemostasis has been investigated in the house sparrow, *Passer domesticus*, baya weaver bird, *Ploceus philippinus*, and common myna, *Acridotheres tristis*, as part of a study of the effects of the pesticide lindane [46]. For control groups, bleeding time was 72.00 ± 4.33, 67.00 ± 3.22, and

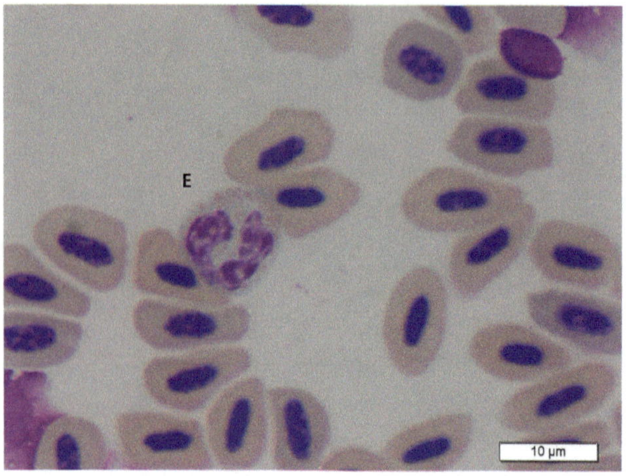

Figure 28.10 Blood smear from a northern cardinal, *Cardinalis cardinalis*, magnified 1000 × and stained with Elitech (formerly Wescor) methanol-based Romanowsky stain. Smudge cells are in the lower left and upper right while an eosinophil is shown centrally.

73.50 ± 3.80 seconds, respectively. Clotting time as measured via the capillary glass tube method was 19.00 ± 2.08, 14.25 ± 1.00 and 21.20 ± 1.88 seconds, respectively [46]. Blood group antigens have received minimal clinical attention in Passeriformes; A, B, AB, and O blood antigens have been identified in passerine birds based on human blood typing methodologies [47]. Cross-matching deserves consideration in these species prior to transfusion [47, 48].

Biochemical Panel

Prospective studies to create reference ranges using current references for biomarkers of health in passerines are rare to nonextant (Table 28.4).

Liver Enzymes

To our knowledge, the diagnostic specificity or sensitivity of enzymes associated with liver health in other species, including bile acids, have not been specifically examined in Passeriforme species. In greenfinches, increased enzyme activities of GOT (glutamate oxaloacetate transaminase), GPT (glutamic pyruvic transaminase), GDH (glutamate dehydrogenase), SDH (sorbitol dehydrogenase), and LDH (lactate dehydrogenase) relative to non-Passeriforme birds are seen. This may be based on the birds' hyperactivity, high metabolic rate, and high tissue blood flow [49].

Muscle Enzymes

In Passeriformes, muscle wasting, subcutaneous fluid therapy, and trauma may increase plasma activities of CK (creatine kinase) and AST (aspartate aminotransferase). Long-distance migration and shivering overnight in winter months can increase plasma activities of CK, LDH, and AST based on muscle catabolism for fuel during long-distance migration or muscle damage shivering for thermogenesis [50].

Renal Enzymes

Increased activities of LDH, AST, and CK (creatine kinase) have been tentatively associated with captivity (and transient physiological harm) during the breeding season in free-ranging passerine birds [51]. As these enzymes occur in multiple internal organs, and normal enzyme activities may be maintained by small amount of renal tissue, renal insufficiency is challenging to definitively diagnose based on biochemical test results alone. Further, in many xeric-adapted Passeriformes, uric acid, plasma osmolality, and BUN may increase based on normal physiologic processes [52]. As passerine birds may deposit amyloid in renal tissues in response to chronic infections, amyloidosis should be included on a list of differentials for renal disease in songbirds [52, 53].

Pancreas

For starch digestion, pancreatic amylase is the key enzyme. In passerine birds, dietary starch content impacts the activity of amylase, maltase, and sucrase [54]. Dietary modulation of pancreatic and intestinal enzyme secretion has been documented in select passerine birds [54–56]. To our knowledge, clinical pancreatitis or diabetes has yet to be diagnosed in a passerine antemortem via clinical signs, enzyme or biochemical markers. Glucose levels in these species tend to be consistent with the relatively increased concentrations, compared to mammals, found in the plasma of other avian species.

Gastrointestinal and Cardiac

Despite commonly being affected by gastrointestinal disease, biomarkers for use in passerine birds remain poorly investigated. Cardiac disease is seldom diagnosed in passerine birds antemortem, and cardiac biomarkers, which could have greater applicability than standard diagnostics because of the diminutive size of these species, awaits investigation. In an Indian hill mynah (*Gracula religiosa*) suffering congestive heart failure, an increased

Table 28.4 Biochemical values for select adult, captive passerine species.

Analyte (abbreviation)	Unit SI (US)	Saffron finch [36] *Sicalis flaveola*	Gouldian finch [36] *Erythrura gouldiae*	Double barred finch [36] *Taeniopygia bichenovii*	Canary [35] *Serinus canaria domestica*	Finch [35]	Mynah [35] *Acridotheres tristis*	Common crow [36, 37] *Corvus brachyrhynchos*
Data		**Mean**	**Mean**	**Mean**	**Mean**	**Range**	**Range**	**Mean [Range] n = 37–90 [37]**
Alkaline (ALP) phosphatase	units/l = (U/l)	216			146–397			259 [36]
Alanine (ALT) aminotransferase	units/l = (U/l)	59						106 [36]
Lactate (LDH) dehydrogenase	units/l = (U/l)	812			120–350		600–1000	447 [36]
Aspartate (AST) Amino-transferase	units/l = (U/l)	220			45–345	150–350	130–350	332 [36] 287 [123–428] [37]
Calcium	mg /dl (mmol/l)	7.7 (0.428)			5.12–13.4 (0.284–0.744)		9–13 (0.5–0.722)	8.3 (0.461) [36] 8.4 [7.1–9.8] [37] 0.467[0.394–0.544] [37]
Creatinine	mg/dl = (μmol/l)				0.12–1.15 (10.61–101.66)		0.12–0.68 (10.61–60.11)	184 [0–398] [37] (16 265.6[0–35 183.20]) [37]
Creatinine (CPK) phosphokinase	units/l = (U/l)	1044 (1044)						297 (297) [36]
Protein, total (TP)	g/dl (g/l)	3.7 (37)	3.0 (30)	4.0 (40)	2–4.5 (20–45)	3–5 (30–50)	2.3–4.5 (23–45)	3.0 (30) [36] 3.7 [2.5–4.8] [37] (37[25–48]) [37]
Phosphorous	mg/dl (μmol /l)	5.1 (450.84)			1.6–5.6 (141.44–495.04)			2.7 (238.68) [36] 2.6 [0–5.6] [37] (229.84[0–495.04]) [37]
Glucose	mg/dl (mmol/l)	431 (23.92)		216 (11.98)	198–396 (11–22)	198–450 (11–25)	189–349 (10.5–19.4)	360 (19.98) [36] 317 [216–416] [37] (17.61[12–23.11]) [37]
Cholesterol	mg/dl (mmol/l)	219 (56.72)						178 [104–249] [37] (9.89 [5.77–13.83]) [37]
Sodium (Na)	mEq/l, *mg /dl* (mmol /l)				*125–154*		*136–152*	159 [144–174] [37] (159 [144–174]) [37]
Potassium (K)	mEq/l, *mg /dl* (mmol/l)				*2.7–4.8*		*3.0–5.1*	3.3[1.2–5.1] [37] (3.3 [1.2–5.1]) [37]
Chloride (Cl)	mEq/l (mmol /l)							120[111–129] [37] (120[111–129]) [37]
Uric acid	mg/dl (μmol /l)	1.44 (24.2)					3.98–10 (237–595)	7.3 [0.0–16.1] [37] (645.32[0–1423.24]) [37]

aspartate aminotransferase (AST) activity [1800 IU/l] was the only biochemical abnormality reported [57].

Lipids

Lipids are seldom determined in captive companion passerine birds but are used to study body condition and the physiology of migration, diet, and stress in free-living and captive passerine birds. Plasma cholesterol and triglyceride concentrations were increased in passerine birds during trans-Saharan migration compared to those obtained from pre-migrants in Germany [58, 59]. Similarly, in a study of the migratory garden warbler, *Sylvia borin,* high fat mass of premigration was associated with increased plasma concentrations of triglycerides, cholesterol, and free fatty acids [3, 59]. In red-winged blackbirds, *Agelaius phoeniceus,* European starlings, *S. vulgaris,* and common grackles, *Quiscalus quiscali,* despite lack of migration or reproductive behavior based on captivity, seasonal changes in lipids and lipoproteins were also observed (Table 28.5) [51]. Handling-induced stress increases the plasmas triglycerides of the captive European starling by 25%–45% independent of photoperiod or time of day [60]. In the white-throated sparrow, *Zonotrichia albicollis,* birds fed a low-protein, high-glucose diet had increased plasma triglyceride concentrations and increased body fat [61]. Thus, while plasma lipids may indicate fattening of birds, diet also affects these analytes [61].

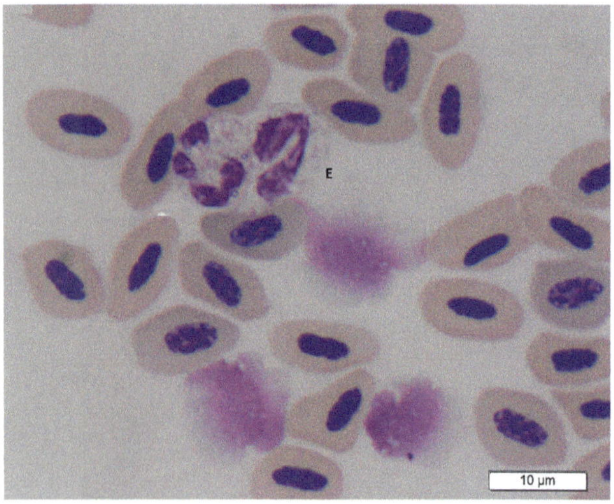

Figure 28.11 Blood smear from a northern cardinal, *Cardinalis cardinalis* magnified 1000 × and stained with Elitech (formerly Wescor) methanol-based Romanowsky stain. Eosinophil labeled E.

Iron

Iron storage disease (hemosiderosis and hemochromatosis) is a nutritional disease of captivity and has not been reported in free-living Passeriformes [62, 63]. Among passerine birds, Indian hill mynas, *G. religiosa,* are most commonly reported as affected; however, birds of paradise, tanagers, crows, Rothschild's starlings, and experimentally the European starling have suffered disease [64]. Idiopathic, heritable causes of iron storage disease and dietary overload are reported [65]. Biochemistry abnormalities which may occur in association with hemosiderosis or hemochromatosis include increased AST, bile acids, and iron. However, in advanced cases with severe liver disease, increase or decrease of liver biomarkers may occur [66].

Table 28.5 Plasma lipids and lipoproteins of select passerine birds based on season (n = 10) [51].

Analyte (abbreviation)	Units SI (US)	Species	Fall	Winter	Spring	Summer
Cholesterol	mmol/l (mg /dl)	Red-winged blackbirds *Agelarius phoeniceus*	5.38 ± 0.21 (208 ± 8)	4.74 ± 0.07 (183 ± 3)	6.47 ± 1.04 (250 ± 40)	3.78 ± 0.16 (146 ± 6)
		European starlings *Sturnus vulgaris*	4.71 ± 0.21 (182 ± 8)	7.07 ± 0.18 (273 ± 7)	6.76 ± 0.23 (261 ± 9)	2.71 ± 0.16 (105 ± 6)
		Common grackles *Quiscalus quiscali*	4.09 ± 0.13 (158 ± 5)	6.22 ± 0.23 (240 ± 9)	5.15 ± 0.13 (199 ± 5)	3.89 ± 0.16 (150 ± 6)
Triglyceride	mmol /l (mg /dl)	Red-winged blackbirds	3.65 ± 0.06 (141 ± 5)	6.22 ± 0.17 (240 ± 15)	6.58 ± 0.14 (254 ± 12)	4.92 ± 0.32 (190 ± 28)
		European starlings	2.82 ± 0.05 (109 ± 4)	3.06 ± 0.05 (118 ± 4)	2.93 ± 0.05 (113 ± 4)	2.49 ± 0.07 (96 ± 6)
		Common grackles	3.16 ± ±0.10 (122 ± 9)	4.48 ± 0.08 (173 ± 7)	3.52 ± 0.04 (136 ± 4)	3.52 ± 0.09 (136 ± 8)

Values expressed as mean ± SEM.

Electrolytes

Values for electrolytes have been reported from relatively few Passeriforme species. Methodology and sample handling may have extreme effects upon electrolytes and may contribute to the wide variation reported for values which should be tightly physiologically controlled, such as potassium and sodium. For the Passeriformes, the effects of sample processing delay, methodology, and sample damage or degradation (RBC lysis) upon electrolytes has not been specifically evaluated. In general, potassium tends to be lower than expected for that of companion mammals in passerine birds. For Passeriformes, concentrations of electrolytes from four species ranged from Na 152–163, Cl 120–132, and K 2.3–4.4 mMol [65]. Differences in electrolytes of Passeriformes which are migratory and nonmigratory have been reported in free-living Passeriformes [20]. Studies of trans-Saharan migrant Passeriformes found increased concentrations of plasma sodium in lean birds, reflective of dehydration from lack of appropriate fat stores to provide metabolic water during their strenuous trek [58].

Blood Proteins

The blood plasma of birds is a complex tissue containing thousands of distinct proteins, which is commonly used to assess health and nutrition in birds [67]. Proteins provide only 0.5% of osmotic pressure in birds [34]. Plasma protein measurement via refractometry in Passeriformes is hindered by physiologic concentrations of lipids, glucose, and beta carotenes. While protein electrophoresis (EPH) remains the gold standard, dry slide analyzer or Biuret methodologies may be a reasonable, although unvalidated, compromise for clinical use in these species. Qualitative examination of starch gel EPH of Passeriformes plasma protein from blood treated with EDTA was studied historically to assess taxonomic relations of avian species. Major differences in protein patterns among closely related passerine species suggests that EPH protein patterns of Passeriformes indicate physiologic status rather than taxonomic relatedness [68].

Prealbumin, albumin, and globulin are the primary plasma proteins reported in Passeriformes. Values (g/L) for total protein vary from 49 to 22 with an average of 36 from 16 species [34]. Values for albumin and globulin fall in the ranges [average] 9.3–20 [13.7] and 7.2–24 [17], respectively, for 10 passerine species. Albumin:globulin ratios in these species are often 1:1 or lower. Wide protein values reported in Passeriformes likely stem not only from species differences but also on varying methodologies used for determination of these analytes. Globulin concentrations were reduced in females with large brood size in the blue tit, *Cyanistes caeruleus* [69]. Increased concentration of heat shock proteins [HSP 60] and decreased humoral and cell mediated responses occur in adult female nesting passerine birds with larger brood size. Nestling house martins, *Delichon urbica*, with ectoparasitism or hemoparasitism had increased HSP 60, and grew more slowly [70]. Heat shock protein determination of birds remains relegated to research use as determination is via Western blot methodology [40, 71].

Blood Gases

Blood gases, lactate, and other acid base analytes are beginning to be evaluated in free-living Passeriformes but have received little attention in captive Passeriformes for clinical assessment of health [20, 72]. These analytes are more commonly determined from venous samples in these diminutive species, based on the difficulty of arterial cannulation. Species, habitat, location elevation and sampling site, and time until sampling may affect these analytes [20, 73]. Sedation of passerine birds with midazolam may change electrolyte concentrations and venous blood gas analytes based on a relative hypoventilation and decreased stress, but sedation is less likely to affect blood pH [74].

Vitamins

Little is known regarding acceptable plasma vitamin concentrations of passerine birds [75]. However, the white-headed munia (the rice bird), which is prone to deficiency, was key in the discovery of thiamine [75]. As species with relatively short gastrointestinal tracts and fast rates of passage, minimal vitamin uptake from intestinal synthesis is likely to occur in these species, this remains, however, to be studied [75].

Many conditions have been reported to affect the Gouldian finch including suspected vitamin D toxicosis resulting in calcification of renal and other tissues, vitamin D deficiency resulting in rickets, calcium deficiency, and selenium/vitamin E deficiency associated with dystocia or egg binding [76]. A single source lists plasma or serum mean values of α-tocopherol for captive passerine birds as (n = 5, 4 species) as 5.5 μg/ml [77]. A study of 13 free-living passerine species, sampled in Michigan in June and July, provides plasma vitamin E concentrations (in absorbance units) considered independent of diet type which range from 5287 in the rose-breasted grosbeak, *Pheucticus ludovicianus*, to 1439 in the red-winged blackbird, *A. phoeniceus* and cedar waxwing, *Bombycilla cedrorum*. The weighted average of vitamin E from the 194 samples was 1649 [78]. In a Gouldian finch suspected of suffering vitamin E deficiency, clinical signs and necropsy findings included acute dyspnea, pulmonary and cerebellar edema, and severe muscular degeneration [79]. In the red-vented bulbul and likely other Passeriformes, the enzyme L-gulonolactone oxidase is lacking, making vitamin C a dietary requirement to avoid signs of deficiency. However, sparrow species do not require dietary vitamin C. The house crow along with multiple mynah species endogenously synthesize vitamin C [75].

Carotenoids may be included in commercial Passeriformes diets and consumed by free-living passerine birds to improve coloration, provide antioxidant and photo protection, and increase breeding potential. They have been used as an indicator of fitness in some free-living Passeriformes. Plasma concentrations considered adequate in Passeriformes are poorly studied as carotenoids are not considered dietary requirements. Captive and free-living Passeriformes which take advantage of these compounds include the Gouldian finch, canary, cedar waxwing, and the northern cardinal. Canthaxanthin and astaxanthin are the most commonly commercially produced supplements in diets provided to captive Passeriformes [75]. Noninvasive methods for determination of carotenoids in free-living Passeriformes as health indicators have received some recent attention [79].

Calcium deficiency may limit reproductive success captive and free-living passerine birds [75]. However, determination of ionized calcium has not been determined in reasonable numbers for these species [20]. Zebra finches' dietary calcium intake changes egg laying amount and quality [80]. In the free-living great tit, acid rain decreases calcium availability of food sources resulting in poor quality eggshells and poor hatchability [81].

Toxins and Metals

Effects of air, soil, and water pollution upon birds including Passeriformes have been studied based on industry (mining and smelting) effects upon these species. Poor calcium metabolism, ataxia, anemia, increased parasitism, organ disease, and decreased breeding/hatching success of passerine birds is associated with heavy metal pollution of air, soil, water, insects, and nesting material [81–84]. Lead toxicity following ammunition exposure at gun ranges occurring in natural habitat affects all body systems [85].

Hormones

Many hormones have received in-depth study in free-living passerine birds based on the physiology of migration, breeding, courtship, and song. Few studies have evaluated hormones in healthy captive Passeriformes as part of clinical diseases processes. Consequently, hormonal assays are seldom available or used by the veterinary practitioner for diagnostic purposes in these species. Below, we have attempted to briefly summarize information which may be of diagnostic value in future for these species, concentrating on common species in captivity when data exist. We have restricted this summary to values for thyroid hormones, corticosterone, and its related binding protein, prolactin, and sex steroids. Other hormones may be of use in future. Methodologies for clinical determination of plasma hormones in Passeriformes are generally dictated by the laboratory chosen; however, recent studies indicate that solid phase extraction may be superior to radioimmunoassay (RIA) or enzyme immunoassay (EIA) for determination of some steroid hormones (dehydroepiandrosterone, corticosterone, and estradiol) from avian plasma based on high and consistent recoveries and separation of interferences [86].

Thyroid Hormones

In Passeriformes, thyroid hormones are associated with molt and with neuron loss and replacement, termed "brain molt." Clinical hypo- or hyperthyroidism has not been reported in captive Passeriformes. However, goiter, presumably based on dietary iodine insufficiency has been anecdotally reported to affect the Gouldian finch [76]. Radioimmunoassay of T4 has been validated and values obtained from the adult zebra finch and the post-fledging white-crowned sparrow, *Zonotrichia leucophrys*, for experimental purposes [37, 87].

Sex and Parental Hormones: Estrogens, Androgens, Luteinizing Hormone, gnRH, and Prolactin

In the altricial canary, plasma prolactin remains increased in females after brood hatch and decreases gradually during continued rearing of the young [88]. In the male canary, which does not incubate or feed the young, plasma prolactin increases only slightly during this time. Thus, in the canary, and likely other passerine birds, prolactin supports parental behavior. Testosterone and its analytes have been studied extensively in songbirds as it supports intraspecific aggression, territoriality, breeding, song, neurodevelopment, and behavior. In exchange, the immune system and parental care are reduced. These analytes are seldom used for clinical diagnosis of Passeriformes [89, 90]. Similarly, estrogens, LH (luteinizing hormone) and GnRH (gonadotropin releasing hormone) have also received primarily scientific attention for similar roles in avian reproduction and behaviors, but validated assays are not routinely available for clinical diagnosis in these species [91–93].

Table 28.6 Urine and plasma values for the sparrow *Zonotrichia capensis* [94].

Analyte	Units SI (US)	30% Dietary protein	70% Dietary protein
Urine osmolality	mOSm/kg (mmol/kg)	786 ± 48 (786 ± 48)	480 ± 184 (480 ± 184)
Plasma osmolality	mOSm /kg (mmol/kg)	382 ± 8 (382 ± 8)	375 ± 10 (375 ± 10)
Hematocrit	% (0.01)	53.17 ± 5.90 (0.53 ± 0.06)	47.2 ± 3.70 (0.47 ± 0.037)
Uric acid	mg/dl (μmol/l)	900 (5547.6)	500 (3082)
Urea	mg /dl (μmol/l)	200 (1232.8)	100 (616.4)
Ammonia	mg/dl	150	75
Total nitrogen	mg/dl (mmol/l)	475 (339.15)	280 (199.92)

Adrenal Hormones: Corticosterone

Corticosteroid binding globulin, CBG, or transcortin, is an α-1 globulin which transports corticosterone, the main adrenocortical hormone in the plasma of Passeriformes including the white-crowned sparrow and the zebra finch [34, 94]. Corticosterone has received extensive study in free-living birds as a stress indicator in association with many other avian behaviors which exhibit physiological increases, such as migration. In several free-living passerine birds, seasonally increased blood concentrations of corticosterone are associated with egg laying (white-crowned sparrow, European starling, western meadowlark) or with brooding (pied flycatcher). To the best of our knowledge, hyper- or hypoadrenocorticism has not been clinically diagnosed via blood assay in captive Passeriformes. Study of the zebra finch revealed maximal stress induced corticosterone levels in control birds of 20 nmol/l [57, 95].

Urinalysis

Based on their small size, urinalysis is not commonly performed in passerine birds, many of which are highly adapted for xeric environments and therefore produce minimal urine sample volume [96]. Increased dietary protein of the omnivorous sparrow, *Zonotrichia capensis,* resulted in increased urine osmolality without marked change of plasma osmolality or hematocrit (Table 28.6) [96]. In the passerine patient with evidence of polyuria, evaluation of a urine/urate sample collected from a clean surface may be of value. Determination of "dip-stick" values as well as microscopic examination of sediment can be performed on small samples within the veterinary practice.

PCR and Serology Useful for Passerine birds

Based on the small size of passerine birds, PCR is often pursued for antemortem and postmortem diagnosis rather than serology. Bacterial and viral disease is a common reason for the presentation of backyard passerine birds exhibiting signs of sepsis and death. PCR may be useful in these cases to assess local infectious disease that may be of public health import such as viral encephalitides (WNV, EEE, etc.), avian influenza, Paramyxoviridae, Salmonellosis, and colibacillosis as well as Passeriforme-specific diseases such as *Mycoplasma* spp. In captive species, Atoxoplasmosis, Polyomavirus, Chlamydiosis, and *Macrorhabdus ornithogaster* may cause morbidity and mortality. Many laboratories offer PCR testing applicable to these species. Nevertheless, it is recommended, especially when testing free-living birds, that the laboratory be consulted prior sample collection and submission to ensure that the most applicable and appropriate results are obtained [97].

Acknowledgements

Special thanks to Dr. Gary Voelker for review of Table 8.1. We would also like to acknowledge Karl Snyder, Lab Section Chief III at the University of Tennessee College of Veterinary Medicine, for contribution of blood smear images.

References

1 Dorrestein, G.M. (1994). Passerine birds. In: *Avian medicine: principles and application, abridged edition* (ed. B.W. Ritchie, G.J. Harrison and L.R. Harrison), 1172. Idaho Falls, ID: Wingers Publishing.

2 Bateson, M. and Feenders, G. (2010). The use of passerine bird species in laboratory research: Implications of Basic Biology for Husbandry and Welfare. *ILAR Journal* 51 (4): 394–408.

3 Bairlein, F. (1998). The effect of diet composition on migratory fueling in garden warblers *Sylvia borin*. *Journal of Avian Biology* 29: 546–551.
4 Brown, M.B. and Brown, C.R. (2009). Blood sampling reduces annual survival in cliff swallows (Petrochelidon pyrrhonota). *The Auk* 126 (4): 853–861.
5 Voss, M., Shutler, D., and Werner, J. (2010). A hard look at blood sampling of birds. *The Auk* 127 (3): 704–708.
6 Hoysak, D.J. and Weatherhead, P.J. (1991). Sampling blood from birds: a technique and an assessment of its effect. *Condor* 1: 746–752.
7 Owen, J.C. (2011). Collecting, processing, and storing avian blood: a review. *Journal of Field Ornithology* 82 (4): 339–354.
8 Heatley, J.J. (2008). Anesthesia. In: *BSAVA manual of raptors, pigeons and passerine birds* (ed. J. Chitty and M. Lierz). British Small Animal Veterinary Association.
9 West, G., Heard, D., and Caulkett, N. (eds.) (2014). *Zoo animal and wildlife immobilization and anesthesia*. Wiley.
10 Hoefer, H.L. (1992). Transfusions in exotic species. *Problems in Veterinary Medicine* 4 (4): 625–635.
11 Van der Heyden, N. (1994). Evaluation and interpretation of the avian hemogram. *Seminars in Avian and Exotic Pet Medicine* 3 (1): 5–13.
12 Palacios, L., Palomeque, J., and Riera, T. (1984). Oxygen transport properties in the starling, *Sturnus vulgaris* L. *Comparative Biochemistry and Physiology Part A: Physiology* 77 (2): 255–260.
13 DeGraw, W.A. and Kern, M.D. (1985). Changes in the blood and plasma volume of Harris' sparrows during postnuptial molt. *Comparative Biochemistry and Physiology Part A: Physiology* 81 (4): 889–893.
14 Ardern, S.L., McLean, I.G., Anderson, S. et al. (1994). The effects of blood sampling on the behavior and survival of the endangered Chatham Island Black Robin (Petroica traversi). *Conservation Biology* 8 (3): 857–862.
15 Kern, M.D. and De Graw, W.A. (1978). Differences in the composition of venous and cardiac blood from white-crowned sparrows. *The Condor* 80 (2): 230–234.
16 Dein, F.J. (1986). Hematology. In: *Clinical avian medicine and surgery* (ed. G.J. Harrison and L.R. Harrison), 174–191. Philadelphia: WB Saunders.
17 Samour, J. (2006). Diagnostic value of hematology. In: *Clinical avian medicine*, vol. 2 (ed. G.J. Harrison and T. Lightfoot), 587–610. Palm beach florida: Spix publishing.
18 Meyer, D.J. and Rich, E.H. (1992). *Veterinary laboratory medicine: interpretation and diagnosis Philadelphia* (ed. L.J. Meyer et al.), 20–30. WB Saunders.
19 Fair, J., Whitaker, S., and Pearson, B. (2007). Sources of variation in hematocrit in birds. *IBIS* 149 (3): 535–552.
20 Heatley, J.J., Cary, J., Russell, K.E., and Voelker, G. (2013). Clinicopathologic analysis of Passeriform venous blood reflects transitions in elevation and habitat. *Veterinary Medicine: Research and Reports* 4: 1–9.
21 Kostelecka-Myrcha, A. (1997). The ratio of amount of haemoglobin to total surface area of erythrocytes in birds in relation to body mass, age of nestlings, and season of the year. *Physiological Zoology* 70 (3): 278–282.
22 Lobato, D.N., Braga, É.M., Belo, N.D., and Antonini, Y. (2011). Hematological and parasitological health conditions of the Pale-breasted Thrush (Turdus leucomelas)(Passeriformes: Turdidae) in southeastern Brazil. *Zoologia (Curitiba)* 28 (6): 771–776.
23 Potti, J., Moreno, J., Merino, S. et al. (1999). Environmental and genetic variation in the haematocrit of fledgling pied flycatchers Ficedula hypoleuca. *Oecologia* 120 (1): 1–8.
24 Simon, A., Thomas, D.W., Bourgault, P. et al. (2005). Between-population differences in nestling size and hematocrit level in blue tits (Parus caeruleus): a cross-fostering test for genetic and environmental effects. *Canadian Journal of Zoology* 83 (5): 694–701.
25 Booth, C.E. and Elliott, P.F. (2002). Hematological responses to hematozoa in North American and neotropical songbirds. *Comparative Biochemistry and Physiology Part A: Molecular & Integrative Physiology* 133 (3): 451–467.
26 Dufva, R. (1996). Blood parasites, health, reproductive success, and egg volume in female Great Tits Parus major. *Journal of Avian Biology* 27: 83–87.
27 Hauptmanova, K., Literak, I., and Bartova, E. (2002). Haematology and leucocytozoonosis of great tits (Parus major L.) during winter. *Acta Veterinaria Brno* 71 (2): 199–204.
28 Hõrak, P., Ots, I., and Murumägi, A. (1998). Haematological health state indices of reproducing Great Tits: a response to brood size manipulation. *Functional Ecology* 12 (5): 750–756.
29 Clemens, D.T. (1990). Interspecific variation and effects of altitude on blood properties of Rosy Finches (Leucosticte arctoa) and House Finches (Carpodacus mexicanus). *Physiological Zoology* 63: 288–307.
30 Ots, I., Murumägi, A., and Horak, P. (1998). Haematological health state indices of reproducing great tits: methodology and sources of natural variation. *Functional Ecology* 12 (4): 700–707.
31 Vaughan, J.A., Mehus, J.O., Brewer, C.M. et al. Theoretical potential of passerine filariasis to enhance the enzootic transmission of West Nile virus. *Journal of Medical Entomology* 49 (6): 1430–1441.
32 Donovan, T.A., Schrenzel, M., Tucker, T.A. et al. (2008). Hepatic hemorrhage, hemocoelom, and sudden death based on Haemoproteus infection in passerine birds: eleven cases. *Journal of Veterinary Diagnostic Investigation* 20 (3): 304–313.

33 Sanchez-Cordon, P.J., Gomez-Villamandos, J.C., and Gutierrez, J. (2007). Atoxoplasma spp. Infection in Captive Canaries (Serinus canaria). *Journal of Veterinary Medicine Series A* 54 (1): 23–26.

34 Scanes, C. (ed.) (2015). Blood Chapter 10. In: *Sturkie's Avian Physiology*, 6e, 167–192. Elsevier.

35 Rosskopf, W.J. Jr., Woerpel, R.W., Rosskopf, G., and Water, D. (1982). *Hematologic and blood chemistry values for common pet avian species*. VM/SAC. Veterinary Medicine and Small Animal Clinician (USA).

36 Teare JA (ed.): 2013, "Genus_species_No_selection_by_gender__All_ages_combined_Standard_International_ Units__2013_CD.html" in ISIS Physiological Reference Intervals for Captive Wildlife: A CD-ROM Resource., International Species Information System, Bloomigton, MN.

37 Tekumalla, P.K., Tontonoz, M., Hesla, M.A. et al. (2002). Effects of excess thyroid hormone on cell death, cell proliferation, and new neuron incorporation in the adult zebra finch telencephalon. *Journal of Neurobiology* 51 (4): 323–341.

38 Ewenson, E.L., Zann, R.A., and Flannery, G.R. (2001). Body condition and immune response in wild zebra finches: effects of capture, confinement and captive-rearing. *Naturwissenschaften* 88 (9): 391–394.

39 LI, Q.J., ZHANG, L., HAO, S.J. et al. (2014). Comparative Studies on Blood Cells of *Fringilla montifringilla* and *Parus major*. *Journal of Liaoning University (Natural Sciences Edition)* 1: 013.

40 Moreno, J., Merino, S., Martinez, J. et al. (2002). Heterophil/lymphocyte ratios and heat-shock protein levels are related to growth in nestling birds. *Ecoscience* 9: 434–439.

41 Cīrule, D., Krama, T., Vrublevska, J. et al. (2012). A rapid effect of handling on counts of white blood cells in a wintering passerine bird: a more practical measure of stress? *Journal of Ornithology* 153 (1): 161–166.

42 Nadolski, J., Skwarska, J., Kaliński, A. et al. (2006). Blood parameters as consistent predictors of nestling performance in great tits (Parus major) in the wild. *Comparative Biochemistry and Physiology Part A: Molecular & Integrative Physiology* 143 (1): 50–54.

43 Kilgas, P., Tilgar, V., and Mänd, R. (2006). Hematological health state indices predict local survival in a small passerine bird, the great tit (Parus major). *Physiological and Biochemical Zoology* 79 (3): 565–572.

44 Ruiz, G., Rosenmann, M., Novoa, F.F., and Sabat, P. (2002). Hematological parameters and stress index in rufous-collared sparrows dwelling in urban environments. *The Condor* 104 (1): 162–166.

45 Vinkler, M., Schnitzer, J., Munclinger, P. et al. (2010). Haematological health assessment in a passerine with extremely high proportion of basophils in peripheral blood. *Journal of Ornithology* 151 (4): 841–849.

46 Mandal, A., Chakraborty, S., and Lahiri, P. (1986). Hematological changes produced by lindane (y-HCH) in six species of birds. *Toxicology* 40 (1): 103–111.

47 Ferrell, G.T. (1966). Variation in blood group frequencies in populations of Song Sparrows of the San Francisco Bay Region. *Evolution* 1: 369–382.

48 Norris, R.A. (1963). *A Preliminary Study of Avian Blood Groups: With Special Reference to the Passeriformes*. Tall Timbers Research Station.

49 Westlake, G.E., Martin, A.D., Stanley, P.I., and Walker, C.H. (1983). Control enzyme levels in the plasma, brain and liver from wild birds and mammals in Britain. *Comparative Biochemistry and Physiology Part C: Comparative Pharmacology* 76 (1): 15–24.

50 Swanson, D.L. and Thomas, N.E. (2007). The relationship of plasma indicators of lipid metabolism and muscle damage to overnight temperature in winter-acclimatized small birds. *Comparative Biochemistry and Physiology Part A: Molecular & Integrative Physiology* 146 (1): 87–94.

51 Hill, E. and Murray, C. (1987). Seasonal variation in diagnostic enzymes and biochemical constituents of captive northern bobwhites and passerine birds. *Comparative Biochemical Physiology* 87B (4): 933–940.

52 Niemuth, J.N., Allgood, J.V., Flowers, J.R. et al. (2013). Ventricular Habronemiasis in Aviary Passerine birds. *Case Reports in Veterinary Medicine* 1–6.

53 Pollock, C. (2006). Diagnosis and treatment of avian renal disease. *The Veterinary Clinics of North America. Exotic Animal Practice* 9 (1): 107–128.

54 Kohl, K.D., Brzek, P., Caviedes-Vidal, E. et al. (2011). Pancreatic and intestinal carbohydrates are matched to dietary starch level in wild passerine birds. *Physiological and Biochemical Zoology* 84 (2): 195–203.

55 Brzek, P., Kohl, K.D., Caviedes-Vidal et al. (2009). Development adjustments of house sparrow (Passer domesticus) nestlings to diet composition. *The Journal of Experimental Biology* 213: 1284–1293.

56 Brzęk, P., Ciminari, M.E., Kohl, K.D. et al. (2013). Effect of age and diet composition on activity of pancreatic enzymes in birds. *Journal of Comparative Physiology B* 183 (5): 685–697.

57 Rosenthal, K. and Stamoulis, M. (1993). Diagnosis of congestive heart failure in an Indian hill mynah bird (Gracula religiosa). *Journal of the Association of Avian Veterinarians* 7 (1): 27–30.

58 Roberts, M.L., Buchanan, K.L., Hasselquist, D., and Evans, M.R. (2007). Effects of testosterone and corticosterone on immunocompetence in the zebra finch. *Hormones and Behavior* 51 (1): 126–134.

59 Bairlein, F. and Totzke, U. (1992). New aspects on migratory physiology of trans-Saharan passerine migrants. *Ornis Scandinavica* 23: 244–250.

60 Totzke, U. and Bairlein, F. (1998). The body mass cycle of the migratory garden warbler (Sylvia borin) is

associated with changes of basal plasma metabolite levels. *Comparative Biochemistry and Physiology Part A: Molecular & Integrative Physiology* 121 (2): 127–133.
61 Remage-Healey, L. and Romero, L.M. (2002). Corticosterone and insulin interact to regulate plasma glucose but not lipid concentrations in molting starlings. *General and Comparative Endocrinology* 129 (2): 88–94.
62 Smith, S.B. and McWilliams, S.R. (2009). Dietary Macronutrients Affect Lipid Metabolites and Body Composition of a Migratory Passerine, the White-Throated Sparrow (Zonotrichia albicollis). *Physiological and Biochemical Zoology* 82 (3): 258–269.
63 Stockdale, B. (2008). Passerine Birds: nutrition and Nutritional diseases. In: *BSAVA Manual of Raptors, Pigeons and Passerines*, vol. 34 (ed. J. Chitty and M. Lierz), 347–355. British Small Animal Veterinary Association.
64 Cork, S.C. (2000). Iron storage diseases in birds. *Avian Pathology* 29 (1): 7–12.
65 Olsen, G.P., Russell, K.P., and Dierenfeld, E. (2006). A comparison of four regimens for treatment of iron storage disease using the European starling (Sturnus vulgaris) as a model. *Journal of Avian Medicine and Surgery* 20 (2): 74–79.
66 Kincaid, A.L. and Stoskopf, M.K. (1987). Passerine dietary iron overload syndrome. *Zoo Biology* 6 (1): 79–88.
67 Kunec, B. (30 June 2014). Proteonomics. In: *Sturkie's avian physiology* (ed. C.G. Scanes), 31. Elevier.
68 Sibley, C.G. and Hendrickson, H.T. (1970). A comparative electrophoretic study of avian plasma proteins. *The Condor* 72 (1): 43–49.
69 Merino, S., Moreno, J., Tomas, G. et al. (2006). Effects of parental effort on blood stress protein HSP60 and immunoglobulins in female blue tits: a brood size manipulation experiment. *Journal of Animal Ecology* 75 (5): 1147–1153.
70 Merino, S., Martínez, J., Barbosa, A. et al. (1998). Increase in a heat-shock protein from blood cells in response of nestling house martins (Delichon urbica) to parasitism: an experimental approach. *Oecologia* 116 (3): 343–347.
71 Morales, J., Moreno, J., Lobato, E. et al. (2006). Higher stress protein levels are associated with lower humoral and cell-mediated immune responses in pied flycatcher females. *Functional Ecology* 20 (4): 647–655.
72 Harms, C.A. and Harms, R.V. (2012). Venous blood gas and lactate values of mourning doves (Zenaida macroura), boat-tailed grackles (Quiscalus major), and house sparrows (Passer domesticus) after capture by mist net, banding, and venipuncture. *Journal of Zoo and Wildlife Medicine* 43 (1): 77–84.
73 Harms, C.A., Jinks, M.R., and Harms, R.V. (2015). Blood gas, lactate and hematology effects of venipuncture timing and location after mist-net capture of Mourning Doves (Zenaida macroura), Boat-tailed grackles (Quiscalus major), and House Sparrows (Passer domesticus). *Journal of Wildlife Diseases* 52 (2s): S54–S64.
74 Heatley, J.J., Cary, J., Kingsley, L. et al. (2015). Midazolam sedates Passeriformes for field sampling but affects multiple venous blood analytes. *Veterinary Medicine: Research and Reports* 6: 61–69.
75 Klasing, K. (ed.) (1998). Vitamins. In: *Comparative Avian Nutrition*. CAB International.
76 Gelis, S. (2003). The gouldian finch (Erythrura gouldiae) in health and disease. *Seminars in Avian and Exotic Pet Medicine* 12 (4): 215–227.
77 Dierenfeld, E.S. and Traber, M.G. (1992). Vitamin E status of exotic animals compared with livestock and domestics. In: *Vitamin E in Health and Disease* (ed. L. Packer and J. Fuchs), 345–370. New York: Marcel Dekker.
78 Cohen, A.A., McGraw, K.J., and Robinson, W.D. (2009). Serum antioxidant levels in wild birds vary in relation to diet, season, life history strategy, and species. *Oecologia* 161 (4): 673–683.
79 Tella, J.L., Negro, J.J., Forero, M.G. et al. (1998). A comparison of spectrophotometry and color charts for evaluating total plasma carotenoids in wild birds. *Physiological and Biochemical Zoology* 71 (6): 708–711.
80 Reynolds, S.J. (2001). The effects of low dietary calcium during egg-laying on eggshell formation and skeletal calcium reserves in the zebra finch Taeniopygia guttata. *IBIS* 143 (2): 205–215.
81 Eeva, T., Tanhuanpaa, C., and Rabergh, S. (2000). Biomarkers and fluctuating asymmetry as indicators of pollution-induced stress in two hole-nesting passerine birds. *Functional Ecology* 14 (2): 235–243.
82 Alvárez, C.R., Moreno, M.J., Alonso, L.L. et al. (2013). Mercury, methylmercury, and selenium in blood of bird species from Doñana National Park (Southwestern Spain) after a mining accident. *Environmental Science and Pollution Research* 20 (8): 5361–5372.
83 Brumbaugh, W.G., Mora, M.A., May, T.W., and Phalen, D.N. (2010). Metal exposure and effects in voles and small birds near a mining haul road in Cape Krusenstern National Monument, Alaska. *Environmental Monitoring and Assessment* 170 (1–4): 73–86.
84 Llacuna, S., Gorriz, A., Sanpera, C., and Nadal, J. (1995). Metal accumulation in three species of passerine birds (Emberiza cia, Parus major, and Turdus merula) subjected to air pollution from a coal-fired power plant. *Archives of Environmental Contamination and Toxicology* 28 (3): 298–303.
85 Fisher, I.J., Pain, D.J., and Thomas, V.G. (2006). A review of lead poisoning from ammunition sources in terrestrial birds. *Biological Conservation* 131 (3): 421–432.

86 Newman, A.E., Chin, E.H., Schmidt, K.L. et al. (2008). Analysis of steroids in songbird plasma and brain by coupling solid phase extraction to radioimmunoassay. *General and Comparative Endocrinology* 155 (3): 503–510.

87 Wingfield, J.C., Smith, J.P., and Farner, D.S. (1980). Changes in plasma levels of luteinizing hormone, steroid, and thyroid hormones during the postfledging development of white-crowned sparrows, *Zonotrichia leucophrys. General and Comparative Endocrinology* 41 (3): 372–377.

88 Goldsmith, A.R. (1982). Plasma concentrations of prolactin during incubation and parental feeding throughout repeated breeding cycles in canaries (*Serinus canarius*). *Journal of Endocrinology* 94 (1): 51–59.

89 Hau, M., Gill, S.A., and Goymann, W. (2008). Tropical field endocrinology: ecology and evolution of testosterone concentrations in male birds. *General and Comparative Endocrinology* 157 (3): 241–248.

90 Voigt, C. and Leitner, S. (2010). No correlation between song and circulating testosterone levels during multiple broods in the domesticated canary (*Serinus canaria*). *Ethology* 116 (2): 113–119.

91 Ball, G.F. and Wingfield, J.C. (1987). Changes in plasma levels of luteinizing hormone and sex steroid hormones in relation to multiple-broodedness and nest-site density in male starlings. *Physiological Zoology* 60 (2): 191–199.

92 Deviche, P. and Sharp, P.J. (2001). Reproductive endocrinology of a free-living, opportunistically breeding passerine (white-winged crossbill, *Loxia leucoptera*). *General and Comparative Endocrinology* 123 (3): 268–279.

93 Deviche, P., Small, T., Sharp, P., and Tsutsui, K. (2006). Control of luteinizing hormone and testosterone secretion in a flexibly breeding male passerine, the Rufous-winged Sparrow, *Aimophila carpalis. General and Comparative Endocrinology* 149 (3): 226–235.

94 Johnson, A.L. (2015). Reproduction in the female. Chapter 28. In: *Sturkie's Avian Physiology*, 6e (ed. C.G. Scanes), 647. Elsevier Publishing.

95 Hodgson, Z.G., Meddle, S.L., Roberts, M.L. et al. (2007). Spatial ability is impaired and hippocampal mineralocorticoid receptor mRNA expression reduced in zebra finches (Taeniopygia guttata) selected for acute high corticosterone response to stress. *Proceedings of the Royal Society of London B: Biological Sciences* 274 (1607): 239–245.

96 Braun, E.J. (2014). Osmoregulatory systems of birds. In: *Sturkie's avian physiology* (ed. C.G. Scanes), 285–300. Elsevier.

97 Powers LV. 2011. Veterinary Care of Passerine birds (songbirds) AAV Proceedings. 135–47.

98 Harr, K. (2006.Table 23.2 Differential Diagnoses based on biochemistry abnormalities). Chapter 23. Diagnostic Value of Biochemistry. In: *Clinical Avian Medicine Volume II* (ed. L. Harrison), 616–617. Palm Beach, FL: Spix Publishing.

99 Sabat, P., Sepulveda-Kattan, E., and Maldonado, K. (2004). Physiological and biochemical responses to dietary protein in the omnivore passerine Zonotrichia capensis (Emberizidae). *Comparative Biochemistry and Physiology* 137 (2): 391–396.

29

Seabirds and Waterfowl

Christine Fiorello DVM, PhD, DACZM

Wildlife Health Center, School of Veterinary Medicine, University of California Davis, Davis, California, USA

Introduction

Seabirds and waterfowl comprise a diverse group of species with a variety of life histories and varying degrees of reliance on aquatic habitats. Although the term "seabirds" is often used to indicate all birds associated with the marine environment, in fact these species are not closely related phylogenetically. For example, pelicans are most closely related to the African shoebill, a nonmarine bird, and grebes may be most closely related to flamingos [1, 2]. For the purposes of this chapter, "seabird" refers to birds in the six orders listed in Table 29.1. "Waterfowl" refers to members of the monophyletic order Anseriformes, and includes ducks, geese, swans, and screamers.

With the exception of pelicans, most seabirds are not often seen in captivity, either in rehabilitation situations or in zoos. Therefore, there is little published information on the clinical pathology of these species [5, 6]. Most analytes have been sampled from free-ranging animals, and thus represent samples from birds captured and sampled only once. The medical history, health status, and sometimes sex and reproductive status are often unknown, so the values reported may not reflect healthy birds, and the effects of gender, age, and reproductive status are unknown.

Sample Collection

Blood collection in seabirds is routine, and common venipuncture sites include the jugular, ulnar, and medial metatarsal veins, although many species lack apterylae, making visualization of the jugular vein challenging. Feathers can be plucked to create a window for venipuncture. However, plucking feathers of free-ranging birds is not recommended because of its impact on waterproofing and thermoregulation. In these situations, jugular venipuncture must be performed using palpation and anatomic landmarks similar to the method employed for mammals (Figures 29.1–29.3).

Most seabirds can be readily bled from the medial metatarsal vein (Figure 29.4). Pelicans can be bled from a vein on the foot that crosses the first phalanx of the second digit (Figure 29.5). For small samples, a 25 gauge (g.) needle can be inserted into the vein, and once the hub is filled, the needle can be withdrawn and the blood collected into microhematocrit tubes.

Venipuncture and sampling are not difficult in waterfowl, and the typical sites used for other birds are easily accessed. Jugular venipuncture is most valuable for larger volumes, while medial metatarsal venipuncture can be used for smaller volumes (Figures 29.6 and 29.7). A surprising amount of blood can be obtained from the medial metatarsal vein of a duck; a warm towel applied over the foot facilitates blood collection in an animal recently removed from cold water.

The results of one comparative study showed that aquatic birds have a higher blood volume than nonaquatic birds [7]. Fatal blood loss in mallard ducks is approximately 60% of blood volume [8]. The maximum recommended amount of blood that can be safely collected from birds at one time for diagnostic purposes or as donors for transfusions is 10% of blood volume.

Sample Handling

Blood from waterfowl and seabirds can be handled similarly to that of other birds. Lithium heparin or EDTA can be used as anticoagulants for complete blood counts (CBCs), although EDTA tends to best preserve cell morphology. Little information on the effect of storage is available for specific analytes, but one study showed that glucose values are reliable for up to 4 h after collection from whole blood in heparin [9].

Exotic Animal Laboratory Diagnosis, First Edition. Edited by J. Jill Heatley and Karen E. Russell.

Table 29.1 Seabird and waterfowl species covered in this chapter [3, 4].

	Order	Family	Common name
Seabirds	Gaviiformes	Gaviidae	Loons
	Podicipediformes	Podicipedidae	Grebes
	Procellariiformes	Procellariidae	Petrels, Fulmars, Shearwaters
		Diomedeidae	Albatrosses
		Hydrobatidae	Storm Petrels
	Charadriiformes	Alcidae	Puffins, Auks, Murres (Guillemots)
		Laridae	Gulls, Kittiwakes
		Sternidae	Terns
		Stercorariidae	Skuas, Jaegers
	Pelecaniformes	Pelecanidae	Pelicans
		Phaethontidae	Tropicbirds
	Suliformes	Anhingidae	Anhingas, Darters
		Sulidae	Gannets, Boobies
		Fregatidae	Frigatebirds
		Phalacrocoracidae	Cormorants, Shags
Waterfowl	Anseriformes	Anatidae	Ducks, Geese, Swans

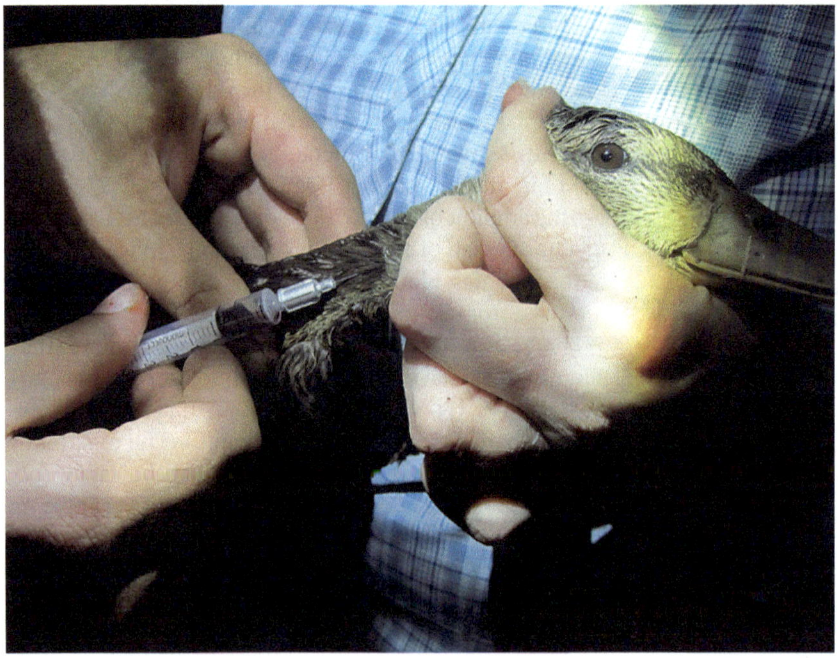

Figure 29.1 Jugular venipuncture of a mottled duck (*Anas fulvigula*).

Specific Analytes

Complete Blood Count (Tables 29.2, 29.3, 29.4, and 29.5; Figures 29.8–29.12)

Indications for and interpretation of CBCs in seabirds and waterfowl are similar to those of other birds. The normal hematocrit of most seabirds is generally between 38% and 48%, although the Alcids (murres, guillemots, auklets, puffins, and murrelets) generally have slightly higher values [22–25]. Mean corpuscular volume (MCV) is higher in diving birds compared to non-diving birds, and often the relatively high MCV is correlated with a relatively low red blood cell (RBC) count [26]. Seabird chicks have lower hematocrits than adults [13, 15, 27–29]. The hematocrit range in waterfowl is similar to that in seabirds [19, 20, 30–34].

As with all vertebrates, the differentials for a decreased hematocrit should consider mechanisms of blood loss,

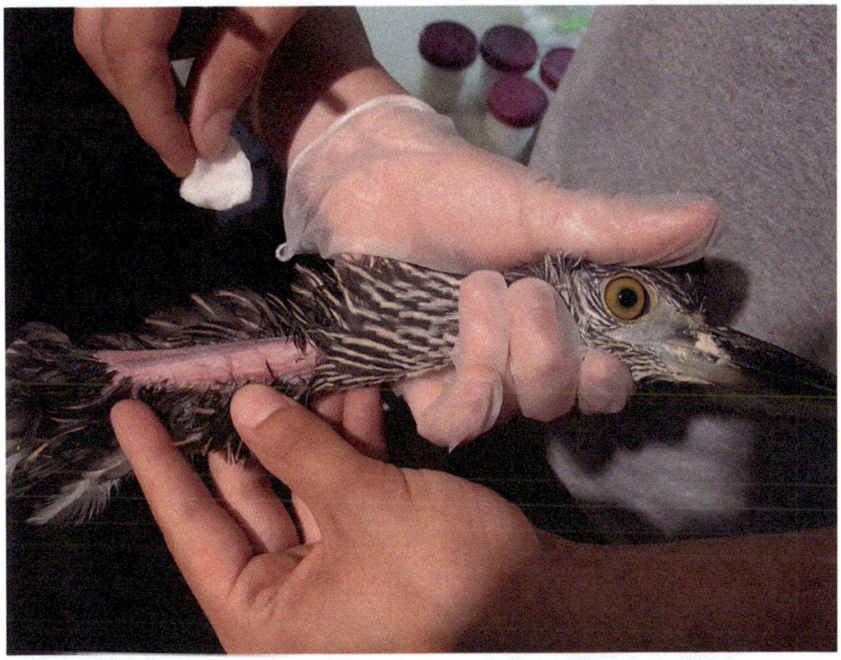

Figure 29.2 Jugular vein of a yellow-crowned night heron (*Nyctasassa violacea*).

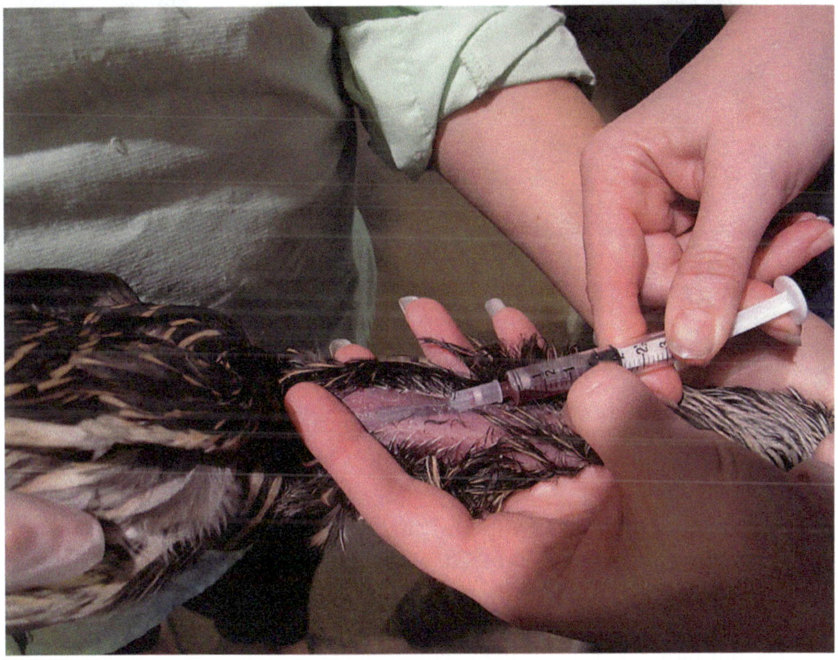

Figure 29.3 Jugular venipuncture of a yellow-crowned night heron (*Nyctanassa violacea*).

decreased production, and increased destruction. Fasting causes a decrease in hematocrit, hemoglobin, and erythrocyte (RBC) counts in herring gulls [35]. Similarly, a drastic food shortage resulted in a decrease of these parameters in free-living black-necked swans [36, 37]. Seabirds in rehabilitation settings are often anemic; it is unknown if this is due to stress related to captivity, underlying disease, or perhaps a physiologic response to lack of physical exertion [38]. Chronic disease, such as aspergillosis, may also result in anemia.

Many toxins can result in anemia. In waterfowl with lead toxicity, hematocrit and hemoglobin begin to decline about three days after exposure, and may fall below 20% and 5 g/dl, respectively [39, 40]. In free-living black ducks with lead poisoning, hemoglobin but not hematocrit decreases [40]. Lead toxicity in free-living albatross chicks did not consistently result in anemia [41]. Hematocrit and hemoglobin drop significantly in seabirds and waterfowl exposed to petroleum via ingestion [42, 43]. In young birds, this may result from Heinz-body hemolytic anemia, and is characterized by a robust regenerative response [42, 44]. Adult birds become anemic after oil exposure but often do not develop Heinz bodies or show evidence of hemolysis; the cause of the anemia is likely

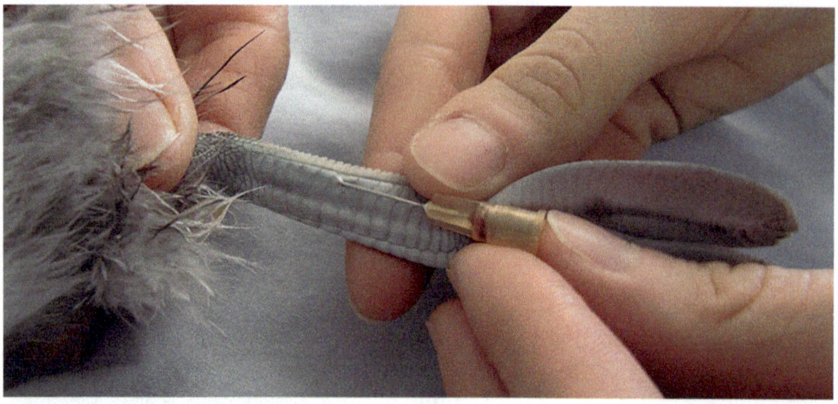

Figure 29.4 Left pelvic limb of a western grebe (*Aechmophorus occidentalis*), demonstrating blood collection from the medial metatarsal vein.

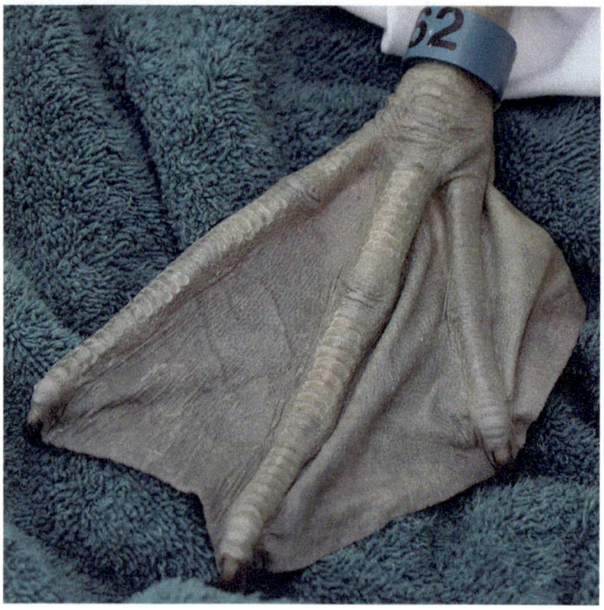

Figure 29.5 The right foot of a pelican; note the vein crossing the proximal aspect of the second digit.

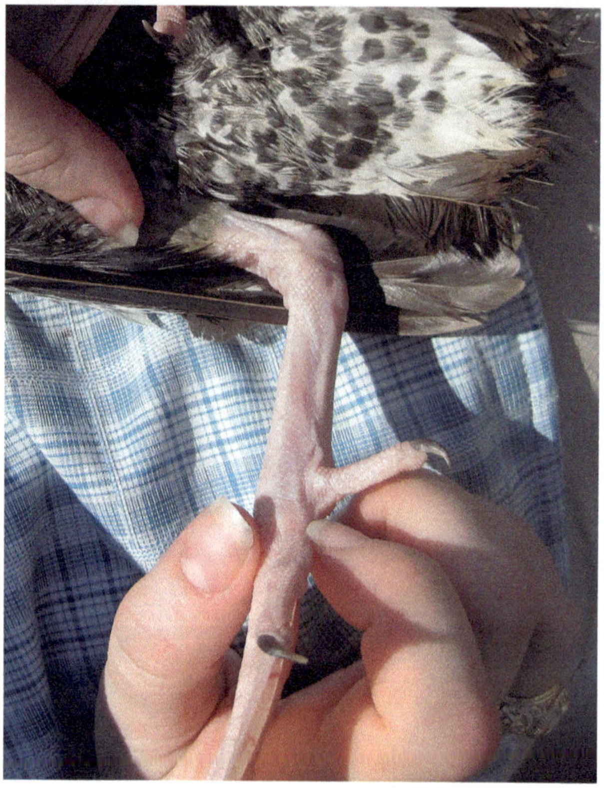

Figure 29.6 Medial metatarsal vein of a black-bellied whistling duck (*Dendrocygna autumnalis*).

multifactorial [38]. In ducks experimentally exposed to red tide toxin, hematocrits increased, while lymphocytes and thrombocytes decreased [45].

The typical leukogram of healthy seabirds varies with species, but most seabirds studied appear to be lymphocytic [10, 12, 24, 26, 46–49]. Pelecaniformes, Suliformes, and Procellariiformes may be lymphocytic or heterophilic depending on species, age, sex, and population [11, 13, 16, 29, 49–52]. Waterfowl also tend to be lymphocytic, although in a study conducted during the breeding season, free-ranging king eider females (but not males) were heterophilic [20, 32, 53–57]. Most seabird adults have lower lymphocyte and total white blood cell counts than chicks, but this varies by species [13, 23, 29, 48, 49]. The leukograms of immature birds should be interpreted with caution, especially if age-specific reference ranges are not available.

As in all birds, leukocytosis is a nonspecific finding associated with inflammatory and infectious disease states. Aspergillosis should be considered in seabirds and waterfowl that have a marked heterophilia [58]. These birds may or may not also have a monocytosis. However, mycobacteriosis, chlamydiosis, and numerous other infections and inflammatory disease states can result in heterophilia, and not all birds with aspergillosis have a heterophilia [58, 59].

Heterophil-to-lymphocyte ratios (H:L) may be higher with disease, stress, or parasitism, but they may also vary

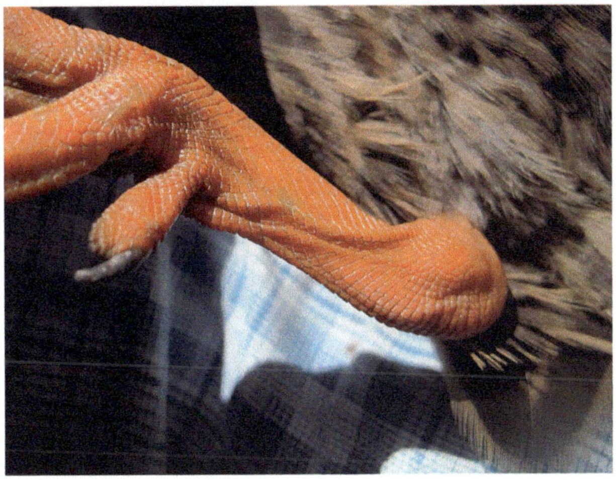

Figure 29.7 Medial metatarsal vein of a mottled duck (*Anas fulvigula*).

with age [11, 23, 46, 50]. A study of the ontogeny of tropicbirds demonstrated that younger chicks have higher H:L ratios than older chicks and adults, and the authors cautioned that this higher ratio should not be interpreted as a sign of disease or stress [60]. In herring gulls, chicks had lower H:L, demonstrating that this parameter likely varies by species [27]. In northern fulmars, the H:L ratio was higher in breeding birds compared to non-breeding birds; however, this was confounded by age as many non-breeding fulmars are simply below the age of sexual maturity [24]. Higher H:L ratios are associated with physiologic stress. A high H:L ratio could indicate an underlying stressor that prompts the bird to opt out of breeding that year. For example, in one study adult Cory's shearwaters that bred had lower pre-breeding H:L than those individuals that did not [61]. A study comparing healthy and "sick" gulls found that the H:L was higher in sick birds [46]. Birds classified as sick were affected by a variety of problems, including crude oil exposure, gunshot wounds, emaciation, and fractures. Experimentally, zinc-intoxicated mallard ducks had higher H:L than control mallards [62]. Black-necked swans experiencing a severe food shortage also had elevated H:L [36].

Hemoparasites

Hemoparasites appear rare in seabirds, with numerous studies failing to find any; this may be partly associated with lack of exposure to arthropod vectors [5, 15, 47, 63–66]. One exception is great frigatebirds; approximately one-third of frigatebirds are infected with *Haemoproteus iwa* [51, 67]. Boobies, gulls, and murres may be infected with *Babesia* spp., but the prevalence of infection is extremely low [68, 69]. In most cases, seabirds with hemoparasites are not clinically affected. Unlike in seabirds, blood parasites are commonly seen in waterfowl [70–72]. *Hemoproteus, Leucocytozoon,* and *Plasmodium* organisms have been reported in various Anseriformes [70, 73, 74]. Morbidity and mortality of waterfowl have been attributed to hemoparasites [75].

Hemostasis

Prothrombin time can be used in birds to assess hemostasis, but its clinical availability is limited. Prolonged prothrombin times have been seen in ducks affected by aflatoxins, and hemorrhages occurred in free-living ducks (but not geese) that died of aflatoxicosis in Texas [76–78]. Infections with the trematode parasite *Sphaeridiotrema globulus* cause increased prothrombin times in mallards [79]. Swan populations have experienced mortalities because of this parasite, and prolonged prothrombin times may be useful in the antemortem diagnosis of sphaeridiotremiasis in swans [79].

Clotting times and coagulation have not been evaluated in seabirds. Fibrinogen, however, is an acute-phase protein in birds and may have value as a prognostic indicator. In a study of oiled common murres, increased fibrinogen concentration was associated with higher mortality after rehabilitation and release [80].

Biochemical Panel (Tables 29.6, 29.7, 29.8, and 29.9)

Liver Enzymes

Alkaline phosphatase is associated with bone growth and healing; therefore, it tends to be higher in immature birds. It may also be higher in females prior to and during egg laying. This enzyme also increases in marine birds exposed to petroleum, and in mallards with high blood lead concentrations [17, 43, 84]. Alanine aminotransferase (ALT) activity may reflect damage to muscle, kidney, or liver cells, and is not considered specific to any one organ in birds [82, 85]. ALT activity may increase in marine waterfowl exposed to petroleum [43]. Aspartate aminotransferase (AST) activity is a sensitive but not specific indicator of hepatocellular damage [85]. Eight years after the Exxon Valdez oil spill, pigeon guillemots from oiled areas had higher AST activities than birds from unoiled areas, which suggests that this enzyme may increase even with sublethal exposure [17]. Most adult seabirds tend to have higher AST activities than chicks [29, 56]. In general, waterfowl have lower AST activity than other avian species, but eiders are an exception [56, 82]. Mallard ducks experimentally intoxicated with zinc had nearly 10-fold higher levels of AST than controls [62].

Muscle Enzymes

Increases in AST and ALT activities may indicate liver or muscle damage, while creatine kinase (CK) is specific to muscle injury in birds [82, 85]. In one study, the

Table 29.2 Hematologic values for free-ranging Procellariiformes [10–13].

Analyte	Units, SI (conventional)	Waved albatross (*Phoebastria irrorata*)	Southern giant petrel (*Macronectes giganteus*)	Northern fulmar (*Fulmarus glacialis*)	Wedge-tailed shearwater (*Puffinus pacificus*)
Packed cell volume (PCV)	Proportion of 1.0 (%)	0.38 ± 0.05 (38.2 ± 5.1)	0.474 ± 0.04 (47.4 ± 4.0)	0.32 ± 0.08 (32 ± 8)	0.48 ± 0.03 (48 ± 3)
White blood cell count (WBC)	$\times 10^9$/l (X 10^3/μl)	5.9 ± 2.4[a] (5.9 ± 2.4)	4.0 ± 1.2 (4.0 ± 1.2)	3.36 ± 0.92[a] (3.36 ± 0.92)	18.18 ± 7.17 (18.18 ± 7.17)
Heterophils	Proportion of 1.0 (%)	0.66 ± 0.30[a] (66.1 ± 30.0)		0.29 ± 0.16 (29 ± 16)	
	$\times 10^9$/l ($\times 10^3$/μl)		2.1 ± 0.7 (2.1 ± 0.7)		4.00 ± 2.09 (4.00 ± 2.09)
Monocytes	Proportion of 1.0 (%)	0.017 ± 0.017[a] (1.7 ± 1.7)		0.02 ± 0.02 (2 ± 2)	
	$\times 10^9$/l ($\times 10^3$/μl)		0.2 ± 0.1 (0.2 ± 0.1)		0.45 ± 0.48 (0.45 ± 0.48)
Lymphocytes	Proportion of 1.0 (%)	0.305 ± 0.15[a] (30.5 ± 15.0)		0.56 ± 0.20 (56 ± 20)	
	$\times 10^9$/l ($\times 10^3$/μl)		1.3 ± 0.5 (1.3 ± 0.5)		12.93 ± 6.21 (12.93 ± 6.21)
Eosinophils	Proportion of 1.0 (%)	0.017 ± 0.017[a] (1.7 ± 1.7)		0.13 ± 0.10 (13 ± 10)	
	$\times 10^9$/l ($\times 10^3$/μl)		0.4 ± 0.2 (0.4 ± 0.2)		0.48 ± 0.51 (0.48 ± 0.51)
Basophils	Proportion of 1.0 (%)	0.0 ± 0.0001[a](0.0–0.01)		0.00 ± 0.01 (0 ± 1)	
	$\times 10^9$/l ($\times 10^3$/μl)		0.006 ± 0.023 (0.006 ± 0.023)		0.31 ± 0.31 (0.31 ± 0.31)

[a] Estimated count.
All data presented as mean ± SD.

Table 29.3 Hematologic values for Gaviiformes, Pelecaniformes, and Podicipediformes [14–16].

Analyte	Units, SI (conventional)	Common loons (*Gavia immer*) [Free-living]	Brown pelicans (*Pelecanus occidentalis*) [Free-living] & [Captive]	Western grebes (*Aechmophorus occidentalis*) [Free-living]
Packed cell volume (PCV)	Proportion of 1.0 (%)	0.47 ± 0.047 (47 ± 4.7)	0.455 ± 0.05 (45.5 ± 5)	0.475 ± 0.05 (47.5 ± 5.5)
Red blood cell (RBC) count	$\times 10^{12}$/l ($\times 10^6$/μl)		2.66 ± 0.4 (2.66 ± 0.4)	2.2 ± 0.2 (2.2 ± 0.2)
White blood cell (WBC) count	$\times 10^9$/l ($\times 10^3$/μl)	17 ± 6.2 (17 ± 6.2)	16.7 ± 4.7 (16.7 ± 4.7)	7.89 ± 3.67[b] (7.89 ± 3.67)
Heterophils	Proportion of 1.0 (%)	0.32 ± 0.11 (32 ± 11)		0.698 ± 0.182) (69.8 ± 18.2)
	$\times 10^9$/l ($\times 10^3$/μl)		8.3 ± 2.1 (8.3 ± 2.1)	6.65 ± 3.88[b] (6.65 ± 3.88)
Monocytes	Proportion of 1.0 (%)			0.043 ± 0.032 (4.3 ± 3.2)
	$\times 10^9$/l ($\times 10^3$/μl)		0.2 ± 0.3 (0.2 ± 0.3)	0.38 ± 0.17[b] (0.38 ± 0.17)
Lymphocytes	Proportion of 1.0 (%)			0.20 ± 0.14 (20.1 ± 14.1)
	$\times 10^9$/l ($\times 10^3$/μl)		7.3 ± 2.2 (7.3 ± 2.2)	1.47 ± 0.83[b] (1.47 ± 0.83)
Mononuclear cells[a]	Proportion of 1.0 (%)	0.37 ± 0.137 (37 ± 13.7)		
Eosinophils	Proportion of 1.0 (%)	0.31 ± 0.115 (31 ± 11.5)		0.048 ± 0.065 (4.8 ± 6.5)
	$\times 10^9$/l ($\times 10^3$/μl)		0.87 ± 1.0 (0.87 ± 1.0)	0.44 ± 0.68[b] (0.44 ± 0.68)
Basophils	Proportion of 1.0 (%)	0	Rarely seen	0.01 ± 0.01 (1.1 ± 1.4)
	$\times 10^9$/l ($\times 10^3$/μl)			0.07 ± 0.12[b] (0.07 ± 0.12)

[a] Monocytes plus lymphocytes.
[b] Estimated count KEY Free-living [Free-living] Captive [Captive].
All data presented as mean ± SD.

endangered marbled murrelet had higher baseline CK activity compared to other seabirds [10].

Renal Analytes

Uric acid is the main nitrogenous waste product of avian metabolism, and is used to assess renal function in birds. It is not as susceptible as blood urea nitrogen (BUN) to changes due to dehydration, but it increases postprandially in faunivorous species and is thus best evaluated after a 24 h fast [85]. As faunivores, seabirds tend to have higher baseline uric acid levels than other birds [10].

Uric acid levels may rise during starvation, as birds begin to catabolize protein as an energy source. Studies of starvation with herring gulls and greater snow geese support this theory [83, 86]. Similarly, free-ranging common eiders studied during incubation fasts had increased uric acid [87]. Experimentally zinc-intoxicated mallards had increased uric acid levels [62]. It is not clear if this was caused by protein catabolism or direct renal injury, but heavy metal intoxication should be considered when presented with a waterfowl species with hyperuricemia. Although not useful for evaluating renal function, BUN is a sensitive indicator of dehydration in birds [86–88].

Pancreas

Glucose metabolism in birds is regulated by insulin and glucagon, but the relative importance of these hormones differs greatly among avian species [85]. While a general guideline is that insulin predominates in faunivorous birds and glucagon predominates in granivorous birds, pancreatic hormones have not been investigated in seabirds or free-living waterfowl. Sodium fluoride tubes are not necessary for collection of avian glucose samples, as avian erythrocytes do not consume glucose [9, 85, 88]. Whole blood in heparin can be stored for up to 4 h without alterations in glucose values [9]. Because faunivorous birds are adapted to a low-carbohydrate diet, these birds are thought to be able to maintain fasting glucose levels longer than granivorous birds [85]. For example, glucose concentrations did not change in herring gulls during an experimental study of starvation [86]. Studies in herbivorous birds indicate that these species tend to become hypoglycemic with food restriction. Greater snow geese maintained their glucose levels for nearly a month during starvation, after which their levels markedly decreased [83]. Black-necked swans, which are largely herbivorous, had steadily decreasing glucose levels during a period of food shortage [89].

Handheld blood glucose monitors consistently underestimate blood glucose levels by an average of 33% compared to results from reference laboratories [9]. Nonetheless, such monitors provide rapid, repeatable results with tiny volumes of blood, so they are a useful tool in avian clinical pathology. Only whole blood or whole blood in heparin should be used with handheld monitors, as whole blood in EDTA results in significantly lower glucose levels [9].

Table 29.4 Hematologic values for free-ranging Charadriiformes [10, 17].

Analyte (abbreviation)	Units, SI (conventional)	Pigeon guillemots (*Cepphus columba*)	Tufted puffins (*Lunda cirrhata*)	Marbled murrelets (*Brachramphus marmoratus*)	Glaucous-winged gulls (*Larus glaucescens*)
Packed cell volume (PCV)	Proportion of 1.0 (%)	0.58 ± 0.06 (58 ± 6)	0.41 ± 0.07 (41 ± 7)	0.41 ± 0.06 (41 ± 6)	0.38 ± 0.08 (38 ± 8)
Red blood cell count (RBC)	$\times 10^{12}$/l ($\times 10^6$/μl)	3.76 ± 0.59 (3.76 ± 0.59)			
Mean (MCV) corpuscular volume	fl	163 ± 10			
Mean (MCHC) corpuscular hemoglobin concentration	g/l (g/dl)	3.32 ± 1.14 (33.2 ± 11.4)			
White blood cell count (WBC)	$\times 10^9$/l ($\times 10^3$/μl)	8 ± 1 (8 ± 1)	3.98 ± 1.87 (3.98 ± 1.87)[a]	5.68 ± 1.99 (5.68 ± 1.99)[a]	5.08 ± 4.47 (5.08 ± 4.47)[a]
Heterophils	Proportion of 1.0 (%)	0.64 ± 0.13 (64 ± 13)	0.37 ± 0.19 (37 ± 19)	0.26 ± 0.21 (26 ± 21)	0.53 ± 0.20 (53 ± 20)
Monocytes	Proportion of 1.0 (%)	0	0.03 ± 0.06 (3 ± 6)	0.01 ± 0.01 (1 ± 1)	0.01 ± 0.01 (1 ± 1)
Lymphocytes	Proportion of 1.0 (%)	0.334 ± 0.121 (33.4 ± 12.1)	0.57 ± 0.18 (57 ± 18)	0.63 ± 14 (63 ± 14)	0.43 ± 0.16 (43 ± 16)
Eosinophils	Proportion of 1.0 (%)	0.0 ± 0.01 (0 ± 1)	0.04 ± 0.08 (4 ± 8)	0.09 ± 0.00 (9 ± 8)	0.03 ± 0.04 (3 ± 4)
Basophils	Proportion of 1.0 (%)	0.03 ± 0.02 (3 ± 2)	0.01 ± 0.02 (1 ± 2)	0.02 ± 0.03 (2 ± 3)	0

[a] Estimated count.
All data presented as mean ± SD.

Table 29.5 Hematologic values for waterfowl [18–21].

Analyte	Units, SI (conventional)	Mallards (*Anas platyrhynchos*) post-molt Ħ ♂	Black ducks (*Anas superciliosa*) ♀	Canada geese (*Branta canadensis leucopareia*) Ħ	Black-necked swans (*Cygnus melanocoryphus*) ♀ ♂
Packed cell volume (PCV)	Proportion of 1.0 (%)	0.39 ± 0.02 (39 ± 2)	0.40 ± 0.04 (40 ± 4)	0.42 ± 0.03 (42 ± 3)	0.41 ± 0.05 (41 ± 5)
Red blood cell count (RBC)	× 10^{12}/l (× 10^6/ml)	2.5 ± 0.03 (2.5 ± 0.03)	2.8 ± 0.2 (2.8 ± 0.2)	2.6 ± 0.4 (2.6 ± 0.4)	1.9 ± 0.4 (1.9 ± 0.4)
Hemoglobin	g/l (g/dl)	134 ± 1 (13.4 ± 0.1)	130 ± 10 (13 ± 1)	132 ± 19 (13.2 ± 1.9)	130 ± 20 (13 ± 2)
Mean corpuscular volume (MCV)	fl	160 ± 1.6	145 ± 10		225 ± 35
Mean corpuscular hemoglobin concentration (MCHC)	g/l (g/dl)	340 ± 3 (34 ± 0.3)	320 ± 10 (32 ± 1)	314 ± 48 (31.4 ± 4.8)	310 ± 20 (31 ± 2)
White blood cell count (WBC)	× 10^9/l (× 10^3/μl)	7.2 ± 0.4 (7.2 ± 0.4)	19.7 ± 6.6 (19.7 ± 6.6)		13.4 ± 1.7 (13.4 ± 1.7)
Heterophils	× 10^9/l (× 10^3/μl)	2.6 ± 0.2 (2.6 ± 0.2)	4.9 ± 1.4 (4.9 ± 1.4)		2.6 ± 1.5 (2.6 ± 1.5)
Monocytes	× 10^9/l (× 10^3/μl)	0.1 ± 0.01 (0.1 ± 0.01)	1.5 ± 1.0 (1.5 ± 1.0)		0.8 ± 0.7 (0.8 ± 0.7)
Lymphocytes	× 10^9/l (× 10^3/μl)	4.0 ± 0.2 (4.0 ± 0.2)	13.0 ± 1.5 (13.0 ± 1.5)		9.9 ± 1.8 (9.9 ± 1.8)
Eosinophils	× 10^9/l (× 10^3/μl)	0.3 ± 0.04 (0.3 ± 0.04)	0.2 ± 0.2 (0.2 ± 0.2)		0.1 ± 0.1 (0.1 ± 0.1)
Basophils	× 10^9/l (× 10^3/μl)	0.3 ± 0.02 (0.3 ± 0.02)	0.2 ± 0.2 (0.2 ± 0.2)		0.1 ± 0.1 (0.1 ± 0.1)

Data presented as mean ± SD.

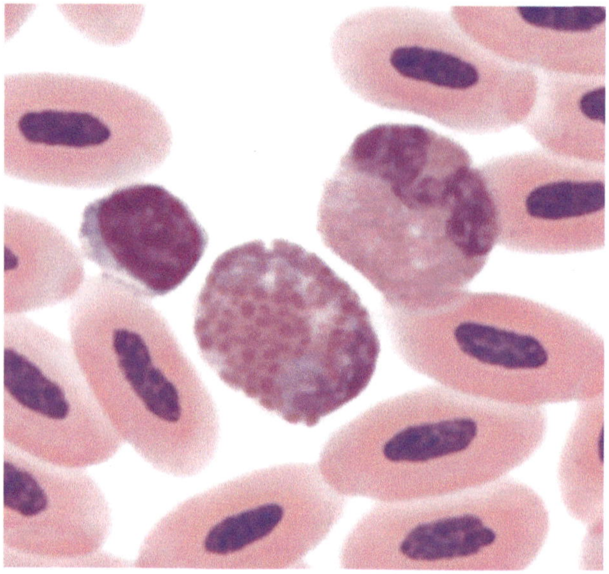

Figure 29.8 Lymphocyte (left), heterophil (center), and eosinophil (right) of a brown pelican *(Pelecanus occidentalis)*.

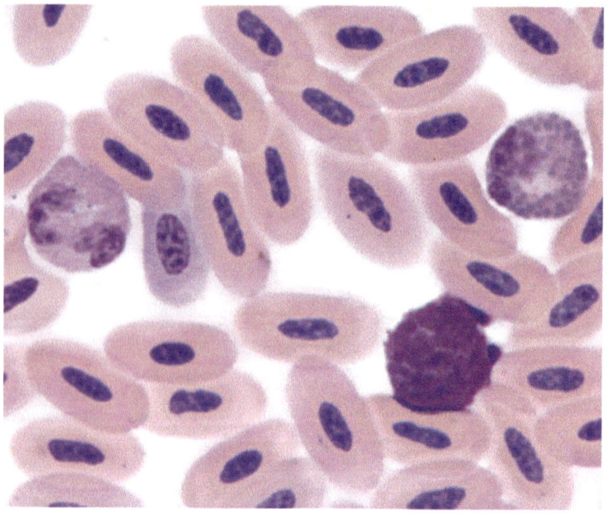

Figure 29.9 Eosinophil (left), basophil (lower right), and heterophil (upper right) of a brown pelican *(Pelecanus occidentalis)*.

Amylase activity has not been extensively studied in birds. It is found in the small intestine and liver as well as in the pancreas, so it may increase with inflammation in any of these visceral organs [88]. In one study of free-living eiders, females had higher activity than males, which the authors attributed to inflammatory changes associated with egg laying [56].

Lipids

Piscivorous birds tend to have higher cholesterol levels compared to granivorous birds such as Psittacines, so it is important to use species-specific reference ranges when evaluating this analyte [88]. Cholesterol levels also change markedly due to age, season, and reproductive activity, with immature birds having higher levels than adults, and females having higher levels than males during the breeding season [29, 85]. Gulls affected by a variety of conditions, including oiling, emaciation, fractures, and gunshot wounds, had lower cholesterol concentrations than clinically healthy birds [46]. In one study,

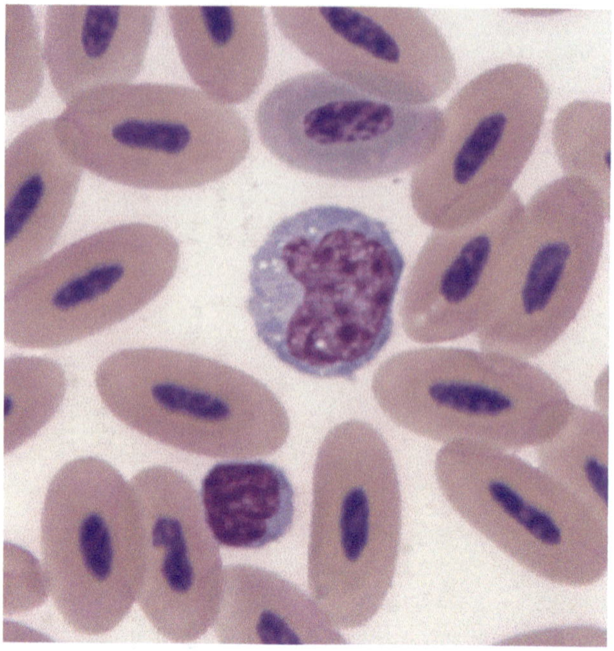

Figure 29.10 Lymphocyte (lower) and monocyte (upper) of a brown pelican *(Pelecanus occidentalis)*.

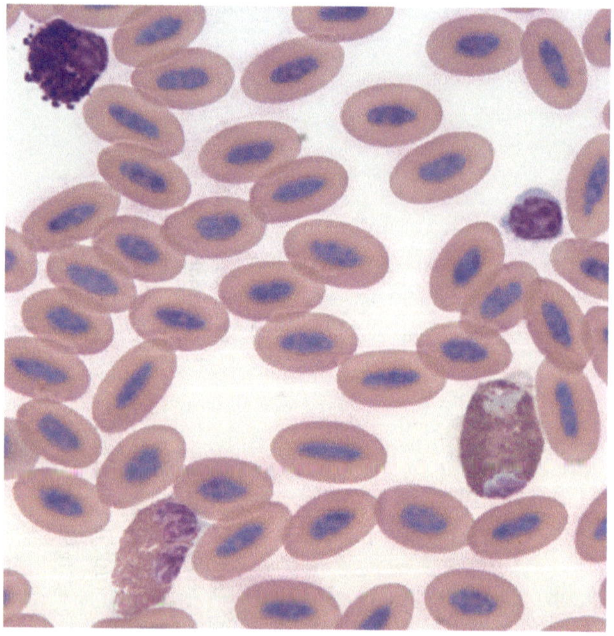

Figure 29.11 Basophil (upper left), lymphocyte (upper right), heterophil (lower right), and eosinophil of a black-bellied whistling duck *(Dendrocygna autumnalis)*.

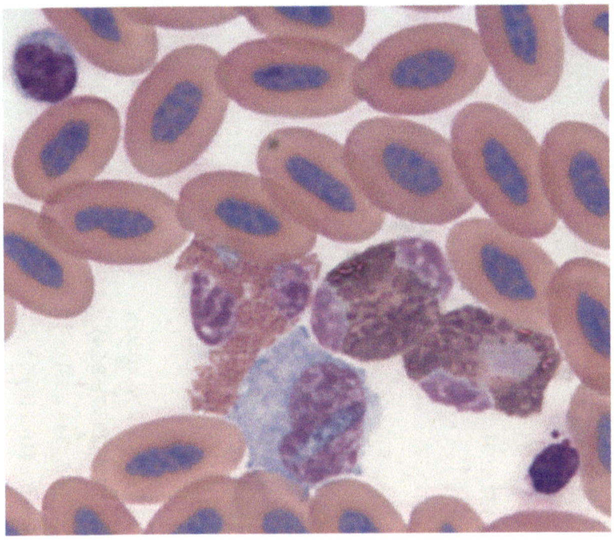

Figure 29.12 From left to right, lymphocyte, eosinophil, monocyte, 2 heterophils, and a thrombocyte from a black-bellied whistling duck *(Dendrocygna autumnalis)*.

captive brown pelicans had higher cholesterol concentrations than free-living pelicans [16].

Triglyceride levels vary during migration and with age and nutritional status and are higher in both males and females of some avian species during breeding [28, 61, 90]. In many species, including brown pelicans, breeding females have significantly higher levels than males [16]. Interestingly, levels remained constant in herring gulls subjected to experimental starvation [86]. In free-living black-necked swans experiencing a severe food shortage, triglyceride levels decreased [36].

Electrolytes

Despite extensive research on the nasal salt gland function of seabirds, little is known of the plasma electrolyte response to disease in seabirds.

Blood Proteins

Total protein (TP) concentration provides information on nutritional and immune status. In brown pelicans, TP levels are normally higher in adults compared to juveniles due to higher globulin concentrations [29]. A significant seasonal effect may be seen on TP levels in pelicans, which is confounded by age and sex. Levels tend to be higher in winter–spring compared to summer–fall [29].

When breeding, female waterfowl tend to have higher TP concentrations compared to males [18, 56]. During physiologically stressful periods, TP and albumin concentrations are likely to decrease. For instance, in free-living food-stressed black-necked swans, levels of both parameters decreased [89]. Similarly, a study of captive bar-headed geese showed that TP was at its lowest level during molt [91]. Male mallards had lower TP levels during and just after molt [92].

Protein electrophoresis (EPH) is a useful tool to detect inflammatory conditions in birds [88, 93, 94]. Elevations in beta and gamma globulins are typical in birds with infectious diseases and have been especially useful as adjuncts in the diagnosis of aspergillosis [93, 94]. Acute-phase protein increases are reflected primarily in increases in alpha and beta globulins, and immunoglobulin increases are reflected in increases in gamma globulins [88]. While it has been hypothesized that molting, an energetically costly process for birds, may result in changes in EPH results that could confound the diagnosis of disease, studies have found that this is unlikely [91, 92]. Although alterations in protein fraction concentrations were documented in molting bar-headed geese and mallards, the changes were small [91, 92].

Fibrinogen is an acute-phase protein that typically increases with infection or inflammation [85, 95]. It may be a sensitive indicator of inflammation in seabirds, as pre-release fibrinogen levels of oiled and rehabilitated common murres were correlated with mortality [80]. Fibrinogen is likely an underutilized diagnostic parameter in avian species.

Vitamins, Minerals, Metals, and Toxins

Calcium and Phosphorous

In birds, calcium levels are generally higher in females than males, and increase in breeding females; seabirds are no exception [10, 16]. However, this effect is species specific, as breeding female brown boobies did not have higher calcium levels than males [49]. In some species, calcium may be correlated with body fat levels in females [10]. This intraindividual variation makes it challenging to develop a reference interval for calcium that is applicable for all seasons and reproductive statuses. In some species, such as the Suliformes (frigates, boobies and gannets), phosphorus is higher in females than in males [49, 51]. It is unknown if this is related to egg-laying physiology or to dietary differences.

Iron

The clinical significance of plasma iron and iron-binding proteins has not been investigated in seabirds. In waterfowl, free-living black-necked swans living in a river polluted with high levels of iron had significantly higher transferrin saturation and significantly lower total iron-binding capacity than a reference population [21]. Interestingly, the plasma iron levels of swans from the polluted river were not higher than those in the reference population [21].

Table 29.6 Biochemical values for free-ranging Procellariiformes [10–13, 81].

Analyte (abbreviation)	Units, SI (conventional)	Waved albatross (*Phoebastria irrorata*)	Southern giant petrel (*Macronectes giganteus*)	Northern fulmar (*Fulmarus glacialis*)	Wedge-tailed shearwater (*Puffinus pacificus*)
Alanine aminotransferase (ALT)	U/l		<4[a]	28 ± 8	
Albumin	g/l (g/dl)	18.0 ± 2.0 (1.8 ± 0.2)	15 ± 3 (1.5 ± 0.3)		15 ± 1 (1.5 ± 0.1)
Alkaline phosphatase (ALP)	U/l		4.3 ± 2.4	219 ± 218	
Amylase	U/l		11.8 ± 16.9		
Aspartate aminotransferase (AST)	U/l	117.6 ± 46.9	93.1 ± 29.6	414 ± 214	258 ± 93
Bile acids	μmol/l (μg/ml)		36.3 ± 13.7 (14.8 ± 5.6)		
Blood urea nitrogen (BUN)	mmol/l (mg/dl)		1.2 ± 0.9 (3.4 ± 2.5)		
Calcium (Ca)	mmol/l (mg/dl = mEq/l)	2.5 ± 0.3 (9.8 ± 1.1)	2.3 ± 0.3 (9.1 ± 1.2)	2.7 ± 0.5 (10.6 ± 2.0)	2.2 ± 0.4 (8.8 ± 1.4)
Chloride (Cl)	mmol/l (mEq/l)	118.0 ± 7.7 (118.0 ± 7.7)	121.3 ± 5.8 (121.3 ± 5.8)		
Cholesterol	mmol/l (mg/dl)	6.5 ± 1.4 (251.8 ± 54.0)		9.4 ± 1.4 (363 ± 53)	
Creatine phosphokinase (CK)	U/l	290.0 ± 173.1	5.7 ± 1.5	2554 ± 1235.5	86 ± 69
Free thyroxine (T_4)	pmol/l (ng/dl)			18.6 ± 7.6 (1.45 ± 0.59)	
Free triiodothyronine (T_3)	pmol/l (pg/dl)			5.1 ± 3.0 (331.2 ± 194.8)	
Globulin	g/l (g/dl)	28.0 ± 5.0 (2.8 ± 0.5)	23 ± 8.6 (2.3 ± 0.86)		18 ± 3 (1.8 ± 0.3)
Glucose	mmol/l (mg/dl)	12.7 ± 2.0 (229.4 ± 35.4)	15.8 ± 2.2 (285 ± 39)	12.5 ± 2.3 (226 ± 42)	13.8 ± 1.6 (248 ± 28)
Lactate dehydrogenase (LDH)	U/l		18.0 ± 9.9	1432 ± 951	
Magnesium (Mg)	mmol/l (ppm)		1.5 ± 0.5 (36.7 ± 12.6)		
Phosphorus (P)	mmol/l (mg/dl)	1.1 ± 0.3 (3.4 ± 0.8)	0.78 ± 0.65 (2.4 ± 2.0)		0.52 ± 0.29 (1.6 ± 0.9)
Potassium (K)	mmol/l (mEq/l)	3.7 ± 0.8 (3.7 ± 0.8)	2.2 ± 0.29 (2.2 ± 0.29)		
Sodium (Na)	mmol/l (mEq/l)	152.7 ± 6.2 (152.7 ± 6.2)	154.5 ± 15.5 (154.5 ± 15.5)		
Total bilirubin	μmol/l (mg/dl)			8.6 ± 5.1 (0.5 ± 0.3)	
Total iron (Fe)	μmol/l (ppm)		15.6–44.9 (1.36 ± 0.57)		
Total protein (TP)	g/l (g/dl)	45.0 ± 6.0 (4.5 ± 0.6)	34 ± 10 (3.4 ± 1.0)	37 ± 10 (3.7 ± 1.0)	34 ± 4 (3.4 ± 0.4)
Total solids (TS) (refractometer)	g/l (g/dl)		62 ± 11 (6.2 ± 1.1)	47 ± 6 (4.7 ± 0.6)	39 ± 4 (3.9 ± 0.4)
Total thyroxine (T_4)	nmol/l (μg/dl)			38.4 ± 12.2 (2.98 ± 0.95)	
Total triiodothyronine (T_3)	nmol/l (ng/dl)			4.6 ± 1.3 (298.7 ± 84.4)	
Triglyceride	nmol/l (mg/dl)			1.6 ± 0.5 (144 ± 48)	
Uric acid	μmol/l (mg/dl)	0.3 ± 0.2 (4.4–2.7)	529.4 ± 136.8 (8.9 ± 2.3)	356.9 ± 416.4 (6 ± 7)	606.7 ± 303.3 (10.2 ± 5.1)

[a] Values below detectable limits.
All values presented as mean ± SD.

Table 29.7 Biochemical values for Suliformes, Pelecaniformes, and Podicipediformes [14, 16, 29, 50].

Analyte (abbreviation)	Units, SI (conventional)	Double-crested cormorants (*Phalacrocorax auritus*) Ħ Ó	Brown pelicans (*Pelecanus occidentalis*) Ħ	Western grebes (*Aechmophorus occidentalis*) ˀ
Alanine (ALT)aminotransferase	U/l		45 ± 18	11.1 ± 13.8
Albumin	g/l (g/dl)	12 ± 3 (1.2 ± 0.3)	20 ± 5 (2.0 ± 0.5)	15 ± 1.5 (1.5 ± 0.15)
Alkaline phosphatase (ALP)	U/l	3690 ± 1113		34.3 ± 27.4
Albumin:globulin (A:G ratio)		0.39 ± 0.17	0.78 ± 0.2	
Alpha$_1$ globulin	g/l (g/dl)		3 ± 1 (0.3 ± 0.1)	
Alpha$_2$ globulin	g/l (g/dl)		6.5 ± 3.0 (0.65 ± 0.3)	
Amylase	U/l		993 ± 119	
Anion gap [Na] + [K]-[Cl]-[tCO_2]	mmol/l (mEq/l)		Freshwater: 50 ± 1[a] (50 ± 1) Seawater: 27 ± 4[a] (27 ± 4)	13.2 ± 2.1 (13.2 ± 2.1)
Aspartate aminotransferase (AST)	U/l	267 ± 94	286 ± 100	473.3 ± 218.4
Beta globulin	g/l (g/dl)		9.2 ± 3.0 (0.92 ± 0.3)	
Bicarbonate	mmol/l (mEq/l)	26 ± 4 (26 ± 4)		25.9 ± 1.8 (25.9 ± 1.8)
Blood urea nitrogen (BUN)	mmol/l (mg/dl)		1.5 ± 0.25 (4.3 ± 0.7)	0.9 ± 0.2 (2.6 ± 0.6)
Calcium (Ca)	mmol/l (mg/dl)	2.89 ± 0.23 (11.6 ± 0.9)	2.5 ± 0.1 ♂ (9.9 ± 0.5) 3.9 ± 0.8 ♀ (15.4 ± 3.3)	2.6 ± 0.3 (10.3 ± 1.1)
Carbon dioxide (CO_2)	mmol/l (mEq/l)		18 ± 3 (18 ± 3)	
Chloride (Cl)	mmol/l (mEq/l)	112 ± 7 (112 ± 7)		118.6 ± 2.1 (118.6 ± 2.1)
Cholesterol	mmol/l (mg/dl)		4.27 ± 1.17 (165 ± 45)	7.86 ± 0.97 (303.6 ± 37.5)
Creatine (CK) phosphokinase	U/l	2047 ± 556	981 ± 545	2329.4 ± 3262.4
Creatinine	μmol/l (mg/dl)	42 ± 8 (0.48 ± 0.09)	61.9 ± 17.7 (0.7 ± 0.2)	
Fibrinogen	μmol/l (mg/dl)			10.3 ± 3.4 (350 ± 116.8)
Gamma globulin	g/l (g/dl)		7.8 ± 4.0 (0.78 ± 0.4)	
Gamma-glutamyl transferase (GGT)	U/l		12 ± 3	
Globulin	g/l (g/dl)			21 ± 1.7 (2.1 ± 0.17)
Glucose	mmol/l (mg/dl)	10.9 ± 1.1 (196 ± 19.8)	12.2 ± 1.6 (220 ± 28)	16.6 ± 3.8 (299.8 ± 69.2)

(Continued)

Table 29.7 (Continued)

Analyte (abbreviation)	Units, SI (conventional)	Double-crested cormorants (*Phalacrocorax auritus*) Ħ Ó	Brown pelicans (*Pelecanus occidentalis*) Ħ₪	Western grebes (*Aechmophorus occidentalis*) ⅋
Lactate dehydrogenase (LDH)	U/l		2352 ± 701	208.0 ± 198.1
Lipase	U/l		49 ± 22	
Phosphorus (P)	mmol/l (mg/dl)	1.97 ± 0.22 (6.1 ± 0.7)	2.1 ± 0.8 (6.4 ± 2.5)	1.1 ± 0.3 (3.5 ± 0.78)
Potassium (K)	mmol/l (mEq/l)	3.2 ± 0.6 (3.2 ± 0.6)	5.1 ± 0.8 (5.1 ± 0.8)	4.1 ± 1.4 (4.1 ± 1.4)
Sodium (Na)	mmol/l (mEq/l)	143 ± 4 (143 ± 4)	147 ± 3 (147 ± 3)	153.5 ± 1.2 (153.5 ± 1.2)
Total bilirubin	µmol/l (mg/dl)			6.8 ± 3.4 (0.4 ± 0.2)
Total protein (TP)	g/l (g/dl)	42 ± 8 (4.2 ± 0.8)	43 ± 7 (4.3 ± 0.7)	36 ± 2.2 (3.6 ± 0.22)
Triglycerides	mmol/l (mg/dl)		0.58 ± 0.44 (51 ± 39) ♂ 6.63 ± 4.72 (587 ± 418) ♀	1.2 ± 0.4 (107.6 ± 30.7)
Uric acid	µmol/l (mg/dl)	1588 ± 394 (26.7 ± 6.6)	731.6 ± 416.4 (12.3 ± 7)	226.0 ± 95.2 (3.8 ± 1.6)

KEY Free-living ⅋, Captive, Ħ Adult ₪, Juvenile Ó, Male ♂, Female ♀.
[a] SE of the mean reported instead of SD.
Data presented as mean ± SD except as indicated.

Toxins

Lead

Lead toxicity is common and well understood in waterfowl, and has been documented in seabirds [40, 41, 96–99]. The "background" level of lead in blood in birds has historically considered to be <20.0 μg/dl, but some scientists are now suggesting that it should be much lower, such <2–5 μg/dl [98, 99]. The environment of the individual bird should be taken into consideration when evaluating lead levels, with lower "background" levels expected in more pristine areas [99]. The Graphite Furnace Atomic Absorption Spectrometry (GFAAS) method is the most commonly used technique for measuring blood lead in birds [100, 101]. The portable ESA LeadCare machine, which has been frequently used for wildlife, systematically but consistently underestimates blood lead concentrations, so the machine must be calibrated with a different technique so that "true" values can be calculated for each species [100].

Delta-aminolevulinic acid dehydratase (ALAD) is an enzyme frequently used in conjunction with lead levels to document lead toxicity because it is highly sensitive and can detect lead exposure at levels before overt clinical signs are seen [102]. Activities of ALAD in blood are negatively correlated with blood lead concentrations in waterfowl [84, 103]. The ALAD ratio, determined by dividing the activity in the sample by the activated activity (obtained by adding zinc sulfate or other activator to the sample), is sometimes preferred as a diagnostic by some authors over the simple enzyme activity [39]. Activity ratios >4 are associated with dietary lead exposure [102].

Petroleum

An immunoassay that detects polyaromatic hydrocarbons (PAH), the main toxic components of crude oil, has been developed that can detect PAH concentrations in blood from 0.2 to 20 ppb [104]. It requires only 50 μl of plasma, making it a useful test for even small seabirds.

Ferritin, an iron storage protein that sequesters iron, typically increases during acute inflammatory reactions and decreases during iron deficiency anemia. In common murres exposed to polycyclic aromatic hydrocarbons, ferritin levels were elevated [44]. Reference ranges for avian ferritin do not exist, but common murres had mean serum ferritin concentrations approximately 10 times higher than those found in broiler chickens (28.6 ± 21.49 ng/ml vs. 2.60 ± 0.78 ng/ml) [44, 105].

Haptoglobin is an acute-phase protein that acts as an antioxidant and that can sequester hemoglobin from lysed RBCs [44]. In the same common murre study, plasma levels of haptoglobin decreased as petroleum levels increased, making it a useful biomarker for Heinz-body anemia and oil exposure [44]. Although exact values that indicate oil exposure have not been determined, the authors suggest that ferritin and haptoglobin can be used together as complementary tests, with the combination of high ferritin and low haptoglobin providing evidence of PAH exposure.

Hormones

Adrenocortical hormone levels, especially corticosterone, are often used to assess stress in birds. Samples taken from free-living birds within 2 min of capture likely reflect pre-capture levels [106]. Corticosterone levels are frequently measured as part of research studies of free-living birds; however, it is unclear how useful this analyte is in clinical avian medicine. Evaluation of this parameter should account for normal seasonal, daily, and reproductive patterns, as well as individual nutritional and metabolic status.

Corticosterone levels in adult red-footed boobies were higher during chick rearing [107]. Nestling storm petrels experienced higher levels of corticosterone as they approached fledging [108]. In herring gulls, food restriction and loss of body condition resulted in higher levels of corticosterone [86]. Handling resulted in increased plasma corticosterone in adult, but not in nestling, Wilson's storm petrels [90]. Corticosterone increased in these nestlings after a storm resulted in several days of fasting [90]. In tufted puffins, corticosterone increased just prior to egg laying and decreased during incubation and brooding [109].

Little information is available on the thyroid hormones of seabirds. In fulmars, pesticide levels did not affect thyroid hormone concentrations [81]. Although birds are thought to have decreased levels of T_3 during fasting, an experimental study in herring gulls found that T_3 levels increased with starvation [86]. Plasma levels of T_3 did not change during the incubation fast of free-living eiders [110].

Serology and PCR

Avian Influenza

Waterfowl and seabirds are the natural reservoir for avian influenza virus, one of the most important zoonotic pathogens of birds. Numerous methods exist to detect infection and exposure to this virus and its many strains. A commercially available reverse-transcriptase PCR test that detects RNA from cloacal and choanal swabs and blood has been validated by the USDA [111]. Virus isolation can also be performed, using embryonated chicken eggs. Interestingly, recent research indicates that birds infected concurrently with avian influenza virus and Newcastle disease virus may have falsely negative results

Table 29.8 Biochemical values for free-ranging Charadriiformes [10, 17].

Analyte	Units, SI (conventional)	Pigeon guillemots (*Cepphus columba*)	Tufted puffins (*Lunda cirrhata*)	Marbled murrelets (*Brachramphus marmoratus*)	Glaucous-winged gulls (*Larus glaucescens*)
Alanine aminotransferase (ALT)	U/l		133 ± 151	102 ± 71	122 ± 5901
Albumin	g/l (g/dl)	26.3 ± 7.1 (2.63 ± 0.71)			
Alkaline phosphatase (ALP)	U/l	137 ± 102	74 ± 61	129 ± 112	252 ± 342
Albumin:globulin (A:G ratio)		0.94 ± 0.27			
$Alpha_1$ globulin	g/l (g/dl)	4.3 ± 2.9 (0.43 ± 0.29)			
$Alpha_2$ globulin	g/l (g/dl)	9.0 ± 4.5 (0.90 ± 0.45)			
Aspartate aminotransferase (AST)	U/l	461 ± 199	437 ± 291	46*	468 ± 298
Beta globulin	g/l (g/dl)	7.1 ± 3.0 (0.71 ± 0.30)			
Bile acids	µmol/l (µg/ml)	2.05 ± 2.6 (0.84 ± 1.06)			
Calcium (Ca)	mmol/l (mg/dl = mEq/l)	2.3 ± 0.3 (9.1 ± 1.2)	5.9 ± 2.5 (11.7 ± 5.0)	5.1 ± 1.5 (10.1 ± 3.0)	4.8 ± 1.2 (9.6 ± 2.3)
Cholesterol	mmol/l (mg/dl)		8.99 ± 1.50 (347 ± 58)	6.37 ± 0.93 (246 ± 36)	6.94 ± 2.38 (268 ± 92)
Creatine phosphokinase (CK)	U/l	375 ± 339	2586 ± 2486	4262 ± 893	1629 ± 1468
Gamma globulin	g/l (g/dl)	10.2 ± 9.7 (1.02 ± 0.97)			
Gamma-glutamyltransferase (GGT)	U/l	10.8 ± 8.2			
Glucose	mmol/l (mg/dl)		15.5 ± 2.5 (279 ± 45)	12.7 ± 3.4 (228 ± 61)	17.8 ± 3.3 (320 ± 60)
Lactate dehydrogenase (LDH)	U/l	915 ± 143	952 ± 403	1342 ± 720	1010 ± 877
Phosphorus (P)	mmol/l (mg/dl)	0.55 ± 0.26 (1.7 ± 0.8)			
Sodium (Na)	mmol/l (mEq/l)	143.8 ± 9.3 (143.8 ± 9.3)			
Total bilirubin	µmol/l (mg/dl)		35.9 ± 22.2 (2.1 ± 1.3)	20.5 ± 15.4 (1.2 ± 0.9)	11.97 ± 8.55 (0.7 ± 0.5)
Total protein (TP)	g/l (g/dl)	56 ± 17 (5.6 ± 1.7)	47 ± 8 (4.7 ± 0.8)	49 ± 10 (4.9 ± 1.0)	34 ± 4 (3.4 ± 0.4)
Total solids (TS) (refractometer)	g/l (g/dl)		53 ± 14 (5.3 ± 1.4)	62 ± 21 (6.2 ± 2.1)	40 ± 8 (4.0 ± 0.8)
Triglycerides	mmol/l (mg/dl)		2.8 ± 3.9 (250 ± 348)	3.2 ± 2.5 (284 ± 223)	1.8 ± 2.0 (163 ± 178)
Uric acid	µmol/l (mg/dl)	868.4 ± 386.6 (14.6 ± 6.5)	1249 ± 833 (21 ± 14)	1784 ± 714 (30 ± 12)	1665 ± 654 (28 ± 11)

All data presented as mean ± SD.

Table 29.9 Biochemical values for waterfowl [18, 31, 55, 82, 83].

Analyte	Units, SI (conventional)	Mallards Ħ₪♀ (*Anas platyrhynchos*)	Canvasback ducks) Ħ (*Aythya valisineria*)	Canada geese Ħ (*Branta canadensis leucopareia*)	Tundra swans (*Cygnus columbianus*) ⅄♀ during molt
	Data format	**Mean ± SD**	**Mean ± SD[a]**	**Mean ± SD**	**Mean ± SE**
Alanine aminotransferase (ALT)	U/l	29.9 ± 9.9	77 ± 31	43 ± 11	
Albumin	g/l (g/dl)	17 ± 2 (1.7 ± 0.2)	16 ± 2 (1.6 ± 0.2)	20 ± 2 (2.0 ± 0.2)	12.7 ± 0.2 (1.27 ± 0.02)
Alkaline phosphatase (ALP)	U/l	44.2 ± 22.7	151 ± 180	72 ± 43	729 ± 47
Alpha$_1$ globulin	g/l (g/dl)		0.8 ± 0.3[b] (0.08 ± 0.03)		
Alpha$_2$ globulin	g/l (g/dl)		1.2 ± 0.6[b] (0.12 ± 0.06)		
Amylase	U/l	2766 ± 684		570 ± 184	4258 ± 141
Aspartate aminotransferase (AST)	U/l	15.8 ± 4.7	80 ± 31	75 ± 19	37.1 ± 4.7
Beta globulin	g/l (g/dl)		4.9 ± 1.2[b] (0.49 ± 0.12)		
Beta$_2$ globulin	g/l (g/dl)		1.9 ± 0.7[b] (0.19 ± 0.07)		
Blood urea nitrogen (BUN)	mmol/l (mg/dl)		1.21 ± 0.89 (3.4 ± 2.5)	1.07 ± 0.71 (3 ± 2)	
Calcium (Ca)	mmol/l (mg/dl)	2.5 ± 0.28 (9.8 ± 1.1)	2.6 ± 0.18 (10.2 ± 0.7)	2.6 ± 0.15 (10.3 ± 0.6)	2.2 ± 0.01 (8.92 ± 0.04)
Chloride (Cl)	mmol/l (mEq/l)		112 ± 5 (112 ± 5)	105 ± 4 (105 ± 4)	
Cholesterol	mmol/l (mg/dl)		5.67 ± 0.77 (219 ± 30)	4.45 ± 0.73 (172 ± 28)	2.84 ± 0.06 (109.5 ± 2.2)
Creatine phosphokinase (CK)	U/l				1775 ± 330
Creatinine	µmol/l (mg/dl)	24.8 ± 6.2 (0.28 ± 0.07)	79.6 ± 26.5 (0.9 ± 0.3)	70.7 ± 26.5 (0.8 ± 0.3)	
Direct bilirubin	µmol/l (mg/dl)	1.20 ± 0.17 (0.07 ± 0.01)	1.03 ± 0.51 (0.06 ± 0.03)	0.71 ± 0.71 (0.01 ± 0.01)	
Fibrinogen	µmol/l (mg/dl)		12.3 ± 5.6[b] (420 ± 190)		
Gamma globulin	g/l (g/dl)		2.2 ± 0.9[b] (0.22 ± 0.09)		
Gamma-glutamyltransferase (GGT)	U/l	8.0 ± 4.8	2.1 ± 1.4	2 ± 3	
Globulin	g/l (g/dl)		27 ± 4 (2.7 ± 0.4)	28 ± 6 (2.8 ± 0.6)	22.2 ± 0.4 (2.22 ± 0.04)
Glucose	mmol/l (mg/dl)	11.9 ± 1.9 (215 ± 34)	12.7 ± 2.8 (229 ± 50)	12.4 ± 2.1 (223 ± 38)	16.2 ± 0.3 (292 ± 5.5)
Iron (Fe)	µmol/l (µg/dl)		37.6 ± 11.8 (210 ± 66)	41.9 ± 12.9 (234 ± 72)	
Magnesium (Mg)	mmol/l (mEq/l)	0.9 ± 0.15 (1.8 ± 0.3)			
Phosphorus (P)	mmol/l (mg/dl)	0.97 ± 0.32 (3.0 ± 1.0)		0.90 ± 0.26 (2.8 ± 0.8)	0.79 ± 0.06 (2.45 ± 0.18)
Potassium (K)	mmol/l (mEq/l)		2.9 ± 0.5 (2.9 ± 0.5)	3.4 ± 0.6 (3.4 ± 0.6)	2.66 ± 0.05 (2.66 ± 0.05)
Lactate dehydrogenase (LDH)	U/l	147 ± 80	310 ± 102	301 ± 80	688 ± 36.8
Sodium (Na)	mmol/l (mEq/l)		148 ± 3 (148 ± 3)	147 ± 4 (147 ± 4)	148 ± 0.2 (148 ± 0.2)
Total bilirubin	µmol/l (mg/dl)	2.74 ± 0.68 (0.16 ± 0.04)	4.79 ± 2.91 (0.28 ± 0.17)	3.42 ± 1.20 (0.20 ± 0.07)	
Total protein (TP)	g/l (g/dl)	42 ± 5 (4.2 ± 0.5)	43 ± 5 (4.3 ± 0.5)	48 ± 7 (4.8 ± 0.7)	34.9 ± 0.5 (3.49 ± 0.05)
Triglycerides	mmol/l (mg/dl)		2.17 ± 0.86 (192 ± 76)	1.71 ± 0.32 (151 ± 28)	
Uric acid	µmol/l (mg/dl)	267.7 ± 107.1 (4.5 ± 1.8)	327.1 ± 124.9 (5.5 ± 2.1)	1189.6 ± 493.7 (20.0 ± 8.3)	453.8 ± 2.4 (7.63 ± 0.04)

KEY Free-living ⅄, Captive Ħ, Adult ₪, Juvenile Ó, Male ♂, Female ♀.

[a] Units not reported in original reference.

[b] System used in this study no longer commercially available.

on virus isolation tests [112]. A serologic test for antibodies is commercially available from IDEXX Laboratories (FlockCheck AI Multi-Screen Antibody Test Kit) and has been used for both seabirds and waterfowl [113, 114]. This test appears to be more sensitive for waterfowl than the agar gel immunodiffusion (AGID) test commonly used for poultry [114].

Avian Paramyxovirus

Avian paramyxovirus type 1, also known as Newcastle disease virus (NDV), is an important zoonotic disease of birds. Similar to avian influenza, NDV has many strains of varying pathogenicity. Pathogenicity varies among avian species; double-crested cormorants are among the most commonly affected free-living birds [115, 116]. As with avian influenza, numerous diagnostic tests are available. Virus isolation can be performed from cloacal swabs, choanal swabs, or feces [115, 117]. Although there is a USDA-validated reverse-transcriptase PCR test for NDV, recent research has shown that rapid evolution of the virus, especially in double-crested cormorant populations, may require the modification of existing PCR tests in order to achieve high sensitivity [116]. Numerous serologic tests for antibodies are also available [115].

Duck Viral Enteritis

Duck viral enteritis, or duck plague, is caused by the alphaherpesvirus Anatid herpesvirus-1. Most waterfowl species appear to be susceptible, but it is most important economically for domestic ducks [118]. The gold standard for diagnosis is virus isolation, but there are numerous serologic tests available for both antigen and antibodies [118]. A PCR test using cloacal swabs is also available and may be helpful for identifying asymptomatic carriers [118].

Fowl Cholera

Avian, or fowl, cholera is caused by the bacterium *Pasteurella multocida* and is most commonly seen in waterfowl. However, most birds are likely susceptible, and species in all the major groups of seabirds have been affected [119]. Antemortem diagnosis of avian cholera is rarely indicated, as death with no premonitory signs is a common presentation [119]. However, culture of nasal, cloacal, and oral swabs is effective for detecting *P. multocida*, and an ELISA for plasma antibodies is also available [119, 120].

Aspergillus

Aspergillosis, caused by *Aspergillus fumigatus*, *A. flavus*, or *A. niger*, is a devastating fungal disease of seabirds and, to a lesser extent, waterfowl. Aquatic birds appear more susceptible than terrestrial species, perhaps because they have less exposure to the organism, both as individuals and as species over evolutionary time [93]. Aspergillosis is challenging to diagnose antemortem, and generally a combination of tests is used, including hematology, serology, and radiology [58, 93, 94]. Although a severe heterophilia, with or without a monocytosis, is a "classic" finding in birds with aspergillosis, this may not be present in seabirds and waterfowl [58, 59, 93]. Protein electrophoresis generally reveals increases in the beta and gamma globulin fractions, but this is a nonspecific finding [58, 94]. A sandwich ELISA for the galactomannan antigen (a component of the fungal cell wall) called Platelia® is relatively sensitive and specific [58, 94]. Another assay, which measures beta-D-glucan, appears to be quite sensitive for fungal infections, but it is not specific for aspergillosis [58]. Antibody testing was not useful for diagnosing aspergillosis in seabirds [58].

References

1 Hackett, S.J., Kimball, R.T., Reddy, S. et al. (2008). A phylogenomic study of birds reveals their evolutionary history. *Science* 320: 1763–1768.

2 Hedges, S.B. and Sibley, C.G. (1994). Molecules vs. morphology in avian evolution: the case of the "pelecaniform" birds. *Proceedings of the National Academy of Sciences* 91: 9861–9865.

3 Bennett, G.F., M. Whiteway, C.B. Woodworth-Lynas. 1982. Host-parasite catalogue of the avian haematozoa. Occasional Papers in Biology No. 5, Memorial University of Newfoundland, Canada.

4 Poole, A. (Editor). 2005. The Birds of North America Online: http://bna.birds.cornell.edu/BNAc. Cornell Laboratory of Ornithology, Ithaca, NY.

5 Barbosa, A. and Palacios, M.J. (2009). Health of Antarctic birds: a review of their parasites, pathogens, and diseases. *Polar Biology* 32: 1095–1115.

6 Mallory, M.L., Robinson, S.A., Hebert, C.E., and Forbes, M.R. (2010). Seabirds as indicators of aquatic ecosystem conditions: a case for gathering multiple proxies of seabird health. *Marine Pollution Bulletin* 60: 7–12.

7 Bond, C.F. and Gilbert, P.W. (1958). Comparative study of blood volume in representative aquatic and nonaquatic birds. *American Journal of Physiology* 194 (3): 519–521.

8 Lichtenberger, M., Orcutt, C., Cray, C. et al. (2009). Comparison of fluid types for resuscitation after acute blood loss in mallard ducks (*Anas platyrhynchos*). *Journal of Veterinary Emergency and Critical Care* 19: 467–472.

9 Lieske, C.L., Ziccardi, M.H., Mazet, J.A.K. et al. (2002). Evaluation of 4 handheld blood glucose monitors for use in seabird rehabilitation. *Journal of Avian Medicine and Surgery* 16: 277–285.

10 Newman, S.H., Piatt, J.F., and White, J. (1997). Hematological and plasma biochemical reference ranges of Alaskan seabirds: their ecological significance and clinical importance. *Colonial Waterbirds* 20 (3): 492–504.

11 Padilla, L.R., Huyvaert, K.P., Merkel, J. et al. (2003). Hematology, plasma chemistry, serology, and *Chlamydophila* status of the waved albatross (*Phoebastria irrorata*) on the Galapagos Islands. *Journal of Zoo and Wildlife Medicine* 34 (3): 278–283.

12 Uhart, M.M., Quintana, F., Karesh, W.B., and Braselton, W.E. (2003). Hematology, plasma biochemistry, and serosurvey for selected infectious agents in southern giant petrels from Patagonia, Argentina. *Journal of Wildlife Diseases* 39: 359–365.

13 Work, T.M. (1996). Weights, hematology, and serum chemistry of seven species of free-ranging tropical pelagic seabirds. *Journal of Wildlife Diseases* 32 (4): 643–657.

14 Fiorello, C.V. 2012. Unpublished raw data.

15 Haefele, H.J., Sidor, I., Evers, D.C. et al. (2005). Hematologic and physiologic reference ranges for free-ranging adult and young common loons (*Gavia immer*). *Journal of Zoo and Wildlife Medicine* 36 (3): 385–390.

16 Zaias, J., Fox, W.P., Cray, C., and Altman, N.H. (2000). Hematologic, plasma protein, and biochemical profiles of brown pelicans (*Pelecanus occidentalis*). *American Journal of Veterinary Research* 61 (7): 771–774.

17 Seiser, P.E., Duffy, L.K., McGuire, A.D. et al. (2000). Comparison of pigeon guillemot, *Cepphus columba*, blood parameters from oiled and unoiled areas of Alaska eight years after the Exxon Valdez oil spill. *Marine Pollution Bulletin* 40: 152–164.

18 Fairbrother, A., Craig, M.A., Walker, K., and O'Loughlin, D. (1990). Changes in mallard (*Anas platyrhynchos*) serum chemistry due to age, sex, and reproductive condition. *Journal of Wildlife Diseases* 26: 67–77.

19 Gee, G.F., Carpenter, J.W., and Hensler, G.L. (1981). Species differences in hematological values of captive cranes, geese, raptors, and quail. *Journal of Wildlife Management* 45 (2): 463–483.

20 Mulley, R.C. (1979). Haematology and blood chemistry of the black duck. *Journal of Wildlife Diseases* 15 (3): 437–441.

21 Norambuena, M.C. and Bozinovic, F. (2009). Mineral metabolism in a black-necked swan (*Cygnus melanocoryphus*) population from southern Chile. *Journal of Zoo and Wildlife Medicine* 40 (4): 617–623.

22 Bearhop, S., Griffiths, R., Orr, K., and Furness, R.W. (1999). The normal haematology of great skuas (*Catharacta skua*) in the wild. *Comparative Haematology International* 9: 107–109.

23 Bradley, L.W. and Threlfall, W. (1974). Blood cell indices of five species of auk (Alcidae) from Newfoundland, Canada. *Journal of Zoology, London* 174: 377–385.

24 Edwards, D.B., Mallory, M.L., and Forbes, M.R. (2006). Variation in baseline haematology of northern fulmars (*Fulmarus glacialis*) in the Canadian high Arctic. *Comparative Clinical Pathology* 14: 206–209.

25 Wanless, S., Barton, T.R., and Harris, M.P. (1997). Blood hematocrit measurements of 4 species of North Atlantic seabirds in relation to levels of infestation by the tick *Ixodes uriae*. *Colonial Waterbirds* 20 (3): 540–544.

26 Melrose, W.D. and Nicol, S.C. (1992). Haematology, red cell metabolism and blood chemistry of the black-faced cormorant *Leucocarbo fuscescens*. *Comparative Biochemistry and Physiology* 102A: 67–70.

27 Grasman, K.A., Scanlon, P.F., and Fox, G.A. (2000). Geographic variation in hematological variables in adult and prefledgling herring gulls (*Larus argentatus*) and possible associations with organochlorine exposure. *Archives of Environmental Contamination and Toxicology* 38: 244–253.

28 Quillfeldt, P., Everaert, N., Buyse, J. et al. (2009). Relationship between plasma leptin-like protein levels, begging, and provisioning in nestling thin-billed prions *Pacyptila belcheri*. *General and Comparative Endocrinology* 161: 171–178.

29 Wolf, S.H., Schreiber, R.W., Kahana, L., and Torres, J.J. (1985). Seasonal, sexual, and age-related variation in the blood composition of the brown pelican (*Pelecanus occidentalis*). *Comparative Biochemistry and Physiology* 82A (4): 837–846.

30 Kocan, R.M. (1972). Some physiologic blood values of wild diving ducks. *Journal of Wildlife Diseases* 8: 115–118.

31 Kocan, R.M. and Pitts, S.M. (1976). Blood values of the canvasback duck by age, sex, and season. *Journal of Wildlife Diseases* 12: 341–346.

32 Mulley, R.C. (1980). Haematology of the wood duck. *Journal of Wildlife Diseases* 16 (2): 271–273.

33 Perry, M.C., Obrecht, H.H. lll, Williams, B.K., and Kuenzel, W.J. (1986). Blood chemistry and hematocrit of captive and wild canvasbacks. *Journal of Wildlife Management* 50: 435–441.

34 Spano, J.S., Pedersoli, W.M., Kemppaninen, R.J. et al. (1987). Baseline hematologic, endocrine, and clinical chemistry values in ducks and roosters. *Avian Diseases* 31: 800–803.

35 Totzke, U., Fenske, M., Huppop, O. et al. (1999). The influence of fasting on blood and plasma composition

of herring gulls (*Larus argentatus*). *Physiological and Biochemical Zoology* 72 (4): 426–437.

36 Artacho, P., Soto-Gamboa, M., Verdugo, C., and Nespolo, R.F. (2007). Using haematological parameters to infer the health and nutritional status of an endangered black-necked swan population. *Comparative Biochemistry and Physiology* 147A: 1060–1066.

37 Norambuena, M.C. and Bozinovic, F. (2009). Health and nutritional status of a perturbed black-necked swan (*Cygnus melanocoryphus*) population: diet quality. *Journal of Zoo and Wildlife Medicine* 40 (4): 607–616.

38 Newman, S.H., Mazet, J.K., Ziccardi, M.H. et al. (1999). Haematological changes and anaemia associated with captivity and petroleum exposure in seabirds. *Comparative Haematology International* 9: 60–67.

39 Pain, D.J. (1989). Haematological parameters as predictors of blood lead and indicators of lead poisoning in the black duck (*Anas rubripes*). *Environmental Pollution* 60: 67–81.

40 Pain, D.J. and Rattner, B.A. (1988). Mortality and hematology associated with the ingestion of one number four lead shot in black ducks, *Anas rubripes*. *Bulletin of Environmental Contamination and Toxicology* 40: 159–164.

41 Sileo, L. and Fefer, S.I. (1987). Paint chip poisoning of Laysan albatross at midway atoll. *Journal of Wildlife Diseases* 23 (3): 432–437.

42 Leighton, F.A., Peakall, D.B., and Butler, R.G. (1983). Heinz-body hemolytic anemia from the ingestion of crude oil: a primary toxic effect in marine birds. *Science* 220: 871–873.

43 Yamato, O., Goto, I., and Maede, Y. (1996). Hemolytic anemia in wild seaducks caused by marine oil pollution. *Journal of Wildlife Diseases* 32 (2): 381–384.

44 Troisi, G., Borjesson, L., Bexton, S., and Robinson, I. (2007). Biomarkers of polycyclic aromatic hydrocarbon (PAH)-associated hemolytic anemia in oiled wildlife. *Environmental Research* 105: 324–329.

45 Forrester, D.J., Gaskin, J.M., White, F.H. et al. (1977). An epizootic of waterfowl associated with a red tide episode in Florida. *Journal of Wildlife Diseases* 13: 160–167.

46 Averbeck, C. (1992). Haematology and blood chemistry of healthy and clinically abnormal great black-backed gulls (*Larus marinus*) and herring gulls (*Larus argentatus*). *Avian Pathology* 21 (2): 215–223.

47 Fiorello, C.V., Nisbet, I.C.T., Hatch, J.J. et al. (2009). Hematology and absence of hemoparasites in breeding common terns (*Sterna hirundo*) from cape cod, Massachusetts. *Journal of Zoo and Wildlife Medicine* 40 (3): 409–413.

48 Travis, E.K., Vargas, R.H., Merkel, J. et al. (2006). Hematology, plasma chemistry, and serology of the flightless cormorant (*Phalacrocorax harrisi*) in the Galapagos Islands, Ecuador. *Journal of Wildlife Diseases* 42 (1): 133–141.

49 Work, T.M. (1999). Weights, hematology, and serum chemistry of free-ranging brown boobies (*Sula leucogaster*) in Johnston atoll, Central Pacific. *Journal of Zoo and Wildlife Medicine* 30 (1): 81–84.

50 Kuiken, T. and Danesik, K.L. (1999). Hematology and serum chemistry of captive juvenile double-crested cormorants (*Phalacrocorax auritus*). *Canadian Veterinary Journal* 40: 493–496.

51 Padilla, L.R., Whiteman, N.K., Merkel, J. et al. (2006). Health assessment of seabirds on Isla Genovesa, Galapagos Islands. *Ornithological Monographs* 60: 86–97.

52 Puerta, M.L., Garcia del Campo, A.L., Huecas, V., and Abelenda, M. (1991). Hematology and blood chemistry of the white pelican (*Pelecanus onocrotalus*). *Comparative Biochemistry and Physiology* 98A: 393–394.

53 Fairbrother, A. and O'Loughlin, D. (1990). Differential white blood cell values of the mallard (*Anas platyrhynchos*) across different ages and reproductive states. *Journal of Wildlife Diseases* 26 (1): 78–82.

54 Gladbach, A., Gladbach, D.J., and Quillfeldt, P. (2010). Variations in leucocyte profiles and plasma biochemistry are related to different aspects of parental investment in male and female upland geese. *Comparative Biochemistry and Physiology* 156A: 269–277.

55 Milani, J.F., Wilson, H., Ziccardi, M. et al. (2012). Hematology, plasma chemistry, and bacteriology of wild tundra swans (*Cygnus columbianus*) in Alaska. *Journal of Wildlife Diseases* 48: 212–215.

56 Scott, C.A., Mazet, J.A.K., and Powell, A.N. (2010). Health evaluation of western Arctic king eiders (*Somateria spectabilis*). *Journal of Wildlife Diseases* 46 (4): 1290–1294.

57 Williams, J.I. and Trainer, D.O. (1971). A hematological study of snow, blue, and Canada geese. *Journal of Wildlife Diseases* 7: 258–265.

58 Burco, J.D. 2010. The Ecology of Aspergillosis in Seabirds. Dissertation. University of California, Davis, 149 pp.

59 Graczyk, T.K., Cranfield, M.R., and Klein, P.N. (1998). Value of antigen and antibody detection, and blood evaluation parameters in diagnosis of avian invasive aspergillosis. *Mycopathologia* 140: 121–127.

60 Dehnhard, N., Quillfeldt, P., and Hennicke, J.C. (2011). Leucocyte profiles and H/L ratios in chicks of red-tailed tropicbirds reflect the ontogeny of the immune system. *Journal of Comparative Physiology B* 181: 641–648.

61 Giudici, A., Navarro, J., Juste, C., and Gonzalez-Solis, J. (2010). Physiological ecology of breeders and

sabbaticals in a pelagic seabird. *Journal of Experimental Marine Biology and Ecology* 389: 13–17.

62 Levengood, J.M., Sanderson, G.C., Anderson, W.L. et al. (2000). Influence of diet on the hematology and serum biochemistry of zinc-intoxicated mallards. *Journal of Wildlife Diseases* 36 (1): 111–123.

63 Jones, H.I., Gallagher, J.M., and Miller, G.D. (2002). Survey of south polar skuas (*Catharacta maccormicki*) for blood parasites in the Vestfold Hills region of Antarctica. *Journal of Wildlife Diseases* 38 (1): 213–215.

64 Jovani, R., Tella, J.L., Forero, M.G. et al. (2001). Apparent absence of blood parasites in the Patagonian seabird community: is it related to the marine environment? *Waterbirds* 24 (3): 430–433.

65 Steadman, D.W., Greiner, E.C., and Wood, C.S. (1990). Absence of blood parasites in indigenous and introduced birds from the Cook Islands, South Pacific. *Conservation Biology* 4 (4): 398–404.

66 Wojczulanis-Jakubas, K., Svoboda, A., Kruszewicz, A., and Johnsen, A. (2010). No evidence of blood parasites in little auks (*Alle alle*) breeding on Svalbard. *Journal of Wildlife Diseases* 46 (2): 574–578.

67 Work, T.M. and Rameyer, R.A. (1996). *Haemoproteus iwa* N.SP. in great frigatebirds (*Fregata minor* [Gmelin]) from Hawaii: parasite morphology and prevalence. *Journal of Parasitology* 82 (3): 489–491.

68 Work, T.M. and Rameyer, R.A. (1997). Description and epizootiology of *Babesia poelea* N.Sp. in brown boobies (*Sula leucogaster* [Boddaert]) on Sand Island, Johnston atoll, Central Pacific. *Journal of Parasitology* 83 (4): 734–738.

69 Yabsley, M.J., Greiner, E., Tseng, F.S. et al. (2009). Description of novel *Babesia* species and associated lesions from common murres (*Uria aalge*) from California. *Journal of Parasitology* 95 (5): 1183–1188.

70 Bennett, G.F., Nieman, D.J., Turner, B. et al. (1982). Blood parasites of prairie anatids and their implications in waterfowl management in Alberta and Saskatchewan. *Journal of Wildlife Diseases* 18 (3): 287–296.

71 Bennett, G.F., Smith, A.D., Whitman, W., and Cameron, M. (1975). Hematozoa of the Anatidae of the Atlantic flyway. II. The maritime provinces of Canada. *Journal of Wildlife Diseases* 11: 280–289.

72 Kloss, C.L., Fedynich, A.M., and Ballard, B.M. (2003). Survey of blood parasites in Ross' and white-fronted geese in southern Texas. *Southwestern Naturalist* 48 (2): 286–289.

73 DeJong, R.J. and Muzzall, P.M. (2000). Hematozoa of waterfowl from Michigan. *Journal of Wildlife Diseases* 36 (4): 767–773.

74 Grim, K.C., McCutchan, T., Sullivan, M., and Cranfield, M.R. (2008). Unidentified *Plasmodium* species in Australian black swans (*Cygnus atratus*) hatched and raised in North America. *Journal of Zoo and Wildlife Medicine* 39 (2): 216–220.

75 Herman, C.M., Barrow, J.H., and Tarshis, I.B. (1975). Leucocytozoonosis in Canada geese at the Seney National Wildlife Refuge. *Journal of Wildlife Diseases* 11: 404–411.

76 Bababummi, E.A. and Bassir, O. (1982). A delay in blood clotting of chickens and ducks induced by aflatoxin treatment. *Poultry Science* 61: 166–168.

77 Ostrowski-Meissner, H.T. (1984). Biochemical and physiological responses of growing chickens and ducklings to dietary aflatoxins. *Comparative Biochemistry and Physiology* 79C: 193–204.

78 Robinson, R.M., Ray, A.C., Reagor, J.C., and Holland, L.A. (1982). Waterfowl mortality caused by aflatoxicosis in Texas. *Journal of Wildlife Diseases* 18: 311–313.

79 Tabery, P., Huffman, J.E., and Fried, B. (1988). Hemolytic and coagulation properties of *Sphaeridiotrema globulus* (Trematoda). *Journal of Parasitology* 74: 730–731.

80 Newman, S.H., R.T. Golightly, E.N. Craig, H.R. Carter, C. Kreuder. 2004. Effects of petroleum exposure and rehabilitation on post-release survival, behavior, and blood health indices: A common murre (Uria aalge) case study following the Stuyvesant petroleum spill. Final Report. Oiled Wildlife Care Network, Wildlife Health Center, University of California, Davis, CA 95616, pp. 1–46.

81 Helgason, L.B., Verreault, J., Braune, B.M. et al. (2010). Relationship between persistent halogenated organic contaminants and TCDD-toxic equivalents on EROD activity and retinoid and thyroid hormone status in northern fulmars. *Science of the Total Environment* 408: 6117–6123.

82 Franson, J.C., Murray, H.C., and Bunck, C. (1985). Enzyme activities in plasma, kidney, liver, and muscle of five avian species. *Journal of Wildlife Diseases* 21 (1): 33–39.

83 Boismenu, C., Gauthier, G., and Larochelle, J. (1992). Physiology of prolonged fasting in greater snow geese (*Chen caerulescens atlantica*). *Auk* 109: 511–521.

84 Martino-Haro, M., Green, A.J., and Mateo, R. (2011). Effects of lead exposure on oxidative stress biomarkers and plasma biochemistry in waterbirds in the field. *Environmental Research* 111: 530–538.

85 Harr, K. (2002). Clinical chemistry of companion avian species: a review. *Veterinary Clinical Pathology* 31: 140–151.

86 Jeffrey, D.A., Peakall, D.B., Miller, D.S., and Herzberg, G.R. (1985). Blood chemistry changes in food-deprived herring gulls. *Comparative Biochemistry and Physiology* 81A (4): 911–913.

87 Hollmen, T., Franson, J.C., Hario, M. et al. (2001). Use of serum biochemistry to evaluate nutritional status and health of incubating common eiders in Finland. *Physiological and Biochemical Zoology* 74: 333–342.

88 Hochleithner, M. (1994). Biochemistries. In: *Avian Medicine: Principles and Applications* (ed. B.W. Ritchie, G.J. Harrison and L.R. Harrison), 223–245. Lake Worth: Wingers Publishing.

89 Artacho, P., Soto-Gamboa, M., Verdugo, C., and Nespolo, R.F. (2007). Blood biochemistry reveals malnutrition in black-necked swans (*Cygnus melanocoryphus*) living in a conservation priority area. *Comparative Biochemistry and Physiology* 146A: 283–290.

90 Quillfeldt, P., Masello, J.F., and Mostl, E. (2004). Blood chemistry in relation to nutrition and ectoparasite load in Wilson's storm-petrels *Oceanites oceanicus*. *Polar Biology* 27: 168–176.

91 Roman, Y., Bomsel-Demontoy, M., Levrier, J. et al. (2009). Influence of molt on plasma protein electrophoretic patterns in bar-headed geese (*Anser indicus*). *Journal of Wildlife Diseases* 45: 661–667.

92 Driver, E.A. (1981). Hematological and blood chemical values of mallard, *Anas p. platyrhynchos*, drakes before, during, and after remige molt. *Journal of Wildlife Diseases* 17: 413–421.

93 Converse, K.A. (2007). Aspergillosis. In: *Infectious Diseases of Wild Birds* (ed. N.J. Thomas, D.B. Hunter and C.T. Atkinson), 360–374. Ames: Blackwell Publishing.

94 Cray, C., Watson, T., Rodriguez, M., and Arheart, K.L. (2009). Application of galactomannan analysis and protein electrophoresis in the diagnosis of aspergillosis in avian species. *Journal of Zoo and Wildlife Medicine* 40: 64–70.

95 Hawkey, C., Hart, M.G., Samour, H.J. et al. (1984). Haematological findings in healthy and sick captive rosy flamingos. *Avian Pathology* 13: 163–172.

96 Finkelstein, M.E., Gwiazda, R.H., and Smith, D.R. (2003). Lead poisoning of seabirds: environmental risks from leaded paint at a decommissioned military base. *Environmental Science and Technology* 37: 3256–3260.

97 Franson, J.C., Hansen, S.P., Creekmore, T.E. et al. (2003). Lead fishing weights and other fishing tackle in selected waterbirds. *Waterbirds* 26: 345–352.

98 Locke, L.N. and Thomas, N.J. (1996). Lead poisoning of waterfowl and raptors. In: *Noninfectious Diseases of Wildlife* (ed. A. Fairbrother, L.N. Locke and G.L. Hoff), 108–117. Ames: Iowa State University Press.

99 Pain, D.J., Fisher, I.J., and Thomas, V.G. (2009). A global update of lead poisoning in terrestrial birds from ammunition sources. In: *Ingestion of Lead from Spent Ammunition: Implications for Wildlife and Humans* (ed. R.T. Watson, M. Fuller, M. Pokras and G. Hunt), 99–118. Boise: The Peregrine Fund.

100 Bedrosian, B., Paris, C.N., and Craighead, D. (2009). Difference between blood lead level detection techniques: analysis within and among three techniques and four avian species. In: *Ingestion of Lead from Spent Ammunition: Implications for Wildlife and Humans* (ed. R.T. Watson, M. Fuller, M. Pokras and G. Hunt), 287–288. The Peregrine Fund: Boise.

101 Brown, C.S., Luebbert, J., Mulcahy, D. et al. (2006). Blood lead levels of wild Steller's eiders (*Polysticta stelleri*) and black scoters (*Mealnitta nigra*) in Alaska using a portable blood lead analyzer. *Journal of Zoo and Wildlife Medicine* 37: 361–365.

102 Scheuhammer, A.M. (1987). Erythrocyte delta-aminolevulinic acid dehydratase in birds. II. Effects of lead exposure *in vivo*. *Toxicology* 45: 165–175.

103 van der Merwe, D., Carpenter, J.W., Nietfeld, J.C., and Miesner, J.F. (2011). Adverse health effects in Canada geese (*Branta canadensis*) associated with waste from zinc and lead mines in the tri-state mining district (Kansas, Oklahoma, and Missouri, USA). *Journal of Wildlife Diseases* 47: 650–660.

104 Troisi, G.M. and Borjesson, L. (2005). Development of an immunoassay for the determination of polyaromatic hydrocarbons in plasma samples from oiled seabirds. *Environmental Science and Technology* 39: 3748–3755.

105 Betini, M.P., R.R. Machado, C.F. Marchini. 2011. Performance and serum iron/ferritin levels in broilers fed organic selenium and zinc, subjected to heat stress. Poultry Industry: XXII Latin American Poultry Congress 2011.

106 Romero, L.M. and Reed, J.M. (2005). Collecting baseline corticosterone samples in the field: is under 3 min good enough? *Comparative Biochemistry and Physiology* 140A: 73–79.

107 Lormee, H., Jouventin, P., Trouve, C., and Chastel, O. (2005). Sex-specific patterns in baseline corticosterone and body condition changes in breeding red-footed boobies *Sula sula*. *Ibis* 145: 212–219.

108 Kozlowski, C.P., Mauck, R.A., O'Reilly, K.M. et al. (2010). Changes in plasma hormone levels correlate with fledging in nestling Leach's storm petrels. *General and Comparative Endocrinology* 169: 91–97.

109 Williams, C.T., Kitaysky, A.S., Kettle, A.B., and Buck, C.L. (2008). Corticosterone levels of tufted puffins vary with breeding stage, body condition index, and reproductive performance. *General and Comparative Endocrinology* 158: 29–35.

110 Criscuolo, F., Raclot, T., Le Maho, Y., and Gabrielsen, G.W. (2003). Do T_3 levels in incubating eiders reflect the cost of incubation among clutch size? *Physiological and Biochemical Zoology* 76: 196–203.

111 Spackmen, E., Senne, D.A., Myers, T.J. et al. (2002). Development of a real-time reverse transcriptase PCR assay for type a influenza virus and the avian H5 and H7 hemagglutinin subtypes. *Journal of Clinical Microbiology* 40: 3256–3260.

112 El Zowalaty, M.E., Chander, Y., Redig, P.T. et al. (2011). Selective isolation of avian influenza virus from cloacal samples containing AIV and Newcastle disease virus. *Journal of Veterinary Diagnostic Investigation* 23: 330–332.

113 Brown, J.D., Luttrell, M.P., Berghaus, R.D. et al. (2010). Prevalence of antibodies to type a influenza virus in wild avian species using two serologic assays. *Journal of Wildlife Diseases* 46: 896–911.

114 Brown, J.D., Stallknecht, D.E., Berghaus, R.D. et al. (2009). Evaluation of a commercial blocking ELISA to detect avian influenza virus antibodies in multiple experimentally infected avian species. *Clinical and Vaccine Immunology* 16: 824–829.

115 Leighton, F.A. and Heckert, R.A. (2007). Newcastle disease and related avian paramyxoviruses. In: *Infectious Diseases of Wild Birds* (ed. N.J. Thomas, D.B. Hunter and C.T. Atkinson), 3–16. Ames: Blackwell Publishing.

116 Rue, C.A., Susta, L., Brown, C.C. et al. (2010). Evolutionary changes affecting rapid identification of 2008 Newcastle disease virus isolated from double-crested cormorants. *Journal of Clinical Microbiology* 48: 2440–2448.

117 Jindal, N., Chander, Y., Chockalingam, A.K. et al. (2009). Phylogenetic analysis of Newcastle disease viruses isolated from waterfowl in the upper Midwest region of the United States. *Virology Journal* 6: 191–200.

118 Hansen, W.R. and Gough, R.E. (2007). Duck plague. In: *Infectious Diseases of Wild Birds* (ed. N.J. Thomas, D.B. Hunter and C.T. Atkinson), 87–107. Ames: Blackwell Publishing.

119 Samuel, M.D., Botzler, R.G., and Wobeser, G.A. (2007). Avian cholera. In: *Infectious Diseases of Wild Birds* (ed. N.J. Thomas, D.B. Hunter and C.T. Atkinson), 239–269. Ames: Blackwell Publishing.

120 Samuel, M.D., Shadduck, D.J., Goldberg, D.R., and Johnson, W.P. (2003). Comparison of methods to detect *Pasteurella multocida* in carrier waterfowl. *Journal of Wildlife Diseases* 39: 125–135.

Index

Page numbers in *italic* indicate tables.

Exotic Animal Laboratory Diagnosis, First Edition. Edited by J. Jill Heatley and Karen E. Russell.

C

i

m

Abbreviations and conversions for common analytes provided in this text

Analyte	Abbreviation	Conventional Unit (USA)	Conversion Factor	SI Units
Alkaline Phosphatase	ALKP	units/L	1.0	U/L
Alanine Amino Transferase	ALT, SGPT	units/L	1.0	U/L
Albumin	ALB	g/dL	10	g/L
Aspartate Amino Transferase	AST, SGOT	units/L	1.0	U/L
Ammonia	NH_3	μg/dL	0.587	μmol/L
Amylase	AMY	units/L	1.0	U/L
Anion Gap	AG	mEq/L	1.0	mmol/L
Bicarbonate	HCO3	mEq/L	1.0	mmol/L
Bilirubin	Bili	mg/dL	17.1	μmol/L
Bile Acids	BA	mg/dl	10	mg/L
Calcium	Ca	mg/dL	0.25	mmol/L
Calcium, Ionized	iCa	mEq/L	0.50	mmol/L
Carbon Dioxide	CO_2	mEq/L	1.0	mmol/L
Chloride	Cl	mEq/L	1.0	mmol/L
Cholesterol	Chol	mg/dL	0.0259	mmol/L
Complete Blood Count	CBC			
Cortisol	Cort	μg/dL	27.59	nmol/L
Creatinine Kinase	CK	units/L	1.0	U/L
Creatinine	Creat	mg/dL	88.4	μmol/L
Fibrinogen		mg/dL	0.0294	μmol/L
Gamma Glutamyl Transferase	GGT	units/L	1.0	U/L
Glucose	Glu	mg/dL	0.0555	mmol/L
Lactate (Lactic Acid)	LAC	mg/dL	0.111	mmol/L
Lactate Dehydrogenase	LDH	units/L	1	U/L
Lead	Pb	μg/dL	0.0483	μmol/L
Hemoglobin	Hgb	g/dL	10.0	g/L
Hematocrit	HCT	%	0.01	Proportion of 1.0
Iron (Total)	Fe	μg/dL	0.179	μmol/L
Iron binding capacity (Total)	TIBC	μg/dL	0.179	μmol/L
Osmolality	OSM	mOsm/kg	1.0	mmol/kg
Packed Cell Volume	PCV	%	0.01	Proportion of 1.0

Partial pressure of carbon dioxide	Pco_2	mm Hg	1.0	mm Hg
pH	pH	pH units	1.0	pH units
Partial pressure of oxygen	Po_2	mm Hg	1.0	mm Hg
Platelets or Thrombocytes		$\times 10^3/\mu L$	1.0	$\times 10^9/L$
Phosphorous	P	mg/dL	0.323	mmol/L
Potassium	K	mEq/L	1.0	mmol/L
Prothrombin Time	PT	s	1.0	s
Protein (Total)	TP	g/dL	10.0	g/L
Red blood cell count	RBC	$\times 10^6/\mu L$	1.0	$\times 10^{12}/L$
Reticulocyte count		% of RBCs	0.01	Proportion of 1.0
Sodium	Na	mEq/L	1.0	mmol/L
Thyrotropin (thyroid stimulating Hormone)	TSH	mIU/L	1.0	mIU/L
Thyroxine, free	T_4	ng/dL	12.87	pmol/L
Triglycerides	Trig	mg/dL	0.0113	mmol/L
Triiodothyronine, Free	Ft3	pg/dL	0.0154	pmol/L
Triiodothyronine, Total	TT3	ng/dL	0.0154	nmol/L
Troponin I (cardiac)	cTnI	ng/mL	1.0	μg/L
Troponin T (cardiac)	cTnT	ng/mL	1.0	μg/L
Vitamin A (retinol)	VitA	μg/dL	0.0349	μmol/L
Vitamin B_6 (pyridoxine)	VitB6	ng/mL	4.046	nmol/L
Vitamin B_{12} (cyanocobalamin)	VitB12	pg/mL	0.738	pmol/L
Vitamin C (ascorbic acid)	VitC	mg/dL	56.78	μmol/L
Vitamin D, 1,25-Dihydroxy	VitD2	pg/mL	2.6	pmol/L
Vitamin D, 25-Hydroxy	VitD3	ng/mL	2.496	nmol/L
Vitamin E	VitE	mg/dL	23.22	μmol/L
Vitamin K	VitK	ng/mL	2.22	nmol/L
Uric Acid	URIC	mg/dL	59.48	μmol/L
Total Solids	TS	g/dL	10.0	g/L
(Blood) Urea Nitrogen	BUN	mg/dL	0.357	mmol/L
White Blood Cell Count, Total, Leukogram	WBC	$\times 10^3/\mu L$	1.0	$\times 10^9/L$
White blood cell differential count	Diff	%	0.01	Proportion of 1.0
Zinc	Zn	μg/dl	0.153	μmol/L

Printed in the USA/Agawam, MA
September 16, 2026
910661.206